2000 UPDATE

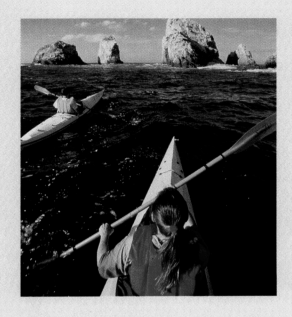

Core Concepts
in Health EIGHTH EDITION

PAUL M. INSEL

WALTON T. ROTH

Stanford University

KIRSTAN PRICE

Developmental Editor

Mayfield Publishing Company

Mountain View, California

London • Toronto

Library of Congress Cataloging-in-Publication Data
Core concepts in health/ [compiled by] Paul M. Insel, Walton T. Roth; Kirstan Price, developmental editor.
   —8th ed.
   p.   cm.
   Includes index.
   ISBN 0-7674-1040-8
   1. Health.   I. Insel, Paul M.   II. Roth, Walton T.
RA776.C83   1999b
613—dc21   99–26823
                                              CIP

Manufactured in the United States of America
10   9   8   7   6   5   4   3   2   1

Mayfield Publishing Company
1280 Villa Street
Mountain View, California 94041

Sponsoring editor, Michele Sordi; *developmental editors,* Kirstan Price, Susan Shook, Kathleen Engelberg, Sue Ewing, and Jeanne Woodward; *production editor,* Julianna Scott Fein; *manuscript editor,* Margaret Moore; *art director and text designer,* Jeanne M. Schreiber; *cover designer,* Laurie Anderson; *design manager,* Jean Mailander; *art editor,* Amy Folden; *illustrators,* Joan Carol, Dale Glasgow, Robin Mouat, Susan Seed, Kevin Somerville, John and Judy Waller, Pamela Drury Wattenmaker; *photo editor,* Brian Pecko; *cover photograph,* © F. Stuart Westmoreland/Natural Selection Stock Photography, Inc.; *proofreader,* Kimberly McCutcheon; *manufacturing manager,* Randy Hurst. This text was set in 10.5/12 Berkeley Book by GTS Graphics, Inc. and printed on 45# Clarendon LG by Banta Book Group.

The Internet addresses listed in the text were accurate at the time of publication. The inclusion of a Web site does not indicate an endorsement by the authors or Mayfield Publishing Company, and Mayfield does not guarantee the accuracy of the information presented at these sites.

TEXT AND PHOTO CREDITS

Text

Pg. 325, "Deciding When to Take Supplements," and pgs. 605, 607–609 adapted from Fahey, T. D., P. M. Insel, and W. T. Roth. 1997. *Fit and Well: Core Concepts and Labs in Physical Fitness and Wellness,* 2nd ed. Mountain View, Calif.: Mayfield. Copyright © 1997 Mayfield Publishing Company. Pgs. 571–574 from Sobel, D., and R. Ornstein. 1996. *The Healthy Mind, Healthy Body Handbook.* DRX. Used with permission. Appendix C from Campbell, J., and M. Keene. 1997. *Mayfield's Quick View Guide to the Internet for Students of Health and Physical Education.* Mountain View, Calif.: Mayfield.

Photo

Title page © 1990 Joel W. Rogers/Offshoot Stock. **Contents** pg. xv, © Bob Daemmrich/The Image Works; pg. xvi, © Esbin-Anderson/The Image Works; pg. xvii, © Laura Dwight/PhotoEdit; pg. xviii, © Rick Browne/Stock Boston; pg. xix, © Bonnie Kamin; pg. xx, © Tim McCarthy/PhotoEdit; pg. xxi, © 1994 Custom Medical Stock Photo Inc. All Rights Reserved; pg. xxiii, © Jim Corwin/Stock Boston; pg. xxv, © John Boykin/PhotoEdit.

Chapter 1   pg. xxviii, © David Madison 1992; pg. 3, © David Young-Wolff/PhotoEdit; pg. 11, © Bob Daemmrich/The Image Works; pg. 16, © Mary Kate Denny/PhotoEdit; pg. 18, © Bob Daemmrich/The Image Works; pg. 20, © Sam Forencich

Chapter 2   pg. 24, © Michelle Bridwell/PhotoEdit; pg. 26, © Michael Grecco/Stock Boston; pg. 30, © Bob Daemmrich/Stock Boston; pg. 36, © John Nordell/The Image Works; pg. 39, © Dorothy Littell Greco/The Image Works; pg. 41, © Tony Freeman/PhotoEdit

Chapter 3   pg. 52, © 1992 Jonathan A. Meyers; pg. 56, © Bob Daemmrich/The Image Works; pg. 58, © Elizabeth Crews; pg. 63, © Mark Antman/The Image Works; pg. 66, © Bob Daemmrich/Stock Boston; pg. 74, © Bob Daemmrich/The Image Works

Chapter 4   pg. 80, © Roberto Soncin Gerometta/Photo 20-20; pg. 83, © Gary A. Conner/PhotoEdit; pg. 87, © R. Lord/The Image Works; pg. 90, © Jennifer Bishop/Actuality, Inc.; pg. 92, © 1996 Phiz Mezey; pg. 97, © Phil Borden/PhotoEdit

Chapter 5   pg. 102, © Esbin-Anderson/The Image Works; pg. 108, © 1997 Phiz Mezey; pg. 111, © Rebecca Cooney/Actuality, Inc.; pg. 117, left, © Tony Freeman/PhotoEdit; pg. 117, right, © Myrleen Ferguson/PhotoEdit; pg. 122, © Starr 1992/Stock Boston; pg. 125, © Michael Siluk/ The Image Works

(Photo credits continue on p. C-1, which constitutes a continuation of the copyright page.)

Preface

Now in its eighth edition, *Core Concepts in Health* has maintained its leadership in the field of health education for over 20 years. Since we pioneered the concept of self-responsibility for personal health in 1976, hundreds of thousands of students have used our book to become active, informed participants in their own health care. Each edition of *Core Concepts* has brought improvements and refinements, but the principles underlying the book have remained the same. Our commitment to these principles has never been stronger than it is today.

OUR GOALS

Our goals in writing this book can be stated simply:

- To present scientifically based, accurate, up-to-date information in an accessible format.
- To involve students in taking responsibility for their health and well-being.
- To instill a sense of competence and personal power in students.

The first of these goals means making expert knowledge about health and health care available to the individual. *Core Concepts* brings scientifically based, accurate, up-to-date information to students about topics and issues that concern them—exercise, stress, nutrition, weight management, contraception, intimate relationships, HIV infection, drugs, alcohol, and a multitude of others. Current, complete, and straightforward coverage is balanced with "user-friendly" features designed to make the text appealing. Written in an engaging, easy-to-read style and presented in a colorful, open format, *Core Concepts* invites the student to read, learn, and remember. Boxes, tables, artwork, photographs, and many other features highlight areas of special interest throughout the book.

The second of our goals is to involve students in taking responsibility for their health. *Core Concepts* uses innovative pedagogy and unique interactive features to get students thinking about how the material they're reading relates to their own lives. We invite them to examine their emotions about the issues under discussion, to consider their personal values and beliefs, and to analyze their health-related behaviors. Beyond this, for students who want to change behaviors that detract from a healthy lifestyle, we offer guidelines and tools, ranging from samples of health journals and personal contracts to detailed assessments and behavior change strategies.

Perhaps our third goal in writing *Core Concepts in Health* is the most important: to instill a sense of competence and personal power in the students who read the book. Everyone has the ability to monitor, understand, and affect his or her own health. Although the medical and health professions possess impressive skills and have access to a huge body of knowledge that benefits everyone in our society, people can help to minimize the amount of professional care they actually require in their lifetime by taking care of their health—taking charge of their health—from an early age. Our hope is that *Core Concepts* will continue to help young people make this exciting discovery—that they have the power to shape their own futures.

ORGANIZATION AND CONTENT OF THE EIGHTH EDITION

The organization of the book as a whole remains essentially the same as in the seventh edition, with some improvements. The book is divided into eight parts. Part One, Establishing a Basis for Wellness, includes chapters on taking charge of your health (Chapter 1), stress (Chapter 2), and psychological health (Chapter 3). Part Two, Understanding Sexuality, opens with an exploration of intimate relationships, including friendship, intimate partnerships, marriage, and family (Chapter 4), and then moves on to discuss physical sexuality (Chapter 5), contraception (Chapter 6), abortion (Chapter 7), and pregnancy and childbirth (Chapter 8). As in previous editions of *Core Concepts,* we devote a separate chapter to abortion to reflect both the importance of this issue and our belief that abortion is not a form of contraception and should not be included in the chapter on that topic.

The order of topics in Part Three, Making Responsible Decisions: Substance Use and Abuse, has been changed for the eighth edition. The part opens with an expanded discussion of addictive behavior and the different classes of psychoactive drugs (Chapter 9), followed by chapters on alcohol (Chapter 10) and tobacco (Chapter 11). The chapters in Part Four, Getting Fit, have also been reordered. Following a detailed discussion of nutrition (Chapter 12), we turn first to exercise (Chapter 13) and then to weight management (Chapter 14). Placing the material on exercise before the coverage of weight management helps emphasize the important role that physical activity plays in maintaining a healthy body weight.

Part Five, Protecting Yourself Against Disease, deals with the most serious health threats facing Americans today—cardiovascular disease (Chapter 15), cancer (Chapter 16), and infectious diseases, including those that are sexually transmitted. The chapters in Part Five have been reordered in the eighth edition so that the discussion of the immune system (Chapter 17) precedes the material on sexually transmitted diseases (Chapter 18). This change will aid students' understanding of the impact of HIV on the immune system.

Part Six, Accepting Physical Limits, explores aging (Chapter 19) and dying and death (Chapter 20). Part Seven, Making Choices in Health Care, provides information about medical self-care (Chapter 21) and the health care system (Chapter 22). And finally, Part Eight, Improving Your Chances: Personal Safety and Environmental Health, expands the boundaries of health to include injury prevention (Chapter 23) and the effects of environment on wellness (Chapter 24). Taken together, the chapters of the book provide students with a complete guide to promoting and protecting their health, now and through their entire lives, as individuals, as participants in a health care community and system, and as citizens of a planet that also needs to be protected if it is to continue providing human beings with the means to live healthy lives.

For the eighth edition, all chapters were carefully reviewed, revised, and updated. The latest information from scientific and health-related research is incorporated in the text, and newly emerging topics and issues are discussed. The following list gives a sample of some of the current concerns addressed in the eighth edition:

- Causes and prevention of violence
- Women's health issues
- Health information on the Internet
- Spiritual wellness
- Progress toward *Healthy People 2000* objectives
- The Surgeon General's 1996 recommendations for physical activity
- HIV treatment and testing
- Binge drinking on college campuses
- Diet and cancer
- Stress and disease
- Addictive behavior
- Genetic testing for cancer
- Safe use of air bags
- Critical thinking and consumer choices

- Emerging infectious diseases
- Physician-assisted death
- Effective communication

For the eighth edition, the coverage of violence has been expanded and moved to Chapter 23, Personal Safety: Protecting Yourself from Unintentional Injuries and Violence. Chapter 23 includes new and expanded sections on factors that contribute to violence, assault, homicide, gangs, hate crimes, family and intimate violence, sexual violence, and the role of firearms in violent injury and death. New boxes help students identify the potential for abusiveness in an intimate partner, prevent date rape, and protect themselves from all types of violent crime. The coverage of unintentional injuries—the leading cause of death for Americans under the age of 45—has also been revised and updated for the eighth edition. The goals of Chapter 23 are to make students more aware of why injuries happen and to give them concrete strategies for keeping themselves safe.

The coverage of HIV infection in Chapter 18, Sexually Transmitted Diseases, has been revised to reflect recent developments in testing and treatment. New illustrations show the effects of HIV on the immune system, the actions of new antiviral drugs, and the relative risk of different types of sexual behaviors. Four boxes address related issues—"HIV Infection Around the World," "Getting an HIV Test," "Talking About Condoms and Safer Sex," and "Preventing HIV Infection." Another box asks students to carefully examine their attitudes and behaviors to determine whether they are putting themselves at risk for HIV infection or another STD.

Chapter 9, The Use and Abuse of Psychoactive Drugs, includes a new opening section on addictive behaviors in general—what they are and how they develop. This section provides specific information on four potentially addictive behaviors: gambling, shopping, sex, and Internet use. The remainder of Chapter 9 covers key psychoactive drugs and includes up-to-date coverage of drug testing, drug legalization, and the social costs of drug use.

Two areas of particular concern—and the subjects of a great deal of recent research—are cardiovascular disease and cancer, the two leading killers of Americans. Chapters 15 and 16 report the latest findings on the roles of diet, exercise, tobacco use, infectious agents, and genetics in determining an individual's risk for developing CVD or cancer. Eleven new boxes address related topics, such as genetic tests for cancer risk, how hormones affect a woman's risk for heart disease, and how personality and social support affect disease risk and outcome.

Core Concepts also takes care to address the health issues and concerns of an increasingly diverse student population. While most health concerns are universal—we all need to eat well, exercise, and manage stress, for example—certain differences among people have important implications for health. These differences can be genetic or cultural, based on factors such as gender, socioeconomic status, age, and ethnicity. Where such differences are important for health, they are discussed in the text or in a type of highlight box called Dimensions of Diversity (discussed in greater detail below). Examples of these discussions include the links between ethnicity and genetic diseases, the relationship between poverty and environmental health, and the effects of gender and ethnicity on body image.

The coverage of health issues for diverse populations has been expanded in the eighth edition, with topics in women's health receiving special attention. The gender gap in medical research has been closing since the establishment of the Office of Research on Women's Health at the National Institutes of Health, and more and more new information has become available as a result of the Women's Health Initiative, the Nurses' Health Study, and other large-scale investigations. New to the eighth edition are discussions of special risks faced by women who smoke or drink, hormonal influences on cardiovascular health and disease, reasons why women are at increased risk for depression and autoimmune disorders, and special dietary challenges faced by women.

The health field is dynamic, with new discoveries, advances, trends, and theories reported every week. Ongoing research—on the role of diet in cancer prevention, for example, or on new treatments for HIV infection—continually changes our understanding of the human body and how it works in health and disease. For this reason, no health book can claim to have the final word on every topic. Yet within these limits, *Core Concepts* does present the latest available information and scientific thinking on innumerable topics.

To aid students in keeping up with rapidly advancing knowledge about health issues, the eighth edition of *Core Concepts* also includes coverage of a key source of up-to-date information—the Internet. Each chapter includes an annotated list of World Wide Web sites that students can use as a launching point for further exploration of important topics. Appendix C, Resources for Self-Care, provides a brief introduction to the Internet, including guidelines for performing Web searches, using newsgroups and mailing lists, and evaluating health information from the Web. Several elements of the supplements package also include Internet resources and activities; see below for more details.

FEATURES OF THE EIGHTH EDITION

This edition of *Core Concepts in Health* builds on the features that attracted and held our readers' interest in the previous editions. One of the most popular features has always been the **boxes,** which allow us to explore a wide range of current topics in greater detail than is possible in the text itself. About half the boxes are new to the eighth edition, and many others have been significantly revised or updated. The boxes are divided into six categories, each marked with a unique icon and label.

 Tactics and Tips boxes distill from each chapter the practical advice students need in order to apply information to their own lives. By referring to these boxes, students can easily find ways to foster friendships, for example; to become more physically active; to improve communication in their relationships; to reduce the amount of fat in their diets; and to help a friend who has a problem with tobacco or drugs or has an eating disorder.

 Critical Consumer boxes, new to the eighth edition, emphasize the key theme of critical thinking. These boxes are designed to help students develop and apply critical thinking skills, thereby allowing them to make sound choices related to health and well-being. Critical Consumer boxes provide specific guidelines for evaluating health news and advertising, using food labels to make dietary choices, choosing and using medical self-tests, avoiding quackery, selecting exercise footwear, making environmentally friendly shopping choices, and so on.

 Dimensions of Diversity boxes are part of our commitment to reflect and respond to the diversity of the student population. These boxes give students the opportunity to identify any special health risks that affect them because of who they are as individuals or as members of a group. They also broaden students' perspectives by exposing them to a wide variety of viewpoints on health-related issues. The different dimensions these boxes reflect include gender, ethnicity, socioeconomic status, and age. The principles embodied by these boxes are described in the first box in the series, "Health Issues for Diverse Populations," which appears in Chapter 1. Topics covered in later chapters include special cardiovascular disease risks for African Americans, exercise for people with disabilities, suicide among older men, ethnic diets and cuisines, links between poverty and poor environmental health, and attitudes toward aging.

In addition, some Dimensions of Diversity boxes highlight health issues and practices in other parts of the world, allowing students to see what Americans share with people in other societies and how they differ. Students have the opportunity to learn about patterns of alcohol use in different cultures, laws and attitudes toward contraception and abortion in other countries, the pattern of HIV infection around the world, and other topics of interest.

Sound Mind, Sound Body boxes explore the close connection between mind and body. Drawn from studies in psychoneuroimmunology and related fields, these boxes focus on total wellness by examining the links between people's feelings and states of mind and their physical health; the boxes emphasize that all the dimensions of wellness must be developed in order for an individual to achieve optimal health and well-being. Included in Sound Mind, Sound Body boxes are topics such as how social support promotes wellness, how stress affects the immune system, how hostility and cardiovascular disease are linked, how intimate relationships improve health, and how exercise fosters psychological and emotional wellness.

 Assess Yourself boxes give students the opportunity to examine their behavior and identify ways that they can change their habits and improve their health. By referring to these boxes, students can examine their eating habits, for example; evaluate their fitness level; discover if they are at increased risk for cancer or cardiovascular disease; evaluate their driving skills; determine what triggers their eating; and examine their drinking and drug-taking behavior.

 A Closer Look boxes highlight current wellness topics of particular interest. Topics include bicycle helmets, diabetes, asthma, genetic testing for cancer, shyness, Prozac, codependency, and physician-assisted death.

In addition to the box program, many new and refined features are included in the eighth edition of *Core Concepts*. Each chapter opens with a new feature called **Test Your Knowledge**—a series of 4–6 multiple choice and true-false questions, with answers. These self-quizzes facilitate learning by getting students involved in a variety of wellness-related issues. The questions emphasize important points, highlight common misconceptions, and spark debate.

Vital Statistics tables and figures highlight important facts and figures in a memorable format that often reveals surprising contrasts and connections. From tables and figures marked with the Vital Statistics label, students can learn about drinking and drug use among college students, health care costs in the United States, world population growth, homicide rates, trends in public opinion about abortion, and a wealth of other information. For students who grasp a subject best when it is displayed graphically, numerically, or in a table, the Vital Statistics feature provides alternative ways of approaching and understanding the text.

The eighth edition also features an expanded program of attractive and helpful **illustrations**. The anatomical art, which has been prepared by medical illustrators, is both visually appealing and highly informative. These illustrations help students understand such important information as how blood flows through the heart, how the process of conception occurs, and how to use a condom. Many of the graphs, charts, and other illustrations have been rendered in a dynamic and appealing new style. New topics illustrated for the eighth edition include the relationship between lifestyle factors and cancer risk, the life cycle of HIV in human cells, the chain of infection, the greenhouse effect, the immune response, and the levels and effects of different sounds. These lively and abundant illustrations will particularly benefit those students who learn best from visual images. Taken together, all the visual elements of the book provide powerful pedagogical tools and create a colorful and inviting look.

Personal Insights are open-ended questions designed to encourage self-examination and heighten students' awareness of their feelings, values, beliefs, thought processes, and past experiences. These questions have been formulated in a nonjudgmental way to foster honest self-analysis. They appear at appropriate points throughout each chapter.

Take Action, appearing at the end of every chapter, suggests hands-on exercises and projects that students can undertake to extend and deepen their grasp of the material. Suggested projects include interviews, investigations of campus or community resources, and experimentation with some of the behavior change techniques suggested in the text. Special care has been taken to ensure that the projects are both feasible and worthwhile.

Journal Entry also appears at the end of each chapter. These entries suggest ways for students to use their Health Journal (which we recommend they keep while using *Core Concepts*) to think about topics and issues, explore and formulate their own views, and express their thoughts in written form. They are designed to help students deepen their understanding of their own health-related behaviors.

Making wise choices about health requires students to sort through and evaluate health information. To help students become skilled evaluators, each chapter contains at least one **Critical Thinking Journal Entry.** These entries help students develop their critical thinking skills, including finding relevant information, separating fact from opinion, recognizing faulty reasoning, evaluating information, and assessing the credibility of sources. Critical Thinking Journal Entry questions do not have right or wrong answers; rather, they ask students to analyze, evaluate, or take a stand on a particular issue.

The **Behavior Change Strategies** that conclude many chapters offer specific behavior management/modification plans relating to the chapter's topic. Based on the principles of behavior management that are carefully explained in Chapter 1, these strategies will help students change unhealthy or counterproductive behaviors.

Included are strategies for dealing with test anxiety, quitting smoking, developing responsible drinking habits, planning a personal exercise program, phasing in a healthier diet, and many other practical plans for change.

Three quick-reference appendixes provide students with resources they can keep and use for years to come:

- Appendix A, "Nutritional Content of Popular Items from Fast-Food Restaurants," provides information on commonly ordered menu items at eight fast-food restaurants.

- Appendix B, "Self-Care Guide for Common Medical Problems," provides information to help students manage common symptoms, including fever, sore throat, indigestion, headache, and cuts and scrapes.

- Appendix C, "Resources for Self-Care," lists books, information centers, hotlines, and electronic sources of wellness-related materials. Guidelines for using the Internet—how to perform searches, how to evaluate online information, and how to use newsgroups, mailing lists, and chat rooms—are also provided.

"First Aid at a Glance" from the Red Cross appears inside the back cover of the text, providing information that can save lives.

LEARNING AIDS

Although all the features of *Core Concepts in Health* are designed to facilitate learning, several specific learning aids have also been incorporated in the text. **Learning Objectives** appear on the opening page of each chapter, identifying major concepts and helping to guide students in their reading and review of the text. Important terms appear in boldface type in the text and are defined in a **running glossary,** helping students handle a large and complex new vocabulary.

Chapter summaries offer students a concise review and a way to make sure they have grasped the most important concepts in the chapter. Also found at the end of every chapter are **Selected Bibliographies** and sections called For More Information. New to the eighth edition, **For More Information** sections contain annotated lists of books, newsletters, hotlines, organizations, and Web sites that students can use to extend and broaden their knowledge or pursue subjects of interest to them. A complete **Index** at the end of the book includes references to glossary terms in boldface type.

TEACHING TOOLS

Available to qualified adopters of the eighth edition of *Core Concepts in Health* is a comprehensive package of supplementary materials that enhance teaching and learning. Included in the package are the following items:

- Instructor's Resource Binder
- Students on Health: Custom Video to Accompany *Core Concepts in Health*
- Transparency Acetates
- Wellness Worksheets
- *Mayfield's Quick View Guide to the Internet for Students of Health and Physical Education*
- *Core Concepts in Health* Presentation Software
- Mayfield Wellness Software
- Student Study Guide
- Computerized Test Bank
- Additional videos, software, and other multimedia

The **Instructor's Resource Binder,** new for the eighth edition, contains a variety of helpful teaching materials in an easy-to-use form. Included in the binder are a comprehensive Instructor's Resource Guide, transparency masters and handouts, an extensive set of examination questions, Wellness Worksheets, a sample color transparency acetate, and complete descriptions and ordering information for special *Core Concepts* packages.

- The **Instructor's Resource Guide** provides a variety of supplementary materials that can be used to direct and facilitate students' learning: extended chapter outlines, learning objectives, classroom activities, additional resources, Internet resources, selected *Healthy People 2000* objectives, and health crossword puzzles.

- **Transparency masters and handouts**—90 in all—are provided as additional lecture resources. The transparency masters include tables, graphs, and key points from the text; illustrations of many body systems are also provided.

- The **examination questions** have been completely revised and updated for the eighth edition by Phyllis D. Murray at Eastern Kentucky University. The test bank contains nearly 3000 multiple choice and true-false questions. The answer key lists the page number in the text where each answer is found.

- The Instructor's Resource Binder also includes a complete set of **Wellness Worksheets,** a student learning aid described below.

Also new for the eighth edition is **Students on Health: Custom Video to Accompany *Core Concepts in Health*.** Filmed exclusively for *Core Concepts* with students at college campuses across the country, this unique video is designed to stimulate critical thinking and class discussion. The 8–10-minute segments focus on key wellness concerns—stress, intimate relationships, alcohol, tobacco, nutrition, exercise, STDs, and personal safety. The accompanying Instructor's Video Guide provides summaries of each segment and discussion questions.

Sixty **transparency acetates,** half in color, provide material suitable for lecture and discussion. The acetates do not duplicate the transparency masters in the Instructor's Resource Binder, and many of them are from sources other than the text.

Wellness Worksheets help students become more involved in their own wellness and better prepared to implement successful behavior change programs. The 90 worksheets developed for the eighth edition include assessment tools that help students learn more about their wellness-related attitudes and behaviors, Internet activities that guide them in finding and using information from the World Wide Web, and knowledge-based reviews of key concepts. Wellness Worksheets are available in an easy-to-use pad (free when shrink-wrapped with the text) and are also found in the Study Guide.

New for the eighth edition is *Mayfield's Quick View Guide to the Internet for Students of Health and Physical Education* by Jennifer Campbell and Michael Keene at University of Tennessee, Knoxville. It provides step-by-step instructions on how to access the Internet and how to find and use information about health. It includes extensive lists of Internet resources for both students and instructors. The *Quick View Guide* also shows students how to evaluate the credibility of online information sources, communicate via e-mail and chat rooms, use listservs and newsgroups, find jobs through the Internet, and even create a Web page.

Also new for the eighth edition is the *Core Concepts in Health* **Presentation Software** package. This helpful lecture aid includes two components. The **CD-ROM Image Bank,** compatible with both IBM and Macintosh computers, contains over 150 images from the eighth edition as an additional lecture resource. The images can be used with LCD overhead projectors and can be imported into PowerPoint® and other presentation software. The **PowerPoint Lecture Outlines** are electronic transparencies that can be customized to fit any lecture.

Easy-to-use **Mayfield Wellness Software** includes instructions and contracts for creating successful behavior change programs, as well as 15 interactive assessment activities. The assessments, which cover fitness, nutrition, stress, weight management, and cardiovascular health, help students pinpoint behaviors they can change to increase wellness. The software is available in both Windows and Macintosh formats and can be networked (free to qualified adopters).

The **Student Study Guide,** prepared by Thomas M. Davis of the University of Northern Iowa, is designed to help students understand and assimilate the material in the text. The Study Guide includes learning objectives, key terms, major points and issues, sample test questions, and the complete set of Wellness Worksheets.

A **computerized test bank** is available to qualified adopters. Microtest III, developed by Chariot Software

Group, allows instructors to design tests using the examination questions included with *Core Concepts in Health* and/or incorporating their own questions. Microtest is available in both Windows and Macintosh formats.

Additional videos, software, and other multimedia—including nutrition, fitness, and health risk appraisal software—are available to qualified adopters. The **Mayfield video library** includes tapes on topics such as stress, intimate relationships, alcohol use, AIDS, nutrition, violence, fitness, and many more. **DINE Healthy software** provides an easy way for students to evaluate the nutritional value of their current diet; it also includes an exercise section that allows students to track their energy expenditures. The **Healthier People Network Health Risk Appraisal** is a self-assessment tool that alerts students to their personal risk areas and advises them on how to improve their risk profile.

If you have any questions concerning the book or teaching package, please call your local Mayfield sales representative or the Marketing and Sales Department at 800-433-1279. You may also reach Mayfield at profservices@mayfieldpub.com.

A NOTE OF THANKS

The efforts of innumerable people have gone into producing this eighth edition of *Core Concepts in Health.* The book has benefited immensely from their thoughtful commentaries, expert knowledge and opinions, and many helpful suggestions. We are deeply grateful for their participation in the project.

Academic Contributors

Stephen Barrett, M.D., Consumer Advocate and Editor, *Nutrition Forum Newsletter*
The Health Care System

Roger Baxter, M.D., Internist and Infectious Disease Specialist, Kaiser Permanente Medical Center, Oakland, California; Associate Clinical Professor, University of California, San Francisco
Immunity and Infection

Virginia Brooke, Ph.D., University of Texas Medical Branch at Galveston
Aging: A Vital Process

Boyce Burge, Ph.D., *Healthline*
Cancer

Christine DeVault, Cabrillo College
Pregnancy and Childbirth

Thomas Fahey, Ed.D., California State University, Chico
Exercise for Health and Fitness

Michael R. Hoadley, Ph.D., University of South Dakota
Personal Safety: Protecting Yourself from Unintentional Injuries and Violence

Paul M. Insel, Ph.D., Stanford University
Taking Charge of Your Health; Stress: The Constant Challenge; Toward a Tobacco-Free Society; Cardiovascular Health

Nancy Kemp, M.D., Sonoma State University
The Responsible Use of Alcohol; Sexually Transmitted Diseases

Charles Ksir, Ph.D., University of Wyoming
The Use and Abuse of Psychoactive Drugs

Joyce D. Nash, Ph.D., Clinical Psychologist in private practice (San Francisco and Palo Alto)
Weight Management

David Quadagno, Ph.D., Florida State University
Sex and Your Body

Walton T. Roth, M.D., Stanford University
Psychological Health

James H. Rothenberger, M.P.H., University of Minnesota
Environmental Health

David Sobel, M.D., M.P.H., Director of Patient Education and Health Promotion, Kaiser Permanente Medical Care Program, Northern California Region
Medical Self-Care: Skills for the Health Care Consumer

Albert Lee Strickland and Lynne Ann DeSpelder, Cabrillo College
Dying and Death

Bryan Strong, Ph.D., University of California, Santa Cruz, and Christine DeVault, Cabrillo College
Intimate Relationships

Mae V. Tinklenberg, R.N., N.P., M.S., *Nurseweek Publications*
Contraception; Abortion

Stella L. Volpe, Ph.D., R.D., F.A.C.S.M., University of Massachusetts–Amherst
Nutrition Basics

Academic Advisers and Reviewers

Dianne A. R. Bartley, Middle Tennessee State University

Dayna S. Brown, Morehead State University

Suzanne M. Christopher, Portland Community College

Paul Finnicum, Arkansas State University

Marianne Frauenknecht, Western Michigan University

Julie Gast, Utah State University

Marie R. Horton, Texas Southern University

Bobby E. Lang, Florida Agricultural and Mechanical University

Rebecca R. Leas, Clarion University of Pennsylvania

Terri Mulkins Manning, University of North Carolina at Charlotte

Juli Miller, Ohio University

M. Sue Reynolds, University of Maryland

N. Heather Savage, University of New Orleans

Martin D. Schwartz, Ohio University

David A. Sleet, National Center for Injury Prevention and Control, Centers for Disease Control and Prevention

Helen M. Welle, Georgia Southern University

Michael A. White, Kings River College

Kathy M. Wood, Butler County Community College

Jenny Kisuk Yi, University of Houston

Technology Focus Group Participants

Ken Allen, University of Wisconsin–Oshkosh

Lisa Farley, Butler University

Barbara Greenburg, Butler University

Bill Johnson, Stephen F. Austin State University

Rita Nugent, University of Evansville

Patricia Dotson Pettit, Nebraska Wesleyan University

Carol Plugge, Lamar University

Steve Sedbrook, Fort Hays State University

Marilyn Strawbridge, Butler University

Finally, the book could not have been published without the efforts of the staff at Mayfield Publishing Company and the *Core Concepts* book team: Serina Beauparlant, Sponsoring Editor; Kirstan Price, Megan Rundel, Susan Shook, and Kate Engelberg, Developmental Editors; Sara Early, Editorial Assistant; Linda Toy, Production Director; Lynn Rabin Bauer, Production Editor; Jeanne M. Schreiber, Art Director; Robin Mouat, Art Editor; Marty Granahan, Permissions Editor; Brian Pecko, Photo Researcher; Randy Hurst, Manufacturing Manager; Ann Marie Hovie, Production Assistant; Michelle Rodgerson, Marketing Manager; Jay Bauer, Marketing Communications. To all we express our deep appreciation.

Paul M. Insel
Walton T. Roth

About the 2000 Update

Because changes in health-related information occur so rapidly, and because we are committed to providing comprehensive, accurate information on the most pressing current issues, we have prepared this updated version of the eighth edition of *Core Concepts in Health*. The overall content, organization, and features of the eighth edition remain in place, but within this framework, key topics and issues have been updated with the most recent information available.

CONTENT AND ORGANIZATION

Coverage has been updated in two general ways:

- Where important new issues or topics have arisen, or where new information has become available in key areas, we have incorporated this information into the text or highlight boxes. Examples of new and updated topics include the draft *Healthy People 2010* objectives, the Dietary Reference Intakes for vitamins and minerals, the new labeling requirements for dietary supplements, the newly approved kits for emergency contraception, physician-assisted suicide laws, hepatitis C, and treatments for breast cancer.

- Wherever more recent statistics have become available, we have replaced older figures with newer ones. For example, we have updated statistics on the incidence of various diseases, including CVD, cancer, and AIDS; on rates of use of tobacco, alcohol, and other drugs; on leading causes of death; on health care spending in the United States; and on worldwide population growth.

For a complete list of changes to the 2000 Update, contact your local Mayfield sales representative or the Marketing and Sales Department (800-433-1279; calpoppy @mayfieldpub.com).

FEATURES AND LEARNING AIDS

All the student-oriented features and learning aids of the eighth edition have been retained and updated: boxes, Learning Objectives, Personal Insights, Vital Statistics tables and figures, Take Action, Journal Entry, Behavior Change Strategies, running glossary, Selected Bibliographies, chapter summaries, and the three appendixes. In every chapter,

For More Information listings of recommended readings, organizations, hotlines, and Web sites have been thoroughly updated; the section in Appendix C on how to locate and evaluate online wellness resources has been expanded. Students can access all the Web sites listed in the book, as well as many others, from the links page of the *Core Concepts in Health* Web site, described in the next section.

The six types of boxes found in the eighth edition have been retained in the 2000 Update—Tactics and Tips, Critical Consumer, Dimensions of Diversity, Assess Yourself, A Closer Look, and Sound Mind, Sound Body. Many of the boxes have been updated with new research findings and new statistics. In addition, new boxes have been added to highlight key current issues:

Health in the Twenty-First Century (Chapter 1)

Major Life Changes, Stress, and Risk of Illness (Chapter 2)

Lifting Depression with Drug Therapy (Chapter 3)

Intercultural Friendships and Intimate Relationships (Chapter 4)

Online Relationships (Chapter 4)

Infertility and Reproductive Technology (Chapter 8)

Using Dietary Supplement Labels (Chapter 12)

Diabetes (Chapter 14)

Calculate and Rate Your Body Mass Index (BMI) (Chapter 14)

Evaluating Fat and Sugar Substitutes (Chapter 14)

Strategies of Successful Weight Managers (Chapter 14)

Complementary and Alternative Medicine (Chapter 22)

Are You an Aggressive Driver? (Chapter 23)

Violence and the News Media: Perception Versus Reality (Chapter 23)

TEACHING TOOLS

For the 2000 Update, the comprehensive package of supplementary materials created for the eighth edition has been updated as needed to match the text:

- Instructor's Resource Binder, including the Instructor's Resource Guide (prepared by Cathy Kennedy and Janna West Kowalski, Colorado State

University), Examination Questions (prepared by Beth Lanning, Baylor University), and Transparency Masters and Handouts

- Transparency Acetates
- Wellness Worksheets (expanded to include 102 worksheets and 28 Internet activities)
- Study Guide
- Computerized Test Bank
- Students on Health: Custom Video to Accompany Core Concepts in Health
- Mayfield's Quick View Guide to the Internet for Students of Health and Physical Education
- Additional videos, software, and other multimedia

In addition, four new supplements have been developed for the 2000 Update. The **Core Concepts in Health Web site** (http://www.mayfieldpub.com/insel) includes resources for both instructors and students. The syllabus builder allows instructors to construct and edit a syllabus that can be accessed online or printed for distribution. An Image Bank, a set of PowerPoint® slides, and the Instructor's Resource Guide can be downloaded from a password-protected portion of the site. For students, there are interactive quizzes that provide immediate feedback and a behavior change workbook that guides them through the process of behavior change. Also included on the Web site is an extensive set of Internet resources, including links for further information, guidelines for finding and evaluating information from the Internet, and Internet activities.

The new **Instructor's CD-ROM** provides a variety of valuable teaching tools for both IBM-compatible and Macintosh computers. The Image Bank contains over 100 full-color images from the book, as well as images from the transparency acetates and masters; the images can be used with LCD projectors and imported into PowerPoint and other presentation software. A complete set of PowerPoint slides, prepared by Steve Sedbrook, Fort Hays State University, is provided as an additional lecture resource. The CD-ROM also contains the text of the Instructor's Resource Guide, which can be customized to fit any course.

Also new is **Core Concepts Interactive**, a CD-ROM designed to help students learn and apply key wellness concepts. It contains interactive quizzes, video segments, a pronunciation guide to many of the text's key terms, electronic versions of the color images from the text, and a link to the *Core Concepts in Health* Web site. The CD-ROM can be used with both IBM-compatible and Macintosh computers.

Finally, the **Nutrition and Weight Management Journal** is also now available for students. This easy-to-use journal guides students in assessing their current diet and making appropriate changes. It includes many valuable tools, including the Food Guide Pyramid, serving-size recommendations, the Dietary Guidelines for Americans, a sample food label, and information about the nutritional content of popular items from fast-food restaurants.

For more information about the teaching tools, contact your local Mayfield representative or contact Mayfield at 800-433-1279 or calpoppy@mayfieldpub.com

ACKNOWLEDGEMENTS

We would like to thank the academic advisers and reviewers for the 2000 Update:

Rick Barnes, East Carolina University

Lois Beach, State University of New York at Plattsburgh

M. Betsy Bergen, Kansas State University

Penny J. Brynildson, Bethel College

Patricia A. Cost, Weber State University

Natalie Erlich, Oklahoma State University

Sally J. Ford, Pima Community College

Daniel S. Gerber, University of Massachusetts–Amherst

Richard Madson, Palm Beach Community College

Bobby C. Martin, Hampton University

La Tonya D. Mouzon, Southern Illinois University at Carbondale

Kerry J. Redican, Virginia Polytechnical Institute and State University

Connie Reynolds, Utah Valley State

Thea Siria Spatz, University of Arkansas at Little Rock

Ladona Tornabene, University of South Dakota

Helen Welle-Graf, Georgia Southern University

Kristin Jacoby Yusko, University of Maryland College Park

Finally, we would like to thank the staff at Mayfield Publishing Company, particularly the members of the *Core Concepts* book team. First, we are indebted to Kirstan Price for her dedication and her extraordinary creative energies, which have helped to make this book such a success. Thanks also go to Michele Sordi, Sponsoring Editor; Susan Shook and Kate Engelberg, Developmental Editors; Bessie Weiss and Catherine New, Editorial Assistants; Linda Toy, Production Director; Julianna Scott Fein, Senior Production Editor; Jeanne M. Schreiber, Art Director; Amy Folden, Art Editor; Marty Granahan, Permissions Editor; Brian Pecko, Photo Editor; Randy Hurst, Manufacturing Manager; Heather Collins, Production Assistant; Michelle Rodgerson, Marketing Manager; Jay Bauer, Marketing Communications Specialist. To all we express our deep appreciation.

Paul M. Insel
Walton T. Roth

Brief Contents

Contents

PART TWO
Understanding Sexuality

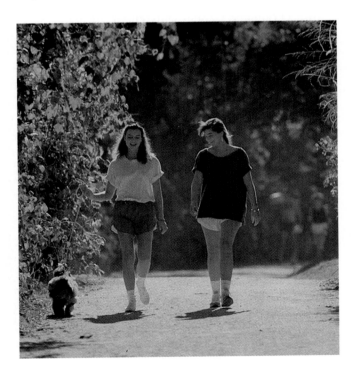

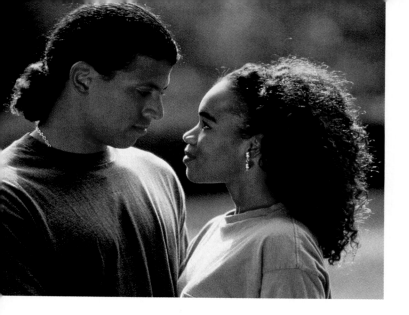

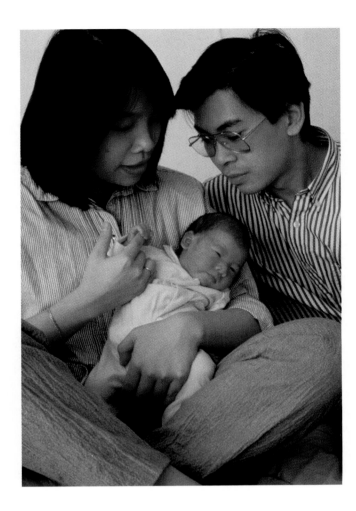

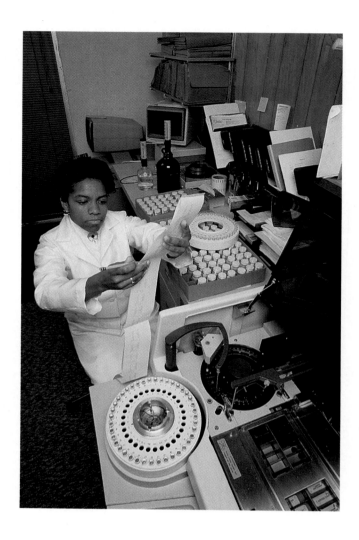

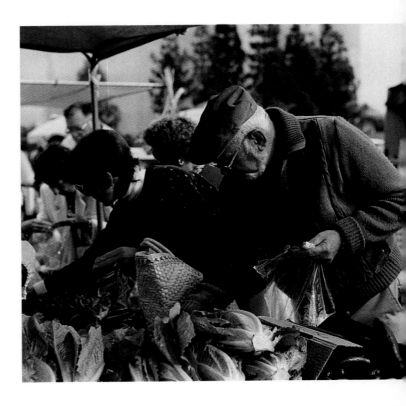

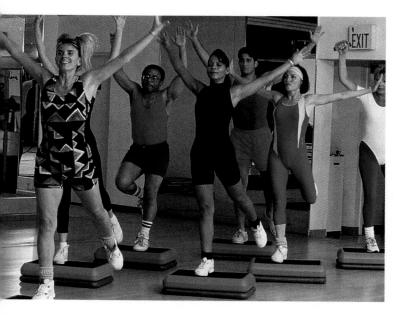

CHAPTER 14
Weight Management   373

CHAPTER 13
Exercise for Health and Fitness   341

PART FIVE
Protecting Yourself from Disease

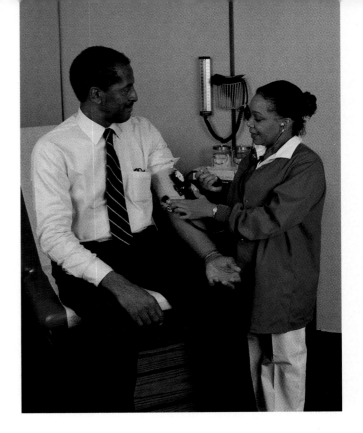

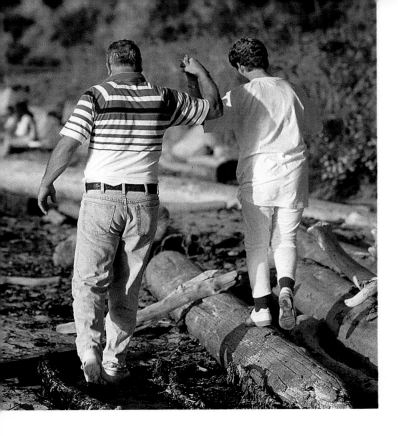

PART SEVEN
Making Choices in Health Care

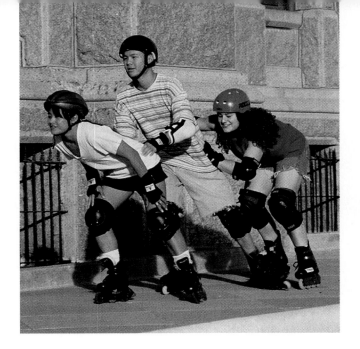

CRITICAL CONSUMER

DIMENSIONS OF DIVERSITY

Note: The health issues and conditions listed here include those that disproportionately influence or affect women or men. For more information, see the index under gender, women, men, and any of the specific topics listed here.

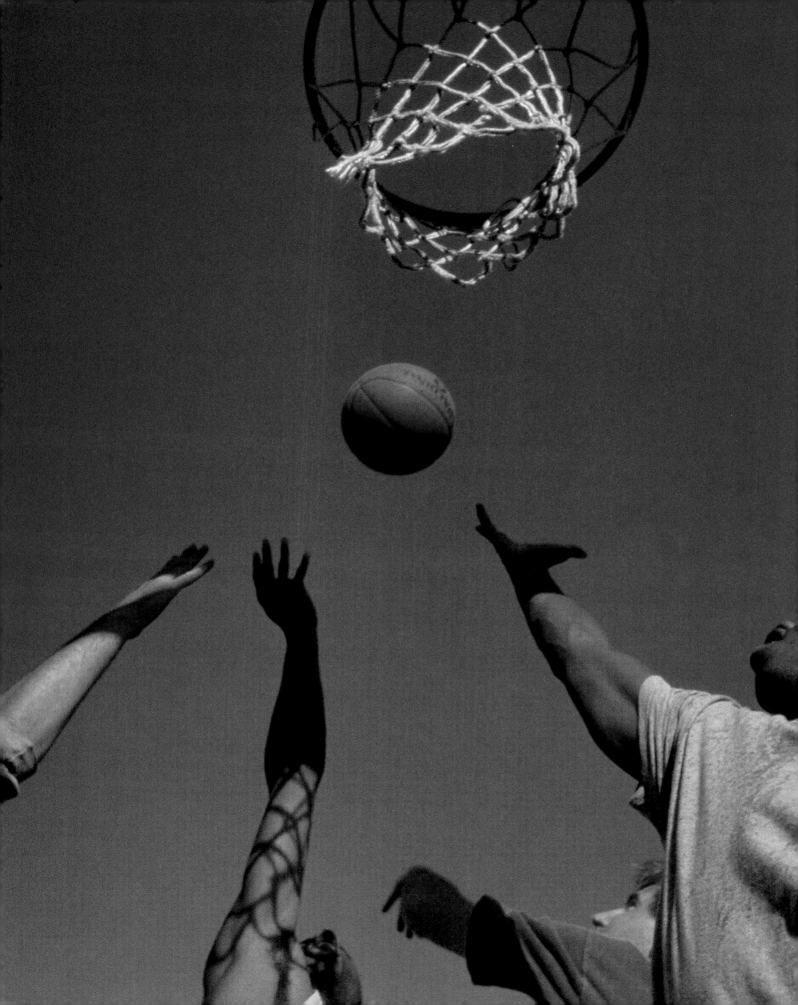

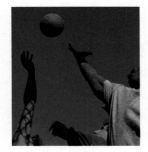

LEARNING OBJECTIVES

After reading this chapter, you should be able to:

- Describe the six dimensions of wellness and a wellness lifestyle.

- Identify major goals of the national Healthy People initiative.

- Explain the importance of personal decision making and behavior change in achieving a wellness lifestyle.

- Create a behavior management plan to change a health-related behavior.

- Describe the influence of gender, socioeconomic status, ethnicity, and age on health.

- Discuss the available sources of health information and how to think critically about them.

Taking Charge of Your Health 1

TEST YOUR KNOWLEDGE

1. Heart disease is the leading cause of death among Americans.
    True or false?

2. If you have a family history of heart disease or cancer, there's not much you can do to lower your risk of getting these diseases.
    True or false?

3. Women tend to live longer than men.
    True or false?

4. Which of the following lifestyle factors contribute(s) to all three leading causes of death for Americans: heart disease, cancer, and stroke?
    a. cigarette smoking
    b. lack of exercise
    c. poor dietary habits

5. More than two-thirds of all college students make which of the following positive lifestyle choices?
    a. use safety belts
    b. do not drink and drive
    c. use contraception (if sexually active)
    d. eat two or fewer high-fat foods per day
    e. do not use tobacco

Answers

1. _True._ Heart disease has been the number-one killer of Americans since 1900.

2. _False._ Lifestyle factors such as diet, exercise, and not smoking play a significant role in preventing these diseases, even for those with a family history of them.

3. _True._ Life expectancy for women is about 6 years longer than for men—79.2 years compared to 73.6 years, for Americans born in 1997.

4. _All three._ Eliminating tobacco use could prevent more than 400,000 deaths annually; improving diet and exercise habits could prevent 300,000 deaths each year.

5. _All five._ However, the majority of students do not exercise regularly, do not wear bicycle helmets, and eat few fruits and vegetables. There are many areas in which college students can change their behavior to improve their health.

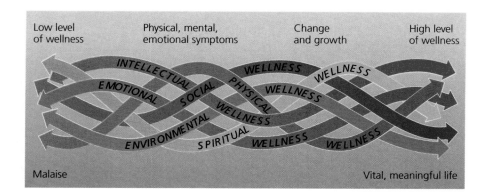

Figure 1-1 The wellness continuum.
Wellness is composed of six interrelated dimensions, all of which must be developed in order to achieve overall wellness.

A first-year college student resolves to meet the challenge of making new friends. A long-sedentary senior starts riding her bike to school every day instead of taking the bus. A busy graduate student volunteers to plant trees in a blighted inner-city neighborhood. What do these people have in common? Each is striving for optimal health and well-being. Not satisfied to be merely free of major illness, these individuals want more. They want to live life actively, energetically, and fully, in a state of optimal personal, interpersonal, and environmental well-being. They have taken charge of their health and are on the path to wellness.

WELLNESS: THE NEW HEALTH GOAL

Wellness is an expanded idea of health. Many people think of health as being just the absence of physical disease. But wellness transcends this concept of health, as when individuals with serious illnesses or disabilities rise above their physical or mental limitations to live rich, meaningful, vital lives. Some aspects of health are determined by your genes, your age, and other factors that may be beyond your control. But true wellness is largely determined by the decisions you make about how to live your life. In this book, we will use the terms "health" and "wellness" interchangeably to mean the ability to live life fully—with vitality and meaning.

The Dimensions of Wellness

No matter what your age or health status, you can optimize your health in each of the following six interrelated dimensions. Wellness in any dimension is not a static goal but a dynamic process of change and growth (Figure 1-1).

TERMS **wellness** Optimal health and vitality, encompassing physical, emotional, intellectual, spiritual, interpersonal, social, and environmental well-being.

Physical Wellness   Optimal physical health requires eating well, exercising, avoiding harmful habits, making responsible decisions about sex, learning about and recognizing the symptoms of disease, getting regular medical and dental checkups, and taking steps to prevent injuries at home, on the road, and on the job. The habits you develop and the decisions you make today will largely determine not only how many years you will live, but the quality of your life during those years.

Emotional Wellness   Optimism, trust, self-esteem, self-acceptance, self-confidence, self-control, satisfying relationships, and an ability to share feelings are just some of the qualities and aspects of emotional wellness. Emotional health is a dynamic state that fluctuates with your physical, intellectual, spiritual, interpersonal and social, and environmental health. Maintaining emotional wellness requires monitoring and exploring your thoughts and feelings, identifying obstacles to emotional well-being, and finding solutions to emotional problems, with the help of a therapist if necessary.

Intellectual Wellness   The hallmarks of intellectual health include an openness to new ideas, a capacity to question and think critically, and the motivation to master new skills, as well as a sense of humor, creativity, and curiosity. An active mind is essential to overall wellness, for learning about, evaluating, and storing health-related information. Your mind detects problems, finds solutions, and directs behavior. People who enjoy intellectual wellness never stop learning. They relish new experiences and challenges and actively seek them out.

Spiritual Wellness   To enjoy spiritual health is to possess a set of guiding beliefs, principles, or values that give meaning and purpose to your life, especially during difficult times. Spiritual wellness involves the capacity for love, compassion, forgiveness, altruism, joy, and fulfillment. It is an antidote to cynicism, anger, fear, anxiety, self-absorption, and pessimism. Spirituality transcends the individual and can be a common bond among people.

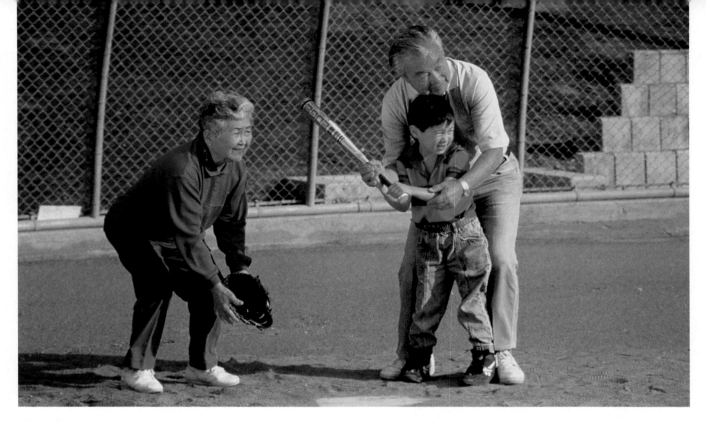

With wellness comes vitality, exuberance, a capacity for joy—and for fun.

Organized religions help many people develop spiritual health. Many others find meaning and purpose in their lives on their own—through nature, art, meditation, political action, or good works.

Interpersonal and Social Wellness Satisfying relationships are basic to both physical and emotional health. We need to have mutually loving, supportive people in our lives. Developing interpersonal wellness means learning good communication skills, developing the capacity for intimacy, and cultivating a support network of caring friends and/or family members. Social wellness requires participating in and contributing to your community, country, and world.

Environmental or Planetary Wellness Increasingly, personal health depends on the health of the planet—from the safety of the food supply to the degree of violence in a society. Other examples of environmental threats to health are ultraviolet radiation in sunlight, air and water pollution, lead in old house paint, and second-hand tobacco smoke in indoor air. Wellness requires learning about and protecting yourself against such hazards—and doing what you can to reduce or eliminate them, either on your own or with others.

The six dimensions of wellness interact continuously, influencing and being influenced by one another. Making a change in one dimension often affects some or all of the others. For example, regular exercise (developing the physical dimension of wellness) can increase feelings of well-being and self-esteem (emotional wellness), which in turn can increase feelings of confidence in social interactions and your achievements at work or school (interpersonal and social wellness). Maintaining good health is a dynamic process, and increasing your level of wellness in one area of life often influences many others.

New Opportunities, New Responsibilities

Wellness is a relatively recent concept. A century ago, people considered themselves lucky just to survive to adulthood. A child born in 1900, for example, could expect to live only about 45 years. Many people died as a result of common infectious diseases and poor environmental conditions (unrefrigerated food, poor sanitation, air and water pollution). However, over the last 100 years, the average life span has nearly doubled, thanks largely to the development of vaccines and antibiotics to prevent and fight infectious diseases, and to public health campaigns to improve environmental conditions.

But a different set of diseases has emerged as our major health threat, and heart disease, cancer, and stroke are now the top three causes of death in the United States. Treating these and other chronic, degenerative diseases has proved enormously expensive and extremely difficult. It has become clear that the best treatment for these diseases is prevention—people having a greater

A study of death rates over the past century illustrates the dramatic changes that have taken place in the nature of health problems and their solutions. The figure below shows overall death rates in the United States from 1885 to the present, with the time at which major medical innovations became available. The dramatic decline in death rates that occurred in the first half of the twentieth century was due primarily to improvements in the environment and in public health policies, including the refrigeration of food, sewage treatment, and limitations on industrial air pollution. The development and widespread use of antibiotics further contributed to this decline. The more gradual downward trend in death rates that has occurred since the 1950s has coincided with the introduction of many medical innovations—vaccines, open-heart surgery, and organ transplantation, for example—as well as with positive lifestyle changes—reduced rates of smoking, lower-fat diets, and increased attention to disease and injury prevention. Although advances in medical technology have not caused an immediate and substantial drop in death rates, their use—and the research underlying them—has paved the way for future developments.

We are currently in the midst of a period of unprecedented technological innovation that promises both to increase life expectancy and to improve quality of life in the twenty-first century. Biotechnology companies are developing ways to process DNA on computer chips, creating a quick profile of an individual's susceptibility to many diseases. Hormones that stimulate the growth of new blood vessels are being studied for use in heart patients as an alternative to surgery for bypassing clogged arteries. Many gene therapies are being developed, including methods to trigger the self-destruct mechanism in cancer cells and to prevent nerve degeneration in stroke patients. Genetic engineering is also being used in other organisms. Scientists are creating bacteria that absorb toxic chemical spills. Corn, soybeans, and other crops are being developed to resist pests. Cows, sheep, and goats are being genetically engineered so that they produce useful drugs in their milk. Innovations in other fields—robotics, electronics, and computer science, to name a few—are being brought into medicine in ways that couldn't have been imagined even 5 years ago.

There may be a downside to some of these spectacular medical developments, however. Treatments based on technological advances are likely to be expensive, taxing the current health care system and increasing the inequities that already exist. And the potential consequences of some of the new technologies, such as cloning, are the subject of active debate. Nevertheless, the drawbacks of many of these new technologies are likely to be outweighed by their tremendous potential benefits.

Perhaps the most important advance of the twenty-first century is the information revolution. A vast amount of health information is now literally at your fingertips, available immediately through the Internet. And new interactive technologies can help you change or reinforce your health-related behaviors. This information explosion puts the responsibility for your own health even more firmly in your own hands. You can choose to make use of all the new information and tools that are available to you—to enhance your well-being and to live a life of health and vitality in the coming era of technological innovation.

SOURCES: National Center for Health Statistics. 1998. *Health, United States, 1998: With Socioeconomic Status and Health Chartbook.* Washington, D.C.: U.S. Government Printing Office, DHHS Pub. (PHS) 98-1232. Vickery, D. M. 1978. *Life Plan for Your Health.* Reading, Mass.: Addison-Wesley.

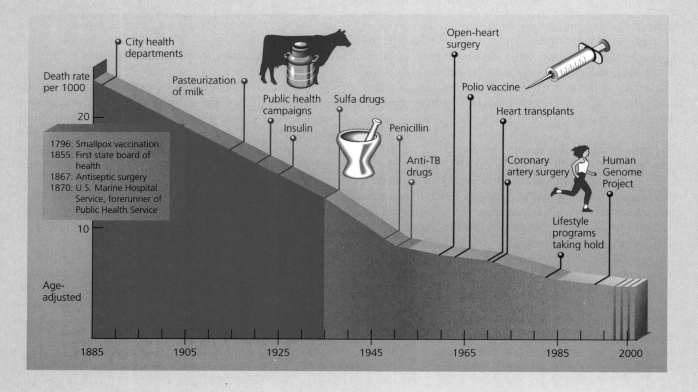

awareness about their own health and about taking care of their bodies.

In recent decades, certain habits and behaviors have been identified as culprits in the development of chronic disease; others have been shown to promote health. Many of these factors—diet, work, play, sexual and reproductive choices, and our environment—turn out to be things that we can control. This knowledge has led to the realization that wellness cannot be prescribed; physicians and other health care professionals can do little more than provide information, advice, and encouragement—the rest is up to each of us. A sense of empowerment regarding our health has thus replaced the fatalism that prevailed in the last century. Today, medical research has given us guidelines we can use to prolong our lives. And beyond that, it has provided us with information we can use to enjoy a quality of life unimagined by our grandparents (see the box "Health in the Twenty-First Century").

National Wellness Goals: The Healthy People Initiative

You may think of health and wellness as personal concerns, goals that you strive for on your own for your own benefit. But the U.S. government also has a vital interest in the health of all Americans. A healthy population is the nation's greatest resource, the source of its vitality, creativity, and wealth. Poor health, in contrast, drains the nation's resources and raises national health care costs. As the embodiment of our society's values, the federal government also has a humane interest in people's health.

The U.S. government's national Healthy People initiative seeks to prevent unnecessary disease and disability and to achieve a better quality of life for all Americans. Healthy People reports, published first in 1980 and revised every decade, set national health goals based on 10-year agendas. Each report includes both broad goals and specific targets in many different areas of wellness. The preliminary version of the latest report, *Healthy People 2010,* proposed two broad national goals:

- *Increase quality and years of healthy life.* The life expectancy of Americans has increased significantly in the past century; however, people can expect poor health to limit their activities and cause distress during the last 15% of their lives (Figure 1-2). "Healthy life" refers to a full range of functional capacity that enables people to work, play, and maintain satisfying relationships. This national goal stresses the importance of health status and nature of life, not just longevity.

- *Eliminate health disparities among Americans.* Many health problems today disproportionately affect certain American populations—for example, ethnic minorities, people of low socioeconomic status or educational attainment, and people with disabilities.

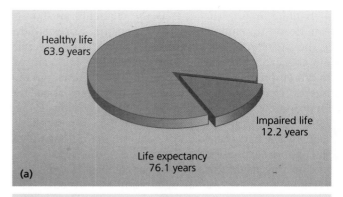

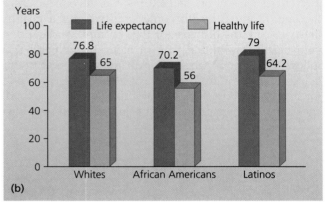

VITAL STATISTICS

Figure 1-2 Quantity of life versus quality of life. (a) Years of healthy life as a proportion of life expectancy in the U.S. population. (b) Years of healthy life versus life expectancy for whites, African Americans, and Latinos in the United States. SOURCE: U.S. Department of Health and Human Services. 1998. *Healthy People 2010 Objectives: Draft for Public Comment.* Washington, D.C.: U.S. Government Printing Office.

Healthy People 2010 calls for eliminating disparities in health status, health risks, and use of preventive services among all population groups within the next decade.

Giving substance to these broad goals are hundreds of specific objectives—measurable targets for the year 2010—in many different priority areas that relate to wellness, including fitness, nutrition, safety, substance abuse, health care, and chronic and infectious diseases. Specific Healthy People targets serve as the basis for national monitoring and tracking of the health status and health risks of Americans and our use of health services. They encompass individual actions as well as larger-scale changes in environment and medical services. Examples of individual health promotion objectives from the 1998 draft of *Healthy People 2010,* as well as estimates of our progress toward these targets, appear in Table 1-1. For more on the Healthy People initiative and the development and publication of the final *Healthy People 2010* objectives, contact the Healthy People office or the Web sites listed in the For More Information section at the end of the chapter.

Healthy People 2010 reflects the changing attitude of Americans: an emerging sense of personal responsibility as the key to good health. This new perspective is seen in our concern about smoking and drug abuse, for example; in our emphasis on physical and emotional fitness; in our interest in good nutrition; and in our concern about the environment. The priority concerns of *Healthy People 2010* are the principal topics covered in this book. In many ways, personal wellness goals are not different from the national aspirations.

The message of this book is that wellness is something everyone can have. Achieving it requires knowledge, self-awareness, motivation, and effort—but the benefits last a lifetime. Optimal health comes mostly from a healthy lifestyle, patterns of behavior that promote and support your health now and as you get older. In the pages that follow, you'll find current information and suggestions you can use to build a better lifestyle. You'll also find tools for assessing yourself, for exploring your inner experiences, and for planning and carrying out specific behavior changes. You can use this book as a guide for taking charge of your health and improving the quality of your life.

CHOOSING WELLNESS

Each of us has the option and the responsibility to decide what kind of future we want—one characterized by zestful living, or one marked by symptoms and declining energy.

Factors That Influence Wellness

Scientific research is continuously revealing new connections between our habits and emotions and the level of health we enjoy. For example, heart disease, the nation's number-one killer, is associated with cigarette smoking, high levels of stress, habitually hostile and suspicious attitudes toward people and the world, a diet high in fat and low in fiber, and a sedentary way of life (Table 1-2). Other habits are beneficial. Regular exercise, for example, can help prevent heart disease, high blood pressure, diabetes, osteoporosis, and depression and may reduce the risk of colon cancer, stroke, and back injury. A balanced and varied diet provides the energy and nutrients we need to live a vital life and also helps prevent many chronic diseases. As we learn more about how our actions affect our bodies and minds, we can make informed choices for a healthier life.

Of course, behavior isn't the only factor involved in wellness. Our heredity, the environment we live in, and whether we have access to adequate health care are other important influences. These factors, which vary for both individuals and groups, can interact in ways that produce either health or disease. For example, a sedentary lifestyle combined with a genetic predisposition for diabetes can greatly increase a person's risk of developing the disease. If this person also lacks adequate health care, he or she is much more likely to suffer dangerous complications from diabetes and have a lower quality of life.

But in many cases, behavior can tip the balance toward good health, even when heredity or environment is a negative factor. For example, breast cancer can run in families, but it also may be associated with being overweight and inactive. A woman with a family history of breast cancer is less likely to develop and die from the disease if she controls her weight, exercises regularly, performs breast self-exams, and has regular mammograms.

Similarly, a young man with a family history of obesity can maintain a normal weight by being careful to balance calorie intake against activities that burn calories. If your life is highly stressful, you can lessen the chances of heart disease and stroke by learning ways to manage and cope with stress. If you live in an area with severe air pollution, you can reduce the risk of lung disease by not smoking. You can also take an active role in improving your environment. Behaviors like these enable you to make a difference in how great an impact heredity and environment will have on your health.

Some of the factors that influence wellness vary with gender, ethnicity, age, socioeconomic status, educational attainment, and other points of difference among groups. In this book, topics and issues in health that affect different American populations are given special consideration. Look for these discussions in the text and in boxes labeled Dimensions of Diversity; the first of these, "Health Issues for Diverse Populations," appears on pp. 8–9. Also discussed in Dimensions of Diversity boxes are health issues and practices in other parts of the world. Explorations beyond the borders of the United States broaden our view, showing us both what we share with people in other societies and how we differ—our common concerns and our divergent solutions. All these discussions are designed to deepen our understanding of the core concepts of wellness in the context of ever-growing diversity.

A Wellness Profile

What does it mean to be healthy today? A basic list of important behaviors and habits includes the following:

- Having a sense of responsibility for your own health, and taking an active rather than a passive stance toward your life.
- Learning to manage stress in effective ways.
- Maintaining high self-esteem and mentally healthy ways of interacting with other people.
- Understanding your sexuality and having satisfying intimate relationships.
- Avoiding tobacco and other drugs; using alcohol responsibly, if at all.

TABLE 1-1　　Selected Healthy People 2010 Objectives

Objective	Estimate of Current Status	Goal
Increase the proportion of people age 18 and older who engage regularly, preferably daily, in sustained physical activity for at least 30 minutes per day.	23%	30%
Increase the proportion of people age 2 and older who meet the Dietary Guidelines' minimum average daily goal of at least five servings of vegetables and fruits.	40%	75%
Increase the prevalence of healthy weight among all people age 20 and older.	41%	60%
Reduce the proportion of adults 18 and older who use tobacco products.	More than 24.7%	13%
Reduce the proportion of college students reporting binge drinking during the past 2 weeks.	38.3%	20%
Increase the proportion of sexually active unmarried people who reported that a condom was used at last sexual intercourse.	40%	46%
Increase the proportion of people who use sunscreens when exposed to sunlight.	29%	75%
Increase the use of safety belts and child restraints by motor vehicle occupants.	69%	At least 93%
Increase the presence of functional smoke alarms to at least one on each habitable floor of all inhabited residential dwellings.	52%	100%
Reduce the proportion of children and adults under 65 without health care coverage.	19%	0%

SOURCE: U.S. Department of Health and Human Services. 1998. *Healthy People 2010 Objectives: Draft for Public Comment.* Washington, D.C.: U.S. Government Printing Office.

VITAL STATISTICS

TABLE 1-2　　Leading Causes of Death in the United States

Rank	Cause of Death	Number of Deaths	Percent of Total Deaths	Female/Male Ratio*	Lifestyle Factors
1	Heart disease	725,790	31.3	50/50	D I S A
2	Cancer	537,390	23.2	48/52	D I S A
3	Stroke	159,877	6.9	61/39	D I S
4	Chronic obstructive lung diseases	110,637	4.8	49/51	S
5	Unintentional injuries	92,191	4.0	35/65	S A
	Motor-vehicle-related	(42,420)	(1.8)	(35/65)	
	All others	(49,772)	(2.2)	(35/65)	
6	Pneumonia and influenza	88,383	3.8	55/45	S
7	Diabetes mellitus	62,332	2.7	55/45	D I S
8	Suicide	29,725	1.3	19/81	A
9	Kidney diseases	25,570	1.1	52/48	D
10	Chronic liver disease and cirrhosis	24,765	1.1	35/65	A
	All causes	2,314,729			

Key: D　Cause of death in which diet plays a part.
I　Cause of death in which an inactive lifestyle plays a part.
S　Cause of death in which smoking plays a part.
A　Cause of death in which excessive alcohol consumption plays a part.

*Ratio of females to males who died of each cause. For example, an equal number of women and men died of heart disease, but only about half as many women as men died of motor-vehicle-related injuries.

SOURCES: National Center for Health Statistics. 1998. Births and deaths: Preliminary data for 1997. *National Vital Statistics Reports* 47(4):7. National Center for Health Statistics. 1998. Births, marriages, divorces, and deaths for 1997. *Monthly Vital Statistics Report* (46)12: 13–14.

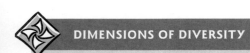

Americans are a diverse people. Our ancestry is European, African, Asian, Pacific Islander, Latin American, and Native American. We live in cities, suburbs, and rural areas, and work at every imaginable occupation. In no other country in the world do so many diverse people live and work together every day. And in no other country is the understanding and tolerance of differences so much a part of the political and cultural ideal. We are at heart a nation of diversity, and, though we often fall short of our goal, we strive for justice and equality among all.

When it comes to health, most differences among people are insignificant; most health issues concern us all equally. We all need to eat well, exercise, manage stress, and cultivate satisfying personal relationships. We need to know how to protect ourselves from heart disease, cancer, sexually transmitted diseases, and injuries. We need to know how to use the health care system.

But some of our differences, as individuals and as members of groups, do have important implications for health. Some of us, for example, have a genetic predisposition for developing certain health problems, such as high cholesterol. Some of us have grown up eating foods that raise our risk of heart disease or obesity. Some of us live in an environment that increases the chance that we'll smoke cigarettes or abuse alcohol. These health-related differences among individuals and groups can be biological—determined genetically—or cultural—acquired as patterns of behavior through daily interactions with our families, communities, and society. Many health conditions are a function of biology and culture combined. A person can have a genetic predisposition for a disease, for example, but won't actually develop the disease itself unless certain lifestyle factors are present, such as stress or a poor diet.

When we talk about health issues for diverse populations, we face two related dangers. The first is the danger of stereotyping, of talking about people as groups rather than as individuals. It's certainly true that every person is an individual with a unique genetic endowment and unique life experiences. But many of these influences are shared with others of similar genetic and cultural background. Statements about these group similarities can be useful; for example, they can alert people to areas that may be of special concern for them and their families.

The second danger is that of overgeneralizing, of ignoring the extensive biological and cultural diversity that exists among peoples who are grouped together. Groups labeled Latino or Hispanic, for example, include Mexican Americans, Puerto Ricans, people from South and Central America, and other Spanish-speaking peoples. Similarly, the population labeled Native American includes hundreds of recognized tribal nations, each with its own genetic and cultural heritage. It's important to

keep these considerations in mind whenever you read about culturally diverse populations.

Health-related differences among groups can be identified and described in the context of several different dimensions.

Gender

Men and women have different life expectancies, different reproductive concerns, and different incidences of many diseases, including heart disease, cancer, stroke, cirrhosis of the liver, and osteoporosis. Men are more likely to develop heart disease in middle age. Women are more affected by issues involving contraception and reproductive choices. They live longer than men. They have lower suicide rates. They are more likely to be poor.

Socioeconomic Status

Many health differences in our society are related to income level. People with low incomes have higher rates of infant mortality, traumatic injury and violent death, and many diseases, including cancer, heart disease, tuberculosis, and HIV infection. They are more likely to eat poorly, be overweight, smoke, drink, and use drugs. They have less access to health care services and medical insurance. They are exposed to more stressors, and they often have less control over the circumstances of their lives. Poverty is a far more important predictor of poor health than any ethnic factor. However, it is often mixed with other factors in a way that makes it difficult to distinguish what causes what. A factor that may be even more closely associated with health status is level of educational attainment.

Ethnicity

Some genetic diseases are concentrated in certain gene pools, the result of each ethnic group's relatively distinct history. Sickle-cell disease occurs almost exclusively among people of African ancestry. Tay-Sachs disease afflicts people of Eastern European Jewish heritage. Cystic fibrosis is more common among Northern Europeans. In addition to biological differences, many cultural differences occur along ethnic lines. Ethnic groups may vary in their traditional diets; their patterns of family and interpersonal relationships; their attitudes toward tobacco, alcohol, and other drugs; and their health beliefs and practices.

Four broad ethnic minority groups are usually distinguished in American society: African Americans (blacks), Latinos, Asian and Pacific Islander Americans, and Native Americans. Each has some special health concerns.

- Eating well, exercising, and maintaining healthy weight.
- Knowing when to treat your illnesses yourself and when to seek help.
- Understanding the health care system and using it intelligently.
- Knowing the facts about cardiovascular disease,

cancer, infections, sexually transmitted diseases, and injuries, and using your knowledge to protect yourself against them.
- Understanding the natural processes of aging and dying, and accepting the limits of human existence.
- Understanding how the environment affects your health, and taking appropriate action to improve it.

African Americans   African Americans are the largest minority group, making up about 12% of the American population. Although African Americans are represented in every socioeconomic group, nearly one-third live below the poverty line. For a poorly understood variety of economic, genetic, and lifestyle reasons, the health status of African Americans lags behind that of the total population in several areas, including life expectancy and incidence of chronic and infectious diseases.

The leading causes of death among African Americans are the same as for the general population: heart disease, cancer, and stroke. But African Americans have a higher infant mortality rate and a lower suicide rate. The age-adjusted death rate for HIV infection and homicide among African American men and women is about four to nine times the rate for white males and females. African American men and women also die from stroke at almost twice the rate of white men and women. Strokes are related to high blood pressure, which is much more common among blacks than in the general population. Also contributing to cardiorespiratory problems is sickle-cell disease.

Cancer is another special concern. African American men have a higher risk of cancer than nonblack men, with a 25% higher risk of all cancers and a 40% higher risk of lung cancer. African American men face a 40% greater risk of prostate cancer than whites, giving them the highest prostate cancer risk of any group in the world.

African Americans also face an increased risk of developing glaucoma and becoming blind as a result. Diabetes is a special concern for black women, especially those who are overweight.

Latinos   Latinos are the second largest and fastest growing minority group in the United States, making up about 11% of the total population. About two-thirds of Latinos are of Mexican descent, 13% are of South or Central American background, 10% are Puerto Rican, and almost 5% are Cuban American. Although many cultural and biological differences exist among the various Latino populations, they are frequently grouped together, often under the umbrella term Hispanic. This label is misleading because many Latinos are of mixed Spanish and American Indian descent, or of mixed Spanish, Indian, and African American descent. Nevertheless, Hispanic is the label most commonly used in studies and statistics to identify Latino populations.

Overall, the leading causes of death for Latinos are the same as those for the general population—heart disease and cancer—but Latinos tend to have lower rates of death from heart disease, and cancer than non-Hispanic whites and African Americans. Latinos have higher rates of death from homicide and infant mortality than non-Hispanic whites, but they have lower rates of death from suicide and cancers of the lung and respiratory system. They also have lower incidences of high cholesterol, high blood pressure, and osteoporosis. Some special concerns are diabetes, gallbladder disease, and obesity, all probably related to American Indian descent. The birth rate among Latinos is higher than that of the general population, and contraceptive use is relatively low.

Asian and Pacific Islander Americans   Like Latinos, this group is characterized by diversity. They represent about 3.5% of the total population. The two oldest and largest groups are Japanese Americans and Chinese Americans. Other groups include Vietnamese, Laotians, Cambodians, Koreans, Filipinos, Asian Indians, Native Hawaiians, and other Pacific Islanders. Numbering over 9 million people, they speak more than 30 different languages and represent a similar number of distinct cultures.

Health differences also exist among these groups. For example, Southeast Asian men have higher rates of lung cancer and liver cancer than the rest of the population, and Hawaiian women have higher than average rates of breast cancer. Diabetes is a concern among Asian Americans; its appearance may be triggered by the American diet. Among recent immigrants from Southeast Asia, tuberculosis and hepatitis B are serious health problems. Smoking is another concern; among some Southeast Asians, over 90% of the men smoke.

Native Americans   Also called American Indians and Alaska Natives, Native Americans represent about 1% of the total population. Most Native Americans embrace a tribal identity, such as Sioux, Navaho, or Hopi, rather than the identity of Native American.

Native Americans have lower rates of death from heart disease, stroke, and cancer than the general population, but they also have high rates of early death. For those under 45, the leading causes of death include unintentional injuries, homicide, suicide, and cirrhosis; many of these problems are linked to alcohol abuse. Diabetes is very prevalent, occurring in over 20% of all adults in some tribes. Many Native Americans have limited access to health care services.

These are just some of the differences among people and groups that can influence wellness. Dimensions of Diversity boxes in later chapters examine special wellness challenges and solutions of diverse population groups in the United States and around the world.

This may seem like a tall order, and in a sense it is the work of a lifetime. But the habits you establish now are crucial: They tend to set lifelong patterns. Some behaviors do more than set up patterns—they produce permanent changes in your health. If you become addicted to drugs or alcohol at age 20, for example, you may be able to kick the habit, but you will always face the struggle of a recovering addict. If you contract gonorrhea, you may discover later that your reproductive organs were damaged without your realizing it, making you infertile or sterile. If you ruin your knees doing the wrong exercises or hurt your back in an automobile crash, you won't have them to count on when you're older. Some things just can't be reversed or corrected.

HOW DO YOU REACH WELLNESS?

Your life may not resemble the one described by the wellness profile at all. You probably have a number of healthy habits and some others that place your health at risk. Maybe your life is more like this:

It's Tuesday. Simon wakes up feeling blue, not really wanting to get out of bed. He wishes he knew what he wanted to do with his life. He wishes he'd meet someone new and fall in love. No time for breakfast, so he grabs a cup of coffee to drink during his first class. He hasn't done the reading and stares blankly at the teacher during the lecture. Later he goes to the student union and has a sugary doughnut and some more coffee; he lights up his first cigarette of the day. Lunch is a fast-food cheeseburger, french fries, and a shake. He spends the afternoon at the library desperately researching a paper that's due the next day, finally quitting at 6:00 and heading to the student union for a beer. He meets up with some buddies and joins them for pizza instead of having dinner at the dorm. By 11:00 he's tired, but he's written only one page of his paper, so he takes an "upper" to keep going. It makes his heart race and floods his head with so many ideas he has difficulty sorting them all out. He works feverishly and finally finishes at 4:00 the next morning. Exhausted, he falls asleep in his clothes. The next thing he knows, it's Wednesday morning, time to start a new day.

This is hardly an ideal lifestyle, but it's not unusual. Simon functions OK, meets his commitments, and shows some self-discipline. On the other hand, time gets away from him, he doesn't get much exercise, doesn't eat as well as he could, and flirts with the dangers of taking drugs. Overall, he is low on energy and has little control over his life. He could be living a lot better.

Simon isn't alone in neglecting or abusing his health; many people fall into a lifestyle that puts their health at risk. Some aren't aware of the damage they're doing to themselves; others are aware but aren't motivated or don't know how to change; still others want to change but can't seem to get started. All of these are very real problems, but they're not insurmountable. If they were, there would be no ex-smokers, recovering alcoholics, or successful graduates of weight-loss programs. People can and do make difficult changes in their lives.

Taking big steps toward wellness may at first seem like too much work, but as you make progress, it gets easier.

At first you'll be rewarded with a greater sense of control over your life, a feeling of empowerment, higher self-esteem, and more joy. These benefits will encourage you to make further improvements. Over time, you'll come to know what wellness feels like—more energy; greater vitality; deeper feelings of curiosity, interest, and enjoyment; and a higher quality of life. To determine whether your current lifestyle promotes wellness, take the quiz in the box "Wellness: Evaluate Your Lifestyle" on pp. 12–13.

How do people go about actually making changes in their health-related behaviors? One theory that has become popular in recent years is the Stages of Change model developed by psychologist James O. Prochaska. Studying thousands of people trying to make changes like quitting smoking or starting an exercise program, he found that we move through six stages as we work to change our behavior: precontemplation, contemplation, preparation, action, maintenance, and termination. In the precontemplation stage, people either deny that a problem exists or believe they have no control over it. Contemplaters recognize the problem and try to understand it but have only vague thoughts about how to solve it. The preparation stage involves making a specific plan of action, such as setting a date to quit smoking, or joining a health club and buying exercise clothes. The action stage requires the most discipline and commitment; this is the phase in which change happens. The maintenance stage begins when a behavior change goal has been reached. A period of struggling against lapses and relapses can last from months to a lifetime. The final stage is reached when the problem and the temptation to relapse no longer exist and the cycle of change is complete. However, people with certain problems, such as drug addiction, may never reach this stage; avoiding relapse may be a lifelong effort. The following sections on behavior change reflect Prochaska's stages and will introduce you to the decisions and challenges involved at each stage of change.

Getting Serious About Your Health

Before you can start changing a health-related behavior, you have to know that the behavior is problematic and that you *can* change it. To make good decisions, you need information about relevant topics and issues (see the box "Evaluating Sources of Health Information," p. 14). You also need knowledge about yourself—how you relate to the wellness profile and what strengths you can draw on to change your behavior and improve your health. While knowledge is a necessary ingredient, it isn't usually enough to make you act. Millions of smokers stick to their habit, for example, even though they know it's bad for their health.

Many people start to consider changing a behavior when they get help from others. An observation from a friend, family member, or physician can help you see yourself as others do, and may get you thinking about your behavior in a new way. For example, Jason has been getting a lot of stomachaches lately. His girlfriend Anna notices other changes as well, and suggests that the stress of classes plus a part-time job and serving as president of the school radio station might be causing some of Jason's problems. Jason never thought much about trying to control the stressors in his life, but with encouragement from Anna he starts noticing what events trigger stress for him.

Landmark events can also get you thinking about behavior change. A birthday, the birth of a child, or the death of someone close to you can be powerful motivators for thinking seriously about behaviors that affect wellness. New information can also help you get started. As you read this text, you may find yourself reevaluating some of your health-related behaviors. This could be a great opportunity to make healthful changes that will stay with you for the rest of your life.

What Does It Take to Change?

As we all know, change doesn't just happen because we want it to. Some people seem to be able to change and grow fairly easily, while others tend to get stuck in problem behaviors for years. What are the secrets of moving toward wellness?

Motivation   Once you recognize that you have an unhealthy behavior, you may consider changing it. But before you can change, you need strong motivation to do so. Although some people are motivated by long-term goals, such as avoiding a disease that may hit them in 20 or 30 years, most are more likely to be moved to action by shorter-term, more personal goals. Looking better, being more popular, doing better in school, getting a good job, improving at a sport, and increasing self-esteem are common sources of motivation.

You can strengthen your motivation by raising your consciousness about your problem behavior. This will enable you to focus on the negatives of the behavior and imagine the consequences if you don't make a change. At the same time, you can visualize the positive results of changing your behavior. Ask yourself: What do I want for myself, now and in the future?

For example, Ruby has never worried much about her smoking because the problems associated with it seem so far away. But lately she's noticed her performance on the volleyball team isn't as good as it used to be. Over the summer she visited her aunt, who has chronic emphysema from smoking and can barely leave her bed. Ruby knows she wants to have children and a career as a teacher someday, and seeing her aunt makes her wonder if her smoking habit could make it difficult for her to reach these goals. She starts to wonder whether her smoking habit is worth the short- and long-term sacrifices.

Social pressures can also increase the motivation to make changes. In Ruby's case, anti-smoking ordinances make it impossible for her to smoke in her dorm and in

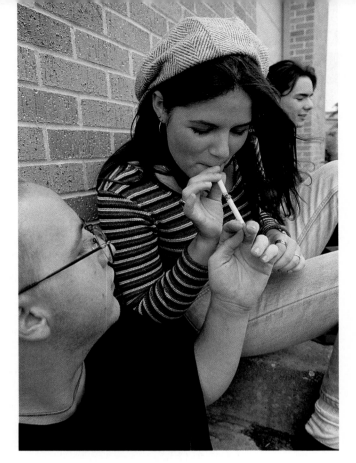

Changing powerful, long-standing habits requires motivation, commitment, and a belief that we are in control of our own behavior. To quit smoking, this young woman must overcome a habit that is supported by her addiction to nicotine and by her social environment.

many public places. The inconvenience of finding a place to smoke—and pressure from her roommate, who doesn't like the smoky smell of Ruby's clothes in their room—add to Ruby's motivation to quit.

Locus of Control   When you start thinking about changing a health behavior, a big factor in your eventual success is whether or not you believe you can change. Who do you believe is controlling your life? Is it your parents, friends, or school? Is it "fate"? Or is it you?

Locus of control refers to the figurative "place" a person designates as the source of responsibility for the events in his or her life. People who believe they are in control of their own lives are said to have an internal locus of control. Those who believe that factors beyond their control—heredity, friends and family, the environment, fate, luck, or other outside forces—are more important in determining the events of their lives are said to have an external locus of control. Most people are not purely "internalizers" or "externalizers"; their locus of control changes in response to the situation.

locus of control   The figurative "place" a person designates   **TERMS**
as the source of responsibility for the events in his or her life.

All of us want optimal health. But many of us do not know how to achieve it. Taking this quiz, adapted from one created by the U.S. Public Health Service, is a good place to start. The behaviors covered in the test are recommended for most Americans.

(Some of them may not apply to people with certain diseases or disabilities, or to pregnant women, who may require special advice from their physician.) After you take the quiz, add up your score for each section.

Tobacco Use

If you never use tobacco, enter a score of 10 for this section and go to the next section.

	Almost Always	Sometimes	Never
1. I avoid using tobacco.	2	1	0
2. I smoke only low-tar/nicotine cigarettes *or* I smoke a pipe or cigars *or* I use smokeless tobacco.	2	1	0

Tobacco Score: _____

Alcohol and Other Drugs

	Almost Always	Sometimes	Never
1. I avoid alcohol *or* I drink no more than 1 (women) or 2 (men) drinks a day.	4	1	0
2. I avoid using alcohol or other drugs as a way of handling stressful situations or problems in my life.	2	1	0
3. I am careful not to drink alcohol when taking medications, such as for colds or allergies, or when pregnant.	2	1	0
4. I read and follow the label directions when using prescribed and over-the-counter drugs.	2	1	0

Alcohol and Other Drugs Score: _____

Nutrition

	Almost Always	Sometimes	Never
1. I eat a variety of foods each day, including five or more servings of fruits and vegetables.	3	1	0
2. I limit the amount of fat and saturated fat in my diet.	3	1	0
3. I avoid skipping meals.	2	1	0
4. I limit the amount of salt and sugar I eat.	2	1	0

Nutrition Score: _____

Exercise/Fitness

	Almost Always	Sometimes	Never
1. I engage in moderate exercise for 20–60 minutes, 3–5 times a week.	4	1	0
2. I maintain a healthy weight, avoiding overweight and underweight.	2	1	0
3. I do exercises to develop muscular strength and endurance at least twice a week.	2	1	0
4. I spend some of my leisure time participating in physical activities such as gardening, bowling, golf, or baseball.	2	1	0

Exercise/Fitness Score: _____

Emotional Health

	Almost Always	Sometimes	Never
1. I enjoy being a student, and I have a job or do other work that I like.	2	1	0
2. I find it easy to relax and express my feelings freely.	2	1	0

For lifestyle management, an internal locus of control is an advantage because it reinforces motivation and commitment. An external locus of control can actually sabotage efforts to change behavior. For example, if you believe you are destined to die of breast cancer because your mother died from the disease, you may view monthly breast self-exams and regular checkups as a waste of time. In contrast, an internal locus of control is an advantage. If you believe you can take action to reduce your hereditary risk of breast cancer, you will be motivated to follow guidelines for early detection of the disease.

People who tend to have an external locus of control can learn to view the events in their lives differently. Examine your attitudes carefully. If you find yourself attributing too much influence to outside forces, gather more information about your health-related behaviors.

	Almost Always	Sometimes	Never
3. I manage stress well.	2	1	0
4. I have close friends, relatives, or others I can talk to about personal matters and call on for help.	2	1	0
5. I participate in group activities (such as church and community organizations) or hobbies that I enjoy.	2	1	0

Emotional Health Score: _____

Safety

	Almost Always	Sometimes	Never
1. I wear a safety belt while riding in a car.	2	1	0
2. I avoid driving while under the influence of alcohol or other drugs.	2	1	0
3. I obey traffic rules and the speed limit when driving.	2	1	0
4. I read and follow instructions on the labels of potentially harmful products or substances, such as household cleaners, poisons, and electrical appliances.	2	1	0
5. I avoid smoking in bed.	2	1	0

Safety Score: _____

Disease Prevention

	Almost Always	Sometimes	Never
1. I know the warning signs of cancer, diabetes, heart attack, and stroke.	2	1	0
2. I avoid overexposure to the sun and use a sunscreen.	2	1	0
3. I get recommended medical screening tests (such as blood pressure checks and Pap tests), immunizations, and booster shots.	2	1	0
4. I practice monthly breast/testicle self-exams.	2	1	0
5. I am not sexually active *or* I have sex with only one mutually faithful, uninfected partner *or* I always engage in safer sex (using condoms) *and* I do not share needles to inject drugs.	2	1	0

Disease Prevention Score: _____

What Your Scores Mean

Scores of 9 and 10   Excellent! Your answers show that you're aware of the importance of this area to wellness. More important, you are putting your knowledge to work for you by practicing good health habits. As long as you continue to do so, this area should not pose a serious health risk. It's likely that you are setting an example for your family and friends to follow. Since you scored high on this part of the quiz, you may want to focus on other areas where your scores indicate room for improvement.

Scores of 6–8   Your health practices in this area are good, but there is room for improvement. Look again at the items you answered with "Sometimes" or "Never." What changes can you make to improve your score? Even a small change can often help you achieve better health.

Scores of 3–5   Your health risks are showing! You may need more information about the risks you're facing and about why it's important for you to change these behaviors. Perhaps you need help in deciding how to successfully make the changes you want.

Scores of 0–2   Your answers show that you may be taking serious and unnecessary risks with your health. Perhaps you are not aware of the risks and what to do about them. You can easily get the information and help you need to improve, if you wish. The next step is up to you.

Make a list of all the ways that making lifestyle changes will improve your health. If you believe you'll succeed, and if you recognize and accept that you are in charge of your life, you're well on your way to wellness.

Choosing a Target Behavior   The worst thing you can do is try to change everything at once—quit smoking, give up high-fat foods, eat a good breakfast, start jogging, plan your study time better, avoid drugs, get enough sleep. Overdoing it leads to burnout. Concentrate on one behavior that you want to change, your **target behavior,** and work on it systematically. Start with something simple, like substituting olive oil for butter in your diet, or

---

target behavior   An isolated behavior selected as the object of a behavior change plan.   **TERMS**

Making sound choices about your own wellness requires critical thinking. In order to choose and implement healthy behaviors, you must be able to identify accurate information about health in general and your own personal risk factors in particular. You must be able to evaluate health-related products and services such as exercise shoes, fast food, health insurance, and medical treatments. Thinking critically is crucial if you are to take advantage of all the opportunities you have to optimize your health and well-being.

A key first step in sharpening your critical thinking skills is to look carefully at your sources of health information. Critical thinking involves knowing where and how to find relevant information, how to separate fact from opinion, how to recognize faulty reasoning, how to evaluate information, and how to assess the credibility of sources. The following strategies can help you sort through the health information you receive from common sources, including television, newspapers, magazines, books, advertisements, and friends and family members.

- *Go to the original source.* Media reports often simplify the results of medical research. Find out for yourself what a study really reported, and determine whether it was based on good science. What type of study was it? Was it published in a recognized medical journal? Did the study include a large number of people? What did the authors of the study actually report in their findings?

- *Watch for misleading language.* Reports that feature so-called "breakthroughs" or "dramatic proof" are probably hype. Some studies will find that a behavior "contributes to" or is "associated with" an outcome; this does not imply a proven cause-and-effect relationship. Information may also be distorted by an author's point of view. Carefully read or listen to information in order to understand its implications.

- *Distinguish between research reports and public health advice.* If a study finds a link between a particular vitamin and can-

cer, that should not necessarily lead you to change your behavior. But if the Surgeon General or the American Cancer Society advises you to eat less fat or quit smoking, you can assume that many studies point in this direction and that this is advice you should follow.

- *Remember that anecdotes are not facts.* Sometimes we do get helpful health information from our friends and family. But just because your cousin Bertha lost 10 pounds on Dr. Amazing's new protein diet doesn't mean it's a safe, effective way for you to lose weight. Before you make a big change in your lifestyle, verify the information with your physician, this text, or other reliable sources.

- *Be skeptical, and use your common sense.* If a report seems too good to be true, it probably is. Be especially wary of information contained in advertisements. The goal of an ad is to sell you something, to create a feeling of need for a product where no real need exists. Evaluate "scientific" claims carefully, and beware of quackery (see Chapter 22).

- *Make choices that are right for you.* Your roommate swears by swimming; you prefer aerobics. Your sister takes a yoga class to help her manage stress; your brother unwinds by walking in the woods. Friends and family members can be a great source of ideas and inspiration, but each of us needs to find a wellness lifestyle that works for us.

You'll find additional strategies for evaluating research studies in Chapter 15. Appendix C includes helpful hints on how to locate and assess health-related information from the Internet.

You will find boxes labeled Critical Consumer throughout the text to help you develop and apply your critical thinking skills. In addition, be sure to work through the Critical Thinking Journal Entry activities at the end of each chapter. Developing the ability to think critically and independently about health issues will serve you well throughout your life.

---

low-fat milk for whole milk. Or concentrate on getting to sleep by 10:00 P.M. Working on even one behavior change will make high demands on your energy.

Developing a Behavior Change Plan

Once you are committed to making a change, it's time to put together a plan of action. Your key to success is a well-thought-out plan that sets goals, anticipates problems, and includes rewards.

1. Monitor Your Behavior and Gather Data   Begin by keeping careful records of the behavior you wish to change (your target behavior) and the circumstances surrounding it. Keep these records in a health journal, a notebook in which you write the details of your behavior along with observations and comments. Note exactly

what the activity was, when and where it happened, what you were doing, and what your feelings were at the time. In a journal for a weight-loss plan, for example, you would typically record how much food you ate, the time of day, the situation, the location, your feelings, and how hungry you were (Figure 1-3). Keep your journal for a week or two to get some solid information about the behavior you want to change.

2. Analyze the Data and Identify Patterns   After you have collected data on the behavior, analyze the data to identify patterns. When are you most hungry? When are you most likely to overeat? What events seem to trigger your appetite? Perhaps you are especially hungry at mid-morning or when you put off eating dinner until 9:00. Perhaps you overindulge in food and drink when you go to a particular restaurant or when you're with certain

Date _____ November 5 _____   Day   M (TU) W TH F SA SU

Time of day	M/S	Food eaten	Cals.	H	Where did you eat?	What else were you doing?	How did someone else influence you?	What made you want to eat what you did?	Emotions and feelings?	Thoughts and concerns?
7:30	M	1 C Crispix cereal 1/2 C skim milk coffee, black 1 C orange juice	110 40 — 120	3	dorm cafeteria	reading newspaper	eating w/ friends, but I ate what I usually eat	I always eat cereal in the morning	a little keyed up & worried	thinking about quiz in class today
10:30	S	1 apple	90	1	library	studying	alone	felt tired & wanted to wake up	tired	worried about next class
12:30	M	1 C chili 1 roll 1 pat butter 1 orange 2 oatmeal cookies 1 soda	290 120 35 60 120 150	2	cafeteria terrace	talking	eating w/ friends; we decided to eat at the cafeteria	wanted to be part of group	excited and happy	interested in hearing everyone's plans for the weekend

M/S = Meal or snack   H = Hunger rating (0–3)

Figure 1-3   Sample health journal entries.

friends. Be sure to note the connections between your feelings and such external cues as time of day, location, situation, and the actions of others around you. Do you always think of having a cigarette when you read the newspaper? Do you always bite your fingernails when you're studying?

3. Set Specific Goals   Whatever your ultimate goal, it's a good idea to break it down into a few small steps. Your plan will seem less overwhelming and more manageable, increasing the chances that you'll stick to it. You'll also build in more opportunities to reward yourself (discussed in step 4), as well as milestones you can use to measure your progress.

If you plan to lose 30 pounds, for example, you'll find it easier to take off 10 pounds at a time. If you want to quit smoking, plan a series of steps that takes you to the day you'll quit, such as asking yourself how ready you are to quit, listing your reasons for quitting, looking at patterns from other times you tried to quit, then cutting your daily smoking in half, and, 3 days later, quitting altogether. Take the easier steps first and work up to the harder steps.

4. Devise a Strategy or Plan of Action   As you write in your health journal, you gather quite a lot of information about your target behavior—the times it typically occurs; the situations in which it usually happens; the ways sight, smell, mood, situation, and accessibility trigger it. You

can probably trace the chain of events that leads to the behavior, and perhaps also identify points along the way where making a different choice would mean changing the behavior.

MODIFY YOUR ENVIRONMENT   You can be more effective in changing behavior if you control the environmental cues that provoke it. This might mean not having cigarettes or certain foods or drinks in the house, not going to parties where you're tempted to overindulge, or not spending time with particular people, at least for a while. If you always get a candy bar at a certain vending machine, change your route so you don't pass by it. If you always end up taking a coffee break and chatting with friends when you go to the library to study, choose a different place to study, such as your room.

It's also helpful to control other behaviors or habits that seem to be linked to the target behavior. You may give in to an urge to eat when you have a beer (alcohol increases the appetite) or when you watch TV. Try substituting some other activities for habits that seem to be linked with your target behavior, such as exercising to music instead of plopping down in front of the TV. Or, if possible, put an exercise bicycle in front of the set and burn calories while you watch your favorite show.

You can change the cues in your environment so they trigger the new behavior you want instead of the old one. Tape a picture of a cyclist speeding down a hill on your TV screen. Leave your exercise shoes in plain view. Put a

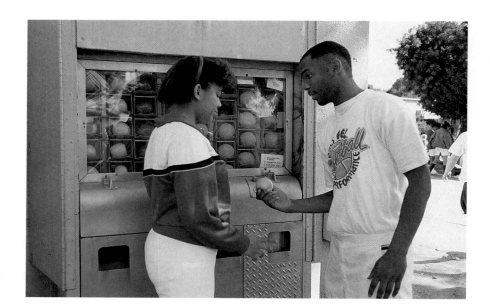

Many actions and behaviors are shaped by cues in the environment. For these softball players, easy access to a vending machine selling fruit, rather than candy, makes it more likely that they will choose a healthy snack.

chart of your progress in a special place at home to make your goals highly visible and inspire you to keep going. When you're trying to change a strong habit, small cues can play an important part in keeping you on track.

REWARD YOURSELF   A second very powerful way to affect your target behavior is by setting up a reward system that will reinforce your efforts. Most people find it difficult to change long-standing habits for rewards they can't see right away. Giving yourself instant, real rewards for good behavior along the way will help you stick with a plan to change your behavior.

Carefully plan your reward payoffs and what they will be. In most cases, rewards should be collected when you reach specific objectives or subgoals in your plan. For example, you might treat yourself to a movie after a week of avoiding extra snacks. Don't forget to reward yourself for good behavior that is consistent and persistent—if you simply stick with your program week after week. Decide on a reward after you reach a certain goal, or mark off the sixth week or month of a valiant effort. Write it down in your health journal and remember it as you follow your plan—especially when the going gets rough.

Make a list of your activities and favorite events to use as rewards. They should be special, inexpensive, and preferably unrelated to food or alcohol. Depending on what you like to do, you might treat yourself to a concert, a ball game, a new CD, a long-distance phone call to a friend, a day off from studying for a long hike in the woods—whatever is rewarding to you.

INVOLVE THE PEOPLE AROUND YOU   Rewards and support can also come from family and friends. Tell them about your plan, and ask for their help. Encourage them to be active, interested participants. Ask them to support

you when you set aside time to go running or avoid second helpings at Thanksgiving dinner. You may have to remind them not to do things that make you "break training" and not to be hurt if you have to refuse something when they forget. To help friends and family members who will be involved in your program respond appropriately, you may want to create a specific list of dos and don'ts. Getting encouragement, support, and praise from important people in your life can powerfully reinforce the new behavior you're trying to adopt.

5. Make a Personal Contract   Once you have set your goals and developed a plan of action, make your plan into a personal contract. A serious personal contract—one that commits your word—can result in a higher chance of follow-through than a casual, offhand promise. Your contract can help prevent procrastination by specifying the important dates and can also serve as a reminder of your personal commitment to change.

Your contract should include a statement of your goal and your commitment to reaching it. Include details of your plan: the date you'll begin, the steps you'll use to measure your progress, the concrete strategies you've developed for promoting change, and the date you expect to reach your final goal. Have someone—preferably someone who will be actively helping you with your program—sign your contract as a witness.

PERSONAL INSIGHT   How do you feel about the idea of putting together and carrying out a plan for changing some part of your behavior? Have you ever taken this kind of deliberate action before? Do you feel uneasy about the idea? Is it exciting?

My Personal Contract for Giving Up Snacking on Candy and Chips

I agree to stop snacking on candy and chips twice every day. I will begin my program on _10/4_ and plan to reach my final goal by _11/15_. I have divided my program into two parts, with two separate goals. For each step in my program, I will give myself the reward listed.

1. I will stop having candy or chips for an afternoon snack on _10/4_.
(Reward: _new CD_)

2. I will stop having candy or chips for an evening snack on _10/25_.
(Reward: _Concert_)

My plan for stopping my snacking includes the following strategies:
1. _Avoiding snack bar by taking a walk or reading at student union._
2. _Eating healthy snacks instead of candy and chips._
3. _Studying at the library instead of at home._

I understand that it is important for me to make a strong personal effort to make this change in my behavior. I sign this contract as an indication of my personal commitment to reach my goal.

Michael Cook   9/28

Witness: _Katie Lim_   9/28

Figure 1-4 A sample behavior change contract.

A Sample Behavior Change Plan Let's take the example of Michael, who wants to break a long-standing habit of eating candy and chips every afternoon and evening. Michael begins by keeping track of his snacking in a journal. He discovers that he always buys candy or a bag of chips at the snack bar on campus between two of his afternoon classes. In the evenings, he eats several candy bars or a large bag of chips while he studies at home.

Next, Michael sets specific goals. He sets a start date and decides to break his plan into two parts. He will begin by cutting out his afternoon snack of candy or chips. Once he successfully reaches this goal, he'll concentrate on his evening snacking. He decides to allow himself 3 weeks for each half of his behavior change plan.

To help increase his chances of success, Michael decides to make several changes in his behavior to help control his urges to buy and eat candy and chips. He plans to bring a healthy snack, such as an apple or orange, to eat between his afternoon classes. He decides to avoid going near the snack bar; instead, he'll spend his between-class break taking a 15-minute walk around campus or reading in the student union. To help break his evening habit, he decides to try studying at the library instead of at home; when he's at home, he'll try studying in a different room. He also plans to stock the refrigerator with healthy snacks that he can have when he feels the urge to snack on candy or chips. Finally, Michael decides on some rewards he'll give himself when he meets his goals, choosing things he likes that aren't too expensive.

After Michael has thought through his plan to stop snacking on candy and chips, he's ready to create and sign a behavior change contract. He decides to enlist one of his housemates as a witness to his contract; he also asks his housemate to check on his progress and offer encouragement (Figure 1-4). Once Michael has signed his contract, he's ready to take action.

Putting Your Plan into Action

The starting date has arrived, and you are ready to put your plan into action. This stage requires commitment, the resolve to stick with the plan no matter what temptations you encounter. Remember all the good reasons you have to make the change—and remember that *you* are the boss.

Use all your strategies to make your plan work. Substituting behaviors are often very important—go for a walk after class instead of eating a bag of chips. Make sure your environment is change-friendly by keeping cues that trigger the problem behavior to a minimum.

Social support can make a big difference as you take action. See if you can find a buddy who wants to make the same changes you do. You can support and encourage each other, as well as exchange information and motivation. For example, an exercise buddy can provide companionship and encouragement for times when you might be tempted to skip that morning jog. Or you and a friend can watch to be sure that you both have only one alcoholic beverage at a party.

Let the people around you know about your plan, and enlist their support in specific ways. Perhaps you know people who have reached the goal you are striving for; they could be role models or mentors for you. Talk to them about how they did it. What strategies worked for them?

Use your health journal to keep track of how well you are doing in achieving your ultimate goal. Record your daily activities and any relevant details, such as how far you walked or how many calories you ate. Each week, chart your progress on a graph and see how it compares to the subgoals on your contract. You may want to track more than one behavior, such as the time you spend exercising each week and your weight.

If you don't seem to be making progress, analyze your plan to see what might be causing the problem. Possible barriers to success are listed in the section "Staying With It," along with suggestions for addressing them. Once you've identified the problem, revise your plan.

Be sure to reward yourself for your successes by treating yourself as specified in your contract. And don't forget to give yourself a pat on the back—congratulate yourself, notice how much better you look or feel, and feel good about how far you've come and how you've gained control of your behavior.

Staying with It

As you continue with your program, don't be surprised when you run up against obstacles; they're inevitable. In fact, it's a good idea to expect problems and give yourself time to step back, see how you're doing, and make some changes before going on again. If you find your program is grinding to a halt, try to identify what it is that's blocking your progress. It may come from one of these sources.

Social Influences   Take a hard look at the reactions of the people you're counting on, and see if they're really supporting you. If they come up short, try connecting and networking with others who will be more supportive.

A related trap is trying to get your friends or family members to change *their* behaviors. The decision to make a major behavior change is something people come to only after intensive self-examination. You may be able to influence someone by tactfully providing facts or support, but that's all. Focus on yourself. If you succeed, you may become a role model for others.

Levels of Motivation and Commitment   You won't make real progress until an inner drive leads you to the stage of change at which you are ready to make a personal commitment to the goal. If commitment is your problem, you may need to wait until the behavior you're dealing with makes your life more unhappy or unhealthy; then your desire to change it will be stronger. Or you may find that changing your goal will inspire you to keep going. If you really want to change but your motivation comes and goes, look at your support system and at your own level

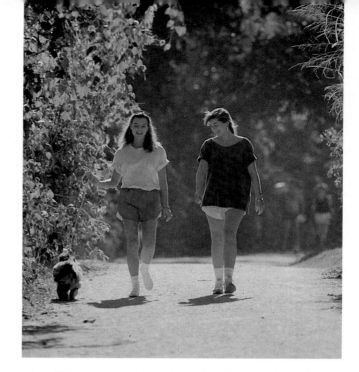

A beautiful day, a spectacular setting, a friendly companion—all contribute to making exercise a satisfying and pleasurable experience for these people. Choosing the right activity and doing it the right way are important elements in a successful health behavior change program.

of confidence. Building these up may be the key to pushing past a barrier. For more ideas, refer to the box "Motivation Boosters."

Choice of Techniques and Level of Effort   Your plan may not be working as well as you thought it would. Make changes where you're having the most trouble. If you've lagged on your running schedule, for example, maybe it's because you really don't like running. An aerobics class might suit you better. There are many ways to move toward your goal. Or you may not be trying hard enough. You do have to push toward your goal. If it were easy, you wouldn't need to have a plan.

Stress Barrier   If you've hit a wall in your program, look at the sources of stress in your life. If the stress is temporary, such as catching a cold or having a term paper due, you may want to wait until it passes before strengthening your efforts. If the stress is ongoing, try to find healthy ways to manage it. For example, taking a half-hour walk after lunch may help. You may even want to make stress management your highest priority for behavior change (see Chapter 2).

Games People Play   Procrastinating, rationalizing, and blaming; even when they want to change, people hold on fiercely to what they know and love (or know and hate). You may have very mixed feelings about the change you're trying to make, and your underlying motives may

Changing behavior takes motivation. But how do you get motivated? The following strategies may help:

- Write down the potential benefits of the change. If you want to lose weight, your list might include increased ease of movement, energy, and self-confidence.

- Now write down the costs of not changing.

- Frequently visualize yourself achieving your goal and enjoying its benefits. If you want to manage time more effectively, picture yourself as a confident, organized person who systematically tackles important tasks and sets aside time each day for relaxation, exercise, and friends.

- Discount obstacles to change. Counter thoughts such as "I'll never have time to shop for and prepare healthy foods" with thoughts such as "Lots of other people have done it and so can I."

- Bombard yourself with propaganda. Subscribe to a self-improvement magazine. Take a class dealing with the change you want to make. Read books and watch talk shows on the subject. Post motivational phrases or pictures on your refrigerator or over your desk. Listen to motiva-

tional tapes in the car. Talk to people who have already made the change you want to make.

- Build up your confidence. Remind yourself of other goals you've achieved. At the end of each day, mentally review your good decisions and actions. See yourself as a capable person, one who is in charge of his or her health.

- Create choices. You will be more likely to exercise every day if you have two or three types of exercise to choose from, and more likely to quit smoking if you've identified more than one way to distract yourself when you crave a cigarette. Get ideas from people who have been successful, and adapt some of their strategies to suit you.

- If you slip, keep trying. Research suggests that four out of five people will experience some degree of backsliding when they try to change a behavior. Only one in four succeeds the first time around. If you retain your commitment to change even when you lapse, you are still farther along the path to change than before you made the commitment. Try again. And again, if necessary.

sabotage your conscious ones if you keep them hidden from yourself. Try to detect the games you might be playing with yourself so that you can stop them.

If you're procrastinating ("It's Friday already; I might as well wait until Monday to begin"), try breaking your plan down into still smaller steps that you can accomplish one day at a time. If you're rationalizing or making excuses ("I wanted to go swimming today, but I wouldn't have had time to wash my hair afterward"), remember that the only one you're fooling is yourself, and that when you "win" by deceiving yourself, it's not much of a victory. If you're wasting time blaming yourself or others ("Everyone in that class talks so much that I don't get a chance to speak"), recognize that blaming is a way of taking your focus off the real problem and denying responsibility for your actions. Try refocusing by taking a positive attitude and renewing your determination to succeed.

Getting Outside Help

Outside help is often needed for changing behavior that may be too deeply rooted for a self-management approach. Alcohol and other drug addictions, excessive overeating, and other conditions or behaviors that put you at a serious health risk fall into this category; so do behaviors that interfere with your ability to function. Many communities have programs to help with these problems—Weight Watchers, Alcoholics Anonymous, Smoke

Enders, and Coke Enders, for example.

On campus, you may find courses in physical fitness, stress management, and weight control. The student health center or campus counseling center may also be a source of assistance. Many communities offer a wide variety of low-cost services through adult education, school programs, health departments, and private agencies. Consult the yellow pages, your local health department, or the United Way; the latter often sponsors local referral services. Whatever you do, don't be stopped by a problem when you can tap into resources to help you solve it.

BEING HEALTHY FOR LIFE

Your first few behavior change projects may never go beyond the planning stage. Those that do may not all succeed. But as you taste success by beginning to see progress and changes, you'll start to experience new and surprising positive feelings about yourself. You'll probably find that you're less likely to buckle under stress. You may begin opening doors to a new world of enjoyable physical and social events. You may accomplish things you never thought possible—winning a race, climbing a mountain, quitting smoking, having a lean, muscular body. Being healthy takes extra effort, but the paybacks in energy and vitality are priceless (see the box "Ten Warning Signs of Wellness," p. 21).

Once you've started, don't stop. Remember that maintaining good health is an ongoing process. Tackle one area at a time, but make a careful inventory of your health strengths and weaknesses and lay out a long-range plan. Take on the easier problems first, then use what you learned to attack more difficult areas. Look over your shoulder to make sure you don't fall into old habits. Keep informed about the latest health news and trends; research is constantly providing new information that directly affects daily choices and habits.

Making Changes in Your World

You can't completely control every aspect of your health. At least three other factors—heredity, health care, and environment—play important roles in your well-being. After you quit smoking, for example, you may still be inhaling smoke from other people's cigarettes. Your resolve to eat better foods may suffer a setback when you can't find any healthy choices in vending machines.

But you can make a difference—you can help create an environment around you that supports wellness for everyone. You can help support nonsmoking areas in public places. You can speak up in favor of more nutritious foods and better physical fitness facilities. You can include nonalcoholic drinks at your parties. You can vote for measures that improve access to health care for all people and support politicians who sponsor them.

You can also work on larger environmental challenges: air and water pollution, traffic congestion, overcrowding and overpopulation, depletion of the atmosphere's ozone layer, toxic and nuclear waste, and many others. These difficult issues need the attention and energy of people who are informed and who care about good health. On every level, from personal to planetary, we can all take an active role in shaping our environment.

What Does the Future Hold?

Sweeping changes in lifestyle have resulted in healthier Americans in recent years and could have even greater effects in the years to come. In your lifetime, you can choose to take an active role in the movement toward increased awareness, greater individual responsibility and control, healthier lifestyles, and a healthier planet. Your choices and actions will have a tremendous impact on your present and future wellness. The door is open, and the time is now—you simply have to begin.

SUMMARY

Wellness: The New Health Goal

- Wellness is the ability to live life fully, with vitality and meaning.

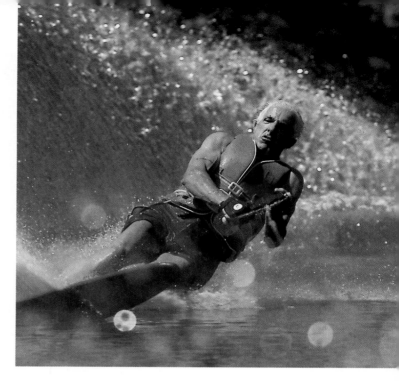

A 60-year-old man who water-skis like a 30-year-old gets his strength from years of vigorous activity. If you want to enjoy vigor and health in *your* middle and old age, begin now to make the choices that will give you lifelong vitality.

- Wellness is dynamic and multidimensional; it incorporates physical, emotional, intellectual, spiritual, interpersonal and social, and environmental dimensions.

- As chronic diseases such as heart disease and cancer have become the leading causes of death in the United States, people have recognized that they have greater control over, and greater responsibility for, their health than ever before.

- The Healthy People initiative seeks to achieve a better quality of life for all Americans. The broad goals of the *Healthy People 2010* report are to increase quality and years of healthy life and to eliminate health disparities among Americans.

Choosing Wellness

- People today have greater control over their health than ever before. Being responsible for one's health means making choices and adopting habits and behaviors that will ensure wellness.

- Although heredity, environment, and health care all play roles in wellness and disease, behavior can mitigate their effects.

- Behaviors and habits that reinforce wellness include (1) taking an active, responsible role in one's health;

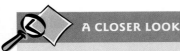

Ten Warning Signs of Wellness

1. The persistent presence of a support network.
2. Chronic positive expectations; the tendency to frame events in a constructive light.
3. Episodic outbreaks of joyful, happy experiences.
4. A sense of spiritual involvement.
5. A tendency to adapt to changing conditions.
6. Rapid response and recovery of stress response systems to repeated challenges.

7. An increased appetite for physical activity.
8. A tendency to identify and communicate feelings.
9. Repeated episodes of gratitude and generosity.
10. A persistent sense of humor.

SOURCE: Ten warning signs of good health. 1996. *Mind/Body Health Newsletter* 5(1). Reprinted by permission.

(2) managing stress; (3) maintaining self-esteem and good interpersonal relationships; (4) understanding sexuality and having satisfying intimate relationships; (5) avoiding tobacco and other drugs and restricting alcohol intake; (6) eating well, exercising, and maintaining healthy weight; (7) knowing about illnesses and how to treat them; (8) understanding and wisely using the health care system; (9) knowing about diseases and injuries and protecting yourself against them; (10) understanding and accepting the processes of aging and dying; and (11) understanding how the environment affects your health, and working to improve the environment.

How Do You Reach Wellness?

- Although it is challenging, people can and do make difficult changes in health-related behaviors.

- In his Stages of Change model, Prochaska describes six stages of change that people move through as they try to change their behavior: precontemplation, contemplation, preparation, action, maintenance, and termination.

- Knowledge about topics in wellness and about yourself is necessary to begin making changes in health-related behavior. Observations by others and landmark events can help get people started on change.

- Strong motivation to change and an internal locus of

control are keys to successful behavior change. It is best to concentrate on one target behavior at a time.

- A specific plan for change can be developed by (1) monitoring behavior by keeping a journal, (2) analyzing the recorded data, (3) setting specific goals, (4) devising strategies for modifying the environment, rewarding yourself, and involving others, and (5) making a personal contract.

- To start and maintain a behavior change program you need commitment, a well-developed and manageable plan, social support, and a system of rewards. It is also important to monitor the progress of your program, revising it as necessary.

- Obstacles sometimes come in the form of unsupportive people, a low level of motivation or commitment, inappropriate techniques, too much stress, and procrastinating, rationalizing, and blaming.

- Taking advantage of outside sources and programs can help; some behavior is too deeply rooted to be changed by self-management techniques alone.

Being Healthy for Life

- Each small success in a behavior change program leads to increased self-esteem and increased motivation to continue.

- Although we cannot control every aspect of our health, we can make a difference in helping create an environment that supports wellness for everyone.

TAKE ACTION

1. Ask some older members of your family (parents and grandparents) what they recall about patterns of health and disease when they were young. Do they remember any large outbreaks of infectious disease? Did any of their friends or relatives die while very young or die of a disease that can now be treated? How have health concerns changed during their lifetime?

2. Choose a person you consider a role model, and interview him or her. What do you admire about this person? What can you borrow from his or her experiences and strategies for success?

1. Purchase a small notebook to use as your health journal throughout this course. At the end of each chapter, we include suggestions for journal entries—opportunities to think about topics and issues, explore and formulate your own views, and express your thoughts in written form. These exercises are intended to help you deepen your understanding of health topics and your own behaviors in relation to them. For your first journal entry, make a list of the positive behaviors that enhance your health (such as jogging and getting enough sleep). Consider what additions you can make to the list or how you can strengthen or reinforce these behaviors. (Don't forget to congratulate yourself for these positive aspects of your life.) Next, list the behaviors that detract from wellness (such as smoking and eating a lot of candy). Consider which of these behaviors you might be able to change. Use these lists as the basis for self-evaluation as you proceed through this book.

2. *Critical Thinking* In this book, several Journal Entry items are designed to help you sharpen your critical thinking skills. For your first Critical Thinking journal entry, write a short essay describing your sources of health information. Do you rely on newspaper or magazine articles? On television? On friends and family? What criteria do you use to evaluate this information, to assess its credibility, and to make decisions about your health?

3. Think about what troubled you most during the past week. In your health journal, write down the names of three or four people who might be able to help you with whatever troubled you. If the problem persists, consider starting at the top of your list and talking to this person about it.

4. Think of the last time you did something you knew to be unhealthy primarily because those around you were doing it. How could you have restructured the situation or changed the environmental cues so that you could have avoided the behavior? In your health journal, describe several possible actions that will help you avoid the behavior the next time you're in a similar situation.

5. Make a list in your health journal of rewards that are meaningful to you. Add to the list as you think of new things to use. Refer to this list of rewards when you're developing plans for behavior change.

FOR MORE INFORMATION

Books

Columbia University's Health Education Program. 1998. *The "Go Ask Alice" Book of Answers.* New York: Henry Holt. *Presents answers to a variety of student-oriented health questions from the popular "Go Ask Alice" Web site.*

Prochaska, J. O., J. C. Norcross, and C. C. DiClemente. 1994. *Changing for Good: The Revolutionary Program That Explains the Six Stages of Change and Teaches You How to Free Yourself from Bad Habits.* New York: Morrow. *Outlines the authors' model of behavior change and offers suggestions and advice for each stage of change.*

Sobel, D. S., and R. Ornstein. 1996. *The Healthy Mind, Healthy Body Handbook.* Los Altos, Calif.: DR$_x$. *Presents concrete strategies for changing behavior, staying well, managing common health problems, and becoming a better consumer of the health care system.*

Swartzberg, J. E., and S. Margen. 1998. *The UC Berkeley Wellness Self-Care Handbook.* New York: Rebus. *Provides information and strategies for promoting health and well-being throughout the life span.*

Newsletters

Consumer Reports on Health, P.O. Box 56356, Boulder, CO 80322.

Harvard Health Letter, P.O. Box 420300, Palm Coast, FL 32142 (http://www.harvardhealthpubs.org).

Harvard Men's Health Watch, P.O. Box 420099, Palm Coast, FL 32142-0099.

Harvard Women's Health Watch, P.O. Box 420068, Palm Coast, FL 32142.

Healthline, 830 Menlo Ave., Suite 100, Menlo Park, CA 94025 (http://www.healthline.com).

HealthNews, P.O. Box 52924, Boulder, CO 80322 (http://www.onhealth.com).

Mayo Clinic Health Letter, P.O. Box 53889, Boulder, CO 80322.

Mind/Body Health, P.O. Box 381069, Cambridge, MA 02238-1069.

University of California at Berkeley Wellness Letter, P.O. Box 420148, Palm Coast, FL 32142.

Organizations, Hotlines, and Web Sites

The Internet addresses (also called uniform resource locators, or URLs) listed here were accurate at the time of publication. Up-to-date links to these and many other wellness-oriented Web sites are provided on the links page of the *Core Concepts in Health* Web site (http://www.mayfieldpub.com/insel). Refer to Appendix C for tips on how to search for and evaluate wellness information from the Internet.

Centers for Disease Control and Prevention. Through phone, fax, and the Internet, the CDC provides a wide variety of information, including materials on HIV infection, national health statistics, travelers' health information, and governmental nutrition recommendations.

404-332-4555 (CDC Infoline); 888-CDC-FAXX (CDC FAX) http://www.cdc.gov

Many other government Web sites provide access to health-related materials:

National Library of Medicine: http://www.nlm.nih.gov
National Institutes of Health: http://www.nih.gov
World Health Organization: http://www.who.org

Go Ask Alice. Sponsored by the Columbia University Health Service, this site provides answers to student questions about stress, sexuality, fitness, and many other wellness topics.

http://www.goaskalice.columbia.edu

Hardin Meta Directory of Internet Health Sources. An index to sites that contain links to other health-related sites.

http://www.lib.uiowa.edu/hardin/md

Healthfinder. A gateway to online publications, Web sites, support and self-help groups, and agencies and organizations that produce reliable health information.

http://www.healthfinder.gov

Healthy People 2000/Healthy People 2010. Provide information on Healthy People objectives and priority areas.

202-205-8583; 301-468-5960.
http://odphp.osophs.dhhs.gov/pubs/hp2000
http://web.health.gov/healthypeople

National Health Information Center (NHIC). Puts consumers in touch with the organizations that are best able to provide answers to health-related questions.

P.O. Box 1133
Washington, DC 20013-1133
800-336-4797
http://nhic-nt.health.org

National Women's Health Information Center. Provides information and answers to frequently asked questions.

800-994-WOMAN
http://www.4woman.org

NOAH: New York Online Access to Health. Provides consumer health information in both English and Spanish.

http://www.noah.cuny.edu

The following are just a few of the many sites that provide consumer-oriented information on a variety of health issues:

American Medical Association Health Insight: http://www.ama-assn.org/consumer.htm
Dr. Koop's Community: http://www.drkoop.com
HealthIndex Health Information Directory: http://www.healthindex.org
InteliHealth: Johns Hopkins Health Information: http://www.intelihealth.com
Mayo Health O@sis: http://www.mayohealth.org
OnHealth: http://www.onhealth.com

The following sites provide daily health news updates:

CNN/Health: http://www.cnn.com/HEALTH
HealthScout: http://www.healthscout.com
New York Times Your Health Daily: http://www.yourhealthdaily.com
Yahoo Health News: http://dailynews.yahoo.com/headlines/hl

See also the listings in Appendix C.

SELECTED BIBLIOGRAPHY

American Cancer Society. 1999. *Cancer Facts and Figures—1999.* Atlanta: American Cancer Society.

American Heart Association. 1999. *1999 Heart and Stroke Statistical Update.* Dallas, TX: American Heart Association.

Casper, R. C. 1998. *Women's Health: Hormones, Emotions, and Behavior.* New York: Cambridge University Press.

Centers for Disease Control and Prevention. Youth Risk Behavior Surveillance: National College Health Risk Behavior Survey—United States, 1995. 1997. *MMWR Surveillance Summary* 46(SS-6): 1–56.

Clark, N. M., and J. A. Dodge. 1999. Exploring self-efficacy as a preditor of disease management. *Health Education Behavior* 26(1): 72–89.

Cole, T. B. 1999. Ebbing epidemic: Youth homicide rate at a 14-year low. *Journal of the American Medical Association* 28(1): 25–26.

Grace, T. W. 1997. Health problems of college students. *Journal of American College Health* 45(6): 243–250.

Laforge, R. G., et al. 1999. Stage distributions for five health behaviors in the United States and Australia. *Preventive Medicine* 28(1): 61–74.

Lantz, P. M., et al. 1998. Socioeconomic factors, health behaviors, and mortality. *Journal of the American Medical Association* 279: 1703–1708.

Lewis, M. A. and K. S. Rook. 1999. Social control in personal relationships: Impact on health behaviors and psychological distress. *Health Psychology* 18(1): 63–71.

Martin, G. and J. Pear. 1999. *Behaviour Modification: What It Is and How to Do It.* 6th ed. Upper Saddle River, N.J.: Prentice Hall.

National Center for Health Statistics. 1997. *Healthy People 2000 Review, 1997.* Hyattsville, Md.: Public Service, DHHS Pub. (PHS) 98-1256.

Riebe, D., and C. Nigg. 1998. Setting the stage for healthy living. *ACSM's Health and Fitness Journal* 2(3): 11–15.

Schank, M. J. 1999. Self-health appraisal: Learning the difficulties of lifestyle change. *Journal of Nursing Education* 38(1): 10–12.

U.S. Bureau of the Census. 1998. *Resident Population of the United States: Estimates, by Sex, Race, and Hispanic Origin* (retrieved September 25, 1998; http://www.census.gov/population/estimates/nation/intfile3-1.txt).

U.S. Department of Health and Human Services. 1998. *Health, United States, 1998: With Socioeconomic Status and Health Chartbook.* Washington, D.C.: U.S. Government Printing Office, DHHS Pub. (PHS) 98-1232.

U.S. Department of Health and Human Services. 1998. *Healthy People 2010 Objectives: Draft for Public Comment.* Washington, D.C.: US. Government Printing Office.

U.S. Department of Health and Human Services. 1990. *Healthy People 2000: National Health Promotion and Disease Prevention Objectives.* Washington, D.C.: U.S. Government Printing Office, DHHS Pub. (PHS) 91-50212.

Vita, A. J., et al. 1998. Aging, health risks, and cumulative disability. *New England Journal of Medicine* 338(15): 1064–1066.

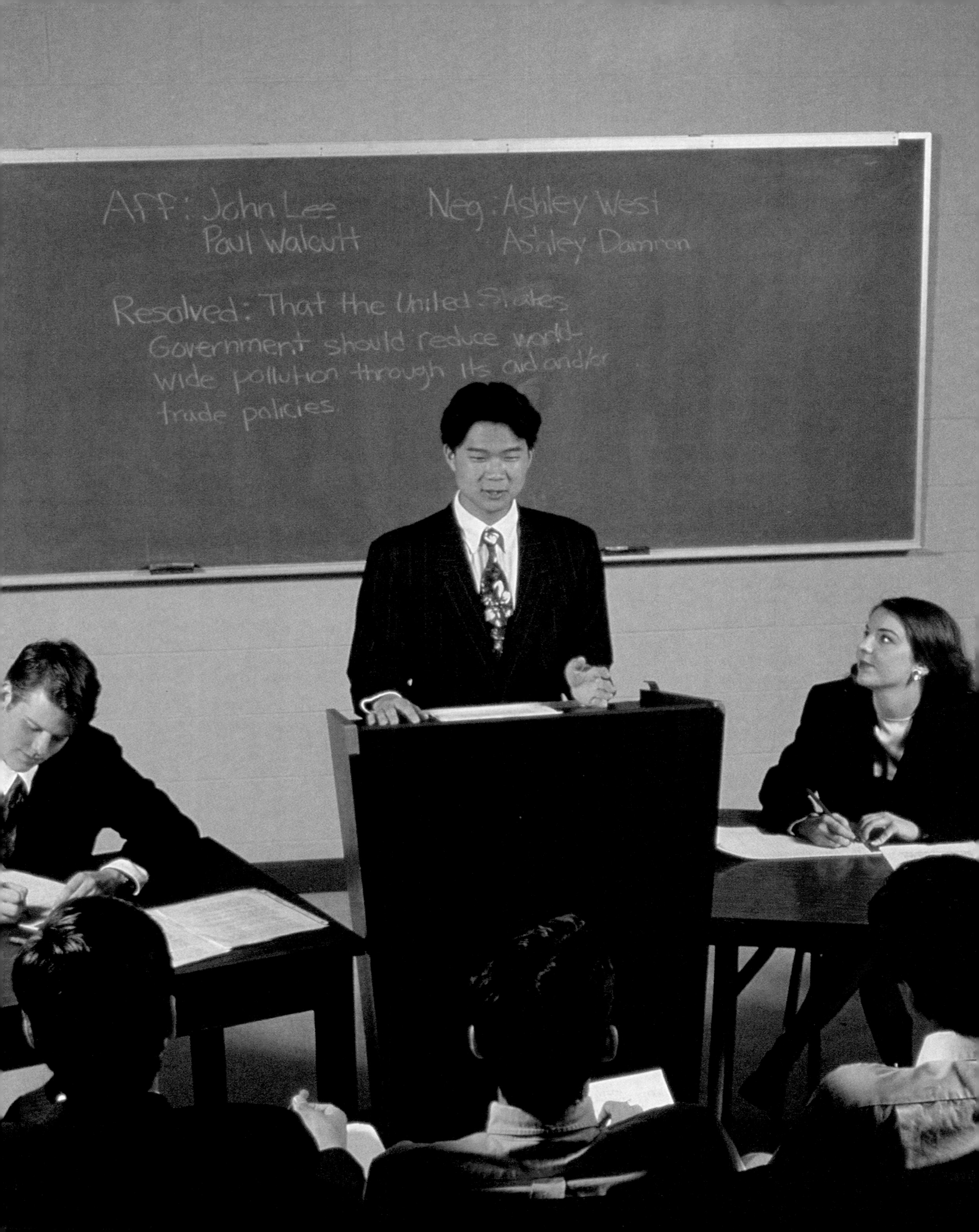
Aff: John Lee
Paul Walcutt
Neg: Ashley West
Ashley Damron
Resolved: That the United States
Government should reduce world-
wide pollution through its aid and/or
trade policies

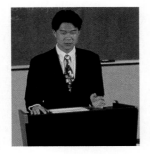

LEARNING OBJECTIVES

After reading this chapter, you should be able to:

- Explain what stress is and how people react to it—physically, emotionally, and behaviorally.

- Describe the relationship between stress and disease.

- List common sources of stress.

- Describe techniques for preventing and managing stress.

- Put together a step-by-step plan for successfully managing the stress in your life.

Stress: The Constant Challenge 2

TEST YOUR KNOWLEDGE

1. Which of the following events can cause stress?
   a. taking out a loan
   b. failing a test
   c. graduating from college
   d. watching a hockey game

2. How many adults experience health problems from stress each year?
   a. 20%
   b. 40%
   c. 60%

3. Which of the following may be caused or aggravated by stress?
   a. headaches
   b. irritable bowel syndrome
   c. insomnia
   d. high blood pressure

4. Vitamins can boost your energy and help you cope with daily stress.
   True or false?

5. About 20% of Americans report that they always feel rushed.
   True or false?

Answers

1. *All four.* Stress-producing factors can be either pleasant or unpleasant, and can include physical challenges and the achievement of personal goals as well as what would commonly be perceived as negative events.

2. *b.* Rates are highest among the economically disadvantaged, women, minorities, single parents, and adults under age 30.

3. *All four.* Stress—interacting with heredity, personality, social environment, and behavior—increases one's vulnerability to many health problems.

4. *False.* Energy comes from calories, and there are no calories in vitamins. Stress does not use up vitamin stores.

5. *False.* Nearly 40% of American adults report that they always feel rushed, and 55% report moderate or high levels of stress. Women are more likely than men to feel rushed and highly stressed.

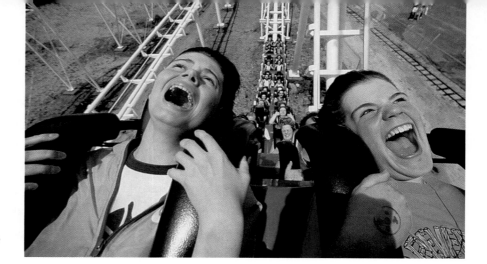

The experience of stress depends on many factors, including the nature of the stressor. Although stress-producing events are commonly thought of as negative, exciting and fun experiences like this amusement park ride can also cause stress.

Everybody talks about stress. People say they're "over-stressed" or "stressed out." They may blame stress for headaches or ulcers, and they may try to combat stress with aerobics classes—or drugs. But what is stress? And why is it important to manage it wisely?

Most people associate stress with negative events: the death of a close relative or friend, financial problems, or other unpleasant life changes that create nervous tension. But stress isn't merely nervous tension. And it isn't something to be avoided at all costs. In fact, only death brings complete freedom from stress. Before we explore more fully what stress is, consider this list of common stressful situations or events:

- Interviewing for a job.
- Running in a race.
- Being accepted to college.
- Going out on a date.
- Watching a basketball game.
- Getting a promotion.

Obviously, stress doesn't arise just from unpleasant situations. Stress can also be associated with physical challenges and the achievement of personal goals. Physical and psychological stress-producing factors can be either pleasant or unpleasant. What's crucial is how the individual responds, whether in positive, life-enhancing ways or in negative, counterproductive ways.

As a college student, you may be in one of the most stressful periods of your life. You may be on your own for the first time, or you may be juggling the demands of college with the responsibilities of a job, a family, or both. Financial pressures may be intense. Housing and transportation may be sources of additional hassles. You're also meeting new people, engaging in new activities, learning new information and skills, and setting a new course for your life. Good and bad, all these changes and challenges are likely to have a powerful effect on you, both physically and psychologically. Respond ineffectively to stress,

and eventually it will take a toll on your sense of wellness. Learn effective responses, however, and you will enhance your health and gain a feeling of control over your life.

How do you know when your stress level is getting dangerously high? How can you develop techniques to cope positively with the stress that is part of your life? This chapter will help you discover answers to these questions.

WHAT IS STRESS?

Just what is stress, if such vastly different situations can cause it? In common usage, "stress" refers to two different things: situations that trigger physical and emotional reactions *and* the reactions themselves. In this text, we'll use the more precise term **stressor** for situations that trigger physical and emotional reactions and the term **stress response** for those reactions. A date and a final exam, then, are stressors; sweaty palms and a pounding heart are symptoms of the stress response. We'll use the term **stress** to describe the general physical and emotional state that accompanies the stress response. A person on a date or taking a final exam experiences stress.

Each individual's experience of stress depends on many factors, including the nature of the stressor and how the stressor is perceived. Responses to stressors include physical changes and emotional and behavioral responses.

Physical Responses to Stressors

Imagine you are waiting to cross a street, perhaps daydreaming about a movie you saw last week. The light turns green and you step off the curb. Almost before you see it, you feel a car speeding toward you. With just a fraction of a second to spare, you leap safely out of harm's way. In that split second of danger, and in the moments following it, you have experienced a predictable series of physical reactions. Your body has gone from a relaxed state to one prepared for physical action to cope with a threat to your life.

Two major control systems in your body are responsible for your physical response to stressors: the nervous system and the endocrine system. Through a variety of rapid chemical reactions affecting almost every part of your body, you are primed to act quickly and appropriately in time of danger.

Actions of the Nervous System   The nervous system consists of the brain, spinal cord, and nerves. Part of the nervous system is under voluntary control, as when you command your arm to reach for a chocolate. The part that is not under conscious supervision, such as what controls the digestion of the chocolate, is known as the **autonomic nervous system.** In addition to digestion, it controls your heart rate, breathing, blood pressure, and hundreds of other functions you normally take for granted.

The autonomic nervous system consists of two divisions. The **parasympathetic division** is in control when you are relaxed; it aids in digesting food, storing energy, and promoting growth. In contrast, the **sympathetic division** is activated when there is an emergency, such as severe pain, anger, or fear. Sympathetic nerves act on many targets—on nearly every organ, sweat gland, blood vessel, and muscle, in fact—to enable your body to handle an emergency. In general, it commands your body to stop storing energy and instead to mobilize all energy resources to respond to the crisis.

Actions of the Endocrine System   One important target of the sympathetic nervous system is the activation of the **endocrine system.** This system of glands, tissues, and cells helps control body functions by releasing **hormones** and other chemical messengers into the bloodstream. These chemicals act on a variety of targets throughout the body. Along with the nervous system with which it closely interacts, the endocrine system helps prepare the body to respond to a stressor.

How do both systems work together in an emergency? Let's go back to your near car collision. As you first sense the car speeding toward you, your sympathetic nervous system prompts the **hypothalamus,** a control center in the brain, to release a chemical messenger to the nearby **pituitary gland.** In turn, the pituitary gland releases **adrenocorticotropic hormone (ACTH)** into the bloodstream. When ACTH reaches the **adrenal glands,** located just above the kidneys, it stimulates them to release **cortisol** and other key hormones into the bloodstream. Simultaneously, sympathetic nerves instruct your adrenal glands to release the hormones **epinephrine,** or adrenaline, and **norepinephrine,** which in turn trigger a series of profound changes as they circulate throughout your body (Figure 2-1, p. 28). Your hearing and vision become more acute.

Bronchi dilate to allow more air into your lungs. Your heart rate accelerates and blood pressure increases to ensure that your blood—and the oxygen, nutrients, and hormones it carries—will be rapidly distributed where needed. Your liver releases extra sugar into your bloodstream to provide an energy boost for your muscles and brain. Your digestion halts. You perspire more to cool your skin. **Endorphins** are released to relieve pain in case of injury. Blood cell production increases. These almost instantaneous changes give you the heightened reflexes and strength you need to dodge the car.

TERMS

stressor   Any physical or psychological event or condition that produces stress.

stress response   The physiological changes associated with stress.

stress   The collective physiological and emotional responses to any stimulus that disturbs an individual's homeostasis.

autonomic nervous system   The branch of the peripheral nervous system that, largely without conscious thought, controls basic body processes; consists of the sympathetic and parasympathetic divisions.

parasympathetic division   A division of the autonomic system that moderates the excitatory effect of the sympathetic division, slowing metabolism and restoring energy supplies.

sympathetic division   A division of the autonomic nervous system that reacts to danger or other challenges by almost instantly accelerating body processes.

endocrine system   The system of glands, tissues, and cells that secrete hormones into the bloodstream to influence metabolism and other body processes.

hormone   A chemical messenger produced in the body and transported by the bloodstream to target cells or organs for specific regulation of their activities.

hypothalamus   A part of the brain that activates, controls, and integrates the autonomic mechanisms, endocrine activities, and many body functions.

pituitary gland   The "master gland," closely linked with the hypothalamus, that controls other endocrine glands and secretes hormones that regulate growth, maturation, and reproduction.

adrenocorticotropic hormone (ACTH)   A hormone, formed in the pituitary gland, that stimulates the outer layer of the adrenal gland to secrete its hormones.

adrenal glands   Two glands, one lying atop each kidney, their outer layer (cortex) producing steroid hormones such as cortisol, and their inner core (medulla) producing the hormones epinephrine and norepinephrine.

cortisol   A steroid hormone secreted by the cortex (outer layer) of the adrenal gland; also called *hydrocortisone.*

epinephrine   A hormone secreted by the medulla (inner core) of the adrenal gland; also called *adrenaline,* the "fear hormone."

norepinephrine   A hormone secreted by the medulla (inner core) of the adrenal gland; also called *noradrenaline,* the "anger hormone."

endorphins   Brain secretions that have pain-inhibiting effects.

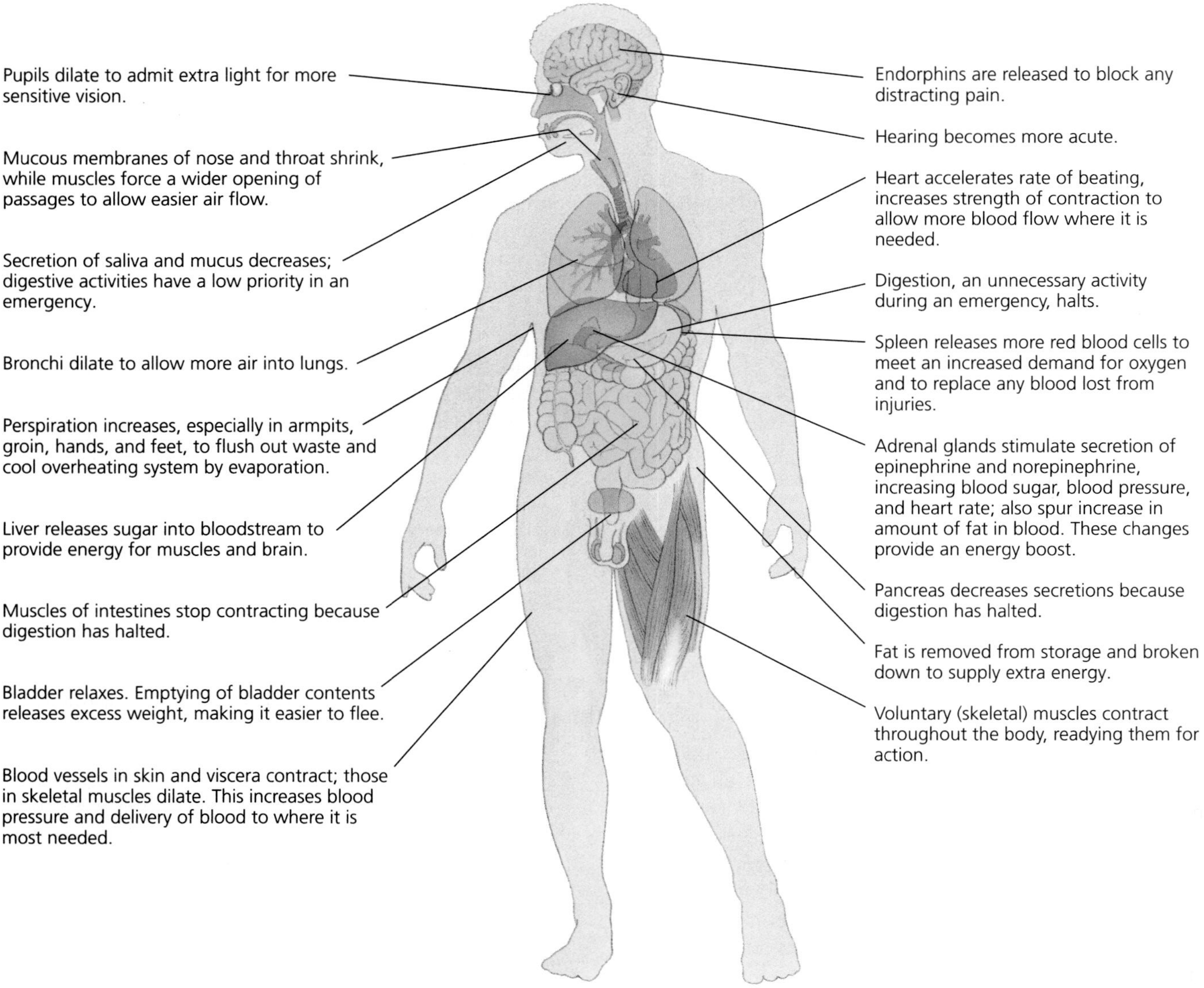

Pupils dilate to admit extra light for more sensitive vision.

Mucous membranes of nose and throat shrink, while muscles force a wider opening of passages to allow easier air flow.

Secretion of saliva and mucus decreases; digestive activities have a low priority in an emergency.

Bronchi dilate to allow more air into lungs.

Perspiration increases, especially in armpits, groin, hands, and feet, to flush out waste and cool overheating system by evaporation.

Liver releases sugar into bloodstream to provide energy for muscles and brain.

Muscles of intestines stop contracting because digestion has halted.

Bladder relaxes. Emptying of bladder contents releases excess weight, making it easier to flee.

Blood vessels in skin and viscera contract; those in skeletal muscles dilate. This increases blood pressure and delivery of blood to where it is most needed.

Endorphins are released to block any distracting pain.

Hearing becomes more acute.

Heart accelerates rate of beating, increases strength of contraction to allow more blood flow where it is needed.

Digestion, an unnecessary activity during an emergency, halts.

Spleen releases more red blood cells to meet an increased demand for oxygen and to replace any blood lost from injuries.

Adrenal glands stimulate secretion of epinephrine and norepinephrine, increasing blood sugar, blood pressure, and heart rate; also spur increase in amount of fat in blood. These changes provide an energy boost.

Pancreas decreases secretions because digestion has halted.

Fat is removed from storage and broken down to supply extra energy.

Voluntary (skeletal) muscles contract throughout the body, readying them for action.

Figure 2-1 The fight-or-flight reaction. In response to a stressor, the autonomic nervous system and the endocrine system cause physical changes that prepare the body to deal with an emergency.

Taken together, these almost instantaneous physical changes are called the **fight-or-flight reaction.** They give you the heightened reflexes and strength you need to dodge the car or deal with other stressors. Although these physical changes may vary in intensity, the same basic set of physical reactions occurs in response to any type of stressor, positive or negative.

The Return to Homeostasis Why doesn't your body remain in a hypervigilant state, perpetually ready for action? Why shouldn't your body always be prepared for a crisis? As you have probably guessed, it would be too exhausting. Your body actually resists dramatic changes. Whenever normal functioning is disrupted, such as during the fight-or-flight reaction, your body strives for **homeostasis,** a state in which blood pressure, heart rate, hormone levels, and other vital functions are maintained within a narrow range of normal.

Once a stressful situation ends, the parasympathetic division of your autonomic nervous system takes command and halts the reaction. It initiates the adjustments necessary to restore homeostasis. Your parasympathetic nervous system calms your body down, slowing a rapid heartbeat, drying sweaty palms, and returning breathing to normal. Gradually, your body resumes its normal "housekeeping" functions, such as digestion and temperature regulation. Damage that may have been sustained during the fight-or-flight reaction is repaired. The day after you narrowly dodge the car, you wake up feeling fine. In this way, your body can grow, repair itself, and acquire reserves of energy. When the next crisis comes, you'll be ready to respond—instantly—again.

The Fight-or-Flight Reaction in Modern Life

The fight-or-flight reaction is a part of our biological heritage, and it's a survival mechanism that has served humankind well. It enables our bodies to quickly prepare to escape from an injury or to engage in a physical battle. In modern life, however, the fight-or-flight reaction is often absurdly inappropriate. Many of the stressors we face in everyday life do not require a physical response—for example, an exam, a mess left by a roommate, or a red traffic light. The fight-or-flight reaction prepares the body for physical action regardless of whether such action is a necessary or appropriate response to a particular stressor.

Emotional and Behavioral Responses to Stressors

The physical response to a stressor may vary in intensity from person to person and situation to situation, but we all experience a similar set of physical changes—the fight-or-flight reaction. Emotionally and behaviorally, however, individuals respond in very different ways to stressors. For example, you may feel confident about taking exams but be nervous about talking to people you don't know, while your roommate may love challenging social situations but be very nervous about taking tests. A poor grade on a group project may prompt you to go for a 10-mile jog, while other members of your project team respond by eating chocolate or getting drunk.

Effective and Ineffective Responses

Our emotional and behavioral responses to stressors are as critical to our overall experience of stress as our physical responses. Common emotional responses to stressors include anxiety, depression, and fear. Although emotional responses are determined in part by inborn personality or temperament, we often can moderate or learn to control them. Coping techniques are discussed in detail later in the chapter.

Our behavioral responses—controlled by the **somatic nervous system,** which manages our conscious actions—are entirely under our control. Effective behavioral responses can promote wellness and enable us to function at our best. Ineffective behavioral responses to stressors can impair wellness and can even become stressors themselves. Depending on the stressor involved, effective behavioral responses may include talking, laughing, exercising, meditating, learning time-management skills, or finding a more compatible roommate. Inappropriate behavioral responses include overeating and using tobacco, alcohol, or other drugs.

Let's consider the different emotional and behavioral responses of two students, Amelia and David, to a common stressor: the first exam of the semester. Both students feel anxious as the exam is passed out. Amelia relaxes her muscles and starts by writing the answers she knows. On a second pass through the exam, she concentrates carefully on the wording of each question. Some material comes back to her, and she makes educated guesses on the remaining items. She spends the whole hour writing as much as she can and checking her answers. She leaves the room feeling calm, relaxed, and confident that she has done well on the exam.

David responds to his initial anxiety with more anxiety. He finds that he doesn't know some of the answers, and he becomes more worried. The more upset he gets, the less he can remember; and the more he blanks out, the more anxious he gets. He begins to imagine the consequences of failing the course and berates himself for not having studied more. David turns in his paper before the hour is up, without checking his answers or going back to the questions he skipped. He leaves feeling depressed and angry at himself.

As you can see, although both Amelia and David experienced the physical stress response as the exam was passed out, their emotional and behavioral responses were quite different—and led to very different outcomes. What determines these differences? Emotional and behavioral responses to stressors depend on a complex set of factors that includes personality, cultural background, gender, past experiences, beliefs and ideas, and coping skills. Let's take a closer look at some of these factors.

Personality and Stress

Some people seem to be nervous, irritable, and easily upset by minor annoyances; others are calm and even-tempered even in difficult situations. Scientists remain unsure just why this is or how the brain's complex emotional mechanisms work. But personality, the sum of behavioral and emotional tendencies, clearly affects how an individual perceives and reacts to stressors. To investigate the links among personality, stress, and overall wellness, researchers have looked at different constellations of characteristics, or "personality types."

TYPE A AND B PERSONALITIES The potential link between stress and heart disease has been the subject of research for many years. Cardiologists Meyer Friedman and Ray Rosenman reported that people with certain personality characteristics had a higher incidence of heart disease than people with other characteristics. They describe peo-

> **TERMS**
>
> **fight-or-flight reaction** A defense reaction that prepares an individual for conflict or escape by triggering hormonal, cardiovascular, metabolic, and other changes.
>
> **homeostasis** A state of stability and consistency in an individual's physiological functioning.
>
> **somatic nervous system** The branch of the peripheral nervous system that governs motor functions and sensory information; largely under our conscious control.

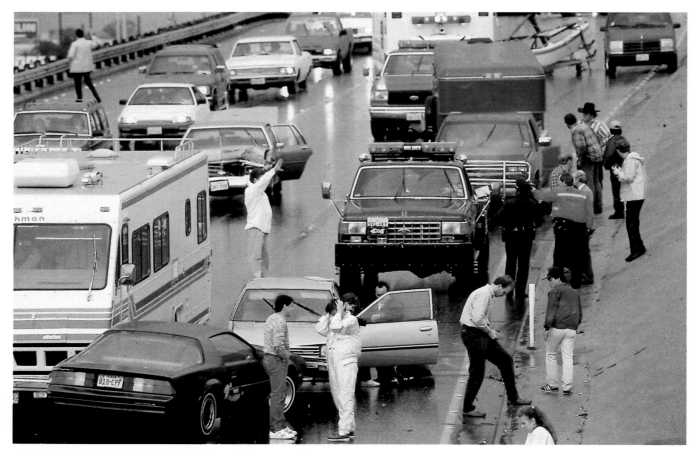

A person's emotional and behavioral responses to stressors depend on many different factors, including personality, gender, and cultural background. Some of the people involved in this series of highway collisions are still unnerved; others reacted more calmly.

ple with "Type A personalities" as ultracompetitive, controlling, impatient, aggressive, and hostile. Type A people tend to react more explosively to stressors, and they are upset by events that others would consider only mild annoyances. On the other hand, Type B individuals are relaxed, contemplative, and much less hurried. They tend to be less frustrated by the flow of daily events and more tolerant of the behavior of others.

Early studies indicated that Type A people have a greater risk of heart disease. However, recent evidence suggests that only particular characteristics of the Type A pattern—anger, cynicism, and hostility—increase the heart disease risk. (The link between hostility and heart disease is discussed further in Chapter 15.) What about Type A traits and other aspects of health? Studies indicate that Type A people may have a higher perceived stress level and more problems coping with stress.

THE HARDY PERSONALITY   Researchers have also looked at personality traits that seem to enable people to deal more successfully with stress. Psychologist Suzanne Kobasa examined "hardiness," a particular form of optimism. She found that people with a hardy personality view potential stressors as challenges and opportunities for growth and learning, rather than as burdens. Hardy people tend to perceive fewer situations as stressful, and their reaction to stressors tends to be less intense. They are committed to their activities, have a sense of inner purpose, and feel at least partly in control over events in their lives.

People with a hardy personality typically have an internal locus of control. As described in Chapter 1, this means that they feel responsible for their own actions and in control over many of the events in their lives. This sense of control helps them cope with stress in a more positive way and put setbacks in proper perspective. People with an external locus of control—a belief that the events in their lives are controlled by outside factors—typically have more difficulties with stress. A person with an external locus of control may feel helpless in a stressful situation and believe it's pointless to make constructive attempts to deal with stressors.

Is there anything people can do to change their personality and become more stress-resistant? It is unlikely that you can change your basic personality. However, you

TABLE 2-1	*Symptoms of Stress*	
Emotional Signs	**Behavioral Signs**	**Physical Signs**
Tendency to be irritable or aggressive	Increased use of alcohol, tobacco, or other drugs	Pounding heart
Tendency to feel anxious, fearful, or edgy	Excessive TV watching	Trembling, with nervous tics
Hyperexcitability, impulsiveness, or emotional instability	Sleep disturbances (e.g., insomnia) or excessive sleep	Grinding of teeth
Depression	Overeating or undereating	Dry mouth
Frequent feelings of boredom	Sexual problems	Excessive perspiration
Inability to concentrate	Crying	Gastrointestinal problems (diarrhea, constipation, indigestion, queasy stomach)
Fatigue	Yelling	Stiff neck or aching lower back
	Job or school burnout	Migraine or tension headaches
	Spouse or child abuse	Frequent colds or low-grade infections
	Panic attacks	Cold hands and feet
		Allergy or asthma attacks
		Skin problems (hives, eczema, psoriasis)

can change your typical behaviors and patterns of thinking and develop positive techniques for coping with stressors. Strategies for successful stress management are described later in the chapter.

Cultural Background   We all know that cultural stereotypes are exaggerations and that a variety of personalities exist within every ethnic group. However, people of various cultures do differ in their values, lifestyles, and what they consider to be acceptable behavior. It's not surprising that dealing with stress is also influenced by the family and the culture in which you are brought up. Even whether you perceive a situation to be stressful or not will depend on your upbringing. Suppose you go out on a date with someone who doesn't say much. You might worry that the person is behaving this way because he doesn't like you, and you may experience stress as a result. If you are quiet by nature and because of your cultural background, you'll probably feel things are going just fine.

Gender   Like cultural background, our **gender role**—the activities, abilities, and behaviors our culture expects of us based on whether we're male or female—also affects our experience of stress. Some behavioral responses to stressors, such as crying or openly expressing anger, may be deemed more appropriate for one gender than the other. Strict adherence to gender roles can thus place limits on how a person responds to stress and can itself become a source of stress. Adherence to traditional gender roles can also affect the perception of a potential stressor. For example, if a man derives most of his sense of self-worth from his work, retirement may be a more stressful life change for him than for a woman whose self-image is based on several different roles.

Past Experiences   Your past experiences significantly influence your response to stressors. For example, if you were unprepared for the first speech you gave in your speech class and performed poorly, you will probably experience greater anxiety in response to future assignments. If you had performed better, your confidence and sense of control would increase, and you would probably experience less stress with future speeches. Effective behavioral responses, such as careful preparation and visualizing yourself giving a successful speech, can help overcome the effects of negative past experiences.

PERSONAL INSIGHT   How do you respond when you're in a frustrating situation, like a traffic jam? Do you find that such situations really bother you at some times but not at others? What else is going on in your life when you stay calm? When you fly off the handle? Do you find that your relationships with others suffer when you're under stress?

The Stress Experience as a Whole

Physical, emotional, and behavioral responses to stressors are intimately interrelated. The more intense the emotional response, the stronger the physical response. Effective behavioral responses can lessen stress; ineffective ones only worsen it. Sometimes people have such intense emotional responses and such ineffective or counterproductive behavioral responses to stressors that they need professional help for learning to cope. (Table 2-1 highlights

gender role   A culturally expected pattern of behavior and attitudes determined by whether a person is male or female.   **TERMS**

some of the danger signals of excess stress.) More often, however, people can learn to handle stressors on their own. Actions you can take to successfully deal with the stress in your life are described later in the chapter.

STRESS AND DISEASE

The role of stress in health and disease is complex, and much remains to be learned about the exact mechanisms by which stress influences health. However, mounting evidence suggests that stress—interacting with a person's genetic predisposition, personality, social environment, and health-related behaviors—can increase vulnerability to numerous ailments. About 40% of people over age 18 experience adverse health effects from stress each year. A variety of related theories have been proposed to explain the relationship between stress and disease.

The General Adaptation Syndrome

Biologist Hans Selye was one of the first scientists to develop a comprehensive theory of stress and disease. Based on his work in the 1930s and 1940s, Selye coined the term **general adaptation syndrome (GAS)** to describe what he believed was a universal and predictable response pattern to all stressors. He recognized that stressors could be pleasant, such as attending a party, or unpleasant, such as a flat tire or a bad grade. He called stress triggered by a pleasant stressor **eustress** and stress triggered by an unpleasant stressor **distress**. The sequence of physical responses associated with GAS is the same for both eustress and distress and occurs in three stages: alarm, resistance, and exhaustion (Figure 2-2).

Alarm This stage includes the complex sequence of events brought on by the activation of the sympathetic nervous system and the endocrine system—the fight-or-flight reaction. During this stage, the body is more susceptible to disease or injury because it is geared up to deal with a crisis. A person in this phase may experience headaches, indigestion, and anxiety. Sleeping and eating patterns may also be disrupted.

Resistance With continued stress, Selye theorized that the body developed a new level of homeostasis in which

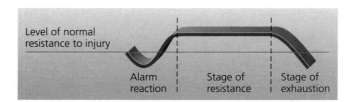

Figure 2-2 The general adaptation syndrome. Selye observed a predictable sequence of responses to stress. During the alarm phase, a lower resistance to injury is evident. With continued stress, resistance to injury is actually enhanced. With prolonged exposure to repeated stressors, exhaustion sets in, with a return of low resistance levels seen during acute stress.

it was more resistant to disease and injury than normal. During the resistance stage, a person can cope with normal life and added stress.

Exhaustion As you might imagine, both the mobilization of forces during the alarm reaction and the maintenance of homeostasis during the resistance stage require a considerable amount of energy. If a stressor persists, or if several stressors occur in succession, general exhaustion results. This is not the sort of exhaustion people complain of after a long, busy day. It's a life-threatening type of physiological exhaustion characterized by such symptoms as distorted perceptions and disorganized thinking.

Allostatic Load

While Selye's model of GAS is still viewed as a key contribution to modern stress theory, some aspects of it are now discounted. For example, increased susceptibility to disease after repeated or prolonged stress is now thought to be due to the effects of the stress response itself rather than to a depletion of resources (Selye's exhaustion state). In particular, long-term overexposure to stress hormones such as cortisol has been linked with health problems. Researchers have termed the long-term wear and tear of the stress response the *allostatic load.* An individual's allostatic load is dependent on many factors, including genetics, life experiences, and emotional and behavioral responses to stressors. A high allostatic load may be due to frequent stressors, poor adaptation to common stressors, an inability to shut down the stress response, or imbalances in the stress response of different body systems. Researchers have linked high allostatic load with heart disease, hypertension, obesity, and reduced brain and immune system functioning.

Psychoneuroimmunology

One of the most fruitful areas of current research into the relationship between stress and disease is **psychoneuroimmunology (PNI)**. PNI is the study of the interac-

Most of us have wondered at one time or another about the connection between mind and body. Can states of mind affect our health? Can negative feelings like fear and anger make us sick? Can positive feelings like hope and a "will to live" help make us well? Recent research seems to indicate that the answer to these questions may be yes.

As described in this chapter, research in the area of psychoneuroimmunology has revealed close connections between physical and emotional responses to stressors and the functioning of the immune system. The fight-or-flight reaction and accompanying feelings of fear and anger can impair the immune response. Other negative emotions that are often related to stress—depression, frustration, despair, and helplessness—also produce negative changes in body chemistry. Positive emotions, on the other hand—love, hope, joy, confidence, determination—may provide a buffer against stress and promote wellness.

Researchers have found numerous other examples of close mind-body connections:

• People with strong social ties live longer and have lower rates of some chronic diseases than people who lack social support.

• Regular exercise improves mood, boosts creativity, and helps maintain mental functioning throughout life.

• People who frequently respond to minor hassles with hostility and aggression have an increased risk of developing heart disease.

• Participation in a support group extends the lives of cancer patients and improves their emotional health.

These and other discoveries have persuaded many medical scientists that the mind and body are best seen not as separate entities but as parts of a fully integrated system—a living, breathing human being. However, the scientific study of mind-body connections is still in its infancy. Some of its findings have been distorted by the popular press, with extravagant and unscientific claims about the "healing powers of the mind." Such claims do a disservice to the research they profess to represent by creating false expectations, and even guilt, in people with life-threatening diseases. More research is needed before we will fully understand the nature and extent of the mind-body connection.

The realization that mind and body are intimately connected gives new meaning to the notion of "a sound mind in a sound body." The implication is that we can't cultivate mental and physical health separately and independently. There is no such thing as a purely psychological event or a purely physical event; the two are inseparable in a living being. For more information on the mind-body connection, look for boxes in this book labeled Sound Mind, Sound Body.

---

tions among the nervous system, the endocrine system, and the immune system. The underlying premise of PNI is that stress, through the actions of the nervous and endocrine systems, impairs the immune system and thereby affects health.

Researchers have discovered a complex network of nerve and chemical connections between the nervous and endocrine systems and the immune system. We have already seen that the hormones and other chemical messengers released during the stress response produce profound physical changes to prepare the body to deal with a stressor. These compounds also affect the immune system. For example, increased levels of cortisol are linked to a decreased number of immune system cells, or lymphocytes. Epinephrine and norepinephrine appear to promote the release of lymphocytes but at the same time reduce their efficiency. Activation of the sympathetic nervous system during the stress response also affects the immune system because certain nervous system fibers directly connect the brain to tissues and organs that produce lymphocytes.

The nervous, endocrine, and immune systems share other connections. Scientists have identified hormone-like substances called neuropeptides that appear to translate emotions into physiological events. Neuropeptides are produced and received by both brain and immune cells, so that the brain and the immune system share a biochemical "language," which also happens to be the language of emotions. The biochemical changes that accompany particular emotions can strongly influence the functioning of the immune system; some emotions may suppress lymphocyte function, while others promote it. The entire lining of the intestines is also equipped with neuropeptide receptors, perhaps accounting for our tendency to experience emotions as "gut feelings."

The degree to which stress affects the immune system and how immune system changes influence health are still being investigated. However, research indicates that stress does affect immunity and health in both the short and long term. Studies of students have found that concentrations of immune cells drop during the period of final exams. Investigators have also found that the long-term stress of caring for someone with Alzheimer's disease is associated with reduced immune function. (For more on the connections among stress, emotions, and health, see the box "The Mind-Body Connection.")

Links Between Stress and Specific Conditions

Although much remains to be learned, it is clear that people who have unresolved chronic stress in their lives or who handle stressors poorly are at risk for a wide range of health problems. In the short term, the problem might just be a cold, a stiff neck, or a stomachache. Over the long term, the problems can be more severe—cardiovascular disease, high blood pressure, or impairment of the immune system.

Cardiovascular Disease

During the stress response, heart rate increases and blood vessels constrict, causing blood pressure to rise. Chronic high blood pressure is a major cause of **atherosclerosis,** a disease in which the lining of the blood vessels becomes damaged and caked with fatty deposits. These deposits can block arteries, causing heart attacks and strokes.

Recent research suggests that certain types of emotional responses increase a person's risk of cardiovascular disease. So-called "hot reactors," people who exhibit extreme increases in heart rate and blood pressure in response to emotional stressors, may face an increased risk of cardiovascular problems. As described earlier in the section on Type A personality, people who tend to react to situations with anger and hostility are more likely to have heart attacks than people with a less explosive, more trusting personality. (For further discussion of heart disease and trust, see Chapter 15.)

Altered Functioning of the Immune System

Sometimes you seem to get sick when you can least afford it—during exam week, when you're going on vacation, or when you have a big job interview. As described earlier regarding PNI, research suggests that this is more than mere coincidence. Some of the health problems linked to stress-related changes in immune function include the following:

- *Colds and other infections.* Stress can leave people more vulnerable to contracting a cold and less able to fight one off.

- *Asthma and allergies.* Stress is a trigger or aggravator of asthma, hives, eczema, and other allergies.

- *Cancer.* One of the functions of the immune system is recognizing and destroying any abnormal cells produced in the body; left unchecked, such cells can develop into cancerous tumors. By compromising the immune system, stress may increase a person's chance of developing cancer and decrease her or his chance of surviving it.

- *Chronic disease flare-ups.* Symptoms of chronic diseases such as genital herpes, HIV infection, and diabetes may flare up during episodes of stress. In addition to decreasing the effectiveness of the immune system, stress may also distract people from their commitment to important disease-management behaviors like eating a healthy diet, exercising, and taking medications.

TERMS **atherosclerosis** The buildup of hard yellow plaques of fatty material in the lining of arteries that have become damaged from advancing age or high blood pressure; a leading cause of heart disease and stroke.

Psychological Problems

The hormones and other chemicals released during the stress response cause emotional as well as physical changes. Moreover, many stressors—a hurricane, for example, or the death of a loved one—are inherently anxiety-producing, depressing, or both. Stress has been found to contribute to such psychological problems as depression, panic attacks, anxiety, eating disorders, and post-traumatic stress disorder (PTSD). PTSD, which afflicts war veterans, rape and child abuse survivors, and others who have suffered or witnessed severe trauma, is characterized by nightmares, flashbacks, and a diminished capacity to experience or express emotion. (For more information on psychological problems, see Chapter 3.)

Other Health Problems

Many other health problems may be caused or worsened by uncontrolled stress, including the following:

- *Digestive problems.* Stress is associated with stomachaches, diarrhea, and constipation, and it may aggravate problems such as irritable bowel syndrome and ulcers.

- *Headaches.* Muscle contractions and changes in blood vessels associated with the stress response can cause tension headaches and trigger migraines.

- *Insomnia and fatigue.* Chemical messengers produced during the fight-or-flight reaction promote alertness and ward off sleep. Sleep disruption in turn can produce fatigue.

- *Injuries.* Stress may distract people and cause them to become less vigilant about key injury prevention behaviors such as wearing a safety belt or bicycle helmet. On-the-job injuries, including repetitive-strain injury (RSI), are also linked to job stress.

- *Endocrine effects and pregnancy complications.* Menstrual irregularities and impotence are both associated with periods of unusual stress. Women who experience significant stress before or during pregnancy may have an increased risk of delivering a premature or low-birth-weight infant.

COMMON SOURCES OF STRESS

We are surrounded by stressors—at home, at school, on the job, and within ourselves. Being able to recognize potential sources of stress is an important step in successfully managing the stress in our lives.

Major Life Changes

Any major change in your life that requires adjustment and accommodation can be a source of stress (see the box "Major Life Changes, Stress, and Risk of Illness"). Early adulthood and the college years are typically associated with many significant changes, such as moving out of the family

Major Life Changes, Stress, and Risk of Illness

Researchers have hypothesized that clusters of life changes may be linked to health problems. Review the list of life changes below; circle the point total next to any life change that you have experienced in the past year.

Health

An injury or illness which	
kept you in bed a week or more,	
or sent you to the hospital	74
was less serious than that	44
Major dental work	26
Major change in eating habits	27
Major change in sleeping habits	26
Major change in your usual type or amount	
of recreation	28

Work

Change to a new type of work	51
Change in your work hours or conditions	35
Change in your responsibilities at work:	
more responsibilities	29
fewer responsibilities	21
promotion	31
demotion	42
transfer	32
Troubles at work:	
with your boss	29
with coworkers	35
with persons under your supervision	35
other work troubles	28
Major business adjustment	60
Retirement	52
Loss of job:	
laid off from work	68
fired from work	79
Correspondence course to help you in	
your work	18

Home and Family

Major change in living conditions	42
Change in residence:	
move within the same town or city	25
move to a different town, city, or state	47
Change in family get-togethers	25
Major change in health or behavior of	
family member	55
Marriage	50
Pregnancy	67
Miscarriage or abortion	65
Gain of a new family member:	
birth of a child	66
adoption of a child	65
a relative moving in with you	59
Spouse beginning or ending work	46
Child leaving home:	
to attend college	41
due to marriage	41
for other reasons	45

Change in arguments with spouse	50
In-law problems	38
Change in marital status of your parents:	
divorce	59
remarriage	50
Separation from spouse:	
due to work	53
due to marital problem	76
Divorce	96
Birth of grandchild	43
Death of spouse	119
Death of other family member:	
child	123
brother or sister	102
parent	100

Personal and Social

Change in personal habits	26
Beginning or ending school or college	38
Change of school or college	35
Change of political beliefs	24
Change in religious beliefs	29
Change in social activities	27
Vacation trip	24
New, close, personal relationship	37
Engagement to marry	45
Girlfriend or boyfriend problems	39
Sexual difficulties	44
"Falling out" of a close personal relationship	47
An accident	48
Minor violation of the law	20
Being held in jail	75
Death of a close friend	70
Major decision about your immediate future	51
Major personal achievement	36

Financial

Major change in finances:	
increased income	38
decreased income	60
investment or credit difficulties	56
Loss or damage of personal property	43
Moderate purchase	20
Major purchase	37
Foreclosure on a mortgage or loan	58

Total score: _____

Add up your points. A total score of anywhere from 250 to 500 or so would be considered a moderate amount of stress. If you score higher than that, you may face an increased risk of illness; if you score lower than that, consider yourself fortunate.

SOURCE: Reprinted from Miller, M. A., and R. H. Rahe. 1997. Life changes scaling for the 1990s. *Journal of Psychosomatic Research* 43(3): 279–292. Copyright © 1997, Elsevier Science Ltd. With permission from Elsevier Science.

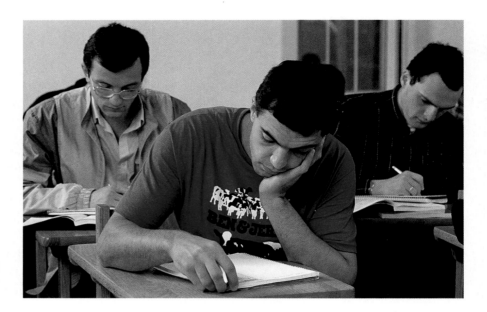

Taking exams is only one of many stressors associated with the college years. College can also be a time of major life events and numerous daily hassles.

home, establishing new relationships, setting educational and career goals, and developing a sense of identity and purpose. Even changes typically thought of as positive—graduation, job promotion, marriage—can be stressful.

Clusters of major life changes may be linked to the development of health problems in some people. Research indicates that some life changes, particularly those that are perceived negatively, can affect health. However, personality and coping skills are important moderating influences. People with a strong support network and a stress-resistant personality are less likely to become ill in response to major life changes than people with fewer internal and external resources.

Daily Hassles

Have you done any of the following in the past week?

- Misplaced your keys, wallet, or an assignment.
- Had an argument with a troublesome neighbor, coworker, or customer.
- Waited in a long line.
- Been stuck in traffic or had another problem with transportation.
- Worried about money.
- Been upset about the weather.

While major life changes are undoubtedly stressful, they seldom occur regularly. Psychologist Richard Lazarus has proposed that minor problems—life's daily hassles—can be an even greater source of stress because they occur much more often. People who perceive hassles negatively are likely to experience a moderate stress response every time they are faced with one. Over time, this can take a significant toll on health. Researchers have found that for some people, daily hassles contribute to a general decrease in overall wellness.

College Stressors

College is a time of major life changes and abundant minor hassles. You will be learning new information and skills and making major decisions about your future. You may be away from home for the first time, or you may be adding extra responsibilities to a life already filled with job and family. Some common sources of stress associated with college are the following:

- *Academic stressors,* such as exams, grades, and choosing a major. (Techniques for overcoming test anxiety, a common stress-related academic problem, are described in the Behavior Change Strategy at the end of the chapter.)
- *Social and interpersonal stressors,* such as establishing new relationships and balancing multiple roles (student, employee, friend, spouse, parent, etc.).
- *Time-related pressures,* caused by accepting too many responsibilities or managing one's time poorly. Time pressures are a problem for most students, but they may be particularly keen for those who also have job and family responsibilities. (Strategies for more effective time management are described in the next section.)
- *Financial concerns,* such as paying tuition, living expenses, and taking out loans.

Job-Related Stressors

In recent surveys, Americans rate their jobs as one of the key sources of stress in their lives. Tight schedules and

Stress is universal, but some groups within the United States face unique stressors and have higher-than-average rates of stress-related physical and emotional problems. These include women, ethnic minorities, the economically disadvantaged, and people with disabilities. Many of the unique stressors that affect special populations stem from prejudice—biased, negative attitudes toward a group of people.

Discrimination occurs when people act according to their prejudices; it can be blatant or subtle. Blatant examples of discrimination are not common, but they are major stressors, akin to significant life changes. Examples include a swastika painted on a Jewish studies house, the defacement of a sculpture honoring the achievements of gay men, and sexual harassment during a fraternity party. More subtle acts may occur much more frequently. For example, an African American student in a mostly white college town feels that shopkeepers are keeping an eye on him, a student using a wheelchair has difficulty with nar-

row aisles and high counters at local stores, and a female business executive finds that restaurants always assume the lunch check should go to her male clients. Some of these social stressors are unique to certain groups, and it may be difficult for other people to understand how serious such stressors can be.

Women and minorities also often face additional job-related stressors because of stereotypes and discrimination. They make less money than white males in comparable jobs and with comparable levels of education. Women are more likely to face sexual harassment on the job. As employment opportunities have expanded for women, they also often find themselves balancing multiple roles—employee, parent, spouse, caregiver to aging parents, and so on. Women who work outside the home still do most of the housework, and time-related stress can be severe. All these types of stressors can contribute to higher levels of stress-related health problems.

overtime contribute to time-related pressures. More than one-third of Americans report that they always feel rushed, and nearly half say they would give up a day's pay for a day off. Worries about job performance, salary, and job security are a source of stress for some people. Interactions with bosses, coworkers, and customers can also contribute to stress. High levels of job stress are also common for people who are left out of important decisions relating to their jobs. When workers are given the opportunity to shape how their jobs are performed, job satisfaction goes up and stress levels go down.

If job-related (or college-related) stress is severe or chronic, the result can be **burnout,** a state of physical, mental, and emotional exhaustion. Burnout occurs most often in highly motivated and driven individuals who come to feel that their work is not recognized or that they are not accomplishing their goals. People in the helping professions—teachers, social workers, caregivers, police officers, and so on—are also prone to burnout. For some people who suffer from burnout, a vacation or leave of absence may be appropriate. For others, a reduced work schedule, better communication with superiors, or a change in job goals may be necessary. Improving time-management skills can also help.

Interpersonal and Social Stressors

Although social support is a key buffer against stress, your interactions with others can also be a source of stress themselves. For many people, the college years are a time of great change in interpersonal relationships. Your relationships with family members and old friends may change as you develop new interests and a new course for your life. You will be meeting new people and establish-

ing new relationships. All of these changes and experiences are potential stressors.

The community and society in which you live can also be major sources of stress. Social stressors include prejudice and discrimination. You may feel stress as you try to relate to people of other ethnic or socioeconomic groups. As a member of a particular ethnic group, you may feel pressure to assimilate into mainstream society. If English is not your first language, you face the added burden of conducting many daily activities in a language with which you may not be completely comfortable. All of these pressures can become significant sources of stress. (For more information on stressors that disproportionately affect people in particular groups, refer to the box "Stress and Diverse Populations.")

Environmental Stressors

Claire loves the food at a certain restaurant, but she always feels "on edge" when eating there because of continuous loud background music. This is an example of an environmental stressor—some condition or event in the physical environment that causes stress. Environmental stressors include things like natural disasters, industrial accidents, and intrusive noises, smells, or sights. Like the loud music that bothers Claire, some environmental stressors are mere inconveniences that are easy to avoid. Others, such as pollen season for a hayfever sufferer or living next to a construction site, may be an unavoidable

---

burnout   A state of physical, mental, and emotional exhaustion.   **TERMS**

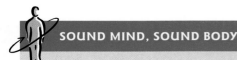

Meaningful connections with others can play a key role in stress management and overall wellness. A sense of isolation can lead to chronic stress, which in turn can increase one's susceptibility to temporary illnesses like colds and to chronic illnesses like heart disease. Although the mechanism isn't clear, social isolation can be as significant to mortality rates as factors like smoking, high blood pressure, and obesity.

There is no single best pattern of social support that works for everyone. However, research suggests that having a variety of types of relationships may be important for wellness. To help determine whether your social network measures up, circle whether each of the following statements is true or false for you.

T F **1.** If I needed an emergency loan of $100, there is someone I could get it from.

T F **2.** There is someone who takes pride in my accomplishments.

T F **3.** I often meet or talk with family or friends.

T F **4.** Most people I know think highly of me.

T F **5.** If I needed an early morning ride to the airport, there's no one I would feel comfortable asking to take me.

T F **6.** I feel there is no one with whom I can share my most private worries and fears.

T F **7.** Most of my friends are more successful making changes in their lives than I am.

T F **8.** I would have a hard time finding someone to go with me on a day trip to the beach or country.

To calculate your score, add the number of true answers to questions 1–4 and the number of false answers to questions 5–8. If your score is 4 or more, you should have enough support to protect your health. If your score is 3 or less, you may need to reach out. There are a variety of things you can do to strengthen your social ties:

- *Foster friendships.* Keep in regular contact with your friends. Offer respect, trust, and acceptance, and provide help and support in times of need. Express appreciation for your friends.

- *Keep your family ties strong.* Stay in touch with the family members you feel close to. Participate in family activities and celebrations. If your family doesn't function well as a support system for its members, create a second "family" of people with whom you have built meaningful ties.

- *Get involved with a group.* Do volunteer work, take a class, attend a lecture series, join a religious group. These types of activities can give you a sense of security, a place to talk about your feelings or concerns, and a way to build new friendships. Choose activities that are meaningful to you and that include direct involvement with other people.

- *Build your communication skills.* The more you share your feelings with others, the closer the bonds between you will become. When others are speaking, be a considerate and attentive listener. (Chapters 3 and 4 include more information on effective communication.)

Individual relationships change over the course of your life, but it's never too late to build friendships or become more involved in your community. Your investment of time and energy in your social network will pay off—in a brighter outlook now, and in better health and well-being for the future.

SOURCE: Friends can be good medicine. 1998. Mind/Body Newsletter 7(1): 3–6. QUIZ SOURCE: Japenga, A. 1995. A family of friends. *Health*, November/December, 94. Adapted with permission. Copyright © 1995 Health.

daily source of stress. For those who live in poor or violent neighborhoods or in a war-torn country, environmental stressors can be major life stressors.

Internal Stressors

Some stressors are found not in our interactions with our environment but within ourselves. We put pressure on ourselves to reach personal goals, and we continuously evaluate our progress and performance. Setting high goals and then striving to reach them can enhance self-esteem if the goals are reasonable. However, unrealistic expectations can be a significant source of stress and a serious blow to self-esteem. Other internal stressors are physical and emotional states such as illness and exhaustion; these can be both a cause and an effect of unmanaged stress.

PERSONAL INSIGHT   What types of stressors are currently of greatest concern to you? Are these stressors new to your life as part of your college experience, or are they the same types of stressors that have given you trouble in the past? How well do you think you are coping with the major stressors in your life?

TECHNIQUES FOR MANAGING STRESS

What can you do about all this stress? A great deal. By shoring up your social support systems; improving your communication skills; developing and maintaining healthy exercise, eating, and sleeping habits; and mastering simple techniques to identify and moderate individ-

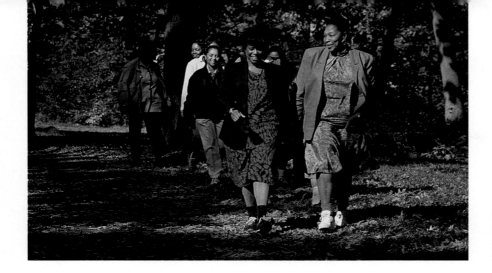

Exercise is a particularly effective antidote to stress. A lunchtime walk gives these coworkers a chance to both exercise and foster friendships.

ual stressors, you can learn to control the stress in your life—instead of allowing it to control you. The effort is well worth the time: People who manage stress effectively not only are healthier, they also have more time to enjoy life and accomplish their goals.

Social Support

People need people. Sharing fears, frustrations, and joys not only makes life richer but also seems to contribute to the well-being of body and mind. Research supports this conclusion: One study of college students living in overcrowded apartments, for example, found that those with a strong social support system were less distressed by their cramped quarters than the "loners" who navigated life's challenges on their own. Other studies have shown that married people live longer than single people and have lower death rates from a wide range of conditions. People with a strong social support system are also better able to withstand the stress of major life changes. The crucial common denominator in all these findings is meaningful connections with others.

Allow yourself time to nourish and maintain a network of people at home, at work, at school, or in your community you can count on for emotional support, feedback, and nurturance. To evaluate your current social support system, and to find strategies for strengthening your social ties, refer to the box "Healthy Connections."

Communication

Do you find yourself often angry at others? Some people express their anger directly by yelling or being aggressive; others indirectly express anger by excessively criticizing others or making cynical comments. A person who is angry with others often has difficulty forming and maintaining successful social relationships. Better communication skills can help: Learn to listen to others and to express your needs and desires nonaggressively. Increase your communication

skills in order to decrease stress in your relationships—at school, at work, and at home.

At the other extreme, you may suppress your feelings and needs entirely. You may have trouble saying no and allow people to take advantage of you. Many businesses encourage employees to take assertiveness training workshops to help them overcome shyness and resistance to communicating their needs. Such communication skills are also valuable in social relationships. (For a fuller discussion of how to enhance communication and resolve interpersonal conflicts, see Chapters 3 and 4.)

PERSONAL INSIGHT   How did people in your family cope with stress when you were growing up? Were their methods successful? Do you use the same methods they did? Are there people around you who use different methods that you could try?

Exercise

One recent study from the National Academy of Sciences found that taking a long walk can help decrease anxiety and blood pressure. Another study found that just a brisk 10-minute walk leaves people feeling more relaxed and energetic for up to 2 hours. Researchers have also found that people who exercise regularly react with milder physical stress responses before, during, and after exposure to stressors. People who took three brisk 45-minute walks a week for 3 months reported that they perceived fewer daily hassles. Their sense of wellness also increased.

It's not hard to incorporate light to moderate exercise into your day. Walk to class or bike to the store instead of driving. Use the stairs instead of the elevator. Take a walk with a friend instead of getting a cup of coffee. Go bowling, play tennis, or roller-skate instead of seeing a movie. Make a habit of taking a brisk after-dinner stroll. Plan

Most people can overcome insomnia by discovering the cause of poor sleep and taking steps to remedy it. Insomnia that lasts for more than 6 months and interferes with daytime functioning requires consultation with a physician. Sleeping pills are not recommended for chronic insomnia because they can be habit-forming; they also lose their effectiveness over time.

If you're bothered by insomnia, here are some tips for getting a better night's sleep:

• Determine how much sleep you need to feel refreshed the next day, and don't sleep longer than that (but do make sure you get enough).

• Go to bed at the same time every night and, more importantly, get up at the same time every morning, 7 days a week, regardless of how much sleep you got. Don't nap during the day.

• Exercise every day, but not too close to bedtime. Your metabolism takes up to 6 hours to slow down after exercise.

• Avoid tobacco (nicotine is a stimulant), caffeine in the later part of the day, and alcohol before bedtime (it causes disturbed, fragmented sleep).

• Have a light snack before bedtime; you'll sleep better if you're not hungry.

• Deal with worries before bedtime. Try writing them down, along with some possible solutions, and then allow yourself to forget about them until the next day.

• Use your bed only for sleep. Don't eat, read, study, or watch television in bed.

• Relax before bedtime with a warm bath (again, not too close to bedtime—allow about 2 hours for your metabolism to slow down afterward), a book, music, or some relaxation exercises. Don't lie down in bed until you're sleepy.

• If you don't fall asleep in 15–20 minutes, or if you wake up and can't fall asleep again, get out of bed, leave the room if possible, and do something monotonous until you feel sleepy.

• Keep a perspective on your plight. Losing a night's sleep isn't the end of the world. Getting upset only makes it harder to fall asleep. Relax, and trust in your body's natural ability to drift off to sleep.

hikes and easy bike outings for the weekends. Play softball or table tennis. Work in your garden.

Consider taking a class in a kind of exercise you've always wanted to try, such as yoga, t'ai chi, square dancing, or fencing. The important thing is to find an activity that you enjoy, so it can become a habit and thereby an effective stress reducer. Once you begin to make sensible exercise a daily part of your life, you may find it hard to live without. (Chapter 13 presents guidelines for creating an exercise program to fit your individual needs and preferences.)

Nutrition

A healthy diet will give you an energy bank to draw on whenever you experience stress. Eating wisely also will enhance your feelings of self-control and self-esteem. Learning the principles of sound nutrition is easy, and sensible eating habits rapidly become second nature when practiced regularly. (For more on sound nutrition, see Chapter 12.)

Avoiding or limiting caffeine is also important in stress management. Although one or two cups of coffee a day probably won't hurt you, caffeine is a mildly addictive stimulant that leaves some people jittery, irritable, and unable to sleep. Tea, cola, some other soft drinks, chocolate, and more than a thousand over-the-counter drugs, including cold remedies, aspirin, and weight-loss preparations, also contain caffeine, sometimes in high doses.

Sleep

Lack of sleep can be both a cause and an effect of excess stress. Without sufficient sleep, our mental and physical processes steadily deteriorate. We get headaches, feel irritable, are unable to concentrate, forget things, and may be more susceptible to illness. Sleep deprivation and fatigue are a major factor in many fatal car, truck, and train crashes. Extreme sleep deprivation can lead to hallucinations and other psychotic symptoms.

Adequate sleep, on the other hand, improves mood, fosters feelings of competence and self-worth, and supports optimal mental and emotional functioning. If you are sleep-deprived, sleeping extra hours may significantly improve your daytime alertness and mental abilities. Sleep requirements vary considerably among individuals; some adults need only 5 hours of sleep, while others need 9 hours or more to feel fully refreshed and alert.

Sleep occurs in two phases: rapid eye movement (REM) and non-REM. Non-REM sleep consists of four stages of successively deeper sleep, during which blood pressure, heart rate, temperature, and breathing rate drop; growth hormone is released; and brain wave patterns become slow and even. REM sleep, during which dreams occur, is characterized by the rapid back-and-forth movement of the sleeper's eyes under closed eyelids. Heart rate, blood pressure, and breathing rate increase; brain activity increases to levels equal to or greater than during waking. Muscles in the limbs relax completely, causing temporary paralysis and preventing the sleeper from acting out her or his dreams. A sleeper goes through several cycles of non-REM and REM sleep each night.

Nearly everyone, at some time in life, has trouble falling asleep or staying asleep—a condition known as insomnia. The most common causes of insomnia are lifestyle factors, such as high caffeine or alcohol intake before bedtime; medical problems, such as a breathing disorder; and psychological stress. If you suffer from sleeping problems, try some of the strategies in the box "Overcoming Insomnia."

Time Management

A surprising number of the stressors in most people's lives relate to time. Many people never seem to have enough time, and they always seem to feel overwhelmed by the pace of their lives. Others have too much time on their hands and are often bored. Learning to manage your time successfully is crucial to coping with the stressors you face every day.

Procrastination—putting something off until later—is a problem for many people. People who put off key tasks and decisions may sabotage personal relationships, college life, careers, and health. Although reasons for procrastination vary, it often camouflages self-doubt, an unreasonable desire for perfection, or a reluctance to make changes. People who set impossibly high standards for themselves may actually protect their self-esteem by procrastinating; if they fail to complete a project, for example, their work will never be evaluated.

If procrastination or another time-related stressor is a problem for you, try some or all of the following strategies for managing your time more productively and creatively:

- *Set priorities.* Divide your tasks into three groups: essential, important, and trivial. Focus on the first two. Ignore the third.
- *Schedule tasks for peak efficiency.* You've undoubtedly noticed you're most productive at certain times of the day (or night). Schedule as many of your tasks for those hours as you can, and stick to your schedule.
- *Set realistic goals, and write them down.* Attainable goals spur you on. Impossible goals, by definition, cause frustration and failure. Fully commit yourself to achieving your goals by putting them in writing.
- *Budget enough time.* For each project you undertake, calculate how long it will take to complete. Then tack on another 10–15%, or even 25%, as a buffer against mistakes, interruptions, or unanticipated problems.
- *Break up long-term goals into short-term ones.* Instead of waiting for or relying on large blocks of time, use short amounts of time to start a project or keep it moving. Say you have a 50-page report due and are about to panic. Divide the assignment into three

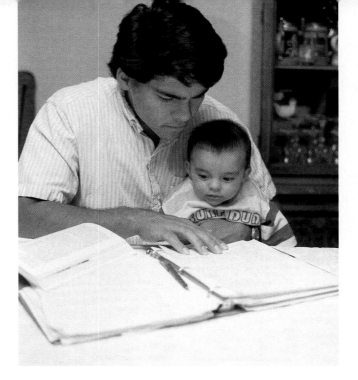

Managing the many commitments of adult life—including work, school, and parenthood—can sometimes feel overwhelming and produce a great deal of stress. Time-management skills, including careful scheduling and prioritizing, help this father cope with busy days.

tasks: research, outlining, and writing. Then budget enough half-hour- or hour-long time slots to complete each task. Your steady progress will make you feel so much better that you'll be encouraged to continue.

- *Visualize the achievement of your goals.* By mentally rehearsing your performance of a task, you will be able to reach your goal more smoothly.
- *Keep track of the tasks you put off.* Analyze the reasons why you procrastinate. If the task is difficult or unpleasant, look for ways to make it easier or more fun. If you hate cleaning up your room, break the work into 10-minute tasks and do a little at a time. If you find the readings for one of your classes particularly difficult, choose an especially nice setting for your reading, then reward yourself each time you complete a section or chapter.
- *Consider doing your least favorite tasks first.* Once you have the most unpleasant ones out of the way, you can work on the projects you enjoy more.
- *Consolidate tasks when possible.* For example, try walking to the store so that you run your errands and exercise in the same block of time.
- *Identify quick transitional tasks.* Keep a list of 5-minute tasks you can do while waiting or between other tasks, such as watering your plants, doing the dishes, or checking a homework assignment.

- *Delegate responsibility.* Asking for help when you have too much to do is no cop-out; it's good time management. Just don't delegate to others the jobs you know you should do yourself, such as researching a paper.

- *Say no when necessary.* If the demands made on you don't seem reasonable, say no—tactfully, but without guilt or apology.

- *Give yourself a break.* Allow time for play—free, unstructured time when you ignore the clock. Don't consider this a waste of time. Play renews you and enables you to work more efficiently.

- *Stop thinking or talking about what you're going to do, and just do it!* Sometimes the best solution for procrastination is to stop waiting for the right moment and just get started. You will probably find that things are not as bad as you feared, and your momentum will keep you going.

Cognitive Techniques

Some stressors arise in our own minds. Ideas, beliefs, perceptions, and patterns of thinking can add to our emotional and physical stress responses and get in the way of effective behavioral responses. Each of the techniques described below can help you change unhealthy thought patterns to ones that will help you cope with stress. As with any skill, mastering these techniques takes practice and patience.

Worry Constructively Worrying, someone once said, is like shoveling smoke. Think back to the worries you had last week. How many of them were needless? Worry only about things you can control. Try to stand aside from the problem, consider the positive steps you can take to solve it, and then carry them out. You've done what you can; you can quit worrying.

Take Control A situation often feels more stressful if you feel you're not in control of it. Time may seem to be slipping away before a big exam, for example. Unexpected obstacles may appear in your path, throwing you off course. When you feel your environment is controlling you instead of the other way around, take charge! Concentrate on what is possible to control, and set realistic goals. Be confident of your ability to succeed.

Problem-Solve When you find yourself stewing over a problem, take a moment to sit down with a piece of paper and go through a formal process of problem solving. Within a few minutes you can generate a plan. Try this approach:

1. Define the problem in one or two sentences.
2. Identify the causes of the problem.
3. Consider alternative solutions; don't just stop with the most obvious one.
4. Make a decision—choose a solution.
5. Make a list of what you will need to do to carry out your decision.
6. Begin to act on your list; if you're unable to do that, temporarily turn to other things.

Modify Your Expectations Expectations are exhausting and restricting. The fewer expectations you have, the more you can live spontaneously and joyfully. The more you expect from others, the more often you will feel let down. And trying to meet the expectations others have of you is often futile.

Monitor Self-Talk If you catch your mind beating up on you—"Late for class again! You can't even cope with college! How do you expect to ever hold down a professional job?"—change your inner dialogue. Talk to yourself as you would to a child you love: "You're a smart, capable person. You've solved other problems; you'll handle this one. Tomorrow you'll simply schedule things so you get to class with a few minutes to spare." (Chapter 3 has more information on self-talk.)

Cultivate Your Sense of Humor When it comes to stress, laughter may be the best medicine. Even a fleeting smile produces changes in your autonomic nervous system that can lift your spirits. And a few minutes of belly laughing can be as invigorating as brisk exercise. Hearty laughter elevates your heart rate, aids digestion, eases pain, and triggers the release of endorphins and other pleasurable and stimulating chemicals in the brain. After a good laugh, your muscles go slack; your pulse and blood pressure dip below normal. You are relaxed. Cultivate the ability to laugh at yourself, and you'll have a handy and instantly effective stress reliever. Try some of the following strategies:

- Keep a humor journal. Write down funny things that you and others say, including unintentional slips of the tongue. Collect funny and clever sayings that make you smile.

- Look at newspaper and magazine cartoons. Cut out those you find particularly funny and add them to your humor journal.

- Collect some funny props—clown noses, "arrow" headbands, Groucho glasses—that you can put on the next time you feel stressed or anxious. Or simply try making funny faces in front of a mirror.

- Watch funny films and television programs. In a study of college students, those who watched an episode of *Seinfeld* prior to giving an impromptu speech were less anxious and had a lower heart rate than those who didn't watch the program.

Weed Out Trivia   You can burden your memory with too much information. A major source of stress is trying to "store" too much data. Forget unimportant details (they will usually be self-evident). Keep your memory free for essential ones.

Live in the Present   Do you clog your mind by reliving past events? Clinging to experiences and emotions, particularly unpleasant ones, can be a deadly business. Clear your mind of the old debris; let it go. Free yourself to enjoy life today.

Go with the Flow   Remember that the branch that bends in the storm doesn't break. Try to flow with your life, accepting the things you can't change. Be forgiving of faults, your own and those of others. Instead of anticipating happiness at some indefinite point in the future, realize that pleasure is integral to being alive. You can create it every day of your life. View challenges as an opportunity to learn and grow. Be flexible. In this way, you can make stress work for you rather than against you, enhancing your overall wellness.

Relaxation Techniques

First identified and described by Herbert Benson of the Harvard Medical School, the **relaxation response** is a physiological state characterized by a feeling of warmth and quiet mental alertness. This is the opposite of the fight-or-flight reaction. When the relaxation response is triggered by a relaxation technique, heart rate, breathing, and metabolism slow down. Blood pressure and oxygen consumption decrease. At the same time, blood flow to the brain and skin increases, and brain waves shift from an alert beta rhythm to a relaxed alpha rhythm. Practiced regularly, relaxation techniques can counteract the debilitating effects of stress. When an Oregon nursing professor taught relaxation techniques to 38 nursing students in one recent study, she found they scored 7 points lower on scales of anxiety and depression after only 3 weeks. A matched group of students who received no training gained 2 points over the same time period.

If you decide to try a relaxation technique, practice it daily until it becomes natural to you, and then use it whenever you feel the need. You may feel calmer and more refreshed after each session. If one technique doesn't seem to work well enough for you after you've given it a good try, try another one. You'll know you've mastered a deep relaxation technique when you start to see subtle changes in other areas of your life: You may notice you've been encountering fewer hassles, working more efficiently, or enjoying more free time. None of the techniques takes long to do—for instance, just a few minutes away from the TV should do the trick.

Progressive Relaxation   Unlike most of the others, this simple method requires no imagination, willpower, or self-suggestion. You simply tense, and then relax, the muscles in your body, group by group. The technique, also known as deep muscle relaxation, helps you become aware of the muscle tension that occurs when you're under stress. When you consciously relax those muscles, other systems of the body get the message and ease up on the stress response.

Start, for example, with your right fist. Inhale as you tense it. Exhale as you relax it. Repeat. Next, contract and relax your right upper arm. Repeat. Do the same with your left arm. Then, beginning at your forehead and ending at your feet, contract and relax your other muscle groups. Repeat each contraction at least once, breathing in as you tense, breathing out as you relax. To speed up the process, tense and relax more muscles at one time—both arms simultaneously, for instance. With practice, you'll be able to relax very quickly and effectively by clenching and releasing only your fists.

Visualization   Also known as using imagery, **visualization** lets you daydream without guilt. Athletes find that the technique enhances sports performance, and visualization is even part of the curriculum at U.S. Olympic training camps. You can use visualization to help you relax, change your habits, or perform well—whether on an exam, a stage, or a playing field.

Next time you feel stressed, close your eyes. Imagine yourself floating on a cloud, sitting on a mountaintop, or lying in a meadow. What do you see and hear? Is it cold out? Or damp? What do you smell? What do you taste? Involve all your senses. Your body will respond as if your imagery were real. An alternative: Close your eyes and imagine a deep purple light filling your body. Now change the color into a soothing gold. As the color lightens, so should your distress.

Visualization can also be used to rehearse for an upcoming event and enhance performance. By preexperiencing an event in your mind, you can practice coping with any difficulties that may arise. Think positively, and you can "psych yourself up" for a successful experience.

Meditation   **Meditation** is a way of telling the mind to be quiet for a while. The need to periodically stop our incessant mental chatter is so great that, from ancient times, hundreds of forms of meditation have developed in cultures all over the world. Because meditation has been

relaxation response   A physiological state characterized by a feeling of warmth and quiet mental alertness. **TERMS**

visualization   A technique for promoting relaxation or improving performance that involves creating or recreating vivid mental pictures of a place or an experience; also called *imagery*.

meditation   A technique for quieting the mind by focusing on a particular word, object (such as a candle flame), or process (such as breathing).

Dr. Herbert Benson developed a simple, practical technique for eliciting the relaxation response.

The Basic Technique

1. Pick a word, phrase, or object to focus on. If you like, you can choose a word or phrase that has a deep meaning for you, but any word or phrase will work. Some meditators prefer to focus on their breathing.

2. Take a comfortable position in a quiet environment, and close your eyes if you're not focusing on an object.

3. Relax your muscles.

4. Breathe slowly and naturally. If you're using a focus word or phrase, silently repeat it each time you exhale. If you're using an object, focus on it as you breathe.

5. Keep your attitude passive. Disregard thoughts that drift in.

6. Continue for 10–20 minutes, once or twice a day.

7. After you've finished, sit quietly for a few minutes with your eyes first closed and then open. Then stand up.

Suggestions

- Allow relaxation to occur at its own pace; don't try to force it. Don't be surprised if you can't tune your mind out for more than a few seconds at a time; it's not a reason for anger or frustration. The more you ignore the intrusions, the easier doing so will get.

- If you want to time your session, peek at a watch or clock occasionally, but don't set a jarring alarm.

- The technique works best on an empty stomach, before a meal or about 2 hours after eating. Avoid times of day when you're tired—unless you want to fall asleep.

- Although you'll feel refreshed even after the first session, it may take a month or more to get noticeable results. Be patient. Eventually the relaxation response will become so natural that it will occur spontaneously, or on demand, when you sit quietly for a few moments.

---

at the core of many Eastern religions and philosophies, it has acquired an "Eastern" mystique that has caused some people to shy away from it. Yet meditation requires no special knowledge or background. We all know how to meditate; we need only discover that we do, and then put our knowledge to use. Whatever philosophical, religious, or emotional reasons may be given for meditation, its power derives from its ability to elicit the relaxation response.

Meditation helps you tune out the world temporarily, relieving you from both internal and external sources of stress. It allows you to transcend past conditioning, fixed expectations, and the trivial pursuits of the psyche; it clears out the mental smog. The "thinker" takes time out to become the "observer"—calmly attentive, without analyzing, judging, comparing, or rationalizing. Regular practice of this quiet awareness will subtly carry over into your daily life, encouraging physical and emotional balance no matter what confronts you. For a step-by-step description of a basic meditation technique, see the box "Meditation and the Relaxation Response."

Deep Breathing Your breathing pattern is closely tied to your stress level. Deep, slow breathing is associated with relaxation. Rapid, shallow, often irregular breathing occurs during the stress response. With practice, you can learn to slow and quiet your breathing pattern, thereby also quieting your mind and relaxing your body. Breathing techniques can be used for on-the-spot tension relief, as well as for long-term stress reduction.

The primary goal of many breathing exercises is to change your breathing pattern from chest breathing to diaphragmatic ("belly") breathing. During the day, most adults breathe by expanding their chest and raising their shoulders rather than by expanding their abdomen. This pattern of chest breathing is associated with stress, a sedentary lifestyle, restrictive clothing, and cultural preferences for a large chest and a small waist. Diaphragmatic breathing, which involves free expansion of the diaphragm and lower abdomen, is the pattern of breathing characteristic of children and sleeping adults. (The diaphragm is a sheet of muscle and connective tissue that divides the chest and abdominal cavities.) Diaphragmatic breathing is slower and deeper than chest breathing. For instructions on how to perform diaphragmatic breathing, refer to the box "Breathing for Relaxation."

Hatha Yoga Yoga is an ancient Sanskrit word referring to the union of mind, body, and soul. The development and practice of yoga are rooted in the Hindu philosophy of spiritual enlightenment. The founders of yoga developed a system of physical postures, called *asanas,* designed to cleanse the body of toxins, calm and clear the mind, bring energy into the body, and raise the level of consciousness.

Hatha yoga, the most common yoga style practiced in the United States, emphasizes physical balance and breathing control. It integrates components of flexibility, muscular strength and endurance, and muscle relaxation; it also sometimes serves as a preliminary to meditation.

A session of hatha yoga typically involves a series of *asanas,* held for a few seconds to several minutes, that stretch and relax different parts of the body. The empha-

Diaphragmatic Breathing

1. Lie on your back with your body relaxed.

2. Place one hand on your chest and one on your abdomen. (You will use your hands to monitor the depth and location of your breathing.)

3. Inhale slowly and deeply through your nose into your abdomen. Your abdomen should push up as far as is comfortable. Your chest should expand only a little and only in conjunction with the movement of your abdomen.

4. Exhale gently through your mouth.

5. Continue diaphragmatic breathing for about 5–10 minutes per session. Focus on the sound and feel of your breathing.

Breathing In Relaxation, Breathing Out Tension

1. Assume a comfortable position, lying on your back or sitting in a chair.

2. Inhale slowly and deeply into your abdomen. Imagine the inhaled, warm air flowing to all parts of your body. Say to yourself, "Breathe in relaxation."

3. Exhale from your abdomen. Image tension flowing out of your body. Say to yourself, "Breathe out tension."

4. Pause before you inhale.

5. Continue for 5–10 minutes or until no tension remains in your body.

Chest Expansion

1. Sit in a comfortable chair, or stand.

2. Inhale slowly and deeply into your abdomen as you raise your arms out to the sides. Pull your shoulders and arms back and lift your chin slightly so that your chest opens up.

3. Exhale gradually as you lower your arms and chin, and return to the starting position.

4. Repeat 5–10 times or until your breathing is deep and regular and your body feels relaxed and energized.

Quick Tension Release

1. Inhale into your abdomen slowly and deeply as you count slowly to four.

2. Exhale slowly as you again count slowly to four. As you exhale, concentrate on relaxing your face, neck, shoulders, and chest.

3. Repeat several times. With each exhalation, feel more tension leaving your body.

SOURCES: Stop stress with a deep breath. 1996. *Health,* October, 53. Breathing for health and relaxation. 1995. *Mental Medicine Update* 4(2): 3–6. When you're stressed, catch your breath. 1995. *Mayo Clinic Health Letter,* December, 5.

---

sis is on breathing, stretching, and balance. There are hundreds of different *asanas,* and they must be performed correctly in order to be beneficial. For this reason, qualified instruction is recommended, particularly for beginners. Yoga classes are offered through many community recreation centers, YMCAs and YWCAs, and private clubs. Regardless of whether you accept the philosophy and symbolism of different *asanas,* the practice of yoga can induce the relaxation response as well as develop body awareness, flexibility, and muscular strength and endurance.

T'ai Chi Ch'uan A martial art that developed in China, t'ai chi ch'uan is a system of self-defense that incorporates philosophical concepts from Taoism and Confucianism. An important part of this philosophy is *chi,* an energy force that surrounds and permeates all things. In addition to serving as a means of self-defense, the goal of t'ai chi ch'uan is to bring the body into balance and harmony with this universal energy, in order to promote health and spiritual growth. It teaches practitioners to remain calm and centered, to conserve and concentrate energy, and to

harmonize with fear. T'ai chi ch'uan seeks to manipulate force by becoming part of it—"going with the flow," so to speak.

T'ai chi ch'uan is considered the gentlest of the martial arts. Instead of using quick and powerful movements, t'ai chi ch'uan consists of a series of slow, fluid, elegant movements, which reinforce the idea of moving *with* rather than *against* the stressors of everyday life. The practice of t'ai chi ch'uan promotes relaxation and concentration as well as the development of body awareness, balance, muscular strength, and flexibility. (An Emory University study found that a group of older adults who completed a t'ai chi ch'uan course reduced their risk of falling by nearly 50% compared with a control group.) It usually takes some time and practice to reap the stress-management benefits of t'ai chi ch'uan, and, as with yoga, it's best to begin with some qualified instruction.

Listening to Music Listening to music is another method of inducing relaxation. It has been shown to influence pulse, blood pressure, and the electrical activity of muscles. Studies of newborns and hospitalized stroke patients have shown that listening to soothing, lyrical music can lessen depression, anxiety, and stress levels. Exposure to rhythmic music has been shown to help people with Parkinson's disease and other physical disabilities walk more steadily. Music therapy, which can involve both listening to music and creating music, has also been shown to be helpful in pain management, including lessening the need for anesthesia during labor.

Although the effects of music are just beginning to be investigated, researchers have found that exposure to soothing music leads to reduced levels of the stress hormone cortisol and causes changes in the electrical activity in the brain. These changes in brain activity may explain the so-called Mozart effect, in which people exposed to music for 10 minutes experienced temporary enhancement of spatial skills (researchers in these studies used the music of Mozart).

To experience the stress-management benefits of music yourself, set aside a time to listen. Choose music that you enjoy and that makes you feel relaxed. If you are interested in learning more about formal music therapy, contact the American Music Therapy Association (see the For More Information section at the end of the chapter).

Biofeedback   **Biofeedback** helps people reduce the stress response by enabling them to become more aware of their level of physiological arousal. It involves mechanical monitoring of some measure of the physiological stress response such as perspiration, heart rate, skin temperature, or muscle tension. A person receives feedback about his or her condition through the use of sound (a tone or music), light, or a meter or dial. For example, as heart rate increases, the tone becomes louder; as it decreases, the tone softens. Through trial and error, people can learn to reduce their physiological stress response through conscious control.

The point of biofeedback training is to teach how relaxation feels, how to induce relaxation, and how to transfer this skill to daily life (without the use of electronic equipment). In addition to monitoring equipment, biofeedback usually also requires the initial help of a therapist, stress counselor, or technician.

Other relaxation techniques include massage, hypnosis and self-hypnosis, and autogenic training. To learn more about these and other techniques for inducing the relaxation response, refer to For More Information at the end of the chapter.

TERMS	**biofeedback** A technique in which monitoring devices are used to help a person become conscious of unconscious body processes, such as body temperature or blood pressure, in order to exert some control over them.

CREATING A PERSONAL PLAN FOR MANAGING STRESS

What are the most important sources of stress in your life? Are you coping successfully with these stressors? No single strategy or program for managing stress will work for everyone, but you can use the principles of behavior management described in Chapter 1 to tailor a plan specifically to your needs. The most important starting point for a successful stress-management plan is to learn to listen to your body. When you learn to recognize the stress response and the emotions and thoughts that accompany it, you'll be in a position to take charge of that crucial moment and handle it in a healthy way.

Identifying Stressors

Before you can learn to manage the stressors in your life, you have to identify them. A strategy many experts recommend is keeping a stress journal for a week or two. Keep a log of your daily activities, and assign a rating to your stress level for every hour. Each time you feel or express a stress response, record the time and the circumstances in your journal. Note what you were doing at the time, what you were thinking or feeling, and the outcome of your response.

After keeping your journal for a few weeks, you should be able to identify your key stressors and spot patterns in how you respond to them. Take note of the people, places, events, and patterns of thought and behavior that cause you the most stress. You may notice, for example, that mornings are usually the most stressful part of your day. Or you may discover that when you're angry at your roommate, you're apt to respond with behaviors that only make matters worse. Once you've outlined the general pattern of stress in your life, you may want to focus on a particularly problematic stressor or on an inappropriate behavioral response you've identified. Keep a stress log for another week or two that focuses just on the early morning hours, for example, or just on your arguments with your roommate. The more information you gather, the easier it will be to develop effective strategies for coping with the stressors in your life.

Designing Your Plan

Earlier in this chapter, you learned about many different techniques for combating stress. Now that you've identified the key stressors in your life, it's time to choose the techniques that will work best for you and create an action plan for change. Finding a buddy to work with you can make the process more fun and increase your chances of success. Some experts recommend drawing up a formal contract with yourself.

Whether or not you complete a contract, it's important

to design rewards into your plan. You might treat yourself to a special breakfast in a favorite restaurant on the weekend (as long as you eat a nutritious breakfast every weekday morning). If you practice your relaxation techique faithfully, you might reward yourself with a long bath or an hour of pleasure reading at the end of the day. It's also important to evaluate your plan regularly and redesign it as your needs change. Under times of increased stress, for example, you might want to focus on good eating, exercise, and relaxation habits. Over time, your new stress-management skills will become almost automatic. You'll feel better, accomplish more, and reduce your risk of disease.

Getting Help

If the techniques discussed so far don't provide you with enough relief from the stress in your life, you might want to read more about specific areas you wish to work on, consult a peer counselor, join a support group, or participate in a few psychotherapy sessions. Excellent self-help guides can be found in bookstores or the library.

Your student health center or student affairs office can tell you whether your campus has a peer counseling program. Such programs are usually staffed by volunteer students with special training that emphasizes maintaining confidentiality. Peer counselors can guide you to other campus or community resources, or can simply provide understanding.

Support groups are typically organized around a particular issue or problem. In your area, you might find a support group for first-year students; for reentering students; for single parents; for students of your ethnicity, religion, or national origin; for people with eating disorders; or for rape survivors. The number of such groups has increased in recent years, as more and more people discover how therapeutic it can be to talk with others who share the same situation.

Short-term psychotherapy can also be tremendously helpful in dealing with stress-related problems. Your student health center may offer psychotherapy on a sliding-fee scale; the county mental health center in your area may do the same. If you belong to any type of religious organization, check to see whether pastoral counseling is available. Your physician can refer you to psychotherapists in your community. Not all therapists are right for all people, so be prepared to have initial sessions with several. Choose the one you feel most comfortable with.

SUMMARY

What Is Stress?

- When confronted with a stressor, the body undergoes a group of physical changes known as the fight-or-flight reaction. The sympathetic nervous system and endocrine system act on many targets in the body to prepare it for action.

- Many physical changes accompany the fight-or-flight reaction: hearing and vision become more acute, heart rate and blood pressure increase, digestion halts, perspiration increases, the liver releases extra sugar into the bloodstream, and endorphins are released.

- The body responds to a stressor with the fight-or-flight reaction even if the situation does not require physical action.

- Emotional and behavioral responses to stressors vary among individuals. Ineffective responses increase stress but can be moderated or changed.

- Factors that influence emotional and behavioral responses to stressors include personality, cultural background, gender, and past experiences.

- Some personality characteristics, including impatience, hostility, and anger, make stress more difficult to handle. Other characteristics, such as optimism, commitment, and an inner locus of control, make an individual more stress-resistant.

- Physical, emotional, and behavioral responses to stressors are closely interrelated.

Stress and Disease

- The general adaptation syndrome (GAS), an early model developed by Hans Selye to describe the relationship between stress and disease, has three stages: alarm, resistance, and exhaustion.

- A high allostatic load characterized by prolonged or repeated exposure to stress hormones can increase a person's risk of health problems.

- Psychoneuroimmunology (PNI) looks at how the physiological changes of the stress response affect the immune system and thereby increase the risk of illness.

- Health problems linked to stress include cardiovascular disease, colds and other infections, asthma and allergies, cancer, flare-ups of chronic diseases, psychological problems, digestive problems, headaches, insomnia, and injuries.

Common Sources of Stress

- A cluster of major life events that require adjustment and accommodation can lead to increased stress and an increased risk of health problems.

- Minor daily hassles increase stress if they are perceived negatively.

- Sources of stress associated with college may be academic, financial, interpersonal, or related to time pressures.

Are you a person who doesn't perform as well as you should on tests? Do you find that anxiety interferes with your ability to study effectively before the test and to think clearly in the test situation? If so, you may be experiencing test anxiety. People suffering from test anxiety often see tests as threatening, feel inadequate to cope with them, concentrate on the negative consequences of doing poorly, and anticipate failure, which becomes a self-fulfilling prophecy. They often feel so helpless that they can't mobilize their resources to deal with the problem.

Behavioral approaches to problems like test anxiety and fear of public speaking operate on the assumption that fear and anxiety are learned behaviors, and that a person can unlearn them by following appropriate procedures. Test anxiety is an ineffective response to a stressful situation, and it can be replaced with more effective responses. Two methods that have proven effective in helping people deal with test anxiety are systematic desensitization and success rehearsal. Both can help people interrupt the cycle of fear that prevents them from doing their best in stressful performance situations. If test anxiety is a problem for you, try one of these methods before taking your next exam.

Systematic Desensitization

Systematic desensitization is based on the premise that you can't feel anxiety and be relaxed at the same time. The method described here has three phases: constructing an anxiety hierarchy, learning and practicing muscle relaxation, and implementing the desensitization program.

Constructing an Anxiety Hierarchy   Begin the first phase by thinking of 10 or more situations related to your fear, such as hearing the announcement of the test date in class, studying for the test, sitting in the classroom waiting for the test to begin, reading the test questions, and so on. Write each situation on an index card, using a brief phrase to describe it on one side of the card. On the other side, list several realistic details or prompts that will help you vividly imagine yourself actually experiencing the situation. For example, if the situation is "hearing that 50%

of the final grade will be based on the two exams," the prompts might include such details as "sitting in the big lecture auditorium in Baily Hall," "taking notes in my blue notebook," "surrounded by other students," and "listening to Professor Smith's voice."

Next, arrange your cards in order, from least-tense to most-tense situation. Rate each situation to reflect the amount of anxiety you feel when you encounter it in real life, to confirm your anxiety hierarchy. Assign ratings on a scale of 0–100, and make sure the distances between items are fairly small and about equal. When you're sure your anxiety hierarchy is a true reflection of your feelings, number the cards.

Learning and Practicing Muscle Relaxation   The second phase of the program involves learning to relax your muscles and to recognize when they are relaxed. A very effective way to do this is through progressive relaxation, which is described in this chapter. Find a quiet, dimly lit setting where you won't be interrupted for 20–30 minutes, and sit or lie on a comfortable couch or bed. It would be ideal to have instructions recorded on tape and to listen to the tape the first several times you practice the relaxation procedure. As you become proficient at relaxing, you'll be able to relax without the tape and ultimately to skip steps and go directly to a deeply relaxed state within a few minutes. When you can do this, you're ready to go on to the next phase of the program.

Implementing the Desensitization Program   Use the quiet place where you practiced your relaxation exercises. Sit comfortably and place your stack of numbered cards within reach. Take several minutes to relax completely, and then look at the first card, reading both the brief phrase and the descriptive prompts. Close your eyes and imagine yourself in that situation for about 10 seconds. Then put the card down and relax completely for about 30 seconds. Look at the card again, imagine the situation for 10 seconds, and relax again for 30 seconds.

At this point, evaluate your current level of anxiety about the situation on the card in terms of the rating scale you devised

- Job-related stress is common, particularly for employees who have little control over decisions relating to their jobs. If stress is severe or prolonged, burnout may occur.

- New and changing relationships, prejudice, and discrimination are examples of interpersonal and social stressors.

- Other sources of stress include environmental stressors such as natural disasters and noise, and internal stressors such as illness, exhaustion, and unrealistically high expectations.

Techniques for Managing Stress

- Social support systems help buffer people against the effects of stress and make illness less likely. Good communication skills foster healthy relationships with others.

- Exercise, nutrition, and sleep are wellness behaviors that reduce stress and increase energy.

- Time management is an effective coping technique for those who tend to procrastinate, take on too many tasks, or organize their time poorly.

earlier. If your anxiety level is 10 or below, relax for two minutes and go on to the second card. If it's higher than 10, repeat the routine with the same card until the anxiety decreases. If you have difficulty with a particular item, go back to the previous item; then try it again. If you still can't visualize it without anxiety, try to construct three new items with smaller steps between them and insert them before the troublesome item.

You should be able to move through about 1–4 items per session. Sessions can be conducted anywhere from twice a day to twice a week and should last no longer than 20 minutes. Keep track of your progress by recording the names and numbers of the items you imagined successfully during each session, the number of times you imagined each one, and the anxiety rating of each item when you first prepared the hierarchy and after you desensitized yourself to it. It's helpful to graph your progress in a way that has meaning for you.

After you have successfully completed your program, you should be desensitized to the real-life situations that previously caused anxiety. If you find that you do experience some anxiety in the real situations, take 30 seconds or a minute to relax completely, just as you did when you were practicing. Remember: Fear and relaxation are incompatible; you can't experience them both at the same time. You have the ability to choose relaxation over fear.

Success Rehearsal

A variation on systematic desensitization is an approach called success rehearsal. To practice this method, take your hierarchy of anxiety-producing situations and vividly imagine yourself successfully dealing with each one. Create a detailed scenario for each situation, and use your imagination to experience genuine feelings of confidence. Recognize your negative thoughts ("I'll be so nervous I won't be able to think straight") and replace them with positive ones ("Anxiety will keep me alert so I can do a good job"). Proceed one step at a time, thinking of strategies for success as you go that you can later implement. These might include the following:

- Before the test, find out everything you can about it—its

format, the material to be covered, the grading criteria. Ask the instructor for practice materials.

- Devise a study plan. This might include forming a study group with one or more classmates, or outlining what you will study, when, where, and for how long.

- Once in the test situation, sit away from possible distractions, listen carefully to instructions, and ask for clarification if you don't understand a direction.

- During the test, answer the easiest questions first. If you don't know an answer and there is no penalty for incorrect answers, guess. If there are several questions you have difficulty answering, review the ones you have already handled. Figure out approximately how much time you have to cover each question.

- For math problems, try to estimate the answer before doing the precise calculations.

- For true-false questions, look for qualifiers such as *always* and *never*. Such questions are likely to be false.

- For essay questions, look for key words in the question that indicate what the instructor is looking for in the answer. Develop a brief outline of your answer, sketching out what you will cover. Stick to your outline, and keep track of the time you're spending on your answer. Don't let yourself get caught with unanswered questions when time is up.

- Remain calm and focused throughout the test. Don't let negative thoughts rattle you. If you start to become nervous, take some deep breaths and relax your muscles completely for a minute or so.

The best way to counter test anxiety is with successful test-taking experiences. The more times you succeed, the more your test anxiety will recede. If you find that these methods aren't sufficient to get your anxiety under control, you may want to seek professional help. But whether you use desensitization, success rehearsal, or another approach, it's wise to take action as early as possible to keep test anxiety from significantly interfering with your education plans and career goals.

- Cognitive techniques for managing stress involve developing new and healthy patterns of thinking, such as worrying constructively, practicing problem solving, monitoring self-talk, cultivating a sense of humor, and going with the flow.

- The relaxation response is the opposite of the fight-or-flight reaction. Techniques that trigger it, including progressive relaxation, imagery, meditation, deep breathing, hatha yoga, t'ai chi ch'uan, listening to music, and biofeedback, counteract the physiological effects of chronic stress.

Creating a Personal Plan for Managing Stress

- A successful individualized plan for coping with stress begins with the use of a stress journal or log to identify and study stressors and inappropriate behavioral responses. Completing a contract and recruiting a buddy can help your stress-management plan succeed.

- Additional help in dealing with stress is available from self-help books, peer counseling, support groups, and psychotherapy.

1. Choose a friend or family member who seems to deal particularly well with stress. Interview that person about his or her methods of managing stress. What strategies does he or she use? What can you learn from that person that can be applied to your own life?

2. Investigate the services available in your community to help people deal with stress, such as peer counseling, support groups, and time-management classes. If possible, visit or gather information on one or more of them. Write a description and evaluation of their services, including your personal reactions.

3. Reread the stress-management techniques described in this chapter, and choose one to try for a week. If possible, select a behavior or strategy, such as regular exercise or systematic time management, that you've never tried before. After a trial period, evaluate the effectiveness of the strategy you chose. Did your stress level decrease during the week? Were you better able to deal with daily hassles and any more severe stressors that you encountered?

1. Watch for the physical changes of the stress response when you're in stressful situations. In your health journal, keep a stress log in which you note how many times in a day you experience the stress response to some degree. Also include a brief description of the circumstances surrounding your stress response. Is your life more or less stressful than you expected?

2. *Critical Thinking* Some techniques for stress management, including meditation and hypnosis, are considered strange or unscientific by some people. Find out more about one such technique through library or Internet research. What evidence can you find to support or oppose the idea that the technique can help people manage stress? Based on your research, write a brief essay in your health journal stating your opinion. As you consider the evidence, be sure to look closely at your sources of information.

3. Think about all the different environments in which you function, including your classrooms, the student union, the dorm, your house. Are some more stressful than others? Make a list of the environments in order from the most stressful to the least stressful. Indicate next to each environment the reasons you think it is stressful or nonstressful. Then start at the top of your list and record three or more ways to reduce the stressful impact these environments have on you.

4. Make a list of the daily hassles you commonly encounter, such as being awakened early by loud neighbors, standing in a long line for lunch, or repeatedly misplacing your keys. Divide your list into two groups: avoidable and unavoidable. For each stressor that is potentially avoidable, describe a strategy for eliminating it from your life. For stressors that are unavoidable, make a list of effective coping mechanisms.

Books and Articles

Davis, M., et al. 1998. *Relaxation and Stress Reduction Workbook*. 4th ed. Ravensdale, Wa.: Idyll Arbor. *Provides step-by-step instructions for many stress-reduction techniques.*

Dement, W. C. 1999. *The Promise of Sleep*. New York: Delacorte. *An exploration of sleep and its effects on wellness by a prominent sleep researcher.* (http://www.stanford.edu/~dement).

Greenberg, J. S. 1999. *Comprehensive Stress Management*. 6th ed. Dubuque, Ia.: Brown and Benchmark. *An easy-to-understand guide to identifying and combatting stressors; includes a separate chapter on college stress.*

Sapolsky, R. M. 1998. *Why Zebras Don't Get Ulcers: An Updated Guide to Stress-Related Diseases and Coping*. New York: W. H. Freeman. *An entertaining look at the effects of stress on the body and the realtionship between stress and disease.*

Seaward, B. L. 1999. *Managing Stress: Principles and Strategies for Health and Wellbeing*. 2nd ed. Boston: Jones and Bartlett. *A comprehensive resource of stress-management strategies.*

Organizations and Web Sites

American Music Therapy Association. Provides information about music therapy and about how to find a certified therapist.
8455 Colesville Rd., Suite 1000
Silver Spring, MD 20910
301-589-3300
http://www.musictherapy.org

American Psychological Association. Provides information on stress management and psychological disorders.
750 First St., N.E.
Washington, DC 20002
202-336-5500; 800-964-2000 (referrals)
http://www.apa.org; http://helping.apa.org

Association for Applied Psychophysiology and Biofeedback. Provides information about biofeedback and referrals to certified biofeedback practitioners.
800-477-8892
http://www.aapb.org

Center for Anxiety and Stress Treatment. A commercial site that also includes an anxiety symptom checklist and a list of stress-busting tips for work stress.

    http://www.stressrelease.com

Duquesne University Stress Links. Provides links to sites with stress-management strategies, many designed especially for college students.

    http://the-duke.duq-duke.duq.edu/special/stress.htm

The Humor Project. A clearinghouse for information and practical ideas related to humor.

    480 Broadway, Suite 210
    Saratoga Springs, NY 12866
    518-587-8770
    http://www.humorproject.com

National Institute of Mental Health (NIMH). Publishes informative brochures about stress and stress management as well as other aspects of mental health.

    6001 Executive Blvd.
    Bethesda, MD 20892
    800-421-4211; 301-443-4513
    http://www.nimh.nih.gov

National Institute for Occupational Safety and Health (NIOSH). Provides information and links on job stress.

    http://www.cdc.gov/niosh/stresshp.html

National Sleep Foundation. Provides information about sleep and how to overcome sleep problems such as insomnia and jet lag; brochures are available from the Web site or via fax.

    729 15th St., N.W., Fourth Floor
    Washington, DC 20005
    888-NSF-SLEEP; 888-FYI-SLEEP (fax service)
    http://www.sleepfoundation.org

Student Counseling Virtual Pamphlet Collection. Links to online pamphlets from student counseling centers at colleges and universities across the country; topics include stress, sleep, and time management.

    http://uhs.uchicago.edu/scrs/vpc/virtulets.html

The following organizations are good resources for audio tapes and books relating to relaxation techniques:

Academy for Guided Imagery
    800-726-2070
    http://www.healthy.net/agi

Mind Body Medical Institute
    617-632-9530

ISHK Book Service
    800-222-4745

New Harbinger Publications
    800-748-6273
    http://www.newharbinger.com

See also the listings for Chapters 1 and 3.

SELECTED BIBLIOGRAPHY

Anshel, M. 1996. Effect of chronic aerobic exercise and progressive relaxation on motor performance and affect following acute stress. *Behavioral Medicine* 21: 186–196.

Cohen, S., et al. 1997. Social ties and susceptibility to the common cold. *Journal of the American Medical Association* 277: 1940–1944.

Dhabhar, F. S., and B. S. McEwen. 1999. Enhancing versus suppressive effects of stress hormones on skin immune function. *Proceedings of the National Academy of Sciences* 96(3): 1059–1064.

Dill, P. L., and T. B. Henley. 1998. Stressors of college: A comparison of traditional and nontraditional students. *Journal of Psychology* 132(1): 25–32.

Fenster, L., et. al. 1999. Psychological stress in the workplace and menstrual function. *American Journal of Epidemiology* 149(2): 127–134.

Glaser, R., et al. 1998. The influence of psychological stress on the immune response to vaccines. *Annals of the New York Academy of Sciences* 840: 656–663.

Horsten, M., et al. 1999. Psychosocial factors and heart rate variability in healthy women. *Psychosomatic Medicine* 61: 49–57.

Infante, J. R., et al. 1998. ACTH and beta-endorphin in transcendental meditation. *Physiology and Behavior* 64(3): 311–315.

Kamarck, T. W., et al. 1998. Effects of task strain, social conflict, and emotional activation on ambulatory cardiovascular activity: Daily life consequences of recurring stress in a multiethnic adult sample. *Health Psychology* 17(1): 17–29.

Maes, M., et. al. 1999. The effects of psychological stress on leukocyte subset distribution in humans: Evidence of immune activation. *Neuropsychobiology* 39(1): 1–9.

Majumdar, B., and S. Ladak. 1998. Management of family and workplace stress experienced by women of colour from various cultural backgrounds. *Canadian Journal of Public Health* 89(1): 48–52.

McEwan, B. S. 1998. Protective and damaging effects of stress mediators. *New England Journal of Medicine* 338(3): 171–179.

McKinney, C. H., et al. 1997. Effects of guided imagery and music (GIM) therapy on mood and cortisol in healthy adults. *Health Psychology* 16(4): 390–400.

National Institute of Occupational Safety and Health (NIOSH). 1999. *Stress . . . at Work.* DHHS (NIOSH) Pub No. 99–101.

National Institutes of Health Technology Assessment Conference Statement. 1995. *Integration of Behavioral and Relaxation Approaches into the Treatment of Chronic Pain and Insomnia* (retrieved October 8, 1998; http://text.nlm.nih.gov/nih/ta/www/017txt.html).

Pashkow, F. J. 1999. Is stress linked to heart disease? The evidence grows stronger. *Cleveland Clinic Journal of Medicine* 66(2): 75–77.

Prasher, D. 1998. Traffic noise increases stress by driving up cortisol. *The Lancet News* 352(9135): 1199.

Rideout, B. E., and J. Taylor. 1997. Enhanced spatial performance following 10 minutes exposure to music: A replication. *Perceptual and Motor Skills* 85(1): 112–114.

Seaward, B. L. 1999. *Managing Stress: Principles and Strategies for Health and Wellbeing,* 2nd ed. Boston: Jones and Bartlett.

Seeman, T. E., et al. 1997. Price of adaptation—allostatic load and its health consequences. *Archives of Internal Medicine* 157(19): 2259–2289.

Young, D. R., et al. 1999. The effects of aerobic exercise and t'ai chi on blood pressure in older people. *Journal of the American Geriatrics Society* 47(3): 277–84.

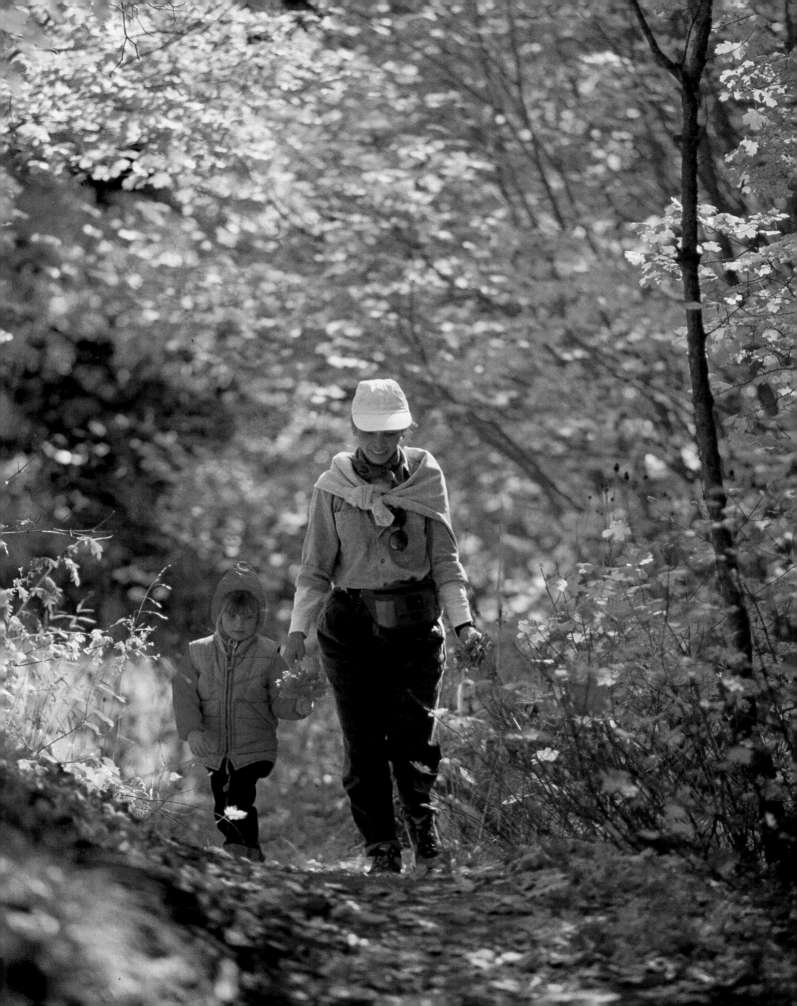

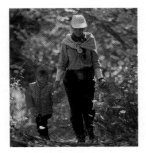

LEARNING OBJECTIVES

After reading this chapter, you should be able to:

- Describe what it means to be psychologically healthy.

- Explain how to develop and maintain a positive self-concept and healthy self-esteem.

- Discuss the importance to psychological health of an optimistic outlook, good communication skills, and constructive approaches to dealing with anger.

- Describe common psychological disorders, and list the warning signs of suicide.

- Explain the different approaches and types of help available for psychological problems.

Psychological Health   3

TEST YOUR KNOWLEDGE

1. Normality is a key component of psychological health.
    True or false?

2. The use of defense mechanisms such as repression and denial is a symptom of mental illness.
    True or false?

3. On television, about 75% of mentally ill characters are depicted as violent. About what percentage of mentally ill people are actually violent?
    a. 7%
    b. 14%
    c. 21%
    d. 28%

4. People who really intend to commit suicide don't talk about it.
    True or false?

5. Which of the following groups has the highest rate of suicide?
    a. youth age 15–19
    b. white males over age 65
    c. African American males

Answers

1. *False.* Normality simply means being close to average, and having unusual ideas or attitudes doesn't mean that a person is mentally ill. The fact that people's ideas are varied makes life interesting and helps people respond in creative ways to life's challenges.

2. *False.* Everyone uses defense mechanisms from time to time. Some of them can be quite useful as coping techniques, as long as they don't keep people from finding lasting solutions to problems.

3. *a.* People who are mentally ill and who have no history of violence are no more likely than members of the general population to become violent. Targets of violence by people with a mental illness are much more likely to be family members or other caregivers than strangers.

4. *False.* Most people who commit suicide have talked about doing it.

5. *b.* The suicide rate for white males over 65 is higher than that for any other group of Americans—more than triple the rate for young people or black males.

What exactly is psychological health? Many people over the centuries have expressed opinions about the nature of psychological (or mental) health. Some even claim that there is no such thing, that psychological health is just a myth. We disagree. We think there is such a thing as psychological health just as there is physical health—and the two are closely interrelated. Just as your body can work well or poorly, giving you pleasure or pain, your mind can also work well or poorly, resulting in happiness or unhappiness. Psychological health is a crucial component of overall wellness. (We are using "mental health" and "psychological health" interchangeably; the latter is the more current term, but it hasn't replaced mental health yet.)

If you feel pain and unhappiness rather than pleasure and happiness, or if you sense that you could be functioning at a higher level, there may be ways you can help yourself—either on your own or with professional help. This chapter will explain how.

WHAT PSYCHOLOGICAL HEALTH IS NOT

Psychological health is not the same as psychological **normality.** Being mentally normal simply means being close to average. You can define normal body temperature because a few degrees above or below this temperature always means physical sickness. But your ideas and attitudes can vary tremendously without losing efficiency or feeling emotional distress. And psychological diversity is valuable; living in a society of people with varied ideas and lifestyles makes life interesting and challenging.

Conforming to social demands is not necessarily a mark of psychological health. If you don't question what's going on around you, you're not fulfilling your potential as a thinking, questioning human being. For example, our society admires the framers of the U.S. Constitution and the abolitionists who rebelled against injustices. If conformity signified mental health, then political dissent would indicate mental illness by definition (and we have seen that definition used by dictators). If such a definition were valid, Galileo would have been mad for insisting that the earth revolved around the sun.

Never seeking help for personal problems does not mean you are psychologically healthy, any more than seeking help proves you are mentally ill. Unhappy people may not want to seek professional help because they don't want to reveal their problems to others, may fear what their friends might think, or may not know whom to ask for help. People who are severely disturbed psychologically or emotionally may not even realize they need help, or they may become so suspicious of other people that they can only be treated without their consent.

We cannot say people are "mentally ill" or "mentally healthy" on the basis of symptoms alone. Life constantly presents problems. Time and life inevitably alter the environment as well as our minds and bodies, and changes present problems. The symptom of anxiety, for example, can help us face a problem and solve it before it gets too big. Someone who shows no anxiety may be refusing to recognize problems or do anything about them. A person who is anxious for good reason is likely to be judged more psychologically healthy in the long run than someone who is inappropriately calm.

Finally, we cannot judge psychological health from the way people look. All too often, a person who seems to be OK and even happy suddenly takes his or her own life. Usually such people lack close friends who might have known of their desperation. At an early age, we learn to conceal and "lie." We may believe that our complaints put unfair demands on others. While suffering in silence can sometimes be a virtue, it can also impede getting help.

DEFINING PSYCHOLOGICAL HEALTH

It is even harder to say what psychological health *is* than what it is *not*. Psychological health can be defined either negatively as the absence of sickness or positively as the presence of wellness. The narrower, negative definition has several advantages: It concentrates attention on the worst problems and on the people most in need, and it tends to avoid value judgments about the best way to lead our lives. However, if we consider everyone to be mentally healthy who is not severely mentally disturbed, we end up ignoring common problems that can be addressed.

A positive definition—psychological health as the presence of wellness—is a more ambitious outlook, one that encourages you to fulfill your own potential. Freedom from disorders is only one factor in psychological wellness. During the 1960s, Abraham Maslow eloquently described an ideal of mental health in his book *Toward a Psychology of Being*. He was convinced that psychologists were too preoccupied with people who had failed in some way. He also disliked the way psychologists tried to reduce human striving to physiological needs or drives.

According to Maslow, there is a *hierarchy of needs,* listed here in order of decreasing urgency: physiological needs, safety, being loved, maintaining self-esteem, and self-actualization (Figure 3-1). When urgent needs like the need for food are satisfied, less urgent needs take priority. Most of us are well fed and feel reasonably safe, so we are driven by higher motives. Maslow's conclusions were based on his study of a group of visibly successful people who seemed to have lived, or be living, at their fullest, including Abraham Lincoln, Henry David Thoreau, Ludwig van Beethoven, Eleanor Roosevelt, and Albert Einstein, as well as some of his own friends and acquaintances. He stated that these people had achieved **self-actualization;** he thought they had fulfilled a good measure of their human potential and suggested that self-actualized people all share certain qualities.

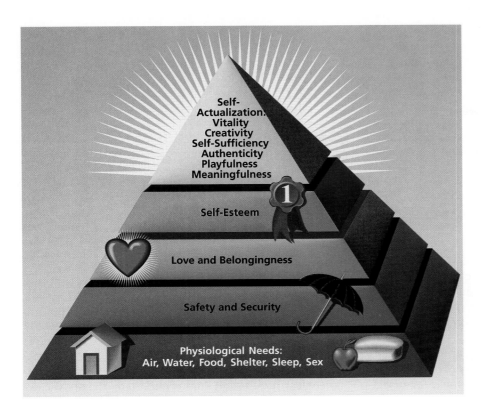

Figure 3-1 Maslow's hierarchy of needs.
SOURCE: Maslow, A. 1970. *Motivation and Personality*, 2nd ed. New York: Harper & Row.

Realism

Self-actualized people are able to deal with the world as it is and not demand that it be otherwise. If you are realistic, you know the difference between what is and what you want. You also know what you can change and what you cannot. Unrealistic people often spend a great deal of time and energy trying to force the world and other people into their ideal picture. Realistic people accept evidence that contradicts what they want to believe, and if it is important evidence, they modify their beliefs.

Acceptance

Psychologically healthy people can largely accept themselves and others. Self-acceptance means having a positive **self-concept** or self-image, or appropriately high **self-esteem.** They have a positive but realistic mental image of themselves, and positive feelings about who they are, what they are capable of, and what roles they play. People who feel good about themselves are likely to live up to their positive self-image and enjoy successes that in turn reinforce these good feelings. A good self-concept is based on a realistic view of personal worth—it does not mean being egocentric or "stuck on yourself."

Being able to tolerate our own imperfections and still feel positive about ourselves helps us tolerate the imperfections of others. Psychologically healthy people tend to

be optimistic about what they can expect from other people, until experience proves their optimism to be unrealistic. Acceptance means being willing to interact with people who are imperfect and unlikely to change.

Autonomy

Psychologically healthy people are able to direct themselves, acting independently of their social environment. **Autonomy** is more than freedom from physical control by something outside the self. Many people, for example, shrink from expressing their feelings because they fear disapproval and rejection. They respond only to what they feel as outside pressure. Behavior such as this is

TERMS

normality The psychological characteristics attributed to the majority of people in a population at a given time.

self-actualization The highest level of growth in Maslow's hierarchy.

self-concept The ideas, feelings, and perceptions one has about oneself; also called *self-image*.

self-esteem Satisfaction and confidence in oneself; the valuing of oneself as a person.

autonomy Independence; the sense of being self-directed.

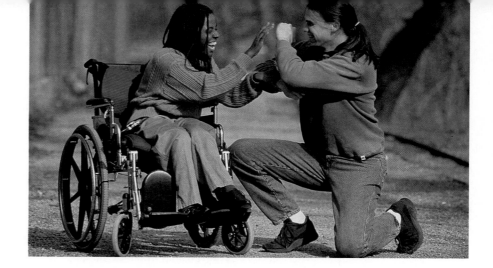

Self-actualized people respond in a genuine, spontaneous way to what happens around them. They are capable of maintaining close interpersonal relationships.

other-directed. In contrast, **inner-directed** people find guidance from within, from their own values and feelings. They are not afraid to be themselves. Psychologically free people act because they choose to, not because they are driven or pressured.

Autonomy can give healthy people certain childlike qualities. Very small children have a quality of being "real." They respond in a genuine, spontaneous way to whatever happens. Someone who is genuine has no pretenses. Being genuine means not having to plan words or actions to get approval or make an impression. It means being aware of feelings and being willing to express them—being unself-consciously oneself. This quality is sometimes called **authenticity**; such people are *authentic,* the "real thing."

A Capacity for Intimacy

Healthy people are capable of physical and emotional intimacy. They can expose their feelings and thoughts to other people. They are open to the pleasure of intimate physical contact and to the risks and satisfactions of being close to others in a caring, sensitive way. Intimate physical contact may mean "good sex," but it also means something more—intense awareness of both your partner and yourself in which contact becomes communication. Chapters 4 and 5 discuss intimacy in more detail.

Creativity

Psychologically healthy people are creative and have a continuing fresh appreciation for what goes on around them. They are not necessarily great poets, artists, or musicians, but they do live their everyday lives in creative ways: "A first-rate soup is more creative than a second-rate painting." Creative people seem to see more and to be open to new experiences; they don't fear the unknown. And they don't need to minimize uncertainty or avoid it; they actually find it attractive.

How did Maslow's group achieve their exemplary psychological health, and (more importantly) how can *we* attain it? Maslow himself did not answer that question, but we have a few suggestions. Undoubtedly it helps to have been treated with respect, love, and understanding as a child, to have experienced stability and to have achieved a sense of mastery. As adults, since we cannot redo the past, we must concentrate on meeting current psychological challenges in ways that will lead to long-term mental wellness.

MEETING LIFE'S CHALLENGES

Life is full of challenges—large and small. Everyone, regardless of heredity and family influences, must learn to cope successfully with new situations and new people. For emotional and mental wellness, each of us must continue to grow psychologically, developing new and more sophisticated coping mechanisms to suit our current lives. We must develop an adult identity that enhances our self-esteem and autonomy. We must also learn to communicate honestly, handle anger appropriately, and avoid being defensive.

Growing Up Psychologically

How we respond to the challenges of life influences the development of our personality and identity. Psychologist Erik Erikson proposed that development proceeds through a series of eight stages, extending throughout the life span. Each stage is characterized by a major crisis or turning point, a time of increased vulnerability as well as increased potential for psychological growth (Table 3-1).

TERMS　**other-directed**　Guided in behavior by the values and expectations of others.

inner-directed　Guided in behavior by an inner set of rules and values.

authenticity　Genuineness.

TABLE 3-1 Erikson's Stages of Development

Age	Conflict	Important People	Task
Birth–1 year	Trust vs. mistrust	Mother or other primary caregiver	In being fed and comforted, developing the trust that others will respond to your needs.
1–3 years	Autonomy vs. shame and self-doubt	Parents	In toilet training, locomotion, and exploration, learning self-control without losing the capacity for assertiveness.
3–6 years	Initiative vs. guilt	Family	In playful talking and locomotion, developing a conscience based on parental prohibitions that is not too inhibiting.
6–12 years	Industry vs. inferiority	Neighborhood and school	In school and playing with peers, learning the value of accomplishment and perseverance without feeling inadequate.
Adolescence	Identity vs. identity confusion	Peers	Developing a stable sense of who you are—your needs, abilities, interpersonal style, and values.
Young adulthood	Intimacy vs. isolation	Close friends, sex partners	Learning to live and share intimately with others, often in sexual relationships.
Middle adulthood	Generativity vs. self-absorption	Work associates, children, community	Doing things for others, including parenting and civic activities.
Older adulthood	Integrity vs. despair	Humankind	Affirming the value of life and its ideals.

SOURCE: Erikson, E. 1963. *Childhood and Society.* New York: Norton.

The successful mastery of one stage is a basis for mastering the next, so early failures can have repercussions in later life. Fortunately, life provides ongoing opportunities for mastering these tasks. For example, although the development of trust begins in infancy, it is refined as we grow older. We learn to trust people outside our immediate family and to limit our trust by identifying people who are untrustworthy.

Developing an Adult Identity A primary task beginning in adolescence is the development of an adult identity: a unified sense of self, characterized by attitudes, beliefs, and ways of acting that are genuinely one's own. People with adult identities know who they are, what they are capable of, what roles they play, and their place among their peers. They have a sense of their own uniqueness but also appreciate what they have in common with others. They view themselves realistically and can assess their strengths and weaknesses without relying on the opinions of others. Achieving an identity also means that one can form intimate relationships with others while maintaining a strong sense of self.

Our identities evolve as we interact with the world and make choices about what we'd like to do and whom we'd like to model ourselves after. Developing an adult identity is particularly challenging in a heterogeneous, secular, and relatively affluent society like ours, in which many roles are possible, many choices are tolerated, and ample time is allowed for experimenting and making up one's mind.

Early identities are often modeled after parents—or the opposite of parents, in rebellion from what they represent. Later, peers, rock stars, sports heroes, and religious figures are added to the list of possible models. In high school and college, people often join cliques that assert a certain identity—the "jocks," the "brains," or the "skaters." Although much of an identity is internal—a way of viewing oneself and the world—it can include such things as styles of talking and dressing, ornaments like earrings, and particular hairstyles.

Early identities are rarely permanent. A student who works for good grades and approval from parents and teachers one year can turn into a dropout devoted to hard rock and wild parties a year later. At some point, however, most of us adopt a more stable, individual identity that ties together the experiences of childhood and the expectations and aspirations of adulthood. Erikson's theory does not suggest that suddenly one day we assume our final identity and never change after that. Life is more interesting for people who continue to evolve into more distinct individuals, rather than being rigidly controlled by their pasts. Identity reflects a lifelong process, and it changes as a person develops new relationships and roles.

Developing an adult identity is an important part of psychological wellness. Without a personal identity, we begin to feel confused about who we are; Erikson called

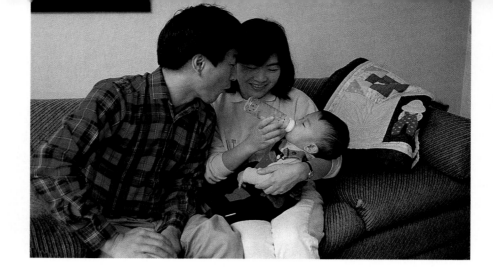

A positive self-concept begins in infancy. Knowing that he's loved and valued by his parents gives this 8-month-old a solid basis for lifelong psychological health.

this situation an *identity crisis*. Until we have "found ourselves," we cannot have much self-esteem because a self is not firmly in place.

How far have you gotten in developing your adult identity? Write down a list of characteristics you think a friend who knows you well would use to describe you. Rank them from the most to the least important. Your list might include elements such as gender, socioeconomic status, ethnic and/or religious identification, choice of college or major, parents' occupations, interests and talents, attitudes toward drugs and alcohol, style of dress, the kinds of people with whom you typically associate, your expected role in society, and aspects of your personality. Which elements of your identity do you feel are permanent and which do you think may change over time? Are there any characteristics missing from your list that you'd like to add?

Developing Intimacy and Purpose in Your Life Erikson's developmental stages don't end with establishing an adult identity. Learning to live intimately with others and finding a productive role for yourself in society are other tasks of adulthood—to be able to love and work.

People with established identities can form intimate relationships and sexual unions characterized by sharing, open communication, long-term commitment, and love. Those who lack a firm sense of self may have difficulty establishing relationships because they feel overwhelmed by closeness and the needs of another person. As a result, they experience only short-term, superficial relationships with others and may remain isolated. As described in Chapter 2, a lack of social support can affect getting both physical and psychological help. (Chapter 4 has more information about intimate relationships.)

A productive role in society means more than just earning enough money for yourself and your family. During middle adulthood, people typically expand their focus beyond personal concerns; self-absorption is replaced by an interest in the next generation and in producing something that will outlive them. People in this

stage of development often express interest in passing on something of value to their own children, to younger friends or relatives, or to younger people at work. Parenting and participation in community activities bring feelings of pride and satisfaction. (For more on developing meaning and purpose in life, see the box "Spiritual Wellness.")

Achieving Healthy Self-Esteem

Having a healthy level of self-esteem means regarding your self, which includes all aspects of your identity, as good, competent, and worthy of love. It is a critical component of wellness.

Developing a Positive Self-Concept Ideally, a positive self-concept begins in childhood, based on experiences within the family and outside it. Children need to develop a sense of being loved and being able to give love and to accomplish their goals. If they feel rejected or neglected by their parents, they may fail to develop feelings of self-worth. They may grow to have a negative concept of themselves.

Another component of self-concept is integration. An integrated self-concept is one that you have made for yourself—not someone else's image of you, or a mask that doesn't quite fit. Important building blocks of self-concept are the personality characteristics and mannerisms of parents, which children may adopt without realizing it. Later, they may be surprised to find themselves acting like one of their parents. Eventually, such building blocks

Spiritual wellness means different things to different people. For many, it involves developing a set of guiding beliefs, principles, or values that give meaning and purpose to life. It helps people achieve a sense of wholeness within themselves and in their relationships with others. Spiritual wellness influences people on an individual level, as well as on a community level, where it can bond people together through compassion, love, forgiveness, and self-sacrifice. For some, spirituality includes a belief in a higher power. Regardless of how it is defined, the development of spiritual wellness is critical for overall health and well-being. Its development is closely tied to the other components of wellness, particularly psychological health.

There are many paths to spiritual wellness. One of the most common in our society is organized religion. Some people object to the notion that organized religion can contribute to psychological health and overall wellness, asserting that it reinforces people's tendency to deny real difficulties and to accept what can and should be changed. Freud criticized religion as wishful thinking; Marx called it an opiate to make the poor accept social injustice. However, many elements of religious belief and practice can promote psychological health.

Organized religion usually involves its members in a community where social and material support is available. Religious organizations offer a social network to those who might otherwise be isolated. The major religions provide paths for transforming the self in ways that can lead to greater happiness and serenity and reduce feelings of anxiety and hopelessness. In Christianity, salvation follows turning away from the selfish ego to God's sovereignty and grace, where a joy is found that frees the believer from anxious self-concern and despair. Islam is the word for a kind of self-surrender leading to peace with God.

Buddhism teaches how to detach oneself from selfish desire, leading to compassion for the suffering of others and freedom from fear-engendering illusions. Judaism emphasizes the social and ethical redemption the Jewish community can experience if it follows the laws of God. Religions teach specific techniques for achieving these transformations of the self: prayer, both in groups and in private; meditation; the performance of rituals and ceremonies symbolizing religious truths; and good works and service to others. Christianity's faith and works are perhaps analogous to the cognitive and behavioral components of a program of behavior change.

Spiritual wellness does not require participation in organized religion. Many people find meaning and purpose in other ways. By spending time in nature or working on environmental issues, people can experience continuity with the natural world. Spiritual wellness can come through helping others in one's community or by promoting human rights, peace and harmony among people, and opportunities for human development on a global level. (The spiritual, psychological, and physical wellness benefits of helping others are discussed further in Chapter 19.) Other people develop spiritual wellness through art or through their personal relationships.

The search for meaning and purpose in life is reflected in Erikson's later stages of development. Particularly in the second half of life, people seem to have an urge to view their activities and consciousness from a transcendent perspective. Perhaps it is the approach of death that makes older people tend to take less interest in material possessions and to devote more time to interpersonal and altruistic pursuits. At every age, however, people seem to feel better if they have beliefs about the ultimate purpose of life and their own place in the universe.

---

should be reshaped and integrated into a new individual personality.

A further aspect of self-concept is stability. Stability depends on the integration of the self and its freedom from contradictions. People who have gotten mixed messages about themselves from parents and friends may have contradictory self-images, which defy integration and make them vulnerable to shifting levels of self-esteem. At times they regard themselves as entirely good, capable, and lovable—an ideal self—and at other times they see themselves as entirely bad, incompetent, and unworthy of love. While at the first pole, they may develop such an inflated ego that they totally ignore other people's needs and see others only as instruments for fulfilling their own desires. At the other pole, they may feel so small and weak that they run for protection to someone who seems powerful and caring. At neither extreme do such people see themselves or others realistically, and their relationships with other people are filled with misunderstandings and ultimately with conflict.

The concepts we have about ourselves and others are

an important part of our personalities. And all the components of our self-concept profoundly influence our interpersonal relationships.

Meeting Challenges to Self-Esteem

As an adult, you sometimes run into situations that challenge your self-concept: People you care about may tell you they don't love you or feel loved by you, or your attempts to accomplish a goal may end in failure. You can react to such challenges in several ways. The best approach is to acknowledge that something has gone wrong and try again, adjusting your goals to your abilities without radically revising your self-concept. Less productive responses are denying that anything went wrong and blaming someone else. While assuming these attitudes may preserve your self-concept temporarily, in the long run they keep you from meeting the challenge. The worst reaction is to develop a lasting negative self-concept in which you feel bad, unloved, and ineffective—in other words, becoming demoralized. Instead of coping, the demoralized person gives up, reinforcing the negative self-concept and setting in motion a cycle of bad self-concept and failure. In people who are genetically predisposed to depression, demoralization can progress to additional symptoms, discussed later in the chapter.

NOTICE YOUR PATTERNS OF THINKING   One method for fighting demoralization is to recognize and test your negative thoughts and assumptions about yourself and others. The first step is to note exactly when an unpleasant emotion—feeling worthless, wanting to give up, feeling depressed—occurs or gets worse, to identify the events or daydreams that trigger that emotion, and to observe whatever thoughts come into your head just before or during the emotional experience. It is helpful to keep a daily journal about such events.

Let's consider the example of Jennifer, a student who went to the college counseling center because she'd been feeling "down" lately. Her social life had not been going well, and she had begun to think she was a boring, uninteresting person. Asked to keep a daily journal, she wrote that she felt let down and discouraged when a date who promised to meet her at 7:30 P.M. was 15 minutes late. The thoughts that occurred to her were: "He's not going to come. It's my fault. He has more important things to do. Maybe he's with someone else. He doesn't like me. Nobody likes me because I don't have anything interesting to say. What if he had a car accident?"

People who are demoralized tend to use all-or-nothing thinking. They overgeneralize from negative events. They overlook the positive and they jump to negative conclusions, minimize their own successes and magnify the successes of others. They take responsibility for unfortunate situations that are not their fault. The minute Jennifer's date was late, she jumped to the conclusion that he was not coming and blamed herself for it. From that point she jumped to more negative conclusions and more unfounded overgeneralizations. Patterns of thinking that make events seem worse than they are in reality are called **cognitive distortions.**

DEVELOP REALISTIC SELF-TALK   Jennifer needs to develop more rational responses. For Jennifer, more rational thinking could be "He's a little late so I'll reread the study questions." If he still hadn't come after 30 minutes, she might have called him to see if something was holding him up, without jumping to any conclusions about the meaning of his lateness.

In your own fight against demoralization, it may be hard to figure out a rational response until hours or days after the event that upset you. But once you get used to

noticing the way your mind works, you may be able to catch yourself thinking negatively and change the thought process before it goes too far.

This approach is not the same as positive thinking—substituting a positive thought for a negative one. Instead, you simply try to make your thoughts as logical and accurate as possible. If Jennifer continues to think she's boring, she should try to collect evidence to prove or disprove that. If she has exaggerated her dullness, as do many demoralized people, her investigations may prove her wrong. For example, she might ask her friends their candid opinions about her personality, and she can observe whether people seem interested in continuing a conversation with her.

Demoralized people can be so tenacious about their negative beliefs that they make them come true in a self-fulfilling prophecy. Jennifer might conclude that she is so boring no one will like her anyway, so she may as well not bother to be involved in what's going on around her. This behavior could help her negative belief become a reality. For additional tips on how to change distorted, negative ways of thinking, see the box "Realistic Self-Talk."

Being Less Defensive

Sometimes our wishes come into conflict with people around us or with our conscience, and we become frustrated and anxious. If we cannot resolve the conflict by changing the external situation, we try to resolve the conflict internally by rearranging our thoughts and feelings. Some standard **defense mechanisms** are listed in Table 3-2. The drawback of many of these coping mechanisms, particularly those at the beginning of the list, is that although they succeed temporarily, they are dead-ends that make finding ultimate solutions much harder. Projection, for example, distorts reality in a way that poisons interpersonal relationships. Repression or denial attempts to banish problems from our life that stubbornly return to haunt us. Daydreaming can be useful insofar as it is a rehearsal for future action, but as a substitute for action it quickly becomes unsatisfying and boring. The mechanisms at the end of the list—such as substitution, sublimation, and humor—can be very useful for coping, as long as they don't keep us from being who we want to be.

Recognizing your favorite defense mechanisms can be difficult, because they've probably become habits, occurring unconsciously. But we each have some inkling about how our mind operates. By remembering the details of conflict situations you have been in, you may be able to figure out which defense mechanisms you used in successful or unsuccessful attempts to cope. Try to look at yourself as an objective, outside observer would, and analyze your thoughts and behavior in a psychologically stressful situation from the past. Having insight into what strategies you typically use can lead to new, less defensive and more effective ways of coping in the future.

TERMS   **cognitive distortion**   A pattern of thinking that makes events seem worse than they are.
defense mechanism   A mental mechanism for coping with conflict or anxiety.

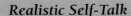

Do your patterns of thinking make events seem worse than they truly are? Do negative beliefs about yourself become self-fulfilling prophecies? Substituting realistic self-talk for negative self-talk can help you build and maintain self-esteem and cope better with the challenges in your life. Here are some examples of common types of distorted negative self-talk, along with suggestions for more accurate and rational responses.

Cognitive Distortion	Negative Self-Talk	Realistic Self-Talk
Focusing on negatives	School is so discouraging—nothing but one hassle after another.	School is pretty challenging and has its difficulties, but there certainly are rewards. It's really a mixture of good and bad.
Expecting the worst	Why would my boss want to meet with me this afternoon if not to fire me?	I wonder why my boss wants to meet with me. I guess I'll just have to wait and see.
Overgeneralizing	(After getting a poor grade on a paper) Just as I thought—I'm incompetent at everything.	I'll start working on the next paper earlier. That way, if I run into problems, I'll have time to consult with the TA.
Minimizing	I won the speech contest, but none of the other speakers was very good. I wouldn't have done as well against stiffer competition.	It may not have been the best speech I'll ever give, but it was good enough to win the contest. I'm really improving as a speaker.
Blaming others	I wouldn't have eaten so much last night if my friends hadn't insisted on going to that restaurant.	I overdid it last night. Next time I'll make different choices.
Expecting perfection	I should have scored 100% on this test. I can't believe I missed that one problem through a careless mistake.	Too bad I missed one problem through carelessness, but overall I did very well on this test. Next time I'll be more careful.
Believing you're the cause of everything	Sarah seems so depressed today. I wish I hadn't had that argument with her yesterday; it must have really upset her.	I wish I had handled the argument better, and in the future I'll try to. But I don't know if Sarah's behavior is related to what I said, or even if she's depressed. In any case, I'm not responsible for how Sarah feels or acts; only she can take responsibility for that.
Thinking in black and white	I've got to score 10 points in the game today. Otherwise, I don't belong on the team.	I'm a good player or else I wouldn't be on the team. I'll play my best—that's all I can do.
Magnifying events	They went to a movie without me. I thought we were friends, but I guess I was wrong.	I'm disappointed they didn't ask me to the movie, but it doesn't mean our friendship is over. It's not that big a deal.

SOURCE: Adapted from Schafer, W. 1995. *Stress Management for Wellness*, 3rd ed. Copyright © 1996 by Holt, Rinehart, and Winston. Reprinted by permission of the publisher.

Being Optimistic

Optimism and pessimism are abstract concepts that might seem to have more to do with philosophy than with psychological health. However, many psychologists believe that pessimism is not just a symptom of everyday depression but an important root cause. Pessimists not only expect repeated failure and rejection, they perversely accept it as deserved. Pessimists do not see themselves as capable of success, and they irrationally dismiss any evidence of their own accomplishments. This negative point of view is learned, typically at a young age from parents and other authority figures. But as an optimist would tell you, that means it also has the potential of being unlearned.

Psychologist Martin Seligman points out that we are more used to refuting negative statements, such as "The problem is going to last forever and ruin everything, and it's all my fault," when they come from a jealous rival rather than from our own mind. But refuting such negative self-statements is exactly what a pessimist must learn to do in order to avoid chronic unhappiness. Pessimists must first recognize, and then dispute, these false, negative predictions they generate about themselves. Seligman points out that learning to be optimistic is easier and more lasting than, for example, learning to eat less.

TABLE 3-2 Defense and Coping Mechanisms

Mechanism	Description	Example
Projection	Reacting to unacceptable inner impulses as if they were from outside the self.	A student who dislikes his roommate feels that the roommate dislikes him.
Repression	Expelling from awareness an unpleasant feeling, idea, or memory.	The child of an alcoholic, neglectful father remembers him as a giving, loving person.
Regression	Acting in childish ways that used to be satisfying and acceptable.	A person in line for movie tickets has a temper tantrum when told the movie is sold out.
Denial	Refusing to acknowledge to yourself what you really know to be true.	A person believes that smoking cigarettes won't harm her because she's young and healthy.
Daydreaming	Escaping, or finding fulfillment, through fantasy.	While waiting for midterms to be passed back, a student fantasizes that he receives the highest score in the class and the professor tells him he's very talented and offers to find him a high-paying job.
Idealization/denigration	Viewing others or self as either all good or all bad, often shifting from one to the other.	A woman believes her husband is perfect and that he will love and care for her forever.
Passive-aggressive behavior	Expressing hostility toward someone by being covertly uncooperative or passive.	A person tells a coworker, with whom she competes for project assignments, that she'll help him with a report, but then never follows through.
Isolation of emotion	Detaching painful feelings from thoughts.	A man feels no emotion when he recalls being beaten and robbed.
Displacement	Shifting one's feelings about a person to another person.	A student who is angry with one of his professors returns home and yells at one of his housemates.
Reaction formation	Covering up a feeling by expressing its opposite.	A young woman tells her roommate that she's a very nice person and a good friend, though in reality she thinks her roommate is inconsiderate.
Rationalization	Giving a false, acceptable reason when the real reason is unacceptable.	A shy young man decides not to attend a dorm party, telling himself he'd be bored.
Avoidance/suppression	Deliberately avoiding tempting actions or thoughts that you think will have an undesirable outcome.	A student decides to skip a fraternity party because he's worried he won't be able to withstand the social pressure to drink.
Substitution	Deliberately replacing a frustrating goal with one that is more attainable.	A student having a difficult time passing courses in chemistry decides to change his major from biology to economics.
Sublimation	Transforming aggressive or sexual impulses into socially approved behavior.	A man who is very angry with his brother goes for a 5-mile jog.
Humor	Finding something funny in unpleasant situations.	A student whose bicycle has been stolen thinks how surprised the thief will be when he or she starts downhill and discovers the brakes don't work.

Unlike refusing foods you love, disputing your own negative thoughts is fun—because doing so makes you feel better immediately.

Maintaining Honest Communication

Another important area of psychological functioning is communicating honestly with others. It can be very frustrating for us and for people around us if we cannot express what we want and feel. Others can hardly respond to our needs if they don't know what those needs are. We must recognize what we want to communicate and then express it clearly. For example, how do you feel about going to the party instead of to the movie? Do you care if your roommate talks on the phone late into the night? Some people know what they want others to do, but don't state it clearly because they fear denial of the request, which they interpret as personal rejection. Such

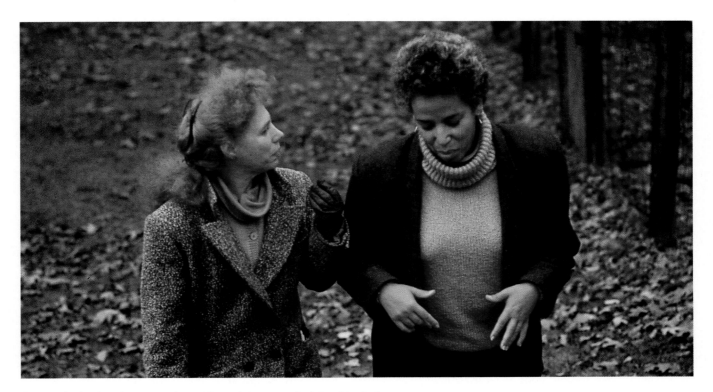

Communication is an important element in any interpersonal relationship. As these women express their thoughts and feelings to each other and listen attentively in response, they enhance their relationship, which in turn supports their psychological well-being.

people might benefit from **assertiveness** training: learning to insist on their rights and to bargain for what they want. Assertiveness includes being able to say no or yes depending on the situation.

Because expressing feelings has become so central to popular psychology, many misconceptions have arisen. Neither "sharing" feelings with everyone on every occasion nor making important decisions based on feelings alone is a legitimate psychological health goal. But communicating your feelings appropriately and clearly *is* important. For example, if you tell people you feel sad, they may have various reactions. If they feel closer to you, they may express an intimate thought of their own. Or they may feel guilty because they think you're implying they have caused your sadness. They may even be angry because they feel obligated to help cheer you up.

Depending on your intention and prediction of how your statement will be taken, you may or may not wish to make it. For example, if you say you feel like staying home tonight, you may also be implying something different. You could really be saying "Don't bother me," or opening a negotiation about what you would be willing to do that evening, given the right event or incentive.

Good communication means expressing yourself clearly. You don't need any special psychological jargon to communicate effectively. (For tips, see the box "Guidelines for Effective Communication" in Chapter 4, p. 88.)

Dealing with Anger

Popular wisdom has said that you should express your anger rather than suppress it. Letting your anger out was thought to be beneficial for both psychological and physical health. However, recent studies have questioned this idea by showing that people who are overtly hostile seem to be at higher risk for heart attacks. Furthermore, angry words or actions won't contribute to psychological wellness if they damage important personal or professional relationships, or produce feelings of guilt or loss of control. Perhaps the best way to resolve this contradiction is to look at the expression of anger in each situation and distinguish between a gratuitous expression of anger and a reasonable level of self-assertiveness.

At one extreme are people who never express anger or any opinion that might offend others, even when their own rights and needs are being jeopardized. They may find themselves in unhealthy relationships, which they can neither change nor escape from. They may be chronically deprived of satisfaction at work and at home. If you have trouble expressing your anger, you might explore training in assertiveness and appropriate expressions of

assertiveness   Expression that is forceful but not hostile.   **TERMS**

anger to help you learn to express your needs, desires, and opinions constructively.

At the other extreme are people whose anger is explosive and misdirected. They protect their self-esteem by angrily rejecting anyone who challenges what they do or say. If you are among these people, the best approach may be to try to learn what triggers your anger and to change the underlying attitudes that lead to outbursts. Until you change these attitudes, you can try to delay the expression of your anger when it wells up—for example, by counting to 10 or 100, if necessary. Or try rethinking a situation in order to diffuse your anger: Thoughts like "There's no need to take it personally" and "Don't act like a jerk just because he did" may help you calm down. Distracting yourself by thinking of other things is another helpful strategy. (See Chapter 15 for more on the relationship between hostility and heart disease and other methods of controlling inappropriate expressions of anger.)

Flexibility—adjusting your behavior based on needs and circumstances—may be the best approach to dealing with anger. Sometimes it may be healthy to let off steam and express your anger in a direct but nonviolent manner. Other times, it may be less damaging to your health and your relationships to hold your anger in.

> **PERSONAL INSIGHT** When you were a child, how were you taught to handle difficult feelings like anger, fear, and sadness? Do you still use the same methods? How are they working now?

PSYCHOLOGICAL DISORDERS

All of us have felt anxious at times, and in dealing with the anxiety, we have thought less rationally than when we were calm. Almost all of us have had periods of feeling down. Such feelings are normal responses to the ordinary challenges of life. But when emotions or irrational thoughts are strong enough to interfere with daily living, they can be regarded as symptoms of a psychological disorder.

Here we focus on anxiety disorders, mood disorders, and schizophrenia. Elsewhere in this book you can learn about other disorders: sexual disorders in Chapter 5, disorders associated with drug and alcohol abuse in Chapters 9 and 10, eating disorders in Chapter 14, and Alzheimer's disease in Chapter 19.

Anxiety Disorders

Fear is a basic and useful emotion. Its value for our ancestors' survival cannot be overestimated; for modern humans, it provides motivation for self-protection and learning to cope with new or potentially dangerous situations. Only when fear is out of proportion to real danger can it be considered a problem. **Anxiety** is another word for fear, especially a feeling of fear that is not directed toward any definite threat. Only when anxiety is experienced almost daily or in life situations that recur and cannot be avoided is it considered a disorder.

The broad concept of anxiety disorders covers a variety of human problems. Following are the main types.

Simple Phobia **Simple phobia** is probably the most common and most understandable anxiety disorder. A phobia is a specific fear—for example, fear of animals or certain locations. Feared animals are usually dogs, snakes, insects, or mice. Frightening locations are high places like tall buildings and closed places like airplanes. Sometimes these fears originate in bad experiences with the feared objects, but often there is no such explanation.

Social Phobia Similar to simple phobia, **social phobia** occurs in interpersonal contexts. People with social phobias fear humiliation or embarrassment while being watched by others. Fear of speaking in public is perhaps the most common social phobia. Extremely shy people can have social fears that extend to almost all social situations (see the box "Shyness").

Panic Disorder **Panic disorder** is characterized by sudden unexpected surges in anxiety, accompanied by symptoms such as rapid and strong heartbeat, shortness of breath, loss of physical equilibrium, and a feeling of losing mental control. Such attacks usually begin in one's early twenties and can lead to fear of being in crowds or closed places or of driving or flying. Sufferers fear that a panic attack will occur in a situation from which escape is difficult (as in an elevator), where the attack could be incapacitating and result in dangerous loss of control (as in driving a car), or where no help is available if needed

TERMS

anxiety A feeling of fear that is not directed toward any definite threat.

simple phobia A persistent and excessive fear of a specific object, activity, or situation.

social phobia An excessive fear of performing in public; speaking in public is the most common example.

panic disorder A syndrome of severe anxiety attacks accompanied by physical symptoms.

obsessive-compulsive disorder (OCD) An anxiety disorder characterized by uncontrollable, recurring thoughts and the performing of senseless rituals.

obsession A recurrent, irrational, unwanted thought or impulse.

compulsion An irrational, repetitive, forced action, usually associated with an obsession.

post-traumatic stress disorder (PTSD) An anxiety disorder characterized by reliving traumatic events through dreams, flashbacks, and hallucinations.

Shyness is a form of social anxiety, a fear of what others will think of one's behavior or appearance. Physical signs include a rapid heartbeat, a nervous stomach, sweating, cold and clammy hands, blushing, dry mouth, a lump in the throat, and trembling muscles. Shy people are often excessively self-critical, and they engage in very negative self-talk. The accompanying feelings of self-consciousness, embarrassment, and unworthiness can be overwhelming.

To avoid situations that make them anxious, shy people may refrain from making eye contact or speaking up in public. They may shun social gatherings. They may avoid college courses or job promotions that demand more interpersonal interaction or public speaking. Shyness is not the same thing as being introverted. Introverts prefer solitude to society. Shy people often long to be more outgoing, but their own negative thoughts prevent them from enjoying the social interaction they desire. The consequences of severe shyness can include social isolation, loneliness, and lost personal and professional opportunities. Very shy people also have higher than average rates of other anxiety and mood disorders and of substance abuse

Shyness is very common, with 40–50% of Americans describing themselves as shy. However, only about 5–10% of adults are so shy that their condition interferes seriously with work, school, daily life, or interpersonal relationships. Shyness is often hidden, and most shy people manage to appear reasonably outgoing, even though they suffer the physical and emotional symptoms of their anxiety. Many shy people do better in structured rather than spontaneous settings.

What causes people to be shy? Research indicates that for some, the trait may be partly inherited. But for shyness, as for many health concerns, biology is not destiny. Many shy children outgrow their shyness, just as others acquire it later in life. Clearly, other factors are involved. The type of attachment between a child and his or her caregiver is important, as are parenting styles. Shyness is more common in cultures where children's failures are attributed to their own actions but successes are attributed to other people or events. People's experiences

during critical developmental transitions, such as starting school and entering adolescence, have also been linked to shyness. For adults, the precipitating factor may be an event such as divorce or the loss of a job.

Recent surveys indicate that shyness rates may be rising in the United States. With the advent of technologies such as ATM machines, video games, voice mail, faxes, and e-mail, the opportunities for face-to-face interaction are diminishing. Electronic media can be a wonderful way for shy people to communicate, but it can also allow them to hide from all social interaction. In fact, one study found that greater use of the Internet was associated with a decline in participants' communication with family members, a reduction in the size of their social circles, and an increase in levels of depression and loneliness. It remains to be seen whether the first generation to have cradle-to-grave access to home computers, faxes, and the Internet will experience higher rates of shyness.

Shyness is often undiagnosed, but help is available. Shyness classes, assertiveness training groups, and public speaking clinics are available (see the Behavior Change Strategy at the end of the chapter). For the seriously shy, effective treatments include cognitive-behavioral therapy and antidepressant drugs.

If you're shy, try to remember that shyness is widespread and that there are worse fates. Some degree of shyness has an up side. Shy people tend to be gentle, supportive, kind, and sensitive; they are often exceptional listeners. People who think carefully before they speak or act are less likely to hurt the feelings of others. Shyness may also facilitate cooperation. For any group or society to function well, a variety of roles is required, and there is a place for quieter, more reflective individuals.

SOURCES: Kraut, R., et al. 1998. Internet paradox: A social technology that reduces social involvement and psychological well-being? *American Psychologist* 53(9): 1017–1031. Lamberg, L. 1998. Social phobia—not just another name for shyness. *Journal of the American Medical Association* 280(8): 685–686. Carducci, B. J., and P. G. Zimbardo. 1995. Are you shy? The problem of shyness. *Psychology Today*, November/December.

(as when a person is alone). People with panic disorder can often function normally if someone trustworthy accompanies them.

Obsessive-Compulsive Disorder

Obsessive-compulsive disorder (OCD) applies to people with obsessions or compulsions or both. **Obsessions** are recurrent, unwanted thoughts or impulses. For example, a parent may have an impulse to kill a beloved child, or a person may brood over whether he or she got HIV from a handshake. **Compulsions** are repetitive, difficult-to-resist actions associated with obsessions. A common compulsion is hand washing, associated with an obsessive fear of contamination by dirt. Other compulsions are counting or repeatedly checking if something has been done—for example, if a door has been locked or a stove turned off.

Post-Traumatic Stress Disorder

Post-traumatic stress disorder (PTSD) is a reaction to severely traumatic events (events that produce a sense of terror and helplessness) such as physical violence to oneself or loved ones. Trauma occurs in personal assaults (rape or military combat), natural disasters (floods, earthquakes), and tragedies like fires and airplane or car crashes. Symptoms include reexperiencing the trauma in dreams and intrusive memories, trying to avoid anything associated with the trauma, and numbing of feelings. Sleep disturbances and other symptoms of anxiety and depression may also occur.

Therapies for anxiety disorders range from medication to psychological interventions that concentrate on a person's thoughts or behavior. As we discuss later, different models of human nature lead to different ideas of causes and appropriate treatments.

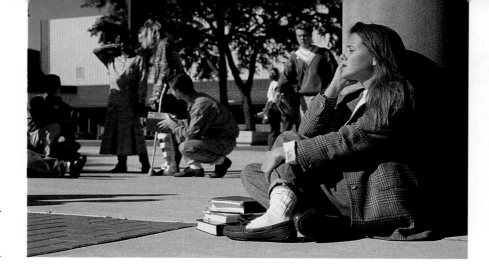

Having a bad day—or seriously depressed? Everyone feels dejected or defeated at times, but pervasive feelings of hopelessness, meaninglessness, or guilt signal deeper emotional problems. A person troubled by these feelings can often benefit from professional help.

Mood Disorders

We all experience ups and downs in our mood, in response to daily events. These temporary mood changes typically don't affect our overall emotional state or level of wellness. A person with a mood disorder, however, experiences emotional disturbances that are intense and persistent enough to affect normal functioning. The two most common mood disorders are depression and bipolar disorder.

Depression The most common mood disorder, **depression** has forms and degrees. It usually involves demoralization and can include the following:

- A feeling of sadness and hopelessness.
- Loss of pleasure in doing usual activities.
- Poor appetite and weight loss.
- Insomnia or disturbed sleep.
- Restlessness or, alternatively, fatigue.
- Thoughts of worthlessness and guilt.
- Trouble concentrating or making decisions.
- Thoughts of death or suicide.

Not all these features are present in every depressive episode. Sometimes instead of poor appetite and insomnia, the opposite occurs—eating too much and sleeping too long. Amazingly, people can have most of the symptoms of depression without feeling sad or hopeless or in a depressed mood, although they usually do experience a loss of interest or pleasure in things (see the box "Are You Depressed?"). In some cases, depression is a clear-cut reaction to specific events, such as the loss of a loved one or failing in school or work, while in other cases no trigger event is obvious.

TERMS **depression** A mood disorder characterized by loss of interest, sadness, hopelessness, loss of appetite, disturbed sleep, and other physical symptoms.

RECOGNIZING THE WARNING SIGNS OF SUICIDE One of the principal dangers of severe depression is suicide. Although a suicide attempt can occur unpredictably and unaccompanied by depression, the chances are greater if symptoms are numerous and severe. Additional warning signs of suicide include the following:

- Expressing the wish to be dead, or revealing contemplated methods.
- Increasing social withdrawal and isolation.
- A sudden, inexplicable lightening of mood (which can mean the person has finally decided to commit suicide).

Certain risk factors increase the likelihood of suicide:

- A history of previous attempts.
- A suicide by a family member or friend.
- Readily available means, such as guns or pills.
- A history of substance abuse or eating disorders.
- Serious medical problems.

The groups in the United States with the highest suicide rates are males age 20–34, Native American males, and white males over age 65. Women attempt three times as many suicides as men, yet men succeed at more than three times the rate of women.

HELPING YOURSELF OR A FRIEND If you are severely depressed or know someone who is, expert help from a mental health professional is essential. Don't try to do it all yourself. If you suspect one of your friends is suicidally depressed, try to get him or her to see a professional.

Don't be afraid to discuss the possibility of suicide with people you fear are suicidal. You won't give them an idea they haven't already thought of (see the box "Myths About Suicide," p. 68). And asking direct questions is the best way to determine whether someone seriously intends to commit suicide. Encourage your friend to talk and to take positive steps to improve his or her situation. If you feel there is an immediate danger of suicide, ensure that the person is not left alone, especially when he or she is

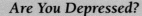

Are You Depressed?

The following test, developed by Lenore Radloff at the Center for Epidemiological Studies of the National Institutes of Mental Health, can help you determine whether you are depressed, relative to other people. Circle the answer that best describes how you have felt over the past week.

	Rarely or none of the time (less than 1 day)	Some or a little of the time (1–2 days)	Occasionally or a moderate amount of the time (3–4 days)	Most or all of the time (5–7 days)
1. I was bothered by things that usually don't bother me.	0	1	2	3
2. I did not feel like eating; my appetite was poor.	0	1	2	3
3. I felt I could not shake off the blues even with help from my family or friends.	0	1	2	3
4. I felt I was just as good as other people.	3	2	1	0
5. I had trouble keeping my mind on what I was doing.	0	1	2	3
6. I felt depressed.	0	1	2	3
7. I felt that everything I did was an effort.	0	1	2	3
8. I felt hopeful about the future.	3	2	1	0
9. I thought my life had been a failure.	0	1	2	3
10. I felt fearful.	0	1	2	3
11. My sleep was restless.	0	1	2	3
12. I was happy.	3	2	1	0
13. I talked less than usual.	0	1	2	3
14. I felt lonely.	0	1	2	3
15. People were unfriendly.	0	1	2	3
16. I enjoyed life.	3	2	1	0
17. I had crying spells.	0	1	2	3
18. I felt sad.	0	1	2	3
19. I felt that people disliked me.	0	1	2	3
20. I could not get going.	0	1	2	3

Scoring and Interpretation

To score the test, simply add up the numbers you circled. If you couldn't decide between two numbers for one item, count the higher of the two. Your score will be between 0 and 60. A score below 10 suggests that you are not depressed. A score of 10–15 indicates mild depression; 16–24, moderate depression; over 24, severe depression. Although occasional mild to moderate symptoms of depression may be normal and not require treatment, more persistent or severe symptoms, especially if accompanied by thoughts of suicide, are a reason to see a mental health professional right away.

It is important not to depend too heavily on any one measure of depression. The subjective experience of depression is highly variable. Some people with few subjective symptoms and normal scores on a depression questionnaire are actually quite depressed and respond markedly to treatment.

SOURCE: Radloff, L. S. 1977. The CES-D scale: A self-report depression scale for research in the general population. *Applied Psychological Measurement* 1: 387. Copyright © 1977 by Sage Publications. Reprinted by permission of the publisher.

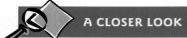
Myth   People who really intend to kill themselves do not let anyone know about it.
Fact   This belief can be an excuse for doing nothing when someone says he or she might commit suicide. In fact, most people who eventually commit suicide *have* talked about doing it.

Myth   People who made a suicide attempt but survived did not really intend to die.
Fact   This may be true for certain people, but people who seriously want to end their life may fail because they misjudge what it takes. Even a pharmacist may misjudge the lethal dose of a drug.

Myth   People who succeed in suicide really wanted to die.
Fact   We cannot be sure of that either. Some people are only trying to make a dramatic gesture or plea for help but miscalculate.

Myth   People who really want to kill themselves will do it regardless of any attempts to prevent them.
Fact   Few people are single-minded about suicide even at the moment of attempting it. People who are quite determined to take their life today may change their minds completely tomorrow.

Myth   Suicide is proof of mental illness.
Fact   Many suicides are committed by people who do not meet ordinary criteria for mental illness, although people with depression, schizophrenia, and other psychological disorders have a much higher than average suicide rate.

Myth   People inherit suicidal tendencies.
Fact   Certain kinds of depression that lead to suicide do have a genetic component. But many examples of suicide running in a family can be explained by factors such as psychologically identifying with a family member who committed suicide, often a parent.

Myth   All suicides are irrational.
Fact   By some standards all suicides may seem "irrational." But many people find it at least understandable that someone might want to commit suicide, for example, when approaching the end of a terminal illness or when facing a long prison term.

---

emotionally upset and more likely to act impulsively. If you must leave your friend alone, have your friend promise not to do anything to harm himself or herself without first calling you. Get qualified help as soon as possible.

If your friend refuses help, you might try to contact your friend's relatives and tell them that you are worried. If the depressed person is a college student, you may need to let someone in your health service or college administration know your concerns. Finally, most communities have emergency help available, often in the form of a hot-line telephone counseling service run by a suicide prevention agency (check the yellow pages).

TREATING DEPRESSION   Although treatments are highly effective, only about 35% of people who suffer from depression currently seek treatment. Treatment for depression depends on its severity and on whether the depressed person is suicidal. The basic treatment is usually some kind of drug therapy, often combined with psychotherapy. "Uppers" such as amphetamines are not good antidepressants. More effective are special drugs that work over a period of 2 or more weeks. Therefore, when suicidal impulses are too strong, hospitalization for a week or so may be necessary. Electroconvulsive therapy (ECT) is effective for severe depression when other approaches have failed.

Mania and Bipolar Disorder   **Mania** is a less common feature of mood disorders. People who are manic are restless, have a lot of energy, need little sleep, and often talk nonstop. They may devote themselves to fantastic projects and spend more money than they can afford. Many manic people swing between manic and depressive states, a syndrome called **bipolar disorder** because of the two opposite poles of mood. Tranquilizers are used to treat individual manic episodes, while special drugs like the salt lithium carbonate taken daily can prevent future mood swings.

Gender Differences   One of the mysteries about mood disorders is the gender gap in the incidence of depression. Although equal numbers of men and women suffer from bipolar disorder, women are twice as likely as men to be clinically depressed. This gender gap starts in adolescence and continues until about age 65. Researchers have looked at both biological and social causative factors.

A genetic basis for depression linked to the female sex chromosome was investigated, but researchers failed to find a strong association. Studies have also not found any correlation between female hormone levels and depression. Neither contraceptive pills nor menopause, both of which modify hormone levels significantly, is clearly linked to depression.

What about social factors? Traditional gender roles make women generally less likely to deal directly and assertively with problems, resulting in stress, economic dependence, and low self-esteem. Researchers have theorized that people with "helpless/hopeless" personalities may be more prone to depression. They have an external locus of control combined with a pessimistic outlook: They expect bad things to happen, feel that negative events are their own fault, and believe there is nothing they can do to prevent them. Some psychologists have suggested that conditions related to women's social roles

—discrimination in the workplace, lack of power in relationships, and role overload—may make women more prone to "learned helplessness," thereby predisposing them to depression. But no specific personality type has been clearly associated with depression, and it is possible that a helpless/hopeless personality is a result rather than a cause of depression.

Schizophrenia

Schizophrenia can be severe and debilitating or quite mild and hardly noticeable. Although people are capable of diagnosing their own depression, they usually don't diagnose their own schizophrenia, because they often can't see that anything is wrong. This disorder is not rare; in fact, one in every 100 people has a schizophrenic episode sometime in his or her lifetime, most commonly starting in adolescence. However, because people who are directly or indirectly affected do not like to talk about schizophrenia, its frequency is not generally appreciated. In addition, schizophrenic people tend to withdraw from society when they are ill, another factor making it seem rarer than it is.

Some general characteristics of schizophrenia include the following:

- *Disorganized thoughts.* Thoughts may be expressed in a vague or confusing way.
- *Inappropriate emotions.* Emotions may be absent or strong but inappropriate.
- *Delusions.* People with delusions—firmly held false beliefs—may think that their minds are controlled by outside forces, that people can read their minds, that they are great personages like Jesus Christ or the president of the United States, or that they are being persecuted by a group like the CIA.
- *Auditory hallucinations.* Schizophrenic people may hear voices when no one is present.
- *Deteriorating social and work functioning.* Social withdrawal and increasingly poor performance at school or work may be so gradual that they are hardly noticed at first.

None of these characteristics is invariably present. Some schizophrenic people are quite logical except on the subject of their delusions. Others show disorganized thoughts but no delusions or hallucinations.

A schizophrenic person needs help from a mental health professional. Suicide is a risk in schizophrenia, and expert treatment can reduce that risk and minimize the social consequences of the illness by shortening the period when symptoms are active. The key element in treatment is regular medication. At times medication is like insulin for diabetes—it makes the difference between being able to function or not. Sometimes hospitalization is temporarily required to relieve family and friends.

PERSONAL INSIGHT When you see people talking to themselves or acting strangely on the street, how do you feel? What do you do? Do you wonder what's going on in their mind? Do you label them as "sick"? What do you think causes them to act so strangely?

MODELS OF HUMAN NATURE AND THERAPEUTIC CHANGE

How people see the world is shaped largely by the model—the picture—of reality they carry in their minds. We will examine four of the most useful models of human nature: the biological, behavioral, cognitive, and psychoanalytic. As a way of understanding these models, let's consider the example of Rob.

Rob is a college student who finds himself so anxious whenever he's about to contribute to a class discussion that he can barely utter a word. In one month, all students in this class are expected to make a brief oral presentation on a special topic. Rob's instructor is beginning to believe that Rob is either uninterested, not doing the assigned reading, or not bright enough for college. Rob has always been a shy person, but until recently he's been able to speak in public situations if he really tries. However, a few weeks ago when he began to answer a question in class, he suddenly felt so nervous he couldn't continue. He started to sweat, lost his breath, and could feel his heart pounding. It was terribly embarrassing to have to stop speaking before he could complete his answer. Now he gets anxious just going into the classroom. All of this depresses him and makes him think about dropping out of school. Rob's mother was a schoolteacher until she died of heart disease a year ago. She was a strict person and often critical of her son. Rob's father is still living. He's an easygoing man who tends to drink too much in the evenings and on weekends. We now present the four principal models, their views on psychological problems, and how they might approach Rob's case.

The Biological Model

The biological model is used more in the context of mental illness than in the context of psychological health. It emphasizes that the mind's activity depends completely

TERMS

mania A mood disorder characterized by excessive elation, irritability, talkativeness, inflated self-esteem, and expansiveness.

bipolar disorder A mental illness characterized by alternating periods of depression and mania.

schizophrenia A psychological disorder that involves a disturbance in thinking and in perceiving reality.

Research over the past 50 years has found that many psychological disorders have a biological basis in disordered brain chemistry. This discovery has led to a revolution in the treatment of many disorders, particularly depression, which affects millions of Americans each year. The new view of depression as based in brain chemistry has also lessened the stigma attached to the condition, leading more people to seek treatment; and antidepressants are now among the most widely prescribed drugs in the United States. The development of effective drugs has provided relief for many people, but wide use of antidepressants has also raised many questions. Are drugs truly the best treatment for all patients? Does psychotherapy also have a role? And should antidepressants be used by people who are not suffering from a psychological disorder?

Antidepressants affect the activity of key neurotransmitters in the brain, including serotonin, dopamine, and noradrenaline. Older types of drugs—heterocyclics and monoamine oxidase inhibitors—are still frequently prescribed. Among the most popular of the newer drugs are the selective serotonin reuptake inhibitors (SSRIs), which include Prozac (fluoxetine), Paxil (paroxetine), and Zoloft (sertraline); Effexor (venlafaxine); and Wellbutrin (bupropion). The herb St. John's wort, used in Germany for mild depression, may also affect serotonin levels and is currently being tested in the United States. As a dietary supplement, however, St. John's wort is not currently regulated, so dosages may vary widely. Anyone who may be suffering from depression should seek a medical evaluation rather than self-treating with a supplement (see Chapter 12 for more on dietary supplements).

Although effective for many people, antidepressants do have side effects and risks. Prozac, for example, may cause nausea and a lessening of sexual pleasure. Several weeks of treatment may be necessary before a medication controls symptoms of depression, and an individual may need to try several drugs to find one that is effective for her or him and has acceptable side effects. For moderate to severe depression, treatment for up to a year may be needed to prevent a relapse.

Given the ability of antidepressants to affect brain chemistry and control symptoms, does psychotherapy still have a role in the treatment of depression? It is almost paradoxical that the emphasis on drug therapy over psychotherapy for mental illness has occurred at the same time as interest has grown in the impact of emotional factors on such physical illnesses as heart disease and cancer. Some mental health professionals worry that health insurance companies, in an effort to save money, will favor drug therapy over psychotherapy for all patients.

Research indicates that for mild cases of depression, psychotherapy and antidepressants are about equally effective. For major depression, combined therapy is significantly more effective than either type of treatment alone. Psychotherapy may be particularly important for people whose depression has a strong psychosocial component. Therapy can help provide insight into factors that precipitated the depression, such as high levels of stress, a history of physical or emotional abuse, unresolved grief, or relationship or financial problems. A therapist can also provide guidance in changing patterns of thinking and behavior that contribute to the problem.

What about the use of antidepressants to treat unwanted personality traits in psychologically healthy people? Anecdotal evidence suggests that Prozac and other SSRIs may help shy or pessimistic people become more outgoing and optimistic, for example. The potential use of antidepressants in this way has sparked ethical debate. Is some degree of vulnerability, anxiety, and sadness an essential part of being human? If antidepressants diminish or eliminate these feelings, will they rob people of the emotional experiences they need to grow and be creative? By masking mental pain, will they interfere with people's connection to reality and to their own emotional experience and expression? This ethical debate extends beyond the question of therapeutic benefits of antidepressants.

---

on an organic structure, the brain, whose composition is genetically determined. The brain can be damaged by infectious agents, such as viruses or bacteria, or by physical trauma, such as that which sometimes accompanies birth. Such damage can produce mental abnormalities. Chemical compounds introduced into the body can induce abnormal mental states that are similar to certain natural psychological disorders; chemicals can also partially reverse such mental symptoms.

Certain abilities and personality characteristics may have a genetic basis. Evidence shows a link between genes and certain kinds of schizophrenia and depression. Genetic explanations of behavior, however, do not mean that the environment has no influence. Genes vary in what is called *penetrance,* the likelihood that they will actually be expressed in the individual. Environmental influences include events surrounding birth and stresses in childhood, adolescence, and adulthood.

What can a biological model say about our student Rob? He is shy, a personality trait that usually begins in early childhood and has a genetic basis. Taking an anti-anxiety medication before going to class might help him overcome his speech inhibitions, but the dose would have to be low or he might get sleepy and have trouble organizing his thoughts. He would have to be careful not to become dependent on such a drug because of his father's tendency toward alcoholism. If Rob inherited this tendency, he might become addicted to tranquilizers. Since Rob had something like a panic attack, he might be suffering from a form of panic disorder, in which case certain antidepressants might be advisable.

Although evidence does not firmly prove the correctness of the biological model for any psychological health problem, it has been useful in motivating scientists to develop new drugs for treating symptoms (see the box "Lifting Depression with Drug Therapy"). Once a drug is proven to be safe and effective, it receives approval from the U.S. Food and Drug Administration (FDA), which allows psychiatrists and other physicians to prescribe it. While these medications have been immensely helpful, it is important to remember that all drugs have side effects. Focusing too narrowly on biology can result in the over-prescribing of drugs. Even those that are not physically addictive can become substitutes for more effective ways of dealing with psychological problems.

The Behavioral Model

The behavioral model focuses on what people do—their overt behavior—rather than on brain structures and chemistry or thoughts and consciousness. This model regards psychological problems as "maladaptive behavior," or bad habits. When and how a person learned bad behavior in the past is less important than what makes it continue in the present. Behaviorists analyze behavior in terms of **stimulus, response,** and **reinforcement.**

The essence of behavior therapy is to analyze an undesirable behavior in terms of the reinforcements that keep it going, then to try to alter those reinforcements. Clients are asked to keep a daily behavior journal to monitor the target behavior and events that precede and follow it (see the snacking example in Chapter 1).

Rob might start a behavioral therapy program by writing down each time he makes a contribution to a classroom discussion and how much time he actually speaks. He would then develop concrete but realistic goals for increasing this amount each week, and contract with himself to reward his successes by spending more time in activities he finds enjoyable. For example, his goals might first be to briefly contribute to class discussions, then to make longer statements, then to volunteer to lead discussions, and finally to give a formal presentation. He can arrange for circumstances that make him more likely to speak, such as adequate preclass preparation or looking at a friendly classmate while speaking, to happen more frequently. Chapter 1 explains other useful measures, such as developing social support for behavior change and using role models.

Exposure is a primary therapeutic method for overcoming the fear of certain places and activities. The treatment program designed for Rob contains the essential ingredient of exposure: practice in speaking in the classroom arranged in assignments of gradually increasing difficulty. Other elements include staying in a feared situation until the fear has abated somewhat. (Leaving when fear is still high causes immediate relief, which acts as a reinforcement of avoidance and escape.) Therapists can have various roles: They help set up the assignments, accompany clients on their assignments, and organize groups of clients to do their assignments together.

Systematic desensitization, which involves imagining the feared object or situation while maintaining relax-

ation, is another behavioral technique for overcoming fears. A model of a desensitization program is given in the Behavior Change Strategy at the end of Chapter 2.

The Cognitive Model

The cognitive model emphasizes the effect of ideas on behavior and feelings. According to this model, behavior results from complicated attitudes, expectations, and motives rather than from simple, immediate reinforcements. When behavioral therapies such as exposure work, it is because they change the way a person thinks about the feared situation and his or her ability to cope with it.

One cognitive theory says that automatically recurring false ideas produce feelings such as anxiety and depression. Identifying and exposing these ideas as false should relieve the painful emotions. When people are anxious, the idea behind the anxiety is "Something bad is going to happen and I won't be able to handle it." The therapist challenges such ideas in three ways: showing that there isn't enough evidence for the idea, suggesting different ways of looking at the situation, and showing that no disaster is going to occur. The therapist does not just *state* his or her position, but encourages clients to examine the logic of their own ideas and then to test the truth of the ideas.

In our example, Rob was afraid to speak up in class and probably harbored such ideas as "If I begin to speak, I'll say something stupid; if I say something stupid, the teacher and my classmates will lose respect for me; then I'll get a low grade, my classmates will avoid me, and life will be hell." In cognitive therapy, Rob would be taught to examine these ideas critically. If he prepares for the presentation, how likely is it that he'll sound stupid? Does Rob actually believe that everything he's going to say will sound stupid, or is he really aiming for an impossible perfection, every sentence exactly correct and beautifully delivered? Will people's opinion of Rob be completely transformed by how he does in one presentation? Do his classmates even care that much about how well he does? And why does *he* care so much about what *they* think? Rob will be taught to notice his thoughts in feared situations and to substitute more realistic ideas for them. The therapist will advise him to speak in front of the class again and test his assumptions.

TERMS

stimulus Anything that causes a response.

response A reaction to a stimulus.

reinforcement Increasing the future probability of a response by following it with a reward.

exposure A therapeutic technique for treating fear, in which the subject learns to come into direct contact with a feared situation.

systematic desensitization A therapeutic technique for treating phobia, in which a phobic stimulus is vividly imagined while relaxation is maintained.

The Psychoanalytic Model

The psychoanalytic model also emphasizes thoughts, but it says that false ideas cannot be fought directly because they are fed by other ideas that are **unconscious.** Sigmund Freud, a Viennese neurologist, developed these revolutionary theories around 1900. He discovered that certain paralyses that had no apparent physical basis and certain losses of sensory function (such as some cases of blindness) were better understood in terms of patients' hidden (unconscious) wishes than in terms of nerve pathways. The ideas that were disturbing behavior were at first hidden from both patient and therapist, but gradually surfaced in dreams, verbal slips, and the patient's behavior toward the therapist. Freud removed the moral stigma from such behavior by saying that patients had no conscious intention to deceive. In fact, such behavior was a medical disorder appropriately studied and treated by physicians. He also refused to make any sharp distinction between the mentally healthy and the mentally ill. We all have irrational ideas, and we can't consciously control all of our own acts.

Therapies based on Freud's ideas do not take symptoms as isolated pieces of behavior but as results of a complex system of secret wishes, emotions, and fantasies hidden by active defenses that keep them unconscious. Defense mechanisms (see Table 3-2) operate unconsciously to conceal the truth so that people can both lie to themselves *and* hide from themselves that they have lied. The concealed truth turns out to derive from wishes, often sexual or aggressive, that are unacceptable to society as well as to the individual's conscience.

Today, the psychoanalytic model is often criticized for being unscientific and therapeutically ineffective. Yet certain of its basic ideas persist. One is that people will become more psychologically healthy if they get to know themselves better, but that self-honesty can be painful. Another idea is that disclosing one's fears and secrets to another person who can be trusted has therapeutic value. Good therapists allow their clients to express themselves as freely as possible.

If Rob received therapy inspired by this model, he would find a therapist interested in not only his public speaking problem but also the totality of his personality. Rob might learn some new things about himself. He would realize that his speaking anxiety was part of a more general problem of shyness and low self-esteem. Standing up in front of others and letting them see him might make him feel as if he were under attack. For example, he might fear others will notice unpleasant traits he thinks he has. And Rob might recall childhood experiences related to his current difficulties, such as being ridiculed by a parent for a stammer he had as a young child and might understand the impact of his critical mother and her recent death. In doing so, he might learn to distance himself from childish ways of thinking and reacting, such as a panicky avoidance of all public speaking.

Implications of the Four Models

The merits of these models are the focus of active debate. Behaviorists and cognitive therapists (usually psychologists) accuse supporters of the biological model (usually psychiatrists) of endangering clients with drug side effects and dependence. They attack psychoanalytically oriented psychotherapists for making a client pay for endless therapy. Psychoanalytically oriented therapists retaliate by accusing adherents of the other models of simplistic thinking, of regarding human beings as machines without rights or responsibilities.

The fact is that each model represents certain truths (see the box "David: A True Story"). Each model can help people deal with specific types of human problems. When two therapies compete to solve the same problem, scientific studies should be conducted to measure rival claims. At present, strong evidence suggests that some therapy is better than no therapy. Effectiveness is hard to demonstrate for therapies that do not focus on specific problems or symptoms, because measuring the changes that occur is difficult, and various therapists' skills come into play. There are important practical considerations, too. Some people and some problems cannot wait long enough for slow-acting treatments to work.

> **PERSONAL INSIGHT**   How do you react when you hear that someone is in therapy? Does it make a difference in how you feel about the person?

GETTING HELP

Knowing when self-help or professional help is required for mental health problems is usually not as difficult as knowing how to start or which professional to choose.

Self-Help

If you have a personal problem to solve, a smart way to begin is finding out what you can do on your own. Some problems are specifically addressed in this book. Behavioral and some cognitive approaches are especially useful for helping yourself. They all involve becoming more aware of self-defeating actions and ideas and combating them in some way: being more assertive; communicating honestly; raising your self-esteem by counteracting thoughts, people, and actions that undermine it; and confronting, rather than avoiding, the things you fear. Get more information by seeing what books are available in

TERMS   **unconscious**   In the mind but out of awareness.

David: A True Story

When a person begins to act strangely in public or with friends or family, others rarely agree about what the behavior means. Opinions vary, based on levels of education or sophistication, and conflicting viewpoints even occur between the best educated and most knowledgeable people. Conflicts between models of psychological health are not just theoretical but have practical results, as this case history illustrates. Only the subject's name and a few details have been changed to maintain confidentiality.

David was a 20-year-old junior at a large, competitive university, majoring in humanities. He had been the best all-around student in his high school class. The high school principal remembered him as brilliant and caring. In college, David maintained an outstanding academic record. Students in his dorm said he was cheerful, outgoing, and "laid back." For 6 months he had been attending meditation classes, had become a vegetarian, and had started to jog daily. He avoided all drugs, including alcohol. Shortly before spring vacation, he told a friend he had been hearing voices and seeing "real" visions. He was convinced that the end of the world—the "Last Judgment"—was coming. He talked of taking his own life because he felt unworthy, and said that his death would help humanity. In contrast to his usual cheerfulness, he became withdrawn and isolated. The worried friend called David's father, who lived far away. The father talked to his son several times by phone and arranged to fly up to see him in a week. The day before they were to meet, David jumped off a high bridge and drowned.

How did different people make sense of what happened? In his father's opinion, David's suicide was a result of spiritual striving—a deep interest in Eastern religions—combined with a drive for perfection in everything he attempted. According to his father, David was totally committed in life and in death. The problem his son had faced was trying to live simultaneously in both a world of reality and a world devoted to spirituality.

His friend took a medical point of view. He thought David's visions and voices sounded schizophrenic. The father agreed only partially. From his phone conversations, he felt something had temporarily snapped in David's mind. Perhaps a biochemical change had altered his mental state. But during the last phone call, the day before the suicide, his son seemed to have become completely lucid and calm again. David assured him he was OK now, that his father could stop worrying. They would see each other soon. His father found consolation in the thought that his son had found a kind of peace at the end. Yet to many who knew David, the story was only a tragedy—a talented, kind young person with most of his life in front of him died before the seriousness of his problems was recognized and treatment could be begun.

There is a strong temptation to lay blame here. Was his father spiritualizing a schizophrenic disorder? Of all people, the father, who had known his son for all of his 20 years, should have recognized that something was wrong. But his father lived far away and was merely empathetically supporting his son's spiritual quest. Religious impulses and spiritual crises are usually not crazy; they can have positive outcomes. And why didn't his friend intervene more actively? He could have contacted a dean, faculty member, or someone at the student health service and insisted that someone in authority step in. Perhaps his respect for David made him hesitate. David might have felt betrayed if he had been hospitalized. And what kind of place was it, where a student could become so troubled yet so few people notice it? But many large universities do not watch students very closely, because they believe students should be treated as adults, with a right to privacy and to living with few rules. Troubled students often keep to themselves; not allowing them to do so would be forcing them to conform.

Thus, we cannot convincingly lay blame, but we can hope that in the future, better informed students, parents, and college administrators will be more sensitive to warning signs like the ones in this case: hearing voices and seeing visions, a major and sudden change in personality, suicidal thoughts, and the ominous false calm that can follow a firm decision to commit suicide.

---

the psychology or self-help sections of libraries and bookstores. But be selective. Watch out for self-help books making fantastic claims that deviate from mainstream approaches.

Some people find it helpful to express their feelings in a journal. Grappling with a painful experience in this way provides an emotional release and can help you develop more constructive ways of dealing with similar situations in the future. Research indicates that using a journal this way can improve physical as well as emotional wellness.

For some people, religious belief and practice may promote psychological health. Religious organizations provide a social network and a supportive community, and religious practices, such as prayer and meditation, offer a path for personal change and transformation.

Peer Counseling and Support Groups

Sharing your concerns with others is another helpful way of dealing with psychological health challenges. Just being able to share what's troubling you with an accepting, empathetic person can bring relief. Comparing notes with people who have problems similar to yours can give you new ideas about coping.

Many colleges offer peer counseling through a health center or through the psychology or education department. Peer counseling is usually done by volunteer students who have received special training that emphasizes confidentiality. Peer counselors may steer you toward an appropriate campus or community resource, or simply offer a sympathetic ear.

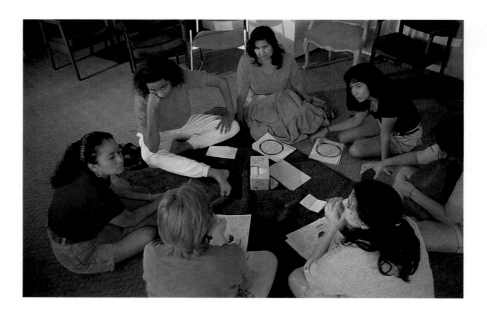

Group therapy is just one of many different approaches to psychological counseling. If you have concerns you would like to discuss with a mental health professional, shop around to find the approach that works for you.

Many self-help groups work on the principle of bringing together people with similar problems to share their experiences and support each other. Support groups are typically organized around a specific issue or problem, such as eating disorders or substance abuse. Self-help groups may be listed in the phone book or campus newspaper.

Professional Help

Sometimes self-help or talking to nonprofessionals is not enough. More objective, more expert, or more discreet help is needed. Many people have trouble accepting the need for professional help, and often those who most need help are the most unwilling to get it. You may someday find yourself having to overcome your own reluctance, or that of a friend, about seeking help.

Determining the Need for Professional Help In some cases, professional help is optional. Some people are interested in improving their psychological health in a general way by going into individual or group therapy to learn more about themselves and how to interact with others. Certain therapies teach people how to adjust the effect of what they say and do on people around them. Clearly, seeking professional help for these reasons is a matter of individual choice. Interpersonal friction among family members or between partners often falls in the middle between necessary and optional. Successful help with such problems can mean the difference between a painful divorce and a satisfying relationship.

It's sometimes difficult to determine whether someone needs professional help, but it is important to be aware of behaviors that may indicate a serious problem. Following are some strong indications that you or someone else needs professional help:

- If depression, anxiety, or other emotional problems begin to interfere seriously with school or work performance, or in getting along with others.
- If suicide is attempted or is seriously considered (refer to the warning signs earlier in the chapter).
- If symptoms such as hallucinations, delusions, incoherent speech, or loss of memory occur.
- If alcohol or drugs are used to the extent that they impair normal functioning during much of the week, if finding or taking drugs occupies much of the week, or if reducing their dosage leads to psychological or physiological withdrawal symptoms.

Choosing a Mental Health Professional Mental health workers belong to several different professions and have different roles. Psychiatrists are medical doctors. They are experts in deciding whether a medical disease lies behind psychological symptoms, and they are usually involved in treatment if medication or hospitalization is required. Clinical psychologists typically hold a Ph.D. degree; they are often experts in behavioral and cognitive therapies. Other mental health workers include social workers, licensed counselors, and clergy with special training in pastoral counseling. In hospitals and clinics, various mental health professionals may join together in treatment teams. For more on finding appropriate help, see the box "Choosing and Evaluating Mental Health Professionals."

PERSONAL INSIGHT   If you were feeling depressed or anxious or were having trouble in a relationship, would you be tempted to see a counselor or therapist? If so, how would you choose among the various therapeutic types?

College students are usually in a good position to find convenient, affordable mental health care. Larger schools typically have both health services that employ psychiatrists and psychologists and counseling centers staffed by professionals and student peer counselors. Resources in the community may include a school of medicine, a hospital, and a variety of professionals who work independently. Although independent practitioners are listed in the telephone book, it's a good idea to get recommendations from physicians, clergy, friends who've been in therapy, or community agencies rather than pick a name at random.

Financial considerations are also important. Find out how much different services will cost and what your health insurance will cover. If you're not adequately covered by a health plan, don't let that stop you from getting help; investigate low-cost alternatives. City, county, and state governments often support mental health clinics for those who can afford to pay little or nothing for treatment. Some on-campus services may be free or offered at very little cost.

The cost of treatment is linked to how many therapy sessions will be needed, which in turn depends on the type of therapy and the nature of the problem. Psychological therapies focusing on specific problems may require eight or ten sessions at weekly intervals. Therapies aiming for psychological awareness and personality change can last months or years.

Deciding whether a therapist is right for you will require meeting the therapist in person. Before or during your first meeting, find out about the therapist's background and training:

- Does she or he have a degree from an appropriate professional school and a state license to practice?

- Has she or he had experience treating people with problems similar to yours?
- How much will therapy cost?

You have a right to know the answers to these questions and should not hesitate to ask them. After your initial meeting, evaluate your impressions:

- Does the therapist seem like a warm, intelligent person who would be able to help you and interested in doing so?
- Are you comfortable with the personality, values, and beliefs of the therapist?
- Is he or she willing to talk about the techniques in use? Do these techniques make sense to you?

If you answer yes to these questions, this therapist may be satisfactory for you. If you feel uncomfortable—and you're not in need of emergency care—it's worthwhile to set up one-time consultations with one or two others before you make up your mind. Take the time to find someone who feels right for you.

Later in your treatment, evaluate your progress:

- Are you being helped by the treatment?
- If you are displeased, is it because you aren't making progress or because therapy is raising difficult, painful issues you don't want to deal with?
- Can you express dissatisfaction to your therapist? Such feedback can improve your treatment.

If you're convinced your therapy isn't working or is harmful, thank your therapist for her or his efforts, and find another.

SUMMARY

What Psychological Health Is Not

- Psychological health encompasses more than a single particular state of normality. Psychological diversity is valuable among groups of people.
- Getting professional help does not necessarily indicate the presence of mental illness. Neither symptoms nor appearances are reliable indicators of an individual's psychological health.

Defining Psychological Health

- A definition of psychological health as the absence of illness focuses attention on the most serious problems and the people in greatest need of help.
- Defining psychological health as the presence of wellness means that to be healthy you must strive to fulfill your potential.
- Maslow's definition of psychological health centered on self-actualization, the highest level in his hierar-

chy of needs. Self-actualized people have high self-esteem and are realistic, inner-directed, authentic, capable of emotional intimacy, and creative.

Meeting Life's Challenges

- Crucial parts of psychological wellness include developing an adult identity, establishing intimate relationships, and finding a sense of meaning and purpose in life.
- A sense of self-esteem develops during childhood as a result of giving and receiving love and learning to accomplish goals. Self-concept is challenged every day; healthy people adjust their goals to their abilities.
- Using defense mechanisms to cope with problems can make finding solutions harder. Analyzing thoughts and behavior can help people develop less defensive and more effective ways of coping.
- A pessimistic outlook can damage psychological well-being; it can be overcome by developing more realistic self-talk.

Everyone is lonely at times, but some people have a harder time meeting new people, initiating friendships, and establishing romantic or sexual relationships than others do. In some cases, the problem is social anxiety, also known as shyness, social inhibition, or interpersonal anxiety. This Behavior Change Strategy describes some of the ways the problem of social anxiety is approached in various programs.

Many programs focus on the variety of subtle social skills needed to initiate and sustain interpersonal relationships. These skills include appropriate eye contact, a sense of humor, facial expression, initiating topics in conversation, and maintaining the flow of conversation by asking questions. One general treatment program assumes a *skills-deficit perspective*. This program teaches college students how to use interpersonal skills to greater personal advantage by means of videotape feedback and modeling (practice exercises). Practice dating programs, in which both partners know that their interaction has been scheduled for practice and self-improvement, help extend modeling well beyond the clinic into actual social settings.

A slightly different approach stems from the belief that people know how to make and keep friends; the problem of social inhibition comes from the anxiety that reduces a person's ability to perform key social skills. Reduced performance produces even greater self-doubt and anxiety, causing a repeating cycle of damaging experiences. With this approach, people for whom anxiety plays a key role receive special training in relaxation skills and other stress-management strategies, perhaps in conjunction with the more complex anxiety-reduction procedure known as *systematic desensitization*.

In most cases, shyness and loneliness are not easily diagnosed as being only a problem of skills or only a problem of anxiety. Most programs assume that *both* skills and anxiety play a role and provide comprehensive treatment that includes modeling, structural practice, and stress-management components.

Programs usually begin with a self-monitoring phase, in which all facets of a person's daily routine are noted in a journal format. The sample Social Activity Journal, shown here, uses a coding scheme (which is noted in the key) to help track the pattern of social contacts, the amount of time spent in effective studying, and the amount of time wasted each day. These patterns are monitored for at least 1 week, to identify general trends.

Depending on the particular program, the shy person is encouraged to make better use of "wasted time," and to begin practicing some of the skills he or she has learned in the class or clinic in the least anxiety-producing situations. This tactic might be translated into an assignment (and behavioral contract) to initiate brief, nonthreatening conversations with classmates on an academic topic (the upcoming midterm or the homework assignment, for example). Once these conversations are successfully accomplished, the next phase of the program could encourage practicing discussions that involve more personal subjects (personal opinions about nonacademic topics). Later assignments might involve social gatherings. The individual steps would form a type of hierarchy, incorporating topics, people, and places, from least to most difficult.

The person would accomplish these steps by using a consistent theme of practice, modeling, and stress-management skills

- Honest communication requires recognizing what needs to be said and the ability to say it clearly. Assertiveness enables people to insist on their rights and to participate in the give-and-take of good communication.

- Dealing successfully with anger involves distinguishing between a reasonable level of assertiveness and gratuitous expressions of anger, and developing a flexible range of responses to anger.

Psychological Disorders

- People with psychological disorders have symptoms severe enough to interfere with daily living.

- Anxiety is a fear that is not directed toward any definite threat. Anxiety disorders include simple phobias, social phobias, panic disorder, obsessive-compulsive disorder, and post-traumatic stress disorder.

- Depression is a common mood disorder; loss of interest or pleasure in things seems to be its most

universal symptom. Severe depression carries a high risk of suicide, and suicidally depressed people need professional help.

- Symptoms of mania include exalted moods with unrealistically high self-esteem, little need for sleep, and rapid speech. Mood swings between mania and depression characterize bipolar disorder.

- Schizophrenia is characterized by disorganized thoughts, inappropriate emotions, delusions, auditory hallucinations, and deteriorating social and work performance.

Models of Human Nature and Therapeutic Change

- The biological model emphasizes that the mind's activity depends on the brain, whose composition is genetically determined.

- The behavioral model focuses on overt behavior and treats psychological problems as bad habits.

- The cognitive model considers how ideas affect behavior and feelings; behavior results from compli-

while moving up the hierarchy. Using these techniques, the person increases social skills and confidence levels, at the same time decreasing anxiety and feelings of insecurity, until social interactions can be sustained with comfort and enjoyment.

To evaluate your own level of social anxiety, examine the following list of statements made by college students identified as lonely in a Stanford University study. These students said that it was difficult for them to:

- Make friends in a simple, natural way.
- Introduce themselves to others at parties.
- Participate in groups.
- Get into the swing of a party.

A sample Social Activity Journal.
Key:
P = Social phone call
I = Social interaction (at least 5 minutes)
A = Social activity
S = Study time
W = Wasted time

- Relax on a date and enjoy themselves.
- Be friendly and sociable with others.
- Make phone calls to others to initiate social activity.

These statements suggest a level of social anxiety and inhibition that interferes with dating and making friends. If they describe you, consider looking into a shyness clinic or treatment program on your campus.

	DATE:	11/16	DATE:		DATE:	
	A.M.	P.M.	A.M.	P.M.	A.M.	P.M.
12		I, I, W				
1		A W				
2		S				
3		S				
4		S				
5		I, I				
6		W				
7		W				
8		S				
9		S, P, P				
10	I, I, S	S				
11	S	W				

cated attitudes, expectations, and motives, not just from simple reinforcements.

- The psychoanalytic model asserts that false ideas are fed by unconscious ideas and cannot be addressed directly.
- Different models lead to different approaches to treatment; each can help people deal with certain types of problems.

Getting Help

- Help is available in a variety of forms, including self-help, peer counseling, support groups, and therapy with a mental health professional. For serious problems, professional help may be the most appropriate.
- Mental health professionals have various forms of training and play different roles in treatment.

TAKE ACTION

1. Investigate the mental health services on your campus and in your community. What services are available? Think about which ones you would feel comfortable using, for either yourself or someone else, should the need ever arise.

2. Many colleges and communities have peer counseling programs, hotline services (for both general problems and specific issues such as rape, suicide, and drug abuse), and other kinds of emergency counseling services. Some programs are staffed by trained volunteers.

Investigate such programs in your school (through the health clinic or student services) or community (look in the yellow pages), and consider volunteering for one. The training and experience can help you understand both yourself and others.

3. Being assertive rather than passive or aggressive is a valuable skill that everyone can learn. To improve your ability to assert yourself appropriately, sign up for a workshop or class in assertiveness training on your campus or in your community.

1. Do you remember incidents or moments from childhood that stand out as wonderful or horrible? Write a short essay about two such incidents, including what your feelings were and what you think you learned from them. Then describe what you would do now in the same situations and why.

2. **Critical Thinking** In the past, some political candidates have dropped out of a race or been defeated after it was revealed that they had undergone psychiatric treatment or some other form of therapy. Do you think a person who has been treated for a mental illness should be excluded from holding a public office or from any other profession? Why or why not? Does your position depend on the type of illness or the treatment the individual received? In your health journal, write a brief essay explaining your position.

3. Think about a person you respect. Describe him or her in writing, listing the qualities you admire. Do you have any of those qualities? What does your list say about the kind of person you want to be?

Books

Fancher, R. 1997. *Cultures of Healing: Correcting the Image of American Mental Health Care.* New York: W. H. Freeman. *A provocative book that explores various schools of mental health theory and treatment, suggesting that they are competing cultures built on ideology and subjective beliefs.*

Francis, A., and M. B. First. 1999. *Your Mental Health: A Layman's Guide to the Psychiatrist's Bible.* New York: Scribner. *A resource-packed reference with information on dozens of mental disorders; based on the APA's DSM-IV.*

Grohol, J. M., and E. L. Zuckerman. 1999. *An Insider's Guide to Mental Health Resources Online.* New York: Guilford Press. *Explains and rates Internet search engines, newsgroups, and Web sites devoted to mental health.*

Jamison, K. R. 1997. *An Unquiet Mind.* New York: Random House. *A psychiatrist describes her own experience with manic-depressive illness.*

Lester, D. 1997. *Making Sense of Suicide: An In-Depth Look at Why People Kill Themselves.* Philadelphia: Charles Press. *An exploration of the reasons why people take their own lives.*

O'Connor, R. 1999. *Undoing Depression.* New York: Berkley Pub. *A guide to help people deal with depression in their thinking, behavior, emotions, and relationships.*

Papolos, D. F., and J. Papolos. 1997. *Overcoming Depression,* 3rd ed. New York: HarperCollins. *Practical advice and up-to-date medical information with a biological orientation that is particularly appropriate for severe mood disorders.*

Rapee, R. M. 1998. *Overcoming Shyness and Social Phobia: A Step-by-Step Guide.* Northvale, N.J.: Jason Aronson. *Practical advice based on proven psychotherapy techniques.*

Seligman, M. E. P. 1998. *Learned Optimism.* New York: Pocket Books. *A discussion of the effects of pessimism, optimism, and learned helplessness, with suggestions for change.*

Slater, L. 1998. *Prozac Diary.* New York: Random House. *A psychologist's insightful account of her own struggles with depression and obsessive-compulsive disorder and her experience with long-term drug therapy.*

Zuercher-White, E. 1998. *An End to Panic,* 2nd ed. Oakland, Calif.: New Harbinger. *Presents a variety of standard self-help techniques, including controlling breathing and developing more realistic self-talk.*

Organizations, Hotlines, and Web Sites

American Psychiatric Association (APA). Provides public information by pamphlet or online about a variety of topics, including depression, anxiety, eating disorders, and psychiatric medications.
> 1400 K St., N.W.
> Washington, DC 20005
> 202-682-6000; 888-357-7924 (fast FAX)
> http://www.psych.org

American Psychological Association Consumer HelpCenter. Provides information about common challenges to psychological health and about how to obtain professional help.
> 800-964-2000
> http://helping.apa.org

Anxiety Disorders Association of America (ADAA). Provides information and resources related to anxiety disorders, including listings of support groups.
> 301-231-9350
> http://www.adaa.org

Internet Mental Health. An encyclopedia of mental health information, including medical diagnostic criteria.
> http://www.mentalhealth.com

Mental Health Net. A comprehensive guide to mental health online, including background information and links for many topics.
> http://www.cmhc.com

NAMI (National Alliance for the Mentally Ill). Provides information and support for people who are affected by mental illness.
> 800-950-NAMI (Help Line)
> http://www.nami.org

National Depressive and Manic-Depressive Association (NDMDA). Provides educational materials and information about support groups and other resources.
> 730 N. Franklin St., Suite 501
> Chicago, IL 60610
> 800-82-NDMDA
> http://www.ndmda.org

National Institute of Mental Health (NIMH). Provides helpful information about anxiety, depression, eating disorders, and other challenges to psychological health.
> 5600 Fishers Ln.
> Rockville, MD 20857

800-421-4211 (NIMH information line); 301-443-4513
http://www.nimh.nih.gov

National Mental Health Association. Provides consumer information on a variety of issues, including how to find help.

1021 Prince St.
Alexandria, VA 22314
800-969-NMHA
http://www.nmha.org

National Mental Health Services Knowledge and Exchange Network (KEN). A one-stop source for information and resources relating to mental health.

800-789-CMHS
http://www.mentalhealth.org

New York University. Psychiatry Information for the General Public. Provides online screening tests for depression, anxiety, personality disorders, and other mental health problems.

http://www.med.nyu.edu/Psych/public.html

Psych Central: Dr. John Grohol's Mental Health Page. A guide to psychology, support, and mental health issues, resources, and people on the Internet.

http://psychcentral.com

Student Counseling Virtual Pamphlet Collection. Provides links to more than 400 pamphlets produced by different student counseling centers; topics range from depression and anxiety to time management and assertiveness.

http://uhs.bsd.uchicago.edu/scrs/vpc/virtulets.html

SELECTED BIBLIOGRAPHY

Agency for Health Care Policy and Research (AHCPR). 1999. *Treatment of Depression—Newer Pharmacotherapies.* Rockville, MD; AHCPR Pub. No. 99-E014.

American Psychiatric Association. 1997 *APA Online Public Information: Psychotherapy* (retrieved October 13, 1998; http://www.psych.org/public_info/psythera.html).

American Psychiatric Association. 1994. *Diagnostic and Statistical Manual of Mental Disorders (DSM-IV),* 4th ed. Washington, D.C.: American Psychiatric Association Press.

Bergin, A. E., and S. L. Garfield. 1994. *Handbook of Psychotherapy and Behavior Change,* 4th ed. New York: Wiley.

Centers for Disease Control and Prevention. 1998. Self-reported frequent mental distress among adults—United States, 1993–1996. *Morbidity and Mortality Weekly Report* 47(16): 325–331.

Chang, E. C., and W. B. Bridewell. 1998. Irrational beliefs, optimism, pessimism, and psychological distress: A preliminary examination of differential effects in a college population. *Journal of Clinical Psychology* 54(2): 137–142.

Dodgson, P. G., and J. V. Wood. 1998. Self-esteem and the cognitive accessibility of strengths and weaknesses after failure. *Journal of Personality and Social Psychology* 75(1): 178–197.

Edwards, J. G. 1998. Long-term pharmacotherapy of depression can reduce relapses and recurrences in major depression. *British Medical Journal* 316(7139): 1180–1181.

Gorman, J. M. 1996. *The New Psychiatry.* New York: St. Martin's Press.

Haney, P., and J. A. Durlak. 1998. Changing self-esteem in children and adolescents: A meta-analytic review. *Journal of Clinical Child Psychology* 27(4): 423–433.

Hick, J. 1989. An *Interpretation of Religion: Human Responses to the Transcendent.* New Haven: Yale University Press.

Hinsie, L. E. 1999. The treatment of schizophrenia: A survey of the literature. *Psychiatric Quarterly* 70(1): 5–26.

Jackson, T. 1999. Differences in psychosocial experiences of employed, unemployed, and student samples of young adults. *Journal of Psychology* 133(1): 49–60.

Kender, K. S., and C. A. Prescott. 1999. A population-based twin study of lifetime major depression in men and women. *Archives of General Psychiatry* 56(1): 39–44.

Kohut, H. 1971. *The Psychology of the Self.* New York: International Universities Press.

Kramer, P. D. 1993. *Listening to Prozac.* New York: Viking.

Lazare, A. 1973. Hidden conceptual models in clinical psychiatry. *New England Journal of Medicine* 288: 345–351.

Leon, A. C., G. L. Klerman, and P. Wickramaratne. 1993. Continuing female predominance in depressive illness. *American Journal of Public Health* 83: 754–757.

Maslow, A. H. 1968. *Toward a Psychology of Being,* 2nd ed. Princeton, N.J.: Van Nostrand Reinhold.

Raikkonen, K., et al. 1999. Effects of optimism, pessimism, and trait anxiety on ambulatory blood pressure and mood during everyday life. *Journal of Personal and Social Psychology* 76(1): 104–113.

Reynolds, C. F., et al. 1999. Nortriptyline and interpersonal psychotherapy as maintenance therapies for recurrent major depression. *Journal of the American Medical Association* 281: 39–45.

Richards, P. S., and A. E. Bergin. 1997. *A Spiritual Strategy for Counseling and Psychotherapy.* Washington, D.C.: American Psychological Association.

Roth, W. T., ed. 1997. *Treating Anxiety Disorders.* San Francisco: Jossey-Bass.

Rustine, G. L., and S. Nolen-Hoeksema. 1998. Regulating responses to anger: Effects of rumination and distraction on angry mood. *Journal of Personality and Social Psychology* 74(3): 790–803.

Stein, M. B., et al. 1998. Paroxetine treatment of generalized social phobia. *Journal of the American Medical Association* 280(8): 708–713.

Stein, M. B., K. L. Jang, and W. J. Livesley. 1999. Heritability of anxiety sensitivity: A twin study. *American Journal of Psychiatry* 156(2): 246–251.

Thase, M. E., et al. 1997. Treatment of major depression with psychotherapy or psychotherapy-pharmacotherapy combinations. *Archives of General Psychiatry* 54(11): 1009–1015.

U.S. Department of Health and Human Services. 1998. *Healthy People 2010 Objectives: Draft for Public Comment.* Washington, D.C.: U.S. Government Printing Office.

U.S. Food and Drug Administration. 1998. Dealing with the depths of depression. *FDA Consumer Magazine,* July/August.

U.S. Pharmacopeia. 1998. *Consumer Information: Hypericum (St. John's Wort)* (retrieved August 31, 1998; http://www.usp.org/did/mgraphs/botanica/hypericum.htm).

Vaillant, G. E. 1977. *Adaptation to Life.* Boston: Little, Brown.

Van Ameringen, M., C. Mancini, and J. M. Oakman. 1998. The relationship of behavioral inhibition and shyness to anxiety disorder. *Journal of Nervous and Mental Disease* 186(7): 425–431.

Wenegrat, W. 1989. *The Divine Archetype: The Sociobiology and Psychology of Religion.* Lexington, Mass.: Lexington Books.

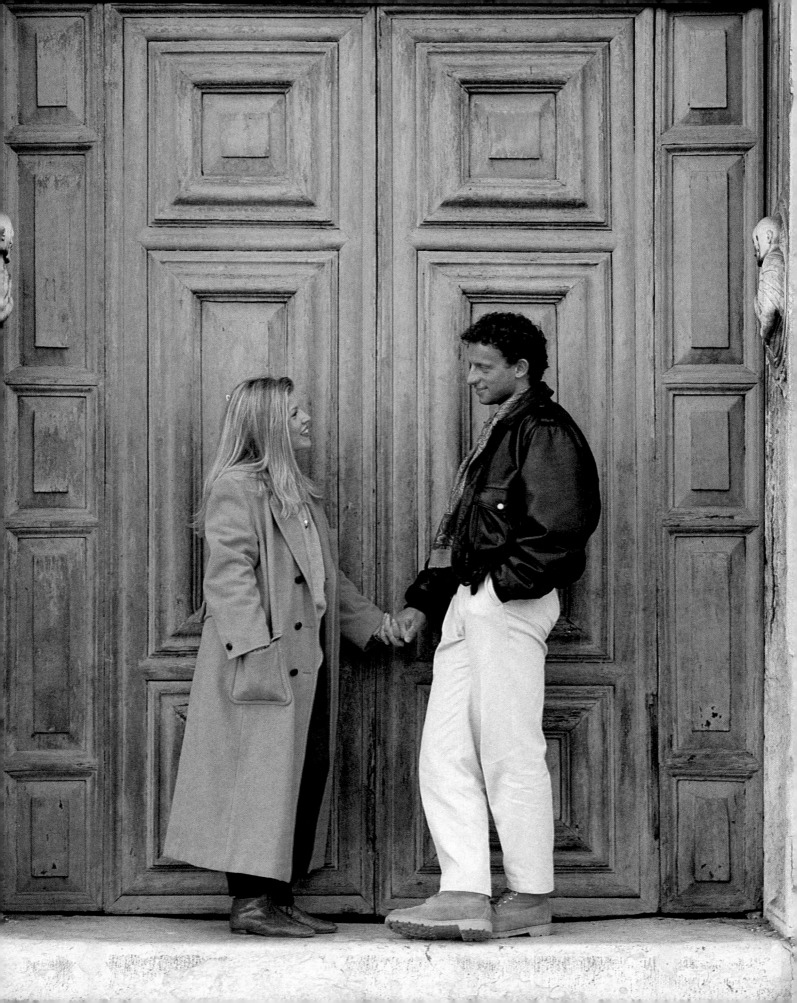

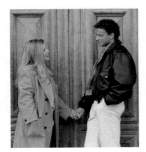

LEARNING OBJECTIVES

After reading this chapter, you should be able to:

- Explain the qualities that help people develop intimate relationships.
- Describe different types of love relationships and the stages they often go through.
- Discuss relationship options available to adults today.
- List some characteristics of successful families and some potential problems families face.
- Explain some of the joys and challenges of being a parent.

Intimate Relationships

4

TEST YOUR KNOWLEDGE

1. Couples who live together before marriage are less likely to get divorced than those who don't.
   True or false?

2. Which of the following is most characteristic of true, lasting love?
   a. jealousy
   b. commitment
   c. wanting to be together most of the time
   d. extreme sexual passion

3. Conflict and fighting are usually signs of trouble in intimate relationships.
   True or false?

4. What is the most common source of conflict for married couples?
   a. sex
   b. money
   c. friends

5. The love that lesbians and gay men experience is similar in quality to that experienced by heterosexuals.
   True or false?

6. What percentage of American households conform to the traditional model of wage-earning father, stay-at-home mother, and children?
   a. 5%
   b. 15%
   c. 30%

Answers

1. *False.* Studies have found that couples who cohabit before they get married are just as likely to divorce as those who don't cohabit.

2. *b.* The key to successful relationships isn't in love's intensity but in transforming passion into a love based on closeness, caring, and the promise of a shared future.

3. *False.* Conflict itself isn't a sign of trouble; it may mean a relationship is growing. What's important is how the partners handle the conflict.

4. *b.* Research indicates that the basic tasks of living together—how to handle money, how to divide housework, and so on—create the most conflict for couples.

5. *True.* Like heterosexual relationships, gay and lesbian partnerships provide intimacy, passion, and security. Most gay men and lesbians experience at least one long-term relationship with a single partner.

6. *b.* Dual-career couples now represent almost half of the U.S. labor force.

81

Human beings need social relationships; we cannot thrive as solitary creatures. Nor could the human species survive if adults didn't cherish and support each other, if we didn't form strong mutual attachments with our infants, and if we didn't create families in which to raise children. Simply put, people need people.

Although people are held together in relationships by a variety of factors, the foundation of many relationships is love. Love in its many forms—romantic, passionate, platonic, parental—is the wellspring from which much of life's meaning and delight flows. In our culture, it binds us together as partners, parents, children, and friends. People devote tremendous energy to seeking mates, nurturing intimate relationships, keeping up friendships, maintaining marriages—all for the pleasure of loving and being loved.

Many human needs are satisfied in intimate relationships: the need for approval and affirmation, for companionship, for meaningful ties and a sense of belonging, for sexual satisfaction. Many of society's needs are fulfilled by relationships, too—most notably, the need to nurture and socialize children. Overall, healthy intimate relationships are an important contributor to the well-being of both individuals and society.

DEVELOPING INTIMATE RELATIONSHIPS

People who develop successful intimate relationships believe in themselves and in the people around them. They are willing to give of themselves—to share their ideas, feelings, time, needs—and to accept what others want to give them.

Self-Concept and Self-Esteem

The principal thing that we all bring to our relationships is our *selves*. To have successful relationships, we must first accept and feel good about ourselves. A positive self-concept and a healthy level of self-esteem help us love and respect others. How and where do we acquire a positive sense of self?

As discussed in Chapter 3, the roots of our identity and sense of self can be found in childhood, in the relationships we had with our parents and other family members. As adults, we probably have a sense that we're basically lovable, worthwhile people and that we can trust others if, as babies and children, we felt loved, valued, and respected; if adults responded to our needs in a reason-

ably appropriate way; and if they gave us the freedom to explore and develop a sense of being separate individuals.

Our personal identity isn't fixed or frozen. According to psychologist Erik Erikson, it continues to develop as we encounter and resolve various crises at each stage of life. The fundamental tasks of early childhood are the development of trust during infancy and of autonomy during toddlerhood. From these experiences and interactions we construct our first ideas about who we are. (For a more detailed discussion of Erikson's developmental theory, see Chapter 3.)

Another thing we learn in early childhood is **gender role**—the activities, abilities, and characteristics our culture deems appropriate for us based on whether we're male or female. In our society, men have traditionally been expected to work and provide for their families; to be aggressive, competitive, and power-oriented; and to use thinking and logic to solve problems. Women have been expected to take care of home and children; to be cooperative, supportive, and nurturing; and to approach life emotionally and intuitively. Although much more egalitarian gender roles are emerging in our society, the stereotypes we absorb in childhood tend to be deeply ingrained.

Our ways of relating to others may also be rooted in childhood. Some researchers have suggested that our adult styles of loving may be based on the style of **attachment** we established in infancy with our mother, father, or other primary caregiver. According to this view, people who are secure in their intimate relationships probably had a secure, trusting, mutually satisfying attachment to their mother, father, or other parenting figure. As adults, they find it relatively easy to get close to others. They don't worry about being abandoned or having someone get too close to them. They feel that other people like them and are generally well-intentioned.

People who are clinging and dependent in their relationships may have had an "anxious/ambivalent" attachment, in which a parent's inconsistent responses made them unsure that their needs would be met. As adults, they worry about whether their partners really love them and will stay with them. They tend to feel that others don't want to get as close as they do. They want to merge completely with another person, which sometimes scares others away.

People who seem to run from relationships may have had an "anxious/avoidant" attachment, in which a parent's inappropriate responses made them want to escape from his or her sphere of influence. As adults, they feel uncomfortable being close to others. They're distrustful and fearful of becoming dependent. Their partners usually want more intimacy than they do.

Even if people's earliest experiences and relationships were less than ideal, however, they can still establish satisfying relationships in adulthood. People can be resilient and flexible. They have the capacity to change their ideas,

TERMS **gender role** A culturally expected pattern of behavior and attitudes determined by whether a person is male or female.

attachment The emotional tie between an infant and his or her caregiver, or between two people in an intimate relationship.

beliefs, and behavior patterns. They can learn ways to raise their self-esteem; they can become more trusting, accepting, and appreciative of others; and they can acquire the communication and conflict resolution skills for maintaining successful relationships. Although it helps to have a good start in life, it may be even more important to begin again, right from where you are.

Friendship

The first relationships we form outside the family are friendships. With members of either the same or the other sex, friendships give people the opportunity to share themselves and discover others. The friendships we form in childhood are important in our development; through them we learn about tolerance, sharing, and trust.

Friendships usually include most or all of the following characteristics:

- *Companionship.* Friends are relaxed and happy in each other's company. They typically have common values and interests, and make plans to spend time together.

- *Respect.* Friends have a basic respect for each other's humanity and individuality. Good friends respect each other's feelings and opinions, and work to resolve their differences without demeaning or insulting each other. They also show their respect by being honest with one another (see the box "Being a Good Friend," p. 84).

- *Acceptance.* Friends accept each other—"warts and all." They feel free to be themselves and express their feelings spontaneously without fear of ridicule or criticism.

- *Help.* Sharing time, energy, and even material goods is important to friendship. Friends know they can rely on each other in times of need. They feel they can ask for help when the going gets tough.

- *Trust.* Friends are secure in the knowledge that they will not intentionally hurt each other. They feel safe confiding in one another.

- *Loyalty.* Friends can count on each other. They stand up for each other in both word and deed.

- *Reciprocity.* Friendships are reciprocal. There is give and take between friends, and the feeling that both share joys and burdens more or less equally over time.

Intimate partnerships are like friendships in many ways, but they have additional characteristics. These relationships usually include sexual desire and expression, a greater demand for exclusiveness, and deeper levels of caring.

Friendships are usually considered more stable and longer lasting than intimate partnerships. Friends are

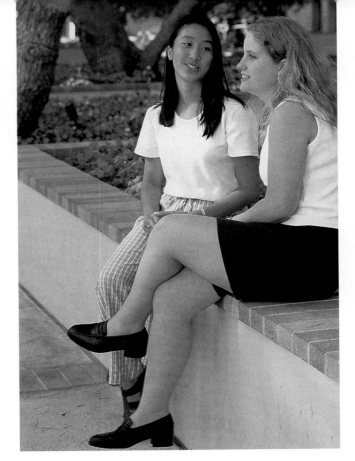

Close relationships without a sexual component are more common than those with sexual activity. Friendship satisfies our need for affection, affirmation, sharing, and companionship.

often more accepting and less critical than lovers, probably because their expectations are different. Like love relationships, friendships bind society together, providing people with emotional support and buffering them from stress.

Love, Sex, and Intimacy

Love is one of the most basic and profound human emotions. It is a powerful force in all our intimate relationships. Love encompasses opposites: affection and anger, excitement and boredom, stability and change, bonds and freedom. Love does not give us perfect happiness, but it does give our lives meaning.

In many kinds of adult relationships, love is closely intertwined with sexuality. In the past, marriage was considered the only acceptable context for sexual activities, but for many people today, sex is legitimized by love. Many couples, both heterosexual and homosexual, live together in committed relationships. We now use personal standards rather than social norms to make decisions about sex. This trend toward personal responsibility results in even more of an emphasis on love than in the past.

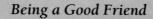
How to Make Friends

- Find people with interests similar to your own. Join a club, participate in sports, do volunteer work, or join a discussion group to meet people with common interests.

- Be a good listener. Take a genuine interest in people. Solicit their opinions, and take time to listen to their problems and ideas.

- Take risks. If you meet someone interesting, ask him or her to join you for a meal or an event you would both enjoy.

How to Be a Good Friend

- Be trustworthy. Honor all confidences, and don't talk about your friend behind his or her back.

- Tell your friend about yourself. Self-disclosure—letting your friend know about your real concerns and joys—signals trust.

- Be supportive and kind. Be there when your friend is going through a rough time. Don't criticize your friend or offer unsolicited advice.

- Develop your capacity for intimacy. Intimate relationships are genuine, spontaneous, and caring.

- Don't expect perfection. Like any relationship, your friendship may go through difficult times. Talk through conflicts as they arise.

For most people, love, sex, and commitment are closely linked ideals in intimate relationships. Love reflects the positive factors that draw people together and sustain them in a relationship. It includes trust, caring, respect, loyalty, interest in the other, and concern for the other's well-being. Sex brings excitement and passion to the relationship. It intensifies the relationship and adds fascination and pleasure. Commitment, the determination to continue, reflects the stable factors that help maintain the relationship. Responsibility, reliability, and faithfulness are characteristics of commitment. Although love, sex, and commitment are related, they are not necessarily connected. One can exist without the others. Despite the various permutations of the three, most of us long for a special relationship that contains them all.

Other elements can be identified as features of love, such as euphoria, preoccupation with the loved one, idealization of the loved one, and so on, but these tend to be temporary. These characteristics may include **infatuation,** which will fade or deepen into something more substantial. As relationships progress, the central aspects of love and commitment take on more importance.

Another way of looking at love has been proposed by psychologist Robert Sternberg. He sees love as being composed of intimacy, passion, and decision/commitment. Intimacy refers to the feelings of warmth and closeness we have with someone we love. Passion refers to romance, attraction, and sexuality. Decision/commitment refers to both the short-term decision that you love someone and the long-term commitment to be in the relationship.

According to Sternberg, these three elements can be enlarged, diminished, or combined in different ways. Each combination gives a different kind of love:

- *Liking* (intimacy only): Love between friends.

- *Infatuation* (passion only): An idealizing, obsessive, all-consuming love, characterized by a high degree of physical and emotional arousal; often unrequited; "love at first sight."

- *Romantic* (intimacy and passion): Love in which commitment may develop over time.

- *Fatuous* (passion and commitment): Deceptive love, the "whirlwind affair"; as passion fades, all that's left is commitment, but without time and intimacy, it's a poor foundation for an enduring relationship.

- *Empty* (decision/commitment only): Dutiful love; also a poor foundation for a relationship.

- *Companionate* (intimacy and commitment): Essentially a committed friendship; often begins as romantic love, but as passion diminishes and intimacy increases, it is transformed into companionate love.

- *Consummate* (all three elements): The love that dreams are made of; difficult to sustain.

Men and women tend to have different views of the relationship between love (or intimacy) and sex (or passion). Numerous studies have found that men can separate love from sex rather easily, although many men find that their most erotic sexual experiences occur in the context of a love relationship. Women generally view sex from the point of view of a relationship. Some people believe you can have satisfying sex without love—with friends, acquaintances, or strangers. Although sex with love is an important norm in our culture, it is frequently disregarded in practice, as the high incidence of extrarelational affairs attests.

The Pleasure and Pain of Love The experience of intense love has confused and tormented lovers throughout history. They live in a tumultuous state of excitement,

Even when a couple starts out with the best of intentions, an intimate relationship may not last. The couple may be mismatched to begin with. Sometimes the relationship doesn't thrive and partners turn elsewhere for satisfaction. Ending an intimate relationship is usually difficult and painful. Both partners may feel attacked and abandoned, but feelings of distress are likely to be more acute for the rejected partner.

If you are involved in a breakup, following these guidelines can make the ending easier:

- *Give the relationship a fair chance before breaking up.* If it's still not working, you'll know you did everything you could.

- *Be fair and honest.* If you're the one initiating the breakup, don't try to make your partner feel responsible.

- *Be tactful and compassionate.* You can leave the relationship without deliberately damaging your partner's self-esteem.

Emphasize your mutual incompatibility, and admit your own contributions to the problem.

- *If you are the rejected person, give yourself time to resolve your anger and pain.* You may go through a process of mourning the relationship, experiencing disbelief, anger, sadness, and finally acceptance. Despite all the romantic talk about your "one and only," remember that there are actually many people with whom you can potentially have an intimate relationship.

- *Recognize the value in the experience.* Ending a close relationship can teach you valuable lessons about your needs, preferences, strengths, and weaknesses. Use your insights to increase your chance of success in your next relationship.

---

subject to wildly fluctuating feelings of joy and despair. They lose their appetite, can't sleep, and can think of nothing but the loved one. Is this happiness? Misery? Or both?

The contradictory nature of passionate love can be understood by recognizing that human emotions have two components: physiological arousal and an emotional explanation for the arousal. (For a discussion of the biochemical and hormonal processes involved in arousal, see the description of the stress response in Chapter 2.) Love is just one of many emotions accompanied by physiological arousal; numerous unpleasant ones can also generate arousal, such as fear, rejection, frustration, and challenge. Although experiences like attraction and sexual desire are pleasant, extreme excitement is similar to fear and is unpleasant. For this reason, passionate love may be too intense to enjoy. Over time, the physical intensity and excitement tend to diminish. When this happens, pleasure may actually increase.

The Transformation of Love   All human relationships change over time, and love relationships are no exception. At first, love is likely to be characterized by high levels of passion and rapidly increasing intimacy. After a while, passion decreases as we become habituated to it and to the person. Generally, increasing the time spent together does not increase arousal.

Sometimes intimacy continues to grow at a deeper, less conscious level; other times, the couple may drift apart. Commitment isn't necessarily diminished or altered by time. It grows more slowly and is maintained as long as we judge the relationship to be successful. If the relationship begins to deteriorate, the level of commitment usually decreases.

The disappearance of romance or passionate love is often experienced as a crisis in a relationship. If a more lasting love fails to emerge, the relationship will likely break up, and each person will search for another who will once again ignite his or her passion. (For guidelines on ending an intimate relationship, see the box "Breaking Up Is Hard to Do.")

Love does not necessarily have to be intensely passionate. When intensity diminishes, partners often discover a more enduring love. They can now move from absorption in each other to a relationship that includes external goals and projects, friends, and family. In this kind of intimate, more secure love, satisfaction comes not just from the relationship itself but also from achieving other creative goals, such as work or child rearing. The key to successful relationships is in transforming passion into an intimate love, based on closeness, caring, and the promise of a shared future. Only with the passage of time can love mature and deepen, allowing us to truly grow both psychologically and spiritually. (To assess your relationship, take the quiz in the box "How Satisfying Is Your Relationship?" on p. 86.)

Jealousy

Jealousy is the angry, painful response to a partner's real, imagined, or likely involvement with a third person.

---

infatuation   An idealizing, obsessive attraction, characterized by a high degree of physical arousal.   **TERMS**

jealousy   An aversive response to another significant person's real, imagined, or likely involvement with or interest in another person.

For each item, circle the number that best reflects your relationship:

1. How well does your partner meet your needs?

1	2	3	4	5
Poorly		Average		Extremely well

2. In general, how satisfied are you with your relationship?

1	2	3	4	5
Unsatisfied		Average		Extremely satisfied

3. How good is your relationship compared to most?

1	2	3	4	5
Poor		Average		Excellent

4. Do you wish you hadn't gotten into this relationship?

1	2	3	4	5
Never		Average		Very often

5. To what extent has your relationship met your original expectations?

1	2	3	4	5
Hardly at all		Average		Completely

6. How much do you love your partner?

1	2	3	4	5
Not much		Average		Very much

7. How many problems are there in your relationship?

1	2	3	4	5
Very few		Average		Very many

Add up your points for all seven items, and find the number closest to your total on the table below.

Score	How satisfying is your relationship compared to the average relationship?
23 or below	Substantially less satisfying
26	Moderately less satisfying
29	About as satisfying as average
32	Moderately more satisfying
35 or above	Substantially more satisfying

SOURCE: Hendrick, S. S. 1988. A generic measure of relationship satisfaction. *Journal of Marriage and the Family* 50(1): 93–98. Copyright © 1988 by the National Council on Family Relations, 3989 Central Ave., N.E., Suite 550, Minneapolis, MN 55421. Reprinted by permission.

Many people think that the existence of jealousy proves the existence of love. We may try to test someone's interest or affection by attempting to make him or her jealous by flirting with another person. If our date or partner becomes jealous, the jealousy is taken as a sign of love. But provoking jealousy proves nothing except that the other person can be made jealous. Making jealousy a test of love is dangerous, for jealousy and love are not necessary companions. Jealousy may be a more accurate yardstick for measuring insecurity or possessiveness than love.

Jealousy can help secure a relationship by guarding its exclusiveness. But in its irrational and extreme forms, it can destroy a relationship by its insistent demands and attempts at control. Jealousy is a factor in precipitating violence in dating relationships among both high school and college students. And abusive spouses often use jealousy to justify their violence. (Violence in relationships is discussed in Chapter 23.)

People with a healthy level of self-esteem are less likely to feel jealous. When jealousy occurs in a relationship, it is important for the partners to communicate clearly with each other about their feelings and needs.

PERSONAL INSIGHT   What are your expectations of love? How much are your expectations shaped by movies and magazines, by what your friends expect, by what you've observed of your parents' relationship? Are there any contradictions among these views? If so, can you reconcile them?

COMMUNICATION

The key to developing and maintaining any type of intimate relationship is good communication. Most of the time, we don't actually think about communicating; we simply talk and behave naturally. But when problems arise—when we feel others don't understand us or when someone accuses us of not listening—we become aware of our limitations or, more commonly, what we think are other people's limitations. Miscommunication creates frustration and distances us from our friends and partners.

Nonverbal Communication

As much as 65% of face-to-face communication is nonverbal. Even when we're silent, we're communicating. We send messages when we look at someone or look away, lean forward or sit back, smile or frown. Especially important forms of nonverbal communication are touch, eye contact, and proximity. If someone we're talking to touches our hand or arm, looks into our eyes, and leans toward us when we talk, we get the message that the person is interested in us and cares about what we're saying. If a person keeps looking around the room while we're talking or takes a step backward, we get the impression the person is uninterested or wants to end the conversation.

The ability to interpret nonverbal messages correctly is important to the success of relationships. It's also important, when sending messages, to make sure our body language agrees with our words. When our verbal and nonverbal messages don't correspond, we send a mixed message.

Communication Skills

Three keys to good communication in relationships are self-disclosure, listening, and feedback.

- *Self-disclosure* involves revealing personal information that we ordinarily wouldn't reveal because of the risk involved. It usually increases feelings of closeness and moves the relationship to a deeper level of intimacy. Friends often disclose the most to each other, sharing feelings, experiences, hopes, and disappointments; married couples sometimes share less because they think they already know everything there is to know about each other.

- *Listening,* the second component of good communication, is a rare skill. Good listening skills require that we spend more time and energy trying to fully understand another person's "story" and less time judging, evaluating, blaming, advising, analyzing, or trying to control. Empathy, warmth, respect, and genuineness are qualities of skillful listeners. Attentive listening encourages friends or partners to share more and, in turn, to be attentive listeners. To connect with other people and develop real emotional intimacy, listening is essential.

- *Feedback,* a constructive response to another's self-disclosure, is the third key to good communication. Giving positive feedback means acknowledging that the friend's or partner's feelings are valid—no matter how upsetting or troubling—and offering self-disclosure in response. If, for example, your partner discloses unhappiness about your relationship, it is more constructive to say that you're concerned or saddened by that and want to hear more about it than to get angry, to blame, to try to inflict pain, or to withdraw. Self-disclosure and feedback can open the door to change, whereas other responses block communication and change. (For tips on improving your skills, see the box "Guidelines for Effective Communication," p. 88.)

Gender and Communication

Some of the difficulties people encounter in relationships can be traced to common gender differences in communication. Many authorities believe that, because of the way they've been raised, men and women generally approach conversation and communication differently. According to this view, men tend to use conversation in a

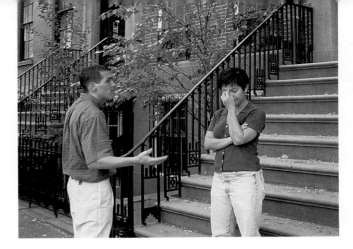

Conflict is an inevitable part of any intimate relationship. Couples need to develop constructive ways of resolving conflicts in order to maintain a healthy relationship.

competitive way, perhaps hoping to establish dominance in relationships. When male conversations are over, men often find themselves in a one-up or a one-down position. Women tend to use conversation in a more *affiliative* way, perhaps hoping to establish friendships. They negotiate various degrees of closeness, seeking to give and receive support. Men tend to talk more—though without disclosing more—and listen less. Women tend to use good listening skills like eye contact, frequent nodding, focused attention, and asking relevant questions.

Although these are generalized patterns, they can translate into problems in specific conversations. Even when a man and a woman are talking about the same subject, their unconscious goals may be very different. The woman may be looking for understanding and closeness, while the man may be trying to demonstrate his competence by giving advice and solving problems. Both styles are valid; the problem comes when differences in styles result in poor communication and misunderstanding.

Sometimes communication is not the problem in a relationship—the partners understand each other all too well. The problem is that they're unable or unwilling to change or compromise. Although good communication can't salvage a bad relationship, it does enable couples to see their differences and make more informed decisions.

Conflict and Conflict Resolution

Conflict is natural in intimate relationships. No matter how close two people become, they still remain separate individuals with their own needs, desires, past experiences, and ways of seeing the world. In fact, the closer the relationship, the more differences and the more opportunities for conflict there will be. Conflict itself isn't dangerous to a relationship; it may simply indicate that the relationship is growing. But if it isn't handled in a constructive way, it will damage—and ultimately destroy—the relationship.

Conflict is often accompanied by anger—a natural

Getting Started

- When you want to have a serious discussion with your partner, find an appropriate time and place. Choose a block of time when you will not be interrupted or rushed, and a place that is private.

- Face your partner and maintain eye contact. Use nonverbal feedback to show that you are interested and involved in the communication process.

Being an Effective Speaker

- State your concern or issue as clearly as you can.

- Use "I" statements—statements about how *you* feel—rather than statements beginning with "You," which tell another person how you think he or she feels. When you use "I" statements, you are taking responsibility for your feelings. "You" statements are often blaming or accusatory and will probably get a defensive or resentful response. The statement "I feel unloved," for example, sends a clearer, less blaming message than the statement "You don't love me."

- Focus on a specific behavior rather than on the whole person. Be specific about the behavior you like or don't like. Avoid generalizations beginning with "You always" or "You never." Such statements make people feel defensive.

- Make constructive requests. Opening your request with "I would like" keeps the focus on your needs rather than your partner's supposed deficiencies.

- Avoid blaming, accusing, and belittling. Even if you are right, you have little to gain by putting your partner down. Studies have shown that when people feel criticized or

attacked, they are less able to think rationally or solve problems constructively.

- Ask for action ahead of time, not after the fact. Tell your partner what you would like to have happen in the future; don't wait for him or her to blow it and then express anger or disappointment.

Being an Effective Listener

- Provide appropriate nonverbal feedback (nodding, smiling, and so on).

- Don't interrupt.

- Develop the skill of reflective listening. Don't judge, evaluate, analyze, or offer solutions (unless asked to do so). Your partner may just need to have you there in order to sort out feelings. By jumping in right away to "fix" the problem, you may actually be cutting off communication.

- Don't give unsolicited advice. Giving advice implies that you know more about what a person needs to do than he or she does; therefore, it often evokes anger or resentment.

- Clarify your understanding of what your partner is saying by restating it in your own words and asking if your understanding is correct.

- Be sure you are really listening, not off somewhere in your mind rehearsing your reply. Try to tune in to your partner's feelings as well as the words.

- Let your partner know that you value what he or she is saying and want to understand. Respect for the other person is the cornerstone of effective communication.

---

emotion, but one that can be difficult to handle. If we express anger, we run the risk of creating distrust, fear, and distance; if we act it out without thinking things through, we can cause the conflict to escalate; if we suppress it, it turns into resentment and hostility. The best way to handle anger in a relationship is to recognize it as a symptom of something that requires attention and needs to be changed. When angry, partners should back off until they calm down, then come back to the issue later and try to resolve it rationally. Negotiation will help dissipate the anger so the conflict can be resolved.

Although the sources of conflict for couples change over time, they primarily revolve around the basic tasks of living together: dividing the housework, handling money, spending time together, and so on. Sexual interaction is also a source of disagreement for many couples.

Although there are numerous theories on, and approaches to, conflict resolution, some basic strategies are generally useful in successfully negotiating with a partner:

1. *Clarify the issue.* Take responsibility for thinking through your feelings and discovering what's really bothering you. Agree that one partner will speak first and have the chance to speak fully while the other listens. Then reverse the roles. Try to understand the other partner's position fully by repeating what you've heard and asking questions to clarify or elicit more information. Agree to talk only about the topic at hand and not get distracted by other issues. Sum up what your partner has said.

2. *Find out what each person wants.* Ask your partner to express his or her desires. Don't assume you know what your partner wants and speak for him or her. Clarify and summarize.

3. *Identify various alternatives for getting each person what he or she wants.* Practice brainstorming to generate a variety of options.

TABLE 4-1 · *Constructive and Destructive Approaches to Conflict Resolution*

Relationship Dimensions	Constructive Approach	Destructive Approach
Issues	Raise and clarify issues.	Bring up old issues.
Feelings	Express both positive and negative feelings.	Express only negative feelings.
Information	Provide complete and honest information.	Provide selective information.
Focus	Focus is on issue rather than person.	Focus is on person rather than issue.
Blame	Accept mutual blame.	Blame other person(s).
Perception	Focus on similarities.	Focus on differences.
Change	Prevent stagnation by facilitating change.	Increase conflict and minimize change.
Outcome	Both win.	One wins and one loses, or both lose.
Intimacy	Resolving conflict increases intimacy.	Escalating conflict decreases intimacy.
Attitude	Trust.	Suspicion.

SOURCE: Olson, D., and J. DeFrain. 2000. *Marriage and the Family*, 3rd ed. Mountain View, Calif.: Mayfield.

4. *Decide how to negotiate.* Work out some agreements or plans for change; for example, one partner will do one task and the other will do another task, or one partner will do a task in exchange for something he or she wants.

5. *Solidify the agreements.* Go over the plan verbally and write it down, if necessary, to ensure that you both understand and agree to it.

6. *Review and renegotiate.* Decide on a time frame for trying out the new plan, and set a time to discuss how it's working. Make adjustments as needed.

To resolve conflicts, partners have to feel safe in voicing disagreements. They have to trust that the discussion won't get out of control, that they won't be abandoned by the other, and that the partner won't take advantage of their vulnerability. Partners should follow some basic ground rules when they argue, such as avoiding ultimatums, resisting the urge to give the silent treatment, refusing to "hit below the belt," and not using sex to smooth over disagreements. Table 4-1 shows some differences between constructive and destructive approaches to conflict resolution.

> **PERSONAL INSIGHT** How did your parents resolve conflicts when you were growing up? How effective were their methods? Has their model influenced the approach to conflict resolution you use in your relationships?

PAIRING AND SINGLEHOOD

Although most people eventually marry, everyone spends some time as a single person, and nearly all make some attempt, consciously or unconsciously, to find a partner. Intimate relationships are as important for singles as for couples.

Choosing a Partner

Most men and women select partners for long-term relationships through a fairly predictable process, although they may not be consciously aware of it. Most people pair with someone who lives in the same geographic area and who is similar in ethnic and socioeconomic background, educational level, lifestyle, physical attractiveness, and other traits. In simple terms, people select partners like themselves.

First attraction is based on easily observable characteristics: looks, dress, social status, and reciprocated interest. Once the euphoria of romantic love winds down, personality traits and behaviors become more significant factors in how the partners view each other. Through sharing and self-disclosure, they gradually gain a deeper knowledge of each other. The emphasis shifts to basic values, such as religious beliefs, political affiliation, sexual attitudes, and future aspirations regarding career, family, and children. At some point, they decide whether the relationship feels viable and is worthy of their continued commitment. If they are compatible, many people gradually discover deeper, more enduring forms of love.

Perhaps the most important question for potential mates is: How much do we have in common? Although differences add interest to a relationship, similarities increase the chances of a relationship's success. If there are major differences, partners should first ask: How accepting of differences are we? Then: How well do we communicate? Acceptance and communication skills go a long way toward making a relationship work, no matter

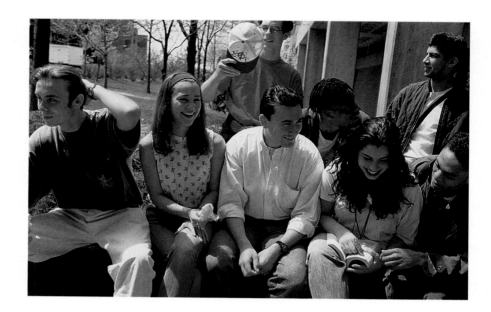

For many college students today, group activities have replaced dating as a way to meet and get to know potential partners.

how different the partners. Areas in which differences can affect the relationship include values, religion, ethnicity, attitudes toward sexuality and gender roles, socio-economic status, familiarity with the other's culture, and interactions with the extended family (see the box "Intercultural Friendships and Intimate Relationships").

Dating

Every culture has certain rituals for pairing and finding mates. Parent-arranged marriages, still the norm in many cultures, are often very stable and permanent. Although the American cultural norm is personal choice in courtship and mate selection, the popularity of dating services (complete with personality tests and videotapes of prospects) and online matchmaking suggests that many people do want help finding a suitable partner (see the box "Online Relationships").

Most Americans—whether single, divorced, widowed, or gay—find romantic partners through some form of dating. They narrow the field through a process of getting to know each other. Dating often revolves around a mutually enjoyable activity, such as seeing a movie or having dinner. In the traditional male-female dating pattern, the man takes the lead, initiating the date, while the woman waits to be called. In this pattern, casual dating might evolve into steady or exclusive dating, then engagement, and finally marriage.

For many young people today, traditional dating has given way to a more casual form of getting together in groups. Greater equality between the sexes is at the root of this change. Rather than strictly as couples, people go out in groups, and each person pays his or her way. A man and woman may begin to spend more time together, but often in the group context. If sexual involvement develops, it is more likely to be based on friendship, respect, and common interests than on expectations related to gender roles. In this model, mate selection may progress from getting together to living together to marriage.

Living Together

According to the U.S. Bureau of the Census, over 4 million heterosexual couples were living together in 1998. In addition, an estimated 1.5 million gay and lesbian couples (who cannot legally marry) live together. Living together, or **cohabitation,** is one of the most rapid and dramatic social changes that has ever occurred in our society. It seems to be gaining acceptance as part of the normal mate selection process. By age 30, about half of all men and women will have cohabited. The only thing separating those who cohabit from those who don't is religion. Several factors are involved in this change, including greater acceptance of premarital sex, increased availability of contraceptives, the tendency for people to wait longer before getting married, and a larger pool of single and divorced individuals.

Cohabitation is more popular among younger people than older, although a significant number of older couples live together without marrying to avoid losing a source of income, such as Social Security benefits, if they were to marry. Living together provides many of the benefits of marriage: companionship; a setting for an enjoyable and meaningful relationship; the opportunity to develop greater intimacy through learning, compromising, and sharing; a satisfying sex life; and a way to save on living costs.

Living together has certain advantages over marriage. For one thing, it can give the partners a greater sense of

TERMS **cohabitation** Living together in a sexual relationship without being married.

Today more than ever we have opportunities to make friends with people from other ethnic groups and cultures. Yet how many of us are encouraged to reach out to those who are different from ourselves? Probably not many. Studies confirm that many families continue to instill negative attitudes toward people of other cultures and ethnicities. For this reason and others, friendships and intimate relationships with people different from ourselves can pose challenges. Yet once these challenges are overcome, these relationships can be mutually fulfilling.

What makes intercultural relationships more challenging? You and a friend from a different cultural background may find that you differ in how you communicate, what you value, and how you view the world. You may encounter disapproval about your relationship from friends and family. And because of these obstacles, you may experience more anxiety during the early stages of your relationship than you would with a friend with a similar cultural background.

Intimate partners with different cultural backgrounds may find that their relationship requires special effort to maintain. They bring two unique worlds to their partnership, and for their relationship to last, they must make room for both of these

worlds. Communication is particularly important—and challenging. Many interethnic couples say that they must explain themselves more frequently, both to each other and to their respective families and communities. If family response to the relationship is negative, an intercultural couple will need to develop their own social support network.

Despite these challenges, increasing numbers of people are establishing friendships and intimate relationships with people outside their own ethnic and cultural heritage. If you develop such a relationship, you and your friend or partner will probably find that it has many special benefits:

- You will get a chance to learn about each other's worlds and unique experiences. You may acquire new skills and information.

- You will build a strong relationship based not only on your similarities but also on your differences.

- You will learn respect, tolerance, and acceptance for people who are different from yourself—key steps in breaking down stereotypes of all kinds.

More and more, people are looking to the Internet to find friends and partners. Communications with others in cyberspace can enable people to be themselves in a relaxed atmosphere, to try out other personas, and to confide in others in a private way. The Internet can also serve as "training wheels" for those who wish to develop their social skills.

The Internet is a good tool for locating people who share your hobbies and interests—whether that's Volkswagens, Sherlock Holmes mysteries, or baseball. You may or may not end up visiting a new contact in person, but if your goal is to communicate with someone about a common interest, e-mail, newsgroups, listservs, and chat rooms are all good options. (Refer to Appendix C for some basic guidelines about finding and using these Internet resources.)

People looking for intimate partners are also using the Internet. By getting to know someone online, you can make that "first impression" in the comfort of your living room. In online relationships, people will respond to you based on who you are rather than on your appearance. And with over 45 million users of the World Wide Web in the United States alone, you have many more people to interact with than on your campus or in your neighborhood.

There are drawbacks to meeting partners online, however. People can misrepresent themselves, pretending to be very different—older or younger or even a different sex—than they really are. Investing time and emotional resources in an unrealistic romance can be painful. There have also been a few

instances in which online romances have become dangerous or even deadly. If you decide to meet someone in person whom you have previously met only online, here are some strategies that can help keep you safe:

- To increase your chances of meeting people interested in you as a person, avoid sexually oriented Internet sites.

- Until you know much more about a cyberfriend, don't give out personal information, including your real full name, school, or place of employment.

- Schedule a phone conversation or a series of phone conversations before deciding whether or not to meet an online friend in person.

- Don't agree to meet someone face to face unless you feel completely comfortable about it. Always meet initially in a very public place—a museum, a coffee shop, a restaurant. Bring along a friend to further increase your safety.

Finally, take care that your pursuit of online relationships does not interfere with your other interpersonal relationships and social activities. As described in Chapter 3, researchers have found that extensive use of the Internet is associated with greater loneliness, less communication with family members, and fewer social contacts. To maximize your emotional and interpersonal wellness, use the Internet to widen your circle of friends, not shrink it.

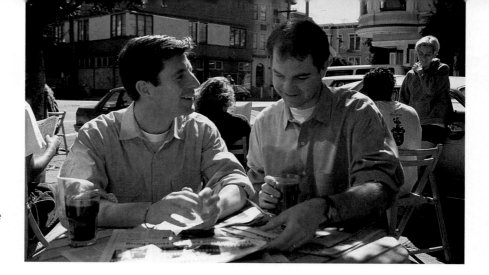

Greater openness has made gay men and lesbians more visible than they used to be, although they still constitute a minority of the population. Most gay men and lesbians have experienced at least one long-term relationship with a single partner.

autonomy. Not bound by the social rules and expectations that are part of the institution of marriage, partners may find it easier to keep their identity and more of their independence. Cohabitation doesn't incur the same obligations as marriage. If things don't work out, the partners may find it easier to leave a relationship that hasn't been legally sanctioned.

But living together has some liabilities, too. In most cases, the legal protections of marriage are absent, such as health insurance benefits and property and inheritance rights. These considerations can be particularly serious if the couple has children, from either former relationships or the current partnership. Since social acceptance of cohabitation is not universal, couples may feel family pressure to marry or otherwise change their living arrangements, especially if they have young children. The general trend, however, is toward legitimizing nonmarital partnerships; for example, some employers and communities now extend benefits to unmarried domestic partners.

Although many people choose cohabitation as a kind of trial marriage, unmarried partnerships tend to be less stable than marriages. In a survey of women age 15 to 44 who had cohabitated, fewer than half were still living—married (37%) or unmarried (10%)—with their first live-in partner; 34% had dissolved the relationship prior to marriage and 21% had married and then divorced their partner. There is little evidence that cohabitation before marriage leads to happier or longer-lasting marriages; in fact, some studies have found slightly less marital satisfaction among couples who had previously cohabited. Researchers speculate that people who have cohabited might have higher expectations for marriage or might be less likely to adapt well to traditional marital roles.

PERSONAL INSIGHT How do you feel about cohabitation? Is it a choice you would make? What influences your attitude?

Gay and Lesbian Partnerships

Regardless of **sexual orientation,** most people look for love in a close, satisfying, committed relationship. Gay and lesbian, or **homosexual,** couples have many similarities with **heterosexual** couples. According to one study, most gay men and lesbians have experienced at least one long-term relationship with a single partner. Like heterosexual relationships, gay and lesbian partnerships provide intimacy, passion, and security.

One difference between heterosexual and homosexual couples is that gay and lesbian couples tend to adopt "best friend" roles in their relationship rather than traditional gender roles. Domestic tasks are shared or split, and both partners usually support themselves financially. Another difference is that gay and lesbian couples often have to deal with societal hostility toward their relationships (in contrast to the social approval given to heterosexual couples). Consequently, community may be more important as a source of identity and social support than it is for heterosexuals.

Singlehood

Despite the prevalence and popularity of marriage, a significant proportion of adults in our society are unmarried. In 1998, about 91 million American adults were single. They are a diverse group, encompassing young people who have not married yet but plan to in the future, people who are living together (gay or heterosexual), divorced and widowed people, and those who would like to marry but haven't found a mate. The category includes people who are single both by choice and by chance. The largest number of unmarried adults have never been married.

Several factors contribute to the growing number of single people. One is the changing view of singlehood, which is increasingly being viewed as a legitimate alternative to marriage. Education and career are delaying the age at which young people are marrying. More young people are living with their parents as they complete their education, seek jobs, or strive for financial independence. Many other single people live together without being married. Gay people who would marry their partners if they were legally permitted to do so are counted among the single population. High divorce rates mean more singles, and people who have experienced divorce in their families may have more negative attitudes about marriage and more positive attitudes about singlehood.

Being single doesn't mean not having close relationships, however. Single people may date, enjoy active and fulfilling social lives, and have a variety of sexual experiences and relationships. Other advantages of being single include more opportunities for personal and career development without concern for family obligations, and more freedom and control in making life choices. Disadvantages include loneliness and a lack of companionship, as well as economic hardships (mainly for single women). Single men and women both experience some discrimination and often are pressured to get married.

Nearly everyone has at least one episode of being single in adult life, whether prior to marriage, between marriages, following divorce or the death of a spouse, or for the entire adult life span. How enjoyable and valuable this single time is depends on several factors, including how deliberately the person has chosen it; how satisfied the person is with social relationships, standard of living, and job; how comfortable the person feels when alone; and how resourceful and energetic the person is about creating an interesting and fulfilling life.

MARRIAGE

Marriage continues to remain popular because it satisfies several basic needs. There are many important social, moral, economic, and political aspects of marriage, all of which have changed over the years. In the past, people married mainly for practical reasons, such as raising children or forming an economic unit. Today, people marry more for personal, emotional reasons. This shift places a greater burden on marriage to fulfill certain expectations that are sometimes unreasonably high. People may assume that all their emotional needs will be met by their partner; they may think that fascination and passion will always remain at high levels; they may simply expect to "live happily ever after." When people enter marriage with such preconceptions, it may be harder for them to appreciate the benefits that marriage really offers.

Benefits of Marriage

The primary functions and benefits of marriage are those of any intimate relationship: affection, personal affirmation, companionship, sexual fulfillment, emotional growth. Marriage also provides a setting in which to raise children, although an increasing number of couples choose to remain childless, and people can also choose to raise children without being married. Marriage is also important for providing for the future. By committing themselves to the relationship, people establish themselves with lifelong companions as well as some insurance for their later years (see the box "Intimate Relationships Are Good for Your Health," p. 94).

Issues in Marriage

Although we might like to believe otherwise, love is not enough to make a successful marriage. Couples have to be strong and successful in their relationship before getting married, because relationship problems will be magnified rather than solved by marriage. The following relationship characteristics appear to be the best predictors of a happy marriage:

- The partners have realistic expectations about their relationship.
- Each feels good about the personality of the other.
- They communicate well.
- They have effective ways of resolving conflicts.
- They agree on religious/ethical values.
- They have an egalitarian role relationship.
- They have a good balance of individual versus joint interests and leisure activities.

Once married, couples must face many adjustment tasks. In addition to providing each other with emotional support, they have to negotiate and establish marital roles, establish domestic and career priorities, manage their finances, make sexual adjustments, manage boundaries and relationships with their extended family, and participate in the larger community.

Marital roles and responsibilities have undergone profound changes in recent years. Many couples no longer accept traditional role assumptions, such as that the husband is solely responsible for supporting the family and the wife is solely responsible for domestic work. Today, many husbands share domestic tasks and many wives work outside the home. In fact, over 50% of married

sexual orientation Sexual attraction to individuals of the opposite sex, same sex, or both.
TERMS

homosexual Sexual preference for members of the same sex.

heterosexual Sexual preference for members of the other sex.

Research studies consistently underscore the importance of strengthening your family and social ties to help maintain emotional and physical wellness. Living alone, or simply feeling alone, can have a negative effect on both your state of mind and your physical health. Married people, on average, live longer than unmarried people—whether single, divorced, or widowed—and they score higher on measures of mental health. Findings suggest that there is something intrinsically beneficial about the long-term commitment that marriage represents.

People with strong social ties are less likely to become ill and tend to recover more quickly if they do. The benefits of intimate relationships have been demonstrated for a range of conditions: People with strong social support are less likely to catch colds. They recover better from heart attacks and live longer with heart disease. Among men with prostate cancer, those who are married live significantly longer than those who are single, divorced, or widowed; women with breast cancer live longer if they participate in a support group.

What is it about social relationships that supports wellness? Friends and partners may encourage and reinforce healthy habits, such as exercising, eating right, and seeing a physician when needed. In times of illness, a loving partner can provide both practical help and emotional support. Feeling loved, esteemed, and valued brings comfort at a time of vulnerability, reduces anxiety, and mitigates the damaging effects of stress.

Although good relationships may help the sick get better, bad relationships may have the opposite effect. The impact of relationship quality on the course of illness may be partly explained by effects on the immune system: A study of married couples whose fighting went beyond normal conflict and into criticism and name-calling found them to have weaker immune responses than couples whose arguments were more civil. (The immune effects were particularly strong among the wives, leading some researchers to postulate that women may be more aware of and affected by relationship problems.)

Marriage, of course, isn't the only support system available. Whether married or single, if you have supportive people in your life, you are likely to enjoy better physical and emotional health than if you feel isolated and alone. So when you start planning lifestyle changes to improve your health and well-being, don't forget to nurture your relationships with family and friends. Relationships are powerful medicine.

women are in the labor force, including women with babies under 1 year of age. Although women still take most of the responsibility for home and children even when they work, and although men still suffer more job-related stress and health problems than women do, the trend is toward an equalization of responsibilities.

PERSONAL INSIGHT What do you think are appropriate roles and activities for husbands and wives? If both husband and wife work full-time, do you think they should share housework and child care equally? What influences your views?

The Role of Commitment

Coping with all these challenges requires that couples be committed to remaining in the relationship through its inevitable ups and downs. They will need to be tolerant of each other's imperfections and keep their perspective and sense of humor. Commitment is based on conscious choice rather than on feelings, which, by their very nature, are transitory. Commitment is a promise of a shared future, a promise to be together, come what may. Committed partners put effort and energy into the relationship, no matter how they feel. They take time to attend to their partner, give compliments, and face conflict when necessary.

Commitment has become an important concept in recent years. We talk about people who are afraid of commitment, or of "making a commitment" to a person or a relationship. To many people, commitment is a more important goal than living together or marriage.

PERSONAL INSIGHT What does commitment mean to you? What would make you feel that a partner was truly committed to your relationship? Have you ever felt a fear of commitment? If so, why?

Separation and Divorce

The high rate of divorce in the United States reflects our extremely high expectations for emotional fulfillment and satisfaction in marriage. It also indicates that we no longer believe in the permanence of marriage.

The process of divorce usually begins with an emotional separation. Often one partner is unhappy and looks beyond the relationship for other forms of validation. Dissatisfaction increases until the unhappy partner decides he or she can no longer stay. Physical separation follows, although it may take some time for the relationship to be over emotionally.

Except for the death of a spouse or family member, divorce is the greatest stress-producing event in life. Both men and women experience turmoil, depression, and lowered self-esteem during and after divorce. People experience separation distress and loneliness for about a

Statistical Trends

- About 95% of all Americans marry at some time in their lives.

- The median age for first marriage is 26.8 for men and 25.0 for women.

- Some 42% of marriageable adults (age 15 and older) are single. There are 118 million married people and 91 million unmarried adults. Never-married persons account for the largest number (58 million) of unmarried adults.

- People marrying today have a 50–55% chance of divorcing.

- Generally, whites are less likely to divorce than blacks; older adults are less likely to divorce than younger people; and those who marry in their twenties are less likely to divorce than those who marry while in their teens.

- Most divorces involve children; about 30% of children under 18 live with one parent.

- Single mothers raising children outnumber single fathers raising children by 5 to 1, but the gap is narrowing.

- Most divorced people eventually remarry; for younger divorced people, remarriage occurs within 5 years of the divorce. Men are slightly more likely to remarry than women, and remarriage is more likely for younger divorced

people than for older divorced ones. Blacks are more likely than whites to remain separated without legally divorcing and are less likely than whites to remarry after divorce.

A Historical Survey

	1960	1998
Median age at first marriage		
Men	22.8	26.7
Women	20.3	25.0
Percentage of all married couples who are interracial	0.36	2.4
Percentage of childbirths outside of marriage	5	32
Percentage of teenage mothers who are unmarried	15	75
Percentage of children living with only one parent	9	28

SOURCES: U.S. Bureau of the Census (http://www.census.gov); National Center for Health Statistics (http://www.cdc.gov/nchswww).

---

year and then begin a recovery period of about 1–3 years. During this time they gradually construct a postdivorce identity, along with a new pattern of life. Most people are surprised by how long it takes to recover from divorce. Children are especially vulnerable to the trauma of divorce, and sometimes counseling is appropriate to help them adjust to the changes in their lives.

Despite the distress of separation and divorce, the negative effects are usually balanced sooner or later by the possibility of finding a more suitable partner, constructing a new life, and developing new aspects of the self. About 75% of all people who divorce remarry, often within 5 years. One result of the high divorce and remarriage rate is a growing number of stepfamilies (discussed in the next section).

FAMILY LIFE

American families are very different today than they were even a few decades ago (see the box "The Changing American Family"). Currently, about half of all families are based on a first marriage; almost one-third are headed by a single parent; the remainder are remarriages or involve some other arrangement. Despite the tremendous variation apparent in American families, certain patterns can still be discerned.

For many young adults, the family life cycle begins with

marriage. This first stage, when newlyweds are learning how to live together, ends abruptly when they have a baby. New parents have a new set of responsibilities, and their roles change profoundly and irreversibly: no more spontaneous outings to see a movie, or leisurely Sunday mornings sipping coffee and browsing through the newspaper. The third member of the family, the new infant, demands round-the-clock attention.

Becoming a Parent

Few new parents have any preparation for the job of parenting, yet they have to assume that role literally overnight. They have to learn quickly how to hold a baby, how to change it, how to feed it, how to interpret its cries. No wonder the birth of the first child is one of the most stressful transitions for any couple.

Even couples with an egalitarian relationship before their first child is born find that their marital roles become more traditional with the arrival of the new baby. The father becomes the principal provider and protector, and the mother becomes the primary nurturer. Most research indicates that mothers have to make greater changes in their lives than fathers do. Although men today spend more time caring for their infants than ever before, women still take the ultimate responsibility for seeing that the baby is fed, clean, and comfortable. In addition, women are usually the ones who make job changes; they may quit working or reduce their hours in order to stay home with the baby for several months or more, or they may try to juggle the multiple roles of mother, homemaker, and employee and feel guilty that they never have enough time to do justice to any of these roles.

Not surprisingly, marital satisfaction often declines after the birth of the first child. The wife who has stopped working may feel she is cut off from the world; the wife who is trying to fulfill duties both at home and on the job may feel overburdened and resentful. The husband may have a hard time adjusting to having to share his wife's love and attention with the baby.

But marital dissatisfaction after the baby is born is not inevitable. Couples who successfully weather the stresses of a new baby seem to have these three characteristics in common:

1. They had developed a strong relationship before the baby was born.

2. They had planned to have the child and want it very much.

3. They communicate well about their feelings and expectations.

Parenting and the Family Life Cycle

Sometimes being a parent is a source of unparalleled pleasure and pride—the first smile (at you), the first word, the first home run. But at other times, parenting can seem like an overwhelming responsibility. How can you be sure you're not making some mistake that will stunt your child's physical, psychological, or emotional growth?

There is really no "right" way to raise children to ensure that they become healthy and happy. Of course, parents must provide for basic physical needs, such as food, shelter, clothing, and medical care. They must also help children develop a positive self-concept, as discussed earlier. But how do parents know how to best accomplish this? Does it mean they must give the child everything he or she wants and never say "No"? Of course not, but there is no set of hard-and-fast rules to guide parents in all situations.

Exactly what a parent does on any given occasion depends on a variety of factors, including values, beliefs, experience, and both the parent's and the child's personalities. Parents should try to remember that raising a child is an ongoing process. No single action is likely to either form or deform a child's personality forever. The important thing is to keep seeking ways to promote satisfaction for all family members—including the parents! It is also important for parents to develop and maintain confidence in their parenting skills, their common sense—and, above all, their love for their children.

At each stage of the family life cycle, the relationship between parents and children changes. And with those changes come new challenges. The parents' primary responsibility to a small, helpless baby is to ensure its physical well-being around the clock. As babies grow into toddlers and begin to crawl and walk and talk, they begin to be able to take care of some of their own physical needs. For parents, the challenge at this stage is to strike a balance between giving children the freedom to explore and setting limits that will keep the children safe and secure. As children grow toward adolescence, parents need to give them increasing independence, and gradually be willing to let them risk success or failure on their own.

Marital satisfaction for most couples tends to decline somewhat while the children are in school. Reasons include the financial and emotional pressures of a growing family and the increased job and community responsibilities of parents in their thirties, forties, and fifties. Once the last child has left home, marital satisfaction usually increases because the couple have time to enjoy each other once more.

Single Parents

Chances are that you know a number of families who haven't followed the traditional family life cycle, or perhaps you're a member of such a family yourself. According to the U.S. Bureau of the Census, in 1998, 28% of all children under 18 were living with only one parent. Today the family life cycle for many women is marriage, motherhood, divorce, single parenthood, remarriage, and widowhood.

In some single-parent families, the traditional family life cycle is reversed and the baby comes before the marriage. In these families, the single parent is usually a teenage mother; she may very well be African American or Latina, and she may never get married or may not marry for several years. In 1998, about 60% of all African American children were living with single parents, as were 33% of Latino children. In single-parent families that are the result of divorce, the mother usually has custody of the children, but about 15% of single-parent families are headed by fathers. About 6% of children under 18 live with grandparents.

Economic difficulties are the primary problem for single mothers, especially for unmarried mothers who have not finished high school and have difficulty finding work. Divorced mothers usually experience a sharp drop in income the first few years on their own, but if they have job skills or education, they usually can eventually support themselves and their children adequately. Other problems for single mothers are the often-conflicting demands of playing both father and mother and the difficulty of satisfying their own needs for adult companionship and affection.

Financial pressures are also a complaint of single fathers, but they do not experience them to the extent that single mothers do. Because they are likely to have less practice than mothers in juggling parental and professional roles, they may worry that they do not spend enough time with their children. Because single fatherhood is not as common as single motherhood, however, the men who choose it are likely to be stable, established, and strongly motivated to be with their children.

Research about the effect on children of growing up in a single-parent family is inconclusive. However, evidence seems to indicate that these children tend to have less success in school and in their careers than children from two-parent families. Nevertheless, two-parent families are not necessarily better if one of the parents spends little time relating to the children or is physically or emotionally abusive.

Stepfamilies

Single parenthood is usually a transitional stage; about three out of four divorced women and about four out of five divorced men will ultimately remarry. Overall, almost half the marriages in the United States are remarriages for the husband, the wife, or both. If either brings children from a previous marriage into the new family unit, a stepfamily (or "blended family") is formed.

Stepfamilies are significantly different from intact families and should not be expected to duplicate the emotions and relationships of an intact family. Research has shown that healthy stepfamilies are less cohesive and more adaptable than healthy intact families; they have a greater capacity to allow for individual differences and accept that biologically related family members will have emotionally closer relationships. Stepfamilies gradually gain more of a sense of being a family as they build a history of shared daily experiences and major life events.

Successful Families

Family life can be extremely challenging. A strong family is not a family without problems; it's a family that copes successfully with stress and crisis. Although there is tremendous variation in American families, researchers have proposed that six major qualities or themes appear in strong families.

1. *Commitment.* The family is very important to its members; sexual fidelity between partners is included in commitment.

2. *Appreciation.* Family members care about one another and express their appreciation. The home is a positive place for family members.

3. *Communication.* Family members spend time listening to one another and enjoying one another's company. They talk about disagreements and attempt to solve problems.

4. *Time together.* Family members do things together, often simple activities that don't cost money.

5. *Spiritual wellness.* The family promotes sharing, love, and compassion for other human beings.

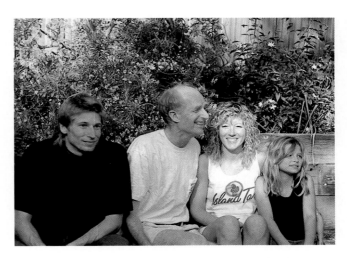

Almost one out of every five American families is a stepfamily, in which parents bring children from a previous marriage into a new family unit.

6. *Coping with stress and crisis.* When faced with illness, death, marital conflict, or other crises, family members pull together, seek help, and use other coping strategies to meet the challenge.

It may surprise some people that members of strong families are often seen at counseling centers. They know that the smartest thing to do in some situations is to get help. Many resources are available for individuals and families seeking counseling; people can turn to physicians, clergy, marriage and family counselors, psychologists, or other trained professionals. To assess your own family, see the box "Rate Your Family's Strengths," p. 98.

Families—and intimate relationships of all kinds—are essential to our overall wellness. A fulfilling life nearly always involves other people. Whether we're single or married, young or old, heterosexual or gay, we continue to need meaningful relationships throughout life.

SUMMARY

- Healthy intimate relationships are an important component of the well-being of both individuals and society. Many intimate relationships are held together by love.

Developing Intimate Relationships

- Successful relationships begin with a positive sense of self and reasonably high self-esteem. Personal identity, gender roles, and styles of attachment are all rooted in childhood experiences.

- Through the friendships we form in childhood, we learn about tolerance, acceptance, and trust. The characteristics of friendship include companionship, respect, acceptance, help, trust, loyalty, and reciprocity.

This Family Strengths Inventory was developed by researchers who studied the strengths of over 3000 families. To assess your family (either the family you grew up in or the family you have formed as an adult), circle the number that best reflects how your family rates on each strength. A 1 represents the lowest rating and a 5 represents the highest.

1. Spending time together and doing things with each other.	1	2	3	4	5
2. Commitment to each other.	1	2	3	4	5
3. Good communication (talking with each other often, listening well, sharing feelings with each other).	1	2	3	4	5
4. Dealing with crises in a positive manner.	1	2	3	4	5
5. Expressing appreciation to each other.	1	2	3	4	5
6. Spiritual wellness.	1	2	3	4	5
7. Closeness of relationship between spouses.	1	2	3	4	5
8. Closeness of relationship between parents and children.	1	2	3	4	5
9. Happiness of relationship between spouses.	1	2	3	4	5
10. Happiness of relationship between parents and children.	1	2	3	4	5
11. Extent to which spouses make each other feel good about themselves (self-confident, worthy, competent, and happy).	1	2	3	4	5
12. Extent to which parents help children feel good about themselves.	1	2	3	4	5

Scoring

Add the numbers you have circled. A score below 39 indicates below-average family strengths. Scores between 39 and 52 are in the average range. Scores above 53 indicate a strong family. Low scores on individual items identify areas that families can profitably spend time on. High scores are worthy of celebration but shouldn't lead to complacency. Families need loving care to remain strong.

SOURCE: Stinnett, N., and J. DeFrain. 1985. *Secrets of Strong Families.* Boston: Little, Brown, 167–169. © 1985 by Nick Stinnett and John DeFrain. By permission of Little, Brown and Company.

- Love, sex, and commitment are closely linked ideals in intimate relationships. Love includes trust, caring, respect, and loyalty. Sex brings excitement, fascination, and passion to the relationship.

- Sternberg sees love as composed of intimacy, passion, and decision/commitment. He defines seven types of love based on various combinations of these elements, ranging from friendship to consummate love.

- Love changes over time, with passion decreasing, intimacy increasing and then leveling off, and commitment increasing or decreasing. The disappearance of passion is often experienced as a crisis, but partners may then discover a more lasting, transforming love.

- Clear communication between partners can help overcome the potentially destructive effects of jealousy.

Communication

- Communication skills are essential to successful relationships. A great deal of communication is non-verbal. The keys to good communication in relationships are self-disclosure, listening, and feedback.

- Cultural differences in how men and women have learned to communicate can create misunderstandings and frustration in relationships.

- Conflict is inevitable in intimate relationships; partners need to have constructive ways to negotiate their differences.

Pairing and Singlehood

- People usually choose partners like themselves. If partners are very different, acceptance and good communication skills are necessary to maintain the relationship.

- Most Americans find partners through dating or getting together in groups.

- Cohabitation is a growing social pattern that allows partners to get to know each other intimately without being married.

- Gay and lesbian partnerships are similar to heterosexual relationships, with some differences. Partners are technically single, since they're not allowed to marry legally; they don't conform to traditional gender roles; and they often experience hostility rather than approval toward their partnerships from society.

- Singlehood is a growing option in our society. Advantages include greater variety in sex partners and more freedom in making life decisions; disadvantages include loneliness and possible economic hardship, especially for single women.

Marriage

- Marriage fulfills many functions for individuals and society. It can provide people with affection, affirmation, and sexual fulfillment; a context for child rearing; and the promise of lifelong companionship.
- Love isn't enough to ensure a successful marriage. Partners have to be realistic, feel good about each other, have communication and conflict resolution skills, share values, and have a balance of individual and joint interests.
- Marital tasks include providing each other with emotional support, establishing domestic and career priorities, managing finances, making sexual adjustments, managing boundaries with parents and extended family, and participating in the community.
- Commitment helps maintain a relationship over time and through difficult changes.

- When problems can't be worked out, people often separate and divorce. Divorce is traumatic for all involved, especially children. The negative effects are usually balanced in time by positive ones. About 75% of all divorced people remarry.

Family Life

- The family life cycle usually begins with marriage; the next stage begins with the arrival of a baby. Becoming a parent profoundly changes the relationship between the partners.
- At each stage of the family life cycle, relationships change. Marital satisfaction may be lower during the child-rearing years and higher later.
- Many families today are single-parent families. Problems for single parents include economic difficulties, conflicting demands, and time pressures.
- Stepfamilies are formed when single or divorced people remarry and create new family units. Stepfamilies gradually gain more of a sense of being a family as they build a history of shared experiences.
- Important qualities of successful families include commitment to the family, appreciation of family members, communication, time spent together, spiritual wellness, and effective methods of dealing with stress. Strong families use outside resources when they need help to resolve problems.

TAKE ACTION

1. Take an informal survey among your friends of what they find attractive in a member of the other sex and what they look for in a romantic partner. Are there substantial differences between people? Do men and women look for different things?

2. Ask your parents what their experiences of dating and courtship were like. How are they different from your experiences? What do your parents think of current customs?

JOURNAL ENTRY

1. What are you looking for in an intimate relationship? In your health journal, make a list of the needs you would like to have met by a partner. Are they needs that you can realistically expect to have satisfied in a relationship?

2. *Critical Thinking* What approach do you take when it comes to communicating your feelings and needs to others? Think of a particular issue that has been bothering you, and write down the statements you would make if you were discussing it. Examine your statements to see whether unrelated feelings or

issues are coming through in them. Devise a strategy for dealing with the issue, using the guidelines given in this chapter on conflict resolution.

3. Make a list of your family's strengths and weaknesses. What do you like best about your family? What would you like to change? Choose one weakness, and develop strategies for dealing with it that you and your family can work on together.

For resources in your area, check your campus directory for a counseling center or peer counseling program, or check the agencies listed in the Mental Health section of the phone book.

Books

Bradshaw, J. E. 1996. *Bradshaw on the Family: A New Way of Creating Solid Self-Esteem.* Rev. ed. Deerfield Beach, Fla.: Health Communications. *A discussion of the dynamics of the family and how problem families can heal themselves.*

Brazelton, T. B. 1994. *Touchpoints: The Essential Reference.* San Francisco: Perseus Press. *A comprehensive guide to children's emotional and behavioral development.*

Gottman, J. M., and N. Silver. 1999. *Seven Principles for Making Marriage Work.* New York: Crown. *Research-based advice for keeping relationships on track.*

Lerner, H. 1997. *Life Preservers: Staying Afloat in Life and Love.* New York: HarperCollins. *Sound advice from a well-known psychologist.*

McKay, M., P. Fanning, and K. Paleg. 1994. *Couple Skills: Making Your Relationship Work.* Oakland, Calif.: New Harbinger. *Practical suggestions for partners who want to improve their communication.*

Olson, D. H., and J. DeFrain. 2000. *Marriage and the Family: Diversity and Strengths.* 3rd ed. Mountain View, Calif.: Mayfield. *A comprehensive look at intimate relationships.*

Ornish, D. 1998. *Love and Survival: The Scientific Basis for the Healing Power of Intimacy.* New York: HarperCollins. *A discussion of the positive health effects of intimate relationships.*

Sternberg, R. J. 1998. *Cupid's Arrow: The Course of Love Through Time.* New York: SIGS Books and Multimedia. *A review of Sternberg's triangular theory of love, with self-help advice.*

Tannen, D. 1998. *The Argument Culture: Moving from Debate to Dialogue.* New York: Random House. *A discussion of the effects of confrontation and argument and a survey of other ways to express disagreement and deal with conflict.*

Visher, E., and J. Visher. 1991. *How to Win as a Stepfamily,* 2nd ed. New York: Brunner/Mazel. *One of the best examinations of the problems confronting parents, stepparents, stepchildren, and stepfamilies in creating a new family.*

Wright, D. E. 1999. *Personal Relationships: An Integrated Perspective.* Mountain View, Calif.: Mayfield. *An interdisciplinary look at the development, maintenance, and functions of friendships and intimate partnerships.*

Organizations and Web Sites

American Association for Marriage and Family Therapy. Provides information on a variety of relationship issues and referrals to therapists.
> 202-452-0109
> http://www.aamft.org

Association for Couples in Marriage Enrichment (ACME). An organization that promotes activities to strengthen marriage; a resource for books, tapes, and other materials.
> P.O. Box 10596
> Winston-Salem, NC 27108
> 800-634-8325
> http://home.swbell.net/tgall/acme.htm

Family Education Network. Provides information about education, safety, health, and other family-related issues.
> http://www.families.com

Go Ask Alice. Professional and peer educators provide answers to questions on many topics relating to interpersonal relationships and communication.
> http://www.goaskalice.columbia.edu

Life Innovations. Provides materials for premarital counseling and marital enrichment.
> Broadway Place West
> 1300 Godward St., Suite 6850
> Minneapolis, MN 55413
> 800-441-1940
> http://www.lifeinnovation.com

Parents Without Partners (PWP). Provides educational programs, literature, and support groups for single parents and their children. Call for a referral to a local chapter.
> 800-637-7974
> http://www.parentswithoutpartners.org

United States Census Bureau. Provides current statistics on births, marriages, and living arrangements.
> http://www.census.gov

Whole Family Center. Provides information on all types of family relationships; the site includes an online magazine and examples of real-life dramas for teens, couples, and parents.
> http://www.wholefamily.com

Yahoo/Lesbians, Gays, and Bisexuals. A Web site and search engine that contains many links to information and support for lesbians and gays.
> http://dir.yahoo.com/society_and_culture/cultures_ and_groups

See also listings for Chapters 3 and 8.

SELECTED BIBLIOGRAPHY

Adams, R., and R. Blieszner. 1994. An integrative conceptual framework for friendship research. *Journal of Social and Personal Relationships* 11(2): 163–184.

Andrews, V. 1999. You've got mail: But you may want it stamped Return to Sender. *Health Scout,* February 12 (retrieved February 18, 1999; http://www.healthscout.com/cig-bin/ WebObjects/af/hsaf.woa?ap=19&id=60996).

Beavers, W., and R. Hampton. 1990. *Successful Families.* New York: Norton.

Berends, P. B. 1997. *Whole Child/Whole Parent,* 4th ed. New York: HarperCollins.

Brown, S., and A. Booth. 1996. Cohabitation versus marriage: A comparison of relationship quality. *Journal of Marriage and the Family* 58: 668–678.

Columbia University Health Education Program. 1997. *Go Ask Alice: Looking for Love on the Information Superhighway* (retrieved September 4, 1998; http://www.goaskalice. columbia.edu/1185.html).

Edmondson, B. 1997. New lifestage: Trial marriage. *American Demographics,* October.

Fehr, B. 1988. Prototype analysis of the concepts of love and commitment. *Journal of Personality and Social Psychology* 55(4): 557–579.

Friends Can Be Good Medicine. 1998. *Mind/Body Health Newsletter* 7(1): 3–6.

Friends may be good for your heart. 1999. *Health News,* January.

Furstenberg, F., and A. Cherlin. 1994. *Divided Families.* Rev. ed. Cambridge, Mass.: Harvard University Press.

Gangon, L., and M. Coleman. 1994. *Remarried Family Relationships.* Newbury Park, Calif.: Sage Publications.

Gottman, J. M. 1994. *What Predicts Divorce? The Relationship Between Marital Processes and Marital Outcomes.* Hillsdale, NJ: Erlbaum.

Hafen, B. Q., et al. 1996. *Mind/Body Health: The Effects of Attitudes, Emotions, and Relationships.* Boston: Allyn & Bacon.

Harter, S., P. Waters, and N. R. Whitesell. 1998. Relational self-worth: Differences in perceived worth as a person across interpersonal contexts among adolescents. *Child Development* 69(3): 756–766.

Hartup, W. 1995. The three faces of friendship. *Journal of Social and Personal Relationships* 12(4): 569–574.

Harvey, E. 1999. Short-term and long-term effects of early parental employment on children of the National Longitudinal Survey of Youth. *Developmental Psychology* 35(2): 445–459.

Horwitz, A. V., J. McLaughlin, and H. R. White. 1998. How the negative and positive aspects of partner relationships affect the mental health of young married people. *Journal of Health and Social Behavior* 39(2): 124–136.

Kate, N. T. 1998. Two careers, one marriage. *American Demographics,* April.

Kayser, K. 1993. *When Love Dies: The Process of Marital Disaffection.* New York: Guilford Press.

Kiecolt-Glaser, J. K., et al. 1998. Marital stress: Immunologic, neuroendocrine, and autonomic correlates. *Annals of the New York Academy of Science* 840: 656-663.

Kiecolt-Glaser, J. K., et al.1997. Marital conflict in older adults: Endocrinological and immunological correlates. *Psychosomatic Medicine* 59(4): 339–349.

Laurenceau, J. P., L. F. Barrett, and P. R. Pietromonaco. 1998. Intimacy as an interpersonal process: The importance of self-disclosure, partner disclosure, and perceived partner responsiveness in interpersonal exchanges. *Journal of Personal and Social Psychology* 74(5): 1238–1251.

Lewis, J. M. 1998. For better or worse: Interpersonal relationships and individual outcome. *American Journal of Psychiatry* 155(5): 582–589.

Lips, H. 1997. *Sex and Gender,* 3rd ed. Mountain View, Calif.: Mayfield.

Lugaila, T. A. 1998. *Current Population Reports: Marital Status and Living Arrangements* (retrieved October 5, 1998; http://www.census.gov/prod/3/98pubs/p20-506.pdf).

Marano, H. E. 1998. Debunking the marriage myth: It works for women, too. *New York Times,* August 4.

Marital status and survival in prostate cancer. 1998. *Harvard Men's Health Watch,* August.

Martin, J. N., and T. K. Nakayama. 1997. *Intercultural Communication in Contexts.* Mountain View, Calif.: Mayfield.

National Center for Health Statistics. 1998. Births and deaths: Preliminary data for 1997. *National Vital Statistics Reports* 47(4).

Olson, D., and J. DeFrain. 2000. *Marriage and the Family,* 3rd ed. Mountain View, Calif.: Mayfield.

Pasley, K., and M. Ihinger-Tallman. 1994. *Remarriage and Stepparenting: Issues in Theory, Research, and Practice,* 2nd ed. Westport, Conn.: Greenwood Press.

Payne, M. 1998. "Waiting for lightning to strike": Social support for interracial couples. In *Readings in Cultural Contexts,* ed. J. N. Martin, T. K. Nakayama, and L. A. Flores. Mountain View, Calif.: Mayfield.

Rice, F. P. 1999. *Intimate Relationships, Marriages, and Families,* 4th ed. Mountain View, Calif.: Mayfield.

Sprecher, S. 1999. "I love you more today than yesterday." Romantic partners' perceptions of changes in love and related affect over time. *Journal of Personal and Social Psychology* 76(1): 46–53.

Sternberg, R., and M. Barnes, eds. 1988. *The Psychology of Love.* New Haven: Yale University Press.

Stinnett, N., and J. DeFrain. 1985. *Secrets of Strong Families.* Boston: Little, Brown.

Strong, B., C. DeVault, and B. Sayad. 1999. *Human Sexuality: Diversity in Contemporary America,* 3rd ed. Mountain View, Calif.: Mayfield.

Strong, B., and C. DeVault. 1995. *The Marriage and Family Experience.* St. Paul, Minn.: West.

Suler, J. 1998. *Online Therapy and Support Groups* (retrieved September 11, 1998; http://www1.rider.edu/~suler/psycyber/therapygroup.html).

Suler, J. 1997. *The Final Showdown Between In-Person and Cyberspace Relationships* (retrieved September 11, 1998; http://www1.rider.edu/~suler/psycyber/showdown.html).

U.S. Bureau of the Census. 1999. *Marital Status of Living Arrangements: March 1998 (Update),* P20-512 (retrieved February 18, 1999; http://www.census.gov/prod/99pubs/p20-514u-pdf).

U.S. Bureau of the Census. 1999. *Marital Status of the Population 15 Years Old and Over, by Sex and Race: 1950 to Present* (retrieved February 18, 1999; http://www.census.gov/populations/socdemo/ms-la/tabms-1.txt).

Wallerstein, J., and J. Kelly. 1996. *Surviving the Breakup: How Children and Parents Cope with Divorce.* New York: Basic Books.

What makes a good marriage? 1998. *Healthline,* July.

Woloshin, S., et al. 1997. Perceived adequacy of tangible social support and health outcomes in patients with coronary artery disease. *Journal of General Internal Medicine* 12(10): 613–618.

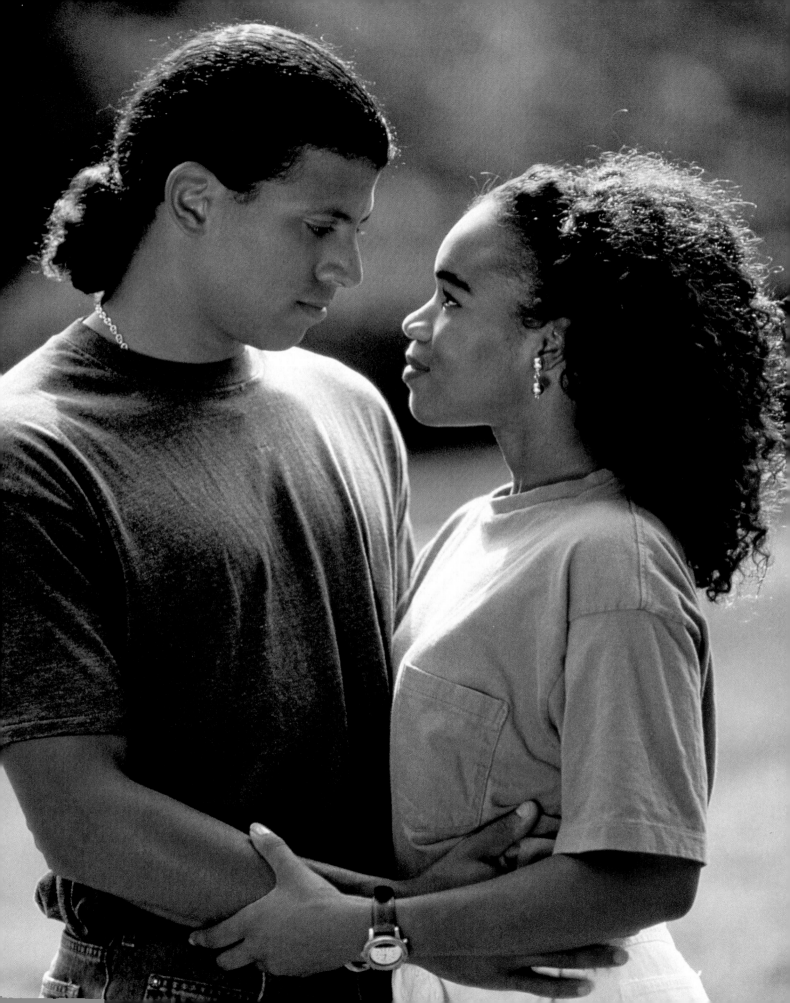

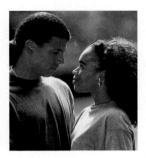

LEARNING OBJECTIVES

After reading this chapter, you should be able to:

- Describe the structure and function of the female and male sex organs.

- Explain the changes in sexual functioning that occur across the life span.

- Describe how the sex organs function during sexual activity, and list common causes of sexual problems.

- Outline the factors that influence sexual behavior and the various ways human sexuality can be expressed.

- Describe guidelines for safe, responsible sexual behavior.

Sex and Your Body

5

TEST YOUR KNOWLEDGE

1. Early in development, all embryos begin as female.
    True or false?

2. Which of the following is the center of sexual arousal in women?
    a. the vagina
    b. the clitoris
    c. the perineum
    d. the hymen

3. Most cases of erectile dysfunction ("impotence") are thought to be due to physical rather than psychological factors
    True or false?

4. Gender roles are determined solely by biological factors.
    True or false?

5. Women's motivations for having sex are usually to express love, while men's motives are usually physical.
    True or false?

6. About how many sexual references, innuendoes, and jokes does a typical teenager view on television each year?
    a. 150
    b. 1500
    c. 15,000

Answers

1. True. Without the influence of sex hormones, all embryos would develop into females.

2. b. While the entire vulva is an erogenous zone for most women, the clitoris has the highest concentration of nerve endings, analogous to the male penis.

3. True. It's estimated that about 70% of cases of erectile dysfunction can be traced to physical factors.

4. False. Although some gender characteristics are determined biologically, many others are defined by society and learned. From birth, children are encouraged to behave in ways that their culture deems appropriate for each gender.

5. False. While this statement is often true for men and women under 40, after age 40, physical gratification becomes the more common motivation for women, while emotional expression becomes more important for men.

6. c. Of these, fewer than 170 deal with abstinence, contraception, sexually transmitted diseases, or pregnancy.

Humans are sexual beings. Sexual activity is the source of our most intense physical pleasures, a central ingredient in many of our intimate emotional relationships, and, of course, the key to the reproduction of our species.

Sexuality is more than just sexual behavior. It includes biological sex (being biologically male or female), gender (masculine and feminine behaviors), sexual anatomy and physiology, sexual functioning and practices, and social and sexual interactions with others. Our individual sense of identity is powerfully influenced by our sexuality. We think of ourselves in very fundamental ways as male or female; as heterosexual or homosexual; as single, attached, married, or divorced. Sexuality is a complex, interacting group of inborn, biological characteristics and acquired behaviors people learn in the course of growing up in a particular family, community, and society.

Sexuality arouses intense feelings, and communicating about it is highly emotionally charged. Because of its basic role in human life, sexual expression is usually regulated with restrictions and taboos—written and unwritten laws specifying which functions and behaviors are acceptable and "normal" and which are unacceptable and "abnormal." Young people growing up in the United States are bombarded with conflicting messages about sex from television, movies, magazines, and popular music. The mass media suggest that the average person is a sexual athlete who continually jumps in and out of bed without using contraception, producing offspring, or contracting

disease. Although parents, educators, and other responsible adults present a more balanced picture, they may convey their own hidden messages as well. Ignorance, confusion, and fear are often the result.

Basic information about the body and about sexual functioning and behavior is vital to healthy adult life. Once we understand the facts, we have a better basis for evaluating the messages we get and for making informed, responsible choices about our sexual activities. If you have questions about aspects of your physical sexuality, this chapter will provide you with some answers.

SEXUAL ANATOMY

In spite of their different appearance, the sex organs of men and women arise from the same structures and fulfill similar functions. Each person has a pair of **gonads;** ovaries are the female gonads, and testes are the male gonads. The gonads produce **germ cells** and **sex hormones.** The female germ cells are ova (eggs); the male germ cells are sperm. Ova and sperm are the basic units of reproduction; their union results in the creation of a new life.

Female Sex Organs

The external sex organs, or genitals, of the female are called the **vulva** (Figure 5-1a). The mons pubis, a rounded mass of fatty tissue over the pubic bone, becomes covered with hair during puberty (biological maturation). Below it are two paired folds of skin called the labia majora (major lips) and the labia minora (minor lips). Enclosed within are the clitoris, the opening of the urethra, and the opening of the vagina. The **clitoris** is highly sensitive to touch and plays an important role in female sexual arousal and orgasm. The clitoris, like the penis, consists of a shaft, glans, and spongy tissue that fills with blood during sexual excitement. The glans is the most sensitive part of the clitoris and is covered by the clitoral hood, or **prepuce,** which is formed from the upper portion of the labia minora.

The female urethra leads directly from the urinary bladder to its opening between the clitoris and the opening of the vagina; it conducts urine from the bladder to the outside of the body. Unlike the male urethra, it is independent of the genitals.

The vaginal opening is partially covered by the hymen. This membrane can be stretched or torn during athletic activity or when a woman has sexual intercourse for the first time. The idea that an intact hymen is the sign of a virgin is a myth.

The **vagina** is the passage that leads to the internal reproductive organs (Figure 5-1b). It is the female structure for heterosexual sexual intercourse and also serves as the birth canal. Its soft, flexible walls are normally in con-

TERMS

sexuality A dimension of personality shaped by biological, psychosocial, and cultural forces and concerning all aspects of sexual behavior.

gonads The primary reproductive organs that produce germ cells and sex hormones; the ovaries and testes.

germ cells Sperm and ova (eggs).

sex hormones Chemical substances that stimulate and promote the development of physical sex characteristics.

vulva The external female genitals, or sex organs.

clitoris The highly sensitive female genital structure.

prepuce The foreskin of the clitoris or penis.

vagina The passage leading from the female genitals to the internal reproductive organs; the birth canal.

cervix The end of the uterus opening toward the vagina.

uterus The hollow, thick-walled, muscular organ in which the fertilized egg develops; the womb.

ovary One of two female reproductive glands that produce ova (eggs) and sex hormones; ovaries are the female gonads.

penis The male genital structure consisting of spongy tissue that becomes engorged with blood during sexual excitement.

scrotum The loose sac of skin and muscle fibers that contains the testes.

testis One of two male gonads, the site of sperm production; plural, *testes.* Also called *testicle.*

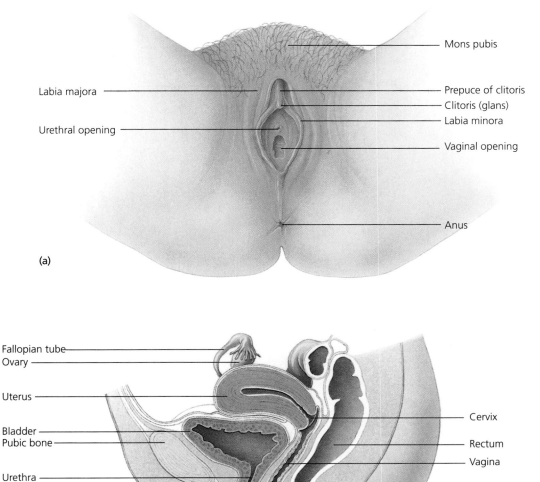

Figure 5-1 The female sex organs. (a) External structures; (b) internal structures.

tact with each other. A cylinder of muscles surrounds the vagina. During sexual excitement, the tension in these muscles increases and the walls of the vagina swell with blood.

Projecting into the upper part of the vagina is the **cervix,** the neck of the uterus. Inside the pear-shaped **uterus,** which slants forward above the bladder, the fertilized egg is implanted and grows into a *fetus.* A pair of *fallopian tubes* (or *oviducts*) extends from the top of the uterus. The end of each oviduct surrounds an **ovary** and guides the mature ovum down into the uterus after the egg bursts from its follicle on the surface of the ovary.

Male Sex Organs

A man's external sex organs, or genitals, are the penis and the scrotum (Figure 5-2a). The **penis** consists of spongy tissue that becomes engorged with blood during sexual excitement, causing the organ to enlarge and become erect. The **scrotum** is a pouch that contains a pair of **testes.** The purpose of the scrotum is to maintain the testes at a temperature approximately 5°F below that of the rest of the body—that is, at about 93.6°F. The process of sperm production is extremely heat-sensitive. In hot temperatures the muscles in the scrotum relax, and the

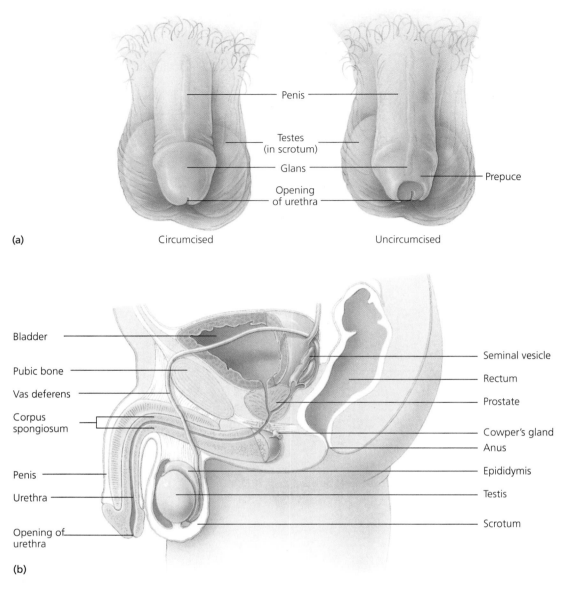

(a)   Circumcised   Uncircumcised

(b)

Figure 5-2   The male sex organs.   (a) External structures; (b) internal structures.

testes move away from the heat of the body. Conversely, in cold temperatures the muscles of the scrotum contract, and the testes move upward toward the body, where they can maintain their 5-degree temperature difference. This ability to regulate the temperature of the testes is important because elevated testicular temperature can interfere with normal sperm production.

Through the entire length of the penis runs a passage called the *urethra,* which can carry both urine and *semen,* the sperm-carrying fluid, to the opening at the tip of the glans (Figure 5-2b). Although urine and semen share a common passage, they are prevented from mixing together by muscles that control their entry into the urethra.

The testes contain tightly packed seminiferous tubules within which sperm are produced. These tubules end in a maze of ducts that flow into a single storage tube called the *epididymis,* on the surface of each testis. This tube leads to the *vas deferens,* a tube that rises into the abdominal cavity. Inside the prostate gland, the two vasa deferentia join the ducts of the two *seminal vesicles,* whose secretions provide nutrients to semen. The *prostate gland* produces some of the fluid in semen that nourishes and transports sperm. The tubes of the seminal vesicle and the vas deferens on each side lead to the *ejaculatory duct,* which joins the urethra. The *Cowper's glands* (bulbourethral glands) are two small structures flanking the urethra. During sexual arousal, these glands secrete a clear, mucuslike fluid that appears at the tip of the penis. The exact purpose of preejaculatory fluid is not known, but it may buffer sperm against any acidic urine in the urethra during ejaculation and help lubricate the urethra to facilitate the passage of sperm. In some men, preejaculatory fluid may contain sperm, so withdrawal of the penis before ejaculation is not a reliable form of contraception.

Circumcision   The smooth, rounded tip of the penis is the highly sensitive **glans,** an important component in sexual arousal. The glans is partially covered by the foreskin, or prepuce, a retractable fold of skin that is removed by **circumcision** in about 60–70% of newborn males in the United States. Circumcision is performed for cultural, religious, and hygienic reasons, and rates of circumcision vary widely among different groups. Worldwide, the rate is about 15%. Most Europeans, Asians, South and Central Americans, and Africans do not perform circumcision; Jews and Muslims are the major groups who circumcise for religious reasons.

The pros and cons of this simple procedure have been widely debated. Proponents argue that it promotes cleanliness and reduces the risk of urinary tract infections in newborns and sexually transmitted diseases (STDs) and sexual dysfunction later in life. Research findings have been mixed; for example, a recent U.S. survey found no relationship between STD risk and circumcision, while international studies have shown a greater risk for STDs among uncircumcised males. Cultural as well as anatomical factors may explain these findings.

Opponents of circumcision state that it is an unnecessary surgical procedure that causes pain and puts a baby at risk for complications. Opponents also argue that by removing the foreskin, circumcision exposes the glans of the penis to constant irritation by clothing, thereby reducing its sensitivity; research into this issue has been inconclusive. The American Academy of Pediatrics takes the position that although circumcision has potential medical benefits, the research is not sufficient to recommend the procedure routinely; and when circumcision is performed, painkilling medication should be provided.

While the debate focuses on medical concerns, most parents make their decision based on social or cultural factors. Fathers tend to want their sons to look like them and their peers. If a father is circumcised, he will most likely want his son to be circumcised, and vice versa. Whether or not to circumcise is a decision each family must make individually.

PERSONAL INSIGHT   Do you ever wonder if you're sexually "normal"? Do you worry about the size, shape, or appearance of any part of your body? Where do you think your ideas of "normal" come from?

HORMONES AND THE REPRODUCTIVE LIFE CYCLE

Many cultural and personal factors help shape the expression of your sexuality. But biology also plays an important role, particularly through the action of *hormones,* chemical messengers that are secreted directly into the bloodstream by the **endocrine glands.** The sex hormones produced by the ovaries or testes have a major influence on the development and function of the reproductive system throughout life.

The sex hormones made by the testes are called **androgens,** the most important of which is *testosterone.* The female sex hormones, produced by the ovaries, belong to two groups: **estrogens** and **progestins,** the most important of which is *progesterone.* The cortex of the **adrenal glands** also produces androgens in both males and females.

The hormones produced by the testes, the ovaries, and the adrenal glands are regulated by the hormones of the **pituitary gland,** located at the base of the brain. This gland in turn is controlled by hormones produced by the **hypothalamus** in the brain. Sex hormones exert their primary developmental influences first in the embryo stage and later during adolescence.

Differentiation of the Embryo

The biological sex of an individual is determined by the fertilizing sperm at the time of conception. All human cells normally contain 23 pairs of **chromosomes.** In 22 of the pairs, the two partner chromosomes match. But in the

TERMS

glans   The rounded head of the penis or the clitoris.

circumcision   Surgical removal of the foreskin of the penis.

endocrine glands   Glands that produce hormones.

androgens   Male sex hormones produced by the testes in males and by the adrenal glands in both sexes.

estrogens   A class of female sex hormones, produced by the ovaries, that bring about sexual maturation at puberty and maintain reproductive functions.

progestins   A class of female sex hormones, produced by the ovaries, that sustain reproductive functions.

adrenal glands   Endocrine glands, located over the kidneys, that produce androgens (among other hormones).

pituitary gland   An endocrine gland at the base of the brain that produces follicle-stimulating hormone (FSH) and luteinizing hormone (LH), among others.

hypothalamus   A region of the brain above the pituitary gland whose hormones control the secretions of the pituitary; also involved in the nervous control of sexual functions.

chromosomes   The threadlike bodies into which the genetic material within the cell nucleus is organized.

twenty-third pair, the **sex chromosomes**, two configurations are possible. Individuals with two matching X chromosomes are female, and individuals with one X and one Y chromosome (a much shorter chromosome carrying specialized genes) are male. Thus, at the time of conception, the genetic sex is established: females are XX and males are XY. The genetic sex will dictate whether the undifferentiated gonads will become ovaries or testes. If a Y chromosome is present, the gonads will become testes; the testes will produce the male hormone **testosterone.** Testosterone circulates throughout the body and causes the undifferentiated reproductive structures to develop into male sex organs (penis, scrotum, and so on). If a Y chromosome is not present, the gonads become ovaries and the reproductive structures develop into female sex organs (clitoris, labia, and so on).

Each male and female reproductive structure develops from the same undifferentiated tissue, so that every structure in one sex has its developmental counterpart in the other. Therefore, the penis corresponds to the clitoris and the scrotum to the labia majora. It is the presence or absence of testosterone that determines which way the tissue will develop.

Female Sexual Maturation

Although humans are fully sexually differentiated at birth, the differences between males and females are accentuated at **puberty,** the period during which the reproductive system matures, secondary sex characteristics develop, and the bodies of males and females come to appear more distinctive. The changes of puberty are induced by testosterone in the male and estrogen and **progesterone** in the female.

Physical Changes   The first sign of puberty in girls is breast development, followed by a rounding of the hips and buttocks. As the breasts develop, hair appears in the pubic region and later in the underarms. Shortly after the onset of breast development, girls show an increase in growth rate. Breast development usually begins between ages 8 and 13, and the time of rapid body growth occurs between ages 9 and 15. Estrogens and progestins from the ovaries, as well as androgens from the adrenal glands, are responsible for the female secondary sex characteristics, the physical changes that occur at puberty.

The Menstrual Cycle   A major landmark of puberty for young women is the onset of the **menstrual cycle,** the monthly ovarian cycle that leads to menstruation (loss of blood and tissue lining the uterus) in the absence of pregnancy. The first *menstrual period,* or menarche, occurs at the average age of 12.8 years in the United States, but it may also normally start several years earlier or later.

The menstrual cycle consists of four phases: (1) menses, (2) the estrogenic phase, (3) ovulation, and (4) the pro-

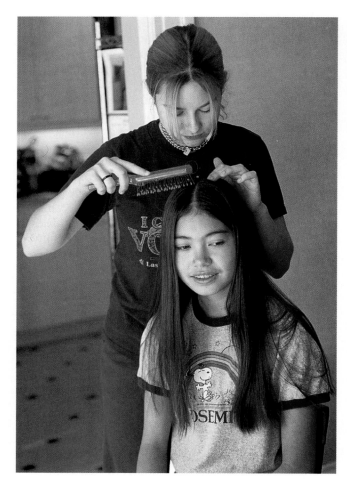

The physical changes of puberty usually begin between the ages of 8 and 13 for girls and 10 and 14 for boys. Once they reach puberty, these adolescents are biologically adults, but it will take another 5–10 years for them to become adults in social and psychological terms.

gestational phase (Figure 5-3). Day 1 of the cycle is considered to be the day of the onset of bleeding. For the purposes of our discussion, a cycle of 28 days will be used; however, normal cycles vary in length.

During menses, characterized by the menstrual flow, hormones from the ovaries and anterior pituitary gland occur in relatively low amounts. This phase of the cycle usually lasts from day 1 to about day 5.

The estrogenic phase begins when the menstrual flow ceases, and the anterior pituitary begins to produce increasing amounts of follicle-stimulating hormone (FSH) and luteinizing hormone (LH). Under the influence of FSH, an egg-containing ovarian *follicle* begins to mature, producing increasingly higher amounts of estrogens. Stimulated by estrogen, the uterine lining, the *endometrium,* thickens with large numbers of blood vessels and uterine glands.

A surge of a potent estrogen called estradiol from the follicle causes the anterior pituitary to release a large burst

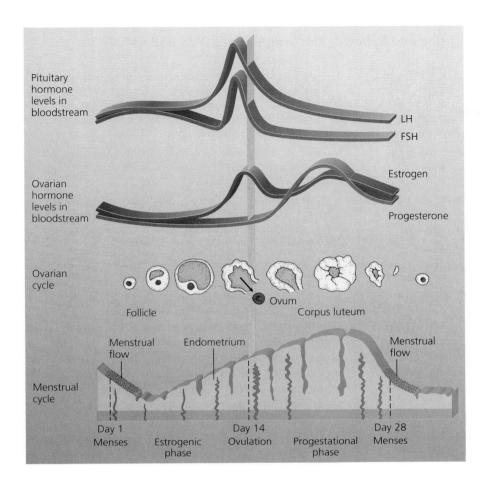

Figure 5-3 The menstrual cycle. The anterior pituitary releases FSH and LH, which stimulate the ovarian follicle to develop and release a mature egg. The ovarian follicle releases estrogen and progesterone, which stimulate the endometrium to continue to develop so that it will be ready to receive and nourish a fertilized egg. Unless pregnancy occurs, ovarian hormone levels fall and the endometrium sloughs off (menses).

of LH and a smaller amount of FSH. The high concentration of LH stimulates the developing follicle to release its ovum. This event is known as *ovulation*. After ovulation, the follicle is transformed into the **corpus luteum**, which produces progesterone and estrogen. Ovulation usually occurs about 14 days prior to the onset of menstrual flow, a fact that can be used to predict the most fertile time during the menstrual cycle, useful in both fertility treatment and natural family planning methods (see Chapter 6).

During the progestational phase of the cycle, the amount of progesterone secreted from the corpus luteum increases and remains high until the onset of the next menses. Under the influence of estrogen and progesterone, the endometrium continues to develop, readying itself to receive and nourish a fertilized ovum. When pregnancy occurs, the fertilized egg produces the hormone human chorionic gonadotropin (HCG), which maintains the corpus luteum. Thus, levels of ovarian hormones remain high and the uterine lining is preserved, preventing menses.

If pregnancy does not occur, the corpus luteum degenerates, and estrogen and progesterone levels gradually fall. Below certain hormonal levels, the endometrium can no longer be maintained, and it begins to slough off, initiating menses. As the levels of ovarian hormones fall, a slight rise in LH and FSH occurs, and a new menstrual cycle begins.

MENSTRUAL PROBLEMS   Menstruation is a normal biological process, but it may cause physical or psychological problems. *Dysmenorrhea* is characterized by cramps in the

sex chromosomes The X and Y chromosomes, which determine an individual's biological sex.

testosterone The most important androgen (male sex hormone); stimulates an embryo to develop into a male, and induces the development of male secondary sex characteristics during puberty.

puberty The period of biological maturation during adolescence.

progesterone The most important progestin (female sex hormone); induces the development of female secondary sex characteristics during puberty, regulates the menstrual cycle, and sustains pregnancy.

menstrual cycle The monthly ovarian cycle, regulated by pituitary and ovarian hormones; in the absence of pregnancy, menstruation occurs.

corpus luteum The part of the ovarian follicle left after ovulation, which secretes estrogen and progesterone during the second half of the menstrual cycle.

TERMS

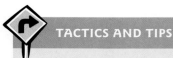

Although no universally effective treatments for PMS and PMDD have been identified, there are lifestyle changes that are often recommended to help prevent or minimize symptoms. The following strategies provide relief for many women, and all of them can contribute to a healthy lifestyle at any time.

- *Limit salt intake.* Salt promotes water retention and bloating. Avoid adding salt to your food, and don't eat salty snacks.

- *Exercise.* Women who exercise experience fewer symptoms both before and after their menstrual periods.

- *Don't use alcohol or tobacco.* Alcohol and tobacco may aggravate certain symptoms of PMS and PMDD.

- *Eat a nutritious diet.* Choose a low-fat diet rich in complex

carbohydrates from vegetables, fruits, and whole-grain breads, cereals, and pasta. Obtain an adequate calcium intake from calcium-rich foods and, if needed, supplements. Minimize your intake of sugar and caffeine; avoid chocolate, which is rich in both.

- *Relax.* Stress reduction is always beneficial, and stressful events can trigger PMS symptoms. Try relaxation techniques during the premenstrual time.

If symptoms persist, keep a daily diary to track both the types of symptoms you experience and their severity. See your physician for an evaluation and to learn more about treatments that are available only with a prescription.

---

lower abdomen, backache, vomiting, nausea, a bloated feeling, diarrhea, and loss of appetite. Some of these symptoms can be attributed to uterine muscular contractions caused by chemicals called prostaglandins. Any drug that blocks the effects of prostaglandins, such as aspirin or ibuprofen, will usually alleviate some of the symptoms of dysmenorrhea.

Many women experience transient physical and emotional symptoms prior to the onset of their menstrual flow. Depending on their severity, these symptoms may be categorized as one of three related conditions: **premenstrual tension, premenstrual syndrome (PMS)**, and **premenstrual dysphoric disorder (PMDD)**. Premenstrual tension symptoms are mild and may include negative mood changes and physical symptoms such as abdominal cramping and backache. More severe symptoms are classified as PMS; very severe symptoms that cause impairment in social functioning and work-related activities are classified as PMDD. All three conditions share a definite pattern: Symptoms appear prior to the onset of menses and disappear within a few days after the start of menstruation. It is estimated that as many as 75% of women report some discomfort prior to the onset of menses, 20–50% of women experience PMS symptoms, and 3–5% meet the criteria for PMDD.

Many symptoms are associated with PMS and PMDD, including physical changes such as breast tenderness, water retention (bloating), headache, and fatigue; insomnia or excessive sleep; appetite changes and food cravings; irritability, anger, and increased interpersonal conflict; mood swings; depression and sadness; anxiety and tearfulness; inability to concentrate; social withdrawal; and the sense that one is out of control or overwhelmed. The key to diagnosing PMS and PMDD is to keep a daily diary of symptoms over several menstrual cycles. PMDD is distinguished from PMS by the severity of symptoms, which in PMDD interfere significantly with work or school and with usual social activities and relationships.

Despite many research studies, the causes of PMS and PMDD are still unknown, and it is unclear why some women are more vulnerable than others. Research has focused on a variety of substances in the body that may fluctuate with the menstrual cycle, including progesterone, prostaglandins, serotonin and other neurotransmitters, calcium, magnesium, and the naturally occurring opiate beta-endorphin. Most researchers feel that PMS is probably caused by a combination of hormonal, nutritional, and psychological factors.

There are no completely effective therapies for PMS and PMDD. Selective serotonin reuptake inhibitors (SSRIs) such as Prozac may be prescribed to maintain serotonin levels and relieve depression and other psychological symptoms (see Chapter 3 for more on SSRIs). An over-the-counter product called PMS Escape has been shown beneficial for some PMS symptoms; it contains a mixture of carbohydrates that increase blood levels of tryptophan, an amino acid the body uses to produce serotonin. Other drug treatments include progesterone, diuretics to minimize water retention, and drugs that block the effects of prostaglandins, such as aspirin, ibuprofen, and more potent prescription prostaglandin inhibitors. A 1998 study found that calcium supplements can relieve some PMS symptoms for some women; prescription calcium channel blockers, which affect the action of calcium in the body, are sometimes also given. Research on the effects of treatment with calcium and magnesium is ongoing. In addition, there are lifestyle measures that may benefit some women; see the box "Preventing and Relieving the Symptoms of PMS and PMDD" for more information.

Male Sexual Maturation

Reproductive maturation of boys occurs about 2 years later than that of girls; it usually begins at about age 10 or 11. Physical changes include enlargement of the testes,

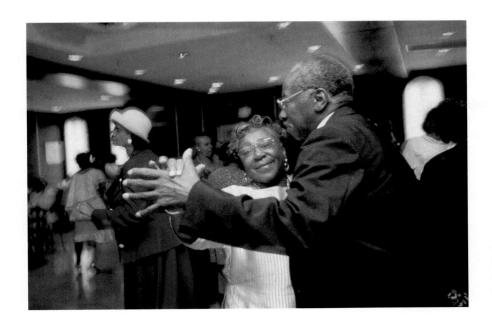

Although sexual physiology changes as people get older, many men and women readily adjust to these alterations. Sexual activity can continue throughout life for people like this healthy and vigorous older couple.

development of pubic hair, growth of the penis, the onset of ejaculation (usually at about age 11 or 12), deepening of the voice, the appearance of facial hair, and a period of rapid growth.

PERSONAL INSIGHT Recall the feelings you had about your sexuality when you went through puberty. Did you feel anxious or overwhelmed by the changes in your body or by feelings—worry, guilt, excitement—you had about your sexuality? Do you still have any of those feelings? Are you satisfied with the adjustment to sexuality you've made so far in your life?

Aging and Human Sexuality

Changes in hormone production and sexual functioning occur as we age. As a woman approaches age 50, her ovaries gradually cease to function and she enters **menopause,** the cessation of menstruation. For some women, the associated drop in hormone production causes symptoms that are troublesome. The most common physical symptoms of menopause are hot flashes, sensations of warmth rising to the face from the upper chest, with or without perspiration and chills. Other symptoms include headaches, dizziness, palpitations, and joint pains. Osteoporosis—decreasing bone density—can develop, making older women more vulnerable to fractures (see Chapter 12). Some menopausal women become moody, even markedly depressed, and they may also experience fatigue, irritability, and forgetfulness. Hormone replacement therapy can significantly relieve most of these symptoms, but it may increase some women's risk of certain types of cancer.

As a result of decreased estrogen production, the vaginal walls become thin, and lubrication in response to sexual arousal diminishes; sexual intercourse may become painful. Hormonal treatment or the use of lubricants during intercourse can minimize these problems.

Some women have a difficult time making the psychological adjustment to this stage of life, associating it with a loss of youth and sexual attractiveness. Others welcome it as a time of increased personal freedom, when the responsibilities of child rearing are over, and sex can be enjoyed without the fear of pregnancy. Today, with longer life expectancies, many women are rejecting the view that the childbearing years are the central period of life, flanked by youth and old age. Instead, they see three equally important periods characterized by different concerns: a time of growing and learning, a time of childbearing and nurturing (or creative expression), and a time of inner growth and repose. Menopause is seen as signaling the end of one phase of life and the beginning of another, equally meaningful one. A 1998 poll of menopausal women found that more than half reported being happier now than in their younger years.

premenstrual tension Mild physical and emotional changes associated with the time before the onset of menses; symptoms can include abdominal cramping and backache.

premenstrual syndrome (PMS) A disorder characterized by physical discomfort, psychological distress, and behavioral changes that begin after ovulation and cease when menstruation begins.

premenstrual dysphoric disorder (PMDD) Severe form of PMS, characterized by symptoms serious enough to interfere with work or school or with social activities and relationships.

menopause The cessation of menstruation, occurring gradually around age 50.

TERMS

In men, testosterone production gradually decreases with age. As they get older, men depend more on direct physical stimulation for sexual arousal. They take longer to get an erection and find it more difficult to maintain; orgasmic contractions are less intense.

Many men go through a period of reassessment and re-adjustment in middle age, which may have repercussions for their sexuality. However, a 1999 study that followed more than 3000 people for 10 years found that far from being a time of dissatisfaction and "midlife crisis," the middle years are a fulfilling time of life characterized by satisfying relationships. As with women, sexual activity can continue to be a source of pleasure and satisfaction for men as they grow older. A 1998 survey found that nearly half of all Americans age 60 or older engage in sexual activity at least once a month.

> **PERSONAL INSIGHT** Many people in their sixties, seventies, and eighties continue to enjoy sex as a vital part of their lives. What are your attitudes toward older people and sex? Where do you think your ideas come from?

SEXUAL FUNCTIONING

In this section, we discuss sexual physiology—how the sex organs function during sexual activity—and problems that can occur with sexual functioning. Sexual activity is based on stimulus and response. Erotic stimulation leads to sexual arousal (excitement), which may culminate in the intensely pleasurable experience of orgasm. But sexual activity should not be thought of only in terms of the sex organs. Responses to sexual stimulation involve not just the genitals but the entire body—and the mind as well.

Sexual Stimulation

Sexual excitement can come from many sources, both physical and psychological. Although physical stimuli have an obvious and direct effect, some people believe psychological stimuli—thoughts, fantasies, desires, perceptions—are even more powerfully erotic. Regardless of the source of erotic stimuli, all stimulation has a physical basis, which is given meaning by the brain.

Physical Stimulation   Physical stimulation comes through the senses: We are aroused by things we see, hear, taste, smell, and feel. It has even been suggested that we may be attracted and aroused by molecules of specific chemicals, called **pheromones**, that are produced by other people's bodies to create sexual excitement. Most often, sexual stimuli come from other people, but they may also come from books, photographs, paintings, songs, films, or other sources.

The most obvious and effective physical stimulation is touching. Even though culturally defined practices vary and individual people have different preferences, most sexual encounters eventually involve some form of touching with hands, lips, and body surfaces. Kissing, caressing, fondling, and hugging are as much a part of sexual encounters as they are of expressing affection.

The most intense form of stimulation by touching involves the genitals. The clitoris and the glans of the penis are particularly sensitive to such stimulation. Other highly responsive areas include the vaginal opening, the nipples, the breasts, the insides of the thighs, the buttocks, the anal region, the scrotum, the lips, and the earlobes.

Such sexually sensitive areas, or **erogenous zones,** are especially susceptible to sexual arousal for most people, most of the time. Often, though, it's not *what* is touched but how, for how long, and by whom that determine the response. Under the right circumstances, touching any part of the body can cause sexual arousal.

Psychological Stimulation   Sexual arousal also has an important psychological component, regardless of the nature of the physical stimulation. Fantasies, ideas, memories of past experiences, and mood can all generate sexual excitement. Erotic thoughts may be linked to an imagined person or situation, or to a sexual experience from the past. Fantasies may involve activities a person doesn't actually wish to experience in reality, usually because they're dangerous, frightening, or forbidden.

Arousal is also powerfully influenced by emotions. How you feel about a person and how the person feels about you matter tremendously in how sexually responsive you are likely to be. Even the most direct forms of physical stimulation carry emotional overtones. Kissing, caressing, and fondling express affection and caring. The emotional charge they give to a sexual interaction is at least as significant to sexual arousal as the purely physical stimulation achieved by touching.

The Sexual Response Cycle

Noted sex researchers William Masters and Virginia Johnson were the first to describe in detail the human sexual response cycle. Men and women respond physiologically with a predictable set of reactions, regardless of the nature of the stimulation (Figure 5-4).

TERMS   **pheromones** Chemical substances produced by animals that are released into the environment and stimulate other animals of the same species; their presence in humans is uncertain.

erogenous zone Any region of the body highly responsive to sexual stimulation.

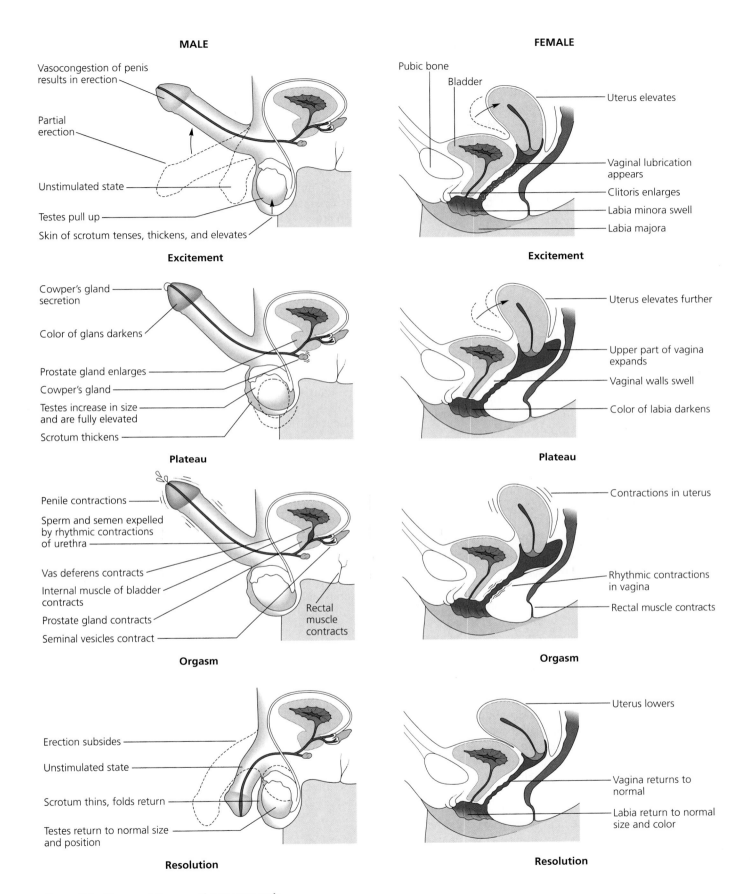

MALE

Vasocongestion of penis results in erection

Partial erection

Unstimulated state

Testes pull up

Skin of scrotum tenses, thickens, and elevates

Excitement

Cowper's gland secretion

Color of glans darkens

Prostate gland enlarges

Cowper's gland

Testes increase in size and are fully elevated

Scrotum thickens

Plateau

Penile contractions

Sperm and semen expelled by rhythmic contractions of urethra

Vas deferens contracts

Internal muscle of bladder contracts

Prostate gland contracts

Seminal vesicles contract

Rectal muscle contracts

Orgasm

Erection subsides

Unstimulated state

Scrotum thins, folds return

Testes return to normal size and position

Resolution

FEMALE

Pubic bone

Bladder

Uterus elevates

Vaginal lubrication appears

Clitoris enlarges

Labia minora swell

Labia majora

Excitement

Uterus elevates further

Upper part of vagina expands

Vaginal walls swell

Color of labia darkens

Plateau

Contractions in uterus

Rhythmic contractions in vagina

Rectal muscle contracts

Orgasm

Uterus lowers

Vagina returns to normal

Labia return to normal size and color

Resolution

Figure 5-4   Stages of the sexual response cycle.

Two physiological mechanisms explain most genital and bodily reactions during sexual arousal and orgasm. These mechanisms are vasocongestion and myotonia. **Vasocongestion** is the engorgement of tissues that results when more blood flows into an organ than is flowing out. Thus, the penis becomes erect on the same principle that makes a garden hose become stiff when the water is turned on. **Myotonia** is increased muscular tension, which culminates in rhythmical muscular contractions during orgasm.

Four phases characterize the sexual response cycle:

1. In the *excitement phase,* the penis becomes erect as its tissues become engorged with blood. The testes expand and are pulled upward within the scrotum. In women, the clitoris and the labia are similarly engorged with blood, and the vaginal walls become moist with lubricating fluid.

2. The *plateau phase* is an extension of the excitement phase. Reactions become more marked: In men, the penis becomes harder, and the testes larger. In women, the lower part of the vagina swells, while its upper end expands and vaginal lubrication increases.

3. In the *orgasmic phase,* or **orgasm,** rhythmic contractions occur along the man's penis, urethra, prostate gland, seminal vesicles, and muscles in the pelvic and anal regions. These involuntary muscular contractions lead to the ejaculation of **semen,** which consists of sperm cells from the testes and secretions from the prostate gland and seminal vesicles. In women, contractions occur in the lower part of the vagina and in the uterus, as well as in the pelvic region and the anus.

4. In the *resolution phase,* all the changes initiated during the excitement phase are reversed. Excess blood drains from tissues, the muscles in the region relax, and the genital structures return to their unstimulated state.

More general physical reactions accompany the genital changes in both men and women. Beginning with the excitement phase, nipples become erect, the woman's breasts begin to swell, and in both sexes the skin of the chest becomes flushed; these changes are more marked in women. The heart rate doubles by the plateau phase, and respiration becomes faster. During orgasm, breathing becomes irregular and the person may moan or cry out. A feeling of warmth leads to increased sweating during the resolution phase. Deep relaxation and a sense of well-being pervade the body and the mind.

Male and female reactions during the sexual response cycle differ somewhat. Generally, the male pattern is more uniform, whereas the female pattern is more varied. For instance, the female excitement phase may lead directly to orgasm, or orgasmic and plateau phases may be fused.

Male orgasm is marked by the ejaculation of semen. After ejaculation, men enter a *refractory period,* during which they cannot be restimulated to orgasm. Women do not have a refractory period, and immediate restimulation to orgasm is possible.

Sexual Problems

Both physical and psychological factors can interfere with sexual functioning. If you are in poor physical health or experiencing high levels of stress or anxiety, sexual functioning may be negatively affected. Difficulties may be caused by infections and other sexual health problems. Disturbances in sexual desire, performance, or satisfaction are referred to as **sexual dysfunctions.**

Common Sexual Health Problems   Some problems with sexual functioning are due to treatable or preventable infections or other sexual health problems. Conditions that affect women include the following:

• *Vaginitis,* inflammation of the vagina, is caused by a variety of organisms: *Candida* (yeast infection), *Trichomonas* (trichomoniasis), and the overgrowth of a variety of bacteria (bacterial vaginosis). Symptoms include vaginal discharge, vaginal irritation, and pain during intercourse. Vaginitis is easily treated with various medications. (See Chapters 17 and 18 for more on yeast infection, trichomoniasis, and bacterial vaginosis.)

• *Endometriosis* is the growth of endometrial tissue (tissue normally found lining the uterus) outside of the uterus. It occurs most often in women of childbearing age, and pain in the lower abdomen and pelvis is the most common symptom. Painful premenstrual intercourse may occur. Endometriosis can cause serious problems if left untreated because the endometrial tissue can scar and partially or completely block the oviducts, causing infertility (difficulty conceiving) or sterility (the inability to conceive). Endometriosis is treated with hormone therapy and/or surgery.

• *Pelvic inflammatory disease (PID)* is an infection of the uterus, oviducts, or ovaries, caused when microorganisms spread to these areas from the vagina. Approximately 50–75% of PID cases are caused by sexually transmitted organisms associated with diseases such as gonorrhea and *Chlamydia* infections. PID can cause scarring of the oviducts, resulting in infertility or sterility. Symptoms include pain in the abdomen and pelvis, fever, and possibly pain during intercourse. Treatment involves bed rest and antibiotic therapy, and prompt treatment reduces the chances of infertility and sterility. (Sexually transmitted diseases are discussed in detail in Chapter 18.)

Sexual health problems that affect men include the following:

• *Prostatitis* is inflammation or infection of the prostate gland. Symptoms are fever, chills, pain in the genital region, frequent urination, and, in some cases, painful ejaculation. More common in men over 40, prostatitis is treated with antibiotics.

- *Testicular cancer* occurs most commonly in men in their twenties and thirties. A rare cancer, it has a very high cure rate if detected early. A testicular self-exam should be performed regularly (see Chapter 16). If any lumps are felt, a physician should be consulted.

Sexual Dysfunctions The term *sexual dysfunction* encompasses disturbances in sexual desire, performance, or satisfaction. A wide variety of physical conditions and drugs may interfere with sexual functioning (diabetes may interfere with the blood and nerve supply to the sex organs, for example); psychological causes and problems in intimate relationships can be important factors in some cases. The same two mechanisms—vasocongestion and myotonia—that are the basis of the sexual response cycle are also at the root of the main forms of sexual disturbance: an inability to become aroused, and problems experiencing orgasm.

COMMON SEXUAL DYSFUNCTIONS Common sexual dysfunctions in men include **erectile dysfunction** (previously called impotence), the inability to have or maintain an erection sufficient for sexual intercourse; **premature ejaculation**, ejaculation before or just on penetration of the vagina or anus; and **retarded ejaculation**, the inability to ejaculate once an erection is achieved. Many men experience occasional difficulty achieving an erection or ejaculating because of excessive alcohol consumption, fatigue, or stress. In fact, it is estimated that 50% of all American men experience occasional bouts of erectile dysfunction and retarded ejaculation.

Two sexual dysfunctions in women are **vaginismus**, in which the woman experiences painful involuntary muscular spasms when sexual intercourse is attempted, and **orgasmic dysfunction**, the inability to experience orgasm. Vaginismus is a conditioned reflex probably related to fear of intercourse. Orgasmic dysfunction has been the subject of a great deal of discussion over the years, as people debated the nature of the female orgasm and what constitutes dysfunction in women. Many women experience orgasm but not during intercourse, or they experience orgasm during intercourse only if the clitoris is directly stimulated at the same time. In general, the inability to experience orgasm under certain circumstances is a problem only if the woman considers it so. If she believes that she has a problem—for example, if she has never experienced orgasm under any circumstances—then she is considered to have orgasmic dysfunction.

TREATING SEXUAL DYSFUNCTION Most forms of sexual dysfunction are treatable. The first step is to have a thorough physical examination to identify any underlying medical condition that may be responsible for the problem. Heart disease and diabetes, for example, may cause erectile dysfunction; in fact, up to 70% of all erectile problems are thought to be due to physical factors, particularly vascular problems. Smoking affects blood vessels and blood flow in the penis and is an independent risk factor for erectile dysfunction. Drugs and medications, especially alcohol and medications used to treat high blood pressure, may also inhibit sexual responses. A sexual dysfunction may disappear when the interfering factor is removed—following treatment for the underlying disease or a change in medication, for example.

If physical problems continue to interfere with sexual response, many treatments are available, particularly for erectile dysfunction. Older treatments include a variety of methods that induce blood flow into the penis—vacuum pumps or drugs that are injected directly into the penis or inserted into the urethra in pellet form—and rigid or inflatable implants. In 1998, Viagra (sildenafil citrate), the first-ever prescription pill for erectile dysfunction, was introduced; it quickly became the most successful new prescription drug in history. Viagra doesn't cause an erection, but it enhances blood flow into the penis, thereby allowing an erection when sexual stimulation occurs. It has been shown to be effective in as many as 70% of men with erectile dysfunction, allowing them to achieve erections comparable for their age group. (In other words, a man of 85 will not have the same erection as when he was 20.) It does not enhance sex drive or sexual response in men who can already achieve an erection.

If no physical problem is found, a sexual dysfunction may be psychosocial in origin. Psychosocial causes of dysfunction include troubled relationships, a lack of sexual skills, irrational attitudes and beliefs, anxiety, and psy-

vasocongestion The accumulation of blood in tissues and organs.   **TERMS**

myotonia Increased muscular tension.

orgasm The discharge of accumulated sexual tension with characteristic genital and bodily manifestations and a subjective sensation of intense pleasure.

semen Seminal fluid, consisting of sperm cells and secretions from the prostate gland and seminal vesicles.

sexual dysfunction A disturbance in sexual desire, performance, or satisfaction.

erectile dysfunction The inability to have or maintain an erection.

premature ejaculation Involuntary orgasm before or shortly after the penis enters the vagina or anus; ejaculation that takes place sooner than desired.

retarded ejaculation The inability to ejaculate when one wishes to during intercourse.

vaginismus Painful, involuntary muscular contractions in the vagina that occur when sexual intercourse is attempted.

orgasmic dysfunction The inability to experience orgasm.

chosexual trauma, such as sexual abuse or rape. Many of these problems can be addressed by sex therapy methods that seek to modify the beliefs and behavior patterns that are interfering with satisfactory sexual relationships. A therapist may recommend books or films to help counter sexual myths and teach sexual skills. A therapist can also promote open discussion between partners and suggest specific activities or techniques. For example, premature ejaculation is often treated by the squeeze technique, in which the tip of the penis is squeezed when the man feels he is about to ejaculate.

Women who seek treatment for orgasmic dysfunction often have not had the chance to learn through trial and error what types of stimulation will excite them and bring them to orgasm. Most sex therapists prefer to treat this problem with **masturbation** (genital self-stimulation). Women are taught about their own anatomy and sexual responses and then are encouraged to experiment with masturbation until they experience orgasm. Once they can masturbate to orgasm, they may need additional treatment to transfer this learning to sexual intercourse with a partner.

Sexual problems are closely tied to emotional and psychological concerns and with a person's perceptions, thoughts, beliefs, values, and relationships with others.

SEXUAL BEHAVIOR

Many behaviors stem from sexual impulses, and sexual expression takes a variety of forms. Probably the most basic aspect of sexuality is reproduction, the process of producing offspring. As important as reproduction is, the intention of creating a child accounts for only a small measure of sexual activity; most people have sex for other reasons as well.

Sexual excitement and satisfaction are aspects of sexual behavior separate from reproduction. The intensely pleasurable sensations of arousal and orgasm are probably the strongest motivators for human sexual behavior. People are infinitely varied in the ways they seek to experience erotic pleasure. In this section, we examine how sexual behavior develops and take a closer look at different sexual behaviors.

The Development of Sexual Behavior

Sexual behavior is a product of many factors, including genetics, physiology, psychology, and social and cultural influences. Our behavior is shaped by the interplay of our biological predispositions and our learning experiences throughout life.

Gender Roles and Gender Identity   The term *gender* is usually used to refer to the state of being male or female; people often use the word *sex* to mean the same thing.

Strictly speaking, *sex* refers only to being biologically male or female, while *gender* encompasses both your biological sex and your masculine or feminine behaviors. As mentioned in Chapter 4, your **gender role** is everything you do in your daily life that expresses your maleness or femaleness to others. Your **gender identity** is your personal, inner sense of being male or female. Gender role and gender identity are usually in agreement, but some people experience conflict between the two. A male who feels trapped in the body of a male and who wants to be a female may exhibit the gender role of a male, but his gender identity is that of a female.

BIOLOGICAL AND CULTURAL INFLUENCES   Some gender characteristics are determined biologically, such as the genitals a person is born with and the secondary sex characteristics that develop at puberty. Others are defined by society and learned in the course of growing up. From birth, children are encouraged to behave in ways their culture deems appropriate for one sex or the other. In our society, parents usually give children gender-specific names, clothes, and toys; and children may model their own behavior after their same-sex parent. People are far more likely to tell a boy why the car is accelerating, and a girl why the cookies aren't chewy. Family and friends create an environment that teaches the child how to act appropriately as a girl or a boy. Teachers, television, books, and even strangers model these gender roles.

Gender roles vary from one society to another and from one time to another. In the United States today, for example, many women shave their legs and wear makeup; in Muslim countries, women wear robes and veils that conceal their face and body. Each set of behaviors expresses some learned aspect of the female gender role in that society, and each set would be inappropriate in the other society. Standards of sexual attractiveness also vary from one culture to another; see the box "Attracting a Partner in Different Cultures," p. 118.

An extreme example of how cultural traditions can affect gender roles and sexual activity is a procedure known as female circumcision. In over 20 African countries, some parts of Asia and the Middle East, and immigrant communities elsewhere, female infants, children, or young women may undergo a circumcision in which parts of the clitoris and labia are removed. In some procedures, only the hood of the clitoris is removed. In others, the entire clitoris, labia minora, and parts of the labia majora are removed. The sides of the labia majora may be sewn together, leaving only a small opening for the passage of urine and menstrual blood. The effects of these painful procedures can include bleeding, infection, the inability to enjoy sex, and infertility.

The practice probably developed as a way of controlling women's sexuality and ensuring that a woman would be a virgin at the time of marriage. Upon marriage, the husband reopens the labia to allow intercourse and child-

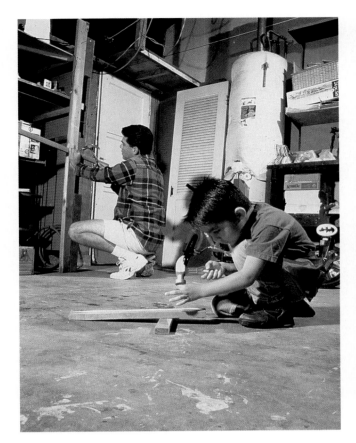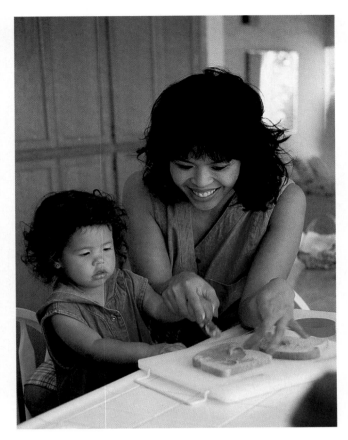

Our sense of gender identity and many of our gender-role behaviors are overwhelmingly influenced by cultural factors. These children are learning gender-specific behaviors by imitating their parents.

birth. It is interesting to note that surgery to remove all or part of the clitoris was practiced by physicians in the nineteenth century in both England and the United States, primarily as a "cure" for masturbation.

Many countries, including the United States, now have laws against female circumcision, and the World Health Organization and other groups are trying to educate people about the negative medical consequences of the procedures. Recently, several women have also sought asylum in the United States and other countries in an attempt to spare themselves or their daughters from the physical and psychological pain of female circumcision.

GENDER-ROLE FLEXIBILITY   Historically, gender roles have tended to highlight and emphasize the differences between males and females, but new gender roles are emerging in our society that reflect more of a mix of male and female characteristics and behaviors. This tendency toward **androgyny** greatly broadens the range of experiences available to both males and females. Many educators, parents, and others have attempted to erase the lines between stereotypically masculine and feminine behaviors for children in hopes of freeing them from the constraints of inflexible gender roles.

Androgynous adults are less stereotyped in their thinking; in how they look, dress, and act; how they divide work in the home; how they think about jobs and careers; and how they express themselves sexually. Women today are able, and even expected, to be much more assertive, competitive, ambitious, and powerful than they were allowed to be in the past; likewise, men can be more sensitive, articulate, nurturing, and emotionally expressive. Children who are exposed to androgynous models are likely to have more choices when they grow up, although many learned gender-role behaviors are so subtle that it's virtually impossible to escape them.

masturbation   Self-stimulation for the purpose of sexual arousal and orgasm.   TERMS

gender role   The different behaviors and attitudes a society expects of women and men.

gender identity   A person's personal, internal sense of maleness or femaleness.

androgyny   A mixing of male and female characteristics and behaviors, especially a lack of stereotyping with respect to gender roles.

While each of us has our own standard of what physical characteristics we consider to be beautiful or handsome, most of us could agree on what is attractive in our culture today. Standards of beauty change over time within a given culture, and standards of attractiveness vary across different cultures. Here's how partners are attracted in two cultures.

A man in the southeastern United States is getting ready for a date. He really wants to impress her tonight, so he puts on his best slacks and new shirt. He dabs on extra after-shave lotion, brushes his teeth for the second time, rinses with mouthwash, and makes sure his well-washed hair is held in place with a bit of hair spray. He's ready.

Thousands of miles away on a remote island in Southeast Asia, another man is getting ready to court a potential mate. He lives on one of the Sulu Islands in the southern Philippines. He has put heavily scented wax on his hair and put white powder on his face. He checks his pinky fingernail and is satisfied that it has grown very long in the past few weeks. He is pleased with the color of nail polish on it. He is dressed in very loose-fitting clothes that reveal his genitals. He's ready.

Back in the United States, a woman is using a multitude of cosmetics—powders, lipstick, hair spray, perfume, eyeliner, and eye shadow—in preparation for her date. She had purchased a nice dress with matching shoes especially for tonight, and her hair is in a new and different style. She's ready.

The potential mate of the man in the Philippines is very excited about meeting him tonight. She will go with other young women and men to the local beach for conversation and the playing of music. Like other women in her culture, she does not wash her hair often, but frequently combs coconut oil through it. Men find this very sexy, and she is happy with the amount of oil in her hair. She puts on some white face powder and perfume, touches up her nail polish, and then puts on lipstick. She is pleased with her appearance and decides to put a spot of lipstick on each cheek. She's ready.

Obviously, each of the cultures described above has its own standard of attractiveness, but it's also clear that there are similarities. In both cases the women use perfume and pay particular attention to their hair. The men also use scent in an attempt to attract a mate. Although cultural standards differ in some ways, we are all intent on securing the most attractive mate, in our own eyes, that we can.

SOURCE: Nimmo, H. A. 1991. Bajau sex and reproduction. In *Human Sexuality: Cross-Cultural Readings,* ed. B. du Toit. New York: McGraw-Hill.

Gender, Sexuality, and the Mass Media   Many of our ideas about sexuality and gender roles are shaped by the mass media. Television, movies, music, magazines, and advertisements are awash with sexual images. These images are usually of young, sexy people promising passionately fulfilling relationships. Women and men are often portrayed in traditional gender roles, with provocatively dressed women in need of protection interacting with aggressive and muscular men.

Media images of sexuality are often more influential than the family in shaping the sexual attitudes and behavior of adolescents and college students. Yet these images are usually unrealistic and help perpetuate stereotypes of women and men in our society. The mass media rarely portray people negotiating safer sex or communicating seriously about other sexual issues.

PERSONAL INSIGHT   What does being a woman or a man mean to you? How much has this idea been shaped by the media? Do you ever feel you can't "measure up" to the people you see on TV or in a magazine?

Childhood Sexual Behavior   The capacity to respond sexually is present at birth. Ultrasound studies suggest that boys experience erections in the uterus. After birth, both sexes have the capacity for orgasm, though many babies may not experience it. As people grow, many discover this capacity through self-exploration. Sexual behaviors gradually emerge in childhood in the form of self-stimulating play. Self-exploration and touching the genitals are common forms of play, observed among infants as young as 6 months. They gradually lead to more deliberate forms of masturbation, with or without orgasm.

Children often engage in sexual play with playmates by exploring each other's genitals. These activities are often part of games like "playing house" or "playing doctor." By age 12, 40% of boys have engaged in sex play; the peak exploration age for girls is 9, by which time 14% have had such experiences. Although parents and teachers actively teach and socialize children, in our culture they largely avoid the task of sex education.

Adolescent Sexuality   A person who has experienced puberty is biologically an adult. But in psychological and social terms, people take 5–10 more years to attain full adult status. This discrepancy between biological and social maturity creates considerable confusion over what constitutes appropriate sexual behavior during adolescence.

Sexual fantasies and dreams become more common and explicit in adolescence than at earlier ages, often as an accompaniment to masturbation. Research has shown that about 80% of teenage boys and 55% of teenage girls masturbate more or less regularly. Once puberty is reached, orgasm in boys is accompanied by ejaculation. Teenage boys also experience **nocturnal emissions** ("wet dreams"). Some girls also have orgasmic dreams. In general, masturbation does not carry the social stigma and imagined perils of former times, but adolescents—and many adults as well—are often still embarrassed by it.

Sexual interaction during adolescence usually takes place between peers in the context of dating. Sexual intimacy is usually expressed in such relationships through petting and necking, which may involve kissing, caressing, and stimulating the breasts and genitals. These activities lead to sexual arousal but may not culminate in orgasm.

Many American teenagers also engage in premarital sexual relations. Recent surveys indicate that the average age of first sexual intercourse is about 17.2 years for girls and 16.6 years for boys; among high school students, 48.8% of males and 47.7% of females report that they have had sexual intercourse. Rates for premarital sex vary considerably from one group to another, however, based on ethnic, educational, religious, geographic, and other factors. Engaging in sexual intercourse for the first time is affected by these same factors, plus psychological readiness, fear of consequences, being in love, going steady, peer pressure, and the need to act like an adult, gain popularity, or rebel. Some people thoughtfully weigh decisions and others plunge recklessly. Teenagers who engage in sexual intercourse or are close to doing so generally value autonomy, have loosened family ties in favor of more reliance on friends, and are more apt to experiment with drugs or alcohol and to engage in political activism than their peers.

Adolescent sexual behaviors are not confined to heterosexual relationships. Beginning in childhood, sex play involves members of one's own sex as well as of the other sex. Homosexual attractions, with or without sexual encounters, are likewise common in adolescence. For many these are youthful experiments and don't mean that participants will ultimately be homosexual. For a minority they may be a factor in adult sexual orientation. Most adult gay men and women trace their preferences to their early years (see Chapter 4).

Adult Sexuality Early adulthood is a time when people make important life choices—a time of increasing responsibility in terms of interpersonal relationships and family life. In recent years, both in the United States and abroad, there has been a definite trend toward marriage at a later age than in past decades. And before marriage, more young adults are driven by an internal need to become sexually knowledgeable. Today, more people in their twenties believe that becoming sexually experienced rather than preserving virginity is an important prelude to selecting a mate. As explained in Chapter 3, according to Erikson, developing the capacity for intimacy is a central task for young adults. Take the quiz in the box "Your Sexual Attitudes" on p. 120 to explore your own beliefs and opinions about sex.

A recent survey investigated women's and men's motivations for engaging in sexual activities. Differing motivations change with age (Figure 5-5). Younger men state that they engage in sex for physical reasons, while women of the same age state that they engage in sex for emotional reasons. As men and women get older, their motives change; men more often engage in sex for emotional reasons, and women more often for physical reasons. In the oldest age groups, women and men actually switch their motives for sex from those of the earliest age groups.

Adult sexuality can include any of the sexual behaviors and practices described in this chapter. In mature love relationships, people ideally can integrate all the aspects of intimacy—physical, sexual, emotional—so that sexuality is a deeply meaningful part of how they express love. People can continue to enjoy sexual activities throughout their entire lives, varying and expanding the scope of their experiences as they gain more understanding of their own and their partners' needs and desires.

Sexuality in Illness and Disability Any disease or disability that affects mobility, well-being, self-esteem, or body image has the potential to affect sexual expression. People with chronic diseases or disabilities often have special needs regarding their sexual behavior. They must also confront widespread myths that they are asexual. In our culture, only people conforming to a narrow standard of youth, attractiveness, and ability are seen as sexual beings. But sexuality is integral to all of us, regardless of our physical status.

The diagnosis of a chronic illness or the onset of a disability usually requires major adjustments in many areas of life, including sexuality. At first, sexual activity may take a low priority because of fear and the loss of self-esteem. Individuals and couples can learn to become creative about sexual expression and develop new approaches based on the limitations of the disability. Developing a positive body image is often a particularly important, and difficult, adjustment for people with physical illness or limitations.

Sexual Decision Making Sharing sexual intimacy can be a source of tremendous pleasure. It can also lead to guilt, confusion, misunderstanding, an unwanted pregnancy, or a sexually transmitted disease. As you consider moving into a sexual relationship, you owe it to yourself and your partner to honestly explore your expectations and responsibilities. Ask yourself questions like the following:

---

nocturnal emissions Orgasm and ejaculation (wet dream) during sleep. **TERMS**

For each statement, circle the response that most closely reflects your position.

	Agree	Not Sure	Disagree
1. Sex education encourages young people to have sex.	1	2	3
2. Homosexuality is a healthy, normal expression of sexuality.	3	2	1
3. Members of the other sex will think more highly of you if you remain mysterious.	1	2	3
4. It's better to wait until marriage to have sex.	1	2	3
5. Abortion should be a personal, private choice for a woman.	3	2	1
6. It's natural for men to have more sexual freedom than women.	1	2	3
7. Condoms should not be made available to teenagers.	1	2	3
8. Pornography should not be restricted for adults.	3	2	1
9. A woman who is raped usually does something to provoke it.	1	2	3
10. Contraception is the woman's responsibility.	1	2	3
11. Feminism has had a positive influence on society.	3	2	1
12. Masturbation is a healthy expression of sexuality.	3	2	1
13. I have many friends of the other sex.	3	2	1
14. Prostitution should be legalized.	3	2	1
15. Women use sex for love; men use love for sex.	1	2	3
16. Our society is too sexually permissive.	1	2	3
17. The man should be the undisputed head of the household.	1	2	3
18. Having sex just for pleasure is OK.	3	2	1

Scoring

Add up the numbers you circled to obtain your overall score.

1–18   Traditional attitude about sexuality.

19–36   Ambivalent or mixed attitude about sexuality.

37–54   Open, progressive attitude about sexuality.

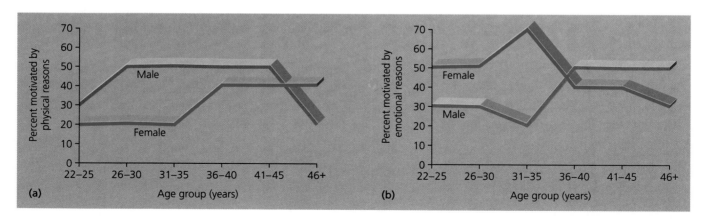

Figure 5-5   Motivations for engaging in sex by age and gender.   (a) The physical motive.
(b) The emotional motive.   SOURCES: Data from Laumann, E., et al. 1994. *The Social Organization of Sexuality: Sexual Practices in the United States.* Chicago: University of Chicago Press. Sprague, J., and D. Quadagno. 1989. Gender and sexual motivation. *Journal of Psychology and Human Sexuality* 2: 57–76.

- *Your background and beliefs.* What are your religious, moral, and/or personal values regarding sexual activity? Will engaging in this activity enhance your self-esteem? How will a sexual relationship fit into the rest of your life? What are your priorities at this time?

- *Your relationship.* How will sexual involvement change the relationship? Do you both want to have sex? Would either one of you feel pressured or guilty about sex? What are your expectations about the future of the relationship?

- *Your health.* Have you and your partner talked about contraception? What contraceptive method will you use? What steps will you take to protect yourself against getting a sexually transmitted disease?

> **PERSONAL INSIGHT** What sexual practices are acceptable to you and what ones are unacceptable? What influences your feelings about them? Are there sexual behaviors that you object to but find arousing anyway? Remember, there's a big difference between what you think and what you do.

Sexual Orientation

Sexual orientation refers to your preference in choosing a sex partner. An individual may be sexually attracted to members of the other sex (heterosexual), the same sex (homosexual), or both sexes (**bisexual**). The terms *straight* and *gay* are often used to refer to heterosexuals and homosexuals, respectively, and female homosexuals are also referred to as *lesbians*.

In a national survey, 2–5% of men had engaged in homosexual sex at some point in their lives, and 1–3% identified themselves as homosexuals. Of the women surveyed, 4% stated that they had engaged in homosexual sex at some point in their lives, and 1.5% identified themselves as homosexuals. These numbers are lower than in past surveys. But do people tell the truth in surveys that probe very sensitive and private aspects of their lives? This question is always an issue.

Heterosexuality The great majority of people are heterosexual. The heterosexual lifestyle usually includes all the behavior and relationship patterns described in Chapter 4: dating, engagement and/or living together, and marriage. Legally recognized and binding marriage is available in our society only to heterosexual couples.

Homosexuality Homosexuality exists in almost all cultures. Although they cannot legally marry, many homosexual couples form long-lasting close and stable ties. (Some religious organizations do solemnize gay and les-

bian unions.) The lifestyle of homosexual people depends largely on whether they are open about their sexual orientation. Those who feel forced to be secretive may lead a double life, one public and one private. Those who have "come out" participate more actively in gay activities and organizations.

The sexual practices of homosexuals resemble those of heterosexuals except for sexual intercourse. Before the AIDS epidemic, research indicated that most homosexual men had more sex partners than most heterosexual men. More recent studies indicate that homosexual men have reduced the number of their sexual contacts, presumably because the risk of HIV infection rises with the number of partners.

Some people are threatened or upset by homosexuality, perhaps because homosexuals are viewed as different or because no one is sure how sexual orientation develops. The "gay liberation" movement of the 1970s and 1980s helped dispel some of the historical prejudice against gays and lesbians, but homosexuality still has not received widespread societal approval. In extreme cases, irrational fear or hatred of homosexuals—known as **homophobia**—causes people to discriminate against or even attack homosexuals.

The major difference between heterosexuals and homosexuals is in their choice of sex partners. Homosexual individuals are as different and varied from each other as are heterosexuals. Just like heterosexuals, lesbians and gay men may be in long-term, committed relationships or they may date different people. They have the same responsibilities and concerns as anyone else. They have job commitments, they raise children, and they seek to fulfill their potential in all areas of their lives. For homosexuals, bisexuals, and heterosexuals, sexual expression is but one facet of human experience.

Bisexuality Some bisexual individuals are involved with partners of both sexes at the same time, while others may alternate between same-sex partners and partners of the other sex ("serial bisexuality"). HIV infection is a risk associated with bisexuality, particularly in cases where bisexual men don't disclose their sexual orientation to their female partners. The largest group of bisexuals are married men who have secret sexual involvements with men but who rarely have female sexual contacts outside marriage.

The Origins of Sexual Orientation Many theories have been proposed to account for the development of sexual orientation. Biological theories have focused on genetic and hormonal influences. One study found structural differences between homosexual and heterosexual men in

bisexual Sexually attracted to people of both sexes.	**TERMS**
homophobia Fear or hatred of homosexuals.	

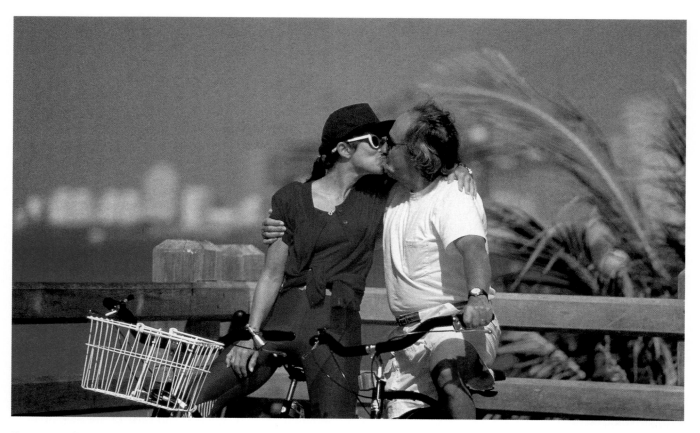

Human sexuality is not just a matter of bodies responding to each other. This couple's physical experiences together will be powerfully affected by their emotions, ideas, and values and by the quality of their relationship.

the brain region that controls sexual behavior. It remains unclear, however, whether this anatomical variation represents a cause or a result of sexual orientation.

Evidence for a genetic basis for sexual orientation was provided by a recent study of 40 families, each with two gay brothers. Researchers found a correlation between homosexuality and a specific piece of DNA on the X chromosome in 64% of the gay brothers in the study. They concluded that this piece of DNA could be linked to homosexuality in some individuals. However, the researchers point out that not everyone who carries the DNA section is gay, nor do all gay men carry this DNA. The DNA segment may affect sexual orientation indirectly, by influencing other personality traits.

In another recent study, researchers looked at 108 sets of female twins in which at least one twin was a lesbian. They found that among the identical twins, both twins were lesbians in 48% of the cases; for the nonidentical twins, both twins were lesbians in 16% of the cases. Among adopted girls with a lesbian sister, only 6% of the adoptive siblings were homosexual. Similar results were obtained in studies of male twins. Although these results may suggest a genetic component to sexual orientation,

other influences must also operate because identical twins do not all share the same orientation. There is no evidence that sexual orientation is determined solely by biological or genetic factors.

Many psychological theories have also been proposed. According to Freud's theory of the Oedipus complex, children are romantically and sexually attracted to the parent of the other sex during the stage of psychosexual development that occurs between ages 3 and 5, but fear of punishment leads the child to renounce the attraction and identify with the parent of the same sex. This identification changes to a heterosexual orientation during adolescence and adulthood, and failure to resolve the Oedipal issues, according to Freud, results in a homosexual orientation. Although many psychologists accept the role of Oedipal relationships in personality development, they question the role of these relationships in the development of sexual orientation.

According to learning theory, behaviors that are rewarded increase in frequency and behaviors that are punished decrease in frequency. Negative experiences with heterosexuality or positive experiences with homosexuality might cause someone to become homosexual. Other research, however, has indicated that sexual orientation has its origin outside of family communication patterns and is not shaped by learning.

Most experts agree that a complex series of interactions—both biological and psychosocial—contribute to sexual orientation.

Varieties of Human Sexual Behavior

Most people express their sexuality in a variety of ways. Some sexual behaviors are aimed at self-stimulation only, such as masturbation, while other practices involve interaction with others in behaviors such as kissing and intercourse. Some people choose not to express their sexuality and practice celibacy instead.

Celibacy   Continuous abstention from sexual activities, termed **celibacy,** can be a conscious and deliberate choice, or it can be necessitated by circumstances. Health considerations—concerns about recurring vaginal infections, sexually transmitted diseases, and particularly the spread of HIV—may contribute to a decision to practice celibacy. Religious and moral beliefs may lead some people to celibacy, particularly until marriage or until an acceptable partner appears.

Celibacy can be practiced temporarily or periodically, for periods of years, or even a lifetime. Some celibates masturbate; others engage in no sexual activities at all. A disadvantage of the celibate life is that it may lack physical contact and affection.

Autoeroticism and Masturbation   The most common form of **autoeroticism** is **erotic fantasy,** creating imaginary experiences that range from fleeting thoughts to elaborate scenarios. Fantasies may be replays of past sexual experiences, or fabrications based on unfulfilled wishes or taken from books, drawings, or photographs.

Masturbation involves manually stimulating the genitals, rubbing them against objects (such as a pillow), or using stimulating devices such as vibrators. Although commonly associated with adolescence, masturbation is practiced by many throughout adult life. It may be used as a substitute for sexual intercourse or as part of sexual activity with a partner. Masturbation gives a person control over the pace, time, and method of sexual release and pleasure. Research indicates that on average, two out of three college students masturbate a few times a week, others do it more or less frequently, and some don't do it at all.

Touching and Foreplay   Tactile stimulation, or touching, is integral to sexual experiences, whether in the form of massage, kissing, fondling, or holding. Our entire body surface is a sensory organ, and touching almost anywhere can enhance intimacy and sexual arousal. As mentioned earlier, some body areas, the erogenous zones, are much more sensitive to touch as a sexual stimulus than others. Touching can convey a variety of messages, including affection, comfort, and a desire for further sexual contact.

During arousal, many men and women manually and orally stimulate each other by touching, stroking, and caressing their partner's genitals. Men and women vary greatly in their preferences for the type, pacing, and vigor of such **foreplay.** Working out the details to accommodate each other's pleasure is a key to enjoying these activities. Direct communication about preferences can enhance sexual pleasure and protect both partners from physical and psychological discomfort.

Oral-Genital Stimulation   **Cunnilingus** (the stimulation of the female genitals with the lips and tongue) and **fellatio** (the stimulation of the penis with the mouth) are quite common practices. A survey of several thousand college students in sexuality classes spanning 15 years revealed that approximately 89% of women and 82% of men had both given and received oral-genital stimulation (although prevalence varied in different populations). Oral sex may be practiced either as part of arousal and foreplay or as a sex act culminating in orgasm. Like all acts of sexual expression between two people, oral sex requires the cooperation and consent of both partners. If they disagree about its acceptability, they need to discuss their feelings and try to reach a mutually pleasing solution.

Anal Intercourse   Another practice, less common but well known, is anal stimulation and penetration by the penis or a finger. About 10% of heterosexuals and 50% of homosexual males regularly practice anal intercourse. In a study of married couples, 25% indicated that they had engaged in anal intercourse at some time. The receiver does not usually reach orgasm from anal intercourse, though men usually experience orgasm while penetrating. Many people have strongly negative attitudes toward anal sex because they consider it unclean, unnatural, or unappealing. Because the anus is composed of delicate tissues that tear easily under such pressure, anal intercourse is one of the riskiest of sexual behaviors associated with the transmission of HIV and the bacteria that cause gonorrhea and syphilis. The use of condoms is highly recommended for anyone engaging in anal sex. Special care and precaution should be exercised if anal sex is

celibacy   Continuous abstention from sexual activity.   **TERMS**

autoeroticism   Behavior aimed at sexual self-stimulation.

erotic fantasy   Sexually arousing thoughts and daydreams.

foreplay   Kissing, touching, and any form of oral or genital contact that stimulates people toward intercourse.

cunnilingus   Oral stimulation of the female genitals.

fellatio   Oral stimulation of the penis.

practiced—cleanliness, lubrication, and gentle entry at the very least. Anything that is inserted into the anus should not subsequently be put into the vagina unless it has been thoroughly washed. Bacteria normally present in the anus can cause vaginal infections.

Sexual Intercourse For most adults, most of the time, **sexual intercourse** is the ultimate sexual experience. Men and women engage in coitus—make love—to fulfill both sexual and psychological needs. The most common heterosexual practice is the man inserting his erect penis into the woman's dilated and lubricated vagina after sufficient arousal.

Much has been written on how to enhance pleasure through various coital techniques, positions, and practices. For a woman, the key factor in physical readiness for coitus is adequate vaginal lubrication, and in psychological readiness, to be aroused and receptive. For a man, the setting and the partner must arouse him to attain and maintain an erection. Personal preferences vary, but most people prefer a safe, private setting. Candlelight and music, for example, can enhance the mood of the occasion. Psychological factors and the quality of the relationship are more important to overall sexual satisfaction than sophisticated or exotic sexual techniques.

Atypical and Problematic Sexual Behaviors

In American culture, many kinds of sexual behavior are accepted. However, some types of sexual expression are considered harmful; they may be against the law or classified as mental disorders, or both. Because sexual behavior occurs on a continuum, it is sometimes difficult to differentiate a behavior that is simply atypical from one that is harmful. When attempting to evaluate an unusual sexual behavior, experts consider the issues of consent between partners and whether physical or psychological harm is done to the individual or to others.

Sexual fantasies and behaviors that are consensual—agreed upon by adult partners—but that are not statistically typical of American sexual behaviors are known as **atypical sexual behaviors.** An example of an atypical

sexual behavior is the consensual use of sex toys. Those behaviors that are classified as mental disorders, or **paraphilias,** are characterized by recurring, intense sexual fantasies and urges that involve nonhuman objects, the suffering or humiliation of oneself or one's partner, or children or other nonconsenting individuals. Examples are peeping into strangers' homes, making obscene phone calls, and having sexual contact with children. The effects of paraphilic behavior on others range from minor upset to serious physical and long-term psychological harm.

The use of force and coercion in sexual relationships is one of the most serious problems in human interactions. The most extreme manifestation of **sexual coercion**—forcing a person to submit to another's sexual desires—is rape, but sexual coercion occurs in many more subtle forms, such as sexual harassment. Sexual coercion—including rape, the sexual abuse of children, and sexual harassment—is discussed in detail in Chapter 23.

Commercial Sex

Conflicting feelings about sexuality are apparent in the attitudes of Americans toward commercial sex: prostitution and sexually oriented materials such as videos, magazines, and books. Our society condemns sexually explicit material and prostitution, but it also provides their customers.

Pornography Derived from the Greek word meaning "the writing of prostitutes," **pornography** is now often defined as obscene literature, art, or movies. A major problem in identifying pornographic material is that different people and communities have different opinions about what is obscene. Differing definitions of obscenity have led to many legal battles over potentially pornographic materials. Currently, the sale and rental of pornographic materials is restricted so that only adults can legally obtain them. The appearance of more than 75,000 sex-related Web sites has made enforcing these laws difficult, however. Additional possible strategies include requiring commercial Web sites to verify the age of customers and developing ways for parents to block children's access to pornographic sites. In any format, materials depicting children in sexual contexts are illegal.

Many people distinguish between "soft porn" and "hard porn" materials. Soft porn, often marketed for couples, typically includes an apparently loving couple having sex in a relaxed setting. There is mutual kissing and touching, and both partners are shown as having a positive experience. In hard porn, there is usually little mutual touching, and only the male appears to enjoy the experience. Hard porn sometimes explicitly depicts sexual violence and exploitation. Hard porn materials tend to be the focus of more criticism than soft porn materials.

Much of the debate about pornography focuses on whether it is harmful. Some people argue that adults who

TERMS

sexual intercourse Sexual relations involving genital union; also called *coitus,* and also known as making love.

atypical sexual behavior Consensual sexual behavior that is not statistically typical within a population.

paraphilia A mental disorder characterized by recurring, intense sexual fantasies and urges that involve nonhuman objects, the suffering or humiliation of oneself or one's partner, or children or other nonconsenting individuals.

sexual coercion The use of physical or psychological force or intimidation to make a person submit to sexual demands.

pornography The explicit or obscene depiction of sexual activities in pictures, writing, or other material.

prostitution The exchange of sexual services for money.

want to view pornographic materials in the privacy of their own homes should be allowed to do so. Others feel that the exposure to explicit sexual material can lead to delinquent or criminal behavior, such as rape or the sexual abuse of children. Currently, there is no reliable evidence that pornography by itself leads to violence or paraphilic behavior, and debate is likely to continue.

Prostitution   **Prostitution** is the exchange of sexual services for money. Prostitutes may be men, women, or children, and the buyer of a prostitute's services is nearly always a man. Except for parts of Nevada, prostitution is illegal in the United States.

Sex with a prostitute provides the customer with sexual release without commitment, the expectation of intimacy, or the fear of rejection. Some men patronize prostitutes to have sex with a different type of partner than usual, or to engage in a type of sex their usual partner will not permit. Most customers are white, middle-class, middle-aged, and married. Although they come from a wide variety of backgrounds, prostitutes are usually motivated to join the profession because of money.

AIDS is a major concern for prostitutes and their customers. Many prostitutes are injecting drug users or are involved with men who are. The rate of HIV infection among prostitutes varies widely, but in some parts of the country it is as high as 25–50%.

Some people are in favor of legalizing prostitution because they consider it to be a victimless crime. They are in favor of a program of licensing and registration by police and health departments. Such systems currently exist in Nevada and parts of Europe. In Nevada, where prostitution is legal in brothels, health officials require prostitutes to use condoms and take monthly HIV tests.

Responsible Sexual Behavior

Healthy sexuality is an important part of adult life. It can be a source of pleasurable experiences and emotions and an important part of intimate partnerships. But sexual behavior also carries many responsibilities, and you need to make choices about your sexuality that contribute to your well-being and that of your partner. Sexual responsibility has many components, several of which are discussed in this section.

Open, Honest Communication   Each partner needs to clearly indicate what sexual involvement means to him or her. Does it mean love, fun, a permanent commitment, or something else? The intentions of both partners should be clear. For strategies on how to talk about sexual issues with your partner, refer to the box "Communicating About Sexuality" on p. 126.

Agreed-Upon Sexual Activities   No one should pressure or coerce a partner. Sexual behaviors should be consistent

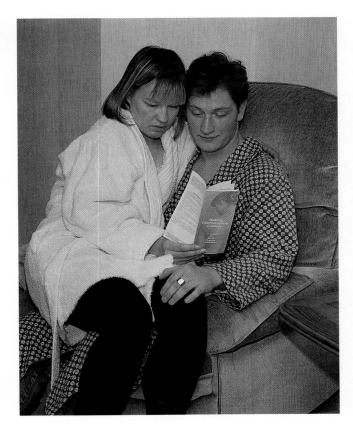

Sexual activity has many potential consequences, including pregnancy, disease, and emotional changes in the relationship. Responsible sexual behavior includes discussing these consequences openly and honestly.

with the sexual values, preferences, and comfort level of both partners. Everyone has the right to refuse sexual activity at any time.

Using Contraception   If pregnancy is not desired, contraception should be used during sexual intercourse. Both partners need to take responsibility for protecting against unwanted pregnancy. Partners should discuss contraception before sexual involvement begins. (See Chapter 6 for more information on contraception.)

Safer Sex   Both partners should be aware of, and practice, safer sex to guard against sexually transmitted diseases (STDs). Many sexual behaviors carry the risk of STDs, including HIV infection. Partners should be honest about their health and any medical conditions and work out a plan for protection. Behaviors that carry no risk of HIV infection are those that don't involve the exchange of body fluids (blood, semen, and vaginal secretions). Anyone who is not in a mutually monogamous relationship with an uninfected partner and who wishes to have sex should always use a condom. (For more information on STDs and safer sex practices, see Chapter 18.)

To talk with your partner about sexuality, follow the general suggestions for effective communication given in Chapter 4. Getting started may be the most difficult part. Some people feel more comfortable if they begin by talking about talking—that is, initiating a discussion about why people are so uncomfortable talking about sexuality. Talking about sexual histories—how partners first learned about sex or how family and cultural background influenced sexual values and attitudes—is another way to get started. Reading about sex can also be a good beginning: Partners can read an article or book and then discuss their reactions.

Be honest about what you feel and what you want from your partner. Cultural and personal obstacles to discussing sexual subjects can be difficult to overcome, but self-disclosure is important for successful relationships. Research indicates that when one partner openly discusses attitudes and feelings, the other partner is more likely to do the same. If your partner seems hesitant to open up, try asking open-ended or either/or questions: "Where do you like to be touched?" or "Would you like to talk about this now or wait until later?"

If something is bothering you about your sexual relationship, choose a good time to initiate a discussion with your partner. Be specific and direct but also tactful. Focus on what you actually observe, rather than on what you think the behavior means. "You didn't touch or hug me when your friends were around" is an observation. "You're ashamed of me around your friends" is an inference about your partner's feelings. Try focusing on a specific behavior that concerns you rather than on the person as a whole—your partner can change behaviors but not his or her entire personality. For example, you could say, "I'd like you to take a few minutes away from studying to kiss me," instead of "You're so caught up in your work, you never have time for me."

If you are going to make a statement that your partner may interpret as criticism, try mixing it with something positive ("I love spending time with you, but I feel annoyed when you . . ."). On the other hand, if your partner says something that upsets you, don't lash back. An aggressive response may make you feel better in the short run, but it will not help the communication process or the quality of the relationship.

If you want to say no to some sexual activity, say no unequivocally. Don't send mixed messages. If you are afraid of hurting your partner's feelings, offer an alternative if it's appropriate—"I am uncomfortable with that. How about. . . ."

If you're in love, you may think that the sexual aspects of a relationship will work out magically without discussion. But partners who never talk about sex deny themselves the opportunity to increase their closeness and improve their relationship.

Taking Responsibility for Consequences   Everyone should be aware of the physical and emotional consequences of their sexual behavior and accept responsibility for them. These primary consequences are pregnancy, STDs, and emotional changes in the relationship between partners.

SUMMARY

Sexual Anatomy

- The female external sex organs are called the vulva; the clitoris plays an important role in sexual arousal and orgasm. The vagina leads to the internal sex organs, including the uterus, oviducts, and ovaries.

- The male external sex organs are the penis and the scrotum; the glans of the penis is an important site of sexual arousal. Internal sexual structures include the testes, vasa deferentia, seminal vesicles, and prostate gland.

Hormones and the Reproductive Life Cycle

- The testes and adrenal glands produce androgens; the ovaries produce estrogens and progestins.

- The fertilizing sperm determines the sex of the individual. Specialized genes on the Y chromosome initiate the process of male sexual differentiation in the embryo.

- Hormones initiate the changes that occur during puberty: The reproductive system matures, secondary sex characteristics develop, and the bodies of males and females become more distinctive.

- Breast development is the first sign of puberty in the female, followed by rapid body growth.

- The menstrual cycle consists of four phases: menses, the estrogenic phase, ovulation, and the progestational phase.

- The reproductive system of boys matures later than that of girls; testosterone triggers most of the male changes of puberty.

- The ovaries gradually cease to function as women approach age 50, and they enter menopause. The pattern of male sexual responses changes with age, and testosterone production gradually decreases.

Sexual Functioning

- Sexual activity is based on stimulus and response. Stimulation may be physical or psychological.

- Vasocongestion and myotonia are the primary physiological mechanisms of sexual arousal.

- The sexual response cycle has four stages: excitement, plateau, orgasm, and resolution.

- Physical and psychological problems can both interfere with sexual functioning.
- A treatment for sexual dysfunction first addresses any underlying medical conditions and then looks at psychosocial problems.

Sexual Behavior

- Some gender characteristics are determined biologically and others are defined by society. Children learn traits and behaviors traditionally deemed appropriate for one sex or the other.
- Gender roles are emerging that reflect a mix of male and female characteristics and behaviors.
- The ability to respond sexually is present at birth. Sexual behaviors emerging in childhood include self-exploration, perhaps leading to masturbation.
- Although puberty defines biological adulthood, people take 5–10 more years to reach social maturity. Sexual fantasies and dreams and nocturnal emissions characterize adolescent sexuality.
- Developing the capacity for intimacy and becoming sexually experienced are important tasks of young adults.

- Decision making about sex should involve a consideration of one's background and beliefs, the relationship, and health.
- A person's sexual orientation can be heterosexual, homosexual, or bisexual. Possible influences include genetics, hormonal factors, and early childhood experiences.
- Human sexual behaviors include celibacy, erotic fantasy, masturbation, touching, cunnilingus, fellatio, anal intercourse, and coitus.
- To evaluate whether an atypical sexual behavior is problematic, experts consider the issues of consent between partners and whether the behavior results in physical or psychological harm.
- Pornography and prostitution are examples of the commercialization of sex, when sexual stimulation is exchanged for money.
- Responsible sexuality includes open, honest communication; agreed-upon sexual activities; using contraception; safer sex practices; and taking responsibility for consequences.

TAKE ACTION

1. Many reputable self-help books about sexual functioning are available in libraries and bookstores. If you're not satisfied with your level of knowledge and understanding, consider consulting some other sources.

2. If you have an intimate sexual relationship with a regular partner, think honestly about what is satisfying about it and what you would like to change. Is there anything you want to discuss with your partner but have been afraid to bring up? Take a chance, and talk with your partner about it.

JOURNAL ENTRY

1. Sexual myths and misconceptions are common in our culture. In your health journal, make a list of statements about sexuality that you've heard but are not sure are accurate. Find out the facts by consulting books and pamphlets mentioned here or available through your school health center or library.

2. *Critical Thinking* Many states have laws prohibiting certain sexual behaviors. How much control do you think society should have over an individual's sexual practices? What types of behaviors do you think should be regulated and why? What behaviors should be left up to the discretion of the individual? Write an essay outlining your position; be sure to explain your reasoning.

3. If you think you may have PMS or PMDD, keep a diary of any physical, emotional, or behavioral symptoms that seem to fluctuate monthly; also keep track of when your period occurs. If you notice a definite cyclical character to your symptoms, consider the tips in the box on p. 110.

4. *Critical Thinking* Consider one or two of your favorite television shows or movies. How are sexuality and sexual behavior presented? How many sexual references occur? What types of sexual behaviors are shown or alluded to? What impression would a viewer have about the typical sexual behaviors of the characters? Are any of the potential emotional or physical consequences of sexual behavior shown? Write a short essay outlining your findings, and state whether or not you think the depiction of sexuality is accurate. In your opinion, can the presentation of sexuality in the programs or movies you chose influence the behavior of viewers? Explain your reasoning.

Books

Borhek, M. 1993. *Coming Out to Parents: A Two-Way Survival Guide for Lesbians and Gay Men and Their Parents,* 2nd ed. Cleveland: Pilgrim Press. *Discusses the concerns and fears of gays as they tell their parents about their homosexuality; also describes parents' reactions and provides suggestions for dealing with the coming-out process.*

Boston Women's Health Book Collective. 1998. *Our Bodies, Ourselves for the New Century.* New York: Simon & Schuster. *Broad coverage of many women's health concerns, with an emphasis on psychological as well as physical factors. A favorite for many years; periodically updated.*

Columbia University's Health Education Program. 1998. *The "Go Ask Alice" Book of Answers: A Guide to Good Physical, Sexual, and Emotional Health.* New York: Henry Holt. *Presents answers to a variety of student-oriented health questions from the popular "Go Ask Alice" Web site.*

Daniluk, J. 1998. *Women's Sexuality Across the Life Span.* New York: Guilford. *Provides information on many aspects of female sexuality, including the interaction of psychological, social, cultural, and biological factors on a woman's sense of herself as a sexual being.*

Men's Health Magazine. 1998. *The Complete Book of Men's Health: The Definitive, Illustrated Guide to Healthy Living, Exercise, and Sex.* Emmaus, Penn.: Rodale. *A comprehensive guide to a healthy lifestyle, including information on communication and sexuality.*

Michael, R., J. Gagnon, E. Laumann, and G. Kolata. 1995. *Sex in America: A Definitive Survey.* New York: Warner Books. *Based on recent research and written for the general public, this book contains a wealth of information about the sex lives of Americans.*

Moe, B. 1998. *Coping with PMS.* New York: Rosen. *A concise, up-to-date book that discusses the possible causes, symptoms, and treatments for PMS; easy to read and understand.*

Strong, B., C. DeVault, and B. Sayad. 1999. *Human Sexuality: Diversity in Contemporary America,* 3rd ed. Mountain View, Calif.: Mayfield. *A comprehensive introduction to human sexuality.*

Organizations and Web Sites

American Association of Sex Educators, Counselors, and Therapists (AASECT). Certifies sex educators, counselors, and therapists and provides listings of local therapists dealing with sexual problems. Send a self-addressed, stamped envelope for information.
P.O. Box 238
Mount Vernon, IA 52314
http://www.aasect.org

The Institute for the Advanced Study of Human Sexuality/Sexology Netline. A Web site containing a large collection of information and answers to frequently asked questions about sexuality.
http://home.netinc.ca/~sexorg

The Kinsey Institute for Research in Sex, Gender, and Reproduction. One of the oldest and most respected institutions doing research on sexuality.
313 Morrison Hall
Indiana University
Bloomington, IN 47405
812-855-7686
http://www.indiana.edu/~kinsey

Male Health Center. A commercial site that provides a variety of information on male sexual health topics.
http://www.malehealthcenter.com

New York University Sexual Disorders Screening. Provides interactive online screening tests for common sexual disorders.
http://www.med.nyu.edu/Psych/screens/sdsm.html (men)
http://www.med.nyu.edu/Psych/screens/sdsf.html (women)

North American Menopause Society (NAMS). Provides general information about menopause and lists of local support groups and menopause clinicians; Web site includes a helpful section with answers to frequently asked questions.
P.O. Box 94527
Cleveland, OH 44101
216-844-8748
http://www.menopause.org

PMS Access/Women's Health America Group. Provides information about PMS and links to other sites dealing with PMS and women's health issues.
429 Gammon Pl.
P.O. Box 259641
Madison, WI 53725
800-222-4767; 800-558-7046
http://www.womenshealth.com

Sexuality Information and Education Council of the United States (SIECUS). Provides information on many aspects of sexuality and has an extensive library and numerous publications.
130 W. 42nd St., Suite 350
New York, NY 10036
212-819-9770
http://www.siecus.org

U.S. Food and Drug Administration/Viagra. Provides information and cautions about the use of sildenafil citrate (Viagra) to treat sexual dysfunction in men.
http://www.fda.gov/cder/consumerinfo/viagra

See also the listings for Chapters 4, 6–8, and 18.

SELECTED BIBLIOGRAPHY

Abma, J. C., et al. 1997. *Fertility, Family Planning, and Women's Health: New Data from the 1995 National Survey of Family Growth.* Hyattsville, Md.: National Center for Health Statistics.

AIDS Knowledge Base Editors. 1998. Factors associated with sexual transmission of HIV. *The AIDS Knowledge Base* (retrieved October 24, 1998; http://hivinsite.ucsf.edu/akb/ 1997/01sextx/toctable2.html).

American Academy of Pediatrics Task Force on Circumcision. 1999. Circumcision Policy Statement. *Pediatrics* 103(3): 686–693.

American Psychiatric Association. 1994. *Diagnostic and Statistical Manual of Mental Disorders (DSM-IV),* 4th ed. Washington, D.C.: American Psychiatric Association Press.

Bailey, M., R. Pillard, M. Neale, and Y. Agyei. 1993. Heritable factors influence sexual orientation. *Archives of General Psychiatry* 50: 217–223.

Burack, R. 1999. Teenage sexual behavior: Attitudes towards and declared sexual activity. *British Journal of Family Planning* 24(4): 145–148.

Centers for Disease Control and Prevention. 1998. Trends in sexual risk behaviors among high school students—United States, 1991–1997. *Morbidity and Mortality Weekly Report* 47(36): 749–752.

Congress bans female genital mutilation in U.S. 1996. *San Francisco Chronicle,* 12 October.

Donovan, P. 1998. Falling teen pregnancy, birthrates: What's behind the declines? *The Guttmacher Report on Public Policy* (1)5 (retrieved October 16, 1998; http://www.agi-usa. org/pubs/journals/gr010506.html).

Goodwin, P. J., et al. 1998. Elevated high-density lipoprotein cholesterol and dietary fat intake in women with cyclic mastopathy. *American Journal of Obstetrics and Gynecology* 179(2): 430–437.

Hatcher, R., et al. 1998. *Contraceptive Technology,* 17th ed. New York: Ardent Media.

Hatzichristou, D. 1998. Current treatment and future perspectives for erectile dysfunction. *International Journal of Impotence Research* 10(Suppl 1): S3–S13.

Heiman, J. R., and C. M. Meston. 1998. Evaluating sexual dysfunction in women. *Clinics in Obstetrics and Gynaecology* 40(3): 616–629.

Korenman, S. G. 1998. New insights into erectile dysfunction: A practical approach. *American Journal of Medicine* 105(2): 135–144.

Kraemer, G. R., and R. R. Kraemer. 1998. Premenstrual syndrome: Diagnosis and treatment experiences. *Journal of Women's Health* 7(7): 893–907.

Krung, R., et al. 1996. Jealousy, general creativity, and coping with social frustration during the menstrual cycle. *Archives of Sexual Behavior* 25: 181–200.

Laan, E., and W. Everaerd. 1995. Habituation of female sexual arousal to slides and films. *Archives of Sexual Behavior* 24: 517–542.

Laumann, E. O., A. Paik, and R. C. Rosen. 1999. Sexual dysfunction in the United States: Prevalence and predictors. *Journal of the American Medical Association* 281: 537–544.

Laumann, E., et al. 1997. Circumcision in the United States: Prevalence, prophylactic effects, and sexual practices. *Journal of the American Medical Association* 277: 1052–1057; *JAMA Letters* 278: 201–203.

Laumann, E., et al. 1994. *The Social Organization of Sexuality: Sexual Practices in the United States.* Chicago: University of Chicago Press.

LeVay, S. 1991. A difference in hypothalamic structure between heterosexual and homosexual men. *Science* 253: 1034–1037.

Moneyyirci-Delale, O., et al. 1998. Sex steroid hormones modulate serum ionized magnesium and calcium levels throughout the menstrual cycle. *Fertility and Sterility* 69: 958–962.

National Council on Aging. 1998. *Half of Older Americans Report They Are Sexually Active; 4 in 10 Want More Sex, Says New Survey* (retrieved September 28, 1998; http://www.ncoa.org/ press/sexsurvey.htm).

New approaches to PMS. 1998. *Harvard Women's Health Watch,* February.

North American Menopause Society. 1998. *Menopause is the Beginning of a New, Fulfilling Stage of Life* (retrieved October 26, 1998; http://www.menopause.org/news.htm#anchor 10312017).

O'Donnell, L., et. al. 1999. The effectiveness of the reach for health community youth service learning program in reducing early and unprotected sex among urban middle school students. *American Journal of Public Health* 89(2): 176–181.

Purifoy, F., A. Grodsky, and L. Giambra. 1992. The relationship of sexual daydreaming to sexual activity for women across the life span. *Archives of Sexual Behavior* 21: 369–386.

Quadagno, D. M., et al. 1991. The menstrual cycle: Does it affect athletic performance? *Physician and Sports Medicine* 19: 121–124.

Rubin, L. 1990. *Erotic Wars.* New York: Farrar, Straus & Giroux.

Sanders, S. A., and J. M. Reinisch. 1999. Would you say you "had sex" if . . .? *Journal of the American Medical Association* 281: 275–277.

Sayegh, R. et al. 1995. The effect of a carbohydrate-rich beverage on mood, appetite, and cognitive function in women with premenstrual syndrome. *Journal of Obstetrics and Gynecology* 86(4): 520–528.

Silence about sexual problems can hurt relationships. 1999. *Journal of the American Medical Association* 281: 210.

Steinberg, S., et al. 1999. A placebo-controlled clinical trial of L-tryptophan in premenstrual dysphoria. *Biological Psychiatry* 45(3): 313–320.

Strasburger, V. C., and E. Donnerstein. 1999. Children, adolescents, and the media: Issues and solutions. *Pediatrics* 103(1): 129–139.

Strong, B., C. DeVault, and B. Sayad. 1999. *Human Sexuality: Diversity in Contemporary America,* 3rd ed. Mountain View, Calif.: Mayfield.

Student, J. 1998. No sex, please . . . we're college graduates. *American Demographics,* February.

Taddio, A., et al. 1997. Efficacy and safety of lidocaine-prilocaine cream for pain during circumcision. *New England Journal of Medicine* 336(17): 1197–1201.

Thys-Jacobs, S., et al. 1998. Calcium carbonate and the premenstrual syndrome: Effects on premenstrual and menstrual symptoms. Premenstrual Syndrome Study Group. *American Journal of Obstetrics and Gynecology* 179(2): 444–452.

Upchurch, D. M., et al. 1998. Gender and ethnic differences in the timing of first sexual intercourse. *Family Planning Perspectives* 30(3): 121–127.

Van de Ven, P., L. Bornholt, and J. Bailey. 1996. Measuring cognitive, affective, and behavioral components of homophobic reaction. *Archives of Sexual Behavior* 25: 155–180.

Waldo, C. R. 1998. Out on campus: Sexual orientation and academic climate in a university context. *American Journal of Community Psychology* 26(5): 745–774.

Wells, J. 1989. Sexual language usage in different interpersonal contexts: A comparison of gender and sexual orientation. *Archives of Sexual Behavior* 18: 127–143.

World Health Organization. 1997. *Fact Sheet: Female Genital Mutilation* (retrieved September 18, 1998; http://www.who. int/inf-fs/en/fact153.html).

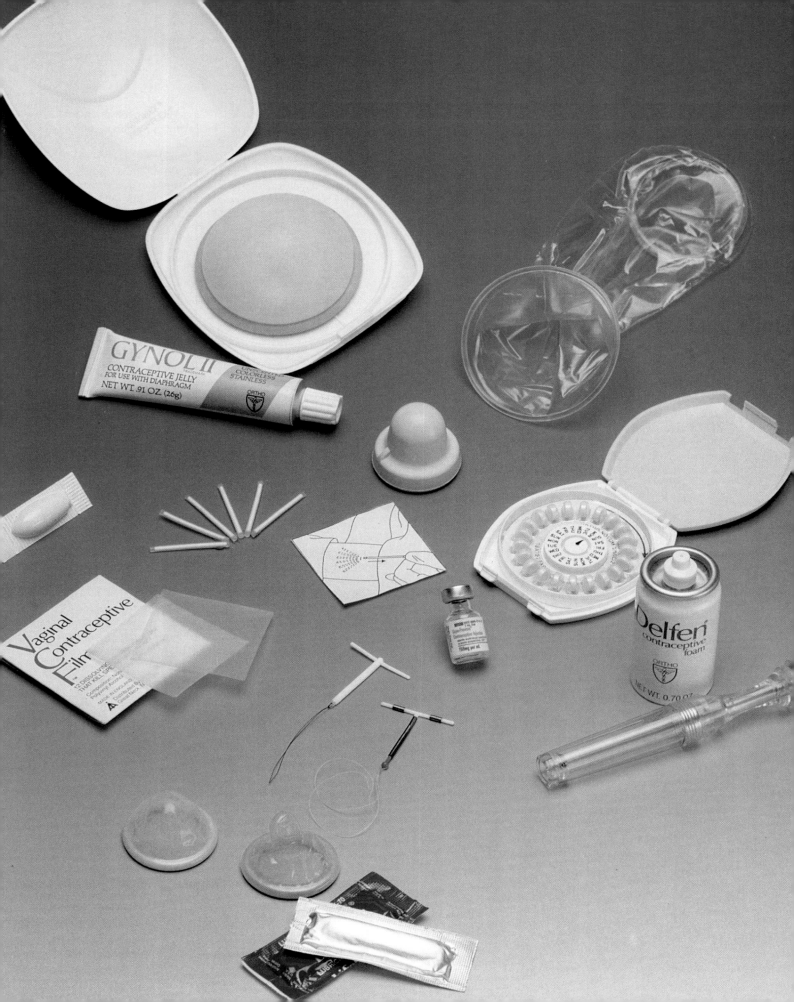

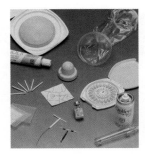

LEARNING OBJECTIVES

After reading this chapter, you should be able to:

- Explain how contraceptives work and how to interpret information about a contraceptive method's effectiveness, risks, and benefits.

- List the most popular contraceptives, and discuss their advantages, disadvantages, and effectiveness.

- Describe research being done to develop new methods of contraception.

- Discuss issues related to contraception, including nonmarital sexual relationships, gender differences, sex education for teenagers, and communication between partners.

- Choose a method of contraception based on the needs of the user and the safety and effectiveness of the method.

Contraception

6

TEST YOUR KNOWLEDGE

1. If a couple, both of whom are of reproductive age, use no contraception for a year, there is a 60% chance the woman will get pregnant.
   True or false?

2. Which of the following contraceptive methods offers the best protection against pregnancy? Which offers the best protection against sexually transmitted diseases?
   a. oral contraceptives
   b. Norplant implants
   c. male condoms
   d. diaphragm with spermicidal foam

3. Hand lotion, Vaseline (petroleum jelly), and baby oil are good choices for condom lubricants.
   True or false?

4. Parents have little influence on an adolescent's decisions about contraception.
   True or false?

5. What percentage of women say they can't trust men to be responsible for contraception?
   a. 25%
   b. 50%
   c. 75%

Answers

1. *False.* There is a 90% chance that the woman will become pregnant. Over 50% of the pregnancies that occur each year are unplanned.

2. *b and c.* Norplant implants are the most effective at preventing pregnancy; male condoms are the most effective against sexually transmitted diseases.

3. *False.* Only water-based lubricants such as K-Y jelly should be used as condom lubricants. Any product that contains mineral oil can cause latex condoms to disintegrate, beginning within 60 seconds of being applied.

4. *False.* A recent study found that adolescents who had frank discussions about condom use with their mothers in the year prior to initiating sexual activity were much more likely to use condoms at first intercourse and regularly thereafter than those who did not have such discussions.

5. *c.* In the same survey, 66% of men agreed with this assessment.

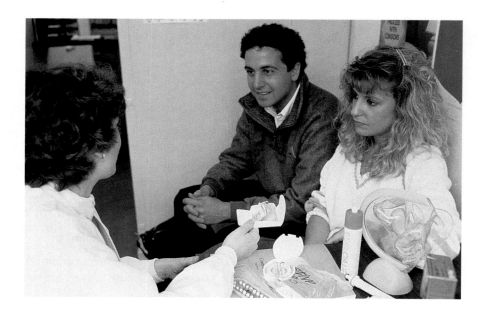

To be effective, contraceptives should be chosen thoughtfully and used correctly. A careful explanation by a health care professional will help this couple choose a method that is right for them.

In her lifetime, the ovaries of an average woman release over 400 eggs, one a month for about 35 years. Each egg is capable of developing into a human embryo if fertilized by one of the millions of sperm a man produces in every ejaculate. Furthermore, unlike most other mammals, humans are capable of sexual activity at any time of the month or year. These facts help explain why people have always had a compelling interest in controlling fertility and in preventing unwanted pregnancies. Historical writings dating back to the fourth century B.C. mention the use of douches, sponges, and crude methods of abortion. Other materials mentioned as potential contraceptives include lemon juice, parsley, seaweed, olive oil, camphor, and opium. Although not fully understood at the time, the underlying principle of these trial-and-error methods was the same as that of today's **contraceptives:** preventing **conception** by blocking the female's egg from uniting with the male's sperm, thereby preventing pregnancy.

Modern contraceptive methods are much more predictable and effective than in the past, and people today have many options when it comes to making decisions about their sexual and contraceptive behavior. (The statistical consequences of these decisions are shown in Table 6-1.) In addition to the primary purpose of preventing pregnancy, many types of contraception play an important role in protecting against **sexually transmitted diseases (STDs).** Being informed about the realities and risks, and making responsible decisions about sexual and contraceptive behavior, are crucial components of lifelong wellness. But because such decisions are emotional, complex, and difficult, people tend to avoid them or deal with them ineffectively.

While biological, social, and media pressures often encourage sexual activity at ever-younger ages, few forces in the United States support a factual, realistic discussion

VITAL STATISTICS

TABLE 6-1	Worldwide Sexual Behavior and Its Consequences

	Estimated Daily Occurrence
Cases of curable STDs	925,000
Pregnancies	550,000
Births	375,000
Abortions	140,000
Cases of HIV infection	16,000
Deaths—from AIDS	6,300
—from childbirth complications	1,600
—from unsafe abortions	200

SOURCES: United Nations Population Fund (http://www.unfpa.org); Interagency Group for Safe Motherhood (http://safemotherhood.org); Population Reference Bureau (http://www.prb.org); Joint United Nations Programme on HIV/AIDS (http://www.unaids.org).

of the importance of either postponing sexual intercourse or using contraception when intercourse is chosen. Our present superficial approaches to education are clearly ineffective: The United States has one of the highest teen pregnancy rates of all developed nations. Because many of the changing roles of women are severely compromised by unplanned child rearing, and since the option of abortion is becoming more restricted, the problem is even worse than the numbers show.

This chapter provides basic information on the various contraceptive methods, including their advantages and disadvantages. The issues raised should encourage you to think about your own beliefs and attitudes about sexual behavior and contraception and to discuss them with oth-

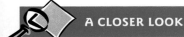
Myth Taking borrowed birth control pills for a few days before having sexual relations gives reliable protection against pregnancy.
Fact Instructions for taking birth control pills must be followed carefully to provide effective contraception. With most pills, this means starting them with a menstrual period and then taking one every day.

Myth Pregnancy never occurs when unprotected intercourse takes place just before or just after a menstrual period.
Fact Menstrual cycles may be irregular, and ovulation may occur at unpredictable times.

Myth During sexual relations, sperm enter the vagina only during ejaculation and never before.
Fact The small amounts of fluid secreted before ejaculation may contain sperm. This is why withdrawing the penis from the vagina just prior to ejaculation is not an effective method of contraception.

Myth If semen is deposited just outside the vaginal entrance, pregnancy cannot occur.
Fact Although sperm usually live about 72 hours within the woman's body, they can live up to 6 or 7 days and are capable of traveling through the vagina and up into the uterus and oviducts.

Myth Douching immediately after sexual relations can prevent sperm from reaching and fertilizing an egg.
Fact During ejaculation (within the vagina), some sperm begin to enter the cervix and uterus. Since they are no longer in the vagina, it is impossible to remove them by douching after sexual relations. Douching may actually push the sperm up farther.

Myth A woman who is breastfeeding does not have to use any contraceptive method to prevent pregnancy.
Fact Frequent and regular breastfeeding may at times prevent ovulation, but not consistently and reliably. Ovulation and pregnancy may occur before the first period after delivering a baby.

Myth Women can't become pregnant the first time they have intercourse.
Fact *Any time* intercourse without protection takes place, sperm may unite with an egg to begin a pregnancy. There is nothing unique about first intercourse to prevent this.

ers. The most critical decisions you will make will involve the time and type of sexual involvement that are best for you, and the commitment to always protect yourself against unwanted pregnancy and STDs.

PRINCIPLES OF CONTRACEPTION

A variety of effective approaches in preventing conception are based on different principles of birth control. **Barrier methods** work by physically blocking the sperm from reaching the egg. Diaphragms, condoms, and several other methods are based on this principle. *Hormonal methods,* such as oral contraceptives (birth control pills), alter the biochemistry of the woman's body, preventing **ovulation** (the release of the egg) and producing changes that make it more difficult for the sperm to reach the egg if ovulation does occur. A variety of so-called *natural methods* of contraception are based on the fact that egg and sperm have to be present at the same time if fertilization is to occur. Finally, *surgical methods*—female and male sterilization—more or less permanently prevent transport of the sperm or eggs to the site of conception.

All contraceptive methods have advantages and disadvantages that make them appropriate for some people but not for others, or at one period of life but not at another. Factors that affect the choice of method include effectiveness, convenience, cost, reversibility, side effects and risks, and protection against STDs. Later in this chapter,

we help you sort through these factors to decide on the method that's best for you. (See the box "Myths About Contraception" to make sure you're not basing your current understanding on common misinformation.)

Effectiveness, one of the factors listed above, requires further explanation. Contraceptive effectiveness is partly determined by the reliability of the method itself—the failure rate if it were always used exactly as directed. This rate cannot be accurately measured, but it can be inferred from studying the most successful users. Effectiveness is also determined by characteristics of the user, including fertility of the individual, frequency of intercourse, and, more importantly, how consistently and correctly the method is used. Because the "method" and "user" variables are difficult to separate out, one overall failure rate

contraceptive Any agent that can prevent conception; condoms, diaphragms, intrauterine devices, and oral contraceptives are examples.   **TERMS**

conception The fusion of ovum and sperm, resulting in a fertilized egg, or zygote.

sexually transmitted disease (STD) Any of several contagious diseases contracted through intimate sexual contact.

barrier method A contraceptive that acts as a physical barrier, blocking the sperm from uniting with the egg.

ovulation The release of the egg (ovum) from the ovaries.

reflecting all variables is generally used. This **contraceptive failure rate** is based on studies that directly measure the percentage of women experiencing an unintended pregnancy in the first year of contraceptive use. For example, the 5% failure rate of oral contraceptives means 5 out of 100 typical users will become pregnant in the first year. This failure rate is likely to be lower for women who are consistently careful in following instructions and higher for those who are frequently careless. Similarly, the 20% failure rate of typical diaphragm use can be decreased or increased significantly by how correct and consistent the woman is in using the device.

Another measure of effectiveness is the **continuation rate**—the percentage of people who continue to use the method after a specified period of time. This measure is important because many unintended pregnancies occur when a method is stopped and not immediately replaced with another. Thus, a contraceptive with a high continuation rate would be more effective at preventing pregnancy than one with a low continuation rate.

We turn now to a description of the various contraceptive methods, discussing first those that are reversible and then those that are permanent.

REVERSIBLE CONTRACEPTIVES

Reversibility is an extremely important consideration for young adults when they choose a contraceptive method, because most people either plan to have children or at least want to keep their options open until they're older. In this section we discuss the reversible contraceptives, beginning with the hormonal methods, then moving to the barrier methods, and finally covering the natural methods.

Oral Contraceptives: The Pill

A century ago or more, a researcher made a key observation: Ovulation does not occur during pregnancy. Further research brought to light the hormonal mechanism: During pregnancy, the corpus luteum secretes progesterone and estrogen in amounts high enough to suppress ovulation. (Refer to Chapter 5 for a complete discussion of the hormonal control of the menstrual cycle.) **Oral contraceptives (OCs)**, or birth control pills, prevent ovulation by mimicking the hormonal activity of the corpus luteum. The active ingredients in OCs are estrogen and progestins, laboratory-made compounds that are closely related to progesterone.

In addition to preventing ovulation, the birth control pill has other backup contraceptive effects. It inhibits the movement of sperm by thickening the cervical mucus, alters the rate of ovum transport by means of its hormonal effects on the oviducts, and may prevent implantation by changing the lining of the uterus, in the unlikely event that a fertilized ovum reaches that area.

The most common type of OC is the combination pill. Each 1-month packet contains 3 weeks of pills that combine varying types and amounts of estrogen and progesterone. Most packets also include a 1-week supply of inactive pills to be taken following the hormone pills; others instruct the woman to simply take no pills at all for 1 week before starting the next cycle. During the week in which no hormones are taken, a light menstrual period occurs. Many different types of combination pills are available today, and if minor problems occur with one brand, women can switch to another.

A second, much less common type of OC is the minipill, a small dose of a synthetic progesterone taken every day of the month. Because the minipill contains no estrogen, it has fewer side effects and health risks, but it also carries a higher risk of pregnancy and irregular bleeding.

A woman is usually advised to start the first cycle of pills with a menstrual period to increase effectiveness and eliminate the possibility of unsuspected pregnancy. She must take each month's pills completely and according to instructions. Taking a few pills just prior to having sexual intercourse will not provide effective contraception.

Hormonal adjustments that occur during the first cycle or two may cause slight bleeding between periods. This spotting is considered normal. Full effectiveness cannot be guaranteed during the first week because maximal levels of hormones haven't yet been reached. A backup method is recommended during the first week and any subsequent cycle in which the woman forgets to take any pills.

Since its approval by the FDA in 1960, the pill has remained a popular contraceptive in the United States. OC use declined temporarily in the late 1970s following publicity regarding possible increased risks of heart attack and stroke. However, these risks have been substantially reduced by the use of lower-dosage pills (those with 50 micrograms or less of estrogen) and the identification of women at higher risk for complications. Today, OCs are the most widely used form of contraception among unmarried women and are second only to sterilization among married women.

Advantages   The main advantage of the oral contraceptive is its high degree of effectiveness in preventing pregnancy. Nearly all unplanned pregnancies result because the pills were not taken as directed. The pill is relatively simple to use and does not require any interruptions that could hinder sexual spontaneity. Most women also enjoy the predictable regularity of periods, as well as the decrease in cramps and blood loss. For young women, the reversibility of the pill is especially important; **fertility**—the ability to reproduce—returns after the pill is discontinued (although not always immediately).

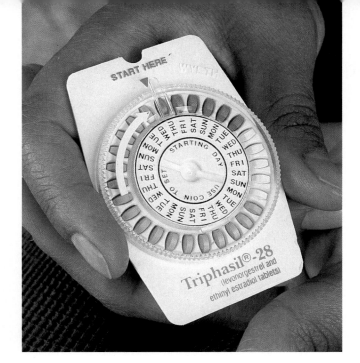

Oral contraceptives are the most popular reversible method of contraception among American women. When used correctly, oral contraceptives are highly effective.

Medical advantages include a decreased incidence of benign breast disease, iron-deficiency anemia, pelvic inflammatory disease (PID), ectopic pregnancy, endometrial cancer (of the lining of the uterus), and ovarian cancer. Women who have never used the pill are twice as likely to develop endometrial or ovarian cancer as those who have taken it for at least 12 months.

Disadvantages   Although oral contraceptives do lower the risk of PID, they do not protect against HIV infection or other STDs in the lower reproductive tract. OCs have been associated with increased cervical chlamydia. Regular condom use is recommended for an OC user, unless she is in a long-term, mutually monogamous relationship with an uninfected partner.

The hormones in birth control pills influence all tissues of the body, and they can lead to a variety of minor disturbances. Symptoms of early pregnancy—morning nausea, weight gain, and swollen breasts, for example—may appear during the first few months of OC use. They usually disappear by the fourth cycle. Other side effects include depression, nervousness, changes in sex drive, dizziness, generalized headaches, migraine, bleeding between periods, and changes in the lining of the walls of the vagina, with an increase in clear or white vaginal discharge. Chloasma, or "mask of pregnancy," sometimes occurs, causing brown "giant freckles" to appear on the face. Acne may develop or worsen, but in most women, using the pill causes acne to clear up, and it is sometimes

prescribed for that purpose. Treatable yeast infections are also more common among OC users.

Serious side effects have been reported in a small number of women. These include blood clots, stroke, and heart attack, concentrated mostly in older women who smoke or have a history of circulatory disease. Recent studies have shown very little, if any, increased risk of stroke or heart attack for healthy young nonsmoking women on lower-dosage pills. OC users may be slightly more prone to high blood pressure, blood clots in the legs and arms, and benign liver tumors that may rupture and bleed. Studies on possible links between OC use and breast and cervical cancer have been inconclusive. Most adverse effects of OCs disappear after pill use is discontinued, and studies show no long-term effect on mortality.

Birth control pills are not recommended for women with a history of blood clots, heart disease or stroke, any form of cancer or liver tumor, or impaired liver function. Women with certain other health conditions or behaviors, including migraines, high blood pressure, cigarette smoking, and sickle-cell disease, require close monitoring.

In trying to decide whether to use oral contraceptives, each woman needs to weigh the benefits against the risks. To make an informed decision, she should seek the help of a health care professional in evaluating the known risk variables that apply to her (see the box "Obtaining a Contraceptive from a Health Clinic or Physician"). A woman can take several steps to lower her risk from OC use:

1. Request a low-dosage pill.
2. Stop smoking.
3. Follow the dosage carefully and consistently.
4. Be alert to preliminary danger signals (severe headaches, problems with vision, severe pain in the abdomen, chest, or legs).
5. Have regular checkups to monitor blood pressure, weight, and urine, and have an annual examination of the thyroid, breasts, abdomen, and pelvis.
6. Have regular **Pap tests** to check for early cervical changes. Because OC use may temporarily increase

contraceptive failure rate   The percentage of women using   **TERMS**
a particular contraceptive method who experience an unintended pregnancy in the first year of use.

continuation rate   The percentage of women who continue to use a particular contraceptive after a specified period of time.

oral contraceptive (OC)   Any of various hormone compounds (estrogen and progestins) in pill form that prevent conception by preventing ovulation.

fertility   The ability to reproduce.

Pap test   A scraping of cells from the cervix for examination under a microscope to detect cancer.

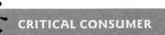

If you are a woman who is considering a method of contraception that requires a prescription or professional fitting or insertion, you'll need to go to a health clinic or a physician to get it. Many of the female methods—including the hormonal methods, IUDs, and the diaphragm and cervical cap—require at least an initial professional visit. The thought of visiting a physician's office or health clinic to discuss and obtain contraception makes many people nervous. Keep in mind that the people in the office are health care professionals who will not pass moral judgment on you. They are dedicated to meeting your health care needs. Knowing what to expect can help you get more from your visit.

Before Your Visit

You can prepare for a more successful visit by doing the following:

1. Pull together your personal and family medical history. Make sure it's accurate and up-to-date.

2. Review the section in this chapter entitled "Which Contraceptive Method Is Right for You?" Carefully consider each topic, and discuss it with your partner if that would be helpful.

3. Write down any questions you have. Clarify in your own mind what you need to find out about your contraceptive options.

4. If you have questions about sexually transmitted diseases or other aspects of sexuality, write those down too.

5. If you like, plan to have your partner, a friend, or a family member accompany you to your appointment.

During Your Visit

When you arrive, you'll probably be asked to fill out forms covering your background and medical history. A physician or staff member will then review the various contraceptive methods with you and answer your questions. She or he can help you evaluate the key factors affecting your choice of method, including health risks, lifestyle factors, cost, and protection against STDs. You may have blood and urine samples taken for lab tests.

The Physical Exam

Your physical exam will probably include a check of your breasts, external genitals, and abdomen, plus a Pap test and possible screening for certain STDs. The exam will help ensure that you can safely use the method you have chosen, as well as protect your overall health. If this is your first pelvic exam and/or you feel nervous or uncomfortable, tell the clinician, and ask her or him to explain each step of the examination.

For the pelvic exam, you will be asked to lie on your back on an examination table, with your feet in metal stirrups and your knees bent. The exam doesn't usually hurt. An instrument called a speculum will be inserted into the vagina to hold it open so the clinician can look at the cervix and vaginal walls. For the Pap test, the clinician will scrape some cells from the cervix and place them on a glass slide. These cells will be analyzed for any signs of cancer. You may feel a slight pressure while the cells are collected. The clinician will also check your internal organs by placing two gloved fingers into the vagina and the other hand on the lower abdomen. He or she will palpate (examine by touching) the uterus and ovaries to check for any abnormalities.

If you're getting a diaphragm or a cervical cap, you will be fitted for it at this time. The clinician will probably try different sizes to find the best fit, then will show you how to insert and remove it.

Following Your Exam

After your exam, a health care worker will either provide you with your contraceptive, arrange for a further appointment (if necessary), or give you a prescription. Make sure you know exactly how to use the method you've chosen. Written instructions and information may be available. Be sure you have a phone number you can call if you have questions later.

---

some women's susceptibility to the STDs chlamydia and gonorrhea, regular screening for those diseases is also recommended, especially when condoms aren't being used.

For most women, the known, directly associated risk of death from taking birth control pills is much lower than the risk of death from pregnancy (Table 6-2).

Effectiveness   Oral contraceptive effectiveness varies substantially because it depends so much on individual factors. If taken exactly as directed, the failure rate is extremely low. However, among average users, lapses such as forgetting to take a pill do occur, and a typical first-year failure rate is 5%. The continuation rate for OCs also varies; the average rate is 71% after 1 year.

Norplant Implants

In December 1990, the Norplant implant, another method of hormonal birth control for women, was approved by the FDA for use in the United States. This and other similar implants have been used for more than 15 years in various countries, including several in South America, Asia, and Scandinavia.

The Norplant implant consists of six flexible, matchstick-sized capsules, each containing progestin, a synthetic progesterone, released in steady doses for up to 5 years. (A newly approved two-capsule implant containing similar hormones is also becoming available for use.) The capsules are placed under the skin, usually on the inside of a woman's upper arm in a fan-shaped configuration. The procedure can be done in less than 15 minutes, with

TABLE 6-2	*Contraceptive Risks*

Contraceptive Method	Risk of Death in Any Given Year
Oral contraceptives	
Nonsmoker	1 in 63,000
Smoker	1 in 16,000
Intrauterine devices (IUDs)	1 in 100,000
Barrier methods (condoms, diaphragm, or cervical cap)	0
Natural methods (abstinence or FAM)	0
Sterilization	
Tubal ligation (laparoscopic)	1 in 67,000
Hysterectomy	1 in 1,600
Vasectomy	1 in 300,000
Pregnancy and childbirth	1 in 14,300

SOURCES: Carlson, K. J., S. A. Eisenstat, and T. Ziporyn. 1996. *The Harvard Guide to Women's Health.* Cambridge, Mass.: Harvard University Press.

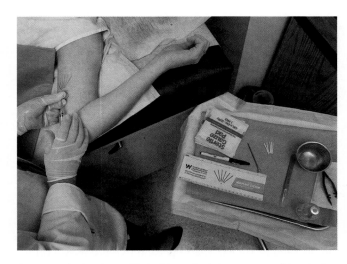

Contraceptive implants, filled with synthetic hormones and inserted under the skin on the arm or leg, can provide 5 years of protection against pregnancy.

a local anesthetic and only one very small incision. No stitches are required.

The progestin in Norplant has several contraceptive effects: Hormonal shifts may inhibit ovulation and affect development of the uterine lining, thickening of cervical mucus inhibits the movement of sperm, and transport of the egg through the fallopian tubes may be slowed.

The use of implants by American women dropped substantially after their first few years of availability because of ongoing lawsuits and related complaints (see "Disadvantages," which follows). This contraceptive option is best suited for women who wish to have continuous and long-term protection against pregnancy.

Advantages Norplant implants are the most effective reversible method of contraception now available. After insertion of the implants, no further action is required for up to 5 years of protection; at the same time, contraceptive effects are quickly reversed upon removal. Because Norplant, unlike the combination pill, contains no estrogen, it carries a lower risk of certain side effects, such as blood clots and other cardiovascular complications. In addition, the progestin is released at a steady rate, in smaller quantities than are found in oral contraceptives. The thickened cervical mucus resulting from Norplant use has a protective effect against PID.

Disadvantages As with the pill, Norplant gives no protection against HIV infection and STDs in the lower reproductive tract. Although the implants are barely visible, their appearance may bother some women. The initial cost can be substantial (but protection is provided for 5 years). Both insertion and removal of implants are procedures

that can be done only by specially trained practitioners. Removal is sometimes difficult, especially if insertion of the implant is deep. Lawsuits that focus on removal difficulties and inadequate warnings about side effects are under way against the maker of Norplant. The manufacturer has responded by issuing a special acknowledgment form to help with patient education and setting up a consumer hotline that offers information on Norplant and the names of practitioners experienced with insertion and removal of the implants (800-934-5556).

The most common side effects of contraceptive implants are menstrual irregularities, including longer menstrual periods, spotting between periods, or having no bleeding at all. The menstrual cycle usually becomes more regular after 1 year of use. Less common side effects include headaches, weight gain, breast tenderness, nausea, acne, and mood swings. Cautions and more serious health concerns are similar to those associated with oral contraceptives, but are less common. Other health factors may also be important, and a complete medical history should be reviewed with a clinician before implants are used.

Effectiveness Typical failure rates are very low (0.05%) in the first year, increasing slowly with each additional year of use. The cumulative failure rate at the end of 5 years is about 3.7%; the continuation rate is about 88%.

Depo-Provera Injections

Contraceptive injections that use long-acting progestins have also received recent FDA approval for use in the United States. Contraceptive injections were developed in the 1960s and are currently being used in at least 80 countries throughout the world. The injectable contraceptive most commonly used in the United States is marketed under the trade name Depo-Provera.

Injected in the arm or buttocks, Depo-Provera is usually given every 12 weeks, although it actually provides effective contraception for a few weeks beyond that. As another progestin-only contraceptive, it prevents pregnancy in the same ways as Norplant implants.

Advantages   The advantages of Depo-Provera are similar to those of Norplant: It is highly effective, requires little action on the part of the user, and has no estrogen-related side effects. In addition, it requires only periodic injections, rather than the minor surgical procedures of implant insertion and removal. Because the injections leave no trace and involve no ongoing supplies, this method allows women almost total privacy in their decision to use contraception.

Disadvantages   Depo-Provera injections provide no protection against HIV infection and STDs in the lower reproductive tract. A woman must visit a health care facility every 3 months to receive the injections. Its side effects are similar to those associated with Norplant use; menstrual irregularities are the most common. After 1 year of using Depo-Provera, many women have no menstrual bleeding at all. After discontinuing use, women may experience infertility for up to 12 months. (It does not lead to permanent infertility.) Other side effects include weight gain, headaches, depression, and dizziness.

Reasons for not using Depo-Provera are similar to those for not using Norplant. Although early animal studies indicated that Depo-Provera increases the risk of breast and other cancers, the FDA has concluded that worldwide studies and years of human use have shown the risk of cancer in humans to be minimal or nonexistent. Recent research suggests that extended use of Depo-Provera may be associated with decreased bone density, a risk factor for osteoporosis (see Chapter 12). Bone density reportedly returned to normal when Depo-Provera was discontinued. More research is needed to clarify Depo-Provera's effect on bone density.

Effectiveness   Typical failure rates with Depo-Provera are 0.3%; the continuation rate is 70%.

Emergency Contraception

Emergency contraception refers to postcoital methods—those used after unprotected sexual intercourse. An emergency contraceptive may be appropriate if a regularly used method has failed (for example, if a condom breaks) or if unprotected sex has occurred. Emergency contraceptives are designed only for emergency use and should not be relied upon as a regular method.

The most frequently used emergency contraceptive is a two-dose regimen of certain oral contraceptives. These pills have been packaged as emergency contraceptives for more than a decade in Great Britain, Germany, and other countries. Although long approved by the FDA as contraceptives and prescribed by some physicians for emergency use, these OCs have only recently been approved specifically for postcoital purposes in the United States. In 1996, an FDA advisory panel concluded that six brands of OCs already available in the United States are safe and effective for emergency contraception, reducing the risk of pregnancy by 75%.

In 1998, the Preven Emergency Contraception Kit became the first FDA-approved product specifically designed for emergency contraception. The kit contains four pills and a pregnancy test. After confirming that she is not pregnant from intercourse earlier in the month or in previous months, a woman takes two of the pills; this dose is followed 12 hours later by a second, two-pill dose. The first dose must be taken within 72 hours after intercourse (the sooner, the better). The most common side effects are nausea, vomiting, and breast tenderness.

Researchers are still uncertain precisely how OCs work as emergency contraceptives. Opponents of their use argue that if they act by preventing implantation of a fertilized egg, they may actually be **abortifacients;** however, recent evidence indicates that prevention of implantation may not be their primary mode of action. Postcoital pills also appear to inhibit or delay ovulation and to alter the transport of sperm and/or eggs.

A specific regimen of the minipill can be used for emergency contraception by women who cannot take combination OCs. In addition, mifepristone, the "abortion pill," is being studied as another possible option (see Chapter 7 for more on mifepristone). Intrauterine devices, discussed in the next section, can also be used for emergency contraception: If inserted within 5 days of unprotected intercourse, they are even more effective than OCs. However, because their use is more complicated, they are not used nearly as frequently.

For more on options for emergency contraception, refer to the resources in the For More Information section at the end of the chapter.

The Intrauterine Device (IUD)

The **intrauterine device (IUD)** is a small plastic device placed in the uterus as a contraceptive. At the height of its popularity in the early 1970s, about 10% of all women using contraceptives in the United States had an IUD. In the late 1970s, however, IUD use began to decline, mostly resulting from publicity about the increased risk of seri-

TERMS   **abortifacient**   An agent or substance that induces abortion.

intrauterine device (IUD)   A plastic device inserted into the uterus as a contraceptive.

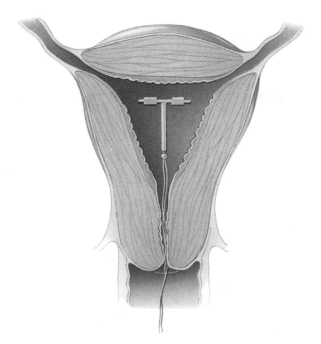

Figure 6-1 An IUD (Copper T-380A) properly positioned in the uterus. The attached threads that protrude from the cervix into the upper vagina allow the woman to check to make sure that the IUD is in place.

ous infections associated with the popular Dalkon Shield and its withdrawal from the market. Two IUDs are now available in the United States: the hormone-releasing Progestasert, which requires replacement every year; and the Copper T-380A (also known as the ParaGard), which gives protection for up to 10 years. A third IUD, the Levonorgestral IUD, may be approved for use in the near future. In the late-1990s, fewer than 1% of all American women who used contraception had IUDs.

Researchers do not know exactly how IUDs prevent pregnancy. Current evidence suggests that they work primarily by preventing fertilization. IUDs may cause biochemical changes in the uterus and affect the movement of sperm and eggs; although less likely, they may also interfere with implantation of fertilized eggs. Progestasert slowly releases very small amounts of progesterone, which impedes fertilization or implantation.

An IUD must be inserted and removed by a trained professional. It can be inserted at any time during the menstrual cycle, as long as the woman is not pregnant. The device is threaded into a sterile inserter, which is introduced through the cervix; a plunger pushes the IUD into the uterus. The threads protruding from the cervix are trimmed so that only 1–1.5 inches remain in the upper vagina (Figure 6-1).

Advantages Intrauterine devices are highly reliable and are simple and convenient to use, requiring no attention except for a periodic check of the string position. They do not require the woman to anticipate or interrupt sexual activity. Usually IUDs have only localized side effects, and in the absence of complications, they are considered a fully reversible contraceptive. In most cases, fertility is restored as soon as the IUD is removed. The long-term expense of using an IUD is low.

Disadvantages Most side effects of IUD use are limited to the genital tract. Heavy menstrual flow and bleeding and spotting between periods may occur. Another side effect is pain, particularly uterine cramps and backache, which seem to occur most often in women who have never been pregnant. Spontaneous expulsion of the IUD happens to 5–10% of women within the first year, most commonly during the first months after insertion. The older the woman is and the more children she has had, the less likely she is to expel the device. In about 1 of 1000 insertions, the IUD punctures the wall of the uterus and may migrate into the abdominal cavity.

A serious complication sometimes associated with IUD use is pelvic inflammatory disease (PID). Most pelvic infections among IUD users are relatively mild and can be treated successfully with antibiotics. However, early and adequate treatment is critical, for a lingering infection can lead to tubal scarring and subsequent infertility.

Some physicians advise against the use of IUDs by young women who have never been pregnant because of the increased incidence of side effects in this group, and the risk of infection with the possibility of subsequent infertility. IUDs are not recommended for women of any age who have a history of pelvic infection or who are at high risk for STDs. They are also unsuitable for women with suspected pregnancy, large tumors of the uterus or other anatomical abnormalities, irregular or unexplained bleeding, a history of ectopic pregnancy, or rheumatic heart disease. No evidence has been found linking IUD use to cancer, but the long-term effects are not well known. IUDs offer no protection against STDs.

Early IUD danger signals are abdominal pain, fever, chills, foul-smelling vaginal discharge, irregular menstrual periods, and other unusual vaginal bleeding. A change in string length should also be noted. An annual checkup is important and should include a Pap test and a blood check for anemia if menstrual flow has increased. (And in the case of Progestasert use, the IUD must be replaced every 12 months.)

Effectiveness The typical failure rate of IUDs during the first year of use is 1–2%. Effectiveness can be increased by periodically checking to see that the device is in place and by using a backup method for the first few months after IUD insertion. If pregnancy occurs, the IUD should be removed to safeguard the health of the woman and to maintain the pregnancy. The continuation rate of IUDs is about 80% after 1 year of use.

Male Condoms

The **male condom** is a thin sheath designed to cover the penis during sexual intercourse. Most brands available in the United States are made of latex, although condoms made of polyurethane are also now available. Condoms prevent sperm from entering the vagina and provide protection against disease. Condoms are the most widely used barrier method and the third most popular of all contraceptive methods used in the United States, after the pill and female sterilization.

Condom sales have increased dramatically in recent years, primarily because they provide some protection against all STDs and are the only method that provides substantial protection against HIV infection. At least one-third of all male condoms are bought by women. This figure will probably increase as more women become aware of the serious risks associated with STDs and assume the right to insist on condom use. Women are more likely to contract an STD from an infected partner than men are. Women also face additional health risks from STDs, including cervical cancer, PID, ectopic pregnancy (which is potentially life-threatening), and infertility. (See Chapter 18 for more information on STDs.)

The man or his partner must put the condom on the penis before it is inserted into the vagina, because the small amounts of fluid that may be secreted unnoticed prior to **ejaculation** often contain sperm capable of causing pregnancy. The rolled-up condom is placed over the head of the erect penis and unrolled down to the base of the penis, leaving a half-inch space (without air) at the tip to collect semen (Figure 6-2). Some brands of condoms have a reservoir tip designed for this purpose. Uncircumcised men must first pull back the foreskin of the penis. Partners must be careful not to damage the condom with fingernails, rings, or other rough objects.

Prelubricated condoms are available containing the **spermicide** nonoxynol-9, the same agent found in many of the contraceptive creams that women use. Spermicide condoms may decrease the risk of pregnancy, but the extent of decreased risk has not been established.

If desired, users can lubricate their own condoms with contraceptive foam, creams, or jelly, or water-based preparations such as K-Y Jelly. Any product that contains mineral or vegetable oil—including baby oil, many lotions, regular Vaseline petroleum jelly, cooking oils (corn oil, Crisco, butter, and so on), and some vaginal lubricants and anti-fungal or anti-itch creams—should

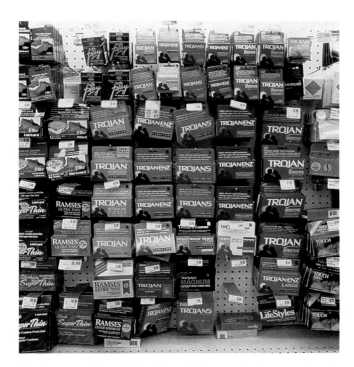

Condoms come in a variety of sizes, textures, and colors; some brands have a reservoir tip designed to collect semen. Used consistently and correctly, condoms provide the most reliable protection available against HIV infection for sexually active people.

never be used with latex condoms; they can cause latex to begin to disintegrate within 60 seconds, thus greatly increasing the chance of condom breakage. (Polyurethane is not affected by oil-based products.)

When the man loses his erection after ejaculating, the condom loses its tight fit. To avoid spilling semen, the condom must be held around the base of the penis as the penis is withdrawn. If any semen is spilled on the vulva, sperm may find their way to the uterus.

Advantages Condoms are easy to purchase and are available without prescription or medical supervision (see the box "Buying and Using Over-the-Counter Contraceptives," p. 142). Simple to use, they provide for greater male participation in contraception. Their effects are immediately and completely reversible. In addition to being free of medical side effects (other than occasional allergic reactions), latex condoms help protect against STDs. Condoms made of polyurethane are appropriate for people who are allergic to latex; they also provide STD protection, but they are not as well-studied as latex condoms, so their exact effectiveness is unknown. (Lambskin condoms permit the passage of HIV and other disease-causing organisms, so they can be used only for pregnancy prevention, not the prevention of STDs.) Except for abstinence, correct and consistent use of latex condoms offers the most reliable available protection against the transmission of HIV.

TERMS **male condom** A sheath, usually made of thin latex (synthetic rubber), that covers the penis during sexual intercourse; used for contraception and to prevent STDs.

ejaculation An abrupt discharge of semen from the penis after sexual stimulation.

spermicide A chemical agent that kills sperm.

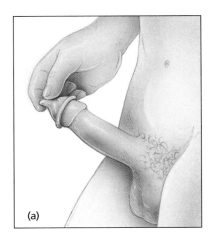

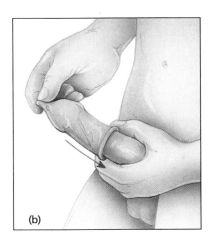

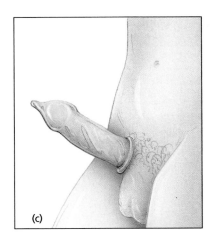

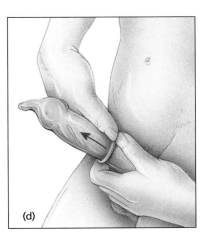

Figure 6-2   Use of the male condom.   (a) Place the rolled-up condom over the head of the erect penis. Hold the top half-inch of the condom (with air squeezed out) to leave room for semen. (b) While holding the tip, unroll the condom onto the penis. Gently smooth out any air bubbles. (c) Unroll the condom down to the base of the penis. (d) To avoid spilling semen after ejaculation, hold the condom around the base of the penis as the penis is withdrawn. Remove the condom away from your partner, taking care not to spill any semen.

Disadvantages   The two most common complaints about condoms are that they diminish sensation and interfere with spontaneity. Although some people find these drawbacks serious, others consider them only minor disadvantages. Many couples learn to creatively integrate condom use into their sexual practices. Indeed, it can be a way to improve communication and share responsibility in a relationship.

Effectiveness   In actual use, the failure rate of condoms varies considerably. First-year rates among typical users average about 14%. At least some pregnancies happen because the condom is carelessly removed after ejaculation. Some may also occur because of a break or a tear, which may happen 1–2 times in every 100 instances of use for latex condoms; some studies have found higher breakage rates for polyurethane condoms. Breakage is more common among inexperienced users. Other contributing factors include poorly fitting condoms, insufficient lubrication, excessively vigorous sex, and improper storage (because heat destroys rubber, latex condoms should not be stored for long periods in a wallet or a car's glove compartment). To help ensure quality, condoms should not be used past their expiration date or more than 5 years past their date of manufacture (2 years for those with spermicide). It is important to note, however, that most condom failures are due to inconsistent or improper use, not problems with condom quality.

If a condom breaks or is carelessly removed, the risk of pregnancy can be reduced somewhat by the immediate use of a vaginal spermicide. If postcoital contraception is an appropriate option, a health care provider should be consulted as soon as possible. The effectiveness of the condom can be greatly improved and approaches that of oral contraceptives if a spermicidal foam is also inserted just *before* intercourse. The most common cause of pregnancy with condom users is "taking a chance"—that is, occasionally not using a condom at all—or waiting to use it until after preejaculate fluid (which may contain some sperm) has already entered the vagina.

PERSONAL INSIGHT   What are your ideas about taking responsibility for contraception? Should one partner be responsible, or should responsibility be shared? Where did you get your ideas? Are they tied to other attitudes you have about gender roles? Are you comfortable with your attitude and the effect it has on your life?

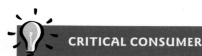
You can buy several types of contraceptives without a prescription. Here are their advantages, especially for college students:

- They are readily accessible and relatively inexpensive.
- They are moderately effective at preventing pregnancy when used correctly.
- They offer some protection against HIV infection and other STDs.

But like all methods, over-the-counter contraceptives work only if they are used correctly. The following guidelines should help.

Male Condoms

- *Buy latex condoms.* If you're allergic to latex, use a polyurethane condom or wear a lambskin condom under a latex one. Lambskin condoms provide no STD protection; polyurethane condoms may provide protection against pregnancy and STDs comparable to latex condoms, but more studies are needed.
- *Buy and use condoms while they are fresh.* Packages have an expiration date or a manufacturing date. Don't use a condom after the expiration date or more than 5 years after the manufacturing date (2 years if it contains spermicide).
- *Try different styles and sizes.* Male condoms come in a variety of textures, colors, shapes, lubricants, and sizes. Shop around until you find a brand that's right for you. Condom widths and lengths vary by about 10–20%. A condom that is too tight may be uncomfortable and more likely to break; one that is too loose may slip off.
- *Use "thinner" condoms with caution.* Condoms advertised as "thinner" are often no thinner than others, and those that really are the thinnest tend to break more easily.
- *Don't remove the condom from an individual sealed wrapper until you're ready to use it.* Open the packet carefully. Don't use a condom if it's gummy, dried out, or discolored.
- *Store condoms correctly.* Don't leave condoms in extreme heat or cold, and don't carry them in a pocket wallet.
- *Use only water-based lubricants.* Never use oil-based lubricants like Vaseline or hand lotion, as they may cause a latex condom to break. Avoid oil-based vaginal products.
- *Use male condoms correctly* (see Figure 6-2). Use a new condom every time you have intercourse. Misuse is by far the leading reason that condoms fail.

Female Condoms

- *Make sure your condom comes with the necessary supplies and information.* The Reality female condom comes individually wrapped. With your condom, you should receive a leaflet of instructions and a small bottle of additional lubricant.
- *Buy and use female condoms while they are fresh.* Check the expiration dates on the condom packet and the lubricant bottle.
- *Buy several condoms.* Buy one or more for practice before using one during sex. Have a backup in case you have a problem with insertion or use.
- *Read the leaflet instructions carefully.* Practice inserting the condom and checking that it's in the proper position.
- *Use the female condom correctly.* Make sure the penis is inserted into the pouch and that the outer ring is not pushed into the vagina. Add lubricant around the outer ring if needed.

Spermicides

- *Try different types of spermicides.* You may find one type easier or more convenient to use. Foams come in aerosol cans and are similar to shaving cream in consistency. Foams are thicker than creams, which are thicker than jellies. Foams, creams, and jellies usually require applicators; spermicidal suppositories and films do not.
- *Read and follow the package directions carefully.* Cans of foam must be shaken before use. Jellies and creams are often inserted with an applicator just outside the entrance to the cervix. Suppositories and film must be placed with the finger.
- *Pay close attention to the timing of use.* Follow the package instructions for inserting the spermicide at the appropriate time before intercourse actually occurs. Spermicides have a fairly narrow window of effectiveness. Be sure to also allow the recommended amount of time for suppositories and films to dissolve.
- *Use an additional full dose for each additional act of intercourse.*
- *Leave the spermicide in place for 8 hours after the last act of intercourse.*
- *Consider using spermicides with another form of birth control.* These include a condom, diaphragm, or cervical cap. Combined use provides greater protection against pregnancy.

Female Condoms

A female condom is a latex or polyurethane pouch that a woman or her partner inserts into her vagina. One brand, Reality, was approved in May 1993 for use in the United States. Although the female condom is preferred in certain situations because it requires less participation on the part of the male partner, its overall popularity remains far below that of the male condom.

The female condom currently available is a disposable device that comes in one size and consists of a soft, loose-fitting polyurethane sheath with two flexible rings (Figure 6-3). The ring at the closed end is inserted into the vagina and placed at the cervix much like a diaphragm. The ring at the open end remains outside the vagina. The walls of the condom protect the inside of the vagina.

The directions that accompany the condom should be followed closely. It can be inserted up to 8 hours before

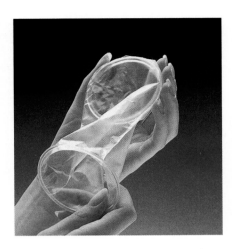

The Reality brand female condom is a poly-urethane sheath about 6.5 inches long. It is held in place by two flexible rings, a closed one placed at the cervix and an open one that hangs outside the body.

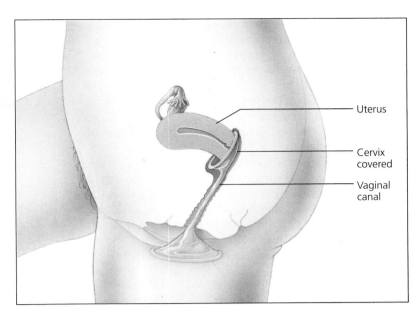

Figure 6-3 **The female condom properly positioned.**

intercourse and should be used with the supplied lubri-cant or a spermicide to prevent penile irritation. As with male condoms, users need to take care not to tear the con-dom during insertion or removal. Following intercourse, the woman should remove the condom immediately, before standing up. By twisting and squeezing the outer ring, she can prevent the spilling of semen. A new con-dom should be used for each act of sexual intercourse. A female condom should not be used with a male condom because when the two are used together, slippage is more likely to occur.

Advantages For many women, the greatest advantage of the female condom is the control it gives them over contraception and STD prevention. Female condoms can be inserted before sexual activity and are thus less disrup-tive than male condoms. Because the outer part of the condom covers the area around the vaginal opening as well as the base of the penis during intercourse, it offers potentially better protection against genital warts or her-pes. The polyurethane pouch can be used by people who are allergic to latex. And because polyurethane is thin and pliable, there is little loss of sensation. When used cor-rectly, the female condom should theoretically provide protection against HIV transmission and STDs compara-ble to that of the latex male condom. However, conclusive evidence is not yet available. Latex male condoms are still recommended as the safest protection.

Disadvantages As with the traditional condom, inter-ference with spontaneity is likely to be a common com-plaint. The outer ring, which hangs visibly outside the vagina, may be bothersome during foreplay; if so, couples

may choose to put the device in just before intercourse. During coitus, both partners must take care that the penis is inserted into the pouch, not outside it, and that the device does not slip inside the vagina. For many couples, initial awkwardness and difficulty are largely eliminated after a few weeks' use. Female condoms, like male con-doms, are made for one-time use. A single female condom costs about four times as much as a single male condom.

Effectiveness The typical first-year failure rate of the female condom is 21%. For women who follow instruc-tions carefully and consistently, the failure rate is consid-erably lower. The effectiveness of the female condom, like that of other barrier contraceptive methods, depends pri-marily on how it is used.

The Diaphragm with Spermicide

Before oral contraceptives were introduced, about 25% of all American couples who used any form of contraception relied on the **diaphragm**. Many former diaphragm users have been won over to the pill or to IUDs, but the diaphragm continues to offer advantages that are impor-tant to some couples. About 1.7% of all women who use contraception use a diaphragm.

The diaphragm is a dome-shaped cup of thin rubber stretched over a collapsible metal ring. When correctly

diaphragm A contraceptive device consisting of a flexible, dome-shaped cup that covers the cervix and prevents sperm from entering the uterus. **TERMS**

used with spermicidal cream or jelly, the diaphragm covers the cervix, blocking sperm from entering the uterus.

A diaphragm can be obtained only by prescription. Because of individual anatomical differences, a diaphragm must be carefully fitted by a trained clinician to ensure both comfort and effectiveness. The fitting should be checked with each routine annual medical examination, as well as after childbirth, abortion, or a weight change of more than 10 pounds.

The woman spreads spermicidal jelly or cream on the diaphragm before inserting it and checking its placement (Figure 6-4). If more than 6 hours elapse between the time of insertion and the time of intercourse, additional spermicide must be applied. The diaphragm must be left in place for at least 6 hours after the last act of coitus to give the spermicide enough time to kill all the sperm.

To remove the diaphragm, the woman simply hooks the front rim down from the pubic bone with one finger and pulls it out. She should wash it with mild soap and water, rinse it, pat it dry, then examine it for holes or cracks. Defects would most likely develop near the rim and can be spotted by looking at the diaphragm in front of a bright light. After inspecting the diaphragm, she should dust it with cornstarch (*not* talcum powder, which may damage it and irritate the vagina) and store it in its case.

Advantages Diaphragm use is less intrusive than condom use because a diaphragm can be inserted up to 6 hours before intercourse. Its use can be limited to times of sexual activity only, and it allows for immediate and total reversibility. The diaphragm is free of medical side effects (other than rare allergic reactions). When used along with spermicidal jelly or cream, it offers significant protection against gonorrhea and possibly chlamydia, STDs that are transmitted only by semen and for which the cervix is the sole site of entry. Diaphragm use can also protect the cervix from semen infected with the human papillomavirus, which has been implicated as an important factor in cellular changes in the cervix that can lead to cancer. However, the diaphragm is unlikely to protect against STDs that can be transmitted through vaginal or vulvar surfaces (in addition to the cervix), including HIV infection, genital herpes, and syphilis.

Disadvantages Diaphragms must always be used with a spermicide, so a woman must keep both of these somewhat bulky supplies with her whenever she anticipates sexual activity. Diaphragms require extra attention, since they must be cleaned and stored with care to preserve their effectiveness. Some women cannot wear a diaphragm because of their vaginal or uterine anatomy. In other women, diaphragm use can cause an increase in bladder infections and may need to be discontinued if repeated infections occur. It has also been associated with a slightly increased risk of **toxic shock syndrome (TSS)**, an occasionally fatal bacterial infection. To diminish the risk of

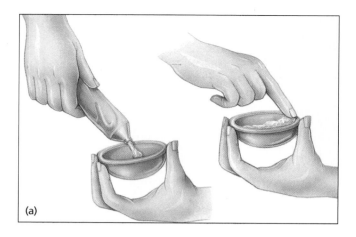

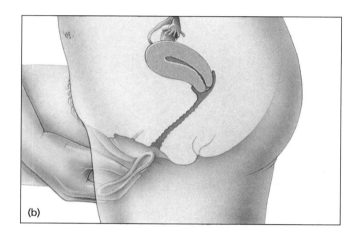

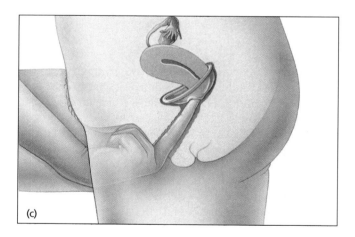

Figure 6-4 Use of the diaphragm. Wash your hands with soap and water before inserting the diaphragm. It can be inserted while squatting, lying down, or standing with one foot raised. (a) Place about a tablespoon of spermicidal jelly or cream in the concave side of the diaphragm, and spread it around the inside of the diaphragm and around the rim. (b) Squeeze the diaphragm into a long narrow shape between the thumb and forefinger. Insert it into the vagina, and push it up along the back wall of the vagina as far it will go. (c) Check its position to make sure the cervix is completely covered and that the front rim of the diaphragm is tucked behind the pubic bone.

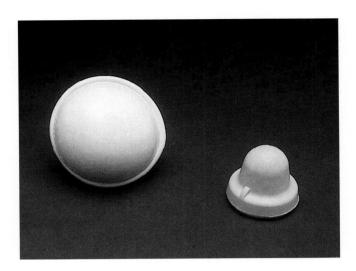

The diaphragm and cervical cap work by covering the mouth of the cervix, blocking sperm from entering the cervix. Both require professional fitting.

TSS, a woman should wash her hands with soap and water before inserting or removing the diaphragm, should not use the diaphragm during menstruation or in the presence of an abnormal vaginal discharge, and should never leave the device in place for more than 24 hours.

Effectiveness   The effectiveness of the diaphragm mainly depends on whether or not it is used properly. In actual practice, women rarely use it correctly every time they have intercourse. Typical failure rates are 20% during the first year of use. The main causes of failure are incorrect insertion, inconsistent use, and inaccurate fitting. Sometimes, too, the vaginal walls expand during sexual stimulation, causing the diaphragm to be dislodged. If a diaphragm slips during intercourse, a woman may choose to contact her physician to discuss use of emergency contraception.

The Cervical Cap

The **cervical cap,** another barrier device, is a thimble-shaped rubber or plastic cup that fits snugly over the cervix and is held in place by suction. The cap comes in various sizes and must be fitted by a trained clinician. It is used in a manner similar to the diaphragm, a small amount of spermicide being placed in the cup before each insertion.

Advantages   Advantages of the cervical cap are similar to those associated with diaphragm use and include partial STD protection. It is an alternative for women who cannot use a diaphragm because of anatomical reasons or recurrent urinary infections. Because the cap fits tightly, it does not require a fresh dose of spermicide with repeated intercourse. It may be left in place for up to 48 hours (compared with 24 hours for the diaphragm).

Disadvantages   Along with most of the disadvantages associated with the diaphragm, difficulty with insertion and removal is more common for cervical cap users. In addition, some studies have indicated that women who use the cap rather than the diaphragm initially have a higher rate of abnormal Pap test results. In most cases, these are due to inflammation or infections of the cervix, conditions that are easily treatable. As a safety precaution, the FDA requires that the cap be prescribed only for women with normal Pap tests, and that a repeat Pap test be done after 3 months of use to confirm that no changes have occurred. Because there may be a slightly increased risk of TSS with prolonged use, the cap should not be left in place for more than 48 hours.

Effectiveness   Studies indicate that for women who have never had children, cervical cap effectiveness is about 20%, similar to that of the diaphragm. For women who have given birth, the failure rate goes up to about 40%.

Vaginal Spermicides

Spermicidal compounds developed for use with a diaphragm have been adapted for use without a diaphragm by combining them with a bulky base. Foams, creams, jellies, and vaginal suppositories are all available. Foam is sold in an aerosol bottle or a metal container with an applicator that fits on the nozzle. Creams and jellies are sold in tubes with an applicator that can be screwed onto the opening of the tube (Figure 6-5).

Foams, creams, and jellies must be placed deep in the vagina near the cervical entrance and must be inserted no more than 30 minutes before intercourse. After an hour, their effectiveness is drastically reduced, and a new dose must be inserted. Another application is also required before each repeated act of coitus. If the woman wants to **douche,** she should wait for at least 8 hours after the last intercourse to make sure that there has been time for the spermicide to kill all the sperm.

The spermicidal suppository is small and easily inserted like a tampon. Because body heat is needed to dissolve and activate the suppository, it is important to wait at least 10 minutes after insertion before having intercourse. The suppository's spermicidal effects are limited in time, and

TERMS

toxic shock syndrome (TSS)   A bacterial disease usually associated with tampon use, but can also occur in men; symptoms include weakness, cold and clammy hands, fever, nausea, and headache. TSS can progress to life-threatening complications, including very low blood pressure (shock) and kidney and liver failure.

cervical cap   A thimble-shaped cup that fits over the cervix, to be used with spermicide.

douche   To apply a stream of water or other solutions to a body part or cavity such as the vagina; not a contraceptive technique.

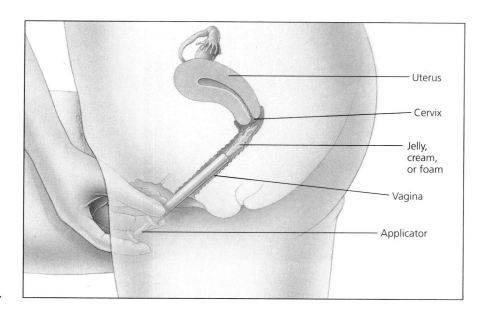

Figure 6-5 The application of spermicide.

coitus should take place within 1 hour of insertion. A new suppository is required for every act of intercourse.

The latest addition to the spermicides is the vaginal contraceptive film (VCF), a paper-thin 2-inch square of film that contains spermicide. It is folded over one or two fingers and placed high in the vagina, as close to the cervix as possible. In about 10 minutes the film dissolves into a spermicidal gel that is effective for about 1.5 hours. A new film must be inserted for each act of intercourse.

Advantages   The use of vaginal spermicides is relatively simple and can be limited to times of sexual activity. They are readily available in most drugstores and do not require a prescription or a pelvic examination. Spermicides allow for complete and immediate reversibility, and the only medical side effects are occasional allergic reactions. Vaginal spermicides may provide limited protection against some STDs, but should never be used instead of condoms for reliable protection, especially when there is any risk of HIV infection.

Disadvantages   When used alone, vaginal spermicides must be inserted shortly before intercourse, so their use may be seen as an annoying disruption. Some women find the slight increase in vaginal fluids after spermicide use unpleasant. Spermicides can alter the balance of bacteria in the vagina. Because this may increase the risk of urinary tract infections, women who are especially prone to these infections may want to avoid spermicides. Overuse of spermicides can irritate vaginal tissues; if this occurs, the risk of HIV transmission may actually increase. The potential risks of long-term use are currently being studied.

Effectiveness   The reported effectiveness rates of vaginal spermicides vary widely, depending partly on how consistently and carefully instructions are followed. The typical failure rate is about 26% during the first year of use. Of the various types of spermicides, foam is probably the most effective, because its effervescent mass forms a more dense and evenly distributed barrier to the cervical opening. Creams and jellies provide only minimal protection unless used with a diaphragm or cervical cap. Spermicide use is generally recommended only in combination with other barrier methods or as a backup with other contraceptives.

> **PERSONAL INSIGHT**   How do you feel about buying contraceptives at the drugstore? About asking for a prescription contraceptive at your health clinic or from your physician? Why do you feel the way you do? Have your feelings changed as you've grown older?

Abstinence and Fertility Awareness

Millions of people throughout the world do not use any of the contraceptive methods we have described, because of religious conviction or cultural prohibitions, or because of poverty or lack of information and supplies. If they use any method at all, they are likely to use one of the following relatively "natural" methods of attempting to prevent conception.

Abstinence   The decision not to engage in sexual intercourse for a chosen period of time, or **abstinence**, has been practiced throughout history for a variety of reasons.

TERMS   **abstinence**   Avoidance of sexual intercourse; a method of contraception.

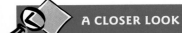 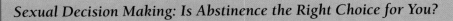

Many approaches have been proposed to address the problems of unintended pregnancy and the spread of sexually transmitted diseases. Abstinence, the avoidance of sexual intercourse, is a solution that is appropriate for some people. Anyone can practice abstinence at any time, including people who are not yet sexually active, those who are beginning a relationship with a new partner, and those who are not currently in a relationship. Consider the reasons for choosing abstinence and the guidelines for making decisions about sex to determine whether abstinence is an appropriate choice for you.

Reasons for Choosing Abstinence

People may choose abstinence for a variety of reasons. The most obvious is that avoiding sexual intercourse is the only sure way to prevent pregnancy and exposure to STDs. Even consistent condom use may fail because condoms can break and may not always cover all infected surfaces.

For some people, the most important reason for choosing abstinence is a moral one, based on cultural or religious beliefs or strongly held personal values. Individuals may feel that sexual intercourse is appropriate only for married couples or for people in serious, committed relationships. Abstinence may also be considered the wisest choice in terms of an individual's emotional needs. A period of abstinence may be useful as a time to focus energies on other aspects of interpersonal or personal growth.

Couples may choose abstinence to allow time for their relationship to grow. A period of abstinence allows partners to get to know each other better and to develop trust and respect for one another. Having intercourse is only one way to express feelings for another person.

There are many reasons for choosing abstinence, and the choice is not as rare as many people think. Recent surveys at Duke University and UCLA found that about 40% of students had not had intercourse; among students under age 21, the figure was closer to 50%.

Making Decisions About Sex

Choosing to have sex can change a relationship and an individual's life. It makes sense to think about it and talk about it. Consider the following issues:

- *Your attitudes, beliefs, and goals.* What are your personal values regarding relationships and sex? What goals or plans do you have for the future? Are you physically, emotionally, and financially ready to accept the potential consequences of the choices you make about sexual activity, including pregnancy or STDs? Consider how you will feel if you act in ways that are not consistent with your values and goals.

- *Your relationship with your partner.* How do you feel about your partner and your relationship? Do you respect and trust your partner? Does he or she respect and trust you? Do you feel comfortable talking about sexual issues, including contraception and safer sex? Have you discussed what you will do if pregnancy occurs? How do you think having intercourse will affect your relationship and how you feel about yourself and your partner? What does having sex mean to each of you?

- *Your reasons for having sex.* Are you feeling pressured to have sex? Are you afraid of losing your partner if you say no? Are you too embarrassed, shy, or insecure to say no or discuss waiting? Think carefully about your reasons for having sex, and be honest with yourself and your partner. Remember that alcohol and drugs affect judgment and may make you act in ways that you'll regret later. Studies show that college students who binge drink are much more likely to engage in unplanned and unprotected intercourse (see Chapter 10). Being drunk or high is not a good reason for having sex.

Your personal decisions about sex should always be respected. You have the right to make your own choices and to do only what you feel comfortable with. What may seem "right" and highly desirable for one person may be unacceptable for another. External pressure alone, either from individuals or from society at large, is not a satisfactory reason for engaging in intercourse. Assertiveness and communication skills are keys to making appropriate choices and sticking to them. When you make choices about sex based on self-respect, along with physical, emotional, and spiritual considerations, you'll be more likely to feel good about your decisions—now and in the future.

SOURCES: The decision to abstain from or engage in sexual activity. 1996. *Duke University Healthy Devil Online* (retrieved April 18, 1997; http://h-devil-www.mc.duke.edu/h-devil/sex/abstain.htm). Abstinence more prevalent than Bruins may think. 1995. *Daily Bruin,* 2 November (retrieved April 18, 1997; http://www.saonet.ucla.edu/health/sexual/abstine.htm). *Teensex? It's Okay to Say: No Way!* 1995. Planned Parenthood Federation of America (retrieved April 18, 1997; http://www.igc.apc.org/ppfa/nowaypub.html).

Until relatively recently, many people abstained because they had no other contraceptive measures. Today, with other methods available, about 2.2% of all American women rely on periodic abstinence as a contraceptive method. To some, other methods simply seem unsuitable. Concern about possible side effects, STDs, and unwanted pregnancy may be factors. (See the box "Sexual Decision Making: Is Abstinence the Right Choice for You?")

Many couples who do choose to abstain from sexual intercourse in the traditional sense turn to other mutually satisfying alternatives. When open communication between partners exists, many new avenues may be explored. These may include dancing, massage, hugging, kissing, petting, mutual masturbation, and oral-genital sex. Sexual

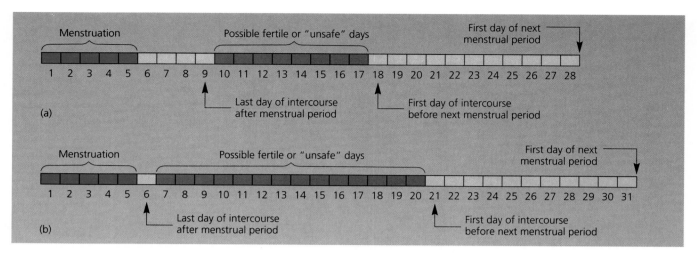

Figure 6-6 The fertility awareness method of contraception. This chart shows the safe and unsafe days for (a) a woman with a regular 28-day cycle and (b) a woman with an irregular cycle, ranging from 25 to 31 days.

feelings and intimacy may be expressed and satisfied through a wide range of activities.

The Fertility Awareness Method The basis for the **fertility awareness method (FAM)** is abstinence from coitus during the fertile phase of a woman's menstrual cycle. Ordinarily only one egg is released by the ovaries each month, and it lives about 24 hours unless it is fertilized. Sperm deposited in the vagina are on average capable of fertilizing an egg for about 6–7 days, so conception can theoretically occur only during 8 days of any cycle. Predicting which 8 days is difficult. It is done by either the calendar method or the temperature method. Information on cyclical changes of the cervical mucus can also help determine the time of ovulation.

The *calendar method* is based on the knowledge that the average woman releases an egg 14–16 days before her next period begins. Few women menstruate with complete regularity, so a record of the menstrual cycle must be kept for 12 months, during which time some other method of contraception must be used. The first day of each period is counted as day 1. To determine the first fertile, or "unsafe," day of the cycle, subtract 18 from the number of days in the shortest cycle (Figure 6-6). To determine the last unsafe day of the cycle, subtract 11 from the number of days in the longest cycle.

The *temperature method* is based on the knowledge that a woman's body temperature drops slightly just before ovulation and rises slightly after ovulation. A woman using the temperature method records her basal (resting) body temperature (BBT) every morning before getting out of bed and before eating or drinking anything. Once the temperature pattern is apparent (usually after about 3 months), the unsafe period for intercourse can be calculated as the interval from day 5 (day 1 is the first day of the period) until 3 days after the rise in BBT. To arrive at a shorter unsafe period, some women combine the calendar and temperature methods, calculating the first unsafe day from the shortest cycle of the calendar chart and the last unsafe day as the third day after a rise in BBT.

The *mucus method* (or Billings method) is based on changes in the cervical secretions throughout the menstrual cycle. During the estrogenic phase, cervical mucus increases and is clear and slippery. At the time of ovulation, some women can detect a slight change in the texture of the mucus and find that it is more likely to form an elastic thread when stretched between thumb and finger. After ovulation, these secretions become cloudy and sticky and decrease in quantity. Infertile, safe days are likely to occur during the relatively dry days just before and after menstruation. These additional clues have been found to be helpful by some couples who rely on the fertility awareness method. One problem that may interfere with this method is that vaginal infections or vaginal products or medication can also alter the cervical mucus.

FAM is not recommended for women who have very irregular cycles—about 15% of all menstruating women. Any woman for whom pregnancy would be a serious problem should not rely on FAM alone, because the failure rate is high—approximately 25% during the first year of use. FAM offers no protection against STDs.

Although sometimes grouped with the so-called natural methods, *withdrawal,* in which the male removes his penis from the vagina just before he ejaculates, is considered a nonmethod by many. It has a high failure rate because the male has to overcome a powerful biological urge; he may also have difficulty judging when to withdraw. In addition, because preejaculatory fluid may contain viable sperm, pregnancy can occur even if the man

TABLE 6-3	*Contraceptive Methods and STD Protection*
Method	**Level of Protection**
Hormonal methods	Do not protect against STDs in lower reproductive tract or HIV; increase risk of cervical chlamydia; provide some protection against PID.
IUD	Does not protect against STDs; associated with PID in first month after insertion.
Latex male condom	Best method for protection against STDs (if used correctly); does not protect against infections from lesions that are not covered by the condom. (Polyurethane condoms should provide protection, but definitive findings are not yet available; lambskin condoms do not protect against STDs.)
Female condom	Theoretically should reduce the risk of STDs, but research results are not yet available.
Diaphragm or cervical cap	Protects against cervical infections and PID. Research results regarding HIV protection are contradictory, but diaphragms and cervical caps are not as effective as male condoms.
Spermicide	Modestly reduces the risk of cervical gonorrhea, chlamydia, and PID; effectiveness against other STDs is uncertain. If vaginal irritation occurs, infection risk may increase.
Abstinence	Complete protection against STDs (as long as all activities that involve the exchange of body fluids are avoided).
FAM	Does not protect against STDs.
Sterilization	Does not protect against STDs.

Abstinence or sex with a mutually monogamous uninfected partner is the surest way to protect yourself against HIV and other STDs. Barring this, correct and consistent use of latex male condoms provides the best protection against STDs.

withdraws prior to ejaculation. Sexual pleasure is often affected because the man must remain in control and the sexual experience of both partners is interrupted.

Combining Methods

Couples can choose to combine the preceding methods in a variety of ways, both to add STD protection and/or to increase contraceptive effectiveness. For example, condoms are strongly recommended along with OCs whenever there is a risk of STDs (Table 6-3). Foam may be added to condom use to increase protection against both STDs and pregnancy. For many couples, and especially for women, the added benefits will far outweigh the extra effort and expense.

Figure 6-7 on p. 150 summarizes the effectiveness of ten reversible contraceptive methods.

PERMANENT CONTRACEPTION: STERILIZATION

Sterilization is permanent, and it provides complete protection. For these reasons, it is becoming an increasingly popular method of contraception. At present it is the most commonly used method in the United States and in the world (see the box "Contraceptive Use Around the World," p. 151). It is especially popular among couples who have been married 10 or more years, as well as cou-

ples who have had all the children they intend. Sterilization provides no protection against STDs.

An important consideration in choosing sterilization is that, in most cases, it cannot be reversed and should be considered permanent. Although the chances of restoring fertility are being increased by modern surgical techniques, such operations are costly, and pregnancy can never be guaranteed. Some couples choosing male sterilization store sperm as a way of extending the option of childbearing.

Some studies indicate that male sterilization is preferable to female sterilization in a variety of ways. The overall cost of a female procedure is about four times that of a male procedure, and women are much more likely than men to experience both minor and major complications following the operation. Furthermore, feelings of regret seem to be somewhat more prevalent in women than in men after sterilization.

Although some physicians will perform surgery for sterilization on request, most require a thorough discussion with both partners before the operation. Most

fertility awareness method (FAM) A method of preventing conception based on avoiding intercourse during the fertile phase of a woman's cycle.   **TERMS**

sterilization Surgically altering the reproductive system to prevent pregnancy. Vasectomy is the procedure in males; tubal sterilization or hysterectomy is the procedure in females.

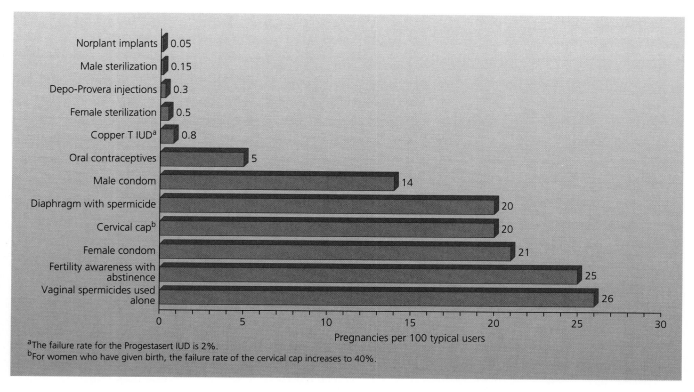

Figures within chart:
Norplant implants — 0.05
Male sterilization — 0.15
Depo-Provera injections — 0.3
Female sterilization — 0.5
Copper T IUD[a] — 0.8
Oral contraceptives — 5
Male condom — 14
Diaphragm with spermicide — 20
Cervical cap[b] — 20
Female condom — 21
Fertility awareness with abstinence — 25
Vaginal spermicides used alone — 26

Pregnancies per 100 typical users

[a]The failure rate for the Progestasert IUD is 2%.
[b]For women who have given birth, the failure rate of the cervical cap increases to 40%.

Figure 6-7   Failure rates of contraceptive methods during the first year of use.
SOURCE: Hatcher, R. A., et al. 1998. *Contraceptive Technology.* 17th rev. ed. New York: Ardent Media.

physicians also recommend that people who have religious conflicts, psychological problems related to sex, or unstable marriages not be sterilized. Young couples who might later change their minds are also frequently advised not to undergo sterilization.

Male Sterilization: Vasectomy

The procedure for male sterilization, **vasectomy**, involves severing the **vasa deferentia**, two tiny ducts that transport sperm from the testes to the seminal vesicles (see Figure 5-2). The testes continue to produce sperm, but the sperm are absorbed into the body. Because the testes contribute only about 10% of the total seminal fluid, the actual quantity of ejaculate is only slightly reduced. Hormone production from the testes continues with very little change, and secondary sex characteristics are not altered.

Vasectomy is ordinarily performed in a physician's office and takes about 30 minutes. A local anesthetic is injected into the skin of the scrotum near the vasa. Small incisions are made at the upper end of the scrotum where it joins the body, and the vas deferens on each side is exposed, severed,

and tied off or sealed by electrocautery. The incisions are then closed with sutures, and a small dressing is applied (Figure 6-8, p. 152). Pain and swelling are usually slight and can be relieved with ice compresses, aspirin, and the use of a scrotal support. Bleeding and infection occasionally develop but are usually easily treated. Fewer complications occur with an alternative procedure involving a midline puncture rather than incisions; this "no-scalpel" technique is used in about 30% of vasectomies performed in the United States. After either procedure, most men are ready to return to work in 2 days.

Men can have sex again as soon as they feel no further discomfort, usually after about a week. Another method of contraception must be used for a few weeks after vasectomy, however, because sperm produced before the operation may still be present in the semen. Microscopic examination of a semen sample can confirm that sperm are no longer present in the ejaculate.

No strong links have been found between vasectomy and chronic diseases like heart disease and prostate cancer. However, research into the long-term health effects of vasectomy is ongoing.

Vasectomy is highly effective. In a small number of cases, a severed vas rejoins itself, so some physicians advise yearly examination of a semen sample. The overall failure rate for vasectomy is 0.15%.

Although some surgeons report pregnancy rates of about 80% for partners of men who have their

TERMS   **vasectomy**   The surgical severing of the ducts that carry sperm to the ejaculatory duct.

vasa deferentia   The two ducts that carry sperm to the ejaculatory duct; singular, vas deferens.

Worldwide, nearly 60% of women and men now use modern contraceptive methods. However, approximately 350 million couples lack information about and access to contraceptives, and 75 million of the 200 million pregnancies that occur each year are unplanned. Sterilization is the most commonly used method, followed by IUDs, oral contraceptives, and condoms. However, striking differences exist between less developed and more developed regions and even between countries of similar levels of development. For example, among developing countries, contraceptive use ranges from 3% in Côte d'Ivoire and Mauritania to 83% in China. Differences in contraceptive use reflect a variety of factors, including the following:

- *Access to services.* How far people have to travel and how long they have to wait to obtain contraceptives are key factors. Geographic barriers can be significant, particularly in developing countries or isolated rural areas.

- *Availability of methods.* Not all methods are available in every country. In the United States, for example, access to IUDs is limited and their popularity is low: Fewer than 1% of American women use IUDs, compared with 26% of women in Sweden and 19% in Germany. In Japan, OCs have been available only in high dosages and only for a few women; this may be one reason condom use is high there (46%). At family planning clinics in developing countries, shortages of condoms, OCs, and IUDs occur frequently. And in many countries, male sterilization is less available than female sterilization, even though male sterilization is medically simpler.

- *Cost.* Studies have found that people are willing to pay moderate amounts for contraceptive supplies; but for many, the price threshold is fairly low. Methods that require replenishing of supplies, such as diaphragms, are less likely to be used in developing countries.

- *Political, cultural, and religious factors.* Government policies can have a strong impact on contraceptive use. China has one of the highest rates of contraceptive use in the world, primarily due to government policies penalizing families with more than one child. Gender roles, power imbalances between women and men, and culturally defined sexual norms are other important factors. A woman seeking contraceptives may encounter opposition from her partner or other family members; in over 70 countries, spousal authorization is required for a woman to have access to some or all contraceptive methods. A large family may be valued as a symbol of virility or fertility or as a source of labor. In some countries, religious traditions and doctrines prohibit contraceptive use. Roman Catholics have opposed national family planning efforts in Mexico, Kenya, and the Philippines. Muslim fundamentalists have done the same in Iran, Egypt, and Pakistan.

Worldwide, the lack of contraceptive use is associated with rapid population growth, poverty, and high mortality rates from unsafe conditions of childbirth, risky illegal abortions, and STDs. This is why family planning is sure to be one of the most pressing—and complex—issues that nations will face in the twenty-first century.

SOURCES: World Health Organization. 1998. *Prevent Unwanted Pregnancy* (retrieved September 18, 1998; http://www.who.org/whday/en/pages1998/whd98_09.html). Piccinino, L. J., and W. D. Mosher. 1998. Trends in contraceptive use in the United States: 1982–1995. *Family Planning Perspectives* (30)1: 4–10. United Nations Population Division. 1997. *The State of World Population 1997. The Right to Choose: Reproductive Rights and Reproductive Health.* New York: United Nations. United Nations Population Division. 1996. Overview of contraceptive use worldwide. *Population Newsletter,* June.

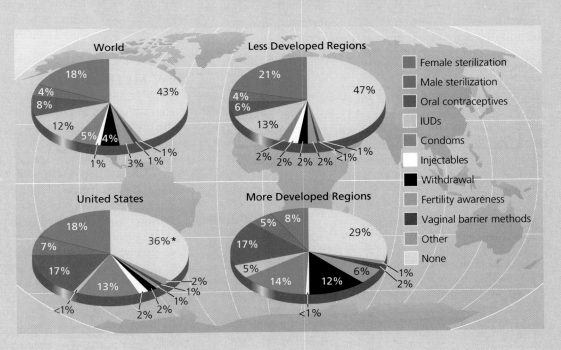

Percentage of couples of reproductive age using each method.

*Of the 36% of American women of reproductive age who are not using a contraceptive method, about 5% are sterile for noncontraceptive reasons, 9% are pregnant or trying to become pregnant, and 17% have never been or are not currently sexually active. The remaining 5% are sexually active but not using any contraceptive; they have nearly half the unintended pregnancies that occur each year in the United States.

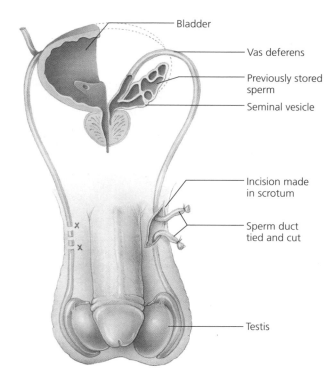

Bladder

Vas deferens

Previously stored sperm

Seminal vesicle

Incision made in scrotum

Sperm duct tied and cut

Testis

Figure 6-8 Vasectomy. This surgical procedure involves severing the vasa deferentia, thereby preventing sperm from being transported and ejaculated.

vasectomies reversed within 10 years of the original procedure, most studies report figures in the 50% range. In at least half of all men who have had vasectomies, the process of absorbing sperm (instead of ejaculating it) results in antisperm antibodies that may interfere with later fertility. Other factors, such as length of time between the vasectomy and the reversal surgery, may also be important predictors of reversal success.

Female Sterilization

The most common method of female sterilization involves severing, or in some manner blocking, the oviducts, thereby preventing the egg from reaching the uterus and the sperm from entering the fallopian tubes (see Figure 5-1). Ovulation and menstruation continue, but the unfertilized eggs are released into the abdominal cavity and absorbed. Although progesterone levels in the blood may

TERMS **tubal sterilization** Severing or in some manner blocking the oviducts, preventing eggs from reaching the uterus.

laparoscopy Examining the internal organs by inserting a tube containing a small light through an abdominal incision.

hysterectomy Total or partial surgical removal of the uterus.

contraceptive sponge A polyurethane device about 2 inches in diameter that fits over the cervix and acts as a barrier, spermicide, and seminal fluid absorbent.

decline slightly, hormone production by the ovaries and secondary sex characteristics are generally not affected.

Tubal sterilization is most commonly performed by a method called **laparoscopy.** A laparoscope, a tube containing a small light, is inserted through a small abdominal incision, and the surgeon looks through it to locate the fallopian tubes. Instruments are passed either through the laparoscope or through a second small incision, and the two fallopian tubes are sealed off with ties or staples or by electrocautery (Figure 6-9). Either a local or a general anesthetic can be used. The operation takes about 15 minutes, and women can usually leave the hospital 2–4 hours after surgery. Tubal sterilization can also be performed shortly after a vaginal delivery, or in the case of cesarean section immediately after the uterine incision is repaired.

Female sterilization is somewhat riskier than male sterilization, with a complication rate of about 0.1–7%. Potential problems include bowel injury, wound infection, and bleeding. Serious complications are rare, and the death rate is low.

The failure rate for tubal sterilization is about 0.5%. When pregnancies do occur, an increased percentage of them are ectopic. Some complaints of long-term abdominal discomfort and menstrual irregularity following tubal sterilization have been reported. Reversibility rates of current methods are about 50–70%. A new method currently being considered for use involves a clip that can be clamped around the fallopian tube; this method may provide a better chance of later reversal.

Hysterectomy, removal of the uterus, is the preferred method of sterilization for only a small number of women, usually those with preexisting menstrual problems. Because of the risks involved, hysterectomy is not recommended unless the woman has serious gynecologic problems, such as disease or damage of the uterus, and future surgery appears inevitable.

NEW METHODS OF CONTRACEPTION

Even with all the improvements of recent years, the best of the present methods of contraception have drawbacks. The search still continues for the ideal method—more effective, safer, cheaper, easier to use, more readily available, easily reversible, and acceptable to more people.

Many people place a high priority specifically on an increase in contraceptive alternatives for men. Throughout history, the responsibility for contraception has been assumed predominantly by women, partly because women have greater personal investment in preventing pregnancy, with its many risks, and childbearing, with the many demands that fall mostly on women. Some women consider complete control to be crucial. More options have been available for women because there are more ways to intervene in the female reproductive system. Another factor may be the continuing underrepresenta-

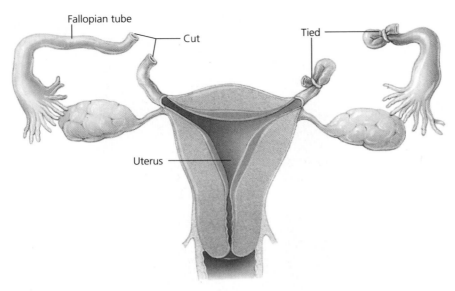

Figure 6-9   Tubal sterilization.   This procedure involves severing or blocking the fallopian tubes, thereby preventing eggs from traveling from the ovaries to the uterus. It is a more complex procedure than vasectomy.

tion of women in medicine, scientific research, pharmaceutical management, the FDA, and other political arenas. Participation by women, and an emphasis on their contraceptive needs, has been limited in these areas.

After years of diminishing contraceptive choice in the United States, several new methods have recently been approved and are now being marketed. Many new methods are widely used in other countries long before they become available in the United States. The U.S. delay is partly due to higher costs of preclinical safety testing, greater liability risk for manufacturers, and lower levels of government funding for contraceptive research.

The contraceptive options most likely to become available soon in the United States are variations of methods already in use: new combinations of hormones in OCs, implants, and injectables; new designs in IUDs, cervical caps, and condoms; and spermicides and microbicides that are more effective in destroying viruses and bacteria as well as sperm. In March 1999, plans to bring back the **contraceptive sponge** were announced. (Although it was previously available, manufacturing problems had led to its discontinuation in 1995.) The sponge is a round, absorbent polyurethane device about 2 inches in diameter with a loop on one side for removal and a dimple on the other side that helps it fit snugly over the cervix. It acts as a barrier to sperm and is also saturated with spermicide. The sponge is for one-time use and is available without a prescription; its effectiveness is similar to that of the cervical cap. Other methods being studied include the following:

* *Biodegradable implants.* As with Norplant capsules, these implants filled with progestin are inserted under

the skin. They provide long-term, effective contraception. Unlike Norplant, the capsules dissolve over time, eliminating the need for surgical removal.

* *Vaginal ring.* The vaginal ring resembles the rim of a diaphragm and is molded with a mixture of progestin and estrogen. The woman inserts the ring herself and wears it for 3 weeks, during which time the hormones are absorbed into her bloodstream, preventing ovulation. Menstruation follows removal, and then a new ring is inserted. Other vaginal rings in development include a contraceptive ring that can be worn for up to 6 months and a ring that can be used for hormone replacement therapy.

* *Chemical contraceptives for men.* Male and female hormones can interfere with sperm development in the male, similar to ovulation suppression in the female. One such hormone under study, testosterone enanthate, has proven quite effective in preventing pregnancy, and it is also readily reversible. However, side effects and the required weekly injections remain a major obstacle. Researchers hope to eventually develop a pill or implant for hormone delivery for men.

* *Injectable microspheres.* A solution containing tiny clusters of molecules, each cluster filled with hormones, is injected into the body. Over a period of 1–6 months, these particles release a fairly constant dose of hormones. This method is being studied for use by both men and women.

* *Contraceptive immunization.* Immunity to fertility has occasionally (though rarely) occurred as a result of a man being nonexperimentally sensitized to his own sperm

cells. He then produces antibodies that inactivate sperm as if they were a disease. In theory, a woman could be purposely sensitized against her own egg cells or against her partner's sperm cells. Another immunocontraceptive under study targets just the zona pellucida (ZP), the protein covering of the egg cell. Immunization against ZP would temporarily block sperm from penetrating the egg without affecting normal egg development.

• *Reversible sterilization.* Present methods of sterilization in both men and women are reversible 50–70% of the time. Several new techniques are being studied in the hope that restoring fertility can be made easier and more predictable. These techniques include injecting liquid silicone into the fallopian tubes, where it solidifies and forms a plug, and placing various types of clips and plugs on the vasa to totally block sperm flow.

• *Prostaglandins.* In pill form and via tampon, **prostaglandins** have been studied extensively as a menses inducer. The pill or the tampon is used regularly at the end of each cycle to induce menstruation, whether or not that cycle had been fertile. Studies show that prostaglandins used in this way are fairly effective in pregnancy prevention, but also cause nausea and diarrhea.

• *Luteinizing hormone-releasing hormone (LHRH).* A naturally occurring compound in both men and women, LHRH acts on the pituitary gland, triggering the release of its hormones, which in turn play an essential role in sperm formation and ovulation. Synthetic versions of LHRH, which are over 100 times as powerful as natural LHRH, are currently available. After they are administered, pituitary hormone levels rise sharply, followed by a drop to subnormal levels, probably because the pituitary gland is overstimulated and exhausted. Once the low levels are established, it appears that in women (on whom most of the studies thus far have been completed) the pituitary-ovary cycle is effectively disrupted, and ovulation and menstruation stop temporarily.

ISSUES IN CONTRACEPTION

The subject of contraception is closely tied to several issues that are currently receiving much attention in the United States—issues like premarital sexual relations, gender differences, and sex education for teenagers.

When Is It OK to Begin Having Sexual Relations?

One issue that strongly affects a society's approach to contraception is the question of at what age it's acceptable to begin having sex. Opinions on this issue often determine

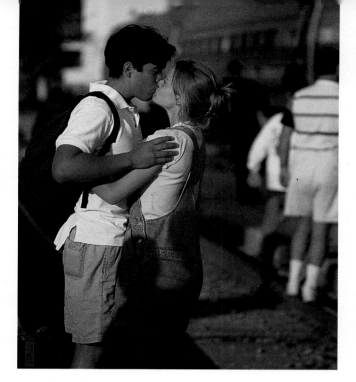

How old should people be when they become sexually active? The answer depends on the personal values, beliefs, and experiences of the individuals involved.

one's views on sex education and contraception accessibility. Americans have a wide range of opinions: only after marriage; when 18 years or older; when in a loving, stable relationship; when the partners have completed their education and/or could support a child; whenever both partners feel ready and are using protection against pregnancy and STDs.

Opinions about appropriate sexual behavior shift from one decade to another. Although attitudes became more liberal during the 1960s and 1970s, people started having more restrictive views in the 1980s and 1990s. Today, the most common reasons for disapproving of sex are the risk of exposure to STDs, the risk of pregnancy, and moral or religious beliefs. According to recent data, most of today's young Americans are somewhat permissive regarding premarital sex. While many approve of sexual relations for couples who are seriously dating or engaged to be married, they are less accepting of sexual intercourse on a first date or at the casual dating stage.

Closely related to the issue of beginning sexual relations is a more personal question: What would you consider the ideal amount of previous sexual experience for you and your partner? Again, opinions vary, especially in terms of what is desirable for men and for women. While limited experience is still more commonly deemed desirable for women, being "sexually experienced" is often valued more highly for men.

As more women consider careers for themselves and therefore often delay childbearing and even marriage, the

TERMS **prostaglandins** Naturally occurring chemicals that stimulate uterine muscle contractions, resulting in cramping.

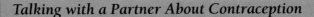
Many people have a difficult time talking about contraception with a potential sex partner. How should you bring it up? And whose responsibility is it, anyway? Talking about the subject may be embarrassing at first, but imagine the possible consequences of *not* talking about it. An unintended pregnancy or a sexually transmitted disease could profoundly affect you for the rest of your life. Talking about contraception is one way of showing that you care about yourself, your partner, and your future.

Before you talk with your partner, explore your own thoughts and feelings. Find out the facts about different methods of contraception, and decide which one you think would be most appropriate for you. If you're nervous about having this discussion with your partner, it may help to practice with a friend.

Pick a good time to bring up the subject. Don't wait until you've started to have sex. A time when you're both feeling comfortable and relaxed will maximize your chances of having

a good discussion. Tell your partner what you know about contraception, how you feel about using it, and talk about what steps you both need to take to get and use a method you can live with. Listen to what your partner has to say, and try to understand his or her point of view. You may need to have more than one discussion, and it may take some time for both of you to feel comfortable with the subject. *But don't have sex until this issue is resolved.*

If you want your partner to be involved but he or she isn't interested in talking about contraception, or if he or she leaves all the responsibility for it up to you, consider whether this is really a person you want to be sexually involved with. If you decide to go ahead with the involvement, you may want to enlist the support of a friend, family member, or health care worker to help you make and implement decisions about the essential issue of contraception.

---

likelihood of sexual activity and the critical need for pregnancy and STD prevention only increase. As a result, making decisions about sexual activity and contraception becomes even more important to those starting college or a career. Unfortunately, however, many individuals in this age group—even those who protect their health in all other areas of their life—end up taking high risks in their sexual behavior. Ambivalence and a lack of communication about who will "take charge" are common and are partly due to the denial of, and hypocrisy about, sexual behavior that exist in our society. (For guidelines on improving your own communication, see the box "Talking with a Partner About Contraception.")

Contraception and Gender Differences

A second issue, one all couples must confront, is the differing significance of contraception to women and men. The consequences of not using contraception are markedly different for men and women. In past years, women have accepted the primary responsibility of contraception, along with related side effects and health risks, partly because of the wider spectrum of methods available to them. Men still have very few contraceptive options, with condoms being the only reversible method. Recently, however, their participation has become critical, since condom use is central to safer sex, even when OCs or other female methods are being used.

Although dependent primarily on the cooperation of the man, condom use and the prevention of STDs has potentially greater consequences for the woman. While men may suffer only local and short-term effects from the most common diseases (not including HIV infection), women face an increased risk of serious long-term effects,

such as cervical cancer and/or pelvic infection with associated infertility, from these same prevalent STDs. In addition, women are more likely to contract HIV from an infected partner than men are. In other words, although dependent on the male, condom use is clearly a more important issue for women. The female condom may offer a helpful alternative, but cooperation of the male partner is still needed to ensure correct use.

The experience of an unintended pregnancy is very different for the two involved partners. While men do suffer emotional stress from such an unexpected occurrence (and sometimes share financial and/or custodial responsibilities), women are much more intimately affected, obviously by the biological process of pregnancy itself, as well as the outcome: abortion, adoption, or parenting. In addition, our societal attitudes are more severely punitive toward the woman and place much greater responsibility and blame on her when an unintended pregnancy occurs; the focus is almost entirely on the "girl who got into trouble" or the "unwed mother," with no mention of the "unwed father." With the current trend of cutting welfare support for single mothers, this increasing number of young women and their children will live with even greater disadvantages.

Fortunately, there is growing interest in the roles and responsibilities of men in family planning. For example, an American Public Health Association (APHA) Task Force on Men in Family Planning and Reproductive Health recently completed a review of available resources in this area. The APHA group concluded that there is a serious lack of both educational materials and clinical programs that focus on male contraception and reproductive health. Men can increase their participation in contraception by initiating and supporting communication regarding contraception and STD protection, buying and using condoms whenever appropriate, helping pay contraceptive costs, and being available for shared responsibility in the resolution of an unintended pregnancy, should one occur.

Sex and Contraceptive Education for Teenagers

A third controversial issue is sex education and pregnancy prevention programs for teenagers. Again, opinion in the United States is sharply divided. Certain religious groups are concerned that more sex education, and especially the availability of contraceptives, will lead to more sexual activity and promiscuity. They maintain that greater access to improved contraception was a key factor contributing to the sexual revolution in the 1960s, and that the ensuing liberal sexual attitudes have been generally more destructive than helpful. They point to an increase in divorces, a dramatic rise in STDs, and a general relaxing of standards of morality as related negative effects.

Many in this group urge that sex education be handled in the home, where parents can instill moral values, including premarital abstinence. According to some in this group, young people should primarily be taught to "just say no." They see most public education about contraception, and especially facilities that make supplies available, as only increasing the problem.

Other groups argue that encouraging the public availability of contraceptive information and supplies does not necessarily result in an increase in promiscuous sexual behavior, pointing to the fact that many young teenagers are already pregnant when they first visit a health care facility. These groups assert that parents are not effectively dealing with the issues, and that a broader, coordinated approach involving public institutions, including schools, is needed, along with parental input. Many current programs focus on postponing sexual involvement, but also emphasize contraceptive use for individuals who are sexually active. An increased availability of contraceptive information and methods is considered a necessary and realistic part of this approach.

Proponents of sex and contraceptive education for teenagers point to countries, such as the Netherlands, that have a far lower incidence of teenage pregnancy than the United States (1.8% and 12.8%, respectively). While Dutch teenagers are just as likely as American teens to engage in sexual intercourse, they are far more likely to use contraception. In the Netherlands, sex and contraceptive education are extensive and quite explicit in radio and television programming, and national health insurance and state-financed clinics provide and fund contraception.

A 1998 study by the Centers for Disease Control and Prevention revealed an encouraging new trend toward safer sexual practices among American high school students. For the first time in the 1990s, more than half of the students surveyed said that they were abstaining from sex. And among those who were sexually active, the rate of condom use was the highest on record for the 1990s: More than 55% of the students reported using a condom the last time they had sex.

While sex and contraceptive education in public facilities remains a volatile issue, there is overall growing support for such programs. Studies show that sexually active students who receive sex education are more likely to use contraceptives, and that those who are not sexually active are not encouraged to initiate having sex. However, these programs are receiving increasing support mainly because of the prevalent fear of HIV infection and other STDs. In fact, in some cases the focus of "sex ed" is almost exclusively on disease prevention. Although not as deadly as the AIDS epidemic, the more than 1 million teenage pregnancies that occur each year in the United States is a serious public health problem and warrants much greater national attention than it has received thus far.

> **PERSONAL INSIGHT**   Did your parents tell you anything about contraception? Are your ideas and needs different from their expectations for you? What will you tell your children about contraception?

WHICH CONTRACEPTIVE METHOD IS RIGHT FOR YOU?

The process of choosing and using a contraceptive method can be complex and varies greatly from one couple to another. Each person must consider many variables in deciding which method is most acceptable and appropriate for her or him. Important considerations include those listed here:

1. *Health risks.* Is there anything in your personal or family medical history that would affect your choice of method? For each method you consider, what are the potential health risks that apply to you? For example, IUDs are not recommended for young women without children because of an increased risk of pelvic infection and subsequent infertility. Hormonal methods should be used only after a clinical evaluation of your medical history. Other methods have only minor and local side effects. If necessary, talk with your physician about the potential health effects of different methods for you.

2. *The implications of an unplanned pregnancy.* How would an unplanned pregnancy affect you and your future? What are your feelings regarding the options—abortion, adoption, or raising a child? If effectiveness is of critical importance to you, carefully consider the ways the effectiveness of each method can be improved. Abstinence is 100% effective, if maintained. If used correctly, hormonal methods offer very good protection against

TABLE 6-4	*Contraceptive Costs*	
Method	**Approximate Unit Cost**	**Approximate Annual Cost**
Oral contraceptives	$21/cycle for pills, $38 annual office visit	$290
Norplant implants	$365 for implants, $333 for insertion	$140 if retained for 5 years
Depo-Provera injectables	$30 for drug, $38 for office visit	$272
Progestasert IUD	$82 for device, $207 for insertion	$289
Copper-T IUD	$184 for device, $207 for insertion	$39 if retained for 10 years
Diaphragm	$18 for device, $38 for fitting, $1 for each application of spermicide	$102 if used for 3 years
Cervical cap	$31 for device, $38 for fitting, $1 for each application of spermicide	$106 if used for 3 years
Male condom	$1 for condom	$83 ($166 if spermicide is used)
Female condom	$3.66 for condom	$303 ($386 if spermicide is used)

Based on costs in a managed-care setting; costs will vary, as will insurance coverage. For comparison, tubal ligation is about $2500; vasectomy, about $750; and pregnancy, about $3800. Withdrawal and fertility awareness are free.

SOURCE: Adapted from Hatcher, R. A., et al. 1998. *Contraceptive Technology*, 17th rev. ed. New York: Ardent Media.

pregnancy. Barrier methods can be combined with spermicides to improve their effectiveness.

3. *STD risk.* How likely are you to be exposed to any sexually transmitted diseases? Have you and your partner been screened for STDs recently? Have you openly and honestly discussed your past sexual behavior? Condom use is of critical importance whenever any risk of STDs is present. This is especially true when you are not in an exclusive, long-term relationship or when you are taking the pill, because cervical changes that occur during hormone use may increase vulnerability to certain diseases. Abstinence or activities that don't involve intercourse or any other exchange of body fluids can be a satisfactory alternative for some people.

4. *Convenience and comfort level.* How do your partner and you view each of the methods? Which would you most likely use consistently? The hormonal methods are generally ranked high in this category, unless there are negative side effects and health risks, or if forgetting to take pills is a problem for you. Some people think condom use disrupts spontaneity and lowers penile sensitivity. (Creative approaches to condom use and improved quality can decrease these concerns.) The diaphragm, cervical cap, contraceptive sponge, female condom, and spermicides can be inserted before intercourse begins, but are still considered a significant inconvenience by some.

5. *Type of relationship.* How easy is it for you to talk with your partner about contraception? How willing is he or she to be involved? Barrier methods require more motivation and a sense of responsibility from *each* partner than hormonal methods do. When the method depends on the cooperation of one's partner, assertiveness is necessary, no matter how difficult. This is especially true in new relationships, when condom use is most important. When sexual activity is infrequent, a barrier method may make more sense than an IUD or one of the hormonal methods.

6. *Ease and cost of obtaining and maintaining each method.* If a physical exam and clinic follow-up is required, how readily accessible is this to you? Can you and your partner afford the associated expenses of the method? Investigate the costs of different methods (Table 6-4). Find out if your insurance covers any of the costs.

7. *Religious or philosophical beliefs.* Are any of the methods unacceptable to you because of your personal beliefs? For some, abstinence and/or FAM may be the only permissible contraceptive methods.

Whatever your needs, circumstances, or beliefs, *do* make a choice about contraception. Not choosing anything is the one method known *not* to work. (To help make a choice that's right for you, take the quiz in the box "Which Contraceptive Method Is Right for You and Your Partner?") This is an area in which taking charge of your health has immediate and profound implications for your future. The method you choose today won't necessarily be the one you'll want to use your whole life or even next year. But it should be one that works for you right now. Contraception is something you can't afford to leave to chance.

If you are sexually active, you need to use the contraceptive method that will work best for you. A number of factors may be involved in your decision. The following questions will help you sort out these factors and choose an appropriate method. Answer yes (Y) or no (N) for each statement as it applies to you and, if appropriate, your partner.

_____ 1. I like sexual spontaneity and don't want to be bothered with contraception at the time of sexual intercourse.
_____ 2. I need a contraceptive immediately.
_____ 3. It is very important that I do not become pregnant now.
_____ 4. I want a contraceptive method that will protect me and my partner against sexually transmitted diseases.
_____ 5. I prefer a contraceptive method that requires the cooperation and involvement of both partners.
_____ 6. I have sexual intercourse frequently.
_____ 7. I have sexual intercourse infrequently.
_____ 8. I am forgetful or have a variable daily routine.
_____ 9. I have more than one sex partner.
_____ 10. I have heavy periods with cramps.
_____ 11. I prefer a method that requires little or no action or bother on my part.
_____ 12. I am a nursing mother.
_____ 13. I want the option of conceiving immediately after discontinuing contraception.
_____ 14. I want a contraceptive method with few or no side effects.

If you answered "yes" to the statements whose numbers are listed in the left columns below, the method in the right columns might be a good choice for you.

1, 3, 6, 10, 11	Oral contraceptives	5, 7, 12, 13, 14	Diaphragm and spermicide
1, 3, 6, 8, 10, 11	Norplant implants	5, 7, 12, 13, 14	Cervical cap
1, 3, 6, 8, 10, 11, 12	Depo-Provera injectables	2, 5, 7, 8, 12, 13, 14	Vaginal spermicides
1, 3, 6, 8, 11, 12, 13	IUD	5, 7, 13, 14	FAM
2, 4, 5, 7, 8, 9, 12, 13, 14	Condoms (male and female)		

Your answers may indicate that more than one method would be appropriate for you. To help narrow your choices, circle the numbers of the statements that are *most* important for you. Before you make a final choice, talk with your partner(s) and your physician. Consider your own lifestyle and preferences, as well as the features of each method (effectiveness, side effects, costs, and so on). For maximum protection against pregnancy and STDs, you might want to consider combining two methods. It's also a good idea to be prepared for change; the method that seems right for you now may be inappropriate if your circumstances become different.

SUMMARY

Principles of Contraception

- Barrier methods of contraception physically prevent sperm from reaching the egg; hormonal methods are designed to prevent ovulation, fertilization, and/or implantation; and surgical methods permanently block the movement of sperm or eggs to the site of conception.

- The choice of contraceptive method depends on effectiveness, convenience, cost, reversibility, side effects and risk factors, and protection against STDs. The concept of effectiveness includes failure rate and continuation rate.

Reversible Contraceptives

- In oral contraceptives (OCs), a combination of estrogen and progestins prevents ovulation, inhibits the movement of sperm, and affects the uterine lining so that implantation is prevented.

- Norplant implants consist of six hormone-filled capsules inserted under the skin that release steady doses of synthetic progesterone, providing effective, reversible protection for up to 5 years.

- Depo-Provera injections contain a long-acting progestin that protects against pregnancy for a period of 3 months.

- The most commonly used emergency contraceptive is a two-dose regimen of OCs.

- How IUDs work is not clearly understood; they may cause biochemical changes in the uterus, affect movement of sperm and eggs, or interfere with the implantation of the egg in the uterus.
- Using condoms has increased dramatically, partly because of their effectiveness against STDs. Advantages include availability and ease of purchase, simplicity of use, immediate reversibility, and freedom from side effects.
- Female condoms consist of a polyurethane or latex sheath that can be inserted well before intercourse. They may be less reliable than male condoms in preventing pregnancy and the transmission of STDs.
- When used correctly, with spermicidal cream or jelly, a diaphragm or cervical cap covers the cervix and blocks sperm from entering.
- Vaginal spermicides come in the form of foams, creams, jellies, suppositories, and film.
- Because of religion, culture, poverty, or lack of information, many people use no contraception at all or use "natural" methods. Abstinence may be chosen out of fear of STDs or because of personal needs.
- The fertility awareness method (FAM) is based on avoiding coitus during the fertile phase of a woman's menstrual cycle. The calendar method, basal body temperature method, or mucus method may be used to determine the fertile period.
- Combining methods can increase contraceptive effectiveness and help protect against STDs.

Permanent Contraception: Sterilization

- Sterilization is considered permanent; reversibility can never be guaranteed. Male sterilization may be preferable to female sterilization because it is less expensive, has fewer complications, and causes fewer feelings of regret.

- Vasectomy—male sterilization—involves severing the vasa deferentia. Female sterilization involves severing or blocking the oviducts so that the egg cannot reach the uterus.

New Methods of Contraception

- Contraceptive techniques currently under investigation include biodegradable implants, the vaginal ring, chemical contraceptives for men, injectable microspheres, contraceptive immunization, reversible sterilization, prostaglandins, and luteinizing hormone-releasing hormone.

Issues in Contraception

- Opinions on when to begin having sexual relations are tied to views on sex education and contraception accessibility. Because women today frequently delay childbearing, decisions about sexual activity and contraception are essential for optimal health.
- Although using condoms depends on male cooperation, the implications of not using them are greater for women, in terms of both pregnancy and the consequences of STDs.
- Opinion in the United States is divided on the issues of sex education and availability of contraceptives for teenagers.

Which Contraceptive Method Is Right for You?

- Issues to be considered in choosing a contraceptive include the individual health risks of each method, the implications of an unplanned pregnancy, STD risk, convenience and comfort level, type of relationship, the cost and ease of obtaining and maintaining each method, and religious or philosophical beliefs.

TAKE ACTION

1.   Make an appointment with a physician or other health care provider to review the health risks of different contraceptive methods as they apply to you. For each method, determine whether any risk factors associated with its use apply to you or your partner.

2.   Visit a local drugstore and make a list of the contraceptives they sell, along with their prices. Next, investigate the costs of prescription contraceptive methods by contacting your physician, medical clinic, and/or pharmacy. Estimate the annual cost of regular use for each method, and rank the methods from most to least expensive.

3.   Devise a public service campaign that will encourage men to become more involved in contraception. Your campaign might use techniques such as TV and print advertisements, radio announcements, and posters. Look at other public service campaigns and advertisements for ideas. What sorts of images do you think would be motivational? What sort of tone and message do you think would be most effective?

1. Consider the different methods of contraception described in this chapter. In your health journal, rank the methods according to how they suit your particular lifestyle. Take into account such considerations as convenience, cost, and how often you have sexual intercourse.

2. In your health journal, list the positive behaviors and attitudes that help you adhere to your beliefs about contraception. (For example, not getting drunk would probably help prevent you from making an unwise choice.) Are there ways you can strengthen these behaviors? Then list behaviors and attitudes that might interfere with your effective use of contraception. Can you do anything to change or improve any of these?

3. *Critical Thinking* What are your feelings about sex education for children and teenagers? Write a brief essay that presents the main arguments, both pro and con. Conclude with a description of the sex education you received and a statement of your own opinion on whether sex education is valuable. Are you satisfied with what you were taught? What effect did it have on your sexual behavior? In general, do you think sex education promotes responsibility or promiscuity? Or neither?

Books

Boston Women's Health Book Collective. 1998. *Our Bodies, Ourselves for the New Century.* New York: Simon & Schuster. *Broad coverage of many women's health concerns, with extensive coverage of contraception.*

Carlson, K. J., S. A. Eisenstat, and T. Ziporyn. 1996. *The Harvard Guide to Women's Health.* Cambridge, Mass.: Harvard University Press. *An inclusive guide to women's health; includes pros and cons of contraceptive options.*

Hatcher, R. A., et al. 1998. *Contraceptive Technology,* 17th rev. ed. New York: Ardent Media. *A compact, reliable source of up-to-date information on contraception.*

Hatcher, R. A., et al. 1997. *Safely Sexual.* New York: Irvington. *Realistic recommendations on the prevention of unplanned pregnancy, as well as HIV infection and other STDs.*

Knowles, J., and M. Ringel. 1998. *All About Birth Control: A Personal Guide.* New York: Three Rivers Press. *Provides detailed descriptions of each contraceptive method.*

Roberson, M., and J. Dubner, eds. 1999. *Getting It On: A Condom Reader.* New York: Soho Press. *An anthology of poetry, short fiction, and comic essays about condoms featuring characters with diverse viewpoints and sexual orientations; authors include Anne Rice, John Irving, and Martin Amis.*

Organizations, Hotlines, and Web Sites

The Alan Guttmacher Institute. A nonprofit institute for reproductive health research, policy analysis, and public education.
120 Wall Street
New York, NY 10005
212-248-1111
http://www.agi-usa.org

Ann Rose's Ultimate Birth Control Links Page. A Web site with information on methods of birth control and decision-making strategies.
http://gynpages.com/ultimate

Association of Reproductive Health Professionals. Offers educational materials about family planning, contraception, and other reproductive health issues; their Web site includes an interactive questionnaire to help people choose contraceptive methods.

2401 Pennsylvania Ave., N.W., Suite 350
Washington, DC 20037
202-466-3825
http://www.arhp.org

Emergency Contraception Hotline. Provides information and referrals.
888-NOT-2-LATE

Emergency Contraception Web site. Provides extensive information about emergency contraception; sponsored by the Office of Population Research at Princeton University.
http://opr.princeton.edu/ec

JAMA Contraception Information Center. Provides patient and professional resources, journal articles, and links.
http://www.ama-assn.org/special/contra/contra.htm

Planned Parenthood Federation of America. Provides information on family planning, contraception, and abortion, and provides counseling services.
810 Seventh Ave.
New York, NY 10019
800-669-0156 (to order publications)
800-230-PLAN (for a list of health centers)
http://www.plannedparenthood.org

Reproductive Health Online (Reproline). Presents information on contraceptive methods currently available and those under study for future use.
http://www.reproline.jhu.edu

The following are some of the many organizations focusing on family planning and reproductive health issues worldwide:

Family Health International
http://www.fhi.org

Global Reproductive Health Forum at Harvard
http://www.hsph.harvard.edu/Organizations/healthnet

International Planned Parenthood Federation
http://www.ippf.org

Safe Motherhood
http://www.safemotherhood.org

United Nations Population Fund
http://www.unfpa.org

See also the listings for Chapters 5, 7, 8, and 18.

Beral, V., et al. 1999. Mortality association with oral contraceptive use: 25 year follow up of cohort of 46,000 women from Royal College of General Practitioners' oral contraception study. *British Medical Journal* 318: 96–100.

Centers for Disease Control and Prevention. 1998. Trends in sexual risk behaviors among high school students—United States, 1991–1997. *Morbidity and Mortality Weekly Report* 47(36): 749–752.

Coukell, A. J., and J. A. Balfour. 1998. Levonorgestrel subdermal implants. A review of contraceptive efficacy and acceptability. *Drugs* 55(6): 861–887.

Critelli, J. W., and D. M. Suire. 1998. Obstacles to condom use: The combination of other forms of birth control and short-term monogamy. *Journal of American College Health* 46(5): 215–219.

Cushman, L. F., et al. 1998. Condom use among women choosing long-term hormonal contraception. *Family Planning Perspectives* 30(5): 240–243.

Davis, M. C. 1999. Oral contraceptive use and hemodynamic, lipid, and fibrinogen responses to smoking and stress in women. *Health Psychology* 18(2): 122–130.

Dull, P., and M. J. Blythe. 1998. Preventing teenage pregnancy. *Primary Care* 25(1): 111–122.

Family Health International. 1998. *The Development of Non-Latex Condoms* (retrieved October 30, 1998; http://www.fhi.org/fp/fpother/conom/conmon15.html).

Fleming, D. 1998. Continuation rates of long-acting methods of contraception: A comparative study of Norplant implants and intrauterine devices. *Journal of the American Medical Association* 279(23): 1851.

Fleming, H. 1998. 1998 may be a turning point in contraception coverage. *Drug Topics* 142(14): 61.

Forste, R., and J. Morgan. 1998. How relationships of U.S. men affect contraceptive use and efforts to prevent STDs. *Family Planning Perspectives* 30(2): 56–62.

Frezieres, R. G., et al. 1998. Breakage and acceptability of a polyurethane condom: A randomized, controlled study. *Family Planning Perspectives* 30(2): 73–78.

Gentile, G. P., et al. 1998. Is there any evidence for a post-tubal-sterilization syndrome? *Fertility and Sterility* 69(2): 179–186.

Glasier, A., and D. Baird. 1998. The effects of self-administering emergency contraception. *New England Journal of Medicine* 339(1): 1–4.

Haignere, C. S., R. Gold, and H. J. McDanel. 1999. Adolescent abstinence and condom use: Are we sure we are really teaching what is safe? *Health Education Behavior* 26(1): 43–54.

Haws, J. M., et al. 1998. Clinical aspects of vasectomies performed in the United States in 1995. *Urology* 52(4): 685–691.

Kirby, D., et al. 1999. The impact of condom distribution in Seattle schools on sexual behavior and condom use. *American Journal of Public Health* 89(2): 182–187.

Kubba, A. A. 1998. Contraception: A review. *International Journal of Clinical Practice* 52(2): 102–105.

Larkin, M. 1998. *Intrauterine Devices: Safe, Effective, and Underutilized* (retrieved October 29, 1998; http://www.ama-assn.org/special/contra/newsline/briefing/iud.htm).

Miller, K. S., et al. 1998. Patterns of condom use among adolescents: The impact of mother-adolescent communication. *American Journal of Public Health* 88(10): 1542–1544.

Nordenberg, T. 1998. Condoms: Barriers to bad news. *FDA Consumer,* March/April.

Piaggio, G., et al. 1999. Timing of emergency contraception with levonorgestrel or the Yuzpe regimen. *Lancet* 353(9154): 721.

Piccinino, L. J., and W. D. Mosher. 1998. Trends in contraceptive use in the United States: 1982–1995. *Family Planning Perspectives* 30(1): 4–10, 46.

Polaneczky, M. 1998. Adolescent contraception. *Current Opinions in Obstetrics and Gynecology* 10(3): 213–219.

Rosen, A. D., and T. Rosen. 1999. Study of condom integrity after brief exposure to over-the-counter vaginal preparations. *Southern Medical Journal* 92(3); 305–307.

Rosenberg, M., and M. S. Waugh. 1999. Causes and consequences of oral contraceptive noncompliance. *American Journal of Obstetrics and Gynecology* 180(2 Pt 2): 276–279.

Sawyer, R. G., et al. 1998. Pregnancy testing and counseling: A university health center's 5-year experience. *Journal of American College Health* 46(5): 221–225.

Sawyer, R. G., and P. J. Pinciaro. 1998. College students' knowledge and attitudes about Norplant and Depo-Provera. *American Journal of Health Behavior* 22(3):163–171.

Schein, A. B. 1999. Pregnancy prevention using emergency contraception: Efficacy, attitudes, and limitations to use. *Journal of Pediatric and Adolescent Gynecology* 12(1): 3–9.

Schwingl, P. J., H. W. Ory, and C. M. Visness. 1999. Estimates of the risk of cardiovascular death attributable to low-dose oral contraceptives in the United States. *American Journal of Obstetrics and Gynecology* 180(1 Pt 1): 241–249.

Sheeran, P., C. Abraham, and S. Orbell. 1999. Psychosocial correlates of heterosexual condom use: a meta-analysis. *Psychological Bulletin* 125(1): 90–132.

Skegg, D. C. G. 1999. Oral contraception and health: Long term study of mortality shows no overall effect in a developed country. *British Medical Journal* 318: 69–70.

Sly, D. F., et al. 1997. Factors associated with use of the female condom. *Family Planning Perspectives* 29(4): 181–184.

Spruyt, A., et al. 1998. Identifying condom users at risk for breakage and slippage: Findings from three international sites. *American Journal of Public Health* 88(2): 239–244.

Task Force on Postovulatory Methods. 1999. Comparison of three single doses of mifepristone as emergency contraception: A randomised trial. *Lancet* 353(9154): 697–702.

Trussell, J., G. Rodriguez, and C. Ellertson. 1998. New estimates of the effectiveness of the Yuzpe regimen of emergency contraception. *Contraception* 57(6): 363–369.

U.S. Food and Drug Administration. 1998. *Preven Emergency Contraceptive Kit Patient Information Book* (retrieved November 2, 1998; http://www.fda.gov/cder/foi/label/1998/20946lbl.pdf).

U.S. Food and Drug Administration. 1998. *Talk Paper: FDA Approves Application for Preven Emergency Contraceptive Kit* (retrieved September 2, 1998; http://www.fda.gov/bbs/topics/ANSWERS/ANS00892.html).

Women's Capital Corporation. 1999. *Women's Capital Corporation Submits NDA for New Emergency Contraceptive* (retrieved February 18, 1999; http://opr.princeton.edu/ec/wcc.html).

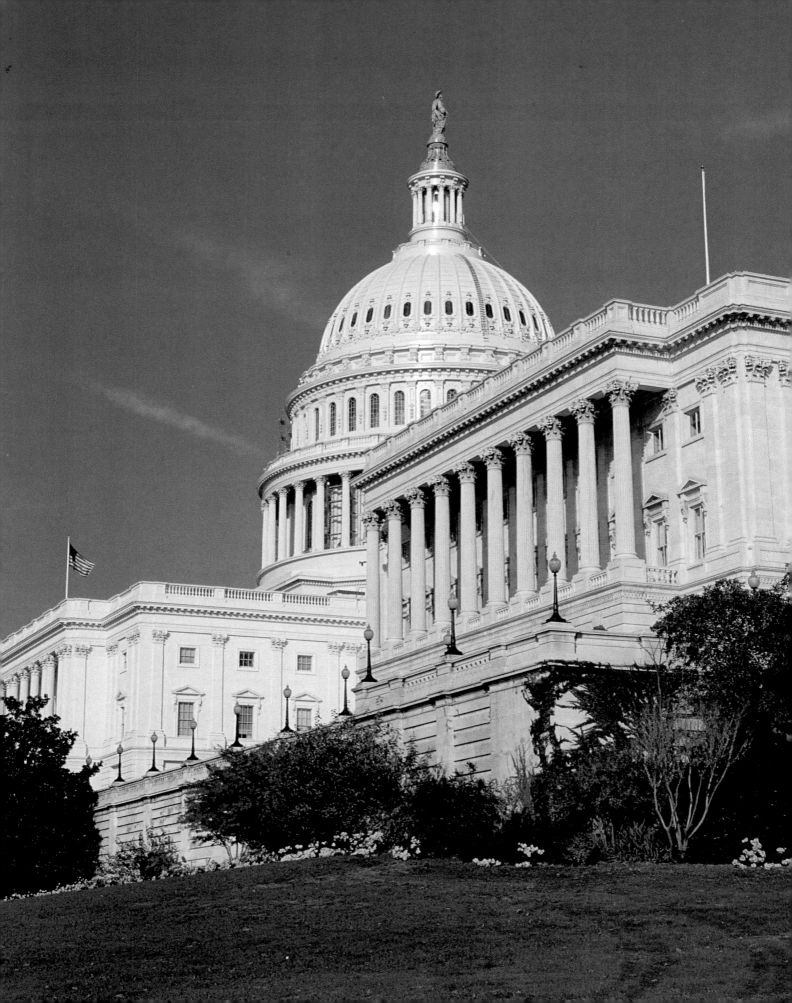

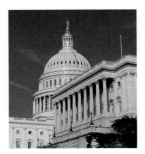

LEARNING OBJECTIVES

After reading this chapter, you should be able to:

- Describe the history and current legal status of abortion in the United States.

- Explain the current debate over abortion, including the main points of the pro-choice and pro-life points of view.

- Describe the methods of abortion available in the United States.

- List possible physical and psychological effects of abortion.

- Discuss the decision-making process a woman and her partner may go through when facing an unintended pregnancy.

Abortion

7

TEST YOUR KNOWLEDGE

1. The rate of abortion in the United States is going up.
   True or false?

2. About what percentage of abortions in the United States take place in the first 12 weeks of pregnancy?
   a. 60%
   b. 70%
   c. 80%
   d. 90%

3. A majority of Americans are in favor of the right to a legal abortion in some circumstances.
   True or false?

4. Most women who have abortions are under 20 years of age.
   True or false?

5. Abortion is more physically dangerous to a woman than carrying and delivering a child.
   True or false?

Answers

1. *False.* The rate of abortion has remained relatively stable since the early 1980s, even declining somewhat between 1990 and 1995.

2. *d.* About 90% of all abortions take place in the first 12 weeks of pregnancy; more than 50% take place in the first 8 weeks.

3. *True.* Current polls indicate that about 23% of Americans favor the right to legal abortion in all circumstances, and an additional 58% favor the right in some circumstances. About 17% of Americans think that abortion should be illegal in all circumstances.

4. *False.* Women in their twenties account for more than half of all abortions; women under 20 account for only about 20%.

5. *False.* The risk of death from an early abortion is 1 in 500,000; for pregnancy and childbirth, the risk of death is 1 in 14,000.

In the United States today, few issues are as complex and emotion-filled as abortion. While most public attention has focused on legal definitions and restrictions, the most difficult aspects of abortion actually take place at a much more personal level. Because the majority of women having abortions are young, many college students have had some type of direct exposure to these more personal experiences of abortion.

On campuses today, as in our society at large, many powerful forces contribute to the high rate of unintended pregnancy and abortion. But at all school levels and in the general public, there is great resistance to confronting these related issues openly and honestly, resulting in a lack of programs to deal with the problem at a preventive level.

College students are in a key position to understand and address the contributing factors as well as the broad effects of unintended pregnancies and abortion. Instead of simply attempting to legislate certain behaviors, they can choose to grapple with the complex human factors that go into the prevention as well as the "treatment" of unintended pregnancy. This chapter will provide basic information on abortion, including the current focuses of controversy. We hope it will act as a springboard for you to form your own views and, more importantly, personal plans for constructive action.

THE ABORTION ISSUE

The following discussion presents various perspectives on abortion. The word **abortion,** by strict definition, means the expulsion of an embryo or fetus from the uterus before it is sufficiently developed to survive. As commonly used, however, abortion refers only to those expulsions that are artificially induced by mechanical means or drugs, and *miscarriage* is generally used for a spontaneous abortion, one that occurs naturally with no causal intervention. In this chapter, abortion will mean a deliberately induced expulsion.

The History of Abortion in the United States

For more than two centuries, abortion policy in the United States followed English common law, which made the practice a crime only when performed after "quickening" (fetal movement that begins at about 20 weeks). There was little public objection to this policy until the early 1800s, when an anti-abortion movement began, led primarily by physicians who questioned the doctrine of quickening and who objected to the growing practice of abortion by untrained persons (in part because it weakened their control of medical services).

TERMS **abortion** The expulsion or removal of an embryo or fetus from the uterus.

This anti-abortion drive gained minimal attention until the mid-1800s, when newspaper advertisements for abortion preparations became common and concern grew that women were using abortion as a means of birth control (and perhaps to cover up extramarital activity). There was much discussion about the corruption of morality among women in the United States, and by the 1900s, virtually all states had anti-abortion laws. These laws stayed in effect until the 1960s, when courts began to invalidate them on the grounds of constitutional vagueness and violation of the right to privacy.

Current Legal Status

In 1973, the U.S. Supreme Court made abortion legal in the landmark case of *Roe v. Wade.* To replace the restrictions most states still imposed at that time, the justices devised new standards to govern abortion decisions. They divided pregnancy into three parts, or trimesters, giving a pregnant woman less choice about abortion as she advances toward full term. In the first trimester, the abortion decision must be left to the judgment of the pregnant woman and her physician. During the second trimester, similar rights remain but a state may regulate factors that protect the health of the woman, such as type of facility where an abortion may be performed. In the third trimester, when the fetus is viable (capable of survival outside of the uterus), a state may regulate and even bar all abortions except those considered necessary to preserve the mother's life or health.

Since 1973, repeated campaigns have been waged to overturn the Supreme Court decision and to ban abortions altogether. Although the Supreme Court has continued to uphold the *Roe* decision, its support for abortion rights has decreased markedly in recent years, with the appointment of several conservative justices.

In July 1989, another legal milestone was reached, when the Supreme Court handed down its decision in *Webster v. Reproductive Health Services.* The Court did not overturn *Roe,* but did let stand several key restrictions on abortions enacted by the Missouri state legislature. The two most severe restrictions forbid the use of all public facilities, resources, and employees for abortion services and require costly and time-consuming tests to determine fetal viability whenever a physician estimates the fetus to be 20 weeks or older. In June 1992, another major Court decision was handed down in *Planned Parenthood of Southeastern Pennsylvania v. Casey.* This ruling continued to uphold a woman's basic right to abortion, but gave the state further power to regulate abortion throughout pregnancy, as long as it does not impose an "undue burden" on women seeking the procedure. The Court decided that the following provisions of the Pennsylvania law did not constitute "undue burden" and therefore let these restrictions stand: Women seeking abortion must be told about fetal development and alternatives to abortion; they must

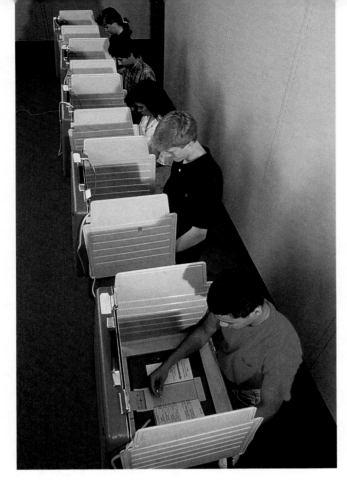

Voting for political candidates with well-defined views on abortion is one way individuals can influence the legal status of abortion in the United States.

states to prohibit all abortion. In the absence of federal legislation, differences in availability, cost, and timing of abortion will continue to exist from one state to another.

Both pro-choice and pro-life groups are likely to remain active at the national level, seeking to advance their positions both by supporting political candidates who share their views and by promoting legislation. Recent political activity on the national level has centered around bills introduced in Congress that would ban certain types of late-term abortions.

> **PERSONAL INSIGHT**   Some people believe that teenagers should have their parents' permission before they can have an abortion and married women should have their husband's permission before they can have an abortion. How do you feel about these views?

Moral Considerations

Along with the legal debates are ongoing arguments between pro-life and pro-choice groups regarding the ethics of abortion (see the two "Opposing Views" boxes). Central to the pro-life position is the belief that the fertilized egg must be valued as a human being from the moment of conception, and that abortion at any time is equivalent to murder. This group holds that any woman who has sexual intercourse knows that pregnancy is a possibility, and should she willingly have intercourse and get pregnant, she is morally obligated to carry the pregnancy through. Pro-life followers encourage adoption for women who feel they are unable to raise the child and point out how many couples are seeking babies for adoption. Pro-lifers do not consider the availability of legal abortion essential to women's well-being, but view it instead as having an overall destructive effect on our traditional morals and values.

By contrast, the pro-choice viewpoint holds that distinctions must be made between the stages of fetal development, and that preserving the fetus early in pregnancy (or *gestation*) is not always the ultimate moral concern. Members of this group maintain that women must have the freedom to decide whether and when to have children; they argue that pregnancy can result from contraceptive failure or other factors out of a woman's control. When pregnancy does occur, pro-choice individuals believe that the most moral decision possible must be determined according to each situation, and that in some cases greater injustice would result if abortion were not an option. If legal abortions were not available, some pro-choice supporters say, "back-alley shops" and do-it-yourself techniques, with their many health risks, as well as the birth of unplanned children, would again grow in number. Others argue that discrimination in health care would result, since wealthy women could more easily

wait at least 24 hours after receiving that information; minors must get permission from a parent or judge; and physicians are required to keep detailed records, subject to public disclosure. The Court turned down a requirement that married women must notify their husbands of their intention to have an abortion.

Because the *Webster* and *Casey* decisions provided few guidelines, legislative activity to limit access to abortion has increased at the state level. In some states, abortion laws have remained unchanged; in others, restrictive measures have been added. While not banning abortion outright, these new regulations have restricted access to abortion for many women, especially those with limited financial resources. In addition, the U.S. Congress bars the use of federal Medicaid funds to pay for abortions except in cases of rape or incest or if the woman's life is in danger; some states use public funds to pay for abortions for poor women, but others do not. Concerns have been raised that a two-tiered system has been created — one for women with means, and another for those without.

The complete overturning of *Roe v. Wade* by the Supreme Court may still occur, as new test cases are brought for consideration. Such a reversal would permit, but not require,

Kate Michelman

Pro-choice is not pro-abortion. Pro-choice is pro-freedom, pro-family, and pro-children. Pro-choice is about the lives, health, and security of women, their children, and their families. It's about freedom—freedom of religion, freedom of conscience, freedom of speech, and the right to privacy. It's about the freedom to choose whether or not to bear a child. No other choice has more impact on our community and our nation.

Reducing the *need* for abortion should be our nation's goal. No one wants an abortion. We all wish we could sail through life without difficult, painful choices. But we live in a complex and uncertain world filled with risk, temptation, illusion, and sometimes terror. No matter how strong the outer protection of love, marriage, income, and stability, each pregnancy comes down to a separate judgment, a different choice.

Women should have the freedom to make that choice.

For most women, the choice of abortion is the hardest choice of all. Abortion is not a choice of convenience. It's a choice wrapped in questions of morality, religion, and ethics. Abortion is filled with wrenching ambivalence and deep matters of the heart. Abortion or not, a woman's right to make this decision should be guaranteed.

In 1973 the question before the Supreme Court in *Roe v. Wade* was: Who should make the deeply personal and profound decision about pregnancy and childbirth? Answer: The woman.

Roe is a compromise that balances the woman and the unborn. It favors one at first and then the other as the pregnancy advances. It chooses the middle ground, the essence of pro-choice. *Roe* is neither libertine nor Draconian. It is neither pro-abortion nor anti-abortion. *Roe* strikes a delicate balance between freedom and responsibility.

For years women have considered the right to choose an abortion to be a basic freedom, no less than freedom of speech or freedom of worship. However, in June 1992 the *Casey* decision imposed restrictions that pushed *Roe* to the very precipice. The Court took the most fundamental American freedom and shattered it into jagged parts.

People once said we shouldn't make choice a political issue. I wish we didn't have to. I wish we could count on the fundamental American right to privacy and dignity. But we've learned the hard way that we can't.

The pro-choice agenda goes beyond the right to choose abortion. It is aimed at creating an America that respects the lives of women, protects the lives of children, and makes whole and happy families.

In a nation with one of the highest rates of unintended pregnancy, we must address the social conditions that force millions of women each year to face the abortion question. Contraception is still hidden behind counters. Expectant mothers still give birth without prenatal care. When it comes to birth control, America is an underdeveloped nation.

America's national policy is fragmented and incoherent. We strongly believe that government has the obligation to pull the pieces together and form a comprehensive reproductive health policy. The central goal of the pro-choice agenda is to reduce abortions. The pro-choice plan seeks to ensure that women who choose to have children can do so in a supportive and healthy environment. We need fundamental and widespread education in human development and sexuality. Our children must understand not just the mechanics of sex and contraception but also the tremendous consequences of pregnancy and birth. It is not enough to counsel abstinence. We've got to foster joint parent/school programs to educate our children about the realities of sex, contraception, and choice. We need to clarify the options and consequences of having children—not just the joys, but the responsibilities; not just the gifts but the costs.

Federal grants to nonprofit organizations for family planning services have been drastically cut. This trend must be reversed. We also urge the federal government to get behind school-linked health clinics. To effectively promote child and teen health, a comprehensive plan must include counseling on pregnancy prevention, drugs, and jobs. Any national reproductive health care plan must guarantee access to prenatal care, treatment for drug-dependent pregnant women, child care, and family and medical leave.

This is not an insurmountable agenda. These are not demands from the political extremes or appeals to break the bank. These are the simple, minimum steps toward a civilized, humane, durable reproductive policy—a policy Americans support.

Kate Michelman is president of the National Abortion and Reproductive Rights Action League. Reprinted by permission of HealthLine.

make the travel arrangements necessary for a legal abortion elsewhere. Still others emphasize that some physicians, because of their strong personal convictions regarding abortion rights, would feel forced into becoming law-breakers.

Some people strongly identify exclusively with either the pro-life or the pro-choice stance, but many have moral beliefs that are blurred, less defined, and in some cases a mixture of the two. A common—but misleading—assumption is that all religious organizations and individuals adhere to the pro-life position.

PERSONAL INSIGHT   How do you define life? When do you think it begins? How does your answer affect your position on abortion?

Public Opinion

In general, U.S. public opinion on abortion seems to change, depending on the specific situation. Many individuals approve of legal abortion as an option when

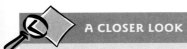 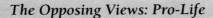
J. C. Willke, M.D.

In considering abortion, the first question to ask is: What is this that grows within the woman? Is this human life? Or, when will it be? If it's not human life, then a case can be made to permit abortion. If, however, this being is fully human, sexed, alive, complete, and intact from the first-cell stage, then a second human life exists and we have a collision of the rights of two humans.

So, first, let's ask: Is this human life? The answer lies in books on biology, embryology, and fetology. In these sciences there is no disagreement on the facts of when human life begins. At the union of sperm and ovum there exists a living, single-celled, complete human organism. It is already male or female, is alive and growing, and is human, as the 46 human chromosomes in the cell's nucleus mark this microscopic being as a member of the human family. This is arguably the most complicated cell in the entire world; it contains more information than could be contained in all of NASA's computers. As this single-celled human organism divides and subdivides, each cell in turn contains progressively less information, is more specialized.

At 1 week of life, this embryonic human attaches to the nutrient lining of the woman's womb and soon sends into her body a hormonal message that stops her period. About 4 days after the time when the woman's period would have begun, the embryo's heart begins to beat. At 40 days, brain waves can be recorded. By 10 weeks, the structure of the body is completely formed. By 3 months, all organ systems are functioning. To deny that fully human life begins at fertilization is to deny the known facts of fetal development and biological science.

Some argue that life existed in the sperm and ovum and will exist in the future. True, but we are not asking about generic life, but rather about this one unique individual's human life, which begins at fertilization and ends at death.

Some would measure the beginning of human life with a theologic yardstick, speaking of soul, God, and creation. In a secular state, however, we cannot use a theologic belief to define when human life begins for the purpose of making laws that either protect or allow the destruction of that life.

Others use various philosophical definitions of when the fullness of humanness exists, such as when cognition and self-consciousness are possible, when love is exchanged, when a being is declared to be "humanized" or "socialized," or when certain biological mileposts are reached. Though these definitions are arrived at by intellectual processes, they cannot be scientifically proven. Open to disagreement among people of good will, these definitions are also beliefs. We should not impose either religious or philosophical beliefs upon others in our culture. If one defines human life from the facts of natural science, then human life, complete and intact, begins at fertilization. That is a fact that we must face and work with.

Because this is human life from the very moment of conception, the issues touching that life are those of civil rights and human rights and the laws protecting those rights.

Let's ask a second question: Should there be equal protection under the law for all living humans? Or, should the law discriminate fatally against entire classes of humans, in this case against those still living in the womb?

Interestingly enough, our nation faced a similar situation once before—slavery. In 1857, the Supreme Court ruled in the Dred Scott case that black people were not legal persons before the law. They were the property of the slave owner, who could buy, sell, or even kill them. Abolitionists' protests were countered: "Now look, you find slavery morally offensive? Well, you don't have to own a slave. But don't force your morality on the owner, for he has the constitutional right to choose to own a slave." In 1973, the Court did it again. In *Roe v. Wade,* also by a 7 to 2 margin, it ruled that unborn people were not legal persons. They were the property of the owner (the mother), who could keep or kill. Pro-lifers objected, to hear the same response. "Look, you find abortion morally offensive. Well, you don't have to have one. But don't force your morality on the owner (the woman), for she now has the constitutional right to choose, to kill."

The *Dred Scott* decision discriminated by skin color; *Roe v. Wade* discriminates by place of residence: still living in the womb. Each is a civil rights outrage.

A woman has a right to her own body, but to say that the little passenger residing within her is a part of her body is to utter a biological absurdity.

But she does not want this child? Since when does anyone's right to live depend upon someone else wanting them? Killing the unwanted is a monstrous evil.

A woman's issue? Women make up the overwhelming majority in the pro-life movement, and opinion polls consistently show more opposition to abortion from females than from males.

So, should a woman have the right to choose? I have a right to free speech, but not to shout "fire" in a theater. A person's right to anything stops when it injures or kills another living human.

No one should minimize the problems of pregnant women. With adequate counseling, informed consent, and the involvement of parents, husbands, and friends, we can help solve most of their problems—but sadly, never all of them. The pivotal question is: Should any civilized nation give to one citizen the absolute legal right to kill another to solve that first person's personal problem? I think not. We must give women far more help, both privately and publicly, than is available today. But we simply cannot continue to solve their personal problems by allowing the ghastly violence of killing tiny, innocent humans.

J. C. Willke is president of the Life Issues Institute and The International Right to Life Federation. Reprinted by permission of HealthLine.

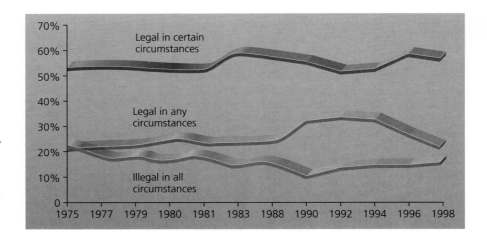

VITAL STATISTICS

Figure 7-1 Public opinion about abortion. This graph represents responses to the question: Do you think abortions should be legal under any circumstances, legal only under certain circumstances, or illegal in all circumstances? SOURCE: Gallup Poll News Service.

destructive health or welfare consequences could result from continuing pregnancy, but they do not advocate abortion as a simple way out of an inconvenient situation. Overall, most adults in the United States continue to approve of legal abortion and are opposed to overturning the basic right to abortion established in *Roe v. Wade* (Figure 7-1). But the amount of public support varies considerably, depending on the circumstances surrounding the abortion request (Table 7-1).

For example, people who feel that abortion should be available in early pregnancy often question at which stage in later pregnancy the fetus's rights should take precedence over the woman's rights. The 1973 U.S. Supreme Court decision considered viability the key criterion in establishing the point beyond which a woman's right to choose abortion becomes markedly restricted. In 1973, viability was generally considered to be about 26–28 weeks. Today it is about 24 weeks, with isolated cases of survival at 23 weeks. Although neonatal intensive care units continue to advance technologically, most experts feel that viability cannot be expected beyond this limit.

Other individuals associate fetal rights not with viability but with earlier developmental characteristics such as the onset of heartbeat, brain size, and nervous system maturity. *The Silent Scream,* a widely shown film that used computer-enhanced ultrasound images, purports to depict a 12-week-old fetus "screaming in pain" during an abortion procedure. Critics contend that the film was manipulated, and experts in fetal medicine have refuted the film's medical premises. Researchers have recently described evidence that minimal nervous system connections necessary for brain function don't develop until after the fifth month of pregnancy.

Still others argue that the embryo becomes a human being at the point of individuation or twinning, which occurs about 2 weeks after conception. (Before that time, the embryo has not yet differentiated into either a single

VITAL STATISTICS

TABLE 7-1	*Views on Abortion*

1. Should a pregnant woman be able to obtain an abortion in the following circumstances?

	Yes
Her own health is seriously endangered by the pregnancy.	88%
There is a strong chance of fetal defect.	75%
The pregnancy results from rape.	84%
The woman has a very low income and cannot afford another child.	43%
A woman is married and does not want any more children.	39%
A woman does not want to marry the man responsible for the pregnancy.	38%

2. Should a woman be permitted to have an abortion during the following stages of pregnancy?

	Yes
In the first 3 months	61%
In the second 3 months	15%
In the last 3 months	7%

	No
3. Should there be a constitutional amendment outlawing abortion?	>75%

SOURCE: Goldberg, C., and J. Elder. 1998. Public still backs abortion, but wants limits, poll says. *New York Times,* January 16.

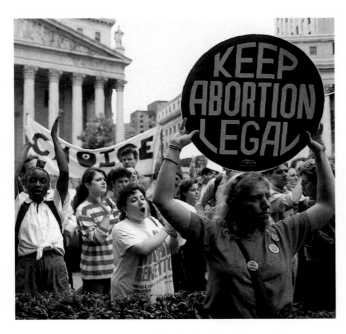

Pro-choice groups believe that the decision to end or continue a pregnancy is a personal matter that should be left up to the individual.

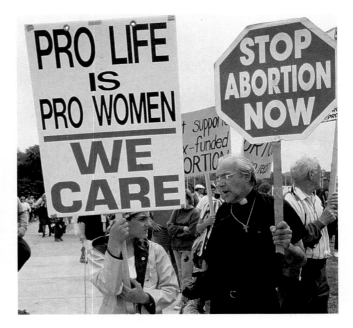

Pro-life groups oppose abortion on the basis of their belief that life begins at the moment of conception.

or an identical twin pregnancy.) Others believe that the moment of conception is the only critical point to consider. For them, all other developmental stages are irrelevant to the abortion debate. As can be seen from such wide variation of opinion, objective measures of humanness and clear-cut guidelines regarding fetal rights are elusive, and decisions ambiguous.

Although opinions vary as to whether, or when, in pregnancy, abortion rights should be tightly regulated by law, most people agree that abortions done later in pregnancy present more difficulties in personal, medical, philosophical, and social terms. Of all abortions done after the 12th week of gestation, more than 35% are performed on teenagers. Possible explanations include teenagers' ignorance, denial, fear, lack of supportive family or friends, and state regulatory hurdles faced by teenagers. Other typical recipients of late abortions include low-income women who may have more difficulty finding suitable facilities as well as necessary funds, and pre-menopausal women who fail to recognize a delayed period as pregnancy. Another small group of women who may seek late abortion are those who have learned through genetic tests that the fetus has a specific abnormality.

Personal Considerations

For the pregnant woman who is considering abortion, the usual legal and moral arguments may sound meaningless as she attempts to weigh the many short- and long-term

ramifications for all lives directly concerned. If she chooses abortion, can she accept that decision in terms of her own religious and moral beliefs? What are her long-range feelings likely to be regarding this decision? What are her partner's feelings regarding abortion, and how will she deal with his responses? Does she have a supportive relative or friend who will help her through this time of emotional adjustment? Which medical facility offering abortions would be most suitable for her? What about transportation and costs? (Figures 7-2 and 7-3 present statistical information about women who choose abortion.)

For the woman who decides against abortion and chooses instead to continue the pregnancy, there are other questions. If she decides to raise the child herself, will she have the critical resources to do it well? Is a supportive, lasting relationship with her partner likely? If not, how does she feel about being a single parent? Are family members available to help with the many demands of child rearing? If she is young, what will the effects be on her own growth? Will she be able to continue with her educational and personal goals? What about the ongoing financial responsibilities?

If the pregnant woman considers adoption, she will have to try to predict what her emotional responses will be throughout the full-term pregnancy and the adoption process. What are her long-range feelings likely to be? What is the best setting for her during her pregnancy? How can she best maintain continuity with the rest of her life and her long-term goals? Which adoption facility is

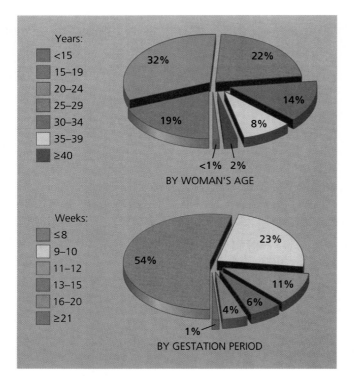

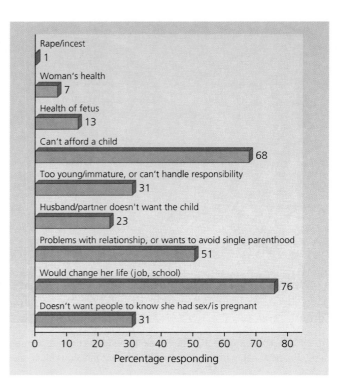

VITAL STATISTICS

Figure 7-2   Distribution of abortions by the woman's age and by the weeks of gestation.   SOURCE: Koonin, L. M., et al. 1998. Abortion surveillance—United States, 1995. *Morbidity and Mortality Weekly Report* 47(SS-2): 31–68.

VITAL STATISTICS

Figure 7-3   The reasons women choose abortions.   The respondents in this study were allowed to give more than one answer. SOURCE: Data from the Alan Guttmacher Institute.

likely to make the most suitable arrangements for her and her baby? A public or a private agency? Is anonymity between the adoptive parents and herself desirable or not? Does she have someone she trusts to help her with these difficult decisions? (The box "Unplanned Pregnancy: Considering Adoption" addresses some of these questions.)

PERSONAL INSIGHT   How would you feel if you discovered that a fetus you were carrying (or your partner was carrying) had a serious genetic defect? Would you be likely to choose abortion? How much would the nature of the defect and its consequences for the baby and you affect your decision?

Current Trends

Clearly, all responses to unintended pregnancy can be difficult, including abortion and especially late abortion. Fortunately, with the increased accessibility to legalized abortion following the mid-1970s, the rate of late abortions dropped steadily, until fewer than 1% of all abortions were performed at more than 20 weeks and fewer

than 11% at more than 12 weeks by the 1990s. The overall abortion *rate* rose during most of the 1970s, leveled off around 1980, and decreased in the early 1990s (Figure 7-4). Possible future influences on the number, rate, and timing of abortions in the United States include the more widespread availability of emergency contraceptives and the introduction of mifepristone, also known as RU-486 or the "abortion pill." (See Chapter 6 for more on emergency contraception; mifepristone is discussed later in this chapter.)

Since the 1989 *Webster* and 1992 *Casey* decisions, many states have imposed additional restrictions on abortion. By 1999, 22 states required mandatory counseling, followed in 14 states by a waiting period; 30 states required parental consent or notification for minors; 11 states banned certain abortion procedures; and 34 states restricted the use of public (Medicaid) funds for abortion except in cases where the woman's life is in danger or the pregnancy is the result of rape or incest; 30 states had three or more restrictions. Research into the effects of these restrictions has been mixed. Some studies indicate that parental consent and notification laws may result in minors traveling out of state to obtain abortions. Mandatory delay laws have been found to influence the number and timing of abortions. Further

Unplanned Pregnancy: Considering Adoption

If you are pregnant and not sure you want to keep the baby, one of the options you may be considering is adoption. There are many people who can help you consider your options—your partner, friends, family members, or a professional counselor. Free counseling is often available at crisis pregnancy centers, family planning clinics, adoption agencies, family service agencies, and mental health centers. No matter where you go, a counselor should always treat you with respect and be willing to discuss all your options with you—keeping the baby, having an abortion, or arranging an adoption. To evaluate a potential counselor, find out what help or services he or she can provide for each of these choices. If you aren't comfortable with a particular counselor, find a different one.

Make sure you explore all possibilities before you make a final choice. The decision to place a child for adoption is a difficult one. It is an act of great courage and love. But adoption is permanent. The adoptive parents will raise your child and have legal authority for his or her welfare. Think about your life now and in the future as you consider your options.

There are two types of adoptions, confidential and open. In confidential adoption, the birth parents and the adoptive parents never know each other. Adoptive parents will be given the information about the birth parents that they would need to help take care of the child, such as medical information. In an open adoption, the birth parents and adoptive parents know something about each other. There are different levels of openness, ranging from reading a brief description of prospective adoptive parents to meeting them and sharing full information.

Another key decision is the amount of contact you would like to have with your child and her or his adoptive family. You may be able to arrange to stay in touch with the family over the years, by visiting, calling, or writing. Some women feel that an open adoption enables them to keep in touch with a baby they will always love; others feel that this would be too difficult and decide against contact with the adoptive family.

In all states, you can work with a licensed child-placing (adoption) agency. In many states, you can also work directly with an adopting couple or their attorney without using an agency; this is called a private or independent adoption. Prospective adoptive parents can be located through personal ads, a physician, adoptive parent support groups, and family members and friends. When you contact an agency or attorney, ask about their rules and procedures.

- Will you receive counseling throughout your pregnancy and following the adoption?

- Will you receive financial help for medical and legal expenses?

- What will you be able to know about the adoptive parents?

- Will you be able to have the amount of contact with the baby that you want?

Find an agency or lawyer who will arrange the type of adoption you want.

As with abortion, there are emotional and physical risks associated with pregnancy, childbirth, and adoption. Throughout the adoption process, make sure that you have the help you need and that you carefully consider all your options. Deciding how to handle an unplanned pregnancy is important, and you have the power to make your own decisions.

SOURCE: Adapted from Smith, D. G. 1992. *NAIC Factsheet: Are You Pregnant and Thinking About Adoption?* Rockville, Md.: National Adoption Information Clearinghouse.

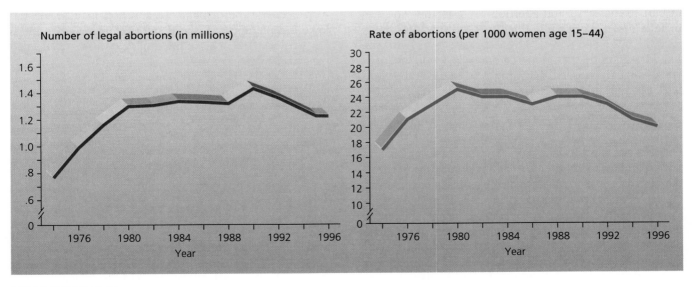

VITAL STATISTICS

Figure 7-4   Abortion rates in the United States.   SOURCE: Centers for Disease Control and Prevention. 1998. Abortion surveillance: Preliminary analysis—United States, 1996. *Morbidity and Mortality Weekly Report* 47 (47): 1025–1029, 1035.

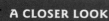
- About 50% of the pregnancies in America are unintended; half of those are terminated by abortion.

- Each year, about 2 out of 100 women age 15–44 have an abortion.

- The majority of women having abortions are young: 52% are under age 25, including about 20% who are teenagers (age 11–19).

- Women age 18–19 have the highest abortion rate.

- The proportion of pregnancies terminated by abortion is higher among unmarried women (51%), women age 40 and over (34%), and teenagers (38%) than among all women (28%).

- Women of low income are about three times more likely than women who are financially better off to have abortions. Nevertheless, 11% of abortions are obtained by women whose household incomes are $50,000 or more.

- Women having no religious affiliation have a higher rate of abortion than women who have some affiliation. Catholic women are about as likely to obtain an abortion as are all women nationally, and Protestants and Jews are less likely.

- About two-thirds of women having an abortion say that they intend to have children in the future.

- Most women who have an abortion after 15 weeks of pregnancy have had problems detecting their pregnancy, and almost half are delayed because of problems, usually financial, in arranging an abortion.

- Among teenagers, 85% of pregnancies are unintended; 40% of women who become pregnant as teenagers choose abortion.

- Of teenagers under age 18 who obtain an abortion, 61% do so with their parents' knowledge; the younger the teenager, the more likely that her parents know.

- At current rates, about 43% of American women will have at least one abortion by the time they are 45 years old.

SOURCE: *Facts in Brief: Induced Abortion.* 1998. New York: Alan Guttmacher Institute.

research is needed to establish whether these types of restrictions constitute an "undue burden" for women seeking abortions.

Adding to the legal restrictions is the growing scarcity of physicians willing to provide abortion services. Currently, 86% of all U.S. counties, 90% of rural counties, and about 30% of metropolitan areas have no abortion providers. This diminishing number of providers is due in part to increased anti-abortion protests and violence, include arson, bombings, threats of anthrax poisoning, and the murders of several physicians and clinic workers. In addition, some states have late-term abortion laws that are so vaguely worded that providers of early abortions fear prosecution and have stopped providing all abortion services.

Women living in areas that have restrictive laws and few abortion providers may continue to obtain abortions, but they are likely to face significant increases in expense and time delays (see the box "Facts About Abortion"). If the constitutional right to abortion is to be maintained, these obstacles need to be carefully considered.

Unless accompanied by a greater effort at preventing unwanted pregnancy, especially among the young single women who make up the majority of those seeking abortions, legal changes alone will probably not dramatically reduce the number of abortions. For a broader perspective, see the box "Abortion Around the World."

We hope the recent surge of public interest in sexual behavior, largely due to the fear of STDs, will lead to more open discussions of sexuality and contraception for individuals who choose to be sexually active. With more communication and a better understanding of one's personal need for intimacy and closeness, individuals and couples can perhaps make informed, responsible decisions about the best way to meet those needs. For those who choose to include sexual intercourse as part of their relationships, contraception should be made readily available and correctly used (see Chapter 6). Other measures that might help decrease the demand for abortion include the following economic and social reforms: increased options for working women, more dual parenting, maternal/paternal leaves, improved child care facilities, and quality prenatal and postnatal care available for all people regardless of socioeconomic status.

PERSONAL INSIGHT Some men feel strongly that they should have a say when their partner is considering abortion. Others feel it's up to the woman. How do you feel about men's roles and rights in decisions about abortion?

METHODS OF ABORTION

Postcoital pills and IUDs inserted immediately after unprotected sexual intercourse are generally not considered abortifacients (agents that produce abortion) from a medical viewpoint, because they act before implantation of the fertilized egg, if one is present (see Chapter 6).

As one would expect, the legal status, availability, and safety of abortion varies widely around the world. Of the 46 million abortions performed each year worldwide, about 26 million are legal and 20 million illegal (see the figure).

- 25% of the world's people live in countries where laws ban abortion entirely or permit it only to save the life of a pregnant woman.

- 14% of the world's people live in countries with somewhat less restrictive laws that permit abortion to protect a pregnant woman's physical or mental health.

- 61% of the world's people live in countries where abortion is permitted either for a wide range or reasons or without restriction as to reason. Many of these countries do have regulations or restrictions such as third-party authorizations, waiting periods, or mandatory counseling, and many place limits on gestational age and the types of facilities where abortions can be performed.

Even in countries where abortion is illegal, women still undergo abortions. In fact, many countries with strict anti-abortion laws have high rates of abortion and, because most procedures are carried out secretly in unsafe conditions, high rates of serious complications. Nearly all of the 80,000 abortion-related deaths that occur each year occur in countries with strict abortion laws. In countries where abortion is legal, widely available at low cost, and performed under safe conditions, abortion rates are relatively low and serious complications rare. (Widespread availability of contraception is another factor associated with low rates of abortion.)

Legal status is not the sole determinant of the availability of safe abortion services, however. How the laws are interpreted and enforced can be just as critical. For example, in some countries that allow abortion for mental health reasons, the law is interpreted to allow the majority of women seeking abortions to obtain them; in other countries with comparable laws, few abortions are allowed. Enforcement also varies. For example, in Mozambique, where abortion is officially banned, women can obtain abortions on request at many hospitals, and abortion-related legal charges are rarely filed. In other countries, laws are strictly enforced, and both women who have abortions and abortion providers are prosecuted. It is estimated that two-thirds of women currently in prison in Nepal have been convicted of undergoing illegal abortions. Strict enforcement of anti-abortion laws tends to disproportionately affect poor women because wealthier women can pay to obtain discreet, safe abortions from private physicians, thus avoiding the more tightly regulated public hospitals.

The attitudes and beliefs of the medical community also influence the availability of abortion services. For example, in Nigeria, many physicians will perform abortions in spite of legal bans because the medical community believes in the need for safe abortion services. On the flip side, major medical associations in Poland and the Republic of Ireland have adopted guidelines that are stricter than their country's laws.

The number and location of abortion providers and the cost of abortion services also influence the true availability of abortion in a particular country, regardless of its actual legal status. Community and physician opposition to abortion has left parts of the United States, Austria, and Germany without abortion providers, despite the fact that abortion is legal in all three countries. In contrast, policies in Denmark go beyond just permitting safe abortion to ensuring that services are widely available: There, each county must have at least one hospital that has the capacity to perform abortions, and services are free t.

SOURCES: Henshaw, S. K., S. Singh, and T. Haas. 1999. The incidence of abortion worldwide. *International Family Planning Perspectives* 25: S30–S38. Rahman, A., L. Katzive, and S. K. Henshaw. 1998. A global review of laws on induced abortion, 1985–1997. *International Family Planning Perspectives* 24(2): 56–64. *Issues in Brief: The Role of Contraception in Reducing Abortion.* 1997. New York: Alan Guttmacher Institute.

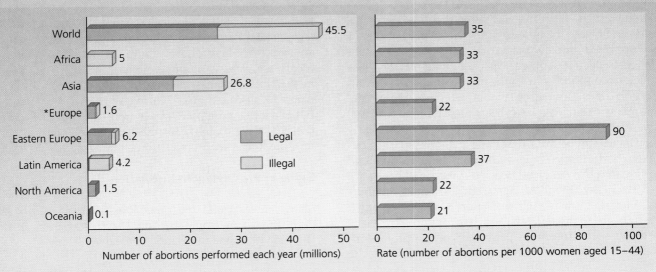

*Excluding Eastern Europe

(During this initial period, the female body naturally washes away an estimated 40% of fertilized eggs.) Therefore, these topics are not discussed here.

Suction Curettage

First developed in China in 1958, **suction curettage** (also called *vacuum aspiration*) is the preferred method for abortions up to the 12th week of pregnancy. It is used in about 90% of all abortions performed in the United States. The procedure can be done quickly, usually on an outpatient basis, and the risk of complications is small.

A sedative may be given, along with a **local anesthetic.** A speculum is inserted into the vagina, and the cervix is cleansed with a surgical solution. The cervix is dilated and a suction curette, a specially designed hollow tube, is then inserted into the uterus (Figure 7-5). The curette is attached to the rubber tubing of an electric pump, and suction is applied. In about 20–30 seconds, the uterus is emptied. Moderate cramping is common during evacuation. To ensure that no fragments of tissue are left in the uterus, the doctor usually scrapes the uterine lining with a metal curette, an instrument with a spoonlike tip. The entire suction curettage procedure takes only 5–10 minutes.

After a few hours in a recovering area, the woman can return home. She is usually instructed not to douche, have intercourse, or use tampons for the first week or two after the abortion and to return for a 2-week postabortion examination. This follow-up exam is important to verify that the abortion was complete and that no signs of infection are present.

Menstrual Extraction

Developed in the early 1970s, **menstrual extraction** is the vacuum aspiration of uterine contents shortly after a missed period. It was originally defined as a procedure to be done up to the 42nd day after the last menstrual period and before the absence or presence of a pregnancy was confirmed. Initially, menstrual extraction was seen as safe, cost-effective, and as especially suitable for those women uncomfortable with the notion of abortion. Complication rates, including incomplete evacuation and continuing pregnancy, have been higher than expected, however (the small amount of tissue present in very early pregnancies can be missed). While some physicians continue to perform menstrual extraction, many recommend waiting until the 7th or 8th week of pregnancy.

With the likelihood of increased restrictions on abortion, interest in menstrual extraction has again emerged in certain groups as a possible self-help option. Physicians warn that such procedures performed by nonprofessionals can be dangerous; complications include missing the fertilized egg, lacerating the cervix, perforating the uterus, and spreading bacterial infection.

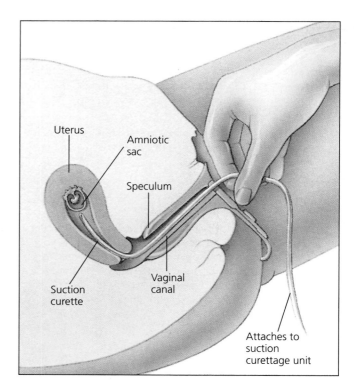

Figure 7-5 Suction curettage. This procedure takes 5–10 minutes and can be performed up to the 12th week of pregnancy.

Dilation and Evacuation

The method most commonly used between the 13th and 15th week of pregnancy and now preferred by some physicians up to and past the 20th week is **dilation and evacuation (D & E).** This procedure combines vacuum aspiration with curettage, in which a curette and forceps (a long grasping instrument) are used to scrape the tissues from the wall of the uterus. Compared with suction curettage, greater cervical dilation and larger suction curettes are required. In late-term abortions, additional instruments are also used. Intravenous fluid that includes a medication to increase uterine contractions and thus limit blood loss is often given during or after the procedure. Either a local, a **regional,** or a **general anesthetic** is used. Both the time required for the D & E and the recovery time are longer than for suction curettage.

Saline or Prostaglandin Instillation

Many centers use D & E procedures after the 15th week of pregnancy, but some use saline or prostaglandin instillation. With saline instillation, a local anesthetic is given, and a long needle is inserted through the abdominal and uterine walls into the **amniotic sac.** Amniotic fluid is drained from the sac and replaced with salt solution. Fetal death, which occurs immediately as a result of the disruption of the chemical balance essential to life, is followed by labor and delivery within a day or two. The uterus is scraped to reduce chances of infection or hemorrhage. The recovery period is slightly longer than for suction curettage, and complications are more frequent.

Prostaglandins, a group of naturally occurring chemicals, also bring on abortion, apparently by stimulating contractions of the uterus. They can be injected into the amniotic sac or inserted through the cervical canal into the uterus. Their major shortcoming is their effect on the muscles of the digestive tract, which produces nausea, vomiting, and diarrhea. Synthetic prostaglandins have fewer side effects than natural ones. Another chemical, urea, is often used in combination with prostaglandins to induce contractions.

Fewer than 1% of abortions performed in the United States use saline or prostaglandin instillation.

Mifepristone

Mifepristone, also known as RU-486, blocks the uterine absorption of progesterone, thereby causing the uterine lining and any fertilized egg to shed. Mifepristone can be administered under medical supervision up to the 49th day following the last menstrual period. A woman takes a dose of mifepristone and follows it up 2 days later with a second drug, the prostaglandin analog misoprostol, which induces contractions. The two-drug regimen has a rate of completed abortion of about 95%; the success rate is highest early in pregnancy. Because it does not involve a surgical procedure, it permits more privacy and costs less than other early abortion options. It also allows a woman to have an abortion earlier in the pregnancy.

Common side effects of the two-drug regimen include nausea, vomiting, diarrhea, and abdominal pain. A few cases of serious cardiovascular problems have been reported, but they occurred almost exclusively in women with preexisting risk factors, such as smokers over age 35. The only other potentially serious side effect is vaginal bleeding. In most cases, bleeding is more prolonged than with surgical abortion, but total blood loss is similar. In a small number of cases, bleeding is heavy, and a follow-up suction curettage is necessary. A disadvantage of mifepristone is that the process takes longer than a surgical abortion, which is usually completed within an hour and can be done under sedation. With mifepristone, abortion can take anywhere from a few hours to several weeks; about 50% of abortions occur with 4 hours and 75% within 24 hours.

Mifepristone has been used extensively in Europe for over 10 years. Large clinical trials completed there and, more recently, studies in the United States have established its safety and efficacy. Although the FDA has granted tentative approval for the drug to be marketed in the United States, legal and manufacturing difficulties have delayed its introduction. With abortion opponents strongly objecting to the use of mifepristone, the controversy surrounding the drug will no doubt continue. (For more on the current status of mifepristone, refer to the resources in the For More Information section at the end of the chapter.)

A second drug, methotrexate, can also be used with prostaglandin for early medical abortion. Methotrexate has been approved by the FDA for cancer treatment since 1953; although not approved specifically for early abortion, it can be, and sometimes is, prescribed for that purpose. Methotrexate stops the embryonic or fetal cells from dividing; it is followed by a dose of prostaglandin in a regimen similar to mifepristone. With this combination of drugs, 80–85% of women will abort within 2 weeks.

COMPLICATIONS OF ABORTION

Along with questions regarding the actual procedure of abortion, many people have concerns about possible aftereffects. In recent years, several detailed and long-term studies have focused on both physical and psychological concerns. More information is gradually being gathered on this important subject.

Possible Physical Effects

The incidence of immediate problems following an abortion (infection, bleeding, trauma to the cervix or uterus, and incomplete abortion requiring repeat curettage) varies widely. The potential for problems is significantly reduced if the woman is in good health, and by early timing of the abortion, use of the suction method and local anesthetic, performance by a well-trained clinician, and the availability and use of prompt follow-up care.

suction curettage Removal of the embryo or fetus by means of suction; also called *vacuum aspiration*. **TERMS**

local anesthetic A drug that blocks the nerves carrying pain sensations to the brain; in abortion and childbirth, the nerves running from the pelvic area to the brain are affected while the woman is left awake and alert.

menstrual extraction The vacuum aspiration of uterine contents shortly after a missed period.

dilation and evacuation (D & E) The method of abortion most commonly used between 13 and 15 weeks of pregnancy. Following dilation of the cervix, both vacuum aspiration and curettage instruments are used as needed.

regional anesthetic A drug that is injected between two of the vertebrae in the spinal column, numbing the body from the waist down.

general anesthetic A drug that produces unconsciousness to relieve pain.

amniotic sac The container of amniotic fluid lining the uterus, which envelopes and protects the fetus.

Problems related specifically to infection can be minimized through preabortion testing and treatment for gonorrhea, chlamydia, and other infections. Some clinicians routinely give antibiotics after an abortion, while others treat only those women who have a history of, or current symptoms of, pelvic infection. Postabortion danger signs are:

- Fever above 100°F.
- Abdominal pain or swelling, cramping, or backache.
- Abdominal tenderness (to pressure).
- Prolonged or heavy bleeding.
- Foul-smelling vaginal discharge.
- Vomiting or fainting.
- Delay in resuming menstrual periods (6 weeks or more).

Some bleeding occurs during and after most abortions. However, excessive bleeding during or after the procedure is rare with early suction curettage. In later pregnancies, the use of uterus-contracting medications reduces the risk significantly. Because aspirin, ibuprofen, and other, nonsteroid anti-inflammatory drugs can increase bleeding, they should be avoided. For pain relief, acetaminophen and a heating pad are safe substitutes.

Cervical trauma or laceration and perforation of the uterus are also uncommon in early abortion with a well-trained clinician. In more advanced pregnancies, slow and careful dilation of the cervix before an abortion can diminish these risks. The use of a local or regional, instead of general, anesthetic also minimizes the risk of uterine perforation, because less relaxation of the uterus occurs.

Incomplete abortion means that some pregnancy tissue has remained in the uterus. With this condition, or when blood clots form in the uterus shortly after an abortion, severe cramping and signs of infection can occur, and a repeat suction curettage is usually needed. On rare occasions, a pregnancy may continue after an incomplete abortion. The recommended follow-up exam is important to establish that the abortion was complete.

Studies on long-term complications—subsequent infertility, spontaneous second abortions, premature delivery, and babies of low birth weight—have not revealed any major risks with the most common abortion methods. The risk of postabortion infertility seems to be very low, especially when any signs of infection are reported and treated promptly.

There is also apparently no effect on the outcome of future pregnancies when an early suction curettage is performed with minimal cervical dilation; with later abortions and with repeated or multiple abortions, there is only a slight risk, if any. For Rh-negative women, dangerous sensitization (the buildup of antibodies) can be minimized by an injection of Rh-immune globulin given within 72 hours of the procedure.

A few studies have reported that women who have abortions have an increased risk of breast cancer. How-

TABLE 7-2	*Abortion Risks*	
		Risk of Death in Any Given Year
Legal abortion		
Before 9 weeks		1 in 500,000
9–12 weeks		1 in 67,000
13–16 weeks		1 in 23,000
After 16 weeks		1 in 8,700
Illegal abortion		1 in 3,000
Pregnancy and childbirth		1 in 14,300

SOURCE: Carlson, K. J., S. A. Eisenstat, and T. Ziporyn. 1996. *The Harvard Guide to Women's Health.* Cambridge, Mass.: Harvard University Press.

ever, a well-designed 1997 study of 1.5 million Danish women found no connection between a woman's abortion history and her risk of breast cancer.

The overall risk of death is low. Mortality rates have decreased substantially since abortion was legalized in 1973 (Table 7-2).

Possible Psychological Effects

After an exhaustive review completed in 1988, then–Surgeon General C. Everett Koop concluded that the available evidence failed to demonstrate either a negative or a positive long-term impact of abortion on mental health. More recent research has resulted in the same general conclusion. The psychological side effects of abortion are less clearly defined than the physical ones. Responses vary and depend on the individual woman's psychological makeup, family background, current personal and social relationships, cultural attitudes, and many other factors. A woman who has specific goals with a somewhat structured life pattern may be able to incorporate her decision to have an abortion as the unequivocally "best" and acceptable course more easily than a woman who feels uncertain about her future.

Although many women experience great relief after an abortion and virtually no negative feelings, some go through a period of ambivalence. Along with relief, they often feel a mixture of other responses, such as guilt, regret, loss, sadness, and/or anger. When a woman feels she was pressured into sexual intercourse or into the abortion, she may feel bitter. If she had strongly believed abortion to be immoral, she may wonder if she is still a good person. Many of these feelings are strongest immediately after the abortion, when hormonal shifts are occurring; such feelings often pass quite rapidly. Others take time and fade only slowly. It is important for a woman to realize that such a mixture of feelings is natural.

Susan

Susan was a first-year college student who was caught up in her new academic and social activities. Bill (another student) and she had been dating for about three months, when one evening she decided to "take a chance" and not use contraception because she had just finished her menstrual period. When her next period was two weeks overdue, she had a pregnancy test. It was positive.

From the moment she found out, Susan considered only one option: abortion. "I couldn't have raised a child," she said. "And I wouldn't bring a child into the world unless I could take the responsibility for it. I think it would be worse to ruin my future and a baby's life because of a mistake." When Bill first learned of the pregnancy, he became distant, but he did agree to help pay for the abortion. Soon, however, he withdrew completely and had no further contact with Susan.

The hardest time for Susan was before the abortion, when she found herself crying frequently. She talked a lot with a close girlfriend, who went with her to the clinic and stayed with her after the abortion. Like all women who have abortions, Susan needed comforting.

After the abortion, Susan felt very strongly that she had made the best decision, but she did occasionally wonder how she would feel in future years. After meeting a new boyfriend with whom she could talk openly, Susan felt more certain than ever that she had made the right choice.

Helen

Helen was attending a junior college and working part-time when she found out she was pregnant. She and Mike had met just a couple of months before the pregnancy. They both planned to become parents at some point in their lives, but this was earlier than either of them had expected. They discussed all the options, and they agreed that getting married and keeping their child was the only acceptable solution.

Helen gave up school for the time being, and Mike took on more hours at work to help pay for the additional expense of a child. Six months after they were married, their daughter was born. Helen and Mike say that it was at this period of their life that they really got to know each other. "Our apartment was so small, we couldn't help but learn everything about each other."

It's now eight years later, and Helen and Mike have two children. Mike works full-time but hopes to return to school and complete his degree in the future. Helen works part-time and attends evening classes twice a week. They'd like to move to a larger apartment and to travel more, but they can't afford to. "We've given up a lot, and it's still a struggle. But we're a happy family, and we know that we made the right choice for us."

Anna

Anna was shocked when she found out she was pregnant. She was sure she wasn't ready to be a parent herself; she was too young, and still hadn't sorted out what she wanted from life. But Anna also felt that having an abortion would be wrong. So she decided to have the baby and put it up for adoption. "I myself am adopted, so adoption seemed a natural choice, and the best one available to me."

Her boyfriend broke up with her when she told him. But her parents were supportive and helped arrange for her baby's placement in a good home. Anna knew she would have to give her baby up as soon as it was born, but during her pregnancy she developed a powerful bond with her child. Anna delivered her son and left the hospital three days later. "I had to just give the baby to the nurse and walk out. My parents and I cried. I spent nine months preparing for that moment, but it was still so painful."

After a year Anna still hurts, but she doesn't regret her decision. "Keeping him would have changed my life completely, and I knew I wasn't ready to be a mother. I couldn't have given my son the kind of life I want him to have." She's proud that she went through her pregnancy. As an adopted child herself, Anna felt she owed her son the same chance that her biological mother gave her.

For a woman who does experience psychological or emotional effects after an abortion, talking with a close friend or family member can be very helpful. Supportive people can help her feel positive about herself and her decision. Although a legal and common procedure in the United States, abortion is still treated very secretively in most of our society, so it is easy for a woman to feel unique, isolated, and alone. Some women may specifically seek out other women who have had an abortion. Many clinical centers that offer abortions make such peer counseling available. Other women find they can identify with case histories in books written on abortion, which can help them deal with their own reactions. In a few cases, unresolved emotions may persist, and a woman should seek professional counseling.

DECISION MAKING AND UNINTENDED PREGNANCY

When faced with an unintended pregnancy, women differ greatly in their approach to decision making (see the box "Personal Decisions About Abortion"). Unprotected sexual intercourse may be followed immediately by a vague sense of anxiety. When symptoms of pregnancy appear, some women—especially young women—respond with denial, ascribing the delayed menstruation and other signs to other causes. Several days or weeks may elapse before the woman finally has the pregnancy confirmed (a major cause of late abortions). After a positive test, women often feel a mixture of anxiety, depression, guilt, and anger, sometimes tinged with some anticipation and

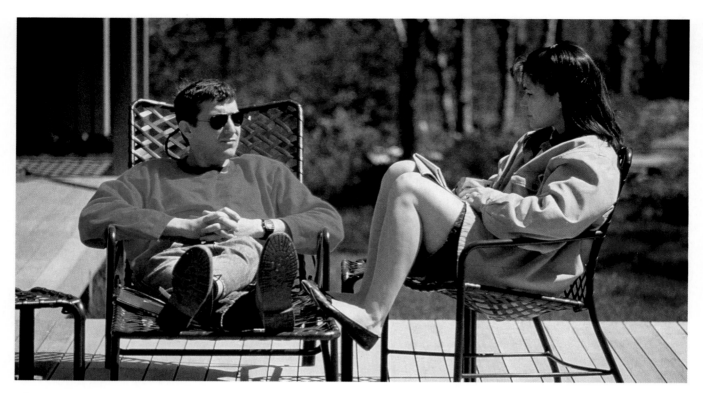

When an unintended pregnancy occurs, both partners can weigh important considerations and help choose an appropriate course of action.

delight. The actual decision making can vary widely. Some women calmly and resolutely make a choice within a very short time, while others, feeling panic and chaos, wrestle with the decision for several weeks. For some women, it is the first time in their lives that they feel unable to find a "right" answer and instead must settle for a "best" but difficult solution.

The response of a woman's partner can have a significant influence on how she experiences an unintended pregnancy. Men's emotional reactions can vary considerably. Some withdraw and choose to remain completely detached; others simply press for the most expedient solution (usually abortion). Still others feel very emotionally involved and wish to play an active role in decision making. Partners can be very helpful, both in weighing important considerations and in actually helping with the chosen course of action. Some couples find that an abortion experience draws them closer together; for others, it's the last straw in an already unstable relationship.

Parents can also be helpful. However, if there are serious disagreements, a stressful situation can become even more difficult. Over half the states have parental consent or notification requirements, although there are "judicial bypass" procedures in which a judge can decide either that a minor is mature and can give informed consent or that an abortion would be in her best interest.

No matter which of the available options to unintended pregnancy is chosen, a series of questions is likely to arise that must be addressed (see the "Personal Considerations" section earlier in the chapter). Although a prompt decision has critical advantages, careful deliberation is important. If there are strong feelings of uncertainty or ambivalence, hasty action should be avoided.

Having a supportive confidant, such as a partner, other close friend, or family member, can be very important in sorting out complex feelings. Along with listening and offering understanding and perspective, supportive people can help find suitable medical personnel and plan financial arrangements. Once a course of action has been chosen, a sense of moving ahead usually follows, and the next step toward resolution can occur.

PERSONAL INSIGHT   Women choose abortion for a wide variety of reasons: the pregnancy threatens their health, having a child would interfere with their educational or career plans, the pregnancy resulted from rape or incest, they can't afford to have a child, they don't want to be single parents, prenatal tests reveal fetal abnormalities, and so on. Under what circumstances (if any) do you think abortion is justified?

SUMMARY

The Abortion Issue

- The common use of the word *abortion* refers only to artificially induced expulsion of the fetus.

- Until the mid-1800s, abortion in the United States was legal if it took place before the 20th week of pregnancy; more restrictive laws passed by the various states remained in effect until they began to be invalidated by courts in the 1960s.

- The 1973 *Roe v. Wade* Supreme Court case devised new standards to govern abortion decisions; based on the trimesters of pregnancy, it limited a woman's choices as her pregnancy advanced.

- Although the Supreme Court continued to uphold its 1973 decision, it gave states further power to regulate abortion in *Webster v. Reproductive Health Services* and *Planned Parenthood of Southeastern Pennsylvania v. Casey*.

- The controversy between pro-life and pro-choice viewpoints focuses on the issue of when life begins. Pro-life groups believe that a fertilized egg is a human life from the moment of conception, and that any abortion is a murder. Pro-choice groups distinguish between stages of fetal development and argue that a woman should make the final decision regarding her pregnancy.

- Overall public opinion in the United States supports legal abortion in at least some circumstances and opposes overturning *Roe v. Wade*. Opinion changes according to individual situations.

- Most people agree that abortions performed late in pregnancy present personal, medical, philosophical, and social problems. The people who most commonly have late abortions include teenagers, poor women, women nearing menopause, and women who have waited for the results of genetic testing.

- The woman considering abortion must think about her own religious and moral beliefs, her long-range reactions, support from others, and the cost and availability of the procedure. The woman who decides against abortion must make decisions about keeping the child, perhaps being a single parent, or choosing adoption.

- Although the overall abortion rate rose during the 1970s, it leveled off around 1980 and has decreased somewhat since then.

Methods of Abortion

- Suction curettage, the preferred method of abortion until the 12th week of pregnancy, uses an electric pump to remove the uterine contents; the physician also scrapes the uterine lining with a metal curette.

- Menstrual extraction is the vacuum aspiration of uterine contents shortly after a missed period; incomplete abortion rates are high, and it is not commonly used in the United States.

- Dilation and evacuation (D & E) extends vacuum aspiration; additional instruments and medications, along with an anesthetic, are typically used. It is the most commonly used method between 13 and 15 weeks of pregnancy.

- Saline or prostaglandin instillation is sometimes used for abortions after the 15th week of pregnancy.

- Mifepristone, also known as RU-486 or the abortion pill, blocks the uterine absorption of progesterone, which causes the uterine lining and any fertilized egg to shed. It can be used up to 49 days following the last menstrual period.

Complications of Abortion

- Physical complications following abortion can be minimized by overall good patient health, early timing, use of the suction method and a local anesthetic, a well-trained physician, and follow-up care.

- The risk of postabortion complications is very low.

- Danger signals include fever, abdominal swelling or tenderness, heavy bleeding, vomiting or fainting, and delay in the resumption of menstruation.

- Psychological aftereffects of abortion vary with the individual. Many women go through a period of ambivalence; the strongest feelings usually occur immediately after the abortion. Having a supportive partner, friend, and/or family member can be helpful.

Decision Making and Unintended Pregnancy

- Women who face unintended pregnancy differ in the way they make decisions; some make their choice calmly and quickly, while others struggle for weeks. It is often a matter of finding the "best," not necessarily the "right," solution.

- The woman's partner can positively influence her experience of an unintended pregnancy, by providing support and helping with the decision. On the other hand, unintended pregnancies often mean the end of an unstable or unsatisfactory relationship.

- Many states mandate parental consent or notification in the case of a minor seeking an abortion.

1. Survey your classmates about their position on the abortion issue. How many people consider themselves pro-choice and how many pro-life? How strong are their opinions? What, if anything, might cause them to change their minds? Do opinions seem to depend on age, gender, or any other factor?

2. Now that you have information about abortion, reevaluate your contraceptive practices. If they aren't adequate to prevent unintended pregnancy, make any changes you consider necessary to protect yourself or your partner.

JOURNAL ENTRY

1. *Critical Thinking* Write a one-page essay presenting your personal opinion on the abortion issue. Include arguments to refute the points typically made by the opposing side. Then write an essay presenting a convincing case for the opposite position. Make sure your arguments are clearly stated and that you can defend them, where appropriate, with facts.

2. Describe in writing the feelings you would have if you were faced with a decision about abortion right now. Decide on a course of action, and then project the consequences of your decision into the future. Describe how your decision might affect the course of your life and how you might feel about it a month from now, a year from now, 10 years from now, and 20 years from now.

FOR MORE INFORMATION

Books

Carlson, K. J., S. A. Eisenstat, and T. Ziporyn. 1996. *Harvard Guide to Women's Health.* Cambridge, Mass.: Harvard University Press. *A comprehensive guide to women's health, including up-to-date information on abortion.*

Kaufmann, K. 1997. *The Abortion Resource Handbook.* New York: Simon & Schuster. *A resource for women seeking abortion, with information on legal, medical, and emotional aspects of abortion.*

National Abortion and Reproductive Rights Action League Foundation. 1999. *Who Decides? A State-by-State Review of Abortion and Reproductive Rights.* Washington, D.C.: NARAL Foundation. *An in-depth annual review of the legal status of reproductive rights in the United States.*

Pojman, L., and F. Beckwith, eds. 1998. *Abortion Controversy: 25 Years after Roe vs. Wade, A Reader,* 2nd ed. Belmont, Calif.: Wadsworth. *Includes academic articles from all perspectives of the abortion debate and abridged versions of key court decisions.*

Rein, M. L., et al., eds. 1998. *Abortion: An Eternal Social and Moral Issue.* Wylie, Tex.: Information Plus. *A brief reference outlining the legal, political, and ethical issues relating to abortion.*

Organizations and Web Sites

Abortion Law Homepage. Includes an overview of the background and state of U.S. abortion law, including the text of major legal decisions.

   http://hometown.aol.com/abtrbng

The Alan Guttmacher Institute. Publishes books and fact sheets on reproductive health issues; their journal, *The Guttmacher Report on Public Policy,* provides timely analysis of national reproductive health policy debates.

   120 Wall St.
   New York, NY 10005
   212-248-1111
   http://www.agi-usa.org

Centers for Disease Control and Prevention Automated Reproductive Health Information Line. Provides information about rates of abortion and teen pregnancy.

   888-232-2306

National Abortion and Reproductive Rights Action League. Provides information on the politics of the pro-choice movement.

   1156 15th St., N.W., Suite 700
   Washington, DC 20005
   202-973-3000
   http://www.naral.org/home.html

National Adoption Information Clearinghouse. Provides resources on all aspects of adoption.

   330 C Street, SW
   Washington, DC 20447
   888-251-0075
   http://www.calib.com/naic

National Right to Life Committee. Provides information on alternatives to abortion and the politics of the pro-life movement.

   419 Seventh St., N.W., Suite 500
   Washington, DC 20004
   202-626-8800
   http://www.nrlc.org

Planned Parenthood Federation of America. Provides information on family planning, contraception, and abortion, and provides counseling services.

   810 Seventh St.
   New York, NY 10019
   800-669-0156 (to order publications)
   800-230-PLAN (for a list of health centers)
   http://www.plannedparenthood.org

Population Council Reproductive Health Products Development Program. Information on the development and testing of mifepristone from the holder of U.S. rights to the drug.

   http://www.popcouncil.org/rhpdev/rhpdev.html

SELECTED BIBLIOGRAPHY

Alan Guttmacher Institute. 1999. *The Status of Major Abortion-Related Laws and Policies in the United States, December 1998* (retrieved February 20, 1999; http://www.agi-usa.org/pubs/abort_law_status.html).

Alan Guttmacher Institute. 1998. *Facts in Brief: Induced Abortion.* New York: Alan Guttmacher Institute.

Alan Guttmacher Institute. 1997. Parental involvement in minors' abortions remains highly salient issue. *State Reproductive Health Monitor* 8(1).

Annas, G. J. 1998. Partial-birth abortion, Congress, and the Constitution. *New England Journal of Medicine* 339(4): 279–283.

Bankole, A., S. Susheela, and T. Haas. 1998. Reasons why women have induced abortions: Evidence from 27 countries. *International Family Planning Perspectives* 24(3): 117–127, 152.

Carbonell, J. L., et al. 1998. Oral methotrexate and vaginal misoprostol for early abortion. *Contraception* 57(2): 83–88.

Carlson, M. 1998. The passive majority: What good is the right to an abortion if extremists can make it unavailable? *Time* 152(1): 60.

Centers for Disease Control and Prevention. 1998. Abortion surveillance: Preliminary analysis—United States, 1996. *Morbidity and Mortality Weekly Report* 47(47): 1025–1028, 1035.

Cohen, S. A. 1998. 25 years after Roe: New technological parameters for an old debate. *The Guttmacher Report on Public Policy* 1(1).

Coleman, P. K., and E. S. Nelson. 1999. Abortion attitudes as determinants of perceptions regarding male involvement in abortion decisions. *Journal of America College Health* 47(4):164–171.

Ellertson, C. 1997. Mandatory parental involvement in minors' abortions: Effects of the laws in Minnesota, Missouri, and Indiana. *American Journal of Public Health* 87(8): 1367–1374.

Grimes, D. A. 1998. The continuing need for late abortions. *Journal of the American Medical Association* 280(8): 747–750.

Henshaw, S. K., S. Singh, and T. Haas. 1999. The incidence of abortion worldwide. *International Family Planning Perspectives* 25: S30–S38.

Henshaw, S. K. 1998. Abortion incidence and services in the United States, 1995–1996. *Family Planning Perspectives* 30(6): 263–270, 287.

Henshaw, S. K. 1998. Unintended pregnancy in the United States. *Family Planning Perspectives* 30(1): 24–29, 46.

Jamieson, M. A., S. P. Hertweck, and J. S. Sanfilippo. 1999. Emergency contraception: Lack of awareness among patients presenting for pregnancy termination. *Journal of Pediatric and Adolescent Gynecology* 12(1): 11–15.

Joyce, T., et al. 1997. The impact of Mississippi's mandatory delay law on abortions and births. *Journal of the American Medical Association* 278(8): 653–658.

Lao, T. T., and L. F. Ho. 1998. Induced abortion is not a cause of subsequent preterm delivery in teenage pregnancies. *Human Reproduction* 13(3): 758–761.

Leo, J. 1998. Taking a right turn. *U.S. News and World Report* 124(7): 13.

Major, B., et al. 1998. Personal resilience, cognitive appraisals, and coping: An integrative model of adjustment to abortion. *Journal of Personality and Social Psychology* 74(3): 735–752.

Melbye, M., et al. 1997. Induced abortion and the risk of breast cancer. *New England Journal of Medicine* 336(2): 81–85.

National Abortion and Reproductive Rights Action League. 1999. *Who Decides? A State-by-State Review of Abortion and Reproductive Rights: Introduction and 1999 Analysis of Key Findings* (retrieved February 20, 1999; http://www.naral.org/publications/who99analysis.html).

National Opinion Research Center. 1998. *Public Opinion on Abortion* (retrieved November 11, 1998; http://www.norc.uchicago.edu/library/abortion.htm).

Parazzini, F., et al. 1998. Induced abortion in the first trimester of pregnancy and risk of miscarriage. *British Journal of Obstetrics and Gynaecology* 105(4): 418–421.

Planned Parenthood. 1999. *State Laws Restricting Access to Abortion 26 Years After* Roe v. Wade (retrieved February 19, 1999; http://www.plannedparenthood.org/library/ABORTION/StateLaws.html).

Planned Parenthood. 1998. *Fact Sheet: Medical Abortion Using Methotrexate and Misoprostol* (retrieved November 13, 1998; http://www.plannedparenthood.org/library/ABORTION/methotrexate.html).

Population Council. 1998. *U.S. Mifepristone Clinical Trial: Summary of Findings* (retrieved November 13, 1998; http://www.popcouncil.org/rhpdev/mifepristone_ustrial.html).

Rahman, A., L. Katzive, and S. K. Henshaw. 1998. A global review of laws on induced abortion, 1985–1997. *International Family Planning Perspectives* 24(2): 56–64.

Randal, J., and L. French. 1998. Mifepristone and misoprostol for termination of early pregnancy. *Journal of Family Practice* 47(2): 96–97.

Russell, S. 1998. U.S. abortions safer but less accessible. *San Francisco Chronicle,* January 22.

Smith, J. P. 1998. Risky choices: The dangers of teens using self-induced abortion attempts. *Journal of Pediatric Health Care* 12(3): 147–151.

Spitz, I. M., et al. 1998. Early pregnancy termination with mifepristone and misoprostol in the United States. *New England Journal of Medicine* 338 (18): 1241–1247.

U.S. Food and Drug Administration. 1996. *FDA Issues Approvable Letter for Mifepristone* (retrieved November 13, 1998; http://www.fda.gov/bbs/topics/ANSWERS/ ANS00758.html)

Waldman, S., et al. 1998. Abortions in America: So many women have them, so few talk about them. *U.S. News and World Report* 124(2): 20–25.

Westfall, J. M., A. O'Brien-Gonzales, and G. Barley. 1998. Update in early medical and surgical abortion. *Journal of Women's Health* 7(8): 991–995.

Winikoff, B., et al. 1998. Acceptability and feasibility of early pregnancy termination by mifepristone-misoprostol. Results of a large multicenter trial in the United States. *Archives of Family Medicine* 7(4): 360–366.

World Health Organization Division of Reproductive Health. 1998. *Fact Sheet: Address Unsafe Abortion.* Geneva: World Health Organization (WHD 98.10).

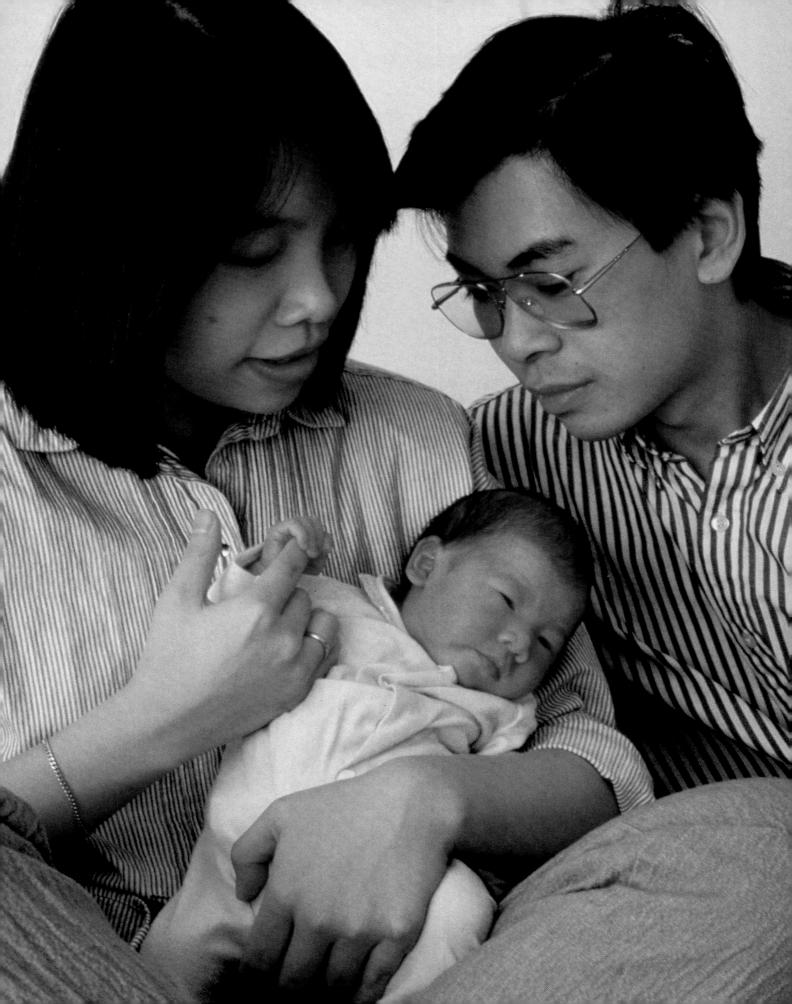

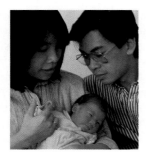

LEARNING OBJECTIVES

After reading this chapter, you should be able to:

- List key issues to consider when deciding about parenthood.
- Explain the process of conception, and describe the most common causes and treatments for infertility.
- Describe the physical and emotional changes a pregnant woman typically experiences.
- Discuss the stages of fetal development.
- List the important components of good prenatal care.
- Describe the process of labor and delivery.

Pregnancy and Childbirth 8

TEST YOUR KNOWLEDGE

1. What is the approximate annual cost of raising a child?
   a. $3,500
   b. $8,500
   c. $15,000

2. Following conception, approximately how many weeks does it take for major body structures to form in a fetus?
   a. 6
   b. 13
   c. 26

3. What is the leading cause of female infertility?
   a. hormone imbalance
   b. growths in the uterus
   c. exposure to radiation
   d. blocked fallopian tubes caused by STDs

4. Adequate intake of the vitamin folic acid before conception and in the early weeks of pregnancy can reduce the risk of birth defects.
   True or false?

5. The position in which babies sleep has a significant impact on their risk of dying from sudden infant death syndrome (SIDS).
   True or false?

Answers

1. b. Depending on a variety of factors, including family income and region of residence, it costs a little more than $8,500 per year to raise a child, for a total of about $153,900 to age 18.

2. b. By the end of the first trimester (week 13), all major body structures are formed, and some systems, including the nervous and circulatory systems, are functioning. The fetus is about 4 inches long and weighs 1 ounce.

3. d. If left untreated, the STDs gonorrhea and chlamydia can lead to tubal scarring and blockage. Leading causes of male infertility include low sperm count and poor sperm motility.

4. True. It is recommended that all reproductive age women consume 400 µg of folic acid from fortified foods and/or supplements each day to reduce the risk of spina bifida and other neural tube defects.

5. True. The rate of SIDS in the United States has dropped by 43% since 1992, when an education campaign called "Back to Sleep" was implemented to teach parents and caregivers to put babies to bed on their back instead of their stomach.

Deciding whether to become a parent is one of the most important decisions you will ever make. Having a child changes your life forever, and deciding not to have children has equally far-reaching implications. Yet many people approach this momentous decision with only the vaguest notion of what is involved in pregnancy and childbirth. An estimated half of the approximately 3.9 million babies born every year in the United States are from unintentional pregnancies.

Today, with changing cultural expectations and increasingly sophisticated contraceptive technology, you have more choice about becoming a parent than people have ever had before. Until recently it was expected that virtually every married couple would have children. Now you can choose whether, when, and how you want to have a child. And you don't have to be part of a couple to have a child; the number of women choosing to have children on their own has risen dramatically. Almost one-third of all U.S. births are to unmarried women.

Pregnancy is a relatively comfortable experience for most women and the outcome predictably happy. Yet for some, problems occur. Some couples who have always planned for children may find that they are unable to conceive; others may face complications during pregnancy. Some problems are impossible to prevent, but you can make choices that minimize the risks and maximize the benefits for yourself, your partner, and your children.

Having a child is one of the most arduous, important, and rewarding enterprises that human beings undertake. The more you know about it—about conception and pregnancy, fetal development and prenatal care, childbirth and parenting—the more capable you will be of making intelligent, informed decisions about it. This chapter presents information you can use both now and later in your life to make the choices about pregnancy and childbirth that are right for you.

PREPARATION FOR PARENTHOOD

Before you decide whether or when to become a parent, you'll want to consider your suitability and readiness. If you make the decision to have a child, there are actions you can take before the pregnancy begins to help ensure a healthy outcome for all.

Deciding to Become a Parent

Many factors have to be taken into account when you are considering parenthood. Following are some questions you should ask yourself and some issues you should consider when making this decision. Some issues are relevant to both men and women; others apply only to women.

- *Your physical health and your age.* Are you in reasonably good health? If not, can you improve your health by changing your lifestyle, perhaps by modifying your diet or giving up cigarettes, alcohol, or drugs? Do you have physical conditions, such as overweight or diabetes, that will require extra care and medical attention during pregnancy? Do you or your partner have a family history of genetic problems that a baby might inherit? Does your age place you or your baby at risk? (Teenagers and women over 35 have a higher incidence of some problems.) Improving your health before pregnancy (discussed in the next section) can help ensure a trouble-free pregnancy and a healthy baby.

- *Your financial circumstances.* Can you afford a child? Will your health insurance cover the costs of pregnancy, delivery, and medical attention for mother and baby before and after the birth, including physicians' fees and hospital costs? Supplies for the baby are expensive, too—diapers, bedding, cribs, strollers, car seats, clothing, food and medical supplies, and child care. Depending on a variety of factors, including age of child, number of children, family income, and region of residence, the annual cost of raising a child averages about $8,550. The cost of raising a child to age 18 averages about $153,900 per child for a middle-class family with two children. If one parent has quit his or her job to care for the child or is on parental leave, the family must live on one income.

- *Your relationship with your partner.* Are you in a stable relationship, and do both of you want a child? Are your views compatible on such issues as child-rearing goals, the distribution of responsibility for the child, and work and housework obligations?

- *Your educational, career, and child care plans.* Have you completed as much of your education as you want right now? Have you established yourself in a career, if that is something you want to do? Have you investigated parental leave and company-sponsored child care? Do you and your partner agree on child care arrangements, and does such child care exist in your community? Some experts advise against full-time child care for babies under 1 year of age, but studies have found no permanent adverse effects of early child care on child development. Some people consider the child care issue the most difficult in parenting.

- *Your emotional readiness for parenthood.* Do you have the emotional discipline and stamina to care for and nurture an infant? Are you prepared to have a helpless baby completely dependent on you all day and all night? Are you willing to change your lifestyle to provide the best conditions for a baby's development, both before and after birth?

- *Your social support system.* Do you have a network of family and friends who will help you with the baby? Are there community resources you can call on for additional assistance? A family's social support system is one of the most important factors affecting their ability to adjust to a baby and cope with new responsibilities.

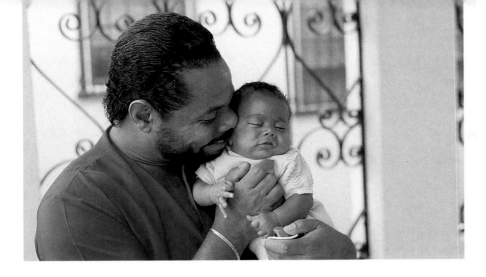

Having a child is one of the most important and rewarding experiences a person can undertake. Careful preparation can help maximize the benefits for both parents and children.

• *Your personal qualities, attitudes toward children, and aptitude for parenting.* Do you like infants, young children, and adolescents? Do you think time with children is time well spent? Do you feel good enough about yourself to love and respect others? Do you have safe ways of handling anger, frustration, and impatience?

• *Your philosophical or religious beliefs.* Some people question the value of bringing more people into an already overcrowded world. They feel that human beings have already fulfilled the biblical directive to be fruitful and multiply, and they choose not to have children.

> **PERSONAL INSIGHT** Do you want to have children? What is the basis for your feelings and desires? Can you distinguish personal reasons from cultural expectations? What do you think people would think of you if you decided not to have children?

Preconception Care

The birth of a healthy baby depends in part on the mother's overall wellness *before* conception. The U.S. Public Health Service recommends that all women receive health care to help them prepare for pregnancy. **Preconception care** should include an assessment of health risks, the promotion of healthy lifestyle behaviors, and any treatments necessary to reduce risk. Following are some of the questions, tests, and treatments you and your partner may encounter during preconception care:

1. Do you have any preexisting medical conditions, such as diabetes, epilepsy, asthma, high blood pressure, or anemia? There may be things you can do to improve the chances of a trouble-free pregnancy and a positive outcome.

2. Are you taking any prescription or over-the-counter medications? Some medications can harm the **fetus,** so you may need to change or discontinue their use to help ensure a healthy pregnancy.

3. Have you had any prior problems with pregnancy and delivery, including miscarriage, premature birth, ectopic pregnancy, or delivery complications? Some problems are due to physical or hormonal difficulties that can be treated.

4. Does your age place you at risk for infertility or health problems during pregnancy, or does it increase the likelihood that your baby may have a genetic or chromosomal disorder? Pregnant teenagers may need special nutritional counseling during pregnancy to meet the needs of their own growing body as well as the baby's. Women under 20 and over 35 have babies with a higher incidence of Down syndrome; genetic testing and counseling may be indicated. Older women may also find that it is harder to become pregnant.

5. Do you smoke, drink, or take other drugs? These habits are dangerous for the baby, and a health care professional can recommend treatment programs. If you are a heavy consumer of caffeine, cutting back before and during pregnancy is recommended.

6. Do you currently have any infections, or do you need any additional vaccinations? Women at risk for hepatitis B or who are not immunized against rubella (German measles) should be vaccinated. Women not immune to parvovirus B19, which causes "fifth disease," or toxoplasmosis, a disease transmitted by animals, especially cats, can find

preconception care Health care in preparation for pregnancy.	**TERMS**

fetus The developmental stage of a human from the 9th week after conception to the moment of birth.

Genes carry the chemical instructions that determine the development of hundreds of individual traits in every human being. Many of these traits are visible—will the baby have blue eyes or brown, be tall or short, be fat or thin? But some important determinants are invisible, such as whether a genetic disease will be passed from the parents to the child.

Two genes, one from each parent, determine a given characteristic. Each of these genes is either more powerful, *dominant*, or less powerful, *recessive*. Dominant genes are expressed in the offspring even if the child inherits only one. Diseases that are carried by dominant genes seldom skip a generation; anyone who carries the gene will probably get the disease.

Recessive genes are expressed as traits only if *both* genes in the pair are positive for the trait. Many common diseases caused by recessive genes occur disproportionately in certain ethnic groups. Prospective parents who come from the same ethnic group can be tested for any recessive diseases found in that group. If both are carriers, each of their children will have about a 25% chance of developing the disease.

Learning all you can about diseases that affect members of your ethnic group can be a lifesaver. Not only can you learn about the risk to your children, you may also discover there are things you can do to manage the disease and reduce its impact.

• *Sickle-cell disease* affects about 1 out of every 500 African Americans and 1 out of every 1200 Latinos. In this disease, the red blood cells, which carry oxygen to the body's tissues, change shape; the normal doughnut-shaped cells become sickle-shaped. These altered cells carry less oxygen and clog small blood vessels.

People who inherit one gene for sickle-cell disease (about 1 in 12 African Americans) experience only mild symptoms; those with two genes become severely, often fatally, ill. Interestingly, people who inherit one sickle-cell gene are far more resistant to malaria than are those without the gene, leading geneticists to conclude that the sickle-cell trait might have developed in tropical regions as an adaptation to the widespread presence of malaria.

If you are at risk for sickle-cell disease, you can:

1. Get genetic counseling to help determine your family's genetic pattern and the degree of risk to you and your potential offspring.

2. Take particular care to reduce stress and respond to minor infections, since red blood cells become sickle-shaped during periods of stress on the body.

3. Get regular checkups and appropriate treatment.

• *Tay-Sachs disease,* another recessive disorder, occurs annually in approximately 1 out of every 1000 Jews of Eastern European ancestry. People with Tay-Sachs disease are unable to metabolize fat properly; as a result, the brain and other nerve tissues deteriorate. Affected children begin by showing weaknesses in their movements and eventually develop blindness and seizures. This disease is fatal, and death usually occurs by age 3 or 4.

If you are of Eastern European Jewish ancestry and are planning to have children, genetic counseling will help you assess the chances that you and your mate will produce a child with Tay-Sachs disease.

• *Cystic fibrosis* occurs in 1 in every 2000 Caucasians per year; about 1 in 20 carry one copy of the cystic fibrosis gene. Because essential enzymes of the pancreas are deficient, thick mucus impairs functioning in the lungs and intestinal tracts of people with this disease. The disease is often fatal in early childhood, but medical treatments are increasingly effective in reducing symptoms and prolonging life. In some cases, symptoms do not appear until early adulthood.

out how to prevent infection during pregnancy (both these diseases can cause miscarriage). Testing for tuberculosis and certain STDs can ensure treatment prior to pregnancy. (See Chapters 17 and 18 for more information about STDs and other infectious diseases.)

7. Are you at risk for HIV infection (see Chapter 18)? If so, you should be tested before you or your partner becomes pregnant. Babies born to HIV-infected mothers can become infected.

8. Do you eat a balanced diet? Are you particularly underweight or overweight? Do you suffer from an eating disorder? Do you have special dietary habits, such as being a vegetarian? Nutritional counseling can help you create a plan for healthy eating, before and during pregnancy. Your physician may also prescribe multivitamins, particularly folic acid. The U.S. Public Health Service recommends that all women of childbearing age take extra folic acid because during the first few weeks of pregnancy it reduces the risk of neural tube defects such as spina bifida (see p. 200).

9. Were you a diethylstilbestrol (DES) baby? Daughters born to women who were given DES during pregnancy to prevent miscarriage—a common practice from the 1940s to the early 1970s—are at risk for a variety of problems with conception and pregnancy. DES daughters may need special monitoring and care to identify and treat problems as soon as they develop. (For more on DES, see Chapter 16.)

10. Do twins or multiple births run in either your or your partner's family? If so, this tendency may increase the likelihood of a multiple birth.

11. Do either you or your partner have a family history of any genetic disease? Have you or any family

If there is a history of cystic fibrosis in your family and you plan to have children, genetic tests and counseling can help in assessing the risk to your prospective offspring.

• *Thalassemia* is a blood disease found most often among Italians, Greeks, and, to a lesser extent, African Americans and Asians. When inherited from one parent, this form of anemia is mild; when two genes are present, the disease is severe and can cause fetal death or, after birth, a condition called Cooley's anemia. Children with this condition require repeated blood transfusions, eventually resulting in a damaging iron buildup. New medical interventions, such as genetic engineering, bone marrow transplants, and chemicals that bind with excess iron and remove it from the body, offer promise.

If you are at risk of carrying thalassemia, you can:

1. Get regular checkups and monitor your health for symptoms.
2. Learn symptom management.
3. Get genetic counseling to assess the risk to your offspring.

• *Lactose intolerance* is a condition affecting about 30–50 million Americans, including a majority of Asian Americans, Native Americans, and African Americans. Although all humans are dependent on milk in the early years, by about age 4 many lose the ability to absorb lactose, the chief nutrient in milk. This lactose intolerance results from an absence of lactase, an enzyme that permits the efficient digestion of milk. When lactose-intolerant people ingest more than 1–2 servings of milk or dairy products, they suffer from gas pains and diarrhea. Studies show that lactose intolerance is especially prevalent in cultures where milk is relatively unimportant after weaning, suggesting that evolutionary adaptation has played a role in its development.

If you suspect lactose intolerance, see your physician for a test. If you are lactose intolerant, use trial and error to determine how many servings of dairy products you can consume without symptoms. If you react to very small amounts of lactose, try lactose-reduced products or lactase drops or tablets.

• *Hemochromatosis* ("iron overload") affects about 1 in 250 Americans; most at risk are people of Northern European (especially Irish), Mediterranean, and Hispanic descent. In people with hemochromatosis, the body absorbs and stores up to 10 times the normal amount of iron. Over time, iron deposits form in the joints, liver, heart, and pancreas. If untreated, hemochromatosis can cause organ failure and death.

Early symptoms are often vague, but early detection and treatment are necessary to prevent damage; routine testing may soon be recommended for all Americans. Treatment involves reducing iron stores by removing blood from the body (a process also known as phlebotomy or "bloodletting").

• *Diabetes* is 55% more common among African Americans than white Americans; Native Americans and Latinos are also at increased risk. Asians have a predisposition for diabetes that may surface with American diets. See Chapter 14 for more on the many steps you can take if you are at risk for diabetes.

• *Osteoporosis* is more likely to develop in light-skinned people of Northern European ancestry than in dark-skinned people. This condition is a gradual loss of bone mass that can result in multiple fractures, crippling, deformity, and constant pain. See Chapter 12 for a detailed discussion of how to reduce your risk of osteoporosis.

Other health problems that have a hereditary component and that disproportionately affect certain ethnic groups include high blood pressure, alcoholism, and certain types of cancer.

member had a child with a birth defect or mental impairment? Genetic testing and counseling can determine whether you are a carrier for a specific disease, what the effects of the disease would be, and whether a baby you conceive can be tested prenatally. Members of certain ethnic groups are at higher risk for genetic disorders that are more prevalent within their groups than in the general population. For more information on these disorders, refer to the box "Ethnicity and Genetic Diseases."

Additional tests or changes in behavior may be recommended if you have recently traveled outside the United States; if you work with chemicals, radiation, or toxic substances; if you participate in physically demanding or hazardous activities or occupations; or if you face significant psychosocial risks, including homelessness, an unsafe home environment, or mental illness.

UNDERSTANDING FERTILITY

Conceiving a child is a highly complex process. Although many couples conceive readily, others can testify to the difficulties that can be encountered.

Conception

The process of **conception** involves the **fertilization** of an egg (ovum) from a woman by a sperm from a man (Figure 8-1). Every month during a woman's fertile years,

conception The fusion of ovum and sperm, resulting in a fertilized egg.

fertilization The initiation of biological reproduction: the union of the nucleus of an egg cell with the nucleus of a sperm cell.

TERMS

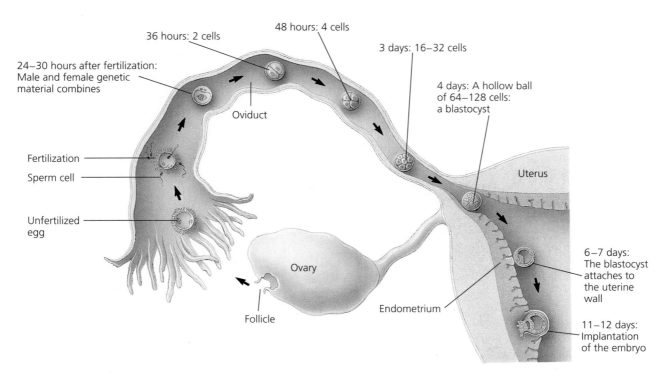

Figure 8-1 Fertilization, and early development of the embryo. The unfertilized egg is released from an ovarian follicle into the oviduct, where it is fertilized by a sperm cell. As the fertilized egg moves through the oviduct toward the uterus, the genetic material from the egg and sperm combine, and the egg begins to divide. When the egg reaches the uterus, it is in the form of a hollow ball of cells called a blastocyst, which becomes implanted in the endometrium.

her body prepares itself for conception and pregnancy. In one of her **ovaries** an egg ripens and is released from its **follicle.** The egg, about the size of a pinpoint, travels through an **oviduct,** or **fallopian tube,** to the **uterus,** in 3–4 days. The lining of the uterus, or **endometrium,** has already thickened for the implantation of a **fertilized egg,** or zygote. If the egg is not fertilized, it lasts about 24 hours and then disintegrates. It is expelled along with the uterine lining during menstruation.

Sperm cells are produced in the man's **testes** and ejaculated from his penis into the woman's vagina during sexual intercourse (except in cases of artificial insemination or assisted reproduction; see p. 191). Sperm cells are much smaller than eggs. The typical ejaculate contains millions of sperm, but only a few complete the journey through the uterus and up the fallopian tube to the egg. Many sperm cells do not survive the acidic environment of the vagina. Once through the cervix and into the uterus, many sperm cells are diverted to the wrong oviduct or get stuck along the way. Of those that reach the egg, only one will penetrate the hard outer layer of the egg. As sperm approach the egg, they release enzymes that soften the outer layer of the egg. Enzymes from hundreds of sperm must be released in order for the egg's outer layers to soften enough to allow one sperm cell to penetrate. The first sperm cell that bumps into a spot that is soft enough can swim into the egg cell. It then merges with the nucleus of the egg, and fertilization occurs. The sperm's tail, its means of locomotion, gets stuck in the outer membrane and drops off, leaving the sperm head inside the egg. The egg then releases a chemical that makes it impenetrable by other sperm.

The ovum carries the hereditary characteristics of the mother and her ancestors; sperm cells carry the hereditary characteristics of the father and his ancestors. Each parent cell—egg or sperm—contains 23 chromosomes, each of which contains **genes,** packages of chemical instructions for the developing baby. Genes specify the infant's sex; whether it will tend to be short, tall, thin, fat, healthy, or sickly; and hundreds of other characteristics. Genes provide the blueprint for a unique individual (see the box "Creating a Family Health Tree," p. 190).

As soon as fertilization occurs, the zygote starts to undergo the cell division that begins the growth process. About 3–4 days after fertilization, the cluster of 16 to 32 cells enters the uterus. Some 6–7 days after fertilization, the cluster attaches itself to the uterine wall, and 4–5 days after that, it becomes implanted in the endometrium.

The usual course of events is that one egg and one sperm unite to produce one fertilized egg and one baby.

But if the ovaries release two (or more) eggs during ovulation, and if both eggs are fertilized, twins will develop. These twins will be no more alike than siblings from different pregnancies, because each will have come from a different fertilized egg. Twins who develop this way are referred to as **fraternal twins;** they may be the same sex or different sexes. Twins can also develop from the division of a single fertilized egg into two cells that develop separately. Because these babies share all genetic material, they will be **identical twins.**

Infertility

Although the main concern for many women and men, especially if they are young and single, is how *not* to get pregnant, the reverse is true for millions of couples who have difficulty conceiving. **Infertility** is usually defined as the inability to conceive after trying for a year or more. It affects about 6 million couples—10% of the reproductive age population of the United States. Over a million couples seek treatment for infertility each year. Although the focus is often on women, 50% of the factors contributing to infertility are male, and in about 15% of infertile couples, both partners have problems. Therefore, it is important that each individual be evaluated.

Female Infertility   The leading cause of infertility in women is blocked fallopian tubes. This blockage is usually the result of *pelvic inflammatory disease (PID),* a serious complication of several different sexually transmitted diseases; most occurrences are associated with untreated cases of chlamydia or gonorrhea. Over 1.5 million cases of PID are treated each year, but physicians estimate that half may go untreated because of an absence of symptoms. Other causes of PID include unsterile abortions, abdominal surgery, and certain types of older IUDs. Surgery may restore fertility if the damage is not too severe.

The second leading cause of infertility in women is *endometriosis.* In this disease, endometrial (uterine) tissue grows outside the uterus, usually in the ovaries, the oviducts (where it may cause blockage), and/or the abdominal cavity. This tissue may bleed each month in response to the hormonal stimulation that controls menstruation. Hormonal therapy and surgery are used to treat endometriosis.

Other causes of infertility in women include benign growths in the uterus and hormonal imbalances that prevent ovulation. Some women develop an allergic response that kills their partner's sperm. Exposure to toxic chemicals or radiation appears to reduce fertility, as does cigarette smoking. Evidence also indicates that the daughters of mothers who took DES during pregnancy have a significantly higher infertility rate. Beginning around age 30, a woman's fertility naturally begins to decline, and by age 35, about one out of four women is infertile.

Male Infertility   The leading causes of infertility among men are low sperm count, lack of sperm motility (the ability to move spontaneously), misshapen sperm, and blocked passageways between the testes and the urethra. Smoking may cause reduced sperm counts and abnormal sperm. The sons of mothers who took DES may have increased sperm abnormalities and fertility problems. Certain prescription and illegal drugs also affect the number of sperm. Large doses of marijuana, for example, cause lower sperm counts and suppress certain reproductive hormones. Other causes of sperm problems include injury to the testicles, infection (especially from mumps during adulthood), birth defects, or subjecting the testes to high temperatures. Some of these problems can be resolved through treatment or by removing the causative factor.

Some studies indicate that sperm counts worldwide have dropped by as much as 50% over the past 30 years. Evidence suggests that toxic substances such as lead, chemical pollutants, and radiation are responsible for this decrease. Recent research has also focused on a class of chemicals known as *endocrine disrupters*—substances found widely in the environment that mimic or interfere with the body's hormones, thereby causing problems with reproduction and development. Examples of hormone mimics include dioxin, PCBs, DDT, and compounds used in some plastics. Animal studies have linked prenatal exposure to endocrine disrupters with feminized genitalia and other reproductive problems in male offspring. Scientists do not yet know, however, what effects endocrine disrupters may have on human health and fertility.

TERMS

ovary   One of the two female reproductive organs that produce ova (eggs) and sex hormones.

follicle   One of many saclike structures on the surface of an ovary in which eggs mature.

oviduct (fallopian tube)   One of two passages through which eggs travel from the ovaries to the uterus; the site of fertilization.

uterus   The hollow, thick-walled, muscular organ in which the fertilized egg develops; the womb.

endometrium   The mucous membrane that forms the inner lining of the cavity of the uterus.

fertilized egg   The egg after penetration by a sperm; a zygote.

testis   One of two male reproductive organs; the testes are the site of sperm production.

gene   A package of chemical instructions, or hereditary material, that defines an individual's unique traits.

fraternal twins   Twins who develop from separate fertilized eggs; not genetically identical.

identical twins   Twins who develop from the division of a single zygote; genetically identical.

infertility   The inability to conceive after trying for a year or more.

The genetic inheritance that each of us receives from our parents—and that our children receive from us—contains more than just physical characteristics, such as eye and hair color. Heredity also contributes to our risk of developing certain diseases and disorders.

For certain uncommon illnesses such as hemophilia and sickle-cell disease, heredity is the primary cause; if your parents pass on the necessary genes, you'll get the disease. But heredity plays a subtler role in many other diseases, which are caused at least in part by environmental influences such as infection, cancer-causing chemicals, or an artery-clogging diet. While your genes alone will not produce those diseases, they can determine how susceptible you are. Researchers have found a genetic influence in many common disorders, including heart disease, diabetes, depression, alcoholism, and certain forms of cancer.

Knowing that a specific disease runs in your family can save your life. It allows you to watch for early warning signs and get screening tests more often than you otherwise would. Changing health habits, too, can be valuable for people with a family history of certain diseases. A smoker with a close relative who had lung cancer, for example, is 14 times more likely to develop lung cancer than other smokers.

In general, the more relatives with a genetically transmitted disease and the closer they are to you, the greater your risk. However, nongenetic factors—such as health habits—can also play a role. Signs of strong hereditary influence include early onset of the disease, appearance of the disease largely or exclusively on one side of the family, onset of the same disease at the same age in more than one relative, and developing the disease despite good health habits.

You can put together a simple family health tree by compiling a few key facts on your primary relatives: siblings, parents, aunts and uncles, and grandparents. Those facts include the date of birth, major diseases, health-related conditions and habits, and, for deceased relatives, the date and cause of death. (For a free family-medical-history form and guidelines on what to ask, contact The March of Dimes; see For More Information

at the end of the chapter.) Once you've collected the information you want, create a tree, using the example here as a guide. Then show your tree to your physician to get a full picture of what the information means for you or your children's health.

A Sample Family Health Tree and What It Means

In this sample family tree, the prostate cancer that killed the man's father means that he should be tested for a prostate tumor at a younger age and more frequently than is generally recommended. His sisters may need to have earlier, more frequent mammograms because of their mother's breast cancer. If they're overweight, they can reduce their risk by losing weight.

One grandmother and one uncle each died of a heart attack. There are several reasons not to worry too much about that: The two relatives were from different sides of the family; both had the attack at a relatively old age; both had two other major risk factors for coronary heart disease—smoking and either diabetes or obesity; and neither of the man's parents had any apparent heart trouble. He should check to see whether either relative had highly elevated cholesterol levels, a possible sign of familial hypercholesterolemia.

The colon cancer that struck another grandmother and uncle is a different story. Two factors suggest a possible hereditary link: They were mother and son, and they both developed the disease at nearly the same comparatively young age. So the man should be screened early and often.

Finally, alcoholism seems to run in the family. The man should be aware that such a history could indicate a hereditary susceptibility to the problem, though the habit might simply have been passed down by example.

SOURCES: Text and art from What's lurking in your family tree? 1996. *Consumer Reports on Health,* September. Copyright 1996 by Consumers Union of U.S., Inc., Yonkers, NY 10703-1057. Reprinted by permission from *Consumer Reports on Health,* Sept. 1996. No photocopying or reproduction permitted. To order a subscription, call 1-800-234-1645.

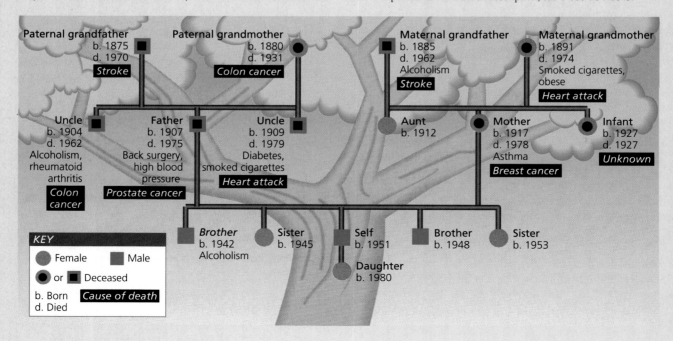

Treating Infertility Some kinds of infertility can be treated; others cannot. About 80% of infertile couples receive a physical diagnosis for their condition; for the remaining 20%, the cause of the infertility remains unexplained. Many techniques are available to help infertile couples conceive a child (see the box "Infertility and Reproductive Technology"). However, most are expensive and emotionally draining, and their success is uncertain. Some infertile couples choose not to try to have children, while others turn to adoption. One measure you can take now to avoid infertility is to protect yourself against STDs, and to treat promptly and completely any disease you do contract.

Emotional Responses to Infertility Couples who seek treatment for infertility have often already confronted the possibility of not being able to become biological parents. Many infertile couples feel they have lost control over a major area of their lives. They may lose perspective on the rest of their lives as they focus more and more on the reasons for their infertility and on treatment. Infertile couples may need to set their own limits on how much treatment they are willing to undergo. Support groups for infertile couples can provide help in this difficult situation, but there are few easy answers to infertility. If treatment is unsuccessful, couples must mourn the loss of the children they will never bear. They must make some kind of decision about their future, whether to pursue plans for adoption or another treatment, or to adjust to childlessness and go on with their lives.

> **PERSONAL INSIGHT** How do you think you would feel if you discovered you were infertile? Would you consider extraordinary measures—artificial insemination or in vitro fertilization, for example—in order to become a parent? Would you consider adoption?

PREGNANCY

Pregnancy is usually discussed in terms of **trimesters**—three periods of about 3 months (or 13 weeks) each. During the first trimester, the mother experiences a few physical changes and some fairly common symptoms. During the second trimester, often the most peaceful time of pregnancy, the mother gains weight, looks noticeably pregnant, and may experience a general sense of well-being if she is happy about having a child. The third trimester is the hardest for the mother because she must breathe, digest, excrete, and circulate blood for herself and the growing fetus. The weight of the fetus, the pressure of its body on her organs, and its increased demands on her system cause discomfort and fatigue and may make the mother increasingly impatient to give birth.

Pregnancy Tests

The earliest tests for pregnancy are chemical tests designed to detect the presence of **human chorionic gonadotropin (HCG)**, a hormone produced by the implanted fertilized egg. These tests may be performed as early as 2 weeks after fertilization. Home pregnancy test kits, which are sold without a prescription in drugstores, come equipped with a small sample of red blood cells coated with HCG antibodies, to which the woman can add a small amount of her own urine. If the concentration of HCG is great enough, it will clump together with the HCG antibodies, indicating that the woman is pregnant. Home pregnancy tests can be very reliable, but the instructions must be followed carefully.

Changes in the Woman's Body

Hormonal changes begin as soon as the egg is fertilized, and for the next 9 months, the woman's body nourishes the fetus and adjusts to its growth. Let's take a closer look at the changes of early, middle, and late pregnancy (Figure 8-2).

Early Signs and Symptoms Early recognition of pregnancy is important, especially for women with physical problems and nutritional deficiencies. The following symptoms are not absolute indications of pregnancy, but they are reasons to visit a gynecologist:

- *A missed menstrual period.* If an egg has been fertilized and implanted in the uterine wall, the endometrium is retained to nourish the embryo. A woman who misses a period after having unprotected intercourse may be pregnant.
- *Slight bleeding.* Slight bleeding may follow implantation of the fertilized egg. Because this happens about the time a period is expected, the bleeding is sometimes mistaken for menstrual flow. It usually lasts only a few days.
- *Nausea.* About two-thirds of pregnant women feel nauseated, probably as a reaction to increased levels of progesterone and other hormones. Often called morning sickness, some women have it all day long. It frequently begins during the 3rd or 4th week and disappears by the 12th week. In some cases, it can last throughout a pregnancy.
- *Breast tenderness.* Some women experience breast tenderness, swelling, and tingling, usually described as different from the tenderness experienced before menstruation.

trimester One of the three 3-month periods of pregnancy. **TERMS**

human chorionic gonadotropin (HCG) A hormone produced by the fertilized egg that can be detected in the urine or blood of the mother within a few weeks of conception.

Most cases of infertility are treated with conventional medical therapies. Surgery can repair oviducts, clear up endometriosis, and correct anatomical problems in both men and women. Fertility drugs can help women ovulate, although they carry the risk of causing multiple births. If these conventional treatments don't work, couples can turn to more advanced techniques. Assisted reproductive technology (ART) has come a long way since the first "test-tube baby" was born in 1978.

Intrauterine Insemination

Male infertility can sometimes be overcome by collecting and concentrating the man's sperm and introducing it by syringe into a woman's vagina or uterus, a procedure known as **artificial (intrauterine) insemination.** The woman is often given fertility drugs to induce ovulation prior to the insemination procedure. The sperm can be provided by the woman's partner or, if there are severe problems with his sperm or he carries a serious genetic disorder, by a donor. Donor sperm is also used by single women and lesbian couples who wish to conceive using artificial insemination. The success rate is about 60%. There are about 30,000 births each year from intrauterine insemination.

In a new technique under development, sperm are sorted by the sex chromosome they carry prior to artificial insemination, thereby enabling couples to select the sex of their infant.

IVF, GIFT, and ZIFT

Three related techniques for overcoming infertility involve removing mature eggs from a woman's ovary. Fewer than 5% of infertile American couples who seek treatment try these techniques. In **in vitro fertilization (IVF),** the harvested eggs are mixed with sperm in a laboratory dish. If eggs are successfully fertilized, one or more of the resulting embryos is inserted into the woman's uterus. IVF is often used by women with blocked oviducts. In **gamete intrafallopian transfer (GIFT)**, eggs and sperm are surgically placed into the fallopian tubes prior to fertilization. In **zygote intrafallopian transfer (ZIFT)**, eggs are fertilized outside the woman's body and surgically introduced into the oviducts after they begin to divide. GIFT and ZIFT can be used by women who have at least one open fallopian tube.

Variations on these three techniques are also becoming available. Donor sperm, donor eggs, and even donor embryos can be used. Extra eggs can be harvested and fertilized and the resulting embryos frozen for later use. In cases of severe male infertility, intracytoplasmic sperm injection (ICSI), in which a single sperm is injected into a mature egg, may be used. In 1996, about 65,000 cycles using these techniques were performed: 68% using IVF (11% of which involved ICSI), 4% using GIFT, 2% using ZIFT, and 15% using frozen embryos.

IVF, GIFT, and ZIFT do have drawbacks. Success rates vary from about 15% to 30%. They cost between $8,000 and $10,000 per procedure and may require five or more cycles to produce one live birth. They also increase the chance of multiple births.

Even more advanced techniques are under development. Researchers are exploring ways to freeze unfertilized eggs as means to extend their fertility or to protect eggs from fertility-damaging cancer treatments. Injecting the cytoplasm (the material in a cell that surrounds the nucleus) from a younger woman's egg into an older woman's egg is being studied as a possible means of reducing genetic errors in the older woman's egg. A related technique under study, known as nuclear transfer, uses **cloning** technology: the nucleus of an older woman's egg is transferred into an egg from a younger woman from which the nucleus has been removed.

Surrogate Motherhood

A controversial approach to infertility is surrogate motherhood. This practice involves a contract between an infertile couple and a fertile woman who agrees to carry a fetus. The surrogate mother agrees to be artificially inseminated by the father's sperm or to undergo IVF with the couple's embryo, to carry the baby to term, and to give it to the couple at birth. In return, the couple pays her for her services. There are thought to be several hundred births to surrogate mothers each year in the United States. Some people think that surrogate motherhood is essentially an arrangement to sell a baby, and they worry about the psychological consequences for children who learn that their mothers "sold" them. Experience has shown, too, that some surrogate mothers have a very difficult time giving up the baby and are unwilling to fulfill the contract after the birth, causing emotional trauma for themselves and the couple.

Ethical challenges

Assisted reproductive technology is a scientific frontier, and legal and ethical issues loom large. The following are just a few of the difficult questions that have been raised:

- Who owns frozen embryos? Should "extra" embryos be donated to other infertile couples, used for research, or destroyed?

- In the case of a multiple pregnancy, should the number of embryos the woman is carrying be reduced to increase the likelihood of a safe and successful pregnancy?

- In the case of IVF involving donor eggs and sperm and a surrogate mother, who are the legal parents of the child?

The potential use of cloning technology is another hotly debated area. Cloning is different from any of the techniques discussed here because it is a form of asexual reproduction: A clone carries the genes of only one person, not two. However, as described above, the cloning technique of nuclear transfer could potentially be used in the treatment of infertility. And although success is uncertain, nuclear transfer could theoretically be used to create a child that is the genetic offspring of two people of the same sex. As technology continues to advance, the ethical and legal issues are likely to become even more complex.

SOURCES: Assisted reproductive technology in the United States. 1999. *Fertility and Sterility* 71(5): 798–807. Centers for Disease Control and Prevention. 1998. *1996 Assisted Reproductive Technology Success Rates.* Atlanta, Ga.: CDC Division of Reproductive Health. American Society for Reproductive Medicine (http://www.asrm.org). Wright, K. 1998. Human in the age of mechanical reproduction. *Discover,* May. Nordenberg, T. 1997. Overcoming infertility. *FDA Consumer,* January/February.

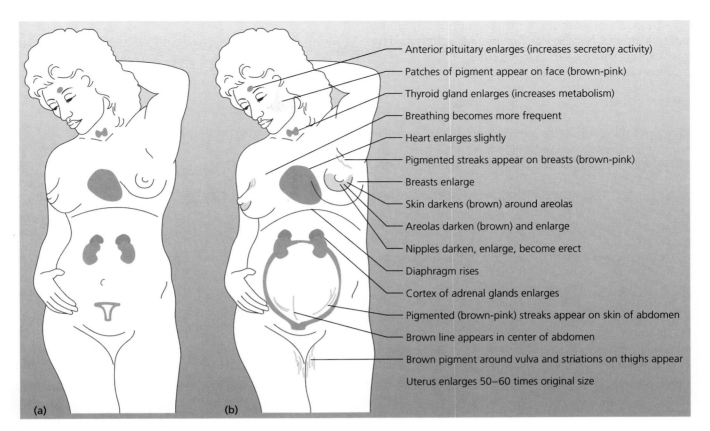

Figure 8-2 Physiological changes during pregnancy. The female body (a) at the time of conception; and (b) after 30 weeks of pregnancy.

Anterior pituitary enlarges (increases secretory activity)
Patches of pigment appear on face (brown-pink)
Thyroid gland enlarges (increases metabolism)
Breathing becomes more frequent
Heart enlarges slightly
Pigmented streaks appear on breasts (brown-pink)
Breasts enlarge
Skin darkens (brown) around areolas
Areolas darken (brown) and enlarge
Nipples darken, enlarge, become erect
Diaphragm rises
Cortex of adrenal glands enlarges
Pigmented (brown-pink) streaks appear on skin of abdomen
Brown line appears in center of abdomen
Brown pigment around vulva and striations on thighs appear
Uterus enlarges 50–60 times original size

- *Sleepiness, fatigue, and emotional upset.* These symptoms result from hormonal changes.

The first reliable physical signs of pregnancy can be distinguished about 4 weeks after a woman misses her menstrual period. A softening of the uterus just above the cervix, called **Hegar's sign,** and other changes in the cervix and pelvis are apparent during a pelvic examination. The labia minora and the cervix may take on a purple color rather than their usual pink hue.

Four weeks after a woman misses her menstrual period, she would be considered to be about 8 weeks pregnant because pregnancy is calculated from the time of a woman's last menstrual period rather than from the time of actual fertilization. (The timing of ovulation and fertilization are often difficult to determine.) Although a woman should see her physician to determine her due date, due dates can be approximated by subtracting three months from the date of the last menstual period and then adding 7 days. For example, a woman whose last menstrual period began on September 20th would have a due date of about June 27th.

Continuing Changes in the Woman's Body The most obvious changes during pregnancy occur in the reproductive organs. During the first 3 months, the uterus en-

larges to about three times its nonpregnant size, but it still cannot be felt in the abdomen. By the fourth month, it is large enough to make the abdomen protrude. By the seventh or eighth month, the uterus pushes up into the rib cage, which makes breathing slightly more difficult. The breasts enlarge and are sensitive; by week 8, they may tingle or throb. The pigmented area around the nipple, the areola, darkens and broadens. After the 10th week,

artificial (intrauterine) insemination The introduction of semen into the vagina by artificial means, usually by syringe.

in vitro fertilization (IVF) Combining egg and sperm outside the body and inserting the fertilized egg into the uterus.

gamete intrafallopian transfer (GIFT) Surgically introducing eggs and sperm into the fallopian tube prior to fertilization.

zygote intrafallopian transfer (ZIFT) Surgically introducing a fertilized egg into the fallopian tube.

cloning Asexual reproduction in which offspring are genetically identical to one parent. DNA from the cell of one animal is transferred to an egg from which DNA has been removed; the egg is then placed in a surrogate and develops as though it were an embryo derived from two parents.

Hegar's sign A softening of the uterus just above the cervix that is an early indication of pregnancy.

TERMS

colostrum, a yellowish fluid, may be squeezed from the mother's nipples, but the secretion of milk is prevented by high levels of estrogen and progesterone.

Other changes are going on as well. Early in pregnancy, the muscles and ligaments attached to bones begin to soften and stretch. The joints between the pelvic bones loosen and spread, making it easier to have a baby but harder to walk. The circulatory system becomes more efficient to accommodate the blood volume, which increases by 50%, and the heart pumps it more rapidly. Much of the increased blood flow goes to the uterus and placenta (the organ that exchanges nutrients and waste between mother and fetus). The mother's lungs also become more efficient, and her rib cage widens to permit her to inhale up to 40% more air. Much of the oxygen goes to the fetus. The kidneys become highly efficient, removing waste products from fetal circulation and producing large amounts of urine by midpregnancy.

How much weight should a woman gain during pregnancy? Women of normal weight gain an average of 18–25% of their initial weight: 20–28 lb for a woman weighing 110; 23–32 lb for a woman weighing 128. (About 90% of women of normal weight lose the weight gained during pregnancy within 24 months of giving birth.) About 60% of weight gained relates directly to the baby—about 7.5 lb for the baby and 8.5 lb for the placenta, amniotic fluid, heavier breasts and uterus—and 40% accumulates over the mother's entire body as fluid (blood, about 4 lb) and fat (4–8 lb). But gains in total pregnancy pounds vary strikingly, and similarities in total weight gain appear to conceal large differences in components of gain. As the woman's skin stretches, small breaks may occur in the elastic fibers of the lower layer of skin, producing stretch marks on her abdomen, hips, breasts, or thighs. Increased pigment production darkens the skin in 90% of pregnant women, especially in places that have stretched.

Sexual activity often changes during pregnancy. Attitudes about sexuality during pregnancy, combined with varying hormone levels and increased sensitivity in the genital area, cause some women to become more interested in sexual activity and others less interested. Intercourse is possible throughout pregnancy, but physical awkwardness in later months may interfere with comfort. Any questions about the safety of sexual activity during pregnancy can be answered by a health care professional. Open communication between the partners is essential.

Changes During the Later Stages of Pregnancy   By the end of the sixth month, the increased needs of the fetus place a burden on the mother's lungs, heart, and kidneys. Her back may ache from the pressure of the baby's weight and from having to throw her shoulders back to keep her balance while standing (Figure 8-3). Her body retains more water, perhaps up to 3 extra quarts of fluid. Her legs, hands, ankles, or feet may swell, and she may be

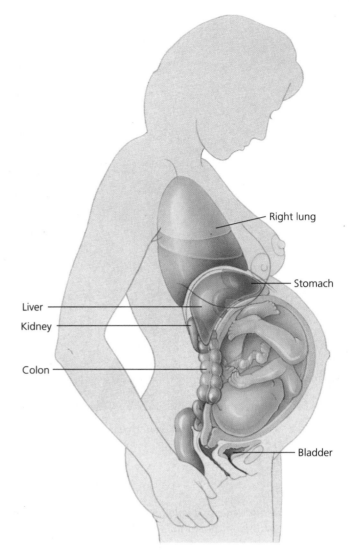

Figure 8-3   The woman and fetus during the third trimester of pregnancy.   Pressure from the rapidly growing fetus on the mother's lungs, bladder, stomach, and other organs may cause shortness of breath, heartburn, and the need for frequent urination. The mother's uterus has expanded to 50–60 times its original size.

bothered by leg cramps, heartburn, or constipation. Despite discomfort, both her digestion and her metabolism are working at top efficiency.

The uterus prepares for childbirth with preliminary contractions, called **Braxton Hicks contractions.** Unlike true labor contractions, these are usually short, irregular, and painless. The mother may only be aware that at times her abdomen is hard to the touch. These contractions become more frequent and intense as the delivery date approaches.

In the ninth month, the baby settles into the pelvic bones, usually head down, fitting snugly. This process, called **lightening,** allows the uterus to sink down about 2 inches, producing a visible change in the mother's profile.

Pelvic pressure increases, and pressure on the diaphragm lightens. Breathing becomes easier; urination becomes more frequent. Sometimes, after a first pregnancy, the baby doesn't settle down into the pelvis until labor begins.

PERSONAL INSIGHT   How do you feel about the changes in a woman's appearance during pregnancy? Do you have an emotional reaction to these changes? Do you think pregnancy makes a woman less or more attractive? Why do you think you feel the way you do?

Emotional Responses to Pregnancy

A woman's feelings during pregnancy will depend on her circumstances—her self-image, how she feels about pregnancy and motherhood, whether the pregnancy was planned, what type of relationship she has with her partner, whether she has a secure home situation, and many other factors. A first pregnancy is especially important because it has traditionally symbolized the transition to maturity and is a major developmental milestone in the lives of mothers—and fathers as well.

Pregnancy is likely to change a couple's relationship. Communication is especially important because people may have preconceived ideas about how they and their partners should feel. Both partners may have fears about the approaching birth, their ability to be good parents, and the ways in which the baby will affect their own relationship. These concerns are normal, and sharing them can deepen and strengthen a relationship. For a woman without a partner or whose partner is not supportive, it's important that she find other sources of support, perhaps from friends, family members, or support groups. The relationships that parents-to-be have with their own parents may also undergo changes. Impending parenthood may encourage them to assert their independence from their parents, but it may also enable them to identify with their parents' own experience of pregnancy, childbirth, and parenting.

Rapid changes in hormone levels can cause a pregnant woman to experience unpredictable emotions. A great part of pregnancy is beyond the woman's control—her changing appearance, her energy level, her variable moods—and some women need extra support and reassurance to keep on an even keel. Hormonal changes can also make women feel exhilarated and euphoric, although for some women such moods are temporary.

Like the physical changes that accompany pregnancy, emotional responses also change as the pregnancy develops. During the first trimester, the pregnant woman may fear that she may miscarry or that the child will not be normal. Education about pregnancy and childbirth, as well as support from her partner, friends, relatives, and health care professionals, are important antidotes to these

fears. During the second trimester, the pregnant woman can feel the fetus move within her, and worries about miscarriages usually begin to diminish. She may look and feel radiantly happy and be delighted as her pregnancy begins to show. However, she may also worry that her increasing size makes her unattractive. Reassurance from her partner can ease these fears.

The third trimester is the time of greatest physical stress during the pregnancy. A woman may find that her physical abilities are limited by her size. Because some women feel physically awkward and sexually unattractive, they may experience periods of depression. But many also feel a great deal of happy excitement and anticipation. The fetus may already be looked upon as a member of the family, and both parents may begin talking to the fetus and interacting with it by patting the mother's belly. The upcoming birth will probably be a focus for both the woman and her partner.

Fetal Development

Now that we've seen what happens to the mother's body during pregnancy, let's consider the development of the fetus (Figures 8-4 and 8-5, pp. 196–197).

The First Trimester   About 30 hours after the egg is fertilized, the cell divides, and this process of cell division repeats many times. As the cluster of cells drifts down the oviduct, several different kinds of cells emerge. The entire set of genetic instructions is passed to every cell, but each cell follows only certain instructions; if this were not the case, there would be no different organs or body parts. For example, all cells carry genes for hair color and eye color, but only the cells of the hair follicles and irises (of the eye) respond to that information.

On about the fourth day after fertilization, the cluster, now about 64–128 cells and hollow, arrives in the uterus; this is a **blastocyst.** On the sixth or seventh day, the blastocyst attaches to the uterine wall, usually along the upper curve. It begins to draw nourishment from the endometrium, the uterine lining.

The blastocyst becomes an **embryo** by the end of the second week after fertilization. The inner cells of the blastocyst separate into three layers. One layer becomes inner

TERMS

colostrum   A yellowish fluid secreted by the mammary glands around the time of childbirth until milk comes in, about the third day.

Braxton Hicks contractions   Uterine contractions that occur during the third trimester of pregnancy, preparing it for labor.

lightening   A process in which the uterus sinks down because the baby's head settles into the pelvic area.

blastocyst   A stage of development, days 6–14, when the cell cluster becomes the embryo and placenta.

embryo   The stage of development between blastocyst and fetus; about weeks 2–8.

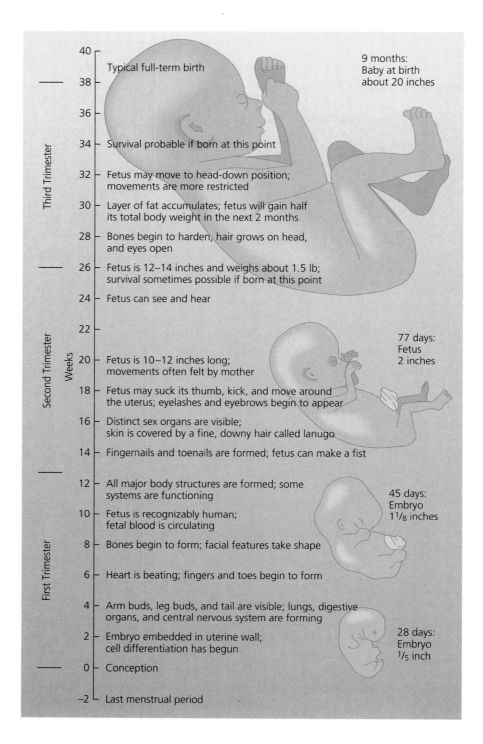

40 — Typical full-term birth

9 months:
Baby at birth
about 20 inches

38 —

36 —

34 — Survival probable if born at this point

32 — Fetus may move to head-down position; movements are more restricted

30 — Layer of fat accumulates; fetus will gain half its total body weight in the next 2 months

28 — Bones begin to harden, hair grows on head, and eyes open

26 — Fetus is 12–14 inches and weighs about 1.5 lb; survival sometimes possible if born at this point

24 — Fetus can see and hear

22 —

77 days:
Fetus
2 inches

20 — Fetus is 10–12 inches long; movements often felt by mother

18 — Fetus may suck its thumb, kick, and move around the uterus; eyelashes and eyebrows begin to appear

16 — Distinct sex organs are visible; skin is covered by a fine, downy hair called lanugo

14 — Fingernails and toenails are formed; fetus can make a fist

12 — All major body structures are formed; some systems are functioning

45 days:
Embryo
1 1/8 inches

10 — Fetus is recognizably human; fetal blood is circulating

8 — Bones begin to form; facial features take shape

6 — Heart is beating; fingers and toes begin to form

4 — Arm buds, leg buds, and tail are visible; lungs, digestive organs, and central nervous system are forming

2 — Embryo embedded in uterine wall; cell differentiation has begun

28 days:
Embryo
1/5 inch

0 — Conception

−2 — Last menstrual period

Weeks

Third Trimester · Second Trimester · First Trimester

Figure 8-4 A chronology of milestones in prenatal development.

body parts, the digestive and respiratory systems; the middle layer becomes muscle, bone, blood, kidneys, and sex glands; and the third layer becomes the skin, hair, and nervous tissue.

The outermost shell of cells becomes the **placenta, umbilical cord,** and **amniotic sac** (Figure 8-6, p. 198). A network of blood vessels called chorionic villi eventually forms the placenta. The human placenta is a two-way exchange of nutrients and waste materials between the mother and the fetus. The placenta brings oxygen and nutrients to the fetus and transports waste products out. The placenta does not provide a perfect barrier between the fetal circulation and the maternal circulation, however. Some blood cells are exchanged and certain substances, such as alcohol, pass freely from the maternal circulation through the placenta to the fetus.

The period between weeks 2 and 9 is a time of rapid differentiation and change. All the major body structures

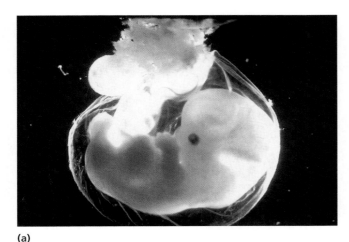

(a)

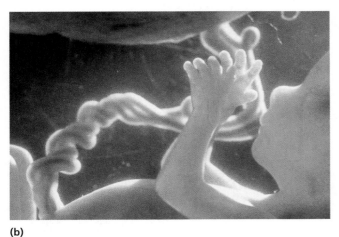

(b)

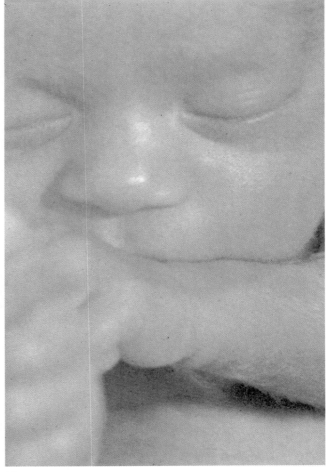

(c)

Figure 8-5 Embryological and fetal development. (a) A 6-week-old embryo has simple internal organs, including a beating heart, and is about 1 inch long. By the end of the first trimester, all the major body structures are formed, and some systems are functioning. (b) By the fourth month, the fetus is growing rapidly and is about 10 inches long. Weighing about 6 ounces, it moves vigorously in the uterus and can suck, frown, and turn its head. (c) At 7 months, the fetus weighs about 3 pounds and has grown to about 15 inches. Although it can now survive if born prematurely, it needs 2 more months in the womb to gain weight and acquire a layer of fat.

are formed during this time, including the heart, brain, liver, lungs, and sex organs; the eyes, nose, ears, arms, and legs also appear. Some organs begin to function—the heart begins to beat and the liver starts producing blood cells. Because body structures are forming, the developing organism is vulnerable to damage from environmental influences such as drugs and infections (discussed in detail in sections that follow).

By the end of the second month, the brain sends out impulses that coordinate the functioning of other organs. The embryo is now a fetus, and most further changes will be in the size and refinement of working body parts. In the third month, the fetus begins to be quite active. By the end of the first trimester, the fetus is about 4 inches long and weighs 1 ounce.

The Second Trimester To grow during the second trimester, to about 14 inches and 2 pounds, the fetus must have large amounts of food, oxygen, and water, which come from the mother through the placenta. All body systems are operating, and the fetal heartbeat can be heard with a stethoscope. Fetal movements can be felt by the

placenta The organ through which the fetus receives nourishment and empties waste via the mother's circulatory system; after birth, the placenta is expelled from the uterus.

umbilical cord The cord connecting the placenta and fetus, through which nutrients pass.

amniotic sac A membranous pouch enclosing and protecting the fetus, containing amniotic fluid.

TERMS

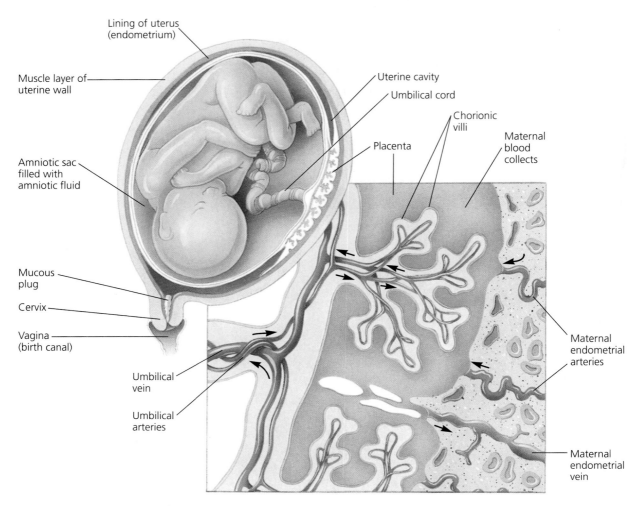

Figure 8-6   A cross-sectional view of the fetus in the uterus, and an enlargement of the placenta.

mother beginning in the fourth or fifth month. Against great odds, a fetus born prematurely at the end of the second trimester might survive.

The Third Trimester   The fetus gains most of its birth weight during the last 3 months. Some of the weight is fatty tissue under the skin that insulates the fetus and supplies food. The fetus must obtain large amounts of calcium, iron, and nitrogen from the food the mother eats. Some 85% of the calcium and iron she consumes goes into the fetal bloodstream.

Although the fetus may live if it is born during the seventh month, it needs the fat layer acquired in the eighth month and time for the organs, especially the respiratory and digestive organs, to develop. It also needs the immunity the mother's blood supplies during the final 3 months. Her blood protects the fetus against many of the diseases to which she has acquired immunity. These immunities wear off within 6 months after birth, but they

can be replenished by the mother's milk if the baby is breastfed.

Diagnosing Fetal Abnormalities   Information about the health and sex of a fetus can be obtained prior to birth through prenatal testing. The most common tests now used are ultrasound, amniocentesis, chorionic villus sampling (CVS), and alpha-fetoprotein (AFP) screening.

Ultrasonography (also called *ultrasound*) uses high-frequency sound waves to create a visual image, or **sonogram,** of the fetus in the uterus. Sonograms show the position of the fetus, its size and gestational age, and the presence of certain anatomical problems. Sonograms can sometimes be used to determine the sex of the fetus. Studies have not identified any problems in humans associated with ultrasound, but high levels of ultrasound have caused problems in animal fetuses.

Amniocentesis involves the removal of fluid from the uterus with a long, thin needle inserted through the ab-

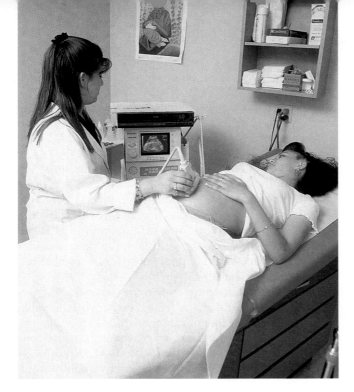

Ultrasonography provides information about the position, size, and physical condition of a fetus in the uterus. This mother-to-be can see her baby move and perhaps tell its sex by watching it on the screen.

dominal wall. It is usually performed between 14 and 18 weeks into the pregnancy, although earlier amniocentesis is becoming available at some centers. A genetic analysis of the fetal cells in the fluid can reveal the presence of chromosomal disorders, such as Down syndrome, and some genetic diseases, including Tay-Sachs disease and spina bifida. The sex of the fetus can also be determined. Most amniocentesis tests are performed on pregnant women over age 35, who have a greater risk of chromosomal abnormalities, or in cases where the fetus is known to be at risk for a particular chromosomal or genetic defect. Amniocentesis carries a slight risk (a 0.5–2% chance of fetal death).

A newer alternative is **chorionic villus sampling (CVS),** which can be performed earlier in pregnancy than amniocentesis, between weeks 10 and 12. This procedure involves removal through the cervix (by catheter) or abdomen (by needle) of a tiny section of chorionic villi, which contain fetal cells that can be analyzed. CVS also carries a slightly higher risk of fetal death than amniocentesis.

Alpha-fetoprotein (AFP), a protein produced by the fetus, is present in the amniotic fluid and in the mother's blood. **Alpha-fetoprotein (AFP) screening,** usually done between 15 and 18 weeks into the pregnancy, involves analysis of AFP levels in a sample of the mother's blood. High levels of AFP may indicate the presence of neural tube defects such as anencephaly (absence of part or all of the brain) and spina bifida; low levels sometimes indicate a chromosomal defect, such as Down syndrome. Because AFP screening is not foolproof, other tests are

done to confirm the results.

Genetic counselors explain the results of the different tests so that parents can understand their implications. If a fetus is found to have a defect, it may be carried to term, aborted, or, in rare instances, treated while still in the uterus. Results of most current screening tests are not available until after week 12 of pregnancy; consequently, if abortion is chosen, it is likely to involve one of the more medically complex and physically difficult methods (see Chapter 7). Researchers are searching for new fetal screening techniques that are less invasive and that can be done earlier in pregnancy. High-resolution ultrasonography and blood tests for combinations of fetal factors are two methods currently under investigation.

The Importance of Prenatal Care

Adequate prenatal care—a nutritious diet, exercise, adequate rest, avoidance of drugs, and regular medical evaluation—is essential to the health of both mother and baby. The pregnant woman cannot help but be responsible for the condition of the baby she carries. Everything she eats, drinks, and does affects the fetus in some respect. The fetus gets its nutrients and oxygen from the mother's bloodstream and has its wastes removed the same way. Many harmful substances can also be passed to the fetus via the placenta and umbilical cord. For these reasons, a mother's caring for her own health during pregnancy is a lifelong investment in her child's health.

Regular Checkups   In the woman's first visit to her obstetrician, she will be asked for a detailed medical history of herself and her family. The physician or midwife will note any hereditary conditions that may assume increased significance during pregnancy. The tendency to develop gestational diabetes (diabetes during pregnancy only), for example, can be inherited; appropriate treatment during pregnancy reduces the risk of serious harm.

The woman is given a complete physical exam and is informed about appropriate diet. She returns for regular checkups throughout the pregnancy, during which her blood pressure and weight gain are measured and tracked and the size and position of the fetus are monitored.

ultrasonography   The use of high-frequency sound waves to   **TERMS** view the fetus in the uterus; also known as *ultrasound.*

sonogram   The visual image of the fetus produced by ultrasonography.

amniocentesis   A process in which amniotic fluid is removed to detect possible birth defects.

chorionic villus sampling (CVS)   Surgical removal of a tiny section of chorionic villi to be analyzed for genetic defects.

alpha-fetoprotein (AFP) screening   Testing the level of AFP in a pregnant woman's blood to detect possible fetal abnormalities.

Regular prenatal visits also give the mother a chance to discuss her concerns and assure herself that everything is proceeding normally. Early advice from physicians, midwives, health educators, and teachers of childbirth classes provides the mother with invaluable information.

Blood Tests   A blood sample is taken during the initial prenatal visit to determine blood type and detect possible anemia or Rh incompatibilities. The Rh factor is a blood protein. If an Rh-positive father and an Rh-negative mother conceive an Rh-positive baby, the baby's blood will be incompatible with the mother's. If some of the baby's blood enters the mother's bloodstream during delivery, she will develop antibodies to it just as she would toward a virus. If she has subsequent Rh-positive babies, the antibodies in the mother's blood, passing through the placenta, will destroy the fetus's red blood cells, possibly leading to jaundice, anemia, mental retardation, or death. This condition is completely treatable with a serum called Rh-immune globulin, which destroys Rh-positive cells as they enter the mother's body and prevents her from forming antibodies to them. (Blood tests can also reveal the presence of some STDs, discussed later in the chapter.)

Prenatal Nutrition   The saying that a pregnant woman needs to "eat for two" is true. A nutritious diet throughout pregnancy is essential for both the fetus and the mother. Not only does the baby get all its nutrients from the mother, it also competes with her for nutrients not sufficiently available to meet both their needs. When a woman's diet is low in iron or calcium, the fetus receives most of it, and the mother may become deficient in the mineral. To meet the increased nutritional demands of her body, a pregnant woman shouldn't just eat more; she should make sure that her diet is adequate in all the basic nutritional categories.

Adequate intake of the B vitamin folic acid before conception and in the early weeks of pregnancy has been shown to decrease the risk of neural tube defects, including spina bifida. It is recommended that any woman capable of becoming pregnant consume at least 400 μg of folic acid daily from fortified foods and/or supplements, in addition to folate from a varied diet. Since 1998, enriched grain products have been fortified with small amounts of folic acid; folate is found naturally in leafy green vegetables, legumes, citrus fruits, and most berries. In the second and third trimesters, requirements increase

for calories and most nutrients, including protein, calcium, iron, magnesium, zinc, the B vitamins, and vitamins A, C, D, and E.

Table 8-1 provides nutritional guidelines for pregnancy; see Chapter 12 for more on individual nutrients and suggestions for planning a healthy diet.

Avoiding Drugs and Other Environmental Hazards   In addition to the food the mother eats, the drugs she takes and the chemicals she is exposed to affect the fetus. Everything the mother ingests may eventually reach the fetus in some proportion. Some drugs harm the fetus but not the mother because the fetus is in the process of developing, and because the proper dose for the mother is a massive dose for the fetus.

During the first trimester, when the major body structures are rapidly forming, the fetus is extremely vulnerable to environmental factors such as viral infections, radiation, drugs, and other **teratogens,** any of which can cause **congenital malformations,** or birth defects. The most susceptible body parts are those growing most rapidly at the time of exposure. The rubella (German measles) virus, for example, can cause a congenital malformation of a delicate system such as the eyes or ears, leading to blindness or deafness, if exposure occurs during the first trimester, but it does no damage later in the pregnancy. Similarly, the tranquilizer thalidomide taken early in pregnancy prevented the formation of arms and legs in fetuses, but taken later, when limbs were already formed, it caused no damage. Other drugs can cause damage throughout prenatal development.

ALCOHOL   Alcohol is a potent teratogen. A high level of alcohol consumption during pregnancy is associated with miscarriages, stillbirths, and, in live babies, **fetal alcohol syndrome (FAS).** A baby born with FAS is likely to suffer from a small head and body size, unusual facial characteristics, congenital heart defects, defective joints, mental impairment, and abnormal behavior patterns. The Centers for Disease Control and Prevention (CDC) estimate that about 1 out of every 1000 infants born in the United States has FAS. The rate is highest among those of low socioeconomic status, African Americans, and Native Americans. Researchers now doubt that any level of alcohol consumption is safe, and they recommend total abstinence during pregnancy. Despite warnings, however, surveys indicate that drinking among pregnant women has increased since the early 1990s (see Chapter 10).

TOBACCO   Pregnant women who smoke should quit, and nonsmoking pregnant women should avoid places where people smoke. Smoking during pregnancy increases the risk of miscarriage, low birth weight, and infant death. If nicotine levels in a mother's bloodstream are high, fetal breathing rate and movement become more rapid; the fetus may also metabolize cancer-causing

TERMS   **teratogen**   An agent or influence that causes physical defects in a developing embryo.

congenital malformation   A physical defect existing at the time of birth, either inherited or caused during gestation.

fetal alcohol syndrome (FAS)   A combination of birth defects caused by excessive alcohol consumption by the mother during pregnancy.

TABLE 8-1 *Nutritional Guidelines for Pregnancy*

Food Group and Daily Requirements[a]	Nutrients Provided	Foods and Serving Sizes[b]
Bread, cereal, rice, and pasta 6–11 servings (9 servings)	Carbohydrate, iron, B vitamins, other vitamins and minerals, fiber	1 slice bread 1 oz ready-to-eat cereal $\frac{1}{2}$ cup cooked cereal, rice, or pasta *Choose whole-grain foods and foods made with little fat or sugar.*
Vegetables 3–4 servings (4 servings)	Carbohydrate, vitamins A and C, folic acid, iron, magnesium, other vitamins and minerals, fiber	1 cup raw leafy vegetables $\frac{1}{2}$ cup other vegetables, cooked or chopped raw $\frac{3}{4}$ cup vegetable juice *Choose dark-green leafy vegetables, deep-yellow vegetables, and legumes often.*
Fruits 2–4 servings (3 servings)	Carbohydrate, vitamins A and C, potassium, fiber	1 medium apple, banana, orange $\frac{1}{2}$ cup chopped, cooked, or canned fruit $\frac{3}{4}$ cup fruit juice *Choose citrus fruits, melons, and berries regularly.*
Milk, yogurt, and cheese 2–3 servings (3 servings)	Protein, calcium, phosphorus, other vitamins and minerals	1 cup milk or yogurt $1\frac{1}{2}$ oz natural cheese 2 oz process cheese *Choose fat-free and lowfat foods often.*
Meat, poultry, fish, dry beans, eggs, and nuts 2–3 servings (3 servings or 6 oz total)	Protein, iron, zinc, B vitamins	2–3 oz cooked lean meat, poultry, or fish (the equivalent of an average hamburger or half a chicken breast) The following are equivalent to 1 oz of meat: 1 egg, $\frac{1}{2}$ cup cooked dry beans, 2 tbsp peanut butter, $\frac{1}{3}$ cup nuts *Choose lean meat, poultry without skin, fish, and dry beans often.*
Fats, oils, and sweets No specific recommendation; use sparingly according to total energy needs	Fats, carbohydrate	Fats and sugar are concentrated in butter, margarine, oils, salad dressing, gravy, mayonnaise, soft drinks, candy, jellies and jams, and sweet desserts
Vitamin and mineral supplements (as directed by physician)	Some physicians may prescribe vitamin and mineral supplements for women who are pregnant or lactating, or who are trying to get pregnant. Supplements may be for a particular nutrient, such as folic acid or iron, or may be a multivitamin and mineral supplement. It is important that a pregnant woman not supplement beyond her physician's advice because some vitamins and minerals are harmful if taken in excess.	

[a]The ranges of servings are from the Food Guide Pyramid; the number of servings in parentheses is the minimum suggested by the American College of Obstetricians and Gynecologists for pregnant women. A woman needs about 300 extra calories per day when pregnant.
[b]For a more detailed discussion of recommended food choices and serving sizes, see Chapter 12.

SOURCES: U.S. Department of Agriculture. 1996. *The Food Guide Pyramid.* Home and Garden Bulletin No. 252. Washington, D.C.: U.S. Government Printing Office. American College of Obstetricians and Gynecologists (ACOG). 1995. *Nutrition During Pregnancy.* Washington, D.C.: ACOG.

byproducts of tobacco. Infants of women who smoke during pregnancy have poorer lung function at birth, and exposure to secondhand smoke after birth increases a baby's susceptibility to pneumonia and bronchitis. If a mother who smokes breastfeeds, her infant will be exposed to tobacco chemicals through breast milk. See Chapter 11 for more on the effects of smoking.

CAFFEINE   Caffeine, a powerful stimulant, should be used conservatively by pregnant women. It puts both mother and fetus under stress by raising the level of the hormone epinephrine. Caffeine also reduces the blood supply to the uterus. Coffee, colas, strong black tea, and chocolate are high in caffeine, as are over-the-counter medications such as Excedrin and NoDōz. A pregnant woman should limit her caffeine intake to no more than the equivalent of 2 cups of coffee per day.

DRUGS AND CHEMICALS   Some prescription drugs can also harm the fetus, so they should be used only under medical supervision. Accutane, a popular anti-acne drug, is thought to be responsible for over 1000 cases of severe birth defects in the 1980s. Vitamins, aspirin, and other over-the-counter drugs should be used only under a physician's direction. Large doses of vitamin A, for example, can cause birth defects. Chemicals and pollutants can also pose a danger to the fetus. Mercury, from fish contaminated by industrial pollution, is known to cause physical deformities. Continuous exposure to lead, found in some paint products and in water from lead pipes, has been implicated as a cause of a variety of learning disorders. Any product containing chemicals—including chemical fertilizers, solvents, and pesticides—should be avoided or used with extreme caution.

STDS AND OTHER INFECTIONS   Infections, including those that are sexually transmitted, are another serious problem for the fetus. If a mother contracts rubella during the first trimester, her child may be born with physical or mental disabilities. Immunization against measles must take place before pregnancy, because the immunization is harmful to the fetus. Syphilis can infect and kill a fetus; if the baby is born alive, it will have syphilis. Penicillin taken by the mother during pregnancy cures syphilis in both mother and fetus. Gonorrhea can infect the baby during delivery and cause blindness. Because gonorrhea is often asymptomatic, in many states the eyes of newborns are routinely treated with silver nitrate or another antibiotic to destroy gonorrheal bacteria. All pregnant women should be tested for hepatitis B, a virus that can pass from the mother to the infant at birth. Infants of infected mothers can be immunized shortly after birth.

Herpes simplex can damage the baby's eyes and brain and cause death, and no cure has yet been discovered for it. About 2000 babies die each year from neonatal herpes. Genital herpes can be transmitted to the baby during delivery if the mother's infection is in the active phase. If this is the case, the baby is delivered by cesarean section. An initial outbreak of herpes can be dangerous if it occurs during pregnancy because the virus may pass through the placenta to the fetus. For this reason, testing for genital herpes is recommended for both expectant parents. Once the baby is born, any caregiver who is experiencing a herpes outbreak should wash his or her hands often and not permit contact between hands or contaminated objects and the baby's mucous membranes (inside of eyes, mouth, nose, penis, vagina, vulva, and rectum).

The human immunodeficiency virus (HIV), which causes AIDS, can be passed to the fetus by an HIV-infected mother during pregnancy, labor and delivery, or breastfeeding. Nationwide, more than 8000 children under age 13 have been diagnosed with AIDS, and many more are infected with HIV. The babies most at risk are those whose mothers inject drugs or are the sex partners of men who inject drugs. HIV testing is critical for any woman at risk for HIV, and some physicians recommend routine testing for all pregnant women. Antiviral drugs, given to an HIV-infected mother during pregnancy and delivery and to her newborn immediately following birth, reduce the rate of HIV transmission from mother to infant from 25% to 8% or less. Of course, women should also take all the necessary precautions against HIV infection during pregnancy. (See Chapter 18 for more on HIV and other STDs.)

Environmental factors affecting fetal or infant development are summarized in Table 8-2.

Prenatal Activity and Exercise   Physical activity during pregnancy contributes to mental and physical wellness. Women can continue working at their jobs until late in their pregnancy, provided the work isn't so physically demanding that it jeopardizes their health. At the same time, pregnant women need more rest and sleep to maintain their own well-being and that of the fetus.

A moderate exercise program during pregnancy does not adversely affect pregnancy or birth; in fact, regular exercise appears to improve a woman's chance of an on-time delivery. The amniotic sac protects the fetus, and normal activities will not harm it. A woman who exercised before becoming pregnant can often continue her program, with appropriate modifications to maintain her comfort and safety. A pregnant woman who hasn't been exercising and wants to start should first consult a physician. Regular cardiorespiratory endurance exercise is recommended. Walking, swimming, and stationary cycling are all good choices; more strenuous activities that could result in a fall, such as skiing, skating, or horseback riding, are best delayed until after the birth. See the box "Exercising During Pregnancy" for more information.

Kegel exercises, to strengthen the pelvic floor muscles, are recommended for pregnant women. These exercises are performed by alternately contracting and releasing

TABLE 8-2 — Selected Environmental Factors Associated with Problems in a Fetus or Infant

Agent or Condition	Potential Effects
Accutane (acne medication)	Small head, mental impairment, deformed or absent ears, heart defects, cleft lip and palate.
Alcohol	Unusual facial characteristics, small head, heart defects, mental impairment, defective joints.
Antiseizure medications	Small head and possible mental impairment, cleft lip and palate, genital and kidney abnormalities, spina bifida.
Chlamydia	Eye infections, pneumonia.
Cigarette smoking	Miscarriage, stillbirth, low birth weight, respiratory problems, sudden infant death.
Cocaine	Miscarriage, stillbirth, low birth weight, small head, defects of genital and urinary tract.
Cytomegalovirus (CMV)	Small head, mental impairment, blindness.
Diabetes (insulin-dependent)	Malformations of the brain, spine, and heart.
Gonorrhea	Eye infection leading to blindness if untreated.
Herpes	Brain damage, death.
HIV infection	Impaired immunity, death.
Lead	Reduced IQ, learning disorders.
Lithium	Heart defects.
Marijuana	Impaired fetal growth; increase in alcohol-related fetal damage.
Mercury	Brain damage.
Propecia (hair loss medication)	Abnormalities of the male sex organs.
Radiation (high dose)	Small head, growth and mental impairment, multiple birth defects.
Rubella (German measles)	Malformation of eyes or ears causing deafness or blindness; small head; mental impairment.
Streptomycin	Deafness.
Syphilis	Fetal death and miscarriage, prematurity, physical deformities.
Tetracycline	Pigmentation of teeth, underdevelopment of enamel.
Toxoplasmosis	Small head, mental impairment, blindness, hearing impairments, seizures, learning disorders.
Vitamin A (excess)	Miscarriage; defects of the head, brain, spine, and urinary tract.

TACTICS AND TIPS — Exercising During Pregnancy

Women can continue to exercise and derive health benefits from exercise during pregnancy. Recommendations for exercising safely during pregnancy include the following:

- Exercise regularly (at least three times a week) rather than intermittently.

- Avoid exercise that has you lying on your back. Research indicates that this position restricts blood flow to the uterus. Also avoid prolonged periods of motionless standing.

- Modify the intensity of your exercise according to how you feel. Stop exercising if you feel fatigued, and don't exercise to exhaustion. You may find that non–weight-bearing exercises such as cycling and swimming are more comfortable than weight-bearing activities in the later months of pregnancy; they also minimize the risk of injury.

- Avoid any type of exercise that has the potential for even mild abdominal trauma.

- Take care when performing any activity in which balance is important, or in which losing balance would be dangerous. Pregnancy shifts your center of gravity.

- Avoid heat stress, particularly during the first trimester, by drinking an adequate amount of fluids, wearing appropriate clothing, and avoiding exercise in hot and humid weather.

- Resume prepregnancy exercise routines gradually. Many of the changes of pregnancy persist for 4–6 weeks after delivery.

- If you experience any unusual symptoms, stop exercising, and consult your physician.

SOURCE: Adapted from American College of Obstetricians and Gynecologists. 1994. Exercise during pregnancy and the postpartum period. *ACOG Technical Bulletin*, 189, February.

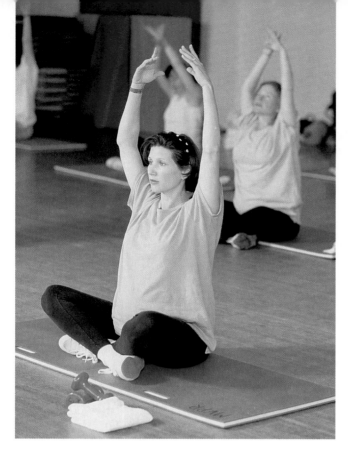

A woman's body changes drastically during pregnancy to accommodate and nourish the growing fetus. Prenatal exercise helps this woman stay healthy while her body works to sustain two lives.

the muscles used to stop the flow of urine. Each contraction should be held for about 5 seconds. Kegel exercises should be done several times a day, for a total of about 50 repetitions daily.

Prenatal exercise classes are valuable because they teach exercises that tone the body muscles involved in birth, especially those of the abdomen, back, and legs. Toned-up muscles aid delivery and help the body regain its nonpregnant shape afterward.

Preparing for Birth　　Hospital childbirth practices have been increasingly challenged over the last 25 years, and many women have chosen to learn techniques to help them deal with the discomfort of labor and delivery without taking pain-relieving drugs. To clear up misunderstandings and dispel fears about childbirth, educators teach prospective parents the details of the birth process, as well as relaxation techniques to use during labor and birth. Several methods of **prepared childbirth** training are used, including the Bradley method and the Lamaze method, all designed to ease birth through knowledge, relaxation, and physical conditioning. Most hospitals and childbirth educators tend to instruct parents in a combination of Lamaze and other relaxation techniques.

Childbirth classes are almost a routine part of the prenatal experience for both mothers and fathers these days. The mother learns and practices a variety of techniques so she will be able to choose what works best for her during labor, when the time comes. The father typically acts as a coach, supporting his partner emotionally and helping her with her breathing and relaxing. He remains with her throughout labor and delivery, even when a cesarean section is performed. It can be an important and fulfilling time for the parents to be together.

Complications of Pregnancy and Pregnancy Loss

Pregnancy usually proceeds without major complications. Sometimes, however, complications may prevent full-term development of the fetus or affect the health of the infant at birth. As discussed earlier in the chapter, exposure to harmful substances, such as alcohol or drugs, can harm the fetus. Other complications are caused by physiological problems or genetic abnormalities.

Ectopic Pregnancy　　In an **ectopic pregnancy,** the fertilized egg implants and begins to develop outside the uterus, usually in an oviduct. Ectopic pregnancies usually occur because the fallopian tube is blocked, most often as a result of pelvic inflammatory disease. The embryo may spontaneously abort, or the embryo and placenta may continue to expand until they rupture the oviduct. Sharp pain on one side of the abdomen or in the lower back, usually in about the 7th or 8th week, may signal an ectopic pregnancy, and there may be irregular bleeding. If bleeding from a rupture is severe, the woman may go into shock, characterized by low blood pressure, a fast pulse, weakness, and fainting. Surgical removal of the embryo and the oviduct may be necessary to save the mother's life, although microsurgery can sometimes be used to repair the damaged oviduct. The incidence of ectopic pregnancy has more than quadrupled in the last 25 years, and it is the leading cause of pregnancy-related death in the United States.

Spontaneous Abortion　　A **spontaneous abortion,** or **miscarriage,** is the termination of pregnancy before the 20th week. It is estimated that 10–40% of pregnancies end this way, some without the woman's awareness that she was even pregnant. Most miscarriages occur between the 6th and 8th weeks of pregnancy, and most—about 60%—are due to chromosomal abnormalities in the fetus. Certain occupations that involve exposure to chemicals may increase the likelihood of a spontaneous abortion.

Vaginal bleeding (spotting) is usually the first sign that a pregnant woman may miscarry. She may also develop pelvic cramps, and her symptoms of pregnancy may disappear. One miscarriage doesn't mean that later pregnancies will be unsuccessful, and about 70–90% of women who miscarry eventually become pregnant again. About 1% of women suffer three or more miscarriages, possibly because of anatomical, hormonal, genetic, or immunological factors.

Toxemia   A potentially serious condition that occasionally develops in the later months of pregnancy (usually not before the 20th week) is **toxemia,** characterized by high blood pressure and fluid retention. The early stages of toxemia, known as **preeclampsia,** can usually be treated through nutritional means. However, if left untreated, blood pressure continues to rise, the woman's face and legs swell, and excess protein appears in her urine. In the later stages, known as **eclampsia,** vision blurs and the head aches continuously, leading eventually to convulsions, coma, and even death. Toxemia is not common and it can be prevented or controlled through diet, rest, and sometimes medication. A woman who notices facial edema (swelling) should see her physician immediately. Changes in blood pressure and the presence of excess protein in the urine are normally noticed and tracked during routine prenatal examinations.

Low Birth Weight   A **low-birth-weight (LBW)** baby usually weighs less than 5.5 pounds at birth. LBW babies may be premature (born before the 37th week of pregnancy) or full-term. Babies who are born small even though they're full-term are referred to as small-for-date babies. Most LBW babies will grow normally, but some will experience problems. Although they are at greater risk than bigger babies for complications during infancy, small-for-date babies tend to have fewer problems than premature infants. The most fundamental problem of prematurity is that many of the infant's organs are not sufficiently developed. Premature infants are subject to respiratory problems and infections. They may have difficulty eating because they may be too small to suck a breast or bottle, and their swallowing mechanism may be underdeveloped. As they get older, premature infants may have problems such as learning difficulties, poor hearing and vision, and physical awkwardness.

Low birth weight affects about 7.5% of infants born each year in the United States. About half of all cases of LBW are related to teenage pregnancy, cigarette smoking, poor nutrition, and poor health of the mother. One study found a sixfold increase in the risk of LBW if the mother had financial problems during the pregnancy. Adequate prenatal care is the best means of preventing LBW.

Infant Mortality   The U.S. rate of infant mortality, the death of a child of less than 1 year of age, is at its lowest point ever; however, it remains far higher than that of most of the developed world. The United States ranks twenty-second among the world's developed countries for low infant mortality, with 7.1 deaths for every 1000 live births in 1997. Poverty and inadequate health care are key causes; in some inner-city areas, the infant mortality rate approaches that of developing countries, with more than 20 deaths per 1000 births.

Other causes of infant death are congenital problems, infectious diseases, and injuries. In the United States, about 3000 infant deaths per year are due to **sudden infant death syndrome (SIDS),** in which an apparently healthy infant dies suddenly while sleeping. The number of SIDS deaths has decreased since 1992, when the "Back to Sleep" campaign was instituted to make people aware that putting babies to bed on their backs rather than on their stomachs significantly reduces the risk of SIDS. Between 1992 and 1997, the number of babies being placed on their stomachs to sleep declined from 70% to 21%, and the number of deaths from SIDS declined by 43%. Other risk factors for SIDS include abnormalities in heart rhythm or in brain receptors controlling breathing; exposing a fetus or infant to tobacco smoke, alcohol, or other drugs; and putting a baby to bed on a soft mattress or with fluffy bedding, pillows, or stuffed toys. Overbundling a baby or keeping a baby's room too warm also increases the risk of SIDS; because of this, the incidence of SIDS tends to rise in the colder months.

Coping with Loss   Parents form a deep attachment to their children even before birth, and those who lose an infant before or during birth usually experience deep grief. Initial feelings of shocked disbelief and numbness may give way to sadness, anger, crying spells, and preoccupation with the loss. Physical sensations such as tightness in the chest or stomach, loss of appetite, and sleeplessness may also occur. For the mother, physical exhaustion and hormone imbalances can compound the emotional and physical stress.

TERMS

prepared childbirth   Methods of preparing for birth, including physical conditioning, instruction in the birth process, and psychological and emotional conditioning.

ectopic pregnancy   A pregnancy in which the embryo develops outside the uterus, usually in the fallopian tube.

spontaneous abortion (miscarriage)   Termination of pregnancy when the uterine contents are expelled; causes include an abnormal uterus, insufficient hormones, and genetic or physical fetal defects.

toxemia   A condition of pregnancy characterized by high blood pressure and edema.

preeclampsia   An early stage of toxemia, characterized by increasingly high blood pressure, edema, and protein in the urine.

eclampsia   A severe, potentially life-threatening form of toxemia, characterized by convulsions and coma.

low birth weight (LBW)   Weighing less than 5.5 lb at birth, often the result of prematurity.

sudden infant death syndrome (SIDS)   The sudden death of an apparently healthy infant during sleep.

Experiencing the pain of loss is part of the healing process, which can take up to a year or more. Keeping active with work or travel can help renew interest in life. A support group or professional counseling is also often helpful. Planning the next pregnancy, with a physician's input, can be an important step toward recovery, as long as the mind and body are given time to heal. If future pregnancies are ruled out, couples can consider other options, such as adoption.

CHILDBIRTH

By the end of the ninth month of pregnancy, most women are tired of being pregnant; both parents are eager to start a new phase of their lives. Most couples find the actual process of birth to be an exciting and positive experience.

Choices in Childbirth

Many couples today can choose the type of practitioner and the environment they want for the birth of their child. A high-risk pregnancy is probably best handled by a specialist physician in a hospital with a nursery, but for low-risk births, many options are available.

Parents can choose to have their baby delivered by a physician (an obstetrician or family practitioner) or by a certified nurse-midwife. Certified nurse-midwives are registered nurses with special training in obstetrical techniques, and they are well qualified for prenatal and postnatal care, routine deliveries, and minor medical emergencies. They are usually much less expensive than physicians, and they are often part of a complete medical team that includes a backup physician in case of emergency. Nurse-midwives can usually participate in births in any setting, although this may vary according to hospital policy, state law, and the midwife's preferences. About 1 in 20 babies each year are delivered by nurse-midwives.

Most babies in the United States are delivered in hospitals or in freestanding alternative birth centers; only about 2% of women choose to have their babies at home. Many hospitals have introduced alternative birth centers in response to criticisms of traditional hospital routines.

Alternative birth centers provide a comfortable, emotionally supportive environment in close proximity to up-to-date medical equipment.

The impersonal, routine quality of hospital birth is increasingly being challenged, and many hospitals and physicians offer a variety of options to parents regarding many aspects of childbirth. It's important for prospective parents to discuss all aspects of labor and delivery with their physician or midwife beforehand, so they can learn what to expect and can state their preferences. For more information, see the box "Making a Birth Plan," p. 208.

> **PERSONAL INSIGHT** If you are a woman and want to have a child, what kind of birth experience do you think you want to have? If you are a man, do you want to participate and have a role in your partner's birth experience or would you rather just leave it to her? Where do you think your ideas come from?

Labor and Delivery

The birth process occurs in three stages (Figure 8-7). **Labor** begins when hormonal changes in both the mother and the baby cause strong, rhythmic uterine **contractions** to begin. These contractions exert pressure on the cervix and cause the lengthwise muscles of the uterus to pull on the circular muscles around the cervix, causing effacement (thinning) and dilation (opening) of the cervix. The contractions also pressure the baby to descend into the mother's pelvis, if it hasn't already. The entire process of labor and delivery usually takes between 2 and 36 hours, depending on the size of the baby, the baby's position in the uterus, the size of the mother's pelvis, and other factors. The length of labor is generally shorter for second and subsequent births.

The First Stage of Labor The first stage of labor averages 13 hours for a first birth, although there is a wide variation among women. Contractions usually last about 30 seconds and occur every 15–20 minutes at first, more often later. The prepared mother relaxes as much as possible during these contractions to allow labor to proceed without being blocked by tension. Early in the first stage, a small amount of bleeding may occur as a plug of slightly bloody mucus that blocked the opening of the cervix during pregnancy is expelled. In some women, the amniotic sac ruptures and the fluid rushes out; this is sometimes referred to as "breaking of the waters."

The last part of the first stage of labor, called **transition,** is characterized by strong and frequent contractions, much more intense than in the early stages of labor. Contractions may last 60–90 seconds and occur every 1–3 minutes. During transition the cervix opens completely, to a diameter of about 10 centimeters. Since the head of the fetus usually measures 9–10 cm, once the cervix has dilated completely, the head can pass through. Many women report that transition, which normally lasts about 30 minutes to an hour, is the most difficult part of labor.

The Second Stage of Labor The second stage of labor begins when the baby's head moves into the birth canal and ends when the baby is born. The baby is slowly pushed down, through the bones of the pelvic ring, past the cervix, and into the vagina, which it stretches open. The mother bears down with the contractions to help push the baby down and out. Some women find this the most difficult part of labor, while others find that the contractions and bearing down bring a sense of euphoria. The baby's back bends, the head turns to fit through the narrowest parts of the passageway, and the soft bones of the baby's skull move together and overlap as it is squeezed through the pelvis. When the top of the head appears at the vaginal opening, the baby is said to be crowning.

As the head of the baby emerges, the physician or midwife will remove any mucus from the mouth and nose, wipe the baby's face, and check to ensure that the umbilical cord is not around the neck. With a few more contractions, the baby's shoulders and body emerge. As the baby is squeezed through the pelvis, cervix, and vagina, the fluid in the lungs is forced out by the pressure on the baby's chest. Once this pressure is released as the baby emerges from the vagina, the chest expands and the lungs fill with air for the first time. The baby will still be connected to the mother via the umbilical cord, which is not cut until it stops pulsating. The baby will appear wet and often is covered with a milky substance. The baby's head may be oddly shaped at first, due to the molding of the soft plates of bone during birth, but it usually takes on a normal appearance within 24 hours.

The Third Stage of Labor In the third stage of labor, the uterus continues to contract until the placenta is expelled. This stage usually takes 5–20 minutes. If the placenta does not come out on its own, the physician or midwife may exert gentle pressure on the abdomen to help with its delivery. It is important that the entire placenta be expelled; if part remains in the uterus, it may cause infection or bleeding. Breastfeeding soon after delivery helps control uterine bleeding because it stimulates the secretion of a hormone that makes the uterus contract; massaging the abdomen may also help.

In the meantime, the physical condition of the baby will be assessed: Heart rate, respiration, color, reflexes, and muscle tone are individually rated with a score of 0–2. The total, called an **Apgar score,** will be at least 7 if the child is healthy. The baby is then usually wrapped tightly in a blanket and returned to the mother, who may begin to nurse the baby right away.

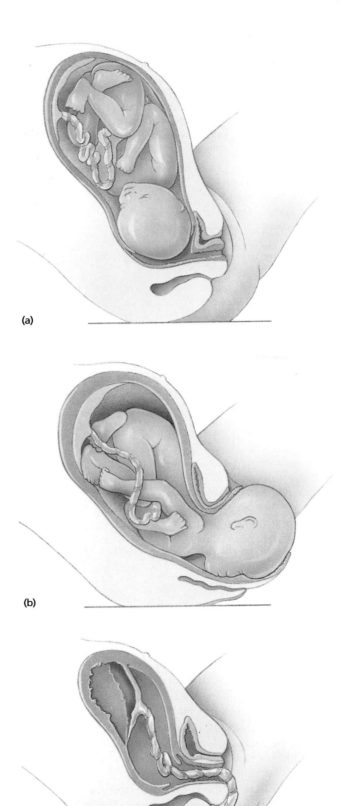

(a)

(b)

(c)

Figure 8-7 Birth: labor and delivery. (a) The first stage of labor; (b) the second stage of labor: delivery of the baby; (c) the third stage of labor: expulsion of the placenta.

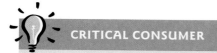
A variety of birth situations can have positive physical and psychological outcomes. Parents should choose what is appropriate for their medical circumstances, and what feels most comfortable to them. Prospective parents should discuss their preferences in the following areas with their physician or midwife:

1. Who will be present at the birth? The father? Friends? Children and other relatives? Will young siblings be allowed to visit the mother and new baby?

2. What type of room will the mother be in during labor, delivery, and recovery? How many times will she be moved?

3. What type of tables, beds, or birthing chairs are available? What type of environment can be created for the birth? Can specific music be played?

4. Will the mother receive any routine preparation, such as an enema, intravenous feeding, or shaving of the pubic area?

5. What is the policy regarding food and drink during labor? Will the mother have the option of walking around or taking a shower or bath during labor?

6. Under what circumstances does the physician or midwife administer drugs to induce or augment labor? The use of these drugs tends to change the course of labor and carries a small risk.

7. Is **electronic fetal monitoring (EFM)** typically used during labor? About 75% of all births are electronically monitored, but there is disagreement among medical authorities about the risks or benefits of EFM. The American College of Obstetricians and Gynecologists recommends periodic monitoring using a stethoscope rather than EFM for low-risk pregnancies.

8. Under what circumstances will an **episiotomy**, an incision at the base of the vaginal opening, be performed? Are any steps taken to avoid it?

9. Under what circumstances will forceps or vacuum extraction be used? In some cases of fetal distress, the use of forceps or vacuum extraction may be necessary to save the infant's life, but some authorities believe these techniques are overused.

10. What types of medications are typically used during labor and delivery? Some form of anesthetic is usually administered during most hospital deliveries, as are hormones that intensify the contractions and shrink the uterus after delivery. Different types of anesthetics, including short-acting narcotics, regional nerve blocks, and local anesthetics, may be available; each has different effects on the mother and the fetus.

11. Under what conditions or circumstances does the physician perform a cesarean section? If prospective parents are concerned, they should research the cesarean frequency rates of different physicians before they make their final choice.

12. Who will "catch" the baby as she or he is born? Who will cut the umbilical cord?

13. What will be done to the baby immediately after birth? What kinds of tests and procedures will be done on the baby, and when?

14. How often will the baby be brought to the mother while they remain in the hospital or birthing center? Can the baby stay in the mother's room rather than in the nursery? This practice is known as **rooming-in.**

15. How will the baby be fed—by breast or bottle? Will feeding be on a schedule or "on demand"? Is there someone with breastfeeding experience available to answer questions if necessary?

Cesarean Deliveries   About 21% of the babies born in the United States are delivered by **cesarean section,** in which the baby is removed through a surgical incision in the abdominal wall and uterus. Cesarean sections are necessary when a baby cannot be delivered vaginally—for example, if the baby's head is bigger than the mother's pelvic girdle, or if the baby is in an unusual position. If the mother has a serious health condition such as high blood pressure, a cesarean may be safer for her than labor and a vaginal delivery. Other reasons for cesarean delivery include abnormal or difficult labor, fetal distress, and the presence of a dangerous infection like herpes that can be passed to the baby during delivery. Repeat cesarean deliveries are also very common; about 72.5% of American women who have had one child by cesarean have subsequent children delivered the same way.

A cesarean section is major surgery and carries some risk, but it is relatively safe. A local anesthetic may be used so the woman can remain conscious during the operation, and the father may be present.

Some people believe cesareans are often performed unnecessarily in the United States. Other countries that have rates of maternal and infant death as low as those in the United States have much lower rates of cesarean section, particularly repeat cesareans. The *Healthy People 2010* report sets a goal for reducing the overall rate of cesarean delivery to no more than 15% and the rate of repeat cesareans to 65%. Several strategies have been suggested to help lower this rate: address physician malpractice concerns; eliminate the financial incentives for cesareans, which are currently more lucrative than vaginal deliveries; publish cesarean rates of individual physicians and hospitals; and increase training in normal vaginal deliveries.

The Postpartum Period

The **postpartum period,** a stage of about 3 months following childbirth, is a time of critical family adjustments.

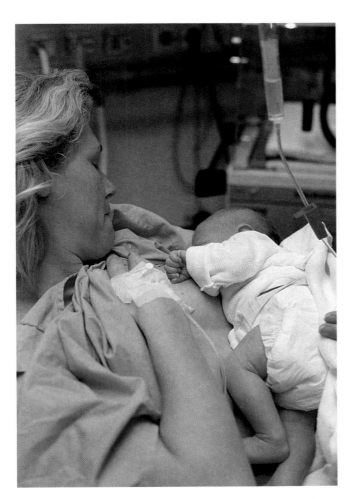

The bond between a mother and her child begins immediately after birth. After having her physical condition checked, this newborn is returned to her mother and begins to breastfeed for the first time.

Parenthood—a job that goes on around the clock without relief—begins literally overnight, and the transition can cause considerable physical and emotional stress.

Following a vaginal delivery, mothers usually leave the hospital within 1–3 days (after a cesarean section, they usually stay 3–5 days). Uterine contractions will occur from time to time for several days after delivery, as the uterus begins to return to its prebirth size. It usually takes 6–8 weeks for a woman's reproductive organs to return to their prebirth condition. She will have a bloody discharge called *lochia* for several weeks after the birth.

Currently, about 60% of mothers breastfeed their infants, up from about 10% in 1970. **Lactation,** the production of milk, begins about 3 days after childbirth. Prior to that time (sometimes as early as the second trimester), colostrum is secreted by the nipples. Colostrum contains antibodies that help protect the newborn from infectious diseases and is also high in protein.

The American Academy of Pediatricians recommends breastfeeding for at least the first year of a baby's life, and or as long after that as a mother and baby desire. Human milk is perfectly suited to the baby's nutritional needs and digestive capabilities, and it supplies the baby with antibodies. There appears to be a dose-response relationship between breast-feeding and risk of illness in the first 6 months of life. Breastfeeding decreases the incidence of infant ear infections, allergies, diarrhea, and bacterial meningitis. One study has even suggested that children who are breastfed do better in school and score higher on standardized tests. Breastfeeding is also beneficial to the mother: It stimulates contractions that help the uterus return to normal more rapidly, contributes to postpregnancy weight loss, and may reduce the risk of ovarian cancer, early breast cancer, and postmenopausal hip fracture. Nursing also provides a sense of closeness and emotional well-being for mother and child. For women who want to breastfeed but have problems, help is available from support groups, books, or a lactation consultant.

For some women, physical problems such as tenderness or infection of the nipples can make breastfeeding difficult. If a woman has an illness or requires drug treatment, she may have to bottlefeed her baby because drugs and infectious agents may show up in breast milk. Breastfeeding can be restrictive, making it especially difficult for working mothers. Employers rarely provide nursing breaks, so bottlefeeding or the use of a breast pump (to express milk for use while the mother is away from her infant) may be the only practical alternatives. Bottlefeeding makes it easier to tell how much milk an infant is taking in, and bottlefed infants tend to sleep longer. Bottlefeeding also allows the father or other caregiver to share in the nurturing process. Both breastfeeding and bottlefeeding can be part of loving, secure parent-child relationships.

When a mother doesn't nurse, menstruation usually begins within about 10 weeks. Breastfeeding can prevent the return of menstruation for as long as 6 months because the hormone prolactin, which aids milk production, suppresses hormones vital to the development of mature eggs. However, ovulation—and pregnancy—can occur before menstruation returns, so breastfeeding is not

electronic fetal monitoring (EFM) The use of an external or internal electronic monitor during labor to measure uterine contractions and fetal heart rate. **TERMS**

episiotomy An incision made to widen the vaginal opening to facilitate childbirth and prevent uncontrolled tearing during delivery.

rooming-in The practice of allowing the mother and baby to remain together in the hospital or birth center after delivery.

cesarean section A surgical incision through the abdominal wall and uterus, performed to extract a fetus.

postpartum period The period of about 3 months after delivering a baby.

lactation The production of milk.

a contraceptive method. If a woman wishes to avoid pregnancy, she should use a reliable method of contraception. If the mother becomes pregnant while still nursing, she should stop nursing to ensure good nutrition for the unborn child.

Many women experience fluctuating emotions during the postpartum period as hormone levels change. The physical stress of labor, as well as dehydration, blood loss, and other physical factors, contribute to lowering the woman's stamina. About 50–80% of new mothers experience "baby blues," characterized by episodes of sadness, weeping, anxiety, headache, sleep disturbances, and irritability. A mother may feel lonely and anxious about caring for her infant. About 10% of new mothers experience **postpartum depression,** a more disabling syndrome characterized by despondency, mood swings, guilt, and occasional hostility. Rest, sharing feelings and concerns with others, and relying on supportive relatives and friends for assistance are usually helpful in dealing with mild cases of the baby blues or postpartum depression, which generally lasts only a few weeks. If the depression is serious, professional treatment may be needed. Some men also seem to get a form of postpartum depression, characterized by anxiety about their changing roles and feelings of inadequacy. Both mothers and fathers need time to adjust to their new roles as parents.

Another feature of the postpartum period is the development of attachment—the strong emotional tie that grows between the baby and the adult who cares for the baby. Parents can foster secure attachment relationships in the early weeks and months by responding sensitively to the baby's true needs. Parents who respond appropriately to the baby's signals of gazing, looking away, smiling, and crying establish feelings of trust in their child. They feed the baby when she's hungry, for example; respond when she cries; interact with her when she gazes, smiles, or babbles; and stop stimulating her when she frowns or looks away. A secure attachment relationship helps the child develop and function well socially, emotionally, and mentally.

For most people, the arrival of a child is one of life's most important events, providing a deep sense of joy and accomplishment. However, adjusting to parenthood requires effort and energy. Talking with friends and relatives about their experiences during the first few weeks or months with a baby can help prepare new parents for the period when the baby's needs may require all the energy that both parents have to expend. But the pleasures of nurturing a new baby are substantial, and many parents look back on this time as one of the most significant and joyful of their lives.

TERMS **postpartum depression** An emotional low that may be experienced by the mother following childbirth.

SUMMARY

Preparation for Parenthood

- Factors to consider when deciding if and when to have a child include physical health and age; financial circumstances; relationship with your partner; educational, career, and child care plans; emotional readiness for parenthood; social support system; personal qualities, attitudes toward children, and aptitude for parenting; and philosophical or religious beliefs.

- Health care before pregnancy can reduce risks for both mother and child. Preconception care examines factors such as preexisting medical conditions, current medications, past history of pregnancy, age of the mother, lifestyle behaviors, infections, nutritional status, and family history of genetic disease.

Understanding Fertility

- Fertilization is a complex process culminating when a sperm penetrates the membrane of the egg released from the woman's ovary.

- Infertility affects about 10% of the reproductive age population of the United States. The leading causes of infertility in women are blocked oviducts and endometriosis. Exposure to toxic substances, the use of certain drugs, injury to the testicles, and infection can all cause infertility in men.

- Some types of infertility can be treated, but advanced techniques are expensive and can be emotionally and physically difficult.

- One way to avoid some forms of infertility is to protect oneself against STDs and to get treatment for any disease contracted.

Pregnancy

- Early pregnancy tests detect the presence of human chorionic gonadotropin (HCG) in the urine or blood of the mother.
- Early signs and symptoms include a missed menstrual period; slight bleeding; nausea; breast tenderness; sleepiness, fatigue, and emotional upset; and a softening of the uterus just above the cervix.
- During pregnancy, the uterus enlarges until it pushes up into the rib cage; the breasts enlarge and may secrete colostrum; the muscles and ligaments soften and stretch; and the circulatory system, lungs, and kidneys become more efficient.
- Pregnancy may lead to either increased or decreased interest in sexual activity. Mood changes are common throughout pregnancy.

- The fetal anatomy is almost completely formed in the first trimester and is refined in the second; during the third trimester, the fetus grows and gains most of its weight, storing nutrients in fatty tissues.

- As the fertilized egg divides, its outer cells develop into the placenta, umbilical cord, and amniotic sac.

- Information about the health and sex of a fetus can be obtained through prenatal tests such as ultrasound, amniocentesis, chorionic villus sampling, and AFP screening.

- Health care during pregnancy includes a complete history and physical at the beginning, followed by regular checkups for blood pressure, weight gain, and size and position of the fetus. Blood tests reveal blood type, anemia, STDs, and Rh incompatibilities.

- Important elements of prenatal care include good nutrition; avoiding drugs, alcohol, tobacco, infections, and other harmful environmental agents or conditions; regular physical activity; and childbirth classes.

- Pregnancy usually proceeds without major complications. Problems that can occur include ectopic pregnancy, spontaneous abortion, toxemia, and low birth weight. The loss of a fetus or infant is deeply felt by most parents, who need time to experience their grief and to heal.

Childbirth

- Couples preparing for childbirth may have many options to choose from, including type of practitioner and facility.

- The first stage of labor begins with contractions that exert pressure on the cervix, causing effacement and dilation. The period of transition is characterized by frequent and intense contractions, and complete dilation of the cervix.

- The second stage of labor begins when the baby's head moves into the birth canal and ends when the baby emerges.

- The third stage of labor is expulsion of the placenta. The umbilical cord is cut, and the baby takes its first breath.

- During the postpartum period, the mother's body begins to return to its prepregnancy state, and she may begin to breastfeed. Both mother and father must adjust to their new roles as parents, as they develop a strong emotional tie to their baby.

TAKE ACTION

1. Interview your parents to find out what your birth was like. What were the cultural conditions like at the time, and what were their personal preferences? Find out as much as you can about hospital procedure, the use of anesthetics, length of hospital stay, and so on. Did your father have a role in your birth? If possible, interview your grandparents or someone of their generation. How was their experience different from that of your parents'?

2. Investigate the childbirth facilities in your community. If possible, visit the maternity wing of a hospital and an alternative birth center. What do you like about them, and what do you not like? What types of childbirth preparation classes do they offer? Which of these do you feel most comfortable with? Why?

JOURNAL ENTRY

1. Would you take advantage of a prenatal diagnostic tool like amniocentesis to find out ahead of time if your child had a genetic abnormality? If such an abnormality was discovered, would you choose to terminate the pregnancy? Write an essay describing what you would do and why. What criteria would you use to make your decision?

2. Do you think you are ready to become a parent? Make a list of the qualities you possess that you think would make you a good parent. Then list those qualities that might be a hindrance to good parenting. Do you think your partner (if you have one) is ready to become a parent? Create the same type of lists based on his or her personal qualities.

3. *Critical Thinking* There have been many legal cases involving the status of sperm or embryos frozen as part of an infertility treatment such as artificial insemination or in vitro fertilization. Research one or more of these cases, and write an essay outlining some of the moral and legal implications of this technology. What guidelines would you suggest for regulating the use and status of frozen sperm and embryos? What evidence can you give to support your position?

Books

Fenwick, L. B. 1998. *Private Choices, Public Consequences: Reproductive Technology and the New Ethics of Conception, Pregnancy, and Family.* New York: E. P. Dutton. *Provides case histories and analyses of a wide range of issues.*

Glazer, E. S., and S. L. Cooper. 1998. *Choosing Assisted Reproduction: Social, Emotional, and Ethical Considerations.* Indianapolis: Perspectives Press. *Support, information, and advice for couples considering assisted reproduction.*

Kluger-Bell, K. 1998. *Unspeakable Losses: Understanding the Experience of Pregnancy Loss, Miscarriage, and Abortion.* New York: Norton. *A sensitive psychological study of the experience of pregnancy loss.*

Milunsky, A., ed. 1998. *Genetic Disorders and the Fetus: Diagnosis, Prevention, and Treatment.* Baltimore: Johns Hopkins Press. *A comprehensive reference covering genetic disorders, prenatal testing, and genetic counseling.*

Nilsson, L., and L. Hamberger. 1993. *A Child Is Born.* New York: DPT/Seymour Lawrence. *The story of birth, beginning with fertilization, told in text and with stunning photographs.*

The following are a few of the many excellent guides to conception, pregnancy, and birth:

American Academy of Pediatrics. 1998. *Caring for Your Baby and Young Child.* New York: Bantam.

Colonero, J. 1998. *With You and Your Baby All the Way: The Complete Guide to Pregnancy, Childbirth, and Early Childcare.* Palo Alto, Calif.: Bull Publishing.

Eisenberg, A., et al. 1996. *What to Expect When You're Expecting.* New York: Workman.

Heinowitz, J. 1999. *Fathering Right from the Start: Straight Talk About Pregnancy, Birth, and Beyond.* San Diego, Calif.: Parents as Partners Press.

Kitzinger, S. 1997. *The Complete Book of Pregnancy and Childbirth.* Rev. ed. New York: Knopf.

Samuels, M., and N. Samuels. 1996. *The New Well Pregnancy Book.* New York: Fireside.

Spencer, P., and the editors of *Parenting Magazine.* 1998. *Parenting Guide to Pregnancy and Childbirth.* New York: Ballantine Books.

Stoppard, M. 1998. *Birth.* New York: DK Publishing.

Organizations and Web Sites

American College of Obstetricians and Gynecologists (ACOG). Provides written materials relating to many aspects of preconception care, pregnancy, and childbirth.
    409 12th St., S.W.
    P.O. Box 96920
    Washington, DC 20090
    202-863-2518
    http://www.acog.org

The American Society for Reproductive Medicine. Provides up-to-date information on all aspects of infertility.
    1209 Montgomery Hwy.
    Birmingham, AL 35216-2809
    205-978-5000
    http://www.asrm.org

Childbirth.Org. Contains medical information and personal stories about all phases of pregnancy and birth.
    http://www.childbirth.org

International Council on Infertility Information Dissemination. A Web site that includes information on current research and treatments for infertility.
    http://www.inciid.org

La Leche League International. Provides advice and support for breastfeeding mothers.
    1400 N. Meacham Rd.
    Schaumburg, IL 60168
    800-LaLeche
    http://www.lalecheleague.org

The March of Dimes. Provides public education materials on many pregnancy-related topics, including preconception care, genetic screening, diet and exercise, and the effects of smoking and drinking during pregnancy.
    1275 Mamaroneck Ave.
    White Plains, NY 10605
    888-MODIMES; 914-428-7100
    http://www.modimes.org

National Institute of Child Health and Human Development. Provides information about reproductive and genetic problems; sponsors the "Back to Sleep" campaign to fight SIDS.
    800-505-CRIB (Back to Sleep hotline)
    http://www.nih.gov/nichd

National Maternal and Child Health Clearinghouse. Distributes publications, posters, and videos relating to maternal, infant, and family health; most items are available free-of-charge.
    703-356-1964
    http://www.nmchc.org

ParentsPlace.com Pregnancy Department. Includes a pregnancy calendar, a due date calculator, and lots of advice on preparing a birth plan and other pregnancy topics.
    http://www.parentsplace.com/pregnancy

Resolve. Provides information, support, and referrals for people facing infertility.
    1310 Broadway
    Somerville, MA 02144
    617-623-0744 (National Helpline)
    http://www.resolve.org

SHARE. Provides information, support, and referrals to parents who have experienced miscarriage, stillbirth, or the death of an infant.
    St. Joseph's Health Center
    300 First Capital Dr.
    St. Charles, MO 63301-2893
    800-821-6819

The following sites include information, graphics, and video clips of fetal development:

Nova/Odyssey of Life
    http://www.pbs.org/wgbh/nova/odyssey/clips

University of Pennsylvania Basic Embryology Review
    http://www.med.upenn.edu/meded/public/berp

Visible Embryo
    http://visembryo.com

SELECTED BIBLIOGRAPHY

A disease of too much iron. 1999. *HealthNews,* January 5.

American Academy of Pediatrics Work Group on Breastfeeding. 1997. Policy statement: Breastfeeding and the use of human milk. *Pediatrics* 100(6): 1035–1039.

American College of Obstetricians and Gynecologists. 1998. *Exercise During Pregnancy.* Washington, D.C.: American College of Obstetricians and Gynecologists.

American Society for Reproductive Medicine. 1998. *Fact Sheet: Infertility* (retrieved September 11, 1998; http://www.asrm.org/fact/infertility.html).

American Society for Reproductive Medicine. 1998. *Frequently Asked Questions About Infertility* (retrieved October 12, 1998; http://www.asrm.org/patient/faqs.html).

Annas, G. J. 1998. The shadowlands—secrets, lies, and assisted reproduction. *New England Journal of Medicine* 339(13): 935–939.

Bastian, L. A., et al. 1998. Diagnostic efficiency of home pregnancy test kits. A meta-analysis. *Archives of Family Medicine* 7(5): 465–469.

Centers for Disease Control and Prevention. 1999. *Parvovirus B19 Infection and Pregnancy* (retrieved April 12,1999; http://www.cdc.gov/ncidod/diseases/parvob19preg.htm).

Centers for Disease Control and Prevention. 1998. Public Health Service Task Force recommendations for the use of antiretroviral drugs in pregnant women infected with HIV-1 for maternal health and for reducing HIV-1 transmission in the United States. *MMWR Recommendations and Reports* 47(RR-2).

Centers for Disease Control and Prevention. 1998. Use of folic acid–containing supplements among women of childbearing age—United States, 1997. *Morbidity and Mortality Weekly Report* 47(7): 131–134.

Chiriboga, C. A., et al. 1999. Dose-response effect of fetal cocaine exposure on newborn neurologic function. *Pediatrics* 103(1): 79–85.

Cooper, P. J., and L. Murray. 1998. Clinical review: Postnatal depression. *British Medical Journal* 316: 1884–1886.

Dejin-Karlsson, E., et al. 1998. Does passive smoking in early pregnancy increase the risk of small-for-gestational-age infants? *American Journal of Public Health* 88: 1523–1527.

Delaney-Black, V., et al. 1998. Prenatal cocaine exposure and child behavior. *Pediatrics* 102(4): 945–950.

Ebrahim, S. H., et al. 1999. Comparison of binge drinking among pregnant and nonpregnant women, United States, 1991–1995. *American Journal of Obstetrics and Gynecology* 180: 1–7.

Gilbert, W. M., T. S. Nesbitt, and B. Danielsen. 1999. Childbearing beyond age 40: Pregnancy outcome in 24,032 cases. *Obstetrics and Gynecology* 93(1): 9–14.

Guzick, D. S., et al. 1999. Efficacy of superovulation and intrauterine insemination in the treatment of infertility. *New England Journal of Medicine* 340: 177–183.

Hakim, R. B., R. H. Gray, and H. Zacur. 1998. Alcohol and caffeine consumption and decreased fertility. *Fertility and Sterility* 70(4): 632–637.

Hatch, M., et al. 1998. Maternal leisure-time exercise and timely delivery. *American Journal of Public Health* 88: 1528–1533.

Herman, W. H., et al. 1999. Diabetes and pregnancy. Preconception care, pregnancy outcomes, resource utilization and costs. *Journal of Reproductive Medicine* 44(1): 33–38.

Hoo, A. F., et al. 1998. Respiratory function among preterm infants whose mothers smoked. *American Journal of Respiratory and Critical Care Medicine* 158(3): 700–705.

Hormone mimics: They're in our food; should we worry? 1998. *Consumer Reports,* June.

Horwood, L. J., and D. M. Fergusson. 1998. Electronic article: Breastfeeding and later cognitive and academic outcomes. *Pediatrics* 101(1): E9 (retrieved September 14, 1998; http://www. pediatrics.org/cgi/content/abstract/101/1/e9).

JAMA patient page: Rock-a-bye baby . . . on their backs. 1998. *Journal of the American Medical Association* 280(4): 722.

Jauniaux, E., et al. 1999. Maternal tobacco exposure and cotinine levels in fetal fluids in the first half of pregnancy. *Obstetrics and Gynecology* 93(1): 25–29.

Latka, M., J. Kline, and M. Hatch. 1999. Exercise and spontaneous abortion of known karyotype. *Epidemiology* 10(1): 73–75.

MacDorman, M. F., and G. K. Singh. 1998. Midwifery care, social and medical risk factors, and birth outcomes in the USA. *Journal of Epidemiology and Community Health* 52(5): 310–317.

March of Dimes. 1997. *Alpha-fetoprotein Screening* (retrieved September 11, 1998; http://www.modimes.org/pub/alpha.htm).

Mascola, M. A., et al. 1998. Exposure of young infants to environmental tobacco smoke: Breast-feeding among smoking mothers. *American Journal of Public Health* 88(6): 893–896.

McBean, L. D., and G. D. Miller. 1998. Allaying fears and fallacies about lactose intolerance. *Journal of the American Dietetic Association* 98(6): 671–676.

National Institute of Child Health and Development. 1999. *News Alert: Incidence of SIDS Increases during Cold Weather* (retrieved February 20, 1999; http://www.nih.gov/nichd/html/news/wintal2.htm).

National Institute on Alcohol Abuse and Alcoholism. 1998. *Drinking and Your Pregnancy* (retrieved November 19, 1998; http://silk.nih.gov/silk/niaaa1/publication/brochure. htm).

Ness, R. B., et al. 1999. Cocaine and tobacco use and the risk of spontaneous abortion. *New England Journal of Medicine* 340: 333–339.

Raisler, J., C. Alexander, and P. O'Campo. 1999. Breast-feeding and infant illness: a dose-response relationship? *American Journal of Public Health* 89: 25–30.

Saidi, J. A., et al. 1999. Declining sperm counts in the United States? A critical review. *Journal or Urology* 16(2): 460–462.

U.S. Bureau of the Census. 1998. *International Data Base: Infant Mortality Rates and Life Expectancy at Birth, by Sex* (retrieved November 18, 1998; http://www.census.gov/cgi-bin/ipc/idbsprd).

U.S. Department of Agriculture. 1998. *USDA Releases Annual Report on the Cost of Raising a Child* (retrieved September 11, 1998; http://www.usda.gov/news/releases/1998/03/0127).

U.S. Department of Health and Human Services. 1998. *Healthy People 2010 Objectives: Draft for Public Comment.* Washington, D.C.: U.S. Government Printing Office.

Williams, R. D. 1999. Healthy pregnancy, healthy baby. *FDA Consumer,* March/April.

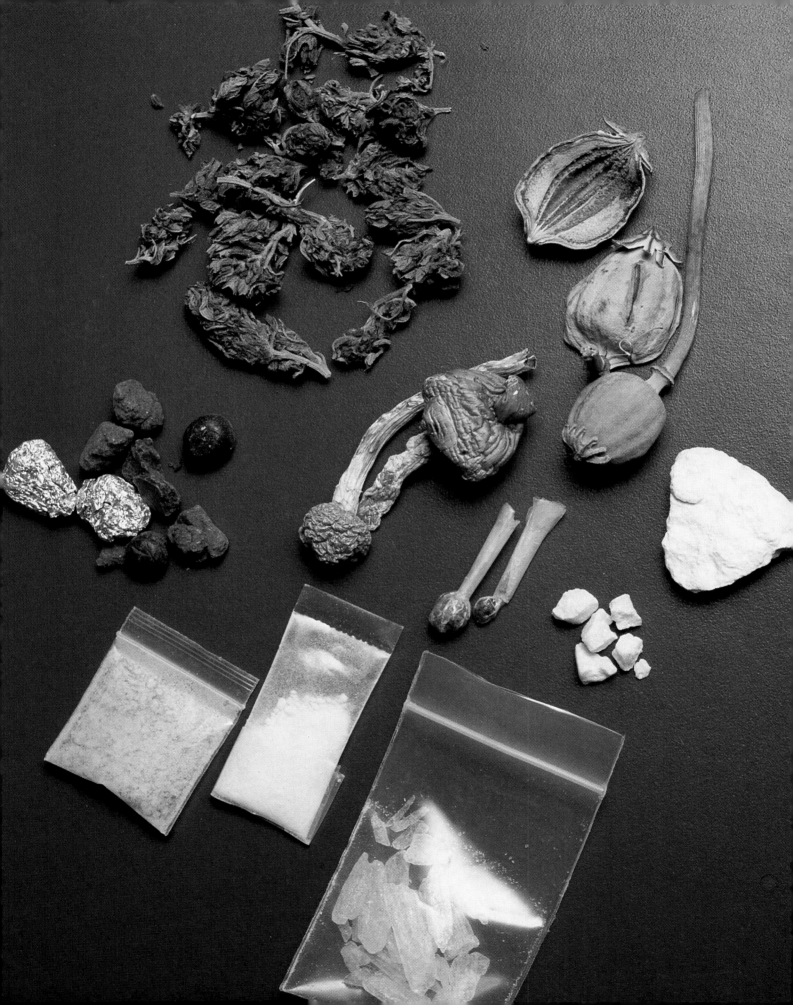

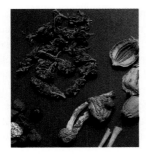

LEARNING OBJECTIVES

After reading this chapter, you should be able to:

- Define and discuss the concepts of addictive behavior, substance abuse, and substance dependence.

- Explain factors contributing to drug use and dependence.

- List the major categories of psychoactive drugs, and describe their effects, methods of use, and potential for abuse and dependence.

- Discuss social issues related to psychoactive drug use and its prevention and treatment.

- Evaluate the role of drugs and other addictive behaviors in your life, and identify your risk factors for abuse or dependence.

The Use and Abuse of Psychoactive Drugs

9

TEST YOUR KNOWLEDGE

1. Which of the following is the most widely used illegal drug in the United States?
   a. heroin
   b. cocaine
   c. marijuana

2. Caffeine use can produce physical dependence.
   True or false?

3. Which of the following drugs is most physically addictive?
   a. heroin
   b. nicotine
   c. Valium
   d. LSD

4. The effects of marijuana are strongly influenced by what the user expects.
   True or false?

5. Drug abuse treatment is available to about what percentage of Americans who are in immediate need of it?
   a. 25%
   b. 50%
   c. 75%

Answers

1. **c.** Marijuana is by far the most popular illegal drug; cocaine is a distant second.

2. **True.** Regular users of caffeine develop physical tolerance, needing more caffeine to produce the same level of alertness. Many also experience withdrawal symptoms, such as headaches and irritability, when they decrease their intake.

3. **b.** Heroin and Valium are also highly addictive; LSD less so. Nicotine is believed to be the most highly addictive psychoactive drug.

4. **True.** Expectations are particularly important at low doses. In studies in which users smoked joints they were told contained no marijuana—but which actually did—the users experienced no effects from the drug.

5. **b.** It is estimated that more than 7 million Americans need drug treatment, including more than 1.5 million injecting drug users. In some instances, addicts who want treatment have to wait a year for placement in a treatment facility.

The use of **drugs** for both medical and social purposes is widespread in American society (Table 9-1). Many people believe that every problem, no matter how large or small, has or should have chemical solutions. For fatigue, many of us turn to caffeine; for insomnia, sleeping pills; for anxiety or boredom, alcohol or other recreational drugs. Advertisements, social pressures, and the human desire for quick fixes to life's difficult problems all contribute to the prevailing attitude that drugs can ease all pain. Unfortunately, using drugs can—and often does—have serious consequences.

The most serious consequences are abuse and addiction. The drugs most often associated with abuse are **psychoactive drugs**—those designed to alter a person's experiences or consciousness. In the short term, psychoactive drugs can cause **intoxication,** a state in which sometimes unpredictable physical and emotional changes occur. A person who is intoxicated may experience potentially serious changes in physical functioning; his or her emotions and judgment may be affected in ways that lead to uncharacteristic and unsafe behavior. In the long term, recurrent drug use can have profound physical, emotional, and social effects.

This chapter focuses primarily on psychoactive drugs: their short- and long-term effects, and their potential for abuse and addiction. Two of the most widely used psychoactive drugs—alcohol and nicotine—will be treated in detail in Chapters 10 and 11. Before turning to the specific types of psychoactive drugs, let's take a closer look at addictive behavior in general.

ADDICTIVE BEHAVIOR

Although addiction is most often associated with drug use, many experts now extend the concept of addiction to other areas. **Addictive behaviors** are habits that have gotten out of control, with a resulting negative impact on a person's health. Looking at the nature of addiction and a range of addictive behaviors can help us understand similar behaviors when they involve drugs.

What Is Addiction?

The word "addiction" tends to be a highly charged one for most people. We may jokingly say we're "addicted to" fudge swirl ice cream or our morning jog, but most of us think of true addiction as a habitual and uncontrollable behavior, usually involving the use of a drug. Some people think of addiction as a moral flaw or a personal weakness. Others think addictions arise from certain personality traits, genetic factors, or socioeconomic influences. Views on the causes of addictions have an impact on our attitudes toward people with addictive disorders, as well as on the approaches to treatment.

Historically, the term *addiction* was applied only when the habitual use of a drug produced chemical changes in the user's body. One such change is physical tolerance, in which the body adapts to a drug so that the initial dose no longer produces the original emotional or psychological effects. This process, caused by chemical changes, means the user has to take larger and larger doses of the drug to achieve the same "high." (Tolerance will be discussed in greater detail later in the chapter.) The concept of addiction as a disease process, one based in brain chemistry, rather than a moral failing, has led to many advances in the understanding and treatment of drug addiction.

Some scientists think that other behaviors may share some of the chemistry of drug addiction. They suggest that activities like gambling, eating, exercising, and sex trigger the release of brain chemicals that cause a pleasurable "rush" in much the same way that psychoactive drugs do. The brain's own chemicals thus become the "drug" that can cause addiction. These theorists suggest that drug addiction and addiction to other pleasurable behaviors have a common mechanism in the brain. In this view, addiction is partly the result of our own natural "wiring."

However, and very importantly, the view that addiction is based in our own brain chemistry does *not* imply that an individual bears no responsibility for his or her addictive behavior. Many experts believe that it is inaccurate and counterproductive to think of all bad habits and excessive behaviors as diseases. They point to other factors, especially lifestyle and personality traits, that play key roles in the development of addictive behaviors. Before we consider what those factors are, let's first look in more detail at what constitutes addictive behavior.

Characteristics of Addictive Behavior

It is often difficult to distinguish between a healthy habit and one that has become an addiction. Experts have identified some general characteristics typically associated with addictive behaviors:

- *Reinforcement.* Addictive behaviors are physically and/or psychologically reinforcing. Some aspect of the behavior produces pleasurable physical and/or emotional states, or relieves negative ones.

- *Compulsion or craving.* The individual feels a strong compulsion—a compelling need—to engage in the behavior, often accompanied by obsessive planning for the next opportunity to perform it.

- *Loss of control.* The individual loses control over the behavior and cannot block the impulse to engage in it. He or she may deny that the behavior is problematic, or may have tried but failed to control it.

- *Escalation.* Addiction often involves a pattern of escalation, in which more and more of a particular

TABLE 9-1	Drug Use Among U.S. College Students	
	Percentage Using the Substance	
Substance	**In the Past Year**	**In the Past 30 Days**
Alcohol	83	68
Cigarettes	44	29
Marijuana	31	19
Spit tobacco	8	5
LSD	7	3
Amphetamines	7	3
Cocaine	4	2
Inhalants	3	1
Tranquilizers	2	<1
Crack	<1	<1
Heroin	<1	<1

SOURCES: National Institute on Drug Abuse; Harvard School of Public Health College Alcohol Study; Core Institute.

substance or activity is required to produce its desired effects. This escalation typically means that a person must give an increasing amount of his or her time, attention, and resources to the behavior.

- *Negative consequences.* The behavior has serious negative consequences, such as problems with academic or job performance, difficulties with personal relationships, health problems, or legal or financial troubles.

PERSONAL INSIGHT Have you ever had a pattern of behavior that you thought might be an addiction? If so, what led you to think you might be addicted? What do you think is the difference between an addiction and a habit?

The Development of Addiction

There is no single cause of addiction. Instead, characteristics of an individual person, of the environment in which the person lives, and of the substance or behavior he or she abuses combine in an addictive behavior. Although addictive behaviors share many common characteristics, the importance of these different factors varies from one case to another, even when the addiction is to the same substance or behavior.

We all engage in activities that are potentially addictive. Some of these activities can be part of a wellness lifestyle if they are done appropriately and in moderation,

but if a behavior starts to be excessive, it may become an addiction. An addiction often starts when a person does something he or she thinks will bring pleasure or help avoid pain. The activity may be drinking a beer, going on the Internet, playing the lottery, or going shopping. If it works, and the behavior does bring pleasure or dull pain, the person is likely to repeat it. He or she becomes increasingly dependent on the behavior, and tolerance develops—that is, the person needs more of the behavior to feel the same effect. Eventually, the behavior becomes a central focus of the person's life, and there is a deterioration in other areas, such as school performance or relationships. The behavior no longer brings pleasure, but it is necessary to avoid the pain of going without it. What started as a seemingly innocent way of feeling good can become a prison.

Many common behaviors are potentially addictive, but most people who engage in them do not develop problems. The reason, again, lies in the combination of factors that are involved in the development of addiction, including personality, lifestyle, heredity, the social and physical environment, and the nature of the substance or behavior in question. For a behavior to become an addiction, these diverse factors must come together in a certain way. For example, nicotine, the psychoactive drug in tobacco, has a very high potential for physical addiction; but a person who doesn't choose to try cigarettes, perhaps because of family influence or a tendency to develop asthma, will never develop nicotine addiction.

Characteristics of People with Addictions

The causes and course of an addiction are extremely varied, but people with addictions do seem to share some characteristics. Many use the substance or activity as a substitute for other, healthier coping strategies. People vary in their ability to manage their lives, and those who have the most trouble dealing with stress and painful emotions may be more susceptible to addiction.

Some people may have a genetic predisposition to addiction to a particular substance; such predispositions may involve variations in brain chemistry. People with addictive disorders usually have a distinct preference for a particular addictive behavior, and they typically expect to

drug Any chemical other than food intended to affect the structure or function of the body.   **TERMS**

psychoactive drug A drug that can alter a person's consciousness or experience.

intoxication The state of being mentally affected by a chemical (literally, a state of being poisoned).

addictive behavior Any habit that has gotten out of control, resulting in a negative effect on one's health.

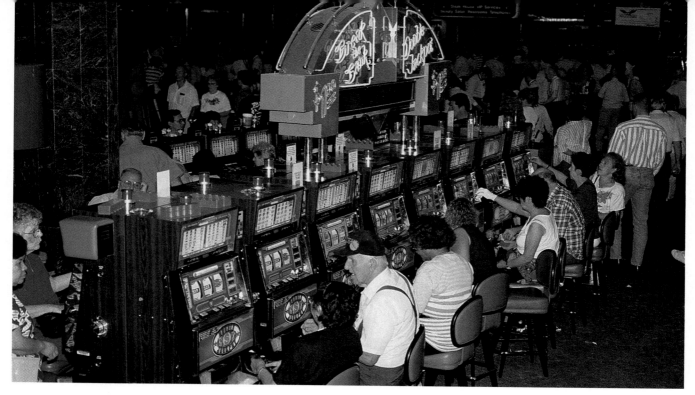

Most people who gamble do so casually and occasionally; but for a few, the habit spins out of control and becomes the central focus of their life. A variety of factors appears to influence whether a habit becomes an addiction, including personality, lifestyle, heredity, social environment, and the nature of the activity.

have a positive experience with it even before they try it. They also often have problems with impulse control and self-regulation and tend to be risk takers.

Examples of Addictive Behaviors

The use and abuse of psychoactive drugs will be explored in detail later in the chapter. In this section, we'll examine some behaviors that are not related to drugs and that can become addictive for some people.

Compulsive or Pathological Gambling   Many people gamble casually by putting a dollar in the office football pool, buying a lottery ticket, or going to the races. But a few become compulsive gamblers, unable to resist or control the urge to gamble, even in the face of financial and personal ruin. Most compulsive gamblers say they are seeking excitement even more than money. Increasingly larger bets are necessary to produce the desired level of excitement. A series of losses can lead to a perceived need to keep placing bets to win back the money. When financial resources become strained, the person may lie or steal to pay off debts. The consequences of compulsive gambling are not just financial; the suicide rate of compulsive gamblers is 20 times higher than that of the general population.

Compulsive gamblers may gamble to relieve negative feelings and become restless and irritable when they are unable to gamble. As with many addictive behaviors,

compulsive gambling may begin or flare up in times of stress. The earlier one starts to gamble, the more likely one is to become a pathological gambler. Gambling is often linked to other risky behaviors, and many compulsive gamblers also have drug and alcohol abuse problems.

The American Psychiatric Association (APA) recognizes pathological gambling as a mental disorder and lists ten characteristic behaviors, including preoccupation with gambling, unsuccessful efforts to cut back or quit, using gambling to escape problems, and lying to family members to conceal the extent of involvement with gambling. Compulsive gambling shares many of these traits with other addictive behaviors, including drug use. An estimated 1.1 million adolescents and 1.9 million adults in the United States may be compulsive gamblers.

Sex and Love Addiction   More controversial is the notion of addiction to sex or love. Some researchers believe that the initial rush of arousal and erotic or romantic "chemistry" produces an effect in the brain comparable to that of taking amphetamines or morphine. After a time, the brain becomes desensitized to those chemicals, and the addict must then seek his or her next "fix" by pursuing a new partner. According to this view, cheating on a partner, having many partners, and sexually victimizing others are behaviors parallel to drug-seeking behavior. Behaviors associated with so-called sex addicts include an extreme preoccupation with sex, a compulsion to have sex repeatedly within a short period of time, spending a great deal of time and energy looking for partners or engaging in sex, using sex as a means of relieving painful feelings, and suffering negative emotional, personal, and professional consequences as a result of sexual activities.

Some experts are reluctant to call compulsive sexual activity a true addiction. However, even therapists who challenge the concept of sex addiction recognize that some people become overly preoccupied with sex, cannot seem to control their sex drive, and act in potentially harmful ways in order to obtain satisfaction. This pattern of sexual behavior does seem to meet the criteria for addictive behaviors discussed earlier.

Compulsive Spending or Shopping   Nearly everyone splurges at the mall or goes into debt once in a while. But a compulsive spender repeatedly gives in to the impulse to buy much more than he or she needs or can afford. For the compulsive shopper, spending may serve to relieve painful feelings like depression or anxiety, or it may produce positive emotions like excitement or happiness. Compulsive spenders usually buy luxury items rather than daily necessities. Men tend to buy cars, exercise equipment, and sporting gear; women are more likely to buy clothes, jewelry, and perfume. Some experts link compulsive shopping with neglect or abuse during childhood; it also seems to be associated with eating disorders, depression, and bipolar disorder. Some compulsive shoppers are helped by antidepressant medications.

Compulsive shoppers are usually significantly distressed by their behavior and its social, personal, and financial consequences. Characteristics of out-of-control spending include shopping in order to "feel better," using money or time set aside for other purposes, hiding spending from others, and spending so much that one goes into debt or engages in illegal activities such as shoplifting or writing bad checks. Like other addictive behaviors, compulsive shopping is characterized by a loss of control over the behavior and significant negative consequences.

Internet Addiction   Some recent research has indicated that surfing the World Wide Web can also be addictive. In order to spend more time online, Internet addicts skip important social, school, or recreational activities, thereby damaging personal relationships and jeopardizing academic and job performance. They may go into debt because of online fees. Despite the negative consequences they are experiencing, they don't feel able to stop. The Internet addicts identified in one study averaged 38 online hours per week.

Internet addicts may feel uncomfortable or be moody or irritable when they are not online. They may be preoccupied with getting back online and may stay there longer than they intend. Like other addictive behaviors described here, online addicts may be using their behavior to alleviate stress or avoid painful emotions.

Other behaviors that can become addictive include exercise, eating, watching TV, and working. Any substance or activity that becomes the focus of a person's life at the expense of other needs and interests can be damaging to health.

We turn now to the substances most commonly associated with addiction: psychoactive drugs.

DRUG USE, ABUSE, AND DEPENDENCE

Drugs are chemicals other than food that are intended to affect the structure or function of the body. They include prescription medicines, such as antibiotics and antidepressants; nonprescription, or over-the-counter (OTC), substances, such as alcohol, tobacco, and caffeine products; and illegal substances, such as cocaine and heroin. The use of drugs is not a new phenomenon in our society; in fact, drug use has a long history.

The Drug Tradition

Using drugs to alter consciousness is an ancient and universal pursuit. People have used alcohol to celebrate and intoxicate for thousands of years. People in all parts of the world have discovered and exploited the psychoactive properties of various local plants, such as the coca plant in South America and the opium poppy in the Middle East and Far East.

In the nineteenth century, chemists were successful in extracting the active chemicals from medicinal plants, such as morphine from the opium poppy and cocaine from the coca leaf. This was the beginning of modern *pharmacy*, the art of compounding drugs, and of *pharmacology*, the science and study of drugs. From this point on, a variety of drugs began to be produced, including morphine, cocaine, codeine, and heroin (Figure 9-1, p. 220).

Initially, the manufacture and sale of these new drugs was not regulated. Pure morphine or cocaine could be purchased by mail order, and the makers of patent medicines and tonics included potentially addictive drugs in their products without informing the consumer of the ingredients or the dangers. The earliest version of the soft drink Coca-Cola contained cocaine, which accounted for the "lift" it provided.

Drug addiction among middle-class Europeans and North Americans was more common by 1900 than at any time before or since. Concerns about drug addiction, and the need to regulate drug sales and manufacture, led in the early 1900s to the passage of U.S. federal drug regulations. Middle-class use of the regulated drugs dropped, and drug use became restricted to, and increasingly identified with, criminal subcultures.

Recreational drug use expanded in the general U.S. population during the 1960s and 1970s, reaching a peak in 1979. After a 12-year decline, marijuana use rose between

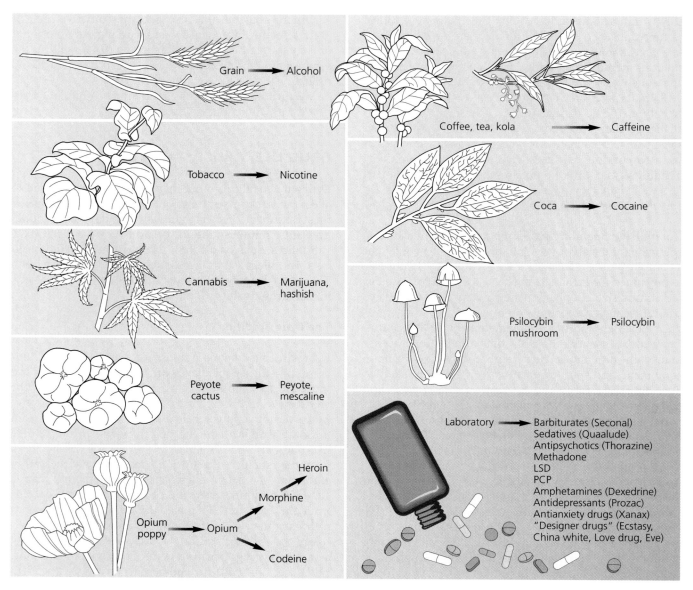

Figure 9-1 *Sources of selected psychoactive drugs.*

1991 and 1997, and then appeared to level off. The use of some other drugs by young people also increased during the 1990s. While it is appropriate for us to be concerned about these increases, no one should lose sight of the fact that the vast majority of young people still do not use marijuana or other illicit drugs.

Drug Abuse and Dependence

The APA's *Diagnostic and Statistical Manual of Mental Disorders* is the authoritative reference for defining all sorts of behavioral disorders, including those related to drugs. The APA has chosen not to use the term *addiction,* in part because it is so broad and has so many connotations.

Instead, they refer to two forms of substance (drug) disorders: substance abuse and substance dependence. Both are maladaptive patterns of substance use that lead to significant impairment or distress. Although the APA's definitions are more precise and more directly related to drug use, they clearly encompass the general characteristics of addictive behavior described in the last section.

Drug Abuse   As defined by the APA, **substance abuse** involves one or more of the following:
- Recurrent drug use, resulting in a failure to fulfill major responsibilities at work, school, or home.
- Recurrent drug use in situations in which it is physically hazardous, such as before driving a car.

- Recurrent drug-related legal problems.
- Continued drug use despite persistent social or interpersonal problems caused by or exacerbated by the effects of the drug.

The pattern of use may be constant or intermittent, and **physical dependence** may or may not be present. For example, a person who smokes marijuana once a week but cuts classes because he or she is high is abusing marijuana, even though he or she is not physically dependent.

Drug Dependence **Substance dependence** is a more complex disorder and is what many people associate with the idea of addiction. The seven specific criteria the APA uses to diagnose substance dependence are listed below. The first two are associated with physical dependence; the final five are associated with compulsive use. To be considered dependent, an individual must experience a cluster of three or more of these seven symptoms during a 12-month period.

1. *Developing tolerance to the substance.* When a person requires increased amounts of a substance to achieve the desired effect or notices a markedly diminished effect with continued use of the same amount, he or she has developed **tolerance.** For example, heavy heroin users may need to take ten times the amount they took at the beginning in order to achieve the desired effect; such a large dose would be lethal to a nonuser. The degree to which tolerance develops varies depending on the drug.

2. *Experiencing withdrawal.* In an individual who has maintained prolonged, heavy use of a substance, a drop in its concentration within the body can result in unpleasant physical and cognitive **withdrawal** symptoms. The person is likely to take the substance to relieve or avoid those symptoms. Withdrawal symptoms are different for different drugs. For example, nausea, vomiting, and tremors are common for alcohol, opioids, and sedatives; for stimulants like amphetamines, cocaine, and caffeine, malaise, fatigue, and irritability may occur. Other drugs have no significant withdrawal symptoms.

3. *Taking the substance in larger amounts or over a longer period than was originally intended.*

4. *Expressing a persistent desire to cut down or regulate substance use.* This desire is often accompanied by many unsuccessful efforts to reduce or discontinue use of the substance.

5. *Spending a great deal of time obtaining the substance, using the substance, or recovering from its effects.*

6. *Giving up or reducing important social, school, work, or recreational activities because of substance use.* A dependent person may withdraw from family activities and hobbies in order to use the substance in private, or to spend more time with substance-using friends.

7. *Continuing to use the substance in spite of recognizing that it is contributing to a psychological or physical problem.* For example, a person might continue to use cocaine despite recognizing that she is suffering from cocaine-induced depression.

If a drug-dependent person experiences either tolerance or withdrawal, he or she is considered physically dependent. However, not everyone who experiences tolerance or withdrawal is drug dependent. For example, a hospital patient who is prescribed therapeutic doses of morphine to relieve pain may develop a tolerance to the drug and experience withdrawal symptoms when the prescription is discontinued. But without showing any signs of compulsive use, this individual would not be considered dependent. Dependence can occur without a physical component, based solely on compulsive use. For example, people with at least three symptoms of compulsive use of marijuana who show no signs of tolerance or withdrawal are suffering from substance dependence. In general, dependence problems that involve physical dependence carry a greater risk of immediate general medical problems and have higher relapse rates.

> **PERSONAL INSIGHT**   Have you ever misused or abused a drug, even coffee or an OTC medication? If so, what were your reasons and motivations? Was it hard to stop? How did the experience affect your current attitudes and behaviors?

Who Uses Drugs?

The use and abuse of drugs occur at all income and education levels, among all ethnic groups, and at all ages.

substance abuse   A maladaptive pattern of use of any substance that persists despite adverse social, psychological, or medical consequences. The pattern may be intermittent, with or without tolerance and physical dependence.

physical dependence   The result of physiological adaptation that occurs in response to the frequent presence of a drug; typically associated with tolerance and withdrawal.

substance dependence   A cluster of cognitive, behavioral, and physiological symptoms that occur in an individual who continues to use a substance despite suffering significant substance-related problems, leading to significant impairment or distress; also known as *addiction*.

tolerance   Lower sensitivity to a drug so that a given dose no longer exerts the usual effect and larger doses are needed.

withdrawal   Physical and psychological symptoms that follow the interrupted use of a drug on which a user is physically dependent; symptoms may be mild or life-threatening.

TERMS

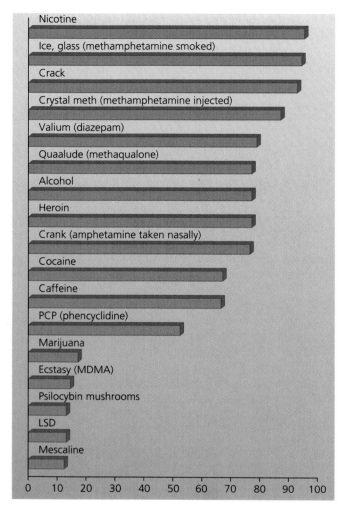

Figure 9-2   **How easy is it to get hooked on drugs?**   The numbers at the bottom of the chart are relative rankings. SOURCE: Hastings, J. 1990. Why do people take drugs? *Health,* November/December. Used with permission of Health Publishing Group.

One reason for our society's concern with the casual or recreational use of illegal drugs is that it is not really possible to know when drug use will lead to abuse or dependence. Some casual users develop substance-related problems; others do not. Some psychoactive drugs are more likely than others to lead to dependence (Figure 9-2). But some users of even heroin or cocaine do not meet the APA's criteria for substance dependence. However, people who begin to use drugs at very young ages have a greater risk for dependence and serious health consequences.

Although we can't accurately predict which drug users will become drug abusers, researchers have identified some characteristics that place young people at higher-than-average risk for *trying* illicit drugs. Being male is one risk factor: Although gender differences in drug use are gradually narrowing, males are still about twice as likely

as females to use illicit drugs. An adolescent who has a poor self-image; lacks self-control; is aggressive, impulsive, or moody; or suffers from attention deficit/hyperactivity disorder (ADHD) may be at increased risk for trying drugs. Internalizing difficult emotions such as depression and anxiety may also increase risk. A thrill-seeking or risk-taking personality is another factor. People who drive too fast or who don't wear safety belts may have this personality type, which is characterized by a sense of invincibility. Such people find it easy to dismiss warnings of danger, whether about drugs or safety belts—"That only happens to other people; it could never happen to me."

A peer group that accepts or rewards drug use is a significant risk factor for trying illicit drugs. Chaotic home environments, dysfunctional families, and parental abuse also increase risk. Children with no parental monitoring after school are more likely to try illicit drugs than those with regular adult supervision. Young people who live in disadvantaged areas are more likely to be offered drugs at a young age, thereby increasing their risk of drug use. Especially at younger ages, the risk of using drugs is higher for people who come from a single-parent family, for those whose parents failed to complete high school, and for those who are uninterested in school and earn poor grades. However, drug use rates among middle-class youths with college-educated parents tend to catch up with, and in some cases outstrip, those of other groups by the time students reach the twelfth grade.

What about people who *don't* use drugs? As a group, nonusers also share some characteristics. Not surprisingly, people who perceive drug use as risky and who disapprove of it are less likely to use drugs than those who believe otherwise. Drug use is also less common among people who have positive self-esteem and self-concept and who are assertive, independent thinkers who are not controlled by peer pressure. Self-control, social competence, optimism, academic achievement, and regular church attendance are also linked to lower rates of drug use.

Home environments are also influential: Coming from a strong family, one that has a clear policy on drug use, is another characteristic of people who don't use drugs. Young people who communicate openly with their parents and feel supported by them are also less likely to use drugs. Although parents may feel they have little effect on their children's drug-related attitudes and behaviors, evidence suggests that they can be a major influence. Some parents may wait too long to express a clear drug policy. Recent surveys indicate that attitudes about drugs and access and exposure to drugs change most dramatically between the ages of 12 and 13. Compared to a 12-year-old, a 13-year-old is about three times more likely to know teens who use and sell drugs and to know where and how to buy drugs. Yet nearly half of 13-year-olds report that their parents have never seriously discussed the dangers of illegal drugs with them.

Why Do People Use Drugs?

The answer to this question depends on both the user and the drug. Young people, especially those from middle-class backgrounds, are frequently drawn to drugs by the allure of the exciting and illegal. They may be curious, rebellious, or vulnerable to peer pressure. They may want to appear to be daring and to be part of the group. They may want to imitate adult models in their lives or in the movies. Most people who have taken illicit drugs have done so on an experimental basis, typically trying the drug one or more times but not continuing. The main factors in the initial choice of a drug are whether it is available and whether other people around are already using it.

Although some people use drugs because they have a desire to alter their mood or are seeking a spiritual experience, others are motivated primarily by a desire to escape boredom, anxiety, depression, feelings of worthlessness, or other distressing symptoms of psychological problems. They use drugs as a way to cope with the difficulties they are experiencing in life. The common practice in our society of seeking a drug solution to every problem is a factor in the widespread reliance on both illicit and prescription drugs.

For people living in poverty in the inner cities, many of these reasons for using drugs are magnified. The problems are more devastating, the need for escape more compelling. Furthermore, the buying and selling of drugs provide access to an unofficial, alternative economy that may seem like an opportunity for success.

> **PERSONAL INSIGHT** What was your family's attitude about drugs when you were growing up? Did your parents discuss drugs with you? Did they set rules or offer advice about how to deal with situations involving drugs? How did their attitudes affect your current values? Do you share your parents' attitudes about drugs, or have you adopted a different position?

Risk Factors for Dependence

Why do some people use psychoactive drugs without becoming dependent, while others aren't as lucky? The answer seems to be a combination of physical, psychological, and social factors. Research indicates that some people may be born with certain characteristics of brain chemistry or metabolism that make them more vulnerable to drug dependence. Other research suggests that people who were exposed to drugs while still in the womb may have an increased risk of abusing drugs themselves later in life. People who suffer from chronic pain, such as those with back injuries, also risk becoming dependent on the medications they take to relieve pain.

Psychological risk factors for drug dependence include difficulty in controlling impulses, and having a strong need for excitement, stimulation, and immediate gratification. Feelings of rejection, hostility, aggression, anxiety, or depression are also associated with drug dependence. People may turn to drugs to blot out their emotional pain.

People with mental illnesses have a very high risk of substance dependence. Research shows that about one-third of people with psychological disorders also have a substance-dependence problem, and about one-third of those have another mental disorder. People with two or more coexisting mental disorders are referred to as having **dual disorders.** Diagnosis of psychological problems among people with substance dependence can be very difficult because drug intoxication and withdrawal can mimic the symptoms of a mental illness.

Social factors that may influence drug dependence include growing up in a family in which a parent or sibling abused drugs, belonging to a peer group that emphasizes and encourages drug abuse, and poverty. Because they have easy access to drugs, health care professionals also have a higher risk. To determine whether you are at risk, take the quiz in the box "Do You Have a Problem with Drugs?" on p. 224.

HOW DRUGS AFFECT THE BODY

The psychoactive drugs discussed in this chapter have complex and variable effects. The same drug may affect different people differently, or the same person in different ways under different circumstances. The effects of a drug depend on three general categories of factors: (1) drug factors—the properties of the drug itself and differences in how it's used, (2) user factors—the physical and psychological characteristics of the user, and (3) social factors.

Drug Factors

When different drugs or dosages produce different effects, the differences are usually caused by one or more of five different drug factors:

1. The **pharmacological properties** of the drug are its overall effects on a person's body chemistry, behavior, and psychology.

> **TERMS**
>
> **dual disorder** The presence of two or more mental disorders simultaneously in the same person; for example, drug dependence and depression.
>
> **pharmacological properties** The overall effects of a drug on a person's behavior, psychology, and chemistry; also, the amount of the drug required to exert various effects, the time course of these effects, and other characteristics, such as the drug's chemical composition.

Answer yes (Y) or no (N) to the following questions:

1. Do you take the drug regularly? _____
2. Have you been taking the drug for a long time? _____
3. Do you always take the drug in certain situations or when you're with certain people? _____
4. Do you find it difficult to stop using the drug? Do you feel powerless to quit? _____
5. Have you tried repeatedly to cut down or control your use of the drug? _____
6. Do you need to take a larger dose of the drug in order to get the same high you're used to? _____
7. Do you feel specific symptoms if you cut back or stop using the drug? _____
8. Do you frequently take another psychoactive substance to relieve withdrawal symptoms? _____
9. Do you take the drug to feel "normal"? _____
10. Do you go to extreme lengths or put yourself in dangerous situations to get the drug? _____
11. Do you hide your drug use from others? Have you ever lied about what you're using or how much you use? _____
12. Do people close to you ask you about your drug use? _____
13. Are you spending more and more time with people who use the same drug as you? _____
14. Do you think about the drug when you're not high, figuring out ways to get it? _____
15. If you stop taking the drug, do you feel bad until you can take it again? _____
16. Does the drug interfere with your ability to study, work, or socialize? _____
17. Do you skip important school, work, social, or recreational activities in order to obtain or use the drug? _____
18. Do you continue to use the drug despite a physical or mental disorder, or despite a significant problem that you know is made worse by drug use? _____
19. Have you developed a mental or physical condition or disorder because of prolonged drug use? _____
20. Have you done something dangerous or that you regret while under the influence of the drug? _____

The more times you answer yes, the more likely it is that you are developing a dependence on the drug. If your answers suggest dependence, talk to someone at your school health clinic or to your physician about taking care of the problem before it gets worse.

2.   The **dose-response function** is the relationship between the amount of drug taken and the type and intensity of the resulting effect. Many psychological effects of drugs reach a plateau in the dose-response function, so that increasing the dose does not increase the effect any further. With LSD, for example, the maximum changes in perception occur at a certain dose, and no further changes in perception take place if higher doses are taken. However, all drugs have more than one effect, and the dose-response functions usually are different for different effects. This means that increasing the dose of any drug may begin to result in additional effects, which are likely to be increasingly unpleasant or dangerous at high doses.

3.   The **time-action function** is the relationship between the time elapsed since a drug was taken and the intensity of its effect. The effects of a drug are greatest when concentrations of the drug in body tissues are changing the fastest, especially if they are increasing.

4.   The person's *drug use history* may influence the effects of a drug. A given amount of alcohol, for example, will generally affect a habitual drinker less than an occasional drinker. Tolerance to some drugs, such as LSD, builds rapidly. To experience the same effect, a user has to abstain from the drug for a period of time before that dosage will again exert its original effects.

5.   The *method of use* has a direct effect on how strong a response a drug produces. Methods of use include ingestion, inhalation, injection, and absorption through the skin or tissue linings. Drugs are usually injected one of three ways: intravenously (IV, or mainlining), intramuscularly (IM), or subcutaneously (SC, or "skin popping").

If a drug is taken by a method that allows the drug to enter the bloodstream and reach the brain rapidly, the effects are usually stronger, and the potential for dependence greater, than when the method involves slower absorption. For example, injecting a drug intravenously

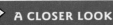

Drugs and HIV/AIDS

The use of contaminated hypodermic needles by injecting drug users is linked to one-third of all cases of AIDS in the United States, including nearly half of those among African Americans and Latinos. Over 60% of the 100,000+ AIDS cases among American women that had been diagnosed by early 1999 could be traced to injecting drug use or sexual contact with injecting drug users. Data gathered from the largest U.S. cities indicate that there are more than 1.5 million injecting drug users, about 14% of whom are infected with HIV. In cities with high rates of injecting drug use, infection rates may be as high as 30%.

No easy solutions are in sight. Most injecting drug users are removed from the social and medical mainstream and lack access to the standard sources of education about health issues. For those dependent on drugs, the physical and psychological cravings for drugs are powerful motivators of behavior, and safety factors alone aren't strong enough to change behavior.

Heroin and other injectable opiates are responsible for much of the spread of HIV infection among injecting drug users. Crack cocaine, even though it is smoked rather than injected, has also played a major role in the spread of HIV among young heterosexuals. Many crack users also engage in injecting drug use, and crack use frequently leads to increased sexual activity. Many users trade sex for drugs or sex for money to buy drugs. Rates of syphilis and other sexually transmitted diseases (STDs) have skyrocketed among crack users, also contributing to the spread of HIV. (The presence of genital sores related to STDs greatly increases the likelihood that a person will contract HIV from an infected sex partner.)

Some public health experts believe free syringe exchange programs (SEPs)—in which injecting drug users turn in a used syringe and get a new, clean one back—could help slow the spread of HIV. One study estimated that implementation of a national SEP early in the AIDS epidemic in the United States could have prevented as many as 20,000 cases of AIDS. Opponents of SEPs argue that supplying addicts with syringes gives them the message that illegal drug use is acceptable and could exacerbate the nation's drug problem. However, a National Academy of Sciences study of SEPs found that well-implemented programs do not increase the use of illegal drugs. Most current SEPs offer AIDS counseling and testing and provide referrals to drug-treatment programs. Despite a ban on federal funding for SEPs, local programs are proliferating and are exchanging nearly 20 million syringes per year.

People on both sides of the SEP debate agree that getting people off drugs is the best solution. But there are far more injecting drug users than treatment facilities can currently handle. Clearly, the spread of HIV among drug users constitutes a medical and social crisis that we will face for years to come.

SOURCES: National Institute on Drug Abuse. 1998. *Drug Abuse and AIDS* (retrieved November 30, 1998; http://www.nida.nih.gov/Infofax/DrugAbuse.html). Centers for Disease Control and Prevention. 1998. Update: Syringe-exchange programs—United States, 1997. *Morbidity and Mortality Weekly Report* 47(31): 652–655. Lurie, P., and E. Drucker. 1997. An opportunity lost: HIV infections associated with lack of a national needle-exchange programme in the USA. *Lancet* 349: 604–608.

---

produces stronger effects than swallowing the same drug. Inhaling a drug, such as when tobacco or crack cocaine is smoked, produces very rapid effects on the brain.

Different methods of drug use are associated with different risks. For example, injecting drugs often involves the sharing of needles, which may be contaminated with disease organisms from another user's blood. For this reason, injecting drug users are at high risk for hepatitis and HIV infection (see the box "Drugs and HIV/AIDS"). The surest way to prevent transmission of disease is never to share needles. Sterilizing needles using bleach may kill HIV, but care must be taken because viruses can be transmitted in very small amounts of blood and can survive in a syringe for a month or more. (See Chapters 17 and 18 for more information about preventing HIV infection and hepatitis.) Other dangers associated with injecting drugs include tetanus, botulism, the collapse of veins, and scarring and abscesses at the site of injection.

User Factors

The second category of factors that determine how a person will respond to a particular drug involves certain physical characteristics. Body mass is one variable. The effects of certain drugs on a 100-pound person will be twice as great as the effect of the same amount of the drug on a 200-pound person. Other variables include general health and various subtle biochemical states, including genetic factors. For example, some people have an inherited ability to rapidly metabolize a cough suppressant called dextromethorphan, which also has psychoactive properties. These people must take a higher-than-normal dose to get a given cough-suppressant effect.

If a person's biochemical state is already altered by another drug, this too can make a difference. Some drugs intensify the effects of other drugs, as is the case with alcohol and sedatives. Some drugs block the effects of other drugs, such as when a tranquilizer is used to relieve

dose-response function The relationship between the amount of a drug taken and the intensity or type of the resulting effect. **TERMS**

time-action function The relationship between the time elapsed since a drug was taken and the intensity of its effect.

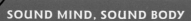
A placebo is a chemically inactive substance or ineffective procedure that a patient believes is an effective medical therapy for his or her condition. Researchers frequently give placebos to the control group in an experiment testing the efficacy of a particular treatment. By comparing the effects of the actual treatment with the effects of the placebo, researchers can judge whether or not the treatment is effective. The so-called placebo effect occurs when a patient improves after receiving a placebo. In such cases, the effect of the placebo on the patient cannot be attributed to the specific actions or properties of the drug or procedure.

Researchers have consistently found that 30–40% of all patients given a placebo show improvement. This result has been observed for a wide variety of conditions or symptoms, including coughing, seasickness, depression, migraines, and angina. For some conditions, placebos have been effective in up to 70% of patients. In some cases, people given a placebo even report having the side effects associated with an actual drug. Placebos are particularly effective when they are administered by a physician whom the patient trusts.

A clear demonstration of the placebo effect occurred in a recent study that examined the effectiveness of a type of beta-blocker, a drug used in the treatment of heart attacks. The men who participated in the study were randomly assigned to one of two groups: One group received the beta-blocker, the other received a placebo (a sugar pill with no chemical effects). Patients did not know to which group they had been assigned. Researchers found that the likelihood of the patient surviving a year was 2.6 times higher among the men who took their pills as prescribed. This may not seem surprising, until you learn that it did not matter which pill they took, the beta-blocker or the sugar pill. The act of taking the pill, regardless of whether it contained the drug, had a greater impact on the health of the patient than the chemical effect of the drug itself.

Placebo-like effects have also been observed in people using psychoactive drugs. People given a punch drink that they had been told contained alcohol reported feeling symptoms of intoxication. A study of people dependent on heroin found that many experienced the expected level of euphoria after injecting a placebo; one participant in the study even exhibited the contraction of the pupils that typically accompanies heroin injection. In another study, regular users of marijuana reported a moderate level of intoxication after using a cigarette that smelled and tasted like marijuana but contained no THC, the active ingredient in marijuana.

The placebo effect does not work for everyone or in all circumstances, and it does not mean you can improve your medical condition if you believe or do just anything, regardless of how irrelevant. Getting well, like getting sick, is a complex process. Anatomy, physiology, mind, emotions, and the environment are all inextricably entwined. But the placebo effect does show that belief can have both psychological and physical effects.

SOURCES: Brown, W. A. 1998. The placebo effect. *Scientific American* 278(1): 90–95. Turner, J. 1995. Placebo effects on pain. *Healthline*, April. The power of hope, 1994. *University of California at Berkeley Wellness Letter*, September.

anxiety caused by cocaine. Interactions between drugs, including many prescription and OTC medications, can be unpredictable and dangerous.

One physical condition that requires special precautions is pregnancy. It can be risky for a woman to use any drugs at all during pregnancy, including alcohol and common OTC preparations like cough medicine. The risks are greatest during the first trimester, when the fetus's body is rapidly forming and even small biochemical alterations in the mother can have a devastating effect on fetal development. Even later, the fetus is more susceptible than the mother to the adverse effects of any drugs she takes. The fetus may even become physically dependent on a drug being taken by the mother and suffer withdrawal symptoms after birth.

Sometimes a person's response to a drug is strongly influenced by the user's expectations about how he or she will react. With large doses, the drug's chemical properties do seem to have the strongest effect on the user's response. But with small doses, psychological (and social) factors are often more important. When people strongly believe that a given drug will affect them a certain way, they are likely to experience those effects regardless of the drug's pharmacological properties. This is an example of the **placebo effect**—when a person receives an inert substance, yet responds as if it were an active drug. (For more information, see the box "The Power of Belief: The Placebo Effect.")

Social Factors

The *setting* is the physical and social environment surrounding the drug use. If a person uses marijuana at home with trusted friends and pleasant music, the effects are likely to be different from the effects if the same dose is taken in an austere experimental laboratory with an impassive research technician. Similarly, the dose of alcohol that produces mild euphoria and stimulation at a noisy, active cocktail party might induce sleepiness and slight depression when taken at home while alone.

Experiments have been conducted in which some subjects smoked small quantities of marijuana while others (unknowingly) smoked a substance that smelled and tasted like marijuana but was not. The intensity of the **high** the subjects experienced was not related to whether or not they had actually smoked marijuana. In other studies, subjects who smoked low doses of real marijuana that they believed to be a placebo experienced no effects from the drug. Clearly, the setting and the user's expectations had greater effects on the smokers than the drug itself.

REPRESENTATIVE PSYCHOACTIVE DRUGS

What are the major psychoactive drugs, and how do they produce their effects? We discuss six different representative groups in this chapter: (1) opioids, (2) central nervous system depressants, (3) central nervous system stimulants, (4) marijuana and other cannabis products, (5) hallucinogens, and (6) inhalants. Some of these drugs are classified according to how they affect the body; others—the opioids and the cannabis products—are classified according to their chemical makeup. (For the sources of selected psychoactive drugs, see Figure 9-1.)

Opioids

Also called *narcotics,* **opioids** are natural or synthetic (laboratory-made) drugs that relieve pain, cause drowsiness, and induce **euphoria.** Opium, morphine, heroin, methadone, codeine, meperidine, and fentanyl are examples of drugs in this category. Opioids tend to reduce anxiety and produce lethargy, apathy, and an inability to concentrate. Opioid users become less active and less responsive to frustration, hunger, and sexual stimulation. These effects are more pronounced in novice users; with repeated use, many effects diminish.

Opioids are typically injected or absorbed into the body from the stomach, intestines, nasal membranes (from snorting or sniffing), or lungs (from smoking). Effects depend on the method of administration: If tissue levels of the drug change rapidly, more immediate effects will result. Although the euphoria associated with opioids is an important factor in their abuse, many people experience a feeling of uneasiness when they first use these drugs. Users also often feel nauseated and vomit, and they may have other unpleasant sensations. Even so, the abuse of opioids often results in dependence. Tolerance can develop rapidly and be pronounced.

Rates of heroin use have always been low, but there are periodic episodes of increased use among some groups. Use among college students remains below 1%; but between 1991 and 1998, heroin use among high school students nearly doubled, mostly due to increased rates of sniffing or smoking the drug. Although these users avoid the special disease risks of injecting drug use, including HIV infection, dependence can readily result from sniffing and smoking heroin. In addition, the potentially high but variable purity of street heroin poses a risk of unintentional overdose. Symptoms of overdose include respiratory depression, coma, and constriction of the pupils; death can result.

Central Nervous System Depressants

Central nervous system **depressants,** also known as **sedative-hypnotics,** slow down the overall activity of the **central nervous system (CNS).** The result can range from mild **sedation** to death, depending on the various factors involved—which drug is used, how it's taken, how tolerant the user is, and so on. CNS depressants include alcohol (discussed in Chapter 10), barbiturates, and other sedatives.

Types The various types of barbiturates are similar in chemical composition and action, but they differ in how quickly and how long they act. Drug users call barbiturates "downers" or "downs" and refer to specific brands by names that describe the color and design of the capsules: "reds" or "red devils" for Seconal; "yellows" or "yellow jackets" for Nembutal. People usually take barbiturates in capsules, but they may also inject them.

Antianxiety agents, also called sedatives or **tranquilizers,** include the benzodiazepines such as Xanax, Valium, Librium, clonazepam (Klonopin), and flunitrazepam (Rohypnol, also called "roofies"). Other CNS depressants include methaqualone (Quaalude), ethchlorvynol (Placidyl), chloral hydrate ("mickey"), and gamma hydroxy butyrate (GHB, or "liquid ecstasy").

Effects CNS depressants reduce anxiety and cause mood changes, impaired muscular coordination, slurring of speech, and drowsiness or sleep. Mental functioning is also affected, but the degree varies from person to person and also depends on the kind of task the person is trying to do. Most people become drowsy with small doses, although a few become more active. Some CNS depressants can also cause anterograde amnesia, the loss of memory of things occurring while under the influence of the drug. Because of this effect, Rohypnol, GHB, and chloral hydrate have been used as "date rape drugs" to incapacitate targets of sexual assault (see Chapter 23).

TERMS

placebo effect A response to an inert or innocuous medication given in place of an active drug.

high The subjectively pleasing effects of a drug, usually felt quite soon after the drug is taken.

opioid Any of several natural or synthetic drugs that relieve pain and cause drowsiness and/or euphoria; examples are opium, morphine, and heroin; also called *narcotic.*

euphoria An exaggerated feeling of well-being.

depressant or sedative-hypnotic A drug that decreases nervous or muscular activity, causing drowsiness or sleep.

central nervous system The brain and spinal cord.

sedation The induction of a calm, relaxed, often sleepy state.

tranquilizer A CNS depressant that reduces tension and anxiety.

Medical Uses Barbiturates, antianxiety agents, and other sedative-hypnotics are widely used to treat insomnia and anxiety disorders and to control seizures. Some CNS depressants are used for their calming properties in combination with **anesthetics** before operations and other medical or dental procedures.

From Use to Abuse People are usually introduced to CNS depressants either through a medical prescription or through drug-using peers. The abuse of CNS depressants by a medical patient may begin with repeated use for insomnia and progress to dependence through increasingly larger doses at night, coupled with a few capsules at stressful times during the day.

Most CNS depressants, including alcohol, can lead to classical physical dependence. Tolerance, sometimes for up to 15 times the usual dose, can develop with repeated use. Tranquilizers have been shown to produce physical dependence even at ordinary prescribed doses. Withdrawal symptoms can be more severe than those accompanying opioid dependence and are similar to the DTs of alcoholism (see Chapter 10). They may begin as anxiety, shaking, and weakness but may turn into convulsions and possible cardiovascular collapse and death.

While intoxicated, people on depressants cannot function very well. They are mentally confused and are frequently obstinate, irritable, and abusive. Even prescription use of benzodiazepines has been associated with an increased risk of automobile crashes. After long-term use, depressants like alcohol can lead to generally poor health and brain damage, with impaired ability to reason and make judgments.

Overdosing with CNS Depressants Too much depression of the central nervous system slows respiration and may stop it entirely. CNS depressants are particularly dangerous in combination with another depressant, such as alcohol. People who combine depressants with alcohol account for thousands of emergency room visits and hundreds of overdose deaths each year. Rohypnol is ten times more potent than Valium and can be fatal if combined with alcohol. GHB is often produced clandestinely, resulting in widely varying degrees of purity; it has been responsible for many poisonings and several deaths.

In recent surveys, about 2% of college students report having used a CNS depressant (other than alcohol) within the past year.

Central Nervous System Stimulants

CNS **stimulants** speed up the activity of the nervous or muscular system. Under their influence, the heart rate accelerates, blood pressure rises, blood vessels constrict, the pupils of the eyes and the bronchial tubes dilate, and gastric and adrenal secretions increase. There is greater muscular tension and sometimes an increase in motor

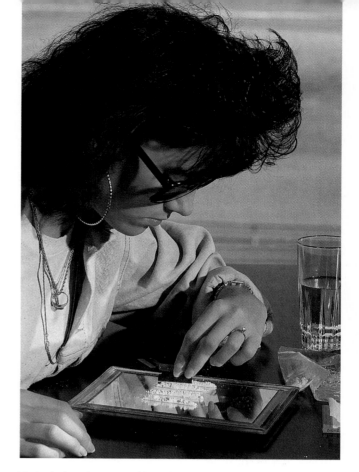

Method of use is one variable in the overall effect of a drug on the body. Sniffing or "snorting" cocaine produces effects in 2–3 minutes. With other methods, such as injecting it intravaneously, inhaling vapors, or smoking crack, the effects of cocaine are felt within seconds.

activity. Small doses usually make people feel more awake and alert, less fatigued and bored. The most common CNS stimulants are cocaine, amphetamine, nicotine (discussed in Chapter 11), ephedrine, and caffeine.

Cocaine Usually derived from the leaves of coca shrubs that grow high in the Andes Mountains in South America, cocaine is a potent CNS stimulant. For centuries, natives of the Andes have chewed coca leaves both for pleasure and to increase their endurance. For a short time during the nineteenth century, some physicians were enthusiastic about the use of cocaine to cure alcoholism and addiction to the painkiller morphine: Enthusiasm waned after the adverse side effects became apparent.

Cocaine—also known as "coke" or "snow"—quickly produces a feeling of euphoria, which makes it a popular recreational drug. Cocaine use surged in popularity during the early 1980s, when the drug's high price made it a "status" drug. The introduction of "crack" cocaine during the 1980s made the drug available in smaller quantities and at lower prices to more people. The typical recreational user shifted rapidly from the wealthy professional snorting (inhaling) powdered cocaine to poor inner-city smokers of crack cocaine. In the general population, cocaine use peaked in 1985 with an estimated 3% of adult Americans reporting use. In 1997, fewer than 1% of adults surveyed reported using cocaine. About 4% of college students report trying cocaine each year.

METHODS OF USE   Cocaine is usually inhaled or injected intravenously, providing rapid increases of the drug's concentration in the blood and therefore fast, intense effects. Another method of use involves processing cocaine with baking soda and water, yielding the ready-to-smoke form of cocaine known as crack. Crack is typically available as small beads or pellets smokable in glass pipes. The tiny but potent beads can be handled more easily than cocaine powder and marketed in smaller, less expensive doses.

EFFECTS   The effects of cocaine are usually intense but short-lived. The euphoria lasts from 5 to 20 minutes and ends abruptly, to be replaced by irritability, anxiety, or slight depression. When cocaine is absorbed via the lungs, by either smoking or inhalation, it reaches the brain in about 10 seconds, and the effects are particularly intense. This is part of the appeal of smoking crack. The effects from IV injections occur almost as quickly—about 20 seconds. Since the mucous membranes in the nose briefly slow absorption, the onset of effects from snorting takes 2–3 minutes. Heavy users who attempt to maintain the effects may inject cocaine intravenously every 10–20 minutes.

The larger the cocaine dose and the more rapidly it is absorbed into the bloodstream, the greater the immediate—and sometimes lethal—effects. Sudden death from cocaine is most commonly the result of excessive CNS stimulation that causes convulsions and respiratory collapse, irregular heartbeat, ischemia (lack of oxygen to the heart), and possibly heart attack or stroke. Although rare, fatalities can occur in young, athletic people who have no underlying health problems.

Cocaine constricts the blood vessels and acts as a local anesthetic. It is still used for minor nose surgery where bleeding is a problem. However, chronic cocaine use produces inflammation of the nasal mucosa, which can lead to persistent bleeding and ulceration of the septum between the nostrils. The use of cocaine may also cause paranoia and/or aggressiveness.

Even as the use of cocaine decreased in the general U.S. population after 1985, cocaine-related deaths and emergency room visits continued to rise into the mid-1990s. This presumably reflects the fact that smoking crack is more toxic than snorting powdered cocaine. Most deaths result from people using cocaine in combination with another substance, such as alcohol or heroin.

ABUSE AND DEPENDENCE   When steady cocaine users stop taking the drug, they experience a sudden "crash," char-acterized by depression, agitation, and fatigue, followed by a period of withdrawal. Their depression can be temporarily relieved by taking more cocaine, so its continued use is reinforced. Cocaine use follows different patterns in different individuals. A binge cocaine user may go for weeks or months without using any cocaine and then take large amounts repeatedly. Although not physically dependent, a binge cocaine user who misses work or school and risks serious health consequences is clearly abusing the drug.

COCAINE USE DURING PREGNANCY   Cocaine rapidly passes from the mother's bloodstream into the placenta and can have serious effects on the fetus. A woman who uses cocaine during pregnancy is at higher risk for miscarriage, premature labor, and stillbirth. She is more likely to deliver a low-birth-weight baby who has a small head circumference. Her infant may be at increased risk for defects of the genitourinary tract, cardiovascular system, central nervous system, and extremities. It is difficult to pinpoint the effects of cocaine because many women who use cocaine also use tobacco and/or alcohol.

Infants whose mothers use cocaine may also be born intoxicated. They are typically irritable, jittery, and do not eat or sleep normally. These characteristics may affect their early social and emotional development because it may be more difficult for adults to interact with them. Cocaine also passes into breast milk, from where it can intoxicate a breastfeeding infant.

Research on the long-term effects of prenatal exposure to cocaine has been inconclusive. Initial findings of devastating effects have not been borne out. Recent studies suggest that prenatal cocaine exposure may cause subtle changes in the brain that affect IQ, language skills, and motor development; behavioral problems—disorganization, poor social skills, and hyperactivity—have also been reported. Although fetal cocaine exposure is an important issue, the type and magnitude of effects produced by nicotine are similar, and there are nearly 20 times more infants exposed to cigarettes than to cocaine.

Amphetamines   Amphetamines are a group of synthetic chemicals that are potent CNS stimulants. Some common amphetamines are dextroamphetamine (Dexedrine), d-1-amphetamine (Benzedrine), and methamphetamine (Methedrine). Popular names for these drugs include "speed," "crank," "crystal," and "meth," and users refer to them all as "uppers."

"Ice," a smokable, high-potency form of methamphetamine, is popular in some cities. Easy to manufacture, ice is cheaper than crack and produces a similar but longer-

anesthetic   A drug that produces a loss of sensation with or without a loss of consciousness.

stimulant   A drug that increases nervous or muscular activity.

TERMS

lasting euphoria. The use of ice can quickly lead to dependence. In a recent survey of high school students, about 5% reported having tried ice at least once.

EFFECTS Small doses of amphetamines usually make people feel more alert and wide-awake and less fatigued or bored. Small doses can produce some improvement in activities that require extreme physical effort or endurance, such as sports and military training. Amphetamines generally increase motor activity but do not measurably alter a normal, rested person's ability to perform tasks calling for challenging motor skills or complex thinking. When amphetamines do improve performance, it is primarily by counteracting fatigue and boredom. Amphetamines in small doses also increase heart rate and blood pressure and change sleep patterns.

Amphetamines are sometimes used to curb appetite, but after a few weeks the user develops tolerance, and higher doses are necessary. When people stop taking the drug, their appetite usually returns, and they gain back the weight they lost unless they have made permanent changes in eating behavior.

FROM USE TO ABUSE Much amphetamine abuse begins as an attempt to cope with a temporary situation. A student cramming for an exam or an exhausted long-haul truck driver can go a little longer by taking amphetamines, but the results can be disastrous. The likelihood of making bad judgments significantly increases. An additional danger is that the stimulating effects may wear off suddenly, and the user may precipitously feel exhausted or fall asleep ("crash").

Another problem is **state dependence,** the phenomenon whereby information learned in a certain drug-induced state is difficult to recall when the person is not in that same physiological state. Test performance may deteriorate when students use drugs to study and then take tests in their normal, nondrug state. (Users of antihistamines may also experience state dependence.)

DEPENDENCE Repeated use of amphetamines, even in moderate doses, often leads to tolerance and the need for increasingly larger doses. The result can be severe disturbances in behavior, including a temporary state of paranoid

psychosis, with delusions of persecution and unprovoked violence. If injected in large doses, amphetamines produce a feeling of intense pleasure, followed by sensations of vigor and euphoria that last for several hours. As these feelings wear off, they are replaced by feelings of irritability and vague uneasiness. Long-term use of amphetamines at high doses can cause paranoia, hallucinations, delusions, and incoherence. Withdrawal symptoms may include muscle aches and tremors, along with profound fatigue, deep depression, despair, and apathy. Chronic high-dose amphetamine use is often associated with pronounced psychological cravings and obsessive drug-seeking behavior.

Women who use amphetamines during pregnancy risk premature birth, stillbirth, and early infant death. Babies born to amphetamine-using mothers have a higher incidence of cleft palate, cleft lip, and missing or deformed limbs. They may also be born dependent on amphetamines. Other hazards of amphetamine use include malnutrition, weight loss, damage to blood vessels, stroke, and other cardiovascular risks. The use of the injection method adds the risk of HIV infection and other blood-borne diseases from contaminated needles.

Ritalin A stimulant with effects similar to amphetamines, Ritalin (methylphenidate) is used to treat attention deficit/hyperactivity disorder. When taken orally at prescribed levels, it has little potential for abuse. When injected or snorted, however, dependence and tolerance can rapidly result. Ritalin abuse among high school and college students began to be reported in the 1990s.

Ephedrine Amphetamine was made in the 1920s by modifying the chemical ephedrine, which was originally isolated from a Chinese herbal tea. Although somewhat less potent than amphetamine, ephedrine does produce stimulant effects. It has been available for many years in OTC weight-loss preparations and has recently been marketed to truck drivers and others seeking a more effective stimulant than caffeine. It is also found in a product known as "herbal ecstasy." Uncontrolled use of ephedrine has been associated with some deaths, and the FDA has proposed regulations for the sale of ephedrine.

Caffeine Caffeine is probably the most popular psychoactive drug and also one of the most ancient. It is found in coffee, tea, cocoa, soft drinks, headache remedies, and OTC preparations like No-Dōz. In ordinary doses, caffeine produces greater alertness and a sense of well-being. It also decreases feelings of fatigue or boredom, and using caffeine may enable a person to keep at physically exhausting or repetitive tasks longer. Such use is usually followed, however, by a sudden letdown. Caffeine does not noticeably influence a person's ability to perform complex intellectual tasks unless fatigue, bore-

TERMS **state dependence** A situation in which information learned in a drug-induced state is difficult to recall when the effect of the drug wears off.

psychosis A severe mental disorder characterized by a distortion of reality; symptoms might include delusions or hallucinations.

depersonalization A state in which a person loses the sense of his or her own reality or perceives his or her own body as unreal.

dom, alcohol, or other factors have already affected normal performance.

Caffeine mildly stimulates the heart and respiratory system, increases muscular tremor, and enhances gastric secretion. Higher doses may cause nervousness, anxiety, irritability, headache, disturbed sleep, and gastric irritation or peptic ulcers. Some people, especially children, are quite vulnerable to the adverse effects of caffeine. They become "wired"—hyperactive and overly sensitive to any stimulation in their environment. In rare instances, the disturbance is so severe that there is misperception of their surroundings—a toxic psychosis.

Drinks containing caffeine are rarely harmful for most individuals, but some tolerance develops, and withdrawal symptoms of irritability, headaches, and even mild depression do occur. Thus, although we don't usually think of caffeine as a dependence-producing drug, for some people it is. People can usually avoid problems by simply decreasing their daily intake of caffeine (Table 9-2).

Marijuana and Other Cannabis Products

Marijuana is the most widely used illegal drug in the United States (cocaine is second). More than 30% of Americans—about 71 million—have tried marijuana at least once; among 18–25-year-olds, more than 40% have tried marijuana. Recent surveys of college students indicate that about 30% used marijuana within the last year.

Marijuana is a crude preparation of various parts of the Indian hemp plant *Cannabis sativa,* which grows in most parts of the world. THC (tetrahydrocannabinol) is the main active ingredient in marijuana. Based on THC content, the potency of marijuana preparations varies widely. Marijuana plants that grow wild often have less than 1% THC in their leaves, whereas when selected strains are cultivated by separation of male and female plants (*sinsemilla*), the bud leaves from the flowering tops may contain 7–8% THC. Hashish, a potent preparation made from the thick resin that exudes from the leaves, may contain up to 14% THC. These various preparations have all been known and used for centuries, so the frequently heard claim that today's marijuana is more potent than the marijuana of the 1970s is not strictly true. However, a greater proportion of the marijuana sold today may be the higher potency (and more expensive) sinsemilla.

Marijuana is usually smoked, but it can also be ingested. The classification of marijuana is a matter of some debate. For this reason, it is treated separately here.

Short-Term Effects and Uses As is true with most psychoactive drugs, the effects of a low dose of marijuana are strongly influenced both by the user's expectations and by past experiences. At low doses, marijuana users typically experience euphoria, a heightening of subjective sensory experiences, a slowing down of the perception of passing

TABLE 9-2	*Common Sources of Caffeine*	
Source	Amount	Typical Caffeine Content (mg)
Coffee		
Filter drip	8 oz	145
Starbucks "Short"	8 oz	140
Automatic percolated	8 oz	130
Instant	8 oz	95
Espresso	2 oz	70
Decaffeinated	8 oz	10
Tea		
Black, leaf or bag	8 oz	50
Green or instant	8 oz	30
Bottled, iced	12 oz	15
Decaffeinated	8 oz	5
Cocoa products		
Chocolate, dark or semisweet	1 oz	20
Chocolate, milk	1 oz	10
Hot chocolate or cocoa	8 oz	5
Cola		
Regular	12 oz	35
Medications*		
Excedrin	2 pills	130
No-Dōz, regular	1 pill	100
Anacin	2 pills	65

*Many weight-loss aids and cold remedies also contain caffeine.

SOURCES: Starbucks brew ha-ha. 1997. *Nutrition Action Healthletter,* January/February. The caffeine corner. 1996. *Nutrition Action Healthletter,* December.

time, and a relaxed, "laid-back" attitude. These pleasant effects are the reason this drug is so widely used. With moderate doses, these effects become stronger, and the user can also expect to have impaired memory function, disturbed thought patterns, lapses of attention, and feelings of **depersonalization,** in which the mind seems to be separated from the body. Decreased driving and workplace safety can also be expected.

The effects of marijuana in higher doses are determined mostly by the drug itself rather than by the user's expectations and setting. Very high doses produce feelings of depersonalization, as well as marked sensory distortion and changes in body image (such as a feeling that the body is very light). Inexperienced users sometimes think these sensations mean they are going crazy and become anxious or even panicky. Such reactions resemble a bad trip on LSD, but they happen much less often, are less severe, and do not last as long.

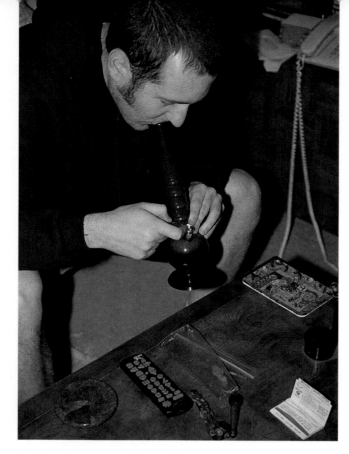

Marijuana is the most widely used illegal drug in the United States. At low doses, marijuana users typically experience euphoria and a relaxed attitude. Further research is needed to determine its precise physiological and psychological effects, particularly for chronic use.

Long-Term Effects   The most probable long-term effect of smoking marijuana is respiratory damage, including chronic bronchial irritation and precancerous changes in the lungs. (These negative effects from smoking marijuana are key reasons why the Institute of Medicine report on medical marijuana recommended the development of alternative methods of delivering the potentially beneficial compounds in marijuana.) Heavy users who are frequently intoxicated experience subtle impairments of attention and memory that may or may not be reversible following long-term abstinence. Long-term use may also decrease testosterone levels and sperm counts and increase sperm abnormalities.

Heavy marijuana use during pregnancy may cause impaired fetal growth and development and low birth weight. Marijuana may act synergistically with alcohol to increase the damaging effects of alcohol on the fetus. THC rapidly enters breast milk and may impair an infant's early motor development.

When we consider the long-term effects of marijuana (and of any other drugs), we should keep in mind the time-lag factor. Tobacco, for example, was long thought to be a "harmless" drug. Widespread marijuana use has been common for only about 25 years, and some effects may take longer than that to appear.

Dependence   Regular users of marijuana can develop tolerance; a few develop dependence. Withdrawal symptoms are generally mild and short-lived; they include restlessness, irritability, insomnia, nausea, and cramping. As with all drugs that relieve "bad" feelings and produce "good" feelings, marijuana can become the focus of the user's life, to the exclusion of other activities. Drug uses appear to be related, and the chronic marijuana user is more likely to be a heavy user of tobacco, alcohol, and other dangerous drugs.

Hallucinogens

Hallucinogens are a group of drugs whose predominant pharmacological effect is to alter the user's perceptions, feelings, and thoughts. Hallucinogens include LSD (lysergic acid diethylamide), mescaline, psilocybin, STP (dimethoxymethyl amphetamine), DMT (dimethyltryptamine), MDMA (3,4-methylene-dioxymethamphetamine), ketamine, and PCP (phencyclidine). These drugs are most commonly ingested or smoked.

LSD   LSD is one of the most powerful psychoactive drugs. Tiny doses will produce noticeable effects in most people, such as an altered sense of time, visual disturbances, an improved sense of hearing, mood changes, and distortions in how people perceive their bodies. Dilation of the pupils and slight dizziness, weakness, and nausea may also occur. With larger doses, users may experience a phenomenon known as **synesthesia**, feel-

Physiologically, marijuana increases heart rate and dilates certain blood vessels in the eyes, which creates the characteristic bloodshot eyes. The user also feels less inclined toward physical exertion.

The question of whether marijuana has any medical uses has been hotly debated. Cannabis preparations were once medically prescribed for a variety of illnesses, but most such uses are no longer supported by research. A legal, prescription form of THC called dronabinol has been available in a capsule for some patients since 1985; however, many patients argue that oral THC is not as effective as smoked marijuana. A 1999 government-commissioned report from the Institute of Medicine concluded that substances in marijuana have potential therapeutical value for pain relief, for control of nausea and vomiting in chemotherapy patients, and for stimulating appetite in people with AIDS-related wasting. Although effective drugs already exist for these conditions, marijuana may be suitable for patients who do not respond to other therapies. The report recommends further studies and the development of alternative methods of drug delivery—inhalers or patches—that would safely deliver set doses of specific compounds in marijuana.

ings of depersonalization, and other alterations in the perceived relationship between self and external reality.

Many hallucinogens induce tolerance so quickly that after only one or two doses, their effects decrease substantially. The user must then stop taking the drug for several days before his or her system can be receptive to it again. These drugs cause little drug-seeking behavior and no physical dependence or withdrawal symptoms.

The immediate effects of low doses of hallucinogens are largely determined by expectations and setting. Many effects are hard to describe because they involve subjective and unusual dimensions of awareness—the **altered states of consciousness** for which these drugs are famous. For this reason, hallucinogens have acquired a certain aura not associated with other drugs. People have taken LSD in search of a religious or mystical experience, or in the hope of exploring new worlds. During the 1960s, some psychiatrists gave LSD to their patients to help them talk about their repressed feelings.

A severe panic reaction, which can be terrifying in the extreme, can result from taking any dose of LSD. It is impossible to predict when a panic reaction will occur. Some LSD users report having hundreds of pleasurable and ecstatic experiences before having a "bad trip," or "bummer." If the user is already in a serene mood and feels no anger or hostility, and if he or she is in secure surroundings with trusted companions, a bad trip may be less likely, but a tranquil experience is not guaranteed.

Even after the drug's chemical effects have worn off, spontaneous flashbacks and other psychological disturbances can occur. **Flashbacks** are perceptual distortions and bizarre thoughts that occur after the drug has been entirely eliminated from the body. Although they are relatively rare phenomena, flashbacks can be extremely distressing. They are often triggered by specific psychological cues associated with the drug-taking experience, such as certain mood states or even types of music.

During the 1970s, researchers claimed that LSD damages chromosomes. But later evidence indicates that LSD in moderate doses, at least the pure LSD produced in the laboratory, does not damage chromosomes, cause detectable genetic damage, or produce birth defects.

Surveys suggest that LSD use may be having a revival. Rates of use among high school students began increasing in 1990. In 1998, more than 13% of high school seniors reported having tried LSD at least once. LSD use among college students also increased. In 1989, 3.4% of college students reported having used LSD within the past year; by the mid-1990s, this figure had risen to 6.9%.

Other Hallucinogens   Most other hallucinogens have the same general effects as LSD, but there are some variations. For example, a DMT or ketamine high does not last as long as an LSD high; an STP high lasts longer. MDMA, known as "ecstasy" or "X," has both hallucinogenic and amphetamine-like properties. Risks of MDMA use include overdose and hyperthermia (dangerously high body temperature brought on by intense physical activity and dehydration). In addition, MDMA has been shown to damage—perhaps permanently—brain nerve cells that produce the key neurotransmitter serotonin. The effects of MDMA on serotonin may help explain why heavy use can lead to persistent problems with verbal and visual memory. Tolerance to MDMA develops quickly, and high doses can cause anxiety, delusions, and paranoia.

PCP, also known as "angel dust," "hog," and "peace pill," reduces and distorts sensory input, especially **proprioception,** the sensation of body position and movement; it creates a state of sensory deprivation. PCP was initially used as an anesthetic, but was unsatisfactory because it caused agitation, confusion, and delirium (loss of contact with reality). Because it can be easily made, PCP is often available illegally and is sometimes used as an inexpensive replacement for other psychoactive drugs. The effects of ketamine, known as "Special K" or "K," are similar to those of PCP—confusion, agitation, aggression, and lack of coordination—but tend to be less predictable. Tolerance to either drug can develop rapidly.

Mescaline (peyote), the ceremonial drug of the Native North American Church, produces an experience different from that caused by LSD. Obtaining mescaline costs far more than making LSD, however, so most street mescaline is LSD that has been highly diluted. Hallucinogenic effects can be obtained from certain mushrooms (*Psilocybe mexicana,* or "magic mushrooms"), certain morning glory seeds, nutmeg, jimsonweed, and other botanical products; but unpleasant side effects, such as dizziness, have limited the popularity of these products.

Inhalants

Inhaling certain chemicals can produce effects ranging from heightened pleasure to delirium. Inhalants fall into three major groups: (1) volatile solvents, which include adhesives and aerosols; (2) nitrites, such as butyl nitrite

---

TERMS

hallucinogen   Any of several drugs that alter perception, feelings, or thoughts; examples are LSD, mescaline, and PCP.

synesthesia   A condition in which a stimulus evokes not only the sensation appropriate to it but also another sensation of a different character; for example, when a color evokes a specific smell.

altered states of consciousness   Profound changes in mood, thinking, and perception.

flashback   A perceptual distortion or bizarre thought that recurs after the chemical effects of a drug have worn off.

proprioception   The sensation of body position and movement, from muscles, joints, and skin.

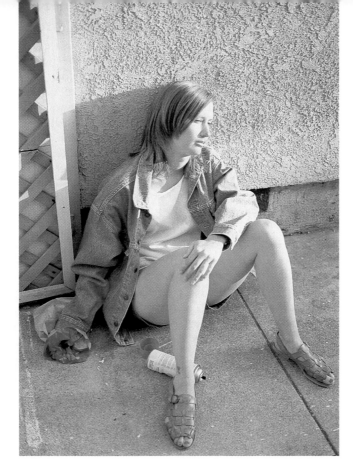

Inhalant use is difficult to monitor and control because inhalants are found in many inexpensive and legal products. Low doses of inhalants may cause a user to feel slightly stimulated; higher concentrations can cause a loss of consciousness, heart failure, and death.

and amyl nitrite; and (3) anesthetics, which include nitrous oxide or "laughing gas." About 15% of all high school seniors have reported using inhalants.

Inhalant use is difficult to control because inhalants are easy to obtain. They are present in a variety of seemingly harmless products, from dessert-topping sprays to under-arm deodorants, that are both inexpensive and legal. Using the drugs also requires no illegal or suspicious paraphernalia. Inhalant users get high by "sniffing," "snorting," "bagging" (inhaling fumes from a plastic bag), or "huffing" (placing an inhalant-soaked rag in the mouth).

Although different in makeup, nearly all inhalants produce effects similar to those of anesthetics, which slow down body functions. Low doses may cause users to feel slightly stimulated; at higher doses, users may feel less inhibited and less in control. Sniffing high concentrations of the chemicals in solvents or aerosol sprays can cause a loss of consciousness, heart failure, and death. High concentrations of any inhalant can also cause death from suffocation by displacing the oxygen in the lungs and central nervous system. Deliberately inhaling from a bag or in a closed area greatly increases the chances of suffocation. Other possible effects of the excessive or long-term use of inhalants include damage to the nervous system (impaired perception, reasoning, memory, and muscular coordination); hearing loss; and damage to the liver, kidneys, and bone marrow.

> **PERSONAL INSIGHT**   What is your attitude toward drug dependence? Do you view it more as a moral violation, a criminal act, or an illness? Where do you think your ideas come from?

DRUG USE: THE DECADES AHEAD

Drug research will undoubtedly provide new information, new treatments, and new chemical combinations in the decades ahead. New psychoactive drugs may present unexpected possibilities for therapy, social use, and abuse. Making honest and unbiased information about drugs available to everyone, however, may cut down on their abuse. Misinformation about the dangers of drugs— "scare tactics"—can lead some people to disbelieve any reports of drug dangers, no matter how soundly based and well documented they are.

Although the use of some drugs, both legal and illegal, has declined dramatically since the 1970s, the use of others has held steady, or increased. Mounting public concern has led to great debate and a wide range of opinions about what should be done. Efforts to combat the problem include workplace drug testing, tougher law enforcement and prosecution, and treatment and education. With drugs entering the country on a massive scale from South America, Southeast Asia, and elsewhere and distributed through tightly controlled drug-smuggling organizations and street gangs, it remains to be seen how effective any program will be.

Drugs, Society, and Families

The economic cost of drug use is staggering. Each year, Americans spend over $50 billion on illegal drugs, with an additional $100 billion going to cover enforcement, prevention, treatment, lost wages, and drug-related injuries and crime. But the costs are more than just financial; they are also paid in human pain and suffering.

The relationship between drugs and crime is complex. The criminal justice system is inundated with people accused of crimes related to drug possession, sale, or use. More than 2 million arrests are made each year for drug and alcohol violations, and over 100,000 people are in jail for violating drug laws. Many assaults and murders occur when people try to acquire or protect drug territories, settle disputes about drugs, or steal from dealers. Violence and the use of guns are more common in neighborhoods where drug trafficking is prevalent. Addicts commit more robberies and burglaries than criminals not on drugs. People under the influence of drugs, especially alcohol, are more likely to commit violent crimes like rape and murder than people who do not use drugs.

Drug use is also a health care issue for society. In the United States, drug abuse leads to more than 500,000 emergency room admissions and over 20,000 deaths annually. While it is in the best interest of society to treat addicts who want help, there is not nearly enough space in treatment facilities to help the estimated 7.1 million Americans severely in need of treatment. Drug addicts who want to quit, especially those among the urban poor, often have to wait a year or more for acceptance into a residential care or other treatment program.

Drug abuse also takes a toll on individuals and families. Children born to women who use drugs like alcohol, tobacco, or cocaine may have long-term health problems. Drug use in families can become a vicious cycle. Observing adults around them using drugs, children assume it is an acceptable way to deal with problems. Other problems like abuse, neglect, lack of opportunity, and unemployment become contributing factors to drug use and serve to perpetuate the cycle.

Legalizing Drugs

Pointing out that many of the social problems associated with drugs are related to prohibition rather than to the effects of the drugs themselves, some people have argued for various forms of drug legalization. Proposals range from making such drugs as marijuana and heroin available by prescription to allowing licensed dealers to sell some of these drugs to adults. Proponents argue that crimes by drug users are usually committed to buy drugs that cost relatively more than alcohol and tobacco because they are produced illegally. By making some currently illicit drugs legal—but putting controls on them similar to those used for alcohol, tobacco, and prescription drugs—many of the problems related to drug use could be eliminated.

Opponents of drug legalization argue that allowing easier access to drugs would expose many more people to possible abuse and dependence. Drugs would be cheaper and easier to obtain, and drug use would be more socially acceptable. Legalizing drugs could cause an increase in drug use among children and teenagers. Opponents point out that alcohol and tobacco are major causes of disease and death in our society, and that they should not be used as models for other practices.

Drug Testing

One of the most controversial issues in American politics is drug testing in the workplace. It has been estimated that as many as 10% of workers use psychoactive drugs

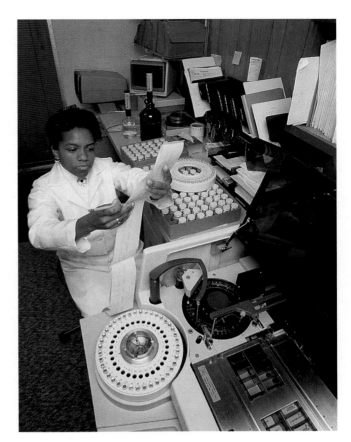

Many companies test current and prospective employees for drug use. Most drug testing involves a urine test that can detect recent use of marijuana, heroin, cocaine, amphetamines, codeine, and many other psychoactive drugs.

on the job. For some occupations, such as air traffic controllers, truck drivers, and train engineers, drug use can create significant hazards, sometimes involving hundreds of people. Some people believe that the dangers are so great that all workers should be tested, and that anyone found with traces of drugs in the blood or urine should be either fired or treated. Others insist that this would violate people's right to privacy and to freedom from unreasonable search, guaranteed by the Fourth Amendment. Opponents point out that most jobs do not involve hazards, so employees who take drugs are not any more dangerous than employees who do not.

Despite the expense, many employers now test their employees, and the U.S. armed forces test military personnel regularly. People in jobs involving transportation—truck drivers, bus drivers, train engineers, airline pilots—are required by federal law to be tested regularly to ensure public safety. The primary criterion leading most companies to use drug testing is the company's liability if an employee under the influence of a drug makes a mistake that could potentially harm others.

Most drug testing involves a urine test; a test for alcohol uses a blood test or a breath test. The accuracy of these tests has been improved in recent years, so there are fewer opportunities for people to cheat, or for the tests to yield inaccurate results. If a person tests positive for drugs, the employer may provide drug counseling or treatment, suspend the employee until he or she tests negative, or fire the individual.

By 1998, the FDA had approved two types of over-the-counter home drug testing kits designed to allow parents to check their children for drug use. For one type, a urine sample is collected at home and sent to a laboratory for analysis; results are available by phone. The other kit provides preliminary results in 10 minutes, but final results also require follow-up laboratory testing.

> **PERSONAL INSIGHT** What do you think about drug testing? Are you in favor of it in some circumstances but not others? How would you feel about being asked to take a drug test as part of a job application process?

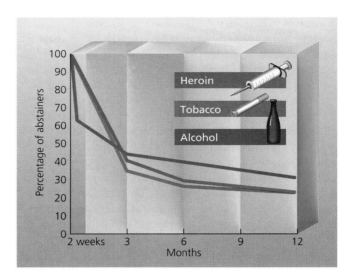

Figure 9-3 Percentage of people who continue to abstain over time, after giving up heroin, tobacco, and alcohol.

Treatment for Drug Dependence

A variety of programs are available to help people break their drug habits, but there is no single best method of treatment, and the relapse rate is high for all types of treatment (Figure 9-3). Nevertheless, numerous studies have shown that being treated is better than not being treated. To be successful, a treatment program must deal with the reasons behind people's drug abuse and help them develop behaviors, attitudes, and a social support system that will help them remain drug-free (see the box "Native American Treatment of Drug Abuse").

Drug Substitution Programs Sometimes a less debilitating drug can be substituted for one with many damaging effects, thus reducing the risks of the drug use. Methadone is a synthetic drug used as a substitute for heroin. When methadone is used, addicts can stop taking heroin without experiencing severe withdrawal reactions. Although methadone is addictive, it decreases the craving for heroin and enables the individual to function normally in social and vocational activities. Methadone maintenance treatment allows many former heroin abusers to live more useful lives. Other heroin substitutes in use or being studied include LAAM (levo-alpha-acetylmethadol) and buprenorphine.

Because they are relatively inexpensive to administer, drug substitution programs are a popular form of treat-

ment. However, the relapse rate is high. Combining drug substitution with psychological and social services improves success rates, underscoring the importance of psychological factors in drug dependence.

Treatment Centers Treatment centers offer a variety of short-term and long-term services, including hospitalization, detoxification, counseling, and other mental health services. A specific type of center is the therapeutic community, a residential program run in a completely drug-free atmosphere. Administered by ex-addicts, these programs use confrontation, strict discipline, and unrelenting peer pressure to attempt to resocialize the addict with a different set of values. "Halfway houses," transitional settings between a 24-hour-a-day program and independent living, are an important phase of treatment for some people. Strategies for evaluating programs are given in the box "Choosing a Drug-Treatment Program," p. 238.

Treatment centers often also offer counseling for those who are close to drug abusers. Drug abuse takes a toll on friends and family members, and counseling can help people work through painful feelings of guilt and powerlessness. Sometimes people close to a drug abuser develop patterns of behavior, known as **codependency,** that help or enable the person to remain drug-dependent (see the box "Codependency," p. 238). Counseling can help people adopt realistic ideas about their role in their loved one's substance dependence and recovery, and identify and change any problematic behavior patterns.

Self-Help Groups and Peer Counseling Groups such as Alcoholics Anonymous (AA) and Narcotics Anonymous (NA) have helped many people. People treated in drug substitution programs or substance-abuse treatment centers are often urged or required to join a self-help group

> **TERMS** **codependency** A relationship in which a non–substance-abusing partner or family member enables the other's substance abuse.

Rates of drug and alcohol abuse among Native Americans and Alaska Natives are much higher than those of the U.S. population as a whole. The death rate from alcoholism among Native Americans is nearly seven times the national average; cirrhosis ranks sixth among the leading causes of death for Native Americans, compared to a tenth-place ranking for the population as a whole. Rates of alcohol- and drug-related suicide, homicide, and unintentional injuries, especially car crashes, are also high. On some reservations, over 80% of young people use drugs or alcohol. Poverty, high unemployment, lack of educational opportunities, and a weakening of cultural values and community ties have all been implicated as causative factors.

To deal with the problem of alcohol and drug abuse, Native American communities have developed unique approaches that incorporate cultural traditions. Many of these programs are funded and operated through the Indian Health Service, a division of the U.S. Public Health Service that provides health care for Native Americans and Alaska Natives living on reservations or with access to reservation health facilities. Other programs are funded by private grants, such as the Robert Wood Johnson Foundation's 6-year "Healthy Nations" initiative, which emphasizes intervention programs for youth. Most locally developed and operated programs incorporate a strong cultural component. In contrast to earlier programs, which were sometimes perceived as imposed by outside agencies, these programs arise from within the community and make sense in the context of Native American traditions and beliefs. Examples of recent programs include the following:

- Wolakota Yukini Wicoti, a prairie camp for teens on the Cheyenne River Reservation in South Dakota. Participants spend a summer traveling on horseback, sleeping outdoors, learning their native language and ceremonies from tribal elders, and even hunting buffalo. By fostering a healthy cultural identity, the program fortifies young people against

personal and social forces that encourage alcohol and drug abuse.

- Four Cedars Medicine Lodge, a program for at-risk youth run by seven tribes in northern Washington. Teens in the program take classes, receive counseling, and participate in traditions such as purification ceremonies. The program helps teens develop pride in themselves and their cultural heritage and provides alternatives to drug and alcohol use.

- Circle of Strength (COS), a partnership of local organizations in the San Francisco Bay Area. Foster care, university programs, and substance-abuse treatment are only a few of the services provided by COS. Recent events have included talking circles, "sweats," and gatherings at Kule Loklo Miwok village, where young people learn traditional crafts and skills.

The effectiveness of these programs is difficult to assess, but many believe that alcoholism and drug abuse among Native Americans has decreased because of traditional approaches. Although still high, the death rate from alcoholism among Native Americans has fallen by about 20% since 1970. Officials in the Indian Health Service say that the community-based programs account for this improvement. In addition to community responsibility, this success can be attributed to the nature of the programs themselves, with their focus on social support, feelings of pride and belonging, and practical alternatives to drugs and alcohol.

SOURCE: Indian Health Service. 1997. *Regional Differences in Indian Health.* Rockville, Md.: Indian Health Service. Circle of Strength project promotes healthy lifestyles for Bay Area Indians. 1997. *Yachá Community Newsletter* 1: 9. Vollers, M. 1996. Indian summer. *Time* 148(10): 36–39. California Native-American coalition seeks integrated services. 1996. *Alcohol and Drug Abuse Week* 8(9): 4. Rauch, K. D. 1992. How Indian youths defeat addictions. *Washington Post Health,* 10 March.

---

as part of their recovery. These groups follow a 12-step program. Group members' first step is to acknowledge that they have a problem over which they have no control. Peer support is a critical ingredient of these programs, and members usually meet at least once a week. Each member is paired with a sponsor to call on for advice and support if the temptation to relapse becomes overwhelming. With such support, thousands of substance-dependent people have been able to recover, remain abstinent, and reclaim their lives. Chapters of AA and NA meet on some college campuses; community-based chapters are listed in the phone book and local newspapers. (Also see the For More Information section at the end of the chapter.)

Many colleges also have peer counseling programs, in which students are trained to help other students who have drug problems. A peer counselor's role may be as limited as referring a student to a professional with expertise in substance dependence for an evaluation, or as

involved as helping arrange a leave of absence from school for participation in a drug-treatment program. Most peer counseling programs are founded on principles of strict confidentiality. Peer counselors may also be able to help students who are concerned about a classmate or loved one with an apparent drug problem (see the box "If Someone You Know Has a Drug Problem . . . ," p. 239). Information about peer counseling programs is usually available from the student health center.

Preventing Drug Abuse

Obviously, the best solution to drug abuse is prevention. Government attempts at controlling the drug problem tend to focus on stopping the production, importation, and distribution of illegal drugs. Creative effort also has to be put into stopping the demand for drugs. Developing persuasive antidrug educational programs offers the best

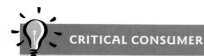
When evaluating different facilities or programs for drug treatment, consider the following issues:

• *What type of treatment or facility is most appropriate?* Intensive outpatient treatment is available through many community mental health centers, as well as through specialized drug-treatment facilities. Such programs typically require several sessions per week, combining individual therapy, group counseling, and attendance at 12-step meetings. Residential, or inpatient, facilities may be associated with a medical facility such as a hospital, or they may be free-standing programs that focus solely on substance-abuse treatment. Some residential treatment programs last longer or cost more per week than many health insurance plans will cover.

• *How will treatment be paid for?* Many health insurance plans limit residential treatment to a maximum of 3 weeks or less. They may also require that you first attempt a less expensive form of treatment before they will approve coverage for a residential facility.

• *Is there likely to be a need for medical support?* Chronic alcoholics or abusers of other CNS depressants may experience life-threatening seizures or other withdrawal symptoms during the first few days of detoxification. Malnutrition is common among substance abusers, and injecting drug users may suffer from local infections and bloodborne diseases such as hepatitis or HIV infection. Medical problems such as these are best handled in an inpatient program with good medical support.

• *What is the level of professional training of the staff?* Is there a medical doctor on site or making frequent visits? Are there trained nurses? Licensed psychologists or social workers? Many successful programs are staffed primarily by recovering alcoholics or drug users. Do those staff members have training and certification as addiction specialists, or some other license or certificate?

• *Can the program provide the names of previous clients who would be willing to talk to you?* The best way to learn about the true nature of a program is to talk with someone who has been through it.

• *Does the program provide related services, such as family and job counseling and post-treatment follow-up?* These types of services are extremely important for the long-term success of drug-abuse treatment.

• *Can you visit the facility and speak with the staff and clients?* A prospective client and his or her family should be allowed to visit any treatment center or program. There used to be a small number of restricted-access programs that isolated clients from their families and demanded total dedication.

Codependency became a trendy term in the late 1980s, and popular authors attributed a long list of personal and social problems to what they termed "codependent behavior." However, the concept is a useful one for looking at the relationships between drug abusers (and people with other types of self-destructive habits) and those close to them. A codependent is a person who is in a continuing relationship with a drug-abusing person and whose actions help or enable that person to remain dependent. Codependency, also called *enabling,* removes or softens the effects of the drug use on the user. People often become enablers spontaneously and naturally. When someone they love becomes dependent on a drug, they want to help, and they assume that their good intentions will persuade the drug user to stop. Unfortunately, substance-dependent people have a system of denial that is strengthened rather than diminished by well-meaning attempts to help.

The habit of enabling inhibits a drug-dependent person's recovery because the person never has to experience the consequences of his or her behavior. Frequently, the enabler is dependent, too—on the patterns of interaction in the relationship. People who need to take care of people often marry people who need to be taken care of. Children in these families often develop the same behavior pattern as one of their parents, by either becoming helpless or becoming a caregiver. This is why treatment programs for drug dependence, such as Alcoholics Anonymous, Narcotics Anonymous, and Cocaine Anonymous, involve the whole family.

Have you ever been an enabler in a relationship? You may have, if you've ever done any of the following:

• Given someone one more chance to stop abusing drugs, then another, and another. . . .

• Made excuses or lied for someone to his or her friends, teachers, or employer.

• Joined someone in drug use and blamed others for your behavior.

• Loaned money to someone to continue drug use.

• Stayed up late waiting for, or gone out searching for, someone who uses drugs.

• Felt embarrassed or angry about the actions of someone who uses drugs.

• Ignored the drug use because the person got defensive when you brought it up.

• Not confronted a friend or relative who was obviously intoxicated or high on a drug.

If you come from a codependent family or see yourself developing codependency relationships, consider acting now to make changes in your patterns of interaction; see the For More Information section for some helpful resources.

TACTICS AND TIPS · *If Someone You Know Has a Drug Problem . . .*

If you notice changes in behavior and mood in someone you know, they may signal a growing dependence on drugs. Signs that a person's life is beginning to focus on drugs include the following:

- Sudden withdrawal or emotional distance.
- Rebellious or unusually irritable behavior.
- A loss of interest in usual activities or hobbies.
- A decline in school performance.
- A sudden change in the chosen group of friends.
- Changes in sleeping or eating habits.
- Frequent borrowing of money or stealing.
- Secretive behavior about personal possessions, such as a backpack or the contents of a drawer.
- Deterioration of physical appearance.

If you believe a family member or friend has a drug problem, obtain information about resources for drug treatment available on your campus or in your community. Communicate your concern, provide him or her with information about treatment options, and offer your support during treatment. If the person continues to deny having a problem, you may want to talk with an experienced counselor about setting up an "intervention"— a formal, structured confrontation designed to end denial by having family, friends, and other caring individuals present their concerns to the drug user. Participants in an intervention would indicate the ways in which the individual is hurting others as well as himself or herself. If your friend or family member agrees to treatment, encourage him or her to attend a support group such as Narcotics Anonymous or Alcoholics Anonymous. And finally, examine your relationship with the abuser for signs of codependency. If necessary, get help for yourself; friends and family of drug users can often benefit from counseling.

TACTICS AND TIPS · *What to Do Instead of Drugs*

- *Bored?* Go for a walk or a run; stimulate your senses at a museum or a movie; challenge your mind with a new game or book; introduce yourself to someone new.
- *Stressed?* Practice relaxation or visualization; try to slow down and open your senses to the natural world; get some exercise.
- *Shy or lonely?* Talk to a counselor; enroll in a shyness clinic; learn and practice communication techniques.
- *Feeling low on self-esteem?* Focus on the areas in which you are competent; give yourself credit for the things you do well. A program of regular exercise can also enhance self-esteem.
- *Depressed or anxious?* Talk to a friend, parent, or counselor.

- *Apathetic or lethargic?* Force yourself to get up and get some exercise to energize yourself; assume responsibility for someone or something outside yourself; volunteer.
- *Searching for meaning?* Try yoga or meditation; explore spiritual experiences through religious groups, church, prayer, or reading.
- *Afraid to say no?* Take a course in assertiveness training; get support from others who don't want to use drugs; remind yourself that you have the right and the responsibility to make your own decisions.
- *Still feeling peer pressure?* Begin to look for new friends or roommates. Take a class or join an organization that attracts other health-conscious people.

hope for solving the drug problem in the future. Indirect approaches to prevention involve building young people's self-esteem, improving their academic skills, and increasing their recreational opportunities. Direct approaches involve giving information about the adverse effects of drugs and teaching tactics that help students resist peer pressure to use drugs in various situations. Developing strategies for resisting peer pressure is one of the more effective techniques.

Prevention efforts need to focus on the different motivations individuals have for using and abusing specific drugs at different ages. For example, grade school children seem receptive to programs that involve their parents or well-known adults like professional athletes. Adolescents in junior or senior high school are often more responsive to peer counselors. Many young adults tend to be influenced by efforts that focus on health education. For all ages, it is important to provide nondrug alternatives that speak to the individual's or group's specific reasons for using drugs, such as recreational facilities, counseling, greater opportunities for leisure activities, and places to socialize (see the box "What to Do Instead of Drugs"). Reminding young people that most people, no matter what age, are *not* users of illegal drugs, do *not* smoke cigarettes, and do *not* get drunk frequently, is a critical part of preventing substance abuse.

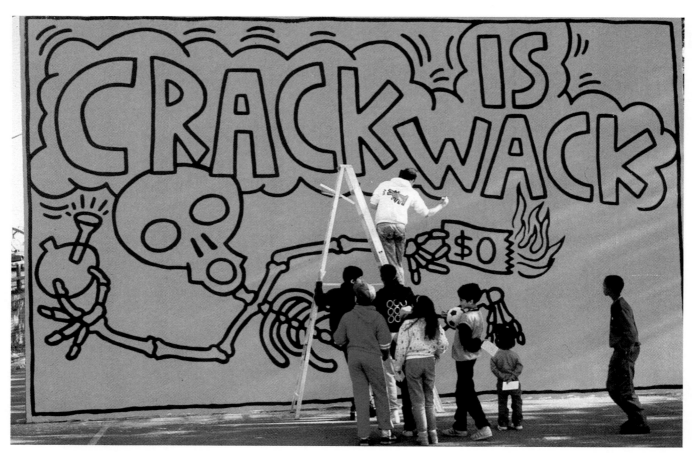

Persuasive antidrug messages may offer the best hope for preventing drug abuse. This playground backboard, painted by the late Keith Haring, attempts to raise awareness among young people about the consequences of crack use.

The Role of Drugs in Your Life

Where do you fit into this complex picture of drug use and abuse? Chances are that you've had experience with OTC and prescription drugs, and you may or may not have had experience with one or more of the drugs described in this chapter. You probably know someone who has used or abused a psychoactive drug. Whatever your experience has been up to now, it's likely that you will encounter drugs at some point in your life. To make sure you'll have the inner resources to resist peer pressure and make your own decision, cultivate a variety of activities you enjoy doing, realize that you are entitled to have your own opinion, and don't neglect your self-esteem.

Before you try a psychoactive drug, consider the following questions:

- *What are the risks involved?* Many drugs carry a immediate risk of injury or death. Almost all involve the longer-term risk of abuse and dependence.

- *Is using the drug compatible with your goals?* Consider how drug use will affect your education and career objectives, your relationships, your future happiness, and the happiness of those who love you.

- *What are your ethical beliefs about drug use?* Consider whether using a drug would cause you to go against your personal ethics, religious beliefs, social values, or family responsibilities.

- *What are the financial costs?* Many drugs are expensive, especially if you become dependent on them.

- *Are you trying to solve a deeper problem?* Drugs will not make emotional pain go away; in the long run, they will only make it worse. If you are feeling depressed or anxious, seek help from a mental health professional instead of self-medicating with drugs.

Like all aspects of health-related behavior, making responsible decisions about drug use depends on information, knowledge, and insight into yourself. Many choices are possible; making the ones that are right for you is what counts.

SUMMARY

Addictive Behavior

- Addictive behaviors are reinforcing. Addicts experience a strong compulsion for the behavior and a loss of control over it; an escalating pattern of abuse with serious negative consequences may result.

- The sources or causes of addiction include heredity, personality, lifestyle, and environmental factors. People may use an addictive behavior as a means of alleviating stress or painful emotions.

- Many common behaviors are potentially addictive, including gambling, shopping, sexual activity, Internet use, exercise, eating, and working.

Drug Use, Abuse, and Dependence

- Risk factors for drug use include being male, being young, having frequent exposure to drugs, and having a risk-taking personality.

- Reasons for using drugs include the lure of the illicit; curiosity; rebellion; peer pressure; and the desire to alter one's mood or escape boredom, anxiety, depression, or other psychological problems.

- Drug abuse is a maladaptive pattern of drug use that persists despite adverse social, psychological, or medical consequences.

- Drug dependence involves taking a drug compulsively, which includes neglecting constructive activities because of it and continuing to use it despite experiencing adverse effects resulting from its use. Tolerance and withdrawal symptoms are often present.

How Drugs Affect the Body

- Drug factors include pharmacological properties, dose-response function, time-action function, the person's drug use history, and method of use.

- User factors include a person's physical and psychological characteristics, such as body mass, general health, and other drugs being taken.

- A person's expectations and the social setting are sometimes more important in determining effects than the drug itself, if low doses are involved.

Representative Psychoactive Drugs

- Opioids relieve pain, cause drowsiness, and induce euphoria; they reduce anxiety and produce lethargy, apathy, and an inability to concentrate.

- CNS depressants slow down the overall activity of the nerves; they reduce anxiety and cause mood changes, impaired muscular coordination, slurring of speech, and drowsiness or sleep. CNS depressants include alcohol; barbiturates; antianxiety agents like Xanax, Valium, and Rohypnol; methaqualone; chloral hydrate; and GHB.

- CNS stimulants speed up the activity of the nerves, causing acceleration of the heart rate, a rise in blood pressure, dilation of the pupils and bronchial tubes, and an increase in gastric and adrenal secretions. CNS stimulants include cocaine, amphetamines, Ritalin, ephedrine, and caffeine.

- Marijuana usually causes euphoria and a relaxed attitude at low doses; very high doses produce feelings of depersonalization and sensory distortion. The long-term effects may include chronic bronchitis and cancer; use during pregnancy may impair fetal growth.

- Hallucinogens alter perception, feelings, and thought. LSD is the most widely known; its effects include an altered sense of time, visual disturbances, and mood changes. Other hallucinogens include DMT, STP, MDMA, PCP, ketamine, and mescaline.

- Inhalants include volatile solvents, nitrites, and anesthetics. They are present in a variety of harmless products; they can cause delirium. Their use can lead to loss of consciousness, heart failure, suffocation, and death.

Drug Use: The Decades Ahead

- Economic and social costs of drug abuse include the financial costs of law enforcement, treatment, and health care, and the social costs of crime, violence, and family problems.

- Some people argue in favor of legalizing drugs to decrease drug-related crime and violence. Opponents argue that legalizing drugs would expose more people, especially teenagers, to possible drug abuse and dependence.

- Drug testing, a controversial issue in American politics, involves a basic conflict between public safety and the individual's right to privacy and freedom from unreasonable search.

- Drug substitution programs using methadone and other drugs attempt to reduce the risks of drug abuse.

- Features of drug-treatment programs include hospitalization, detoxification, counseling, and other psychiatric services. Counseling for friends and relatives of drug abusers is also often available.

- Self-help groups and peer counseling are helpful forms of treatment for some drug abusers.

- Persuasive antidrug educational programs are necessary; especially important is helping students develop strategies for resisting peer pressure.

This behavior change strategy focuses on one of the most commonly used drugs—caffeine. If you are concerned about your use of a different drug, or another type of addictive behavior, you can devise your own plan based on this one and on the steps outlined in Chapter 1.

Because caffeine supports certain behaviors that are characteristic of our culture, such as sedentary, stressful work, you may find yourself relying on coffee (or tea, chocolate, or cola) to get through a busy schedule. Such habits often begin in college. Fortunately, it's easier to break a habit before it becomes entrenched as a lifelong dependency.

When you are studying for exams, the forced physical inactivity and the need to concentrate even when fatigued may lead you to overuse caffeine. But caffeine doesn't "help" unless you are already sleepy. And it does not relieve any underlying condition (you are just more tired when it wears off). How can you change this pattern?

Self-Monitoring

Keep a log of how much caffeine you eat or drink. Use a measuring cup to measure coffee or tea. Using Table 9-2, convert the amounts you eat or drink into an estimate expressed in milligrams of caffeine. Be sure to include all forms, such as chocolate bars and OTC medications, as well as caffeine candy, colas, cocoa or hot chocolate, chocolate cake, tea, and coffee.

Self-Assessment

At the end of the week, add up your daily totals and divide by 7 to get your daily average in milligrams. How much is too much? At more than 250 mg per day, you may well be experiencing some adverse symptoms. If you are experiencing at least five of the following symptoms, you may want to cut down.

- Restlessness
- Nervousness
- Excitement
- Insomnia
- Flushed face
- Excessive sweating

- Gastrointestinal problems
- Muscle twitching
- Rambling thoughts and speech
- Irregular heartbeat
- Periods of inexhaustibility
- Excessive pacing or movement

Set Limits

Can you restrict your caffeine intake to a daily total, and stick to this contract? If so, set a cutoff point, such as one cup of coffee. Pegging it to a specific time of day can be helpful, because then you won't confront a decision at any other point (and possibly fail). If you find you cannot stick to your limit, you may want to cut out caffeine altogether; abstinence can be easier than moderation for some people. If you experience caffeine withdrawal symptoms (headache, fatigue), you may want to cut your intake more gradually.

Find Other Ways to Keep Your Energy Up

If you are fatigued, it makes sense to get enough sleep or exercise more, rather than drowning the problem in coffee or tea. Different people need different amounts of sleep; you may also need more sleep at different times, such as during a personal crisis or an illness. Also, exercise raises your metabolic rate for hours afterward—a handy fact to exploit when you want to feel more awake and want to avoid an irritable caffeine jag. And if you've been compounding your fatigue by not eating properly, try filling up on complex carbohydrates such as whole-grain bread or potatoes instead of candy bars.

Tips on Cutting Out Caffeine   Here are some more ways to decrease your consumption of caffeine:

- Keep some noncaffeined drinks on hand, such as decaffeinated coffee, herbal teas, mineral water, bouillon, or hot water.

- Alternate between hot and very cold liquids.

- Fill your coffee cup only halfway.

- Avoid the office or school lunchroom or cafeteria and the chocolate sections of the grocery store. (Often people drink coffee or tea and eat chocolate simply because they're available.)

- Read labels of over-the-counter medications to check for hidden sources of caffeine.

1. Find out what types of services are available on your campus or in your community to handle drug dependence and other addictive behaviors. If there are none, what services are needed? Locate the school official and public health agency responsible for your campus and community, and ask why these needs aren't being met.

2. Survey three older adults and three young students about their attitudes toward legalizing marijuana.

Are there any differences? If so, what accounts for these differences? What kinds of reasons do they give for their positions?

3. Look at a current movie or television program, paying special attention to how drug use is portrayed. What messages are being conveyed? If possible, compare a recent movie with a movie made 10–15 years ago. Has the presentation of drug use changed? If so, how?

1. Keep track of your own drug use for a week, noting in your health journal the name of the drug, the approximate dosage, the time of day, and what you think your reasons were for taking each dose. Don't forget to include coffee, soft drinks, and OTC medications. What types of drugs are you taking? Are there any patterns? Are there any signs of abuse or dependence? If you'd like to cut down, begin by making a list of alternative behaviors you could substitute for drug use.

2. *Critical Thinking* Does a woman have an obligation to avoid alcohol and other drugs during pregnancy? What about smoking cigarettes and eating junk food? If she doesn't follow her physician's advice, should she be held legally responsible for the effects on her child? What rights do the mother and child have in this situation? In your health journal, write an essay stating your opinion; be sure to defend your position.

3. *Critical Thinking* Do you think there is such a thing as the responsible use of illegal psychoactive drugs? Are they a legitimate recreational activity? Would you change any of the current laws governing drugs? If so, how would you draw the line between legitimate and illegitimate use? Write an essay explaining your position.

FOR MORE INFORMATION

Books

Beattie, M. 1997. *Codependent No More and Beyond Codependency.* New York: Fine Communications. *A straightforward discussion of codependency by the writer who first popularized the concept.*

Columbia University's Health Education Program. 1998. *The "Go Ask Alice" Book of Answers: A Guide to Good Physical, Sexual, and Emotional Health.* New York: Henry Holt. *Includes a separate section with answers to college students' frequently asked questions about drugs; based on the popular Web site (http://www.goaskalice.columbia.edu).*

Fanning, P. 1996. *The Addiction Workbook: A Step-by-Step Guide to Quitting Alcohol and Drugs.* Oakland, Calif.: New Harbinger. *Includes questionnaires and other tools to help addicts understand their addiction and move toward recovery.*

Hales, D., R. E. Hales, and A. Frances. 1996. *Caring for the Mind: A Comprehensive Guide to Mental Health.* New York: Bantam. *An easy-to-understand reference that includes separate chapters on substance-abuse problems and impulse-control disorders, including compulsive gambling and shopping.*

Kuhn, C., et al. 1998. *Buzzed: The Straight Facts About the Most Used and Abused Drugs from Alcohol to Ecstasy.* New York: W. W. Norton. *An accurate, straightforward guide to commonly used drugs.*

Rudgley, R. 1999. *Encyclopedia of Psychoactive Substances.* New York: St. Martins. *Describes the physiological and psychological effects of psychoactive drugs and provides a historical and cultural perspective on their use.*

Schaler, J. A., ed. 1998. *Drugs: Should We Legalize, Decriminalize, or Deregulate?* Amherst, N.Y.: Prometheus. *Reviews the ongoing debate over the legal status of drugs.*

Schuckit, M. A. 1998. *Educate Yourself About Alcohol and Drugs: A People's Primer.* Rev. ed. New York: Plenum Press. *A guide to the physical, emotional, and social effects of drug abuse and to resources that are available to help users stop.*

Twerski, A. J. 1997. *Addictive Thinking: Understanding Self-Deception.* Center City, Minn.: Hazelden. *Describes the complicated and contradictory patterns of thinking associated with addiction.*

Organizations, Hotlines, and Web Sites

Center for On-Line Addiction. Contains information about Internet addiction for both professionals and online addicts.
http://netaddiction.com

Center for Substance Abuse Research (CESAR)/University of Maryland–College Park. Researches and analyzes substance-abuse issues; Web site has overviews of key topics, a substance-abuse bulletin board, and an online student risk assessment.
http://www.cesar.umd.edu

Do It Now Foundation. Provides youth-oriented information about drugs.
http://www.doitnow.org

DrugHelp Hotlines. A 24-hour service that provides confidential information and referrals.
800-DRUGHELP; 800-COCAINE; 800-RELAPSE
http://www.drughelp.org

Habitsmart. Contains information about addictive behavior, including tips for effectively managing problematic habitual behaviors, a self-scoring alcohol check-up, and links.
http://www.habitsmart.com

Higher Education Center for Alcohol and Other Drug Prevention. Provides nationwide support for campus alcohol and illegal drug prevention efforts. The Web site gives information about alcohol and drug abuse on campus and links to related sites; it also has an area designed specifically for students.
http://www.edc.org/hec

Indiana Prevention Resource Center. A clearinghouse of information and links on substance-abuse topics, including specific psychoactive drugs and issues such as drug testing and drug legalization.
http://www.drugs.indiana.edu

Join Together Online. Provides resources and a meeting place for communities working to reduce substance abuse and gun violence.
http://www.jointogether.org

Life Education Center. A sponsor of child education programs designed to prevent drug abuse, violence, and AIDS; its Web site includes information on specific drugs and on the worldwide manufacture and distribution of drugs.

http://www.lec.org

Narcotics Anonymous (NA). Similar to Alcoholics Anonymous, NA sponsors 12-step meetings and provides other support services for drug abusers.

19737 Nordhoff Place
Chatsworth, CA 91311
818-773-9999
http://www.na.org

There are also 12-step programs that focus on specific drugs:

Cocaine Anonymous
http://www.ca.org
Marijuana Anonymous
http://www.marijuana-anonymous.org

National Center on Addiction and Substance Abuse (CASA) at Columbia University. Provides information about the costs of substance abuse to individuals and society.

http://www.casacolumbia.org

National Clearinghouse for Alcohol and Drug Information. Provides statistics, information, and publications on substance abuse, including resources for people who want to help friends and family members overcome substance-abuse problems.

P.O. Box 2345
Rockville, MD 20847
800-729-6686; 301-468-2600
http://www.health.org

National Drug Information, Treatment, and Referral Hotlines. Sponsored by the SAMHSA Center for Substance Abuse Treatment, these hotlines provide information on drug abuse and on

HIV infection as it relates to substance abuse; referrals to support groups and treatment programs are available.

800-662-HELP
800-729-6686 (Spanish)
800-487-4889 (TDD for hearing impaired)

National Institute on Drug Abuse. Develops and supports research on drug abuse prevention programs; fact sheets on drugs of abuse are available on the Web site or via recorded phone messages, fax, or mail.

6001 Executive Blvd.
Bethesda, MD 20892
888-644-6432 (Infofax)
http://www.nida.nih.gov

Office of National Drug Control Policy (ONDCP). Provides information on national and international drug-related topics, including U.S. policies relating to prevention, education, treatment, and enforcement.

http://www.whitehousedrugpolicy.gov

Substance Abuse and Mental Health Services Administration (SAMHSA). Provides statistics, information, and other resources relating to substance-abuse prevention and treatment.

301-443-8956
http://www.samhsa.gov

Web of Addictions. Provides a wealth of information about substance abuse and dependence, including fact sheets, contact information for relevant agencies and organizations, and links to related sites.

http://www.well.com/user/woa

See also the listings for Chapters 10 and 11.

SELECTED BIBLIOGRAPHY

Abdala, N., et al. 1999. Survival of HIV-1 in syringes. *Journal of Acquired Immune Deficiency Syndromes and Human Retrovirology* 20(1): 73–80.

American Psychiatric Association. 1994. *Diagnostic and Statistical Manual of Mental Disorders,* 4th ed. (*DSM-IV*). Washington, D.C.: American Psychiatric Association.

Arendt, R., et al. 1999. Motor development of cocaine-exposed children at age two years. *Pediatrics* 103(1): 86–92.

Aytaclar, S., et al. 1999. Association between hyperactivity and executive cognitive functioning in childhood and substance use in early adolescence. *Journal of the American Academy of Child and Adolescent Psychiatry* 38(2): 172–178.

Barsky, S. H., et al. 1998. Histopathologic and molecular alterations in bronchial epithelium in habitual smokers of marijuana, cocaine, and/or tobacco. *Journal of the National Cancer Institute* 90(16): 1198–1205.

Battaglia, G., and T. C. Napier. 1998. The effects of cocaine and the amphetamines on brain and behavior. A conference report. *Drug and Alcohol Dependence* 52(1): 41–48.

Belcher, H. M. E., and H. E. Shinitzky. 1998. Substance abuse in children: Prediction, protection and prevention. *Archives of Pediatrics and Adolescent Medicine* 152: 952–960.

Bolla, K. I., U. D. McCann, and G. A. Ricaurte. 1998. Memory impairment in abstinent MDMA ("Ecstasy") users. *Neurology* 51(6): 1532–1537.

Brenner, V. 1998. Psychology of computer use: XLVII. Parameters of Internet use, abuse and addiction: The first 90 days of the Internet Usage Survey. *Psychological Reports* 80 (3 Pt 1): 879–882.

Center on Addiction and Substance Abuse. 1998. *Press Release: CASA 1998 Back to School Teen Survey* (retrieved September 2, 1998; http://www.casacolumbia.org/media/press/090198.htm).

Centers for Disease Control and Prevention. 1999. Adverse events associated with the ingestion of gamma-butyrolactone—Minnesota, New Mexico, and Texas, 1998–1999. *Morbidity and Mortality Weekly Report* 48(7): 137–140.

Chin, R. L., et al. 1998. Clinical course of gamma-hydroxybutyrate overdose. *Annals of Emergency Medicine* 31(6): 716–722.

Core Institute. 1998. *Recent Statistics on Alcohol and Other Drug Use on American College Campuses* (retrieved November 5, 1998; http://www.siu.edu/departments/coreinst/public_html/recent.html).

Delaney-Black, V., et al. 1998. Prenatal cocaine exposure and child behavior. *Pediatrics* 102(4): 945–950.

Doyle, R. 1999. Privacy in the workplace. *Scientific American,* January.

Duncan, S. C., T. E. Duncan, and H. Hops. 1998. Progressions of alcohol, cigarette, and marijuana use in adolescence. *Journal of Behavioral Medicine* 21(4): 375–388.

Gold, S. N., and C. L. Heffner. 1998. Sexual addiction: Many conceptions, minimal data. *Clinical Psychology Review* 18(3): 367–381.

Goldman, D., and A. Bergen. 1998. General and specific inheritance of substance abuse and alcoholism. *Archives of General Psychiatry* 55(11): 964–965.

Gurley, R. J., R. Aranow, and M. Katz. 1998. Medicinal marijuana: A comprehensive review. *Journal of Psychoactive Drugs* 30(2): 137–147.

Hales, D., and R. E. Hales. 1995. *Caring for the Mind: The Comprehensive Guide to Mental Health.* New York: Bantam.

Hall, W., and N. Solowij. 1998. Adverse effects of cannabis. *Lancet* 352: 1611–1616.

Institute of Medicine. 1999. *Marijuana and Medicine: Assessing the Science Base.* Washington, D.C.: National Academy Press.

Lester, B. M., L. L. LaGasse, and R. Siefer. 1998. Cocaine exposure and children: The meaning of subtle effects. *Science* 282(5389): 633–634.

Marwick, C. 1998. Challenging report on pregnancy and drug abuse. *Journal of the American Medical Association* 280: 1039–1040.

McCann, U. D., et al. 1998. Positron emission tomographic evidence of toxic effect of MDMA ("Ecstasy") on brain serotonin neurons in human beings. *Lancet* 352: 1433–1437.

Meng, I. D., et al. 1998. An analgesia circuit activated by cannabinoids. *Nature* 395: 381–385.

Monitoring the Future Study. 1998. *Drug Statistics Table* (retrieved January 7, 1999; http://www.isr.umich.edu/src/mtf/pr98t1aa.html).

Monitoring the Future Study. 1998. *Tables Including College Students and Young Adults, 1991–1997* (retrieved December 1, 1998; http://www.isr.umich.edu/src/mtf/t2_1a1.html).

Monroe, J. 1996. What is addiction? *Current Health,* January, 16–19.

National Institute on Alcohol Abuse and Alcoholism. 1998. *The Economic Costs of Alcohol and Drug Abuse in the United States* (retrieved November 5, 1998; http://www.health.org/pressrel/sept98/csat-study.html).

National Institute on Drug Abuse. 1998. *NIDA Infofax: Nationwide Trends* (retrieved November 30, 1998; http://www.nida.nih.gov/Infofax/nationtrends.html).

National Institute on Drug Abuse. 1998. *NIDA Media Advisory: New Research Helps Explain Ritalin's Low Abuse Potential When Taken as Prescribed* (retrieved November 30, 1998; http://www.nida.nih.gov/MedAdv/98/MA-929.html).

National Research Council. 1999. *Pathological Gambling.* Washington, D.C.: National Academy Press.

Ness, R. B., et al. 1999. Cocaine and tobacco use and the risk of spontaneous abortion. *New England Journal of Medicine* 340(5): 333–339.

Office of National Drug Control Policy. 1998. *Drug Use Trends: Youth* (retrieved December 1, 1998; http://www.whitehousedrugpolicy.gov/drugfact/drugtrends/youth.html).

Parker, J. 1998. *Club Drugs: Destination "X."* Tempe, Ariz.: Do It Now Foundation.

Patock-Peckham, J. A., et al. 1998. Effect of religion and religiosity on alcohol use in a college student sample. *Drug and Alcohol Dependence* 49(2): 81–88.

Ray, O. S., and C. Ksir. 1996. *Drugs, Society and Human Behavior,* 7th ed. St. Louis: Mosby.

Rickert. V. I., C. M. Wiemann, and A. B. Berenson. 1999. Prevalence, patterns and correlates of voluntary flunitrazepam use. *Pediatrics* 103(1): E6. (retrieved January 8, 1999; http://www.pediatrics.org/cgi/content/full/103/1/e6).

Rogers, J. E. 1994. Addiction: A whole new view. *Psychology Today.* September/October.

Schwartz, R. H. 1998. Adolescent heroin use: A review. *Pediatrics* 102(6): 1461–1466.

Soderstrom, C. A., P. C. Dischinger, and T. J. Kerns. 1998. Benzodiazepine use and crash risk in older patients. *Journal of the American Medical Association* 279(2): 114–115.

Substance Abuse and Mental Health Services Administration. 1998. *Preliminary Estimates from the 1997 Household Survey on Drug Abuse.* Washington, D.C.: U.S. Public Health Service.

Substance Abuse and Mental Health Services Administration. 1998. *Preliminary Estimates from the Drug Abuse Warning Network.* Washington, D.C.: U.S. Public Health Service.

U.S. Department of Health and Human Services. 1998. *Healthy People 2010 Objectives: Draft for Public Comment.* Washington, D.C.: U.S. Government Printing Office.

U.S. Drug Enforcement Agency. 1998. *Flunitrazepam (Rohypnol) "Roofies"* (retrieved November 30, 1998; http://www.usdoj.gov/dea/programs/diverson/divpub/substanc/roofies.htm).

U.S. Drug Enforcement Agency. 1997. *Ketamine Abuse Increasing* (retrieved November 30, 1998; http://www.usdoj.gov/dea/programs/diverson/divpub/substanc/ketamine.htm).

U.S. Food and Drug Administration. 1998. *FDA Talk Paper: FDA Clears New Home Drug Screening Test* (retrieved October 16, 1998; http://www.fda.gov/bbs/topics/ANSWERS/ANS00917.html).

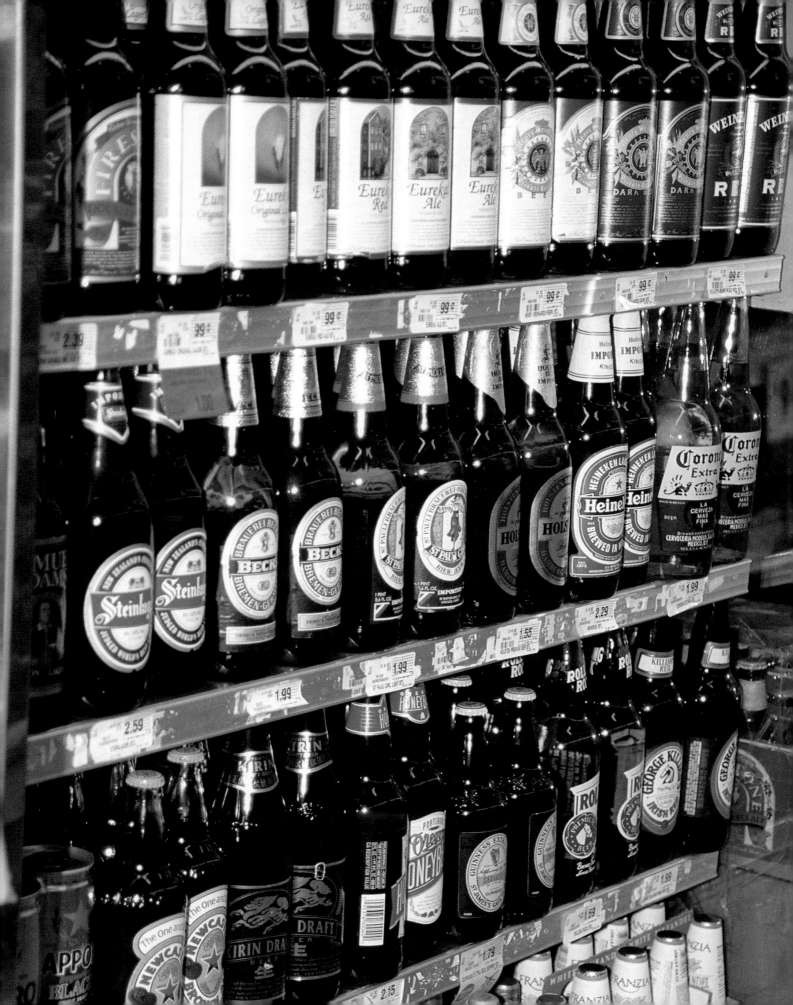

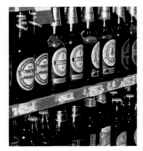

LEARNING OBJECTIVES

After reading this chapter, you should be able to:

- Explain how alcohol is absorbed and metabolized by the body.

- Describe the immediate and long-term effects of drinking alcohol.

- Define alcohol abuse, binge drinking, and alcoholism, and discuss their effects on the drinker and others.

- Evaluate the role of alcohol in your life, and list strategies for using it responsibly.

The Responsible Use of Alcohol

10

TEST YOUR KNOWLEDGE

1. "Moderate drinking" is having three or fewer drinks per day.
   True or false?

2. If a man and a woman of the same weight drink the same amount of alcohol, the woman will become intoxicated more quickly than the man.
   True or false?

3. How many Americans are injured in alcohol-related automobile crashes every year?
   a. 50,000
   b. 250,000
   c. 500,000

4. Drinking coffee will help you sober up.
   True or false?

5. Alcohol use is associated with academic problems and lower grades.
   True or false?

6. How many calories does a typical can of beer contain?
   a. 50
   b. 100
   c. 150
   d. 200

Answers

1. *False.* Moderate drinking is no more than one drink per day for women and no more than two drinks per day for men.

2. *True.* Women usually have a higher percentage of body fat than men and a less active form of a stomach enzyme that breaks down alcohol. Both factors cause them to become intoxicated more quickly and to a greater degree.

3. *c.* Even small amounts of alcohol can affect a person's ability to drive. Many people are significantly impaired after one drink and legally intoxicated after two.

4. *False.* Once alcohol has been absorbed by the body, nothing speeds its metabolism. All you can do to sober up is wait until the alcohol in your body is metabolized.

5. *True.* On average, A students consume fewer than three alcoholic beverages a week; D students drink more than twice that amount.

6. *c.* Three beers have about the same number of calories as a Big Mac.

Alcohol is probably the oldest drug in the world. It has been used in religious ceremonies, in feasts and celebrations, and as a medicine for thousands of years. Throughout history, alcohol has been more popular than any other drug in the Western world, despite numerous prohibitions against it. In fact, forbidding the use of alcohol seems only to make it more popular.

Alcohol has a somewhat contradictory role in human life. Most of us think of alcohol the way it is portrayed in advertisements, on television, and in movies—as part of good times at the beach, social occasions, and elegant gatherings. Used in moderation, alcohol can enhance social occasions by loosening inhibitions and creating a pleasant feeling of relaxation. For some people, alcohol is an integral part of celebrations and special events. But the use of alcohol can also be an unhealthy adaptation. Like other drugs, alcohol has definite physiological effects on the body that can impair functioning in the short term and cause devastating damage in the long term. For some people, alcohol becomes an addiction, leading to a lifetime of recovery or, for a few, to debilitation and death. Many of our slang expressions for intoxication reflect its less positive aspects; we say we're "smashed," "bombed," "wasted."

About 64% of Americans over the age of 12 drink alcohol in some form. If the total amount of alcohol consumed in the United States in a year were evenly divided among drinkers, each would consume the equivalent of 4 gallons of whiskey, 20 gallons of wine, or 50 gallons of beer. But heavy drinkers, who constitute about 8.5% of the American drinking population, account for over half of all the alcohol consumed, as well as a disproportionate amount of the social, economic, and medical costs of alcohol abuse (estimated at $170 billion per year). And through unintentional injuries, especially automobile crashes, alcohol is the leading cause of death among people between the ages of 15 and 24.

The use of alcohol is a complex issue, one that demands conscious thought and informed decisions. In our society, some people choose to drink in moderation, some choose not to drink at all, and others realize too late that they've made an unwise choice—when they become dependent on alcohol, are involved in an alcohol-related car crash, or simply wake up to discover they've done something they regret. This chapter discusses the complexities of alcohol use and provides information that will help you make the choices that are right for you.

PERSONAL INSIGHT   How was alcohol used in your family when you were growing up, and what are your associations with it? Was it used for family celebrations? Was there alcohol abuse in your family? If so, how did you react at the time? How do you feel about it now?

THE NATURE OF ALCOHOL

How does alcohol affect people? Does it affect some people differently than others? Can some people "handle" alcohol? Is it possible to drink a safe amount of alcohol? Many of the misconceptions about the effects of alcohol can be cleared up by taking a closer look at the chemistry of alcohol and how it is absorbed and metabolized by the body.

The Chemistry of Alcohol

Ethyl alcohol is the common psychoactive ingredient in all alcoholic beverages. Beer, a mild intoxicant brewed from a mixture of grains, usually contains 3–6% alcohol by volume. Ales and malt liquors are 6–8% alcohol by volume. Wines are made by *fermenting* the juices of grapes or other fruits. The concentration of alcohol in table wines is about 9–14%. *Fortified wines,* so named because alcohol has been added to them, contain about 20% alcohol; these include sherry, port, and Madeira. Stronger alcoholic beverages, called *hard liquors,* are made by *distilling* brewed or fermented grains or other products. These beverages, including gin, whiskey, brandy, rum, and liqueurs, usually contain 35–50% alcohol.

The concentration of alcohol in a beverage is indicated by the **proof value,** which is two times the percentage concentration. For example, if a beverage is 100 proof, it contains 50% alcohol. Two ounces of 100-proof whiskey contain 1 ounce of pure alcohol. The proof value of hard liquors can usually be found on the bottle labels. When alcohol consumption is discussed, "one drink" refers to a 12-ounce bottle of beer, a 5-ounce glass of table wine, or a cocktail with 1.5 ounces of 80-proof liquor. Each of these different drinks contains approximately the same amount of alcohol: 0.6 ounce.

There are a number of different kinds of alcohol. In this book, the term **alcohol** refers to ethyl alcohol, which is the only kind of alcohol that can be consumed. Other kinds of alcohol such as methanol (wood alcohol) and isopropyl alcohol (rubbing alcohol) are highly toxic and can cause blindness and other serious problems when consumed even in low doses.

Absorption

When a person ingests alcohol, about 20% is rapidly absorbed from the stomach into the bloodstream. About 75% is absorbed through the upper part of the small intestine. Any remaining alcohol enters the bloodstream further along the gastrointestinal tract. The rate of absorption is affected by a variety of factors. For example, the carbonation in a beverage like champagne increases the rate of alcohol absorption. Food in the stomach slows the rate of absorption, as does the drinking of highly concentrated alcoholic beverages such as hard liquor. But

Alcohol Intake and Blood Alcohol Concentration

Blood alcohol concentration (BAC), a measure of intoxication, is determined by the amount of alcohol consumed and by individual factors such as body weight and amount of body fat. In most cases, a smaller person develops a higher BAC than a larger person after drinking the same amount of alcohol. This is because a smaller person has less overall body tissue into which alcohol can be distributed. A person with a higher percentage of body fat will usually develop a higher BAC than a more muscular person who weighs the same. This is because alcohol does not concentrate as much in fatty tissue as in muscle and most other tissues, in part because fat has fewer blood vessels. Women generally have higher BACs than men after consuming the same amount of alcohol because they usually have a higher percentage of body fat than men, and because the stomach enzyme that breaks down alcohol before it enters the bloodstream is four times more active in men than in women.

BAC also depends on the balance between the rate of alcohol absorption and the rate of alcohol metabolism. A man who weighs 154 pounds and has normal liver function metabolizes about 0.3–0.5 ounce of alcohol per hour, the equivalent of slightly less than a 12-ounce bottle of beer or a 5-ounce glass of wine.

The rate of alcohol metabolism varies among individuals and is largely determined by genetic factors and drinking behavior. (Chronic drinking activates enzymes that metabolize alcohol in the liver, so people who drink frequently metabolize alcohol at a more rapid rate than nondrinkers.) Contrary to popular myths, this metabolic rate cannot be influenced by exercise, breathing deeply, eating, drinking coffee, or taking other drugs. The rate of alcohol metabolism is the same whether a person is asleep or awake (see the box "Myths About Alcohol").

If a person absorbs slightly less alcohol each hour than he or she can metabolize in an hour, the BAC remains low. People can drink large amounts of alcohol this way over a long period of time without becoming noticeably intoxicated; however, they do run the risk of significant long-term health hazards (described later in the chapter). If a person is absorbing alcohol more quickly than it can be metabolized, the BAC will steadily increase, and he or she will become more and more drunk (Table 10-1).

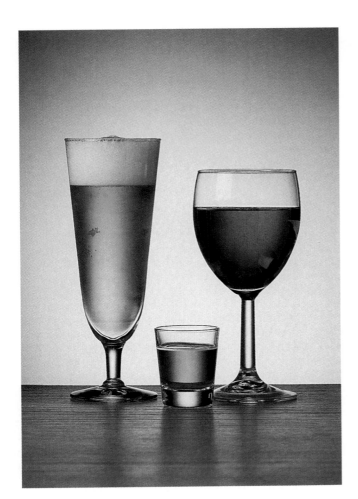

Ethyl alcohol is the common psychoactive drug found in all alcoholic beverages. One drink—a 12-ounce beer, a 1.5-ounce cocktail, or a 5-ounce glass of wine—contains about 0.6 ounce of ethyl alcohol.

remember: *All* alcohol a person consumes is eventually absorbed.

Metabolism and Excretion

Alcohol is quickly transported throughout the body by the blood. Because alcohol easily moves through most biological membranes, it is rapidly distributed throughout most body tissues. The main site of alcohol **metabolism** is the liver, though a small amount of alcohol is metabolized in the stomach. (See the box "Metabolizing Alcohol: Our Bodies Work Differently" for more information.)

About 2–10% of ingested alcohol is not metabolized in the liver or other tissues, but is excreted unchanged by the lungs, kidneys, and sweat glands. Excreted alcohol causes the telltale smell on a drinker's breath and is the basis of breath and urine analyses for alcohol levels. Although such analyses do not give precise measurements of alcohol concentrations in the blood, they do provide a reasonable approximation if done correctly.

proof value Two times the percentage of alcohol by volume; **TERMS** a beverage that is 50% alcohol by volume is 100 proof.

alcohol The intoxicating ingredient in fermented liquors; a colorless, pungent liquid.

metabolism The chemical transformation of food and other substances in the body into energy and wastes.

blood alcohol concentration (BAC) The amount of alcohol in the blood in terms of weight per unit volume; used as a measurement of intoxication.

Do you notice that you react differently to alcohol than some of your friends do? If so, you may be noticing genetic differences in alcohol metabolism that are associated with gender or ethnicity. Alcohol is metabolized mainly in the liver, but some alcohol is broken down in the stomach before it can be sent into the bloodstream and on to the liver. Once it's circulating in the bloodstream, alcohol produces the well-known feelings of intoxication. Studies have shown that women metabolize less alcohol in the stomach than men do, so they release more unmetabolized alcohol into the bloodstream. (The stomach enzyme that breaks down alcohol before it enters the blood-stream is less active in women than in men.) The same amount of alcohol will have more effect on a woman than on a man—she will feel the effects sooner and more strongly.

Other differences in alcohol metabolism are associated with ethnicity. Alcohol is broken down in the liver by an enzyme called alcohol dehydrogenase, producing a by-product called acetaldehyde (see the figure). Acetaldehyde is responsible for many of the unpleasant effects of alcohol abuse. Another enzyme, acetaldehyde dehydrogenase, breaks this product down further. Some people, including many of Asian descent, have genetic information that causes them to produce somewhat different forms of the two enzymes that metabolize alcohol. The result is high concentrations of acetaldehyde in the brain and other tissues, producing a host of unpleasant symptoms. When people with these enzymes drink alcohol, they experience a physiological reaction referred to as *flushing syndrome*. Their skin feels hot, their heart and respiration rates increase, and they may get a headache, vomit, or break out in hives. Drinking makes some people so uncomfortable that it's unlikely they could ever become addicted to alcohol. The body's response to acetaldehyde is the basis for treating alcohol abuse with the drug disulfiram (Antabuse), which inhibits the action of acetaldehyde dehydrogenase. When a person taking disulfiram ingests alcohol, acetaldehyde levels increase rapidly, and he or she develops an intense flushing reaction along with weakness, nausea, vomiting, and other disagreeable symptoms.

How people behave in relation to alcohol is influenced in complex ways by many factors, including social and cultural ones. But in these two cases at least, individual choices and behavior are strongly influenced by a specific genetic characteristic.

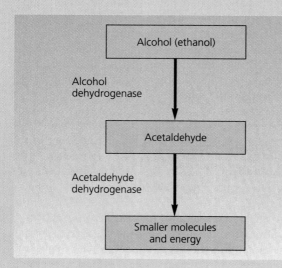

Myth   You can speed up the metabolism of alcohol by exercising, drinking coffee or taking other CNS stimulants, or by breathing fresh air.
Fact   Once alcohol is absorbed, there are no ways of appreciably accelerating its breakdown.

Myth   Getting drunk on the weekend is normal for many people and does not cause any lasting harm.
Fact   Binge drinking results in many deaths from injuries and crimes. Alcohol poisoning can result in death. A single heavy binge can result in pancreatitis (inflammation of the pancreas), causing severe abdominal pain and requiring hospitalization.

Myth   Alcoholics can "handle their alcohol" better than non-alcoholics.
Fact   In the early stages of alcoholism, this is sometimes true. However, in later stages of alcoholism, tolerance to alcohol often decreases. In some severe alcoholics, tolerance fluctuates from day to day: On one day, a liter of wine has little behavioral effect; on another day, one glass of wine causes intoxication.

Myth   When you are under the influence of alcohol, you are so relaxed you are less likely to get hurt in a car crash or fall.
Fact   Alcohol slows protective reflexes and impairs coordination. People under the influence of alcohol have a much greater risk of injury (and death) from car crashes and falls.

Myth   Most alcoholics are consciously aware of drinking too much.
Fact   Denial, the unconscious psychological process that blocks awareness of reality, is an almost universal characteristic of alcoholics and other drug abusers. There is a clinical adage: "The two hallmarks of alcoholism are drinking too much and denying that you drink too much."

Myth   An alcoholic must want help before he or she will respond to it.
Fact   Many alcoholics respond to coercive intervention—to save their relationships, their careers, or their driver's licenses—even though they continue to deny their drinking problems.

Myth   Only an alcoholic can understand and help another.
Fact   Recovering alcoholics do have something unique to offer: a positive, encouraging example. But most of us have experienced, and can empathize with, the feelings associated with excessive drinking—anxiety, depression, loneliness, remorse.

Myth   An alcoholic must "hit bottom" before he or she is ready to stop drinking.
Fact   Alcoholics do not have to lose all before they are motivated to stop. People vary markedly in what induces them to change their behavior. For some, the first blackout or alcohol-related automobile crash fosters abstinence.

TABLE 10-1	The Effects of Alcohol	
BAC (%)	**Common Behavioral Effects**	**Hours Required to Metabolize Alcohol**
0.00–0.05	Slight change in feelings, usually relaxation and euphoria. Decreased alertness.	2–3
0.05–0.10	Emotional instability, with exaggerated feelings and behavior. Reduced social inhibitions. Impairment of reaction time and fine motor coordination. Increasingly impaired during driving. Legally drunk at 0.08% in many states and 0.10% in others.	4–6
0.10–0.15	Unsteadiness in standing and walking. Loss of peripheral vision. Driving is extremely dangerous.	6–10
0.15–0.30	Staggering gait. Slurred speech. Pain and other sensory perceptions greatly impaired.	10–24
More than 0.30	Stupor or unconsciousness. Anesthesia. Death possible at 0.35% and above. Can result from rapid or binge drinking with few earlier effects.	More than 24

ALCOHOL AND HEALTH

The effects of alcohol consumption on health depend on the individual, the circumstances, and the amount of alcohol consumed.

The Immediate Effects of Alcohol

BAC is a primary factor determining the effects of alcohol (see Table 10-1). At low concentrations, alcohol tends to make people feel relaxed and jovial, but at higher concentrations people are more likely to feel angry, sedated, or sleepy. Alcohol is a CNS depressant, and its effects vary because body systems are affected to different degrees at different BACs. At any given BAC, the effects of alcohol are more pronounced when the BAC is rapidly increasing compared to when it is slowly increasing, steady, or decreasing. The effects of alcohol are more pronounced if a person drinks on an empty stomach, because alcohol is absorbed more quickly and the BAC rises more quickly.

Low Concentrations of Alcohol   The effects of alcohol can first be felt at a BAC of about 0.03–0.05%. These effects may include light-headedness, relaxation, and a release of inhibitions. Most drinkers experience mild euphoria and become more sociable. When people drink in social settings, alcohol often seems to act as a stimulant, enhancing conviviality or assertiveness. This apparent stimulation occurs because alcohol depresses inhibitory centers in the brain.

Higher Concentrations of Alcohol   At higher concentrations, the pleasant effects tend to be replaced by more nega-

tive ones: interference with motor coordination, verbal performance, and intellectual functions. The drinker often becomes irritable and may be easily angered or given to crying. When the BAC reaches 0.1%, most sensory and motor functioning is reduced, and many people become sleepy. Vision, smell, taste, and hearing become less acute. At 0.2%, most drinkers are completely unable to function, either physically or psychologically, because of the pronounced depression of the central nervous system, muscles, and other body systems. Coma usually occurs at a BAC of 0.35%, and any higher level can be fatal.

Shakespeare accurately described the effects of alcohol on sexual functioning. He said (in *Macbeth*) that "it stirs up desire, but it takes away the performance." Small doses may improve sexual functioning for individuals who are especially anxious or self-conscious, but higher doses usually have a negative effect. Excessive alcohol use can result in reduced erection response and reduced vaginal lubrication. Testicular atrophy (shrinking) may result from the long-term overuse of alcohol.

Alcohol causes blood vessels near the skin to dilate, so drinkers often feel warm; their skin flushes, and they may sweat more. Flushing and sweating contribute to heat loss, and so the internal body temperature falls. High doses of alcohol may impair the body's ability to regulate temperature, causing it to drop sharply, especially if the surrounding temperature is low. Drinking alcoholic beverages to keep warm in cold weather does not work, and it can even be dangerous.

Drinking alcohol, particularly in large amounts, disturbs normal sleep patterns. Alcohol may facilitate falling asleep more quickly, but the sleep is often light, punctuated with awakenings, and unrefreshing. Even after the

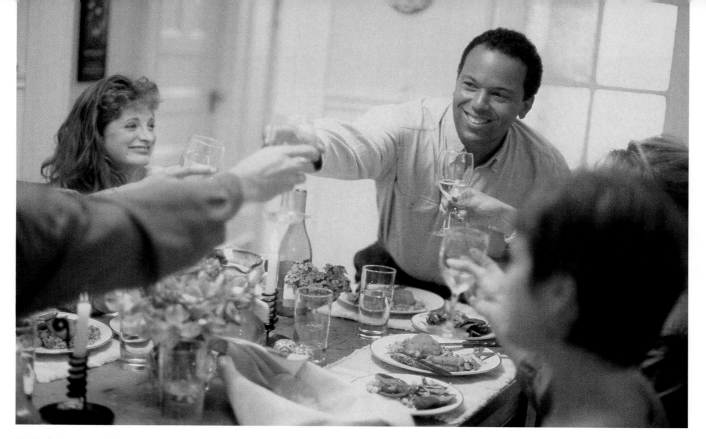

Alcoholic beverages like beer and wine are an integral part of social occasions for many people. A central nervous system depressant, alcohol loosen inhibitions; when used in moderation, it tends to make people feel more relaxed and sociable.

habitual drinker stops drinking, his or her sleep may be altered for weeks or months. Users of alcohol frequently awaken with a "hangover"—headache, nausea, stomach distress, and generalized discomfort.

Alcohol Poisoning   Acute alcohol poisoning occurs much more frequently than most people realize, and all too often it can cause death. Drinking large amounts of alcohol over a short period of time can rapidly raise the BAC into the lethal range. Alcohol, either alone or in combination with other drugs, is probably responsible for more toxic overdose deaths than any other drug. A common scenario for alcohol poisoning occurs when inexperienced drinkers try to outdo each other by consuming glass after glass of alcohol as rapidly as possible. Coma and death can result before the participants in this game have any awareness of how dangerous this kind of "alcohol roulette" can be. Children are at especially high risk for alcohol poisoning. Even a partially empty glass of liquor carelessly left out after a party can result in serious poisoning, or even death, if consumed by a toddler or small child.

Death from alcohol poisoning may be caused either by central nervous system and respiratory depression or by inhaling fluid or vomit into the lungs. The amount of alcohol it takes to make a person unconscious is danger-ously close to a fatal dose. If you come into contact with a person who has been drinking and becomes unconscious, do not assume he or she is just "sleeping it off." The person should be placed on his or her side (to minimize the possibility of choking if vomiting occurs) and watched. If the person's breathing is slow (less than 8 breaths per minute or lapses of 10 seconds or more between breaths) or if the person looks pale or bluish or the skin feels clammy, call 911 immediately. If you aren't sure, call 911 for help.

Using Alcohol with Other Drugs   Combining alcohol and other legal and illegal drugs can be extremely dangerous. Alcohol-drug combinations are the number-one cause of drug-related deaths in this country. Many people are simply unaware that combining alcohol with certain common drugs can be deadly.

Using alcohol while taking any other drug that can cause CNS depression increases the effects of both drugs, potentially leading to coma, respiratory depression, and death. Examples of common drugs that can result in oversedation when combined with alcohol include barbiturates, Valium-like drugs, narcotics such as codeine, antidepressants such as Prozac, and OTC antihistamines like Benadryl. For people who consume 3 or more drinks per day, use of OTC pain relievers like aspirin, ibuprofen, or acetaminophen increases the risk of stomach bleeding or liver damage. Some antibiotics and diabetes medications can also interact dangerously with alcohol.

Many illegal drugs are especially dangerous when combined with alcohol. Life-threatening overdoses occur at much lower doses when heroin and other narcotics are combined with alcohol. When cocaine and alcohol are used together, a toxic substance called cocaethylene is formed; this substance is responsible for more than half of all cocaine-related deaths.

The safest strategy is to avoid combining alcohol with any other drug—prescription, over-the-counter, or illegal. If in doubt, ask your pharmacist or physician before using any drug in combination with alcohol, or just don't do it.

Alcohol-Related Injuries and Violence   The combination of impaired judgment, weakened sensory perception, reduced inhibitions, impaired motor coordination, and, often, increased aggressiveness and hostility that characterize alcohol intoxication can be dangerous or even deadly. Through homicide, suicide, automobile crashes (discussed in the next section), and other incidents, alcohol kills over 100,000 Americans each year. Alcohol use contributes to over 50% of all murders, assaults, and rapes, and alcohol is frequently found in the bloodstream of both perpetrators and victims. Nearly 80% of people who attempt suicide have been drinking, and about half of all successful suicides are alcoholics. Alcohol use more than triples the chances of fatal injuries during leisure activities such as swimming and boating, and more than half of all fatal falls and serious burns occur to people who have been drinking. Being drunk is clearly hazardous to your health.

PERSONAL INSIGHT   Have you ever said or done anything while under the influence of alcohol that you regretted later? If so, how did you deal with the consequences? Did you change your behavior so it didn't happen again?

Drinking and Driving

Drunk driving continues to be one of the most serious public health and safety problems in the United States. Every year, about 500,000 people are injured in alcohol-related automobile crashes—an average of *one person every minute*. Nearly half of the more than 40,000 crash fatalities each year are alcohol-related.

As introduced in Chapter 9, the *dose-response function* is the relationship between the amount of alcohol or drug consumed and the type and intensity of the resulting effect. Higher doses of alcohol are associated with a much greater probability of automobile crashes (Figure 10-1). A person driving with a BAC of 0.14% is more than 40 times more likely to be involved in a crash than someone with no alcohol in his or her blood. For those with a BAC

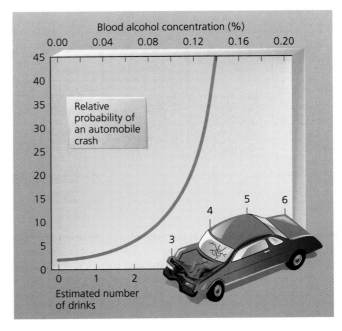

VITAL STATISTICS

Figure 10-1   The dose-response relationship between BAC and automobile crashes.

above 0.14%, the risk of a fatal crash is estimated to be 380 times higher. The risks for young drivers are even greater than indicated in Figure 10-1, especially at very low BACs. Younger drivers have less experience with both driving and alcohol, which results in significant impairment even with BACs as low as 0.02%.

In addition to an increased risk of injury and death, driving while intoxicated can have serious legal consequences. Drunk driving is against the law. The legal limit for BAC is 0.08% in some states and 0.10% in others. Under "zero tolerance" laws in many states, drivers under age 21 who have consumed *any* alcohol may have their licenses suspended. There are stiff penalties for drunk driving, including fines, loss of license, confiscation of vehicle, and jail time. Many cities have checkpoints where drivers are stopped and checked for intoxication.

The number of drinks it takes the average person to reach various BACs is shown in Figure 10-2, p. 254. Even more important than understanding BAC levels is the knowledge that any amount of alcohol can impair your ability to drive safely. If you are going to drink, designate a nondrinking driver or find an alternative means of transportation. Remember, you risk more than your own life. Causing serious injury or death because of driving after drinking results in lifelong feelings of sadness and guilt for the driver and tremendous grief for the friends and families of the victims. While you can do something about your own drinking, it's harder to protect yourself against someone else; the box "Protecting Yourself on the Road," p. 255, provides some guidelines.

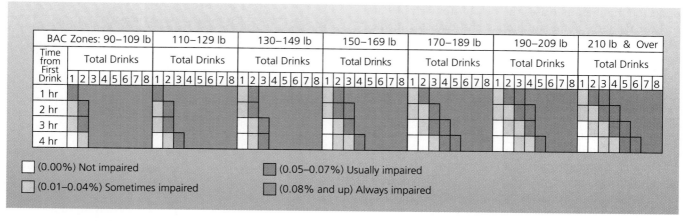

BAC Zones:	90–109 lb								110–129 lb								130–149 lb								150–169 lb								170–189 lb								190–209 lb								210 lb & Over							
Time from First Drink	Total Drinks								Total Drinks								Total Drinks								Total Drinks								Total Drinks								Total Drinks								Total Drinks							
	1	2	3	4	5	6	7	8	1	2	3	4	5	6	7	8	1	2	3	4	5	6	7	8	1	2	3	4	5	6	7	8	1	2	3	4	5	6	7	8	1	2	3	4	5	6	7	8	1	2	3	4	5	6	7	8
1 hr																																																								
2 hr																																																								
3 hr																																																								
4 hr																																																								

☐ (0.00%) Not impaired   ☐ (0.05–0.07%) Usually impaired

☐ (0.01–0.04%) Sometimes impaired   ☐ (0.08% and up) Always impaired

Figure 10-2 Approximate blood alcohol concentration and body weight. This chart illustrates the BAC an average person of a given weight would reach after drinking the specified number of drinks in the time shown. The legal limit for BAC is 0.08% in some states and 0.10% in most others. For drivers under 21 years of age, many states have "zero tolerance" laws that set BAC limits of 0.01% or 0.02%.

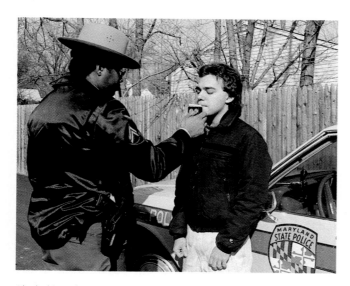

Alcohol interferes with judgment, perception, coordination, and other areas of mental and physical functioning, and it is a factor in a majority of all fatal automobile crashes. This driver is lucky that he was stopped by a suspicious police officer before a crash occurred. He is being given a breath test to determine his blood alcohol concentration.

The Effects of Chronic Use

Because alcohol is distributed throughout most of the body, it can affect many different organs and tissues (Figure 10-3, p. 256). Problems associated with chronic, or habitual, use of alcohol include diseases of the digestive and cardiovascular systems and some cancers. Drinking during pregnancy risks the health of both the woman and the developing fetus.

The Digestive System Even in relatively small amounts, alcohol can alter the normal functioning of the liver. With continued alcohol use, liver cells are damaged and then progressively destroyed. The destroyed cells are often replaced by fibrous scar tissue, a condition known as **cirrhosis of the liver.** As cirrhosis develops, a drinker may gradually lose his or her capacity to tolerate alcohol, because there are fewer and fewer healthy cells remaining in the liver to metabolize it. Alcohol-precipitated cirrhosis is the tenth leading cause of death in the United States.

As with most health hazards, the risk of cirrhosis depends on an individual's susceptibility, largely genetically determined, and the amount of alcohol consumed over time. Some people show signs of cirrhosis after a few years of consuming three or four drinks per day. Women generally develop cirrhosis at lower levels of alcohol consumption than men. Early signs of cirrhosis include jaundice (a yellowing of the skin and white part of the eyes) and the accumulation of fluid in the abdomen and lower extremities. Treatment for cirrhosis includes a balanced diet and complete abstinence from alcohol. People with cirrhosis who continue to drink have only a 50% chance of surviving 5 or more years.

Alcohol can inflame the pancreas, causing nausea, vomiting, abnormal digestion, and severe pain. Acute alcoholic pancreatitis generally occurs in binge drinkers. Unlike cirrhosis, which usually occurs after years of fairly heavy alcohol use, pancreatitis can occur after just one or two severe binge-drinking episodes. Acute pancreatitis is often fatal and can also develop into a chronic condition.

Acute or chronic overuse of alcohol can cause violent vomiting and tear blood vessels in the wall of the esophagus. Alcohol also irritates the lining of the stomach. Potentially life-threatening bleeding can result.

Protecting Yourself on the Road

People who drink and drive are unable to drive responsibly because their judgment is impaired, their reaction time is slower, and their coordination is reduced. Some of the skills involved in driving are affected at BACs of 0.02% and lower; at 0.05%, visual perception, reaction time, and certain steering tasks are all impaired. No one can drive skillfully and safely when under the influence of alcohol.

What can you do to protect yourself against alcohol-related automobile crashes? If you are out of your home and drinking, follow the practice of having a *designated driver,* an individual who refrains from drinking in order to provide safe transportation home for others in the group. The responsibility can be rotated for different occasions.

To reduce your chances of being involved in a crash caused by someone else, learn to be alert to the erratic driving that signals an impaired driver. Warnings signs include wide, abrupt, and illegal turns; straddling the center line or lane marker; driving on the shoulder; weaving, swerving, or nearly striking an object or another vehicle; following too closely; erratic speed; driving with headlights off at night; and driving with the window down in very cold weather.

If you see any of these warning signs, what should you do?

- If the driver is ahead of you, maintain a safe following distance. Do not try to pass, because the driver may swerve into your car.
- If the driver is behind you, turn right at the nearest intersection, and let the driver pass.
- If the driver is approaching your car, move to the shoulder and stop. Avoid a head-on collision by sounding your horn or flashing your lights.
- When approaching an intersection, slow down and expect the unexpected.
- Make sure your safety belt is fastened, children are in approved safety seats, and your doors are locked.
- Report suspected impaired drivers to the nearest police station by phone. Give a description of the vehicle, license number, location, and direction the vehicle is headed.

SOURCES: Adapted from National Institute on Alcohol Abuse and Alcoholism. 1996. *Drinking and Driving.* No. 31 PH 362. The designated driver: Being a friend. 1986. *Healthline,* December.

The Cardiovascular System The effects of alcohol on the cardiovascular system depend on the amount of alcohol consumed. Moderate doses of alcohol—less than one drink a day for women and two drinks a day for men—may reduce the risk of heart disease and heart attack in some people. (The possible health benefits of alcohol are discussed later in this chapter.) However, higher doses of alcohol have harmful effects on the cardiovascular system. In some people, more than two drinks a day will elevate blood pressure, making stroke and heart attack more likely. Some alcoholics show a weakening of the heart muscle, a condition known as **cardiac myopathy.** Binge drinking can cause "holiday heart," a syndrome characterized by serious abnormal heart rhythms, which usually appear within 24 hours of a binge episode.

Although the relationships between alcohol and cardiovascular disease are multiple and complex, it is clear that excessive drinking increases the risk of disease. These health risks progressively increase as the amount of excessive drinking increases.

Cancer Alcoholics have a cancer rate about ten times higher than that of the general population. They are particularly vulnerable to cancers of the throat, larynx, esophagus, upper stomach, liver, and pancreas. Drinking three or more alcoholic beverages per day doubles a woman's risk of developing breast cancer. Some studies have linked even moderate drinking to increased risk for cancers of the breast, mouth, throat, and esophagus.

Mortality As an ancient proverb states, "Those who worship Bacchus [the god of wine] die young." Excessive alcohol consumption is a factor in five of the ten leading causes of death for Americans. Average life expectancy among alcoholics is about 58 years; heavy drinkers may die in their 20s or 30s.

The Effects of Alcohol Use During Pregnancy

Studies of animals and humans indicate that alcohol ingested during pregnancy can harm the fetus. Alcohol and its metabolic product acetaldehyde quickly cross the placenta. As with many drug hazards, the effects of alcohol on the fetus are dose-related. Below-normal birth weights occur when pregnant mothers consume as few as two alcoholic drinks a day. With heavier drinking, a collection of birth defects known as **fetal alcohol syndrome (FAS)** becomes increasingly likely. These children have a characteristic mixture of deformities that include a small head, flat nasal bridge, short nose, and long upper lip. They are

cirrhosis of the liver A disease in which the liver is severely damaged by alcohol, other toxins, or infection. TERMS

cardiac myopathy Weakening of the heart muscle through disease.

fetal alcohol syndrome (FAS) A characteristic group of birth defects caused by excessive alcohol consumption by the mother, including facial deformities, heart defects, and physical and mental impairments.

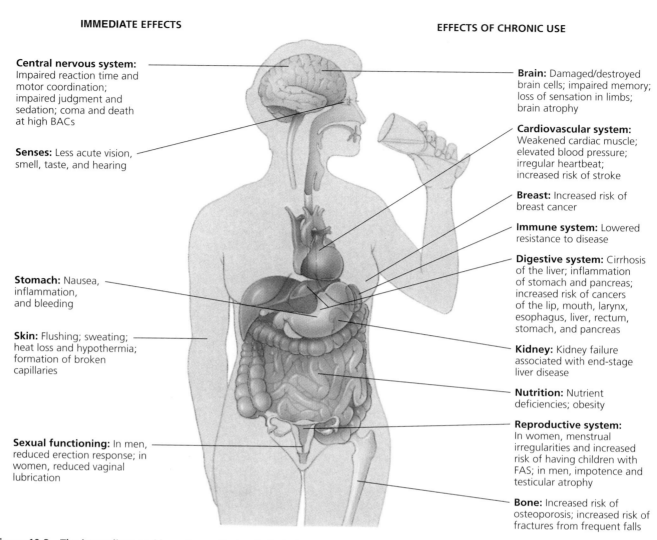

Central nervous system: Impaired reaction time and motor coordination; impaired judgment and sedation; coma and death at high BACs

Senses: Less acute vision, smell, taste, and hearing

Stomach: Nausea, inflammation, and bleeding

Skin: Flushing; sweating; heat loss and hypothermia; formation of broken capillaries

Sexual functioning: In men, reduced erection response; in women, reduced vaginal lubrication

Brain: Damaged/destroyed brain cells; impaired memory; loss of sensation in limbs; brain atrophy

Cardiovascular system: Weakened cardiac muscle; elevated blood pressure; irregular heartbeat; increased risk of stroke

Breast: Increased risk of breast cancer

Immune system: Lowered resistance to disease

Digestive system: Cirrhosis of the liver; inflammation of stomach and pancreas; increased risk of cancers of the lip, mouth, larynx, esophagus, liver, rectum, stomach, and pancreas

Kidney: Kidney failure associated with end-stage liver disease

Nutrition: Nutrient deficiencies; obesity

Reproductive system: In women, menstrual irregularities and increased risk of having children with FAS; in men, impotence and testicular atrophy

Bone: Increased risk of osteoporosis; increased risk of fractures from frequent falls

Figure 10-3   The immediate and long-term effects of alcohol use.

usually small and may have heart defects, as well as many other physical abnormalities. Even with the best of care, their physical and mental growth rates are slower than normal during childhood. In adolescence they sometimes catch up with their age mates in terms of physical size, but not usually in mental abilities. Most remain mentally impaired, with IQs in the 40–80 range (normal is 90–110). FAS effects also include subtle changes in fine motor coordination and behavioral and learning problems. The U.S. incidence of FAS is estimated to be 1 or 2 in every 1000 live births. It is the most common preventable cause of mental impairments in the Western world.

There is no precise BAC level above which damage occurs and below which there is no danger. Instead, the frequency and severity of defects progressively increase as the amount of drinking increases. Exposing the fetus to alcohol or other drugs during the first 12 or 13 weeks of

pregnancy is particularly hazardous because during this time the critical formation of the central nervous system, heart, and other organs occurs. Even a moderate intake of alcohol, too low to cause full-blown FAS, has been shown to cause significant abnormalities in children's psychomotor development. Women who drink five or more drinks per occasion are at a higher risk of having a baby with a cleft palate or lip; babies born to alcoholic mothers may also experience withdrawal symptoms. The safest course of action is abstinence from alcohol during pregnancy.

Any alcohol consumed by a nursing mother quickly enters the breast milk. What impact this has on the child or on the mother's milk production is a matter of controversy. Dosage may again be the key issue. However, many physicians advise nursing mothers to abstain from drinking alcohol because of the belief that any amount may have subtle negative effects on the baby's brain development.

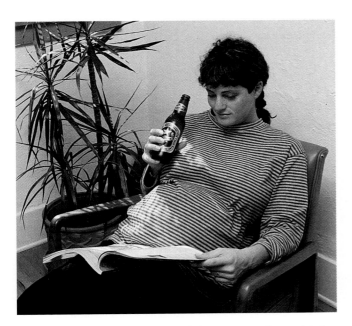

A high level of alcohol consumption during pregnancy is associated with miscarriage, stillbirth, and a cluster of birth defects known as fetal alcohol syndrome. Total abstinence from alcohol during pregnancy is recommended.

Possible Health Benefits of Alcohol

The relationship between alcohol use and health is complex and still under investigation. Both abstainers and moderate drinkers live longer than heavy drinkers, but people who drink moderately—no more than one drink a day for women and two drinks a day for men—live longer than those who abstain completely. Moderate drinking appears to lower the risk for heart attack and some strokes by raising blood levels of HDL, the beneficial form of cholesterol, and reducing the risk of dangerous blood clots. (Alcohol makes platelets, cell fragments found in blood, less likely to stick together and form clots.) Some evidence also suggests that moderate drinkers may be less likely to develop a variety of other conditions, including diabetes, arterial blockages in the legs, Alzheimer's disease, and benign prostate enlargement.

Moderate drinking is not without risk, however. It increases the risk of dying from unintentional injuries, violence, and certain types of cancer. In women, moderate drinking may increase the risk of breast cancer; those who are at risk for breast cancer should discuss the potential risks and benefits of alcohol with their physician. There is also a risk that moderate drinking will not stay moderate. People who avoid alcohol because they or family members have had problems with dependence in the past should not start drinking for their health. People with conditions such as peptic ulcer, diabetes, or depression that are worsened by alcohol use should probably avoid even moderate drinking. Nor should drinkers use this information as an excuse to overindulge. In addition, there are many situations in which consuming any amount of alcohol is unwise, including during pregnancy, while taking medication that may interact with alcohol, and when driving or engaging in another activity that requires alertness.

The bottom line is that limited, regular consumption of alcohol appears to be beneficial for some adults; but there is a narrow window of benefit, and excessive drinking causes serious health problems. The *Dietary Guidelines for Americans,* published by the U.S. Department of Agriculture (USDA), recommend that if you drink alcoholic beverages, you do it in moderation, with meals, at times when consumption does not put you or others at risk.

ALCOHOL ABUSE AND DEPENDENCE

Abuse and dependence on alcohol affect more than just the drinker. Friends, family members, coworkers, strangers that drinkers encounter on the road, and society as a whole pay the physical, emotional, and financial costs of the misuse of alcohol.

Alcohol Abuse

As explained in Chapter 9, the American Psychiatric Association's *Diagnostic and Statistical Manual of Mental Disorders* makes a distinction between substance abuse and substance dependence. **Alcohol abuse** is recurrent alcohol use that has negative consequences, such as drinking in dangerous situations (such as before driving), or drinking patterns that result in academic, professional, interpersonal, or legal difficulties. **Alcohol dependence,** or **alcoholism,** involves more extensive problems with alcohol use, usually involving physical tolerance and withdrawal. Alcoholism is discussed in greater detail later in the chapter.

Other authorities use different definitions to describe problems associated with drinking. The important point is that one does not have to be an alcoholic to have problems with alcohol. The person who drinks only once a month, perhaps after an exam, but then drives while intoxicated is an alcohol abuser.

TERMS

alcohol abuse The use of alcohol to a degree that causes physical damage, impairs functioning, or results in behavior harmful to others.

alcohol dependence A pathological use of alcohol, or impairment in functioning due to alcohol; characterized by tolerance and withdrawal symptoms; alcoholism.

alcoholism A chronic psychological disorder characterized by excessive and compulsive drinking.

TABLE 10-2	The Effects of Binge Drinking on College Students

| | Percent of Students Experiencing Problem | | |
Alcohol-Related Problem	Non–Binge Drinkers	Infrequent Binge Drinkers	Frequent Binge Drinkers
Drove after drinking alcohol	20	43	59
Did something they regretted	18	41	66
Missed a class	10	33	65
Argued with friends	10	24	47
Engaged in unplanned sex	10	24	45
Got behind in schoolwork	9	25	48
Had unprotected sex	5	10	24
Got hurt or injured	3	11	27
Got into trouble with police	2	5	15
Had five or more of these problems since school year began	4	17	52

SOURCE: Wechsler, H., et al. 1998. Change in binge drinking and related problems among American college students between 1993 and 1997. *Journal of American College Health* 47: 57–68.

How can you tell if you are beginning to abuse alcohol or if someone you know is doing so? Look for the following warning signs:

- Drinking alone or secretively.

- Using alcohol deliberately and repeatedly to perform or get through difficult situations.

- Feeling uncomfortable on certain occasions when alcohol is not available.

- Escalating alcohol consumption beyond an already established drinking pattern.

- Consuming alcohol heavily in risky situations, such as before driving.

- Getting drunk regularly or more frequently than in the past.

- Drinking in the morning or at other unusual times.

Binge Drinking

A common form of alcohol abuse on college campuses is known as **binge drinking**. In surveys of students on over 100 college campuses, 43% reported binge drinking, defined as having five drinks in a row for men or four in a row for women on at least one occasion in the 2 weeks prior to the survey. Some 21% of all students were found to be frequent binge drinkers, defined as having at least three binges during the 2-week period. Students living at fraternity or sorority houses had the highest rate of binge drinking, 81%. Men were more likely to binge than women, and white students had higher rates of binge drinking than students of other ethnicities. Nineteen percent of students abstained from alcohol.

Binge drinking has a profound effect on students' lives. Frequent binge drinkers were found to be 3–9 times more likely than non–binge drinkers to engage in unplanned or unprotected sex, to drive after drinking, and to get hurt or injured (Table 10-2). Binge drinkers were also more likely to miss classes, get behind in schoolwork, and argue with friends. The more frequent the binges, the more problems the students encountered. Despite their experiences, fewer than 1% of the binge drinkers identified themselves as problem drinkers.

Binge drinking also affects non-bingeing students. At schools with high rates of binge drinking, the non-bingers were up to three times as likely to report being bothered by the alcohol-related behaviors of others than students at schools with lower rates of binge drinking. These problems included having sleep or studying disrupted; having to take care of a drunken student; being insulted or humiliated; experiencing unwanted sexual advances; and being pushed, hit, or assaulted.

The draft *Healthy People 2010* report sets the goals of reducing the rate of binge drinking to 18% among 18–25-year-olds and 15% among 26–34-year-olds. Binge drinking is a difficult problem to address because many students arrive at college with drinking patterns already established (binge drinking during high school is a strong predictor of binge drinking during the college years). Many colleges have drinking "cultures" that perpetuate the pattern of binge drinking. On many campuses, drinking behavior that would be classified as abuse in another setting may be viewed as socially acceptable or even attractive. This is despite the evidence that such behavior leads to automobile crashes, injuries, violence, suicide, and high-risk sexual behavior (see the box "Facts About Drinking Among College Students").

- About 8 out of 10 college students drink alcohol—an estimated 70% of students consume alcohol every month, and 4% drink every day. More than three times as many male students as female students drink daily.

- The average yearly consumption of alcoholic beverages per student is over 34 gallons. As a group, American college students consume almost 4 billion cans of beer each year.

- About 40% of students' academic problems and 28% of dropouts are related to alcohol use.

- In national surveys, 20% of students reported doing poorly on a test or assignment and nearly 30% said they had missed class in the prior year because of alcohol or other drug use. Frequent binge drinkers were more than six times more likely to miss class than students who didn't binge drink.

- There is a negative relationship between college grades and amount of alcohol consumed. Among students at two-year colleges, those with an A average have about 2.5 drinks per week; B students have 3.5; C students, 4; and D or F students, 6. A similar pattern is seen among students at four-year colleges.

- Between 50% and 80% of all violence on college campuses is alcohol-related. Drinking alcohol increases the risk that a student will commit or be a victim of a crime. Nearly 70% of perpetrators and 80% of victims of sexual assault are under the influence of alcohol at the time of the attack.

- One-half to two-thirds of undergraduates have driven while intoxicated or have been a passenger in a car when the driver was intoxicated.

- In a survey of nearly 100,000 college students, half reported that alcohol and drug use by fellow students had interfered with their quality of life.

SOURCES: Higher Education Center for Alcohol and Other Drug Prevention (http://www.edc.org/hec). Wechsler, H., et al. 1998. Changes in binge drinking and related problems among American college students between 1993 and 1997. *Journal of American College Health* 47: 57–68. Eigin, L. D. 1991. *Alcohol Practices, Policies, and Potentials of American Colleges and Universities.* Washington, D.C.: U.S. Department of Health and Human Services.

Alcoholism

As mentioned earlier, alcoholism, or alcohol dependence, is usually characterized by tolerance to alcohol and withdrawal symptoms. Everyone who drinks—even nonalcoholics—develops tolerance after repeated alcohol use. As described in Chapter 9, *tolerance* means that a drinker needs more alcohol to achieve intoxication or the desired effect, that the effects of continued use of the same amount of alcohol are diminished, or that the drinker can function adequately at doses or a BAC that would produce significant impairment in a casual user. Heavy users of alcohol may need to consume about 50% more than they originally needed in order to experience the same degree of intoxication.

Withdrawal occurs when someone who has been using alcohol heavily for several days or more suddenly stops drinking or markedly reduces her or his intake. Symptoms of withdrawal include trembling and nervousness, and sometimes even **hallucinations** and seizures.

Patterns and Prevalence   Alcoholism occurs among people of all ethnic groups and at all socioeconomic levels. The stereotype of the alcoholic skid row bum actually accounts for fewer than 5% of all alcohol-dependent people, and usually represents the final stage of a drinking career that began years earlier. There are different patterns of alcohol dependence, including these four common ones:

1. *Regular daily intake of large amounts.* This continuous pattern is the most common adult pattern of excessive consumption in most countries.

2. *Regular heavy drinking limited to weekends.* This pattern of binge drinking is often followed by teenagers and college students.

3. *Long periods of sobriety interspersed with binges of daily heavy drinking lasting for weeks or months.* This episodic or "bender" pattern is common in the United States but quite uncommon in France, although the per capita consumption of alcohol is higher in France.

4. *Heavy drinking limited to periods of stress.* This "reactive" pattern is associated with periods of anxiety or depression, such as at times of test or other performance fears, interpersonal problems, or school or work pressures.

Once established, alcoholism often exhibits a pattern of exacerbations and remissions. The person may stop drinking and abstain from alcohol for days or months after a frightening problem develops. After a period of abstinence, an alcoholic often attempts controlled drinking, which almost inevitably leads to an escalation in drinking

binge drinking   Periodically drinking alcohol to the point of severe intoxication.

hallucination   A false perception that does not correspond to external reality, such as seeing visions or hearing voices that are not there.

TERMS

About 1 out of 8 Americans grows up in an alcoholic household. For these children, life is a struggle to deal with constant stress, anxiety, and embarrassment. They may be victims of violence, abuse, or neglect in the home. Family life centers on the drinking parent, and children's needs are often ignored.

Children in alcoholic households often cope by learning patterns of interaction that help them survive childhood but that don't support their own healthy development. Many adult children of alcoholics fear losing control, and they try to control their own feelings and behavior and those of people around them. They may fear emotions, even pleasant feelings such as happiness and joy. They avoid conflict and are easily upset by criticism from authority figures. Other common traits include an overdeveloped sense of responsibility and hypersensitivity to the needs of others. Children of alcoholics often feel guilty if they stand up for themselves and acknowledge their own needs. All these characteristics can be stumbling blocks to forming healthy relationships.

Children of alcoholics are more likely than other children to become alcoholic themselves and to marry alcoholics. An estimated 13–25% of children of alcoholics will become alcoholic at some point in their lives. They are more likely to abuse other drugs and develop an eating disorder. They are also particularly prone to stress-related medical illnesses.

If you are the child of an alcoholic, be aware, first, that you are not alone. Millions of people have been through the same problem and have dreamed of having a happy family life in which drinking is not an issue. Realize, too, that other people can understand what you have been through and can help. Find a person you can trust, and confide in her or him. It may seem safer to keep your feelings secret, but talking about the problem is the first step toward a healthy readjustment. Many adult children of alcoholics benefit greatly from therapy with a counselor who is experienced in treating people who have been affected by an alcoholic family. Individual or group therapy can be a critical step in recovery. (The For More Information section at the end of this chapter lists agencies that can provide help and referrals.)

Finally, acknowledge that your parent's alcoholism is not your fault. Many children of alcoholics carry a burden of guilt from early childhood, when they could not understand that they weren't the cause of their parent's behavior. This unexamined assumption is often part of the emotional pain experienced by children of alcoholics.

and more problems. Alcoholism is not hopeless, however; many alcoholics do achieve permanent abstinence.

The 1997 National Household Survey on Drug Abuse revealed that 11 million Americans were heavy drinkers and 32 million were binge drinkers. Studies suggest that the lifetime risk of alcoholism in the United States is about 10% for men and about 3% for women. The risk for women has been increasing in recent years, as women's roles in our society have expanded.

Health Effects   Tolerance and withdrawal can have a serious impact on health. An alcoholic requires increasingly larger amounts to produce the desired effects, and these larger doses increase the chance of adverse physical effects. When alcoholics stop drinking or sharply decrease their intake, they experience withdrawal. Symptoms include trembling hands ("shakes" or "jitters"), a rapid pulse and accelerated breathing rate, insomnia, nightmares, anxiety, and gastrointestinal upset. These symptoms usually begin 5–10 hours after alcohol intake is decreased and improve after 4–5 days. After a week, most people feel much better; but occasionally anxiety, insomnia, and other symptoms can persist for 6 months or more.

More severe withdrawal symptoms occur in about 5% of alcoholics. These include seizures (sometimes called "rum fits"), confusion, and hallucinations. Still less common is **DTs (delirium tremens)**, a medical emergency characterized by severe disorientation, confusion, multiple seizures, and vivid hallucinations, often of vermin and small animals. The mortality rate from DTs can be as high as 15%, especially in very debilitated people with preexisting medical illnesses.

Because alcohol is distributed throughout the body's organs and tissues, alcoholism takes a heavy physical and psychological toll. Alcoholics face all the physical health risks associated with intoxication and chronic drinking described earlier in the chapter. Some of the damage is worsened by nutritional deficiencies that often accompany alcoholism. Some people develop alcoholic **paranoia,** characterized by delusions, jealousy, suspicion, and mistrust. Other mental problems associated with alcoholism include profound memory gaps (commonly known as "blackouts"), which are sometimes filled by conscious or unconscious lying.

The specific health effects of alcoholism tend to vary from person to person. One individual may suffer primarily from problems with memory and CNS defects while having no liver or gastrointestinal problems. Another person with a similar drinking and nutritional history may have advanced liver disease but no memory gaps.

Social and Psychological Effects   Alcohol use causes more serious social and psychological problems than all other forms of substance abuse combined. For every person who is an alcoholic, another three or four people are directly affected (see the box "Children of Alcoholics"). In a 1997 Gallup poll, almost a third of Americans reported that alcohol had been a source of trouble in their family—

the highest rate recorded since Gallup began asking the question in 1950.

Alcoholics frequently suffer from *dual disorders,* mental disorders in addition to their substance dependence. Alcoholics are much more likely than nonalcoholics to suffer from clinical depression, panic disorder, schizophrenia, and antisocial personality disorders. People with anxiety or panic attacks may try to use alcohol to lessen their anxiety, even though alcohol often makes these disorders worse. About two-thirds of alcoholics entering treatment have symptoms resembling anxiety disorders, but most of these symptoms subside after withdrawal ends and the individual has been sober for several weeks or months. In true dual disorders, symptoms of the mental disorder will persist even after the person has been sober for many weeks.

Alcoholics also often have other substance-abuse problems. About 90% of all cocaine abusers also abuse alcohol. Recovering alcoholics need to be very careful about the use of both illegal and legal drugs because they are at greater risk for substance dependence than people who have never had a drinking problem.

An estimated 4 million Americans age 14–17 show signs of potential alcohol dependence. These numbers are far greater than those associated with cocaine, heroin, or marijuana use. The social and psychological consequences of excessive drinking in young people are more difficult to measure than the risks to physical health. One of the consequences is that excessive drinking interferes with learning the interpersonal and job-related skills required for adult life. Excessive drinkers sometimes narrow their circle of friends to other heavy drinkers and thus limit the range of people they can learn from. Perhaps most important is that people who were excessive drinkers in college are more likely to have social, occupational, and health problems 20 years later. Despite media attention on cocaine and other drugs, alcohol abuse remains our society's number-one drug problem.

Causes of Alcoholism   The precise causes of alcoholism are unknown, but many factors are probably involved. Recent studies of twins and adopted children clearly demonstrate the importance of genetics. If one of a pair of fraternal twins is alcoholic, then the other has about twice the chance of becoming alcoholic. For the identical twin of an alcoholic, the risk of alcoholism is about four times that of the general population. These risks persist even when the twins have little contact with each other or their biological parents. Similarly, adoption studies show an increased risk for children of alcoholics, even if they were adopted away at birth into nondrinking families. Alcoholism in adoptive parents, on the other hand, does not make individuals either more or less likely to become alcoholic. Some studies suggest that as much as 50% of a person's risk for alcoholism is determined by genetic factors.

Not all children of alcoholics become alcoholic, however, and it is clear that other factors are involved. A person's risk of developing alcoholism may be increased by certain personality disorders, having been subjected as a child to destructive child-rearing practices, and imitating the alcohol abuse of peers and other role models. People who begin drinking excessively in their teens are especially prone to alcoholism later in life. Common psychological features of individuals who abuse alcohol are denial ("I don't have a problem") and rationalization ("I drink because I need to socialize with my customers"). Certain social factors have also been linked with alcoholism, including urbanization, disappearance of the extended family, a general loosening of kinship ties, increased mobility, and changing values. For more on the social influences on drinking behavior, see the box "Cultural Variations in Alcohol Use," p. 262.

Treatment   Some alcoholics recover without professional help. How often this occurs is unknown, but possibly as many as 25% stop drinking on their own or reduce their drinking enough to eliminate problems. Often these spontaneous recoveries are linked to an alcohol-related crisis, such as a health problem or the threat of being fired.

Most alcoholics, however, require a treatment program of some kind in order to stop drinking. Many different kinds of programs exist. No single treatment works for everyone, so a person may have to try different programs before finding the right one. Over 1 million Americans enter treatment for alcoholism every year.

Although not all alcoholics can be successfully treated, considerable optimism has replaced the older view that nothing could be done. Many alcoholics have patterns of drinking that fluctuate widely over time. These fluctuations indicate that their alcohol abuse is a response to environmental factors, such as life stressors or social pressures, and therefore may be influenced by treatment.

One of the oldest and best-known recovery programs is Alcoholics Anonymous (AA). AA consists of self-help groups that meet several times each week in most communities and follow a 12-step program. Important steps for people in these programs include recognizing that they are "powerless over alcohol" and must seek help from a "higher power" in order to regain control of their lives. By verbalizing these steps, the alcoholic directly addresses the denial that is often prominent in alcoholism and other addictions. Many AA members have a sponsor

DTs (delirium tremens)   A state of confusion brought on by the reduction of alcohol intake in an alcohol-dependent person; other symptoms are sweating, trembling, anxiety, hallucinations, and seizures.   **TERMS**

paranoia   A mental disorder characterized by persistent delusions—fixed, false beliefs that would not be accepted by the individual's culture.

Burukutu, saki, tzuika, arrack—these are the names of some local favorite alcoholic beverages around the world. Alcohol is used in most cultures, but patterns of use and rates of abuse vary widely. Some cultures seem to promote a moderate use of alcohol, while others have a larger percentage of alcoholics. Some of the factors that contribute to the rate of alcohol use and abuse in any given culture are social and religious traditions, genetic factors, history, economic factors, and even climate.

Residents of the Mediterranean countries in southern Europe have a long tradition of moderate drinking as part of their cultures. Italy and France are major wine-producing nations, and many people in these countries regularly drink wine with lunch and dinner. Children are given small amounts of wine with meals. A moderate use of alcohol is the norm, and excessive drinking is not tolerated. In Greece, alcohol has long been a important part of social occasions, but it is considered unacceptable to become intoxicated. The consumption of alcohol per person in these countries is relatively high, but rates of death from cirrhosis of the liver are fairly low.

In contrast, some cultures of northern Europe have strong traditions of heavy drinking. In Ireland and Russia, children and adolescents are often forbidden to drink in the home, while adult men are expected to drink large quantities of distilled spirits. Much of the drinking occurs in bars and pubs, away from family influences. One theory is that cultures that view alcohol as "forbidden fruit" and have ambiguous social attitudes about alcohol use tend to have higher rates of alcoholism. In these cultures, alcohol use is associated with virility, and alcohol use rates are much higher among young men than in the rest of the population.

In most Asian cultures, rates of alcohol abuse have traditionally been quite low. One reason for this is that about half of all Asian people carry a gene that causes uncomfortable side effects from drinking alcohol, such as facial flushing, sweating, and nausea. In spite of this common reaction, heavy drinking has been on the rise in much of Asia as Western habits become fashionable. Getting intoxicated is becoming an important business ritual in Japan and Korea; mixed drinks are even available from vending machines on the street. South Korea is now reported to have the highest per-person consumption of distilled spirits in the world.

In many cultures today, traditional patterns of alcohol use are being undermined by advertising and the media. The developing world is being targeted by the alcohol industry as a new source of consumers, and rates of alcoholism are on the rise. Meanwhile, alcohol use has declined in the United States and other Western countries in the last decade, as people have become aware of the health and safety hazards associated with excessive drinking.

---

of their choosing who is available by phone 24 hours a day for individual support and crisis intervention. AA convincingly shows the alcoholic that abstinence can be achieved and also provides a sober peer group of people who share the same identity—that of recovering alcoholics.

Alcoholics Anonymous is generally recognized as an effective mutual help program, but not everyone responds to its style and message, and other recovery approaches are available. Some, like Rational Recovery and Women for Sobriety, deliberately avoid any emphasis on higher spiritual powers. Even people who are helped by AA often find that it works best in combination with counseling and medical care.

A companion program to AA is Al-Anon, which consists of groups for families and friends of alcoholics. In Al-Anon, spouses and others explore how they enabled the alcoholic to drink by denying, rationalizing, or covering up his or her drinking and how they can change this codependent behavior.

Employee assistance programs and school-based programs represent another approach to alcoholism treatment that works for some people. One of the advantages of these programs is that they can deal directly with work and campus issues, often important sources of stress for the alcohol abuser. These programs sometimes encourage learning effective coping responses for internal and external sources of distress. Individuals might also benefit from learning new cognitive concepts, such as a self-identity that does not involve drinking.

Inpatient hospital rehabilitation is useful for some alcoholics, especially if they have serious medical or mental problems, or if life stressors threaten to overwhelm them. When the person returns to the community, however, it is critical that there be some form of active, continuing, long-term treatment. Patients who return to a spouse or family often require ongoing treatment on issues involving those significant others, such as establishing new routines and planning shared recreational activities that do not involve drinking.

There are also some pharmacological treatments for alcoholism. One involves the use of disulfiram (trade name Antabuse), which inhibits the metabolic breakdown of acetaldehyde (see the box "Metabolizing Alcohol: Our Bodies Work Differently" on p. 250). Disulfiram causes patients to become violently ill when they drink and thus theoretically prevents impulse drinking. However, it is potentially dangerous and must be combined with ongoing therapy to be useful over time. In 1995, the FDA approved the drug naltrexone for the treatment of alcohol dependence. In contrast to Antabuse, naltrexone reduces the craving for alcohol and decreases the pleasant, reinforcing effects of alcohol without making the user ill. Naltrexone works most effectively in combination with counseling and other forms of psychosocial treatment.

In people who abuse alcohol and have significant depression or anxiety, the use of antidepressant or anti-anxiety medication can improve both mental health and drinking behavior. In addition, drugs such as diazepam (Valium) are sometimes prescribed to replace alcohol during initial stages of withdrawal. Most therapists feel that such chemical substitutes are useful for only a week or so, because alcoholics are at particularly high risk of developing dependence on Valium and other similar medications. Drug therapy is usually only a small component of an alcohol-treatment plan. Counseling and peer-group support are generally the most essential elements of alcoholism treatment.

Alcohol-treatment programs are successful in achieving an extended period of sobriety for about half of those who participate. Success rates of conventional treatment programs are about the same for men and women and for people from different ethnic groups. Women, minorities, and the poor often face major economic and social barriers to receiving treatment. Most inpatient treatment programs are financially out of reach for people of low income or those without insurance coverage. AA remains the mainstay of treatment for most people and is often a component of even the most expensive treatment programs. Special AA groups exist in many communities for young people, women, gay men and lesbians, non–English speakers, and a variety of interest groups. You can find out about AA meetings in your community by looking in the phone book, or consult the For More Information section at the end of the chapter.

> **PERSONAL INSIGHT** What is your attitude about alcoholism? Do you think of it as a disease, a weakness, an affliction, a choice? What is the basis for your attitude?

Gender and Ethnic Differences

Alcohol abusers come from all socioeconomic levels and cultural groups, but there are notable differences in patterns of drinking between men and women and among different ethnic groups.

Men Among white American men, excessive drinking often begins in the teens or twenties and progresses gradually through the thirties, until the individual is clearly identifiable as an alcoholic by the time he is in his late thirties or early forties. Other men remain controlled drinkers until later in life, sometimes becoming alcoholic in association with retirement, the inevitable losses of aging, boredom, illness, or psychological disorders.

Women The progression of alcoholism in women is usually different. Women tend to become alcoholic at a later age and with fewer years of heavy drinking. It is not unusual for women in their forties or fifties to become alcoholic after years of controlled drinking. Women alcoholics develop cirrhosis and other medical complications somewhat more often than men. Women alcoholics may have more medical problems because they are less likely to seek early treatment. In addition, there may be an inherently greater biological risk for women who drink (see the box "Women and Alcohol," p. 264).

African Americans Alcohol abuse is a serious problem for African Americans. Although as a group they use less alcohol than most other groups (including whites), they face disproportionately high levels of alcohol-related birth defects, cirrhosis, cancer, hypertension, and other medical problems. In addition, blacks are more likely than members of other ethnic groups to be victims of alcohol-related homicides, criminal assaults, and injuries. African American women are more likely to abstain from alcohol use than white women; but among black women who drink, there is a higher percentage of heavy drinkers. Urban black males commonly start drinking excessively and develop serious neurological illnesses at an earlier age than urban white males. They also have a higher rate of alcoholism-related suicide.

AA groups of predominantly African Americans have been shown to provide effective treatment, perhaps because essential elements of AA—sharing common experiences, mutual acceptance of one another as human beings, and trusting a higher power—are already a part of African American culture. Treatment efforts that use the extended family and include occupational training are also especially effective.

Latinos Drinking patterns among Latinos vary significantly, depending on their specific cultural background and how long they and their families have lived in the United States. Drunk driving and cirrhosis are the most common causes of alcohol-related death and injury among Hispanic men. Hispanic women are more likely to abstain from alcohol than white or black women, but those who do drink are at special risk for problems. Treating the entire family as a unit is an important part of treatment because family pride, solidarity, and support are important aspects of Latino culture. Some Hispanics do better during treatment if treatment efforts are integrated with the techniques of *curanderos* (folk healers) and *espiritistas* (spiritists).

Asian Americans As a group, Asian Americans and Pacific Islanders have lower-than-average rates of alcohol abuse. However, acculturation may somewhat weaken the generally strong Asian taboos and community sanctions against alcohol use. For many Asian Americans,

Whether a woman is a "social drinker," a binge drinker, or a heavy daily user, the impact of alcohol on her will be different, and generally greater, than comparable use in a man. Women become intoxicated at lower doses of alcohol because of their smaller size, greater proportion of body fat, and less active form of an alcohol-metabolizing stomach enzyme. Hormonal fluctuations may also affect the rate of alcohol metabolism, making a woman more susceptible to high BACs at certain times during her menstrual cycle (usually just prior to the onset of menstruation).

Like men, women are more likely to be the perpetrator or victim of a crime when they have been drinking. Sexual assaults of all types, and date rape in particular, are more likely to occur if a woman has been drinking. Alcohol use makes women much less likely to practice safer sex, leaving them especially vulnerable to significant and lasting health problems as a result of sexually transmitted diseases and unintended pregnancy.

Women tend to experience the adverse physical effects of chronic drinking sooner and at lower levels of alcohol consumption than men. Female alcoholics have death rates 50–100% higher than those of male alcoholics. They develop alcohol liver disease after a comparatively shorter period of heavy drinking and at a lower level of daily drinking than men. They have higher death rates from cirrhosis. Other alcohol-related health problems that are unique to women include an increased risk for breast cancer, menstrual disorders, infertility, and, in pregnant women, giving birth to a child suffering from FAS. Because of the social stigma attached to problem drinking, women are also less likely to seek early treatment.

About one-third of all problem drinkers in the United States are women. Women from all walks of life and all ethnic groups can develop alcohol problems, but those who have never married or are divorced are more likely to drink heavily than married or widowed women. Women who have multiple life roles are less vulnerable to alcohol problems than women who have fewer roles.

though, the genetically based physiologic aversion to alcohol remains a deterrent to abuse. For those needing treatment, ethnic agencies, health care professionals, and ministers seem to be the most effective sources.

Native Americans and Alaska Natives Alcohol abuse is one of the most widespread and severe health problems among Native Americans and Alaska Natives, especially for adolescents and young adults. Excessive drinking varies from tribe to tribe but is generally high in both men and women. The rate of alcoholism among Native Americans is twice that of the general population, and the death rate from alcohol-related causes is about eight times higher. Treatment programs may be more effective if they reflect Native American values. Some healers have incorporated aspects of Native American religions into the therapeutic process, using traditional sweat houses, prayers, and dances.

Helping Someone with an Alcohol Problem

Helping a friend or relative with an alcohol problem requires skill and tact. One of the first steps is making sure you are not an enabler or codependent, perhaps unknowingly allowing someone to continue excessively using alcohol. Enabling takes many forms. One of the most common is making excuses or covering up for the alcohol abuser—for example, saying "he has the flu" when it is really a hangover. Whenever you find yourself minimizing or lying about someone's drinking behavior, a warning bell should sound (see the box "Codependency" in Chapter 9). Another important step is open, honest labeling—"I think you have a problem with alcohol."

Such explicit statements usually elicit emotional rebuttals and may endanger a relationship. In the long run, however, you are not helping your friends by allowing them to deny their problems with alcohol or other drugs. Even when problems are acknowledged, there is usually reluctance to get help. Your best role might be to obtain information about the available resources, and persistently encourage their use.

DRINKING BEHAVIOR AND RESPONSIBILITY

The responsible use of alcohol means drinking in such a way that you keep your BAC low, so that your behavior is always under your control. In addition to controlling your own drinking, there are things you can do to promote responsible alcohol use in others.

Examine Your Drinking Behavior

When you want to drink responsibly, it's helpful to know, first of all, why you drink. The following are common reasons given by college students:

- "It lets me go along with my friends."
- "It makes me less self-conscious and more social."
- "It makes me less inhibited in thinking, saying, or doing certain things."
- "It relieves depression, anxiety, tension, or worries."
- "It enables me to experience a different state of consciousness."

How can you tell whether you, or someone close to you, may have a drinking problem? Completing the CAGE screening test can help you find out. Answer yes or no to the following questions:

Have you ever felt you should....... **C**ut down on your drinking?

Have people................................. **A**nnoyed you by criticizing your drinking?

Have you ever felt bad or.............. **G**uilty about your drinking?

Have you ever had an................... **E**ye-opener (a drink first thing in the morning to steady your nerves or get rid of a hangover)?

One "yes" response suggests a possible alcoholic problem. If you answered yes to more than one question, it is highly likely that a problem exists. In either case, it is important that you see your physician or other health care provider right away to discuss your responses to these questions. He or she can help you determine whether you have a drinking problem and, if so, recommend the best course of action for you.

Even if you answered no to all of the above questions, if you are encountering drinking-related problems with your job, academic performance, relationships, or health, or with the law, you should still seek professional help. The effects of alcohol abuse can be extremely serious—even fatal—both to you and to others.

SOURCE: National Institute on Alcohol Abuse and Alcoholism. 1996. *Alcoholism: Getting the Facts.* NIH Publication No. 96-4153. Bethesda, Md.: National Institute on Alcohol Abuse and Alcoholism.

If you drink alcohol, what are your reasons for doing so? Are you attempting to meet underlying needs that could best be addressed by other means?

After examining your reasons for drinking, take a closer look at your drinking behavior. Is it moderate and responsible? Or do you frequently overindulge and suffer negative consequences? (See the box "Do You Have a Drinking Problem?") The Behavior Change Strategy at the end of the chapter explains how to keep and analyze a record of your drinking.

Drink Moderately and Responsibly

Sometimes people lose control when they misjudge how much they can drink. Other times, they set out deliberately to get drunk. Following are some strategies for keeping your drinking and your behavior under control.

Drink Slowly   Learn to sip your drinks rather than gulp them. Do not drink alcoholic beverages to quench your thirst. Avoid drinks made with carbonated mixers, especially if you're thirsty; you'll be more likely to gulp them down.

Space Your Drinks   Learn to drink nonalcoholic drinks at parties, or alternate them with alcoholic drinks. Learn to refuse a round: "I've had enough for right now." Parties are easier for some people if they hold a glass of something nonalcoholic that has ice and a twist of lime floating in it so it looks like an alcoholic drink.

Eat Before and While Drinking   Avoid drinking on an empty stomach. Food in your stomach will not prevent the alcohol from eventually being absorbed, but it will slow down the rate somewhat, and thus often lower the peak BAC. In restaurants, order your food before you order a drink. Try to have something to eat before you go out to a party where alcohol will be served.

Know Your Limits and Your Drinks   Learn how different BACs affect you. In a safe setting such as your home, with your roommate or a friend, see how a set amount—say, two drinks in an hour—affects you. A good test is walking heel to toe in a straight line with your eyes closed, or standing with your feet crossed and trying to touch your finger to your nose with your eyes closed.

But be aware that in different settings your performance, and especially your ability to judge your behavior, may change. At a given BAC, you will perform less well when surrounded by activity and boisterous companions than you will in a quiet test setting with just one or two other people. This impairment results partially because alcohol reduces your ability to perform when your brain is bombarded by multiple stimuli. It is useful to discover the rate at which you can drink without increasing your BAC. Be able to calculate the approximate amount a given drink increases your BAC.

Promote Responsible Drinking in Others

Although you cannot completely control the drinking behavior of others, there are things you can do to help promote responsible drinking.

Encourage Responsible Attitudes   Our society teaches us attitudes toward drinking that contribute to alcohol-related problems. Many of us have difficulty expressing disapproval about someone who has drunk too much, and we are amused by the antics of the "funny" drunk. We accept the alcohol industry's linkage of drinking with virility or sexuality (see the box "Alcohol Advertising"). We treat nondrinkers as nonconformists.

Dominic and Jason are watching the Super Bowl on television, when the ads come on and a different set of football "players" line up for a play. A team of helmet-clad Budweiser beer bottles matches skill with the opposing Bud Light team. The young men laugh; Jason roots for the Bud team, while Dominic pulls for Bud Light. They follow the progress of the Bud Bowl through a series of commercials that run during the Super Bowl. "The Bud Bowl is better than the real game," says Jason.

To be a careful and informed health consumer, you need to carefully consider the effects that advertisements have on you. Are alcohol ads, such as the Bud Bowl, harmless fun? Or can they have more serious effects? How do such ads affect you?

Alcohol manufacturers spend $2 billion every year on advertising. They claim that the purpose of their advertising is to persuade adults who already drink to choose a certain brand. But in reality, ads like the Bud Bowl cleverly engage young people and children—never overtly suggesting that young people should drink, but clearly linking alcohol and good times. Alcohol ads are common during televised sporting events and other shows popular with teenagers. By age 18, the average American teen will have seen 100,000 TV beer commercials. Studies show that the more TV adolescents watch, the more likely they are to take up drinking in their teens.

Alcohol manufacturers also reach out to young people at youth-oriented activities like concerts and sporting events. Product logos are heavily marketed through sales of T-shirts, hats, and other items. Many colleges allow alcohol manufacturers to advertise at campus events in exchange for sponsorship.

What is the message of all these advertisements? Think about the alcohol ads you've seen. Many give the impression that drinking alcohol is a normal part of everyday life and good times. This message seems to work well on the young, many of whom believe that heavy-duty drinking at parties is normal and fun. The use of famous athletes or actors in commercials increases the appeal of alcohol by associating it with fame, wealth, and popularity. What ads don't show is the darker side of drinking. You never see hangovers, car crashes, slipping grades, or violence. Although some ads include a brief message such as "know when to say when," the impact of such cautions is small compared to the image of happy, attractive young people having fun while drinking.

The next time you see an advertisement for alcohol, take a critical look. What is the message of the ad? What audience is being targeted, and what is the ad implying about alcohol use? Be aware of its effect on you.

We need to recognize that the choice to abstain is neither odd nor unusual. About 20% of adults do not drink at all or drink very infrequently. Most adults are capable of enjoying their leisure time without alcohol or drugs. In hazardous situations, such as driving or operating complicated machinery, abstinence is the only appropriate choice.

Be a Responsible Host   When you are the host, serve nonalcoholic beverages as well as alcohol. Popular nonalcoholic choices include soft drinks, sparkling water, fruit juice, and alcohol-free wine, beer, and mixers. Serve only enough alcohol for each guest to have a moderate number of drinks. Don't put out large kegs of beer, as these invite people to overindulge.

Always serve food along with alcohol, and stop serving alcohol an hour or more before people will leave. If possible, arrange carpools with designated nondrinking drivers in advance. Remind your guests who are under 21 about the new "zero tolerance" laws in many states—even a single drink can result in an illegal BAC. Insist that a guest who drank too much take a taxi, ride with someone else, or stay overnight rather than drive.

Plan social functions with no alcohol at all. Outdoor parties, hikes, and practically every other type of social occasion can be enjoyable without alcohol. If that doesn't seem possible to you, then examine your drinking patterns and attitudes toward alcohol. If you can't have fun without drinking, you may have a problem with alcohol.

Hold the Drinker Responsible   When any alcohol is consumed, the individual must take full responsibility for his or her behavior. Pardoning unacceptable behavior fosters the attitude that the behavior is due to the drug. The drinker is thereby excused from responsibility and learns to expect minimal adverse consequences for his or her behavior. Research indicates that the opposite approach —holding the individual fully accountable for his or her behavior—is a more effective policy. For example, alcohol-impaired drivers who receive legal penalties have fewer subsequent rearrests than those who receive only mandatory treatment. Restrictions on public smoking gained momentum after nonsmokers learned about the dangers that environmental tobacco smoke posed to them. Other people's drunkenness can impinge on your living or study environment. Speak up—and insist on your rights.

Learn About Prevention Programs   What alternatives are being developed on your campus or in your community to "keg parties" and other events where heavy drinking occurs? Are programs available for students who are at high risk for alcohol abuse, such as those whose parents abused alcohol? Are counseling or self-help programs like AA available?

Take Community Action   Consider joining an action group such as Students Against Drunk Driving (SADD).

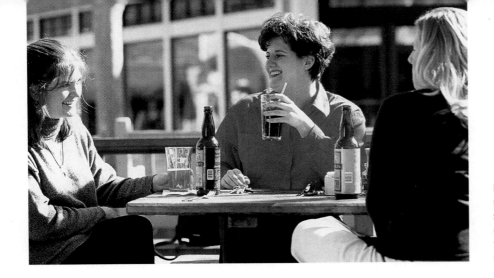

People who choose to drink should do so responsibly—in moderation and when doing so does not put themselves or others in danger. By choosing a designated driver, these women help ensure themselves a safe trip home.

The goal of SADD is to save students' lives by changing their beliefs and attitudes about alcohol. Lesson plans, peer counseling, and the promotion of better communication between students and parents are all used to help protect students from the dangers of drinking and driving.

> **PERSONAL INSIGHT**   How do you perceive a nondrinker in a social situation where others are drinking? Does it seem like an acceptable choice to you? What is the basis for your attitude?

SUMMARY

- Although alcohol has been a part of human celebrations for a long time, it is a psychoactive drug capable of causing addiction.

The Nature of Alcohol

- After being absorbed into the bloodstream in the stomach and small intestine, alcohol is transported throughout the body. The liver metabolizes alcohol as blood circulates through it.
- If people drink more alcohol each hour than their body can metabolize, blood alcohol concentration (BAC) increases.
- The rate of alcohol metabolism depends on a variety of individual factors, including gender, body weight, and percentage of body fat.

Alcohol and Health

- Alcohol is a CNS depressant. At low doses, it tends to make people feel relaxed.
- At higher doses, alcohol interferes with motor and mental functioning; at very high doses, alcohol

poisoning, coma, and death can occur. Effects may be increased if alcohol is combined with other drugs.

- Alcohol use increases the risk of injury and violence; drinking before driving is particularly dangerous, even at low doses.
- Continued alcohol use has negative effects on the digestive and cardiovascular systems and increases cancer risk and overall mortality.
- Women who drink while pregnant risk giving birth to children with a cluster of birth defects known as fetal alcohol syndrome (FAS).
- Moderate drinking may decrease the risk of coronary heart disease in some people.

Alcohol Abuse and Dependence

- Alcohol abuse involves drinking in dangerous situations or drinking to a degree that causes academic, professional, interpersonal, or legal difficulties.
- Alcohol dependence, or alcoholism, is characterized by more extensive problems with alcohol, usually involving tolerance and withdrawal.
- Binge drinking is a common form of alcohol abuse on college campuses that has negative effects on both drinking and nondrinking students.
- Physical consequences of alcoholism include the direct effects of tolerance and withdrawal, as well as all the problems associated with chronic drinking. Psychological problems include paranoia, memory loss, and dual disorders.
- Alcoholism causes many social problems; it especially affects children of alcohol abusers.
- Possible causes of alcoholism include genetic, personality, and social factors.
- Treatment approaches include mutual support

How much do you drink? Is it the right amount for you? You may know the answer to this question already, or you may not have given it much thought. Many people learn through a single unpleasant experience how alcohol affects their bodies or minds. Others suffer ill effects but choose to ignore or deny them.

To make responsible, informed choices about using alcohol, consider, first, whether there is any history of alcohol abuse in your family. If someone in your family is dependent on alcohol, you have a higher-than-average likelihood of becoming dependent too. Second, consider whether you are dependent on other substances or behaviors. Do you smoke, drink strong coffee every day, or use other drugs regularly? Does some habit control your life? Some people have more of a tendency to become addicted than others, and a person with one addiction is often likely to have other addictions as well. If this is the case for you, again, you may need to be more cautious with alcohol.

Keep a Record

Once you have answered these questions, find out more about your alcohol-related behavior by keeping track of your drinking for 2 weeks in your health journal. Keep a daily alcohol behavior record like the one illustrated in Chapter 1 for eating behavior. Include information on

- *The drinking situation,* including type of drink, time of day, how fast you drank it, where you were, and what else you were doing.

- *Your internal state,* including what made you want to drink and your feelings, thoughts, and concerns at the time. Note how others influenced you.

- *The consequences of drinking,* including any changes in your feelings or behavior while or after you were drinking, such as silliness, assertiveness, aggressiveness, or depression.

Analyze Your Record

Next, analyze your record to detect patterns of feelings and environmental cues. Do you always drink when you're at a certain place or with certain people? Do you sometimes drink just to be sociable, when you don't really want a drink and would be satisfied with a nonalcoholic beverage? Refer to the list of warning signs of alcohol abuse given in the text. Are any of them true for you? For example, do you feel uncomfortable in a social situation if alcohol is *not* available?

Set Goals

Now that you've analyzed your record, think about whether you want to change any of your behaviors. This might be the case if you tend to drink too much, even without driving, because alcohol damages your body. It should definitely be the case if you drink and drive, or if you're becoming dependent on alcohol. Decide on goals that will give you the best health and safety returns, such as a beer or a glass of wine with dinner, one drink per hour at a party, or no alcohol at all.

Devise a Plan

Refer to your health journal to see what kinds of patterns your drinking falls into and where you can intervene to break the behavior chain. You may be able to make changes in your environment, such as by stocking your refrigerator with alternative beverages like juices or sparkling water. If you feel self-conscious about ordering a nonalcoholic drink when you're out with a group, try recruiting a friend to do the same. If it's impossible to avoid drinking in some situations, such as at a bar or beer party, you may decide to avoid those situations for a period of time.

Instead of drinking, you can try other activities that produce the same effect. For example, if you drink to relieve anxiety or tension, try adding 20–30 minutes of exercise to your schedule to help you manage stress. Or try doing a relaxation exercise or going for a brisk walk to help reduce anxiety before a party or date. If you drink to relieve depression or to stop worrying, consider finding a trustworthy person (perhaps a professional counselor) to talk to about the problem that's bothering you. If you drink to feel more comfortable sexually, consider ways to improve communication with your partner so you can deal with sexual issues more openly. When these activities are successful, they will reinforce your responsible drinking decisions, and make it more likely that you'll make the same decisions again in the future.

For other ways to monitor and control your drinking behavior, see the suggestions in the section "Drinking Behavior and Responsibility."

Reward Yourself and Monitor Your Progress

If changing your drinking behavior turns out to be difficult, it may be a clue that drinking was becoming a problem for you— all the more reason to get it under control now. Be sure to reward yourself as you learn to drink responsibly (or not at all). You may lose weight, look better, feel better, and have higher self-esteem as a result of limiting your drinking. Keep track of your progress in your health journal, and use the strategies described in Chapter 1 for maintaining your program. Remember, when you establish sensible drinking habits, you're planning not just for this week or month—but for your whole life.

groups like AA, job- and school-based programs, inpatient hospital programs, and pharmacological treatments.

- Helping someone who abuses alcohol means avoiding being an enabler, and obtaining information about available resources and persistently encouraging their use.
- Alcohol abuse affects people from all ethnic groups at all socioeconomic levels. However, different drinking patterns and problems are more common among some groups.

Drinking Behavior and Responsibility

- Strategies for keeping drinking under control include examining drinking behavior, drinking slowly, spacing drinks, eating before and while drinking, and knowing one's limits.
- Strategies for promoting responsible drinking in others include encouraging responsible attitudes, being a responsible host, holding the drinker responsible for his or her actions, learning about prevention programs, and taking community action.

TAKE ACTION

1. Interview some of your fellow students about their drinking habits. How much do they drink, and how often? Are they more likely to drink on certain days or in certain circumstances? Are there any habits that seem to be common to most students? How do your own drinking habits compare to those of people you interviewed?

2. Some AA groups encourage visitors. If your local chapter does so, attend a meeting to see how the organization functions. What behavioral techniques are used to help people stop drinking? How effective do these techniques seem to be? If there is a local codependent or Al-Anon group, attend one of their meetings. What themes are emphasized? Do any themes apply to your relationships?

3. Plan an alcohol-free party. What would you serve to eat and drink? What would you tell people about the party when you invite them?

JOURNAL ENTRY

1. In your health journal, list the positive behaviors that help you drink responsibly. Consider how you can strengthen these behaviors. Then list the behaviors that interfere with responsible drinking for you. Which ones can you change?

2. Write a list of statements or questions you might use to talk with (1) a person you think is developing a drinking problem; (2) a person planning to drive under the influence of alcohol, with and without you in the car; and (3) a person you want to ask about your own behavior when you drink. Condsider using statements from your list when an appropriate situation arises.

3. *Critical Thinking*   Look at advertisements for alcoholic beverages in magazines and on billboards. Analyze several of these ads. What psychological techniques are used to sell the products? What are the hidden messages? Write an essay outlining your opinion of alcohol advertising and marketing. Do you think it's ethical to sell a potentially dangerous substance by appealing to people's desires and vulnerabilities? Do you think liquor manufacturers ought to be held responsible for the damage alcohol inflicts on some people? Explain your reasoning.

FOR MORE INFORMATION

Books

Alcoholics Anonymous, 3rd ed. 1976. New York: Alcoholics Anonymous World Services. *The "Big Book," the basic text for AA; includes the founding tenets of AA and vivid histories of recovering alcoholics.*

Braun, S. 1997. *Buzz: The Science and Lore of Alcohol and Caffeine.* New York: Penguin. *An introduction to the chemical and biological effects of alcohol and caffeine.*

Dimeff, L. A., et al. 1999. *Brief Alcohol Screening and Interventions for College Students (BASICS). A Harm Reduction Approach.* New York: Guilford. *Presents a model designed to help students reduce their alcohol consumption and the risks they face from heavy drinking; includes handouts and assessment forms.*

From Survival to Recovery: Growing Up in an Alcoholic Home. 1994. New York: Al-Anon Family Group Headquarters. *First-person accounts of life with an alcoholic and the 12-step healing process.*

Kinney, J., and G. Leaton. 1995. *Loosening the Grip: A Handbook of Alcohol Information*, 5th ed. St. Louis: Mosby. *A fascinating book about alcohol, including information on physical effects, abuse, alcoholism, and cultural aspects of alcohol use.*

Knapp, C. 1997. *Drinking: A Love Story.* Baltimore: Delta. *A memoir that describes the special risks facing women drinkers and the struggles involved in overcoming addiction.*

Schuckit, M. A. 1998. *Educating Yourself About Alcohol and Drugs: A People's Primer.* Rev. ed. New York: Plenum. *Provides basic information about how alcohol and drug abuse affects peo-*

ple, how to recognize substance-abuse problems, and how to choose a treatment program.

Valverde, M. 1999. *Disease of the Will: Alcohol and the Dilemmas of Freedom.* New York: Cambridge University Press. *A historical and sociological look at alcohol use.*

West, J. 1997. *The Betty Ford Center Book of Answers.* New York: Simon and Schuster. Straightforward answers to commonly asked questions about alcoholism and other addictions.

Organizations, Hotlines, and Web Sites

Al-Anon Family Group Headquarters. Provides information and referrals to local Al-Anon and Alateen groups. The Web site includes a self-quiz to determine if you are affected by someone's drinking.

> 1600 Corporate Landing Parkway
> Virginia Beach, VA 23454
> 800-344-2666; 757-563-1600
> http://www.al-anon.alateen.org

Alcoholics Anonymous (AA) World Services. Provides general information on AA, literature on alcoholism, and information about AA meetings. The Web site provides an excellent introduction to the many support services offered to alcoholics and their families by AA and related 12-step organizations.

> P.O. Box 459
> New York, NY 10163
> 212-870-3400
> http://www.alcoholics-anonymous.org

Alcohol and Drug Helpline. Provides referrals to local treatment facilities.

> 800-821-4357

Alcohol Treatment Referral Hotline. Provides referrals to local intervention and treatment providers.

> 800-ALCOHOL

Bacchus and Gamma Peer Education Network. An association of college- and university-based peer education programs that focus on prevention of alcohol abuse.

> http://www.bacchusgamma.org

The College Alcohol Study. Harvard School of Public Health. Provides information about and results from the recent studies of binge drinking on college campuses.

> http://www.hsph.harvard.edu/cas

Habitsmart. Contains an online self-scoring alcohol-use assessment, tips for outsmarting cravings, and links to related sites.

> http://www.habitsmart.com

Higher Education Center for Alcohol and Other Drug Prevention. Provides support for campus alcohol and illegal drug pre-

vention efforts; a Web site gives information about alcohol and drug abuse on campus and links to related sites and also has an area designed specifically for students.

> http://www.edc.org/hec

Intoximeters Drink Wheel Blood Alcohol Test. Calculate your approximate BAC based on body weight, gender, and amount of alcohol consumed.

> http://www.intox.com

Mothers Against Drunk Driving (MADD). Supports efforts to develop solutions to the problems of drunk driving and underage drinking; provides news, information, and brochures about many topics, including a guide for giving a safe party.

> http://www.madd.org

National Association for Children of Alcoholics (NACoA). Provides information and support for children of alcoholics.

> 11426 Rockville Pike, Suite 100
> Rockville, MD 20852
> 888-554-COAS; 301-468-0985
> http://www.health.org/nacoa

National Clearinghouse for Alcohol and Drug Information/Prevention Online. Provides statistics, information, and publications on alcohol abuse, including resources for people who want to help friends and family members overcome alcohol-abuse problems.

> P.O. Box 2345
> Rockville, MD 20847-2345
> 800-729-6686; 301-468-2600
> http://www.health.org

National Council on Alcoholism and Drug Dependence (NCADD). Provides information on alcoholism and counseling referrals.

> 212-206-6770; 800-NCA-CALL (24-hour Hope Line)
> http://www.ncadd.org

National Institute on Alcohol Abuse and Alcoholism (NIAAA). Provides booklets and other publications on a variety of alcohol-related topics, including fetal alcohol syndrome, alcoholism treatment, and alcohol use and minorities.

> 6000 Executive Blvd.
> Bethesda, MD 20892-7003
> 301-443-3860
> http://www.niaaa.nih.gov

The Trauma Foundation/Alcohol-Related Injury and Violence. Provides fact sheets, literature reviews, and other resources about alcohol-related injuries.

> http://www.traumafdn.org/alcohol/ariv

See also the listings for Chapter 9.

SELECTED BIBLIOGRAPHY

American Psychiatric Association. 1994. *Diagnostic and Statistical Manual of Mental Disorders,* 4th ed. *(DSM-IV).* Washington, D.C.: American Psychiatric Association.

Burge, S. K., and F. D. Schneider. 1999. Alcohol-related problems: Recognition and intervention. *American Family Physician* 59(2): 361–370, 372.

Centers for Disease Control and Prevention. 1998. Identification of children with fetal alcohol syndrome and referral of their mothers for primary prevention. *Morbidity and Mortality Weekly Report* 47(40): 861–864.

Centers for Disease Control and Prevention. 1997. Alcohol-

related traffic fatalities involving children—United States, 1985–1996. *Morbidity and Mortality Weekly Report* 46(48): 1130–1133.

Coutelle, C. et al. 1997. Laryngeal and oropharyngeal cancer, and alcohol dehydrogenase 3 and glutathione S-transferase M1 polymorphisms. *Human Genetics* 99(3): 319–325.

Davidson, D., et al. 1999. Effects of naltrexone on alcohol self-administration in heavy drinkers. *Alcoholism, Clinical and Experimental Research* 23(2): 195–203.

Ebrahim, S. H., et al. 1999. Comparison of binge drinking among pregnant and nonpregnant women, United States,

1991–1995. *American Journal of Obstetrics and Gynecology* 180(1 Pt 1): 1–7.

Feldman, L., et al. 1999. Alcohol use beliefs and behaviors among high school students. *Journal of Adolescent Health* 24(1): 48–58.

Figueredo, V. M. 1997. The effects of alcohol on the heart: Detrimental or beneficial? *Postgraduate Medicine* 101(2): 165–168, 171–172, 175–176.

Food and Drug Administration. 1998. *FDA Announces New Alcohol Warnings for Pain Relievers and Fever Reducers* (retrieved October 24, 1998; http://www.fda.gov/bbs/topics/NEWS/NEW00659.html).

Higher Education Center for Alcohol and Other Drug Prevention. 1997. *Factsheet: College Academic Performance and Alcohol and Other Drug Use* (retrieved November 5, 1998; http://www.edc.org/hec/pubs/factsheets/fact_sheet2.html).

Higher Education Center for Alcohol and Other Drug Prevention. 1997. *Factsheet: Sexual Assault and Alcohol and Other Drug Use* (retrieved November 5, 1998; http://www.edc.org/hec/pubs/factsheets/fact_sheet1.html).

Insurance Institute for Highway Safety. 1998. *1998 State Law Facts: DUI/DWI Laws* (retrieved November 5, 1998; http://www.hwysafety.org/facts/dui.htm).

Laroque, B. 1995. Moderate prenatal alcohol exposure and psychomotor development at preschool age. *American Journal of Public Health* 85(12): 1654.

Litten, R. Z., and J. P. Allen. 1999. Medications for alcohol, illicit drug, and tobacco dependence. An update of research findings. *Journal of Substance Abuse Treatment* 16(2): 105–112.

McAneny, L. 1997. *Gallup Poll: Drinking a Cause of Family Problems for Three Out of Ten Americans* (retrieved October 26, 1998; http://www.gallup.com/POLL_ARCHIVES/1997/970927.htm).

National Institute on Alcohol Abuse and Alcoholism. 1998. *NIH News Release: Age of Drinking Onset Predicts Future Alcohol Abuse and Dependence* (retrieved September 15, 1998; http://silk.nih.gov/silk/niaaa1/releases/aging.htm).

National Institute on Alcohol and Alcoholism. 1998. *The Economic Costs of Alcohol and Drug Abuse in the United States* (retrieved November 5, 1998; http://www.health.org/pressrel/sept98/csat-study.html).

National Institute on Alcohol Abuse and Alcoholism. 1997. *Alcohol Alert: Alcohol Metabolism* (retrieved October 20, 1998; http://silk.nih.gov/silk/niaaa1/publication/aa35.htm).

National Institute on Alcohol Abuse and Alcoholism. 1996. *How to Cut Down on Your Drinking.* NIH Publication No. 3770. Bethesda, Md.: National Institute on Alcohol Abuse and Alcoholism.

Power, C., B. Rodgers, and S. Hope. 1998. U-shaped relation for alcohol consumption and health in early adulthood and implications for mortality. *Lancet* 352(9131): 877.

Robinson, T. N., H. L. Chen, and J. D. Killen. 1998. Television and music video exposure and risk of adolescent alcohol use. *Pediatrics* 102(5): e54 (retrieved November 2, 1998; http://www.pediatrics.org/cgi/content/abstract/102/5/e54).

Sacco, R. L., et al. 1999. The protective effect of moderate alcohol consumption on ischemic stroke. *Journal of the American Medical Association* 281(1): 53–60.

Seppä, K., and P. Sillanaukee. 1999. Binge drinking and ambulatory blood pressure. *Hypertension* 33: 79–82.

Shaw, G. M., and E. J. Lammer. 1999. Maternal periconceptional alcohol consumption and risk for orofacial clefts. *Journal of Pediatrics* 134(3): 298–303.

Students Who Use Drugs or Alcohol Found More Likely to Suffer Violence. 1998. *The Chronicle of Higher Education,* February 20.

Thun, M. J., et al. 1997. Alcohol consumption and mortality among middle-aged and elderly U.S. adults. *New England Journal of Medicine* 337(24): 1705–1714.

U.S. Department of Health and Human Services. 1998. *1997 National Household Survey on Drug Abuse.* Substance Abuse and Mental Health Services Administration.

U.S. Department of Health and Human Services. 1998. *Healthy People 2010 Objectives: Draft for Public Comment.* Washington, D.C.: U.S. Government Printing Office.

U.S. Department of Transportation. 1998. *Alcohol-Related Traffic Deaths Dropped to a Record Low in 1997* (retrieved November 9, 1998; http://www.nhtsa.dot.gov/nhtsa/announce/press/pressdisplay.dbm?year=1998&filename=pr051498.html).

U.S. Treasury Department. Bureau of Alcohol, Tobacco, and Firearms. 1999. *Treasury Announces Actions Concerning Labeling of Alcoholic Beverages* (retrieved February 6, 1999; http://www.atf.treas.gov/press/label_ab.htm).

Wechsler, H., et al. 1998. Changes in binge drinking and related problems among American college students between 1993 and 1997. Results of the Harvard School of Public Health College Alcohol Study. *Journal of American College Health* 47: 57–68.

Windle, M., and R. C. Windle. 1999. Adolescent tobacco, alcohol, and drug use: Current findings. *Adolescent Medicine* 10(1): 153–163.

Wright, S. W., et al. 1998. Alcohol on campus: Alcohol-related emergencies in undergraduate college students. *Southern Medical Journal* 91(10): 909–913.

Zhang, Y., et al. 1999. Alcohol consumption and risk of breast cancer: The Framingham Study revisited. *American Journal of Epidemiology* 149(2): 93–101.

Zwerling, C., and M. P. Jones. 1999. Evaluation of the effectiveness of low blood alcohol concentration laws for younger drivers. *American Journal of Preventive Medicine* 16(1 Suppl): 76–80.

SILVER CITY

WE ARE TOTALLY NON-SMOKING

HOT DOGS 99¢

WELCOME

ENTRANCE

WELCOME TO A TOTALLY SMOKE-FREE ENVIRONMENT

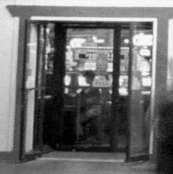
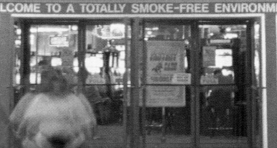
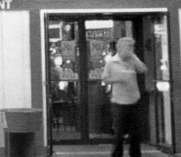

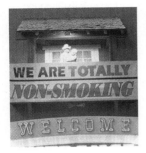

LEARNING OBJECTIVES

After reading this chapter, you should be able to:

- List the reasons people start using tobacco and why they continue to use it.

- Explain the short- and long-term health risks associated with tobacco use.

- Discuss the effects of environmental tobacco smoke on nonsmokers.

- Describe the social costs of tobacco, and list actions that have been taken to combat smoking in the public and private sectors.

- Prepare plans to stop using tobacco and to avoid environmental tobacco smoke.

Toward a Tobacco-Free Society

11

TEST YOUR KNOWLEDGE

1. The average age for starting smoking is 16.
   True or false?

2. Which of the following substances is found in tobacco smoke?
   a. arsenic (poison)
   b. hydrogen cyanide (gas chamber poison)
   c. naphthalene (active ingredient in mothballs)
   d. formaldehyde (body tissue and fabric preservative)

3. More than 80% of nonsmokers are exposed to environmental ("secondhand") tobacco smoke.
   True or false?

4. Cigarette smoking increases the risk for which of the following conditions?
   a. facial wrinkling
   b. miscarriage
   c. impotence
   d. automobile crashes

5. The rate of smoking among college students is declining.
   True or false?

Answers

1. *False.* The average age for starting smoking is 13; for smokeless tobacco users, it is 10.

2. *All four.* Tobacco contains thousands of chemical substances, including many that are poisonous or linked to the development of cancer.

3. *True.* In one study, 88% of nonsmokers had measurable blood levels of a compound that indicates recent nicotine exposure.

4. *All four.* Cigarette smoking reduces the quality of life and is the greatest preventable cause of death in the United States.

5. *False.* The rate of smoking among college students has increased by 25% since 1993 and is now higher than the national average.

Once considered a glamorous and sophisticated habit, smoking is now viewed with increasing disapproval. The recognition of the health risks of smoking is a primary cause of this change in public opinion, and it has led to significant changes in the behavior of many Americans. Over the past four decades, the proportion of cigarette smoking among adults in the United States has dropped 30%. Private businesses and all levels of government have jumped on the nonsmoking bandwagon: Almost every state now restricts smoking in public places, and several have introduced statewide smoking bans for indoor workplaces. The U.S. Surgeon General has proposed that America become completely smoke-free.

Despite such progress, tobacco use remains widespread. About one in four American adults smokes, and each year more than 400,000 Americans die from the effects of cigarette smoking (Table 11-1). Nonsmokers also suffer: Exposure to environmental tobacco smoke (ETS) causes more than 50,000 annual deaths among nonsmokers. Smoking by pregnant women is responsible for about 10% of all infant deaths in this country. Spit (smokeless) tobacco and cigars are regaining popularity. The use of spit tobacco products has tripled since 1972; cigar smoking has increased 50% since 1993.

Given the overwhelming evidence against tobacco, why would anyone today begin using it? How does it exercise its hold over users? What can smokers and nonsmokers do to help achieve a tobacco-free society? In this chapter, we explore answers to these and other questions.

WHY PEOPLE USE TOBACCO

About 47 million American adults and 4 million adolescents smoke. Two-thirds of adult smokers believe that they'll die of tobacco-related causes if they don't quit. Yet each day, 6000 young people try cigarettes and 3000 become regular smokers. This section examines the personal and societal forces that induce people to start smoking and encourage them to continue.

Nicotine Addiction

The primary reason people continue to use **tobacco** despite the health risks is that they have become addicted to a powerful psychoactive drug: **nicotine**. Although the tobacco industry long maintained that there was insufficient evidence about the addictiveness of nicotine, scientific evidence overwhelmingly supports the conclusion that nicotine is highly addictive. In fact, many researchers consider nicotine to be the most physically addictive of all the psychoactive drugs.

Recent neurological studies indicate that nicotine acts on the brain in much the same way as cocaine and heroin. Nicotine reaches the brain via the bloodstream seconds after it is inhaled or, in the case of smokeless tobacco,

VITAL STATISTICS

TABLE 11-1	*Causes of Death in the United States*

Cause	Approximate Number of Deaths Per Year
Tobacco	430,000
Diet and activity habits	300,000
Alcohol	100,000
Microbial agents	90,000
Toxic agents	60,000
Secondhand tobacco smoke	50,000
Motor vehicle crashes	40,000
Firearms	35,000
Sexual behavior	30,000
Illegal drug use	20,000

SOURCES: American Heart Association. Centers for Disease Control and Prevention. 1998. Births and deaths: Preliminary data for 1997. *National Vital Statistics Report* 47(4). CDC TIPS. 1998. *Targeting Tobacco Use* (retrieved November 22, 1998; http://www.cdc.gov/nccdphp/osh/oshaag.htm). McGinnis, J. M., and W. H. Fóege. 1993. Actual causes of death in the United States. *Journal of the American Medical Association* 270: 2207–2212.

absorbed through membranes of the mouth or nose. It triggers the release of powerful chemical messengers in the brain, including epinephrine, norepinephrine, and dopamine. But unlike street drugs, most of which are used to achieve a high, nicotine's primary attraction seems to lie in its ability to modulate everyday emotions.

At low doses, nicotine acts as a stimulant: It increases heart rate and blood pressure and can enhance alertness, concentration, rapid information processing, memory, and learning. People type faster on nicotine, for instance. At high doses, on the other hand, nicotine appears to act as a sedative; it can reduce aggressiveness and alleviate the stress response. Tobacco users may be able to fine-tune nicotine's effects and regulate their moods by increasing or decreasing their intake of the drug. Studies have shown that smokers experience milder mood variation than nonsmokers while performing long, boring tasks or while watching emotional movies, for example.

All tobacco products contain nicotine, and the use of any of them can lead to addiction (see the box "Nicotine Dependence: Are You Hooked?"). Nicotine addiction fulfills the criteria for substance dependence described in Chapter 9, including loss of control, tolerance, and withdrawal.

Loss of Control Three out of four smokers want to quit but find they cannot. Of the 60–80% of people who kick cigarettes at stop-smoking clinics, 75% start smoking again within a year—a relapse rate similar to rates for alcoholics and heroin addicts. Some evidence suggests quitting is even harder for smokeless users: In one study, only 1 of 14 spit tobacco users who participated in a

Nicotine Dependence: Are You Hooked?

Answer each question in the list below, giving yourself the appropriate points.

		1 point	2 points	
___ 1.	How soon after you wake up do you smoke your first cigarette?	After 30 minutes	Within 30 minutes	—
___ 2.	Do you find it difficult to refrain from smoking in places where it is forbidden, such as the library, a theater, or a doctor's office?	No	Yes	—
___ 3.	Which of all the cigarettes you smoke in a day is the most satisfying?	Any other than the first one in the morning	The first one in the morning	—
___ 4.	How many cigarettes a day do you smoke?	1–15	16–25	26+
___ 5.	Do you smoke more during the morning than during the rest of the day?	No	Yes	—
___ 6.	Do you smoke when you are so ill that you are in bed most of the day?	No	Yes	—
___ 7.	Does the brand you smoke have a low, medium, or high nicotine content?	Low	Medium	High
___ 8.	How often do you inhale the smoke?	Never	Sometimes	Always
___ Total				

Scoring

More than 6 points—very dependent
Less than 6 points—low to moderate dependence.

SOURCE: American Lung Association: Fagerstom Test.

tobacco-cessation clinic was able to stop for more than 4 hours.

Regular tobacco users live according to a rigid cycle of need and gratification. On average, they can go no more than 40 minutes between doses of nicotine; otherwise, they begin feeling edgy and irritable and have trouble concentrating. If ignored, nicotine cravings build until getting a cigarette or some spit tobacco becomes a paramount concern, crowding out other thoughts. Tobacco users become adept, therefore, at keeping a steady amount of nicotine circulating in the blood and going to the brain. In one experiment, smokers were given cigarettes that looked and tasted alike but varied in nicotine content. The subjects automatically adjusted their rate and depth of inhalation so that they absorbed their usual amount of nicotine. In other studies, heavy smokers were given nicotine without knowing it, and they cut down on their smoking without a conscious effort. Spit tobacco users maintain blood nicotine levels as high as those of cigarette smokers.

Tolerance and Withdrawal Using tobacco builds up tolerance. Where one cigarette may make a beginning smoker nauseated and dizzy, a long-term smoker may have to chain-smoke a pack or more to experience the same effects. For most regular tobacco users, sudden abstinence from nicotine produces predictable withdrawal symptoms as well. These symptoms, which come on several hours after the last dose of nicotine, can include severe cravings, insomnia, confusion, tremors, difficulty concentrating, fatigue, muscle pains, headache, nausea, irritability, anger, and depression. Users undergo measurable changes in brain waves, heart rate, and blood pressure, and they perform poorly on tasks requiring sustained attention. While most of these symptoms pass in 2–3 days, many ex-smokers report intermittent, intense urges to smoke for years after quitting.

Addiction occurs at an early age, despite many teenagers' beliefs that they will be able to stop when they wish to. A 1996 ABC News poll found that about one in three teenagers who tried smoking continued to smoke as a habit. Some 75% stated they wished they had never started. Another survey revealed that only 5% of high school smokers predicted they would definitely be smoking in 5 years; in fact, close to 75% were smoking 7–9 years later.

TERMS

tobacco The leaves of cultivated tobacco plants prepared for smoking, chewing, or use as snuff.

nicotine A poisonous, addictive substance found in tobacco and responsible for many of the effects of tobacco.

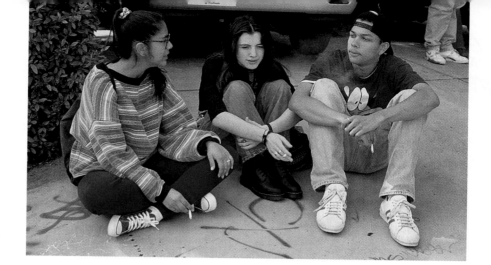

The average age of new smokers is 13, and most adult smokers began as teenagers. In polls, about 75% of teen smokers state they wish they had never started.

Social and Psychological Factors

Why do tobacco users have such a hard time quitting even when they want to? Social and psychological forces combine with physiological addiction to maintain the tobacco habit. Many people, for example, have established habits of smoking while doing something else—while talking, working, drinking, and so on. The smokeless tobacco habit is also associated with certain situations—studying, drinking coffee, or playing sports. It is difficult for these people to break their habits because the activities they associate with tobacco use continue to trigger their urge. Such activities are called **secondary reinforcers;** they act together with the physiological addiction to keep the user dependent on tobacco.

Why Start in the First Place?

A junior high school girl takes up smoking in an attempt to appear older. A high school boy uses smokeless tobacco in the bullpen, emulating the major league ball players he admires. An overweight first-year college student turns to cigarettes, hoping they will curb her appetite. Although smoking rates among American youth declined throughout the 1980s, they rose steadily during the 1990s. The largest increase was among 13- and 14-year-olds. Children and teenagers constitute 90% of all new smokers in this country: Every day, an estimated 3000 adolescents become regular cigarette smokers, while hundreds of others take up snuff or chewing tobacco. The average age for starting smokers is 13; for smokeless tobacco users, 10. Meanwhile, children—especially girls—are beginning to experiment with tobacco at ever-younger ages. The trends are particularly worrisome because the earlier people begin smoking, the more

likely they are to become heavy smokers—and to die of tobacco-related disease.

Rationalizing the Dangers Making the decision to smoke requires minimizing or denying both the health risks of tobacco use and the tremendous pain, disability, emotional trauma, family stress, and financial expense involved in tobacco-related diseases such as cancer and emphysema. A sense of invincibility, characteristic of many adolescents and young adults, also contributes to the decision to use tobacco. These young people may persuade themselves they are too intelligent, too lucky, or too robustly healthy to be vulnerable to tobacco's dangers. "I'm not dumb enough to get hooked," they may argue. "I'll be able to quit before I do myself any real harm." Other typical rationalizations: "My grandmother smoked and she lived to be 80" and "You can get killed just by crossing the street."

Listening to Advertising Advertising is another influence. The tobacco industry spends nearly $6 billion each year on ads—more than the entire annual budget for Puerto Rico. These ads link tobacco products with desirable traits such as confidence, popularity, sexual attractiveness, and slenderness. Young people are a prime target of these ads. Once a teen begins smoking, nicotine addiction can lead to a lifetime of smoking. As one teenager said, "It may have been my decision to smoke my first cigarette, and maybe even my second. But now *needing* to smoke is no longer a choice."

One measure of the effectiveness of advertising can be seen in the fact that 86% of teens prefer the three most heavily advertised brands (Marlboro, Camel, Newport); these three are preferred by just 32% of adults, who tend to favor cheap generic brands. Joe Camel, the former advertising image of Camel cigarettes, had become more familiar to children than Mickey Mouse. In surveys, more than 90% of 6-year-olds recognized him and associated him with cigarettes. In the 3 years following the introduction of the Joe Camel ad campaign, the Camel market

TERMS **secondary reinforcers** Stimuli that are not necessarily pleasurable in themselves, but that are associated with other stimuli that are pleasurable.

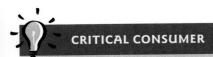
In order to maintain current sales, the tobacco industry must "capture" about 5000 new smokers every day to replace those smokers who die or quit. Since people who don't start smoking before the age of 20 are unlikely to do so, it is not surprising that young people are a big target for tobacco advertisements.

The tobacco industry spends nearly $6 billion every year to convince you to start smoking if you don't already. If you do smoke, they want to sell you on the image of their brand. Many people are not aware of the power advertising has over them. But you can start to resist the influence of tobacco ads by critically evaluating them.

- If you smoke or use other tobacco products, what brand do you use? Why do you use this brand?
- Think of two tobacco ads you have seen lately. Write down as many details as you can remember about each ad; see if you can sketch it. What makes these ads memorable?

- If you think of the ad as telling a story, what story does it tell?
- What characteristics does the ad associate with its product? Here are some common ones to get you started: fun, sex appeal, success, independence, popularity, satisfaction, rebellion, wealth.
- Which of these messages might you be particularly susceptible to; that is, which ads promise their cigarettes will help you meet your personal goals?
- Based on the information in this chapter, will using tobacco really deliver on these promises?
- What role do you think advertising has played in your use or nonuse of tobacco? Why do you think campaigns like those for Marlboro and Camel have been so successful? Can you remember any anti-smoking public service ads you've seen? Were they effective?

share among underage smokers quadrupled. In part because of criticism and a lawsuit brought by the Federal Trade Commission, the R. J. Reynolds Tobacco Company discontinued the Joe Camel campaign in July 1997.

Young people are not the only group targeted. Certain brands are designed to appeal primarily to men, women, or particular ethnic groups. For example, Virginia Slims tries to appeal to women by associating the brand with confidence and sexual attractiveness. Magazines that are targeted at African American audiences receive proportionately more revenues from cigarette advertising than do other consumer magazines. Billboards advertising tobacco products are placed in African American communities four or five times more often than in primarily white communities.

Tobacco advertising extends beyond magazines and billboards. Sponsorship of sports or racing events may result in millions of people, many of them children, viewing the name of a brand or company for hours. Brand names are also advertised on free caps, gym bags, and other products that appeal to youths. Virginia Slims introduced a line of clothing designed to appeal to young women and girls that can be purchased with proofs of purchase from cigarette packages.

The government began regulating tobacco advertising in 1967. Under the Fairness Doctrine, the Federal Communications Commission (FCC) required broadcasters to air anti-smoking messages along with industry-sponsored cigarette advertisements on television and radio. Anti-smoking ad campaigns can be extremely effective. Ads featuring unattractive older people smoking or cigarettes used as coffin nails counteract the glamorous images that appear in tobacco ads. Between 1967 and 1971, when anti-smoking messages were first broadcast, per-capita cigarette consumption declined by 7%—one of the largest declines ever. Cigarette advertising on television and radio was banned altogether in 1971. In 1996, the FDA issued strict advertising regulations designed to reduce the exposure and access of tobacco advertising and products to minors; whether or not these regulations go into effect depends on legal appeals and possible congressional legislation.

In November 1998, controls on advertising were enacted as part of the deal to settle lawsuits brought against the tobacco industry by the attorneys general of 39 states (see pp. 287–288 for more information). This settlement limits or bans billboard and transit advertising of tobacco products; cartoon characters in advertisements and packaging; tobacco logos on T-shirts, hats, and other promotional items; brand-name sponsorship of sporting events; and payments for product placement in movies, television, and concerts. Some health officials are worried about potential loopholes in the settlement deal; and even if the deal results in a dramatic change in advertising patterns, it will be many years before the positive image of smoking promoted in tobacco ads fades from the public's mind. For current information on the tobacco settlement deal and other legal actions, call or visit the Web site of one of the tobacco control advocacy groups listed in the For More Information section at the end of the chapter.

If you wonder how advertising might be affecting your attitudes toward smoking, try analyzing some ads using the strategies in the box "Evaluating Tobacco Advertising."

PERSONAL INSIGHT   Did people in your family smoke when you were growing up? Do you think it has affected your feelings and attitudes about smoking today? If so, how?

Who Uses Tobacco?

Not all young people are equally vulnerable to the lure of tobacco. Research suggests that the more of the following characteristics that apply to a child or adolescent, the more likely he or she is to use tobacco:

- A parent or sibling uses tobacco.
- Peers use tobacco.
- The child comes from a blue-collar family.
- The child comes from a low-income home.
- The family is headed by a single parent.
- The child performs poorly in school.
- The child drops out of school.
- The child has positive attitudes about tobacco use.

In 1995, about 27% of men and 23% of women smoked cigarettes (Table 11-2). Rates of smoking varied, based on gender, age, ethnicity, and education level. Adults with less than a twelfth-grade education were more than twice as likely to smoke cigarettes as those with a college degree. The reverse is true for cigars: Cigar smoking is most common among the affluent and those with high educational attainment.

Although all states ban the sale of tobacco to anyone under 18 years of age, at least 500 million packs of cigarettes and 26 million containers of chewing tobacco are consumed by minors each year. Among high school students, about 36% smoke cigarettes at least occasionally and 22% smoke cigars. An estimated 9%, including 20% of white male students, use spit tobacco. Male college athletes and professional baseball players report even higher rates of spit tobacco use.

Drug addicts are another major group of tobacco users. Some studies have found that over 90% of heroin addicts and 80% of alcoholics are heavy cigarette smokers. Other recent studies suggest that smokers are more likely than nonsmokers to have suffered from depression. Such findings lead some researchers to suggest that underlying psychological or physiological traits may predispose people to drug use, including tobacco.

PERSONAL INSIGHT How do you think you would feel if you found your 12-year-old brother or sister smoking? Would your feelings depend on whether you yourself were a smoker or a nonsmoker?

HEALTH HAZARDS

Tobacco adversely affects nearly every part of the body, including the brain, stomach, mouth, and reproductive organs.

TABLE 11-2 *Who Smokes?*

	Percentage of Smokers		
	Men	Women	Total
Ethnic group (all ages)			
White	27	24	26
Black	29	24	26
Asian/Pacific Islander	29	4	17
American Indian/ Alaska Native	37	35	36
Latino	22	15	18
Education, in years (age ≥ 25)			
≤ 8	28	18	23
9–11	42	34	38
12	34	26	30
13–15	25	23	24
≥ 16	14	14	14
Total	27	23	25

SOURCE: Centers for Disease Control and Prevention. 1997. Cigarette smoking among adults—United States, 1995. *Morbidity and Mortality Weekly Report* 46(51): 1217–1220.

Tobacco Smoke: A Poisonous Mix

Tobacco smoke contains hundreds of damaging chemical substances (Table 11-3). Smoke from a typical unfiltered cigarette contains about 5 billion particles per cubic millimeter—50,000 times as many as are found in an equal volume of smoggy urban air. These particles, when condensed, form the brown, sticky mass called **cigarette tar.**

At least 43 chemicals in tobacco smoke are linked to the development of cancer. Some, such as benzo(a)pyrene and urethane, are **carcinogens;** that is, they directly cause cancer. Other chemicals, such as formaldehyde, are **co-carcinogens;** they do not themselves cause cancer but combine with other chemicals to stimulate the growth of certain cancers, at least in laboratory animals. Other substances in tobacco cause health problems because they damage the lining of the respiratory tract or decrease the lungs' ability to fight off infection.

Tobacco also contains poisonous substances, including arsenic. In addition to being an addictive psychoactive drug, nicotine is also a poison and can be fatal in high doses. Many cases of nicotine poisoning occur each year in toddlers and infants who pick up and eat cigarette butts they find at home or on the playground.

Cigarette smoke contains carbon monoxide, the deadly gas in automobile exhaust, in concentrations 400 times greater than is considered safe in industrial workplaces. Not surprisingly, smokers often complain of breathlessness when they require a burst of energy to run across campus for their next class. Carbon monoxide displaces oxygen in red blood cells, depleting the body's supply of

TABLE 11-3	Selected Substances in Cigarette Smoke

Cancer-Causing Agents

Nitrosamines	Polonium
Crysenes	Nickel
Cadmium	Toluidine
Benzo(a)pyrene	Urethane

Metals

Aluminum	Gold
Zinc	Silver
Magnesium	Titanium
Mercury	Lead

Other Substances

Chemical	Typical Use or Source
Acetone	Nail polish remover
Ammonia	Floor/toilet cleaner
Arsenic	Poison
Butane	Cigarette lighter fluid
Cadmium	Rechargeable batteries
Carbon monoxide	Car exhaust fumes
DDT/dieldrin	Insecticides
Ethanol	Alcohol
Formaldehyde	Body tissue and fabric preserver
Hexamine	Lighter fluid
Hydrogen cyanide	Gas chamber poison
Methane	Swamp gas
Methanol	Rocket fuel
Naphthalene	Mothballs
Nicotine	Insecticide, addictive drug
Nitrous oxide phenols	Disinfectant
Stearic acid	Candle wax
Toluene	Industrial solvent
Vinyl chloride	Makes PVC

SOURCE: Health Partnership Project/California Medical Association Foundation, 1995. Used with permission.

life-giving oxygen for extra work. Carbon monoxide also impairs visual acuity, especially at night.

All smokers absorb some gases, tar, and nicotine from cigarette smoke, but smokers who inhale bring most of these substances into their bodies and keep them there. In 1 year, a typical pack-a-day smoker takes in 50,000–70,000 puffs. Smoke from a cigarette, pipe, or cigar directly assaults the mouth, throat, and respiratory tract. The nose, which normally filters about 75% of foreign matter we breathe, is completely bypassed.

In a cigarette, the unburned tobacco itself acts as a filter. As a cigarette burns down, there is less and less filter. Thus, more chemicals are absorbed into the body during the last third of a cigarette than during the first. A smoker can cut down on the absorption of harmful chemicals by not smoking cigarettes down to short butts. Any gains, of course, will be offset by smoking more cigarettes, inhaling more deeply, or puffing more frequently.

Some smokers switch to low-tar, low-nicotine, or filtered cigarettes because they believe them to be healthier alternatives that expose the smoker to fewer harmful chemicals. But there is no such thing as a "safe" cigarette. Low-tar or low-nicotine cigarettes may reduce some health risks. However, smokers who switch to a low-nicotine brand often compensate by smoking more cigarettes or inhaling more deeply to maintain their previous nicotine levels. Some filtered brands deliver even more carbon monoxide than unfiltered brands. And smokers sometimes offset the effects of the filters by knowingly or unknowingly blocking them.

Concerns have also been raised about menthol cigarettes, which are heavily favored by African American smokers. Studies have found that blacks absorb more nicotine than other groups and metabolize it more slowly. The anesthetizing effect of menthol, which may allow smokers to inhale more deeply and hold smoke in their lungs for a longer period, may be partly responsible for this difference. Further research is needed to determine if chemical effects of menthol and differences in smoking behavior can help explain the higher rates of smoking-related diseases seen among blacks.

The Immediate Effects of Smoking

The beginning smoker often has symptoms of mild nicotine poisoning: dizziness; faintness; rapid pulse; cold, clammy skin; and sometimes nausea, vomiting, and diarrhea. The seasoned smoker occasionally suffers these effects of nicotine poisoning, particularly after quitting and returning to a previous level of consumption. The effects of nicotine on smokers vary, depending greatly on the size of the nicotine dose and how much tolerance previous smoking has built up. Nicotine can either excite or tranquilize the nervous system, depending on dosage.

Nicotine has many other immediate effects. It stimulates the part of the brain called the **cerebral cortex.** It also stimulates the adrenal glands to discharge adrenaline. And it inhibits the formation of urine; constricts the blood vessels, especially in the skin; accelerates the heart rate; and elevates blood pressure. Higher blood pressure, faster heart rate, and constricted blood vessels require the heart to pump more blood. In healthy people, the heart can usually meet this demand, but in people whose

cigarette tar A brown sticky mass created when the chemical particles in tobacco smoke condense.

carcinogen Any substance that causes cancer.

cocarcinogen A substance that works with a carcinogen to cause cancer.

cerebral cortex The outer layer of the brain, which controls complex behavior and mental activity.

TERMS

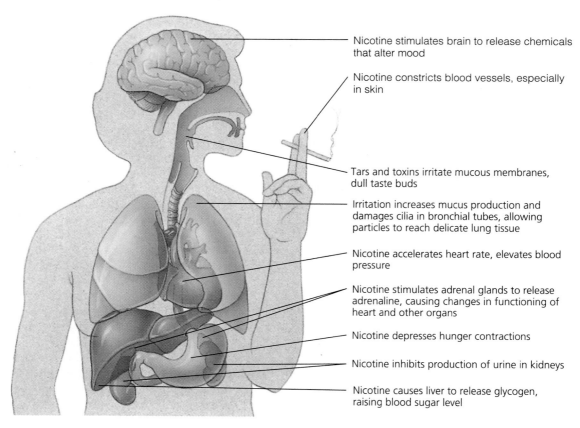

Figure 11-1 The short-term effects of smoking a cigarette.

Nicotine stimulates brain to release chemicals that alter mood

Nicotine constricts blood vessels, especially in skin

Tars and toxins irritate mucous membranes, dull taste buds

Irritation increases mucus production and damages cilia in bronchial tubes, allowing particles to reach delicate lung tissue

Nicotine accelerates heart rate, elevates blood pressure

Nicotine stimulates adrenal glands to release adrenaline, causing changes in functioning of heart and other organs

Nicotine depresses hunger contractions

Nicotine inhibits production of urine in kidneys

Nicotine causes liver to release glycogen, raising blood sugar level

coronary arteries are damaged enough to interfere with the flow of blood, the heart muscle may be strained.

Smoking depresses hunger contractions and dulls the taste buds; smokers who quit often notice that food tastes much better. Smoking is not useful for weight loss, however. (Smoking for decades may lessen or prevent age-associated weight gain for some smokers; but for people under 30, smoking is not associated with weight loss.) Figure 11-1 summarizes these immediate effects.

The Long-Term Effects of Smoking

Smoking is a dangerous habit that is linked to many deadly and disabling diseases. Research indicates that the total amount of tobacco smoke inhaled is a key factor contributing to disease. People who smoke more cigarettes per day, inhale deeply, puff frequently, smoke cigarettes down to the butts, or begin smoking at an early age run a greater risk of disease than do those who smoke more moderately or who do not smoke at all. Many diseases have already been linked to smoking, and as more research is done, even more diseases associated with smoking are being uncovered. The most costly ones—to society as well as to the individual—are cardiovascular

diseases, respiratory diseases such as emphysema and lung cancer, and other cancers.

Cardiovascular Disease Although cancer tends to receive the most publicity, one form of cardiovascular disease, **coronary heart disease (CHD),** is actually the most widespread single cause of death for cigarette smokers. CHD often results from **atherosclerosis,** a condition in which fatty deposits called **plaques** form on the inner walls of heart arteries, causing them to narrow and stiffen. A 1998 study found that smoking and exposure to ETS permanently accelerate the rate of plaque accumulation in the coronary arteries—50% for smokers, 25% for ex-smokers, and 20% for people regularly exposed to ETS. The crushing chest pain of **angina pectoris,** a primary symptom of CHD, results when the heart muscle, or *myocardium,* does not get enough oxygen. Sometimes a plaque forms at a narrow point in a main coronary artery. If the plaque completely blocks the flow of blood to a portion of the heart, that portion may die. This type of heart attack is called a **myocardial infarction.**

CHD can also interfere with the heart's electrical activity, resulting in disturbances of the normal heartbeat rhythm. Sudden and unexpected death is a common result of CHD, particularly among smokers. (See Chapter 15 for a more extensive discussion of cardiovascular disease.)

Smokers have a 70% higher death rate from CHD than nonsmokers. Deaths from CHD associated with cigarette smoking are most common in people age 40–50. (By contrast, deaths from lung cancer caused by smoking are most likely to occur in 60–70-year-olds.) Cigar and pipe smokers run a lower risk than cigarette smokers.

We do not completely understand how cigarette smoking increases the risk of CHD, but researchers are beginning to shed light on the process. Smoking reduces the amount of "good" cholesterol (high-density lipoprotein, or HDL) in the blood, thereby promoting plaque formation in artery walls. Smoking may also increase tension in heart muscle walls, speeding up the rate of muscular contraction and accelerating the heart rate. The workload of the heart thus increases, as does its need for oxygen and other nutrients. Carbon monoxide produced by cigarette smoking combines with hemoglobin in the red blood cells, displacing oxygen and thus providing less oxygen to the heart.

The risks of CHD decrease rapidly when the person stops smoking, particularly in younger smokers whose coronary arteries have not yet been extensively damaged. Cigarette smoking has also been linked to other cardiovascular diseases, including:

- *Stroke,* a sudden interference with the circulation of blood in a part of the brain, resulting in the destruction of brain cells.
- *Aortic aneurysm,* a bulge in the aorta caused by a weakening in its walls.
- *Pulmonary heart disease,* a disorder of the right side of the heart, caused by changes in the blood vessels of the lungs.

Lung Cancer and Other Cancers

Cigarette smoking is the primary cause of lung cancer. A recent study identified the precise mechanism: Benzo(a)pyrene, a chemical found in tobacco smoke, causes genetic mutations in lung cells that are identical to those found in many patients with lung cancer. Those who smoke two or more packs of cigarettes a day have lung cancer death rates 12–25 times greater than nonsmokers. The dramatic rise in lung cancer rates among women clearly parallels the increase of smoking in this group; lung cancer now exceeds breast cancer as the leading cause of cancer deaths among women. The risk of developing lung cancer increases with the number of cigarettes smoked each day, the number of years smoking, and the age at which the person started smoking.

While cigar and pipe smokers have a higher risk of lung cancer than nonsmokers do, the risk is lower than that for cigarette smokers. Smoking filter-tipped cigarettes slightly reduces health hazards, unless the smoker compensates by smoking more, as is often the case.

Evidence suggests that after 1 year without smoking, the risk of lung cancer decreases substantially. After 10 years, the risk of lung cancer among ex-smokers is 50% of that of continuing smokers. The sooner one quits, the better: If smoking is stopped before cancer has started, lung tissue tends to repair itself, even if cellular changes that can lead to cancer are already present.

Research has also linked smoking to cancers of the trachea, mouth, pharynx, esophagus, larynx, pancreas, bladder, kidney, cervix, stomach, liver, and colon. For more information on cancer, see Chapter 16.

Chronic Obstructive Lung Disease

The lungs of a smoker are constantly exposed to dangerous chemicals and irritants, and they must work harder to function adequately. The stresses placed on the lungs by smoking can permanently damage lung function and lead to *chronic obstructive lung disease (COLD),* also known as chronic obstructive pulmonary disease. COLD is the fourth leading cause of death in the United States. This progressive and disabling disorder consists of several different but related diseases; emphysema and chronic bronchitis are two of the most common.

Cigarette smokers are up to 18 times more likely than nonsmokers to die from emphysema and chronic bronchitis. (Pipe and cigar smokers are more likely to die from COLD than are nonsmokers, but they have a smaller risk than cigarette smokers.) The risk of developing COLD rises with the number of cigarettes smoked and falls when smoking ceases. For most Americans, cigarette smoking is a more important cause of COLD than air pollution, but exposure to both is more dangerous than exposure to either by itself.

EMPHYSEMA   Smoking is the primary cause of **emphysema,** a particularly disabling condition in which the walls of the air sacs in the lungs lose their elasticity and are gradually destroyed. The lungs' ability to obtain oxygen and remove carbon dioxide is impaired. A person with emphysema is breathless, is constantly gasping for

coronary heart disease (CHD)   Cardiovascular disease caused by hardening of the arteries that supply oxygen to the heart muscle; also called *coronary artery disease.*

atherosclerosis   Cardiovascular disease caused by the deposit of fatty substances in the walls of the arteries.

TERMS

plaque   A deposit on the inner wall of blood vessels; blood can coagulate around plaque and form a clot.

angina pectoris   Chest pain due to coronary heart disease.

myocardial infarction   A heart attack caused by the complete blockage of a main coronary artery.

emphysema   A disease characterized by a loss of lung tissue elasticity and breakup of the air sacs, impairing the lungs' ability to obtain oxygen and remove carbon dioxide.

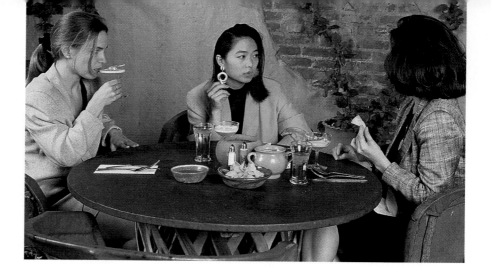

Cigarette smoke contains many toxic and carcinogenic chemicals that affect both the person smoking and the people breathing the environmental tobacco smoke. A growing body of evidence links ETS with lung cancer and respiratory and cardiovascular diseases.

air, and has the feeling of drowning. The heart must pump harder and may become enlarged. People with emphysema often die from a damaged heart. There is no known way to reverse this disease. In its advanced stage, the victim is bedridden and severely disabled.

CHRONIC BRONCHITIS   Persistent, recurrent inflammation of the bronchial tubes characterizes **chronic bronchitis.** When the cell lining of the bronchial tubes is irritated, it secretes excess mucus. Bronchial congestion is followed by a chronic cough, which makes breathing more and more difficult. If smokers have chronic bronchitis, they face a greater risk of lung cancer, no matter how old they are or how many (or few) cigarettes they smoke. Chronic bronchitis seems to be a shortcut to lung cancer.

Other Respiratory Damage   Even when the smoker shows no signs of lung impairment or disease, cigarette smoking damages the respiratory system. Normally the cells lining the bronchial tubes secrete mucus, a sticky fluid that collects particles of soot, dust, and other substances in inhaled air. Mucus is carried up to the mouth by the continuous motion of the cilia, hairlike structures that protrude from the inner surface of the bronchial tubes (Figure 11-2). If the cilia are destroyed or impaired, or if the pollution of inhaled air is more than the system can remove, the protection provided by cilia is lost.

Cigarette smoke first slows, then stops the action of the cilia. Eventually it destroys them, leaving delicate membranes exposed to injury from substances inhaled in cigarette smoke or from the polluted air in which the person lives or works. Special cells, *macrophages,* a type of white blood cell, also work to remove foreign particles from the

respiratory tract by engulfing them. Smoking appears to make macrophages work less efficiently. This interference with the functioning of the respiratory system often leads rapidly to the conditions known as smoker's throat and smoker's cough, as well as to shortness of breath. Even smokers of high school age show impaired respiratory function, compared with nonsmokers of the same age. Other respiratory effects of smoking include a worsening of allergy and asthma symptoms and an increase in the smoker's susceptibility to colds.

Although cigarette smoking can cause many respiratory disorders and diseases, the damage is not always permanent. Once a person stops smoking, steady improvement in overall lung function usually takes place. Chronic coughing subsides, mucus production returns to normal, and breathing becomes easier. The likelihood of lung disease drops sharply. People of all ages, even those who have been smoking for decades, improve after they stop smoking. If given a chance, the human body has remarkable powers of restoring itself.

Additional Health, Cosmetic, and Economic Concerns

- *Ulcers.* People who smoke are more likely to develop peptic ulcers and are more likely to die from them (especially stomach ulcers), because smoking impairs the body's healing ability.

- *Impotence.* Smoking affects blood flow in the veins and arteries of the penis, and it is an independent risk factor for impotence. Smokers are about 50% more likely than nonsmokers to suffer from persistent impotence.

- *Reproductive health problems.* Smoking is linked to reduced fertility in both men and women. A study of 18-year-old smoking men found that they had a significantly higher proportion of abnormally shaped sperm and sperm with genetic defects compared with nonsmokers. In women, smoking can contribute to menstrual disorders, early menopause,

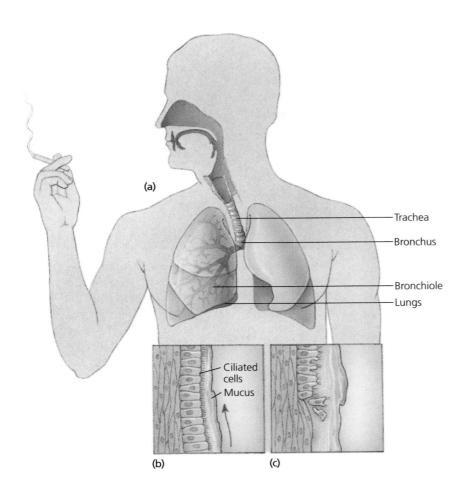

(a)

Trachea

Bronchus

Bronchiole

Lungs

Ciliated
cells

Mucus

(b)   (c)

**Figure 11-2   Damage to the lungs
caused by smoking.**   (a) The respiratory
system. (b) The inside of a bronchiole of a
nonsmoker. Foreign particles are collected by
a thin layer of sticky mucus and transported
out of the lungs, up toward the mouth, by
the action of cilia. (c) The inside of a bronchiole of a smoker. Smoking irritates the lung
tissue and causes increased mucus production, which can overwhelm the action of the
cilia. A smoker develops a chronic cough as
the lungs try to rid themselves of foreign
particles and excess mucus. Eventually the
cilia are destroyed, leaving the delicate
lung tissue exposed to injury from foreign
substances.

and complications of pregnancy (see pp. 286–287
for more on the effects of smoking during pregnancy).

- *Dental diseases.* Smoking is linked to tooth decay
  and gum and periodontal diseases.

- *Diminished physical senses.* Smoking dulls the senses
  of taste and smell. Over time, it increases the risk for
  hearing loss and cataracts (a serious eye condition
  that can result in partial or total blindness).

- *Injuries.* Smokers have higher rates of motor vehicle
  crashes and fire-related injuries.

- *Cosmetic concerns.* Smoking can cause premature
  skin wrinkling, premature baldness, stained teeth,
  discolored fingers, and a persistent tobacco odor in
  clothes and hair.

- *Economic costs.* A pack-a-day habit costs an average
  of $1000 per year. Other financial costs include
  higher health and home insurance premiums; more
  frequent cleaning of clothes, teeth, home, office, and
  car; and repair of burnt clothing, upholstery, and
  carpeting.

In addition, smoking contributes to osteoporosis, increases
the risk of complications from diabetes, and accelerates

the course of multiple sclerosis. Further research may link
tobacco use to still other disorders.

Cumulative Effects   The cumulative effects of tobacco
use fall into two general categories. The first category is
reduced life expectancy. A male who takes up smoking
before age 15 and continues to smoke is only half as likely
to live to age 75 as a male who never smokes. If he inhales
deeply, he risks losing a minute of life for every minute of
smoking. Females who have similar smoking habits also
have a reduced life expectancy. On average, smokers live
8 years less than nonsmokers.

The second category involves quality of life. A national
health survey begun in 1964 shows that smokers spend
one-third more time away from their jobs because of illness than nonsmokers. Female smokers spend 17% more
days sick in bed than female nonsmokers. Lost work days
due to smoking number in the millions.

Both men and women smokers show a greater rate of
acute and chronic disease than those who have never
smoked. The U.S. Public Health Service estimates that if
all people had the same rate of disease as those who never
smoked, there would be 1 million fewer cases of chronic

bronchitis, 1.8 million fewer cases of **sinusitis,** and 1 million fewer cases of peptic ulcers in the country every year.

Other Forms of Tobacco Use

Many smokers have switched from cigarettes to other forms of tobacco, such as cigars, pipes, clove cigarettes, and spit (smokeless) tobacco. However, each of these alternatives is far from safe.

Spit (Smokeless) Tobacco More than 5 million adults and nearly 10% of all high school students are current spit tobacco users. Spit tobacco use has increased in recent years and is especially common among Native Americans, adolescent males (especially white males), male college athletes, and professional baseball players. About 80% of users start by the ninth grade.

Spit tobacco comes in two major forms—snuff and chewing tobacco ("chew"). In snuff, the tobacco leaf is processed into a coarse, moist powder and mixed with flavorings. Snuff is usually sold in small tins. Users place a "pinch," "dip," or "quid" between the lower lip or cheek and gum and suck on it. In chewing tobacco, the tobacco leaf may be shredded ("leaf"), pressed into bricks or cakes ("plugs"), or dried and twisted into ropelike strands ("twists"). Chew is usually sold in pouches. Users place a wad of tobacco in their mouth and then chew or suck it to release the nicotine. All types of smokeless tobacco cause an increase in saliva production, and resulting tobacco juice is spit out or swallowed.

The nicotine in spit tobacco—along with flavorings and additives—is absorbed through the gums and lining of the mouth. Holding an average-size dip in the mouth for 30 minutes delivers about the same amount of nicotine as two or three cigarettes. Because of its nicotine content, spit tobacco is highly addictive. Some users keep it in their mouth even while sleeping.

Although not as dangerous as cigarettes, the use of spit tobacco carries many health risks. Changes can occur in the mouth after only a few weeks of use: Gums and lips become dried and irritated and may bleed. White or red patches may appear inside the mouth; this condition, known as *leukoplakia,* can lead to oral cancer (see below). A 1998 study of major league baseball players found dangerous mouth lesions in 83 out of the 141 spit tobacco–using players who were examined. Other studies have found even higher rates of oral sores. About 25% of regular spit tobacco users have *gingivitis* (inflammation) and recession of the gums and bone loss around the teeth, especially where the tobacco is usually placed. The senses of taste and smell are usually dulled. In addition, many people find the presence of wads of tobacco in the mouth, stained teeth, bad breath, and behaviors such as frequent spitting to be unpleasant.

One of the most serious effects of smokeless tobacco is an increased risk of oral cancer—cancers of the lip,

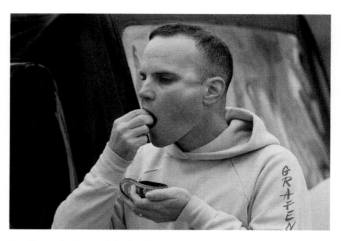

Nearly one in five male high school seniors uses smokeless tobacco, a habit linked to oral cancer, dental problems, dulling of the senses of taste and smell, and possibly cardiovascular problems.

tongue, cheek, throat, gums, roof and floor of the mouth, and larynx. Spit tobacco contains at least 28 chemicals known to cause cancer, and long-term snuff use may increase the risk of oral cancer by as much as 50 times. Surgery to treat oral cancer is often disfiguring and may involve removing parts of the face, tongue, cheek, or lip.

Data on the incidence of heart disease among spit tobacco users have not yet been collected. But it is known that dipping and chewing tobacco produce blood levels of nicotine similar to those in cigarette smokers. High blood levels of nicotine have dangerous effects on the cardiovascular system, including elevation of blood pressure, heart rate, and blood levels of certain fats. Other chemicals in spit tobacco are believed to pose risks to developing fetuses.

Cigars and Pipes After more than two decades of decline, cigar smoking has increased by nearly 50% since 1993. The popularity of cigars is highest among white males age 18–44 with higher than average income and education, but women are also smoking cigars in record numbers. Cigar use is also growing among young people: In the latest government surveys, 22% of high school students reported having smoked at least one cigar in the previous month. An estimated 2% of Americans, mostly males who also smoke cigarettes, are pipe smokers.

Cigars are made from rolled whole tobacco leaves; pipe tobacco is made from shredded leaves and often flavored. Because cigar and pipe smoke is more alkaline than cigarette smoke, users of cigars and pipes do not need to inhale in order to ingest nicotine; instead, they absorb nicotine through the gums and lining of the mouth. Cigars contain more tobacco than cigarettes and so contain more nicotine and produce more tar when smoked. Large cigars may contain as much tobacco as a whole pack of cigarettes and take 1–2 hours to smoke.

The smoke from cigars contains many of the same toxins and carcinogens as the smoke from cigarettes, some in much higher quantities. The health risks of cigars depend on the number of cigars smoked and whether or not the smoker inhales. Because most cigar and pipe users do not inhale, they have a lower risk of cancer and cardiovascular and respiratory diseases than cigarette smokers. However, their risks are substantially higher than those of nonsmokers. For example, compared to nonsmokers, people who smoke one or two cigars per day without inhaling have six times the risk of cancer of the larynx. The risks are much higher for cigar smokers who do inhale: They have 27 times the risk of oral cancer and 53 times the risk of cancer of the larynx compared to nonsmokers, and their risk of heart and lung diseases approaches that of cigarette smokers. Smoking a cigar immediately impairs the ability of blood vessels to dilate, reducing the amount of oxygen delivered to tissues, including heart muscle, especially during times of stress. Pipe and cigar smoking are also risk factors for pancreatic cancer, which is almost always fatal.

Nicotine addiction is another concern. Most adults who smoke cigars do so only occasionally, and there is little evidence that use of cigars by adults leads to addiction. The recent rise in cigar use among teens has raised concerns, however, because nicotine addiction almost always develops in the teen or young adult years. More research is needed to determine if cigar use by teens will develop into nicotine addiction and frequent use of either cigarettes or spit tobacco.

Clove Cigarettes and Bidis   Clove cigarettes, also called "kreteks" or "chicartas," are made of tobacco mixed with chopped cloves; they are imported primarily from Indonesia and Pakistan. Clove cigarettes contain almost twice as much tar, nicotine, and carbon monoxide as conventional cigarettes and so have all the same health hazards. Some chemical constituents of cloves may also be dangerous. For example, eugenol, an anesthetic compound found in cloves, may impair the respiratory system's ability to detect and defend against foreign particles. There have been a number of serious respiratory injuries and deaths from the use of clove cigarettes.

Bidis, or "beadies," are small cigarettes imported from India that contain species of tobacco different from those used by U.S. cigarette manufacturers. The tobacco in bidis is hand-rolled in Indian ebony leaves (tendu) and then often flavored; clove, mint, chocolate, and fruit varieties are available. Bidis contain up to four times more nicotine and twice as much tar as U.S. cigarettes. Use of bidis has been growing among teens, possibly because of the flavorings they contain or because they look and smell somewhat like marijuana cigarettes ("joints"); they do not have the same effects as marijuana, however.

Neither clove cigarettes nor bidis is a safe or healthy alternative to conventional tobacco cigarettes.

THE EFFECTS OF SMOKING ON THE NONSMOKER

In a watershed decision in 1993, the U.S. Environmental Protection Agency (EPA) designated **environmental tobacco smoke (ETS)** a Class A carcinogen—an agent known to cause cancer in humans. This designation put ETS in the same category as notorious cancer-causing agents like asbestos. Every year, ETS causes thousands of deaths from lung cancer and heart disease and is responsible for hundreds of thousands of respiratory infections in young children. For the U.S. tobacco industry, the EPA's report was the worst blow since 1964 when the Surgeon General first declared that smoking causes cancer. The EPA report gave new momentum to efforts to limit or ban smoking in public and in the workplace.

Environmental Tobacco Smoke

Environmental tobacco smoke, commonly known as *secondhand smoke,* consists of mainstream smoke and sidestream smoke. Smoke exhaled by smokers is referred to as **mainstream smoke. Sidestream smoke** enters the atmosphere from the burning end of a cigarette, cigar, or pipe. Undiluted sidestream smoke, because it is not filtered through either a cigarette filter or a smoker's lungs, has significantly higher concentrations of the toxic and carcinogenic compounds found in mainstream smoke. For example, compared to mainstream smoke, sidestream smoke has (1) twice as much tar and nicotine; (2) three times as much benzo(a)pyrene, a carcinogen; (3) almost three times as much carbon monoxide, which displaces oxygen from red blood cells and forms *carboxyhemoglobin,* a dangerous compound that seriously limits the body's ability to use oxygen; and (4) three times as much ammonia.

Nearly 85% of the smoke in a room where someone is smoking comes from sidestream smoke. Of course, sidestream smoke is diffused through the air, so nonsmokers don't inhale the same concentrations of toxic chemicals that the smoker does. Still, the concentrations can be considerable. In rooms where people are smoking, levels of carbon monoxide, for instance, can exceed those permitted by Federal Air Quality Standards for outside air.

sinusitis Inflammation of the sinus cavities; symptoms include headache, fever, and pain.   **TERMS**

environmental tobacco smoke (ETS) Smoke that enters the atmosphere from the burning end of a cigarette, cigar, or pipe, as well as smoke that is exhaled by smokers; also called *secondhand smoke.*

mainstream smoke Smoke that is inhaled by a smoker and then exhaled into the atmosphere.

sidestream smoke Smoke that comes from the burning end of a cigarette, cigar, or pipe.

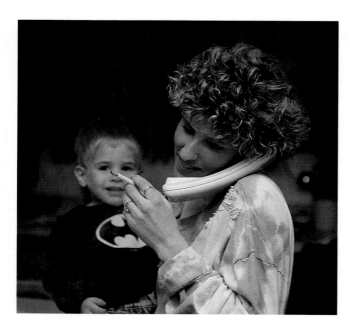

It is estimated that 9 million American children are regularly exposed to environmental tobacco smoke. ETS can trigger respiratory infections, cause or aggravate asthma, contribute to middle-ear infections, and impair development.

In a typical home with the windows closed, it takes about 6 hours for 95% of the airborne cigarette smoke particles to clear.

The secondhand smoke from a cigar can be even more dangerous than that from cigarettes. The EPA has found that the output of carcinogenic particles from a cigar exceeds that of three cigarettes, and cigar smoke contains up to 30 times more carbon monoxide.

ETS Effects   Studies show that up to 25% of nonsmokers subjected to ETS develop coughs, 30% develop headaches and nasal discomfort, and 70% suffer from eye irritation. Other symptoms range from breathlessness to sinus problems. People with allergies tend to suffer the most. The odor of tobacco smoke clings to skin and clothes—another unpleasant effect of ETS.

But ETS causes more than just annoyance and discomfort. The EPA estimates that ETS causes 3000 lung cancer deaths annually. People who live, work, or socialize among smokers face a 24–50% increase in lung cancer risk. ETS is also responsible for about 50,000 deaths from heart disease each year. As described earlier, exposure to ETS is associated with a 20% increase in the progression of atherosclerosis. ETS also aggravates asthma, an increasing cause of sudden death in otherwise healthy adults. Scientists have been able to measure changes that contribute to lung tissue damage and potential tumor promotion in the bloodstreams of healthy young test subjects who spend just 3 hours in a smoke-filled room. And nonsmokers can still be affected by the harmful effects of ETS hours after they have left a smoky environment. Carbon monoxide,

for example, lingers in the bloodstream 5 hours later. See the box "Avoiding Environmental Tobacco Smoke" for strategies on protecting yourself against ETS.

Infants, Children, and ETS   Recent studies have shown that infants exposed to smoke from more than 21 cigarettes a day are more than 23 times more likely to die of sudden infant death syndrome (SIDS) than babies not exposed to ETS. A 1996 British study estimated that more than 60% of all SIDS deaths are due to cigarette exposure. Children under 5 whose primary caregiver smokes 10 or more cigarettes per day have measurable blood levels of nicotine and tobacco carcinogens. Chemicals in tobacco smoke also show up in breast milk, and breastfeeding may pass more chemicals to the infant of a smoking mother than direct exposure to ETS.

The EPA estimates that environmental tobacco smoke triggers 150,000–300,000 cases of bronchitis, pneumonia, and other respiratory infections in infants and toddlers up to 18 months of age each year, resulting in 7500–15,000 hospitalizations. Older children suffer, too. The EPA has labeled ETS a risk factor for asthma in children who have not previously displayed symptoms of the disease, and has blamed ETS for aggravating the symptoms of the 200,000 to 1 million children who already have asthma. The EPA also links ETS to reduced lung function and identifies it as a cause of fluid buildup in the middle ear, a contributing factor in middle-ear infections, a leading reason for childhood surgery.

Why are infants and children so vulnerable? Because they breathe faster than adults, they inhale more air—and more of the pollutants in the air. Because they also weigh less, they inhale three times more pollutants per unit of body weight than adults do. And because their young lungs are still growing, this intake can impair optimal development. The problem is widespread. The American Academy of Pediatrics estimates that some 9 million American children are exposed to ETS.

Smoking and Pregnancy

Smoking almost doubles a pregnant woman's chance of having a miscarriage, and it significantly increases her risk of ectopic pregnancy (see the box "Special Risks for Women Who Smoke"). Maternal smoking causes an estimated 4600 infant deaths in the United States each year, primarily due to premature delivery and smoking-related problems with the placenta. Maternal smoking is a major factor in low birth weight, which puts newborns at high risk for infections and other serious problems. If a nonsmoking mother is regularly exposed to ETS, her infant is also at greater risk for low birth weight.

Babies born to mothers who smoke more than two packs a day perform poorly on developmental tests in the first hours after birth, compared to babies of nonsmoking mothers. Later in life, hyperactivity, short attention span, and lower scores on spelling and reading tests all occur more frequently in children whose mothers smoked during pregnancy than in those born to nonsmoking mothers. Males born to smoking mothers have higher rates of adolescent and adult criminal activity, suggesting that maternal smoking may cause brain damage that increases the risk of criminal behavior. Nevertheless, about 14% of pregnant women smoke throughout pregnancy; *Healthy People 2010* sets a goal of reducing this to 2%.

The Cost of Tobacco Use to Society

A 1998 study estimated the health care costs associated with smoking at $73 billion per year. If the cost of lost

productivity from sickness, disability, and premature death is included, the total is closer to $125 billion. This works out to $5 per pack of cigarettes, far more than the average $0.39 per pack tax collected by states to offset tobacco-related medical costs.

In order to recoup public health care expenditures, 43 state attorneys general filed suit against tobacco companies. In March 1997, Liggett Group settled its part of the suit by agreeing to turn over internal documents and to pay a portion of its profits to cover tobacco-related medical expenses and anti-smoking campaigns. A preliminary deal reached with the larger tobacco companies in June 1997 failed to obtain the necessary congressional approval. In November 1998, a new agreement was reached that would settle 39 state lawsuits and apply to seven states that never filed suit. (Four states—Florida, Minnesota, Mississippi, and Texas—settled their suits separately for a total of $40 billion). The 1998 settlement requires the tobacco companies to pay states $206 billion over 25 years; it also limits or bans certain types of advertising, promotions, and lobbying. Many of the provisions of the deal are designed to limit youth exposure and access to tobacco. In exchange, the tobacco industry settles the state lawsuits and is protected from future suits by states, counties, towns, and other public entities. The 1998 version of the settlement does not need overall congressional approval because it does not contain any provision for FDA regulation of tobacco products. However, further congressional action and additional lawsuits are expected; for current information on political and legal activities, call or visit the Web site of one of the tobacco control advocacy groups listed in the For More Information section at the end of the chapter.

WHAT CAN BE DONE?

In 1967, John F. Banzhaf III, outraged by a TV commercial that equated smoking with masculinity, submitted a petition to the FCC. In it, Banzhaf, then fresh out of law school, demanded that foes of cigarettes be given a chance to air their side. On June 2, 1967, the FCC issued a landmark decision agreeing with him. The agency ordered broadcasters to provide free air time for anticigarette announcements. Four years later, Congress banned all cigarette advertising from TV and radio.

In 1993, shortly after he heard that the EPA had declared ETS to be a carcinogen, W. D. "Bill" Landis vowed to stop smoking around his newborn grandson. But he didn't stop there. Landis, a deputy sheriff and city councilman in Pleasanton, California, launched a drive to force others in his town to do the same. He proposed a citywide ban on smoking in all public and private workplaces, including restaurants, and a ban on cigarette vending machines. The ordinance passed unanimously.

In both cases, individuals acted on their own to combat tobacco use, arguably the deadliest plague of our time. Every hour, 60 Americans die from preventable smoking-related diseases. Today there are more avenues than ever before for individual and group action against this major public health threat.

Action at the Local Level

Before the EPA issued its report, most efforts to limit smoking focused on enacting local laws and ordinances. Tobacco interests have been able to block actions at the national and state levels through lobbying and political contributions. However, during the 1980s and 1990s, tobacco restrictions were passed by local school boards, town councils, and county boards of supervisors, over which the tobacco industry has little or no influence.

There are now thousands of local ordinances across the nation that restrict or ban smoking in restaurants, stores, and workplaces. Since the EPA classification of environmental tobacco smoke as a carcinogen, local governments and businesses have become bolder about protecting nonsmokers. Even public outdoor areas are not exempt from regulations: Sharon, Massachusetts, has banned smoking at all beaches and playgrounds. Honolulu, Hawaii, has also banned smoking at the beach, but for a different reason—to protect sea turtles from being poisoned by eating cigarette butts.

As local no-smoking rules proliferate, evidence is mounting that such restrictions encourage smokers to quit. The smoking rate dropped from one in three adults in 1980 to one in four in 1996.

> **PERSONAL INSIGHT** How do you feel when someone near you lights up a cigarette? What knowledge or experience influences your feelings? If it bothers you, but you have difficulty asserting yourself, what feelings are making you uncomfortable? Can you think of ways to deal with them?

Action at the State and Federal Levels

The EPA report fundamentally changed the politics of tobacco by declaring that smokers not only shorten their own lives, they kill bystanders. It became harder for politicians who are sympathetic to the tobacco industry—and who often accept sizable contributions from tobacco interests—to argue that anti-tobacco laws constitute unwarranted intrusions into voters' private lives.

Following the EPA report, state legislatures passed many tough new anti-tobacco laws. A statewide ban on smoking in almost all indoor workplaces, including restaurants, passed the California legislature in 1994 after a defeat there just a year earlier; in 1998, California became the first state to ban smoking in bars. In 1997, voters in Alaska approved an increase in the tax on cigarettes, bringing that state's tax to a national high of $1.00 per pack.

The EPA report also set off a flurry of federal activity. Smoking is banned on virtually all domestic airplane flights. Former FDA commissioner David Kessler concluded that cigarettes and smokeless tobacco are delivery devices for nicotine, an addictive drug, and thus subject to FDA regulation. The FDA issued stringent guidelines regarding the advertising and sale of tobacco products to minors; enactment of the guidelines depends on the outcome of legal appeals and/or the passage of legislation.

The federal government is also acting to protect nonsmokers from environmental tobacco smoke. The U.S. Defense Department has banned smoking at all military work sites, and the Labor Department proposed a ban at its indoor work sites. And the U.S. Occupational Safety

The National Cancer Institute recommends a "Four A's" approach for physicians who want to help patients quit tobacco. The approach can be adapted for anyone who wants to help a tobacco user quit.

1. *Ask* about tobacco use. Has your younger brother ever dipped snuff? How long has your roommate smoked? How many cigarettes a day is your friend up to?

2. *Advise* tobacco users to stop. "As your friend, I hate to see you jeopardize your health. I've noticed you cough a lot already and your voice is raspy. You should stop." Studies show the cumulative messages tobacco users get about quitting do help motivate them to stop.

3. *Assist* the tobacco user who is willing to stop. To coincide with your friend's quit date, invite him or her on a camping trip, hike, or other outing far from any stores selling tobacco. Be tolerant if the quitter is irritable and unpleasant. Introduce

the quitter to restaurants that don't allow smoking. Offer to be an exercise partner; exercise can increase a quitter's chance of success. Call the quitter once a day to offer encouragement and help. Bring gifts of low-calorie snacks or crafts that occupy the hands. Offer to take a relaxation course with him or her. If the quitter lapses, be encouraging. A lapse doesn't have to become a relapse.

4. *Arrange* follow-up. Maintaining abstinence is an ongoing process. Every month or so, congratulate quitters again on their success. Note how much better their cars and rooms smell, how they get winded less easily and cough less often, and how much you appreciate not having to breathe their smoke. Continue to engage quitters in exercise and to help them find new ways to enjoy life that don't revolve around tobacco.

and Health Administration considered nationwide rules that would, in effect, ban smoking on the job except in specially ventilated areas.

International Action

Many countries are following the United States' lead in restricting smoking. Smoking is now banned on many international air flights, as well as in many restaurants and hotels and on public transportation in some countries. The World Health Organization and the International Olympic Committee are cosponsors of the annual World No-Tobacco Day, an event that increases the awareness of governments and individuals about the hazards of tobacco use. On this day, people are encouraged to refrain from using tobacco for at least 24 hours.

Action in the Private Sector

The EPA report also shook up the private sector, giving employers reason to fear worker's compensation claims based on exposure to workplace smoke. The year after the report was issued, businesses including McDonald's and Taco Bell banned smoking in thousands of their restaurants across the country. By 1995, 70% of the nation's shopping malls were smoke-free.

Such local, state, national, and international efforts represent progress, but health activists warn that tobacco industry influence remains strong. The tobacco industry contributes heavily to sympathetic legislative officeholders and candidates. Many states have relatively weak antismoking laws that are backed by the tobacco industry and include clauses that prevent the passage of stricter local ordinances. Tobacco companies spent $43 million during

the first half of 1998 in attempts to block the passage of strict national tobacco control legislation.

Individual Action

When a smoker violates a no-smoking designation, complain. If your favorite restaurant or shop doesn't have a nonsmoking policy, ask the manager to adopt one. If you see children buying tobacco, report this illegal activity to the facility manager or the police. Learn more about addiction and tobacco cessation so you can better support the tobacco users you know (see the box "How You Can Help a Tobacco User Quit"). Vote for candidates who support anti-tobacco measures; contact local, state, and national representatives to express your view.

Cancel your subscriptions to magazines that carry tobacco advertising; include a note to the publisher explaining your decision. Voice your opinion about other positive representations of tobacco use. (A 1999 study found that more than two-thirds of children's animated feature films have featured tobacco or alcohol use with no clear message that such practices were unhealthy.) Volunteer with the American Lung Association, the American Cancer Society, or the American Heart Association.

These are just some of the many ways individuals can help support tobacco prevention and stop-smoking efforts. Nonsmokers not only have the right to breathe clean air, but they also have the right to take action to help solve one of society's most serious public health threats (Figure 11-3).

Controlling the Tobacco Companies

With their immensely profitable industry shrinking, tobacco companies are concentrating on appealing to

Nonsmoker's Bill of Rights

NONSMOKERS HELP PROTECT THE HEALTH, COMFORT, AND SAFETY OF EVERYONE BY INSISTING ON THE FOLLOWING RIGHTS:

THE RIGHT TO BREATHE CLEAN AIR
Nonsmokers have the right to breathe clean air, free from harmful and irritating tobacco smoke. This right supersedes the right to smoke when the two conflict.

THE RIGHT TO SPEAK OUT
Nonsmokers have the right to express—firmly but politely—their discomfort and adverse reactions to tobacco smoke. They have the right to voice their objections when smokers light up without asking permission.

THE RIGHT TO ACT
Nonsmokers have the right to take action through legislative means—as individuals or in groups—to prevent or discourage smokers from polluting the atmosphere and to seek the restriction of smoking in public places.

Figure 11-3 The Nonsmoker's Bill of Rights.

narrower and narrower market segments with an ever-increasing array of brands and styles—over 350 in all. As tobacco use has declined among better-educated, wealthier segments of the American population, tobacco companies have redirected their marketing efforts toward minorities, the poor, and young women, populations among whom smoking rates are still high. This practice of targeting specific segments of the market has become controversial, especially when the segment has an unusually high risk for fatal diseases caused by tobacco use.

With cigarette sales falling in the United States, tobacco companies have begun focusing on increasing the export of cigarettes, particularly to developing nations (see the box "Exporting the Nicotine Habit Around the World"). As companies compete for customers in the years ahead, the need to exercise public pressure to keep the powerful tobacco companies in check will persist.

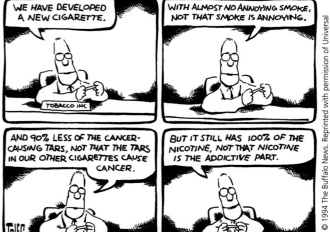

HOW A TOBACCO USER CAN QUIT

Since 1964, over 50% of all adults who have ever smoked have quit. Giving up tobacco is a long-term, intricate process. Heavy smokers who say they have just stopped "cold turkey" don't tell of the thinking and struggling and other mental processes that contributed to their final conquest over this powerful addiction. Olympic diver Greg Louganis, who began smoking at the age of 8, has said that he considers quitting, at the age of 23, the greatest accomplishment of his life.

Research shows that tobacco users move through predictable stages—from being uninterested in stopping, to thinking about change, to making a concerted effort to stop, to finally maintaining abstinence. But most attempt to quit several times before they finally succeed. Relapse is a normal part of the process.

The Benefits of Quitting

Giving up tobacco provides immediate health benefits to men and women of all ages (Table 11-4). People who quit smoking find that food tastes better. Their sense of smell is sharper. Circulation improves, heart rate and blood pressure drop, and lung function and heart efficiency increase. Ex-smokers can breathe more easily, and their capacity for exercise improves. Many ex-smokers report feeling more energetic and alert. They experience fewer headaches. Even their complexion may improve. Quitting also has a positive effect on long-term disease risk. From the first day without tobacco, ex-smokers begin to decrease their risk of cancer of the lung, larynx, mouth, pancreas, bladder, cervix, and other sites. Risk of heart attack, stroke, and other cardiovascular diseases drops quickly, too.

Since the 1964 Surgeon General's report confirmed the risks of smoking, tobacco use in the United States has steadily declined. There are now about as many ex-smokers in the United States as there are current smokers. To compensate for the loss in revenues, the U.S. tobacco industry, the world's number-one tobacco exporter, has increased its effort to sell to foreign markets, especially those in developing nations. Cigarette exports by U.S. companies have more than tripled since 1980 and now represent a large portion of domestic production. Worldwide, about 1.1 billion people smoke. Smoking currently causes about 4 million deaths per year, but the annual toll is expected to rise to 10 million by 2025, with 70% of the deaths occurring in developing countries. The World Health Organization has expressed particular concern about China, which has more than 300 million smokers, mostly men; by 2050, it's estimated that smoking will kill 3 million Chinese men per year.

Developing countries are particularly vulnerable to the efforts of tobacco companies. They tend to have fewer, if any, restrictions on advertising, and tobacco companies use marketing techniques that have long been banned in the United States. In Poland, for example, cigarette billboards can be found adjacent to elementary schools; in Japan, tobacco ads appear even during children's TV shows. Since the trade embargo with Vietnam ended in 1994, heavily advertised foreign brands have captured 16% of the market there, despite the fact that they cost more than domestic brands. Tobacco critics point to the launch of the Virginia Slims brand in Hong Kong, where less than 2% of women currently smoke, as proof that the industry hopes to create new smokers through advertising.

Developing countries have recently begun to take action against the tobacco companies. China passed a law requiring the printing of tar levels and a health warning on all packs of cigarettes. (Exported cigarettes often lack health warnings, and they typically contain more tar and nicotine than those sold in the United States.) China also banned TV and radio tobacco advertisements and placed limits on smoking in public places. The Thailand Ministry of Public Health proposed regulations requiring companies to reveal the type and amount of all cigarette additives. Several governments, including those of Guatemala, Panama, and British Columbia, have filed suits against the tobacco industry similar to those filed by the U.S. state attorneys general. Despite these efforts, smoking continues to increase globally, and half a billion people now living will die from using tobacco products.

SOURCES: Lopez, A. D. 1998. Counting the dead in China: Measuring tobacco's impact in the developing world. *British Medical Journal* 317(7170): 1399. Headden, S. 1998. The Marlboro man lives! Restrained at home, tobacco firms step up their marketing overseas. *U.S. News & World Report* 125(11): 58–59. Jenkins, C. N. H., et al. 1997. Tobacco use in Vietnam: Prevalence, predictors, and the role of the transnational tobacco corporations. *Journal of the American Medical Association* 277: 1726–1731.

TABLE 11-4	*Benefits of Quitting Smoking*

Within 20 minutes of your last cigarette:
- You stop polluting the air
- Blood pressure drops to normal
- Pulse rate drops to normal
- Temperature of hands and feet increases to normal

8 hours:
- Carbon monoxide level in blood drops to normal
- Oxygen level in blood increases to normal

24 hours:
- Chance of heart attack decreases

48 hours:
- Nerve endings adjust to the absence of nicotine
- Ability to smell and taste things is enhanced

72 hours:
- Bronchial tubes relax, making breathing easier
- Lung capacity increases

2–3 months:
- Circulation improves
- Walking becomes easier
- Lung function increases up to 30%

1–9 months:
- Coughing, sinus congestion, fatigue, and shortness of breath all decrease
- Cilia regrow in lungs, reduce infection
- Body's overall energy level increases

1 year:
- Heart disease death rate is halfway back to that of a nonsmoker

5 years:
- Stroke risk drops nearly to the risk for nonsmokers

10 years:
- Lung cancer death rate drops to 50% of that of continuing smokers
- The incidence of other cancers (mouth, larynx, esophagus, bladder, kidney, and pancreas) decreases

15 years:
- Risk of lung cancer is about 25% of that of continuing smokers
- Risks of heart disease and stroke are close to those for nonsmokers

SOURCES: Will you pay for your past as a smoker? 1998. *Harvard Health Letter,* June. Health Partnership Project/California Medical Association, 1995. Used with permission.

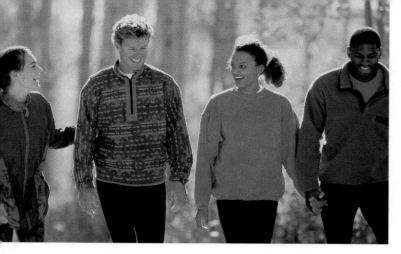

Quitting smoking improves the quality of life. In addition to reducing their long-term disease risks, these ex-smokers have more energy and an improved capacity for exercise.

The younger people are when they stop smoking, the more pronounced the health improvements. And these improvements gradually but invariably increase as the period of nonsmoking lengthens. It's never too late to quit, though. According to a U.S. Surgeon General's report, people who quit smoking, regardless of age, live longer than people who continue to smoke. Even smokers who have already developed chronic bronchitis or emphysema show some improvement when they quit.

Options for Quitting

The 70% of tobacco users who want to quit now have many options. No single method works for everyone, but each does work for some people some of the time. As with any significant change in health-related behavior, giving up tobacco requires planning, sustained effort, and the support of friends and family. It is an ongoing process, not a one-time event. For more on quitting, see the box "Choosing How to Quit" and the Behavior Change Strategy at the end of the chapter.

SUMMARY

- Smoking is the largest preventable cause of ill health and death in the United States. Nevertheless, millions of Americans continue to use tobacco.

Why People Use Tobacco

- Regular tobacco use causes physical dependence on nicotine, characterized by loss of control, tolerance, and withdrawal. Habits can become associated with tobacco use and trigger the urge for a cigarette or other tobacco product.

- People who begin smoking are usually imitating others or responding to seductive advertising. They often deny or minimize the risks of smoking. Smoking is associated with low education level and the use of other drugs.

Health Hazards

- Tobacco smoke is made up of particles of several hundred different chemicals, including some that are carcinogenic or poisonous or that damage or irritate the respiratory system.

- Depending on dosage, nicotine acts on the nervous system as a stimulant or a depressant. Nicotine can cause blood pressure and heart rate to increase, straining the heart.

- Cardiovascular disease is the most widespread cause of death for cigarette smokers. Cigarette smoking has been linked to stroke, aortic aneurysm, and pulmonary heart disease; it is the primary cause of lung cancer; and it is linked to many other cancers.

- Smoking can permanently damage lung function and lead to chronic obstructive lung disease (COLD), emphysema, and chronic bronchitis.

- Cigarette smoking decreases lung function, damages the cilia in the bronchial tubes, and impairs the functioning of macrophages.

- Cigarette smoking is linked to ulcers, impotence, reproductive health problems, dental diseases, and other conditions. Tobacco use leads to lower life expectancy and to a diminished quality of life.

- The use of spit tobacco leads to nicotine addiction and is linked to oral cancers.

- Cigars, pipes, and clove cigarettes are not safe alternatives to cigarettes.

The Effects of Smoking on the Nonsmoker

- Environmental tobacco smoke (ETS) contains high concentrations of toxic chemicals and can cause headaches, eye and nasal irritation, and sinus problems. Long-term exposure to ETS can cause lung cancer and heart disease.

- Infants and young children inhale more air than adults do and therefore take in more pollutants; children whose parents smoke are especially susceptible to respiratory diseases.

- Smoking during pregnancy increases the risk of miscarriage, stillbirth, congenital abnormalities, premature birth, and low birth weight. SIDS and long-term impairments in physical and intellectual development are also risks.

Quitting on Your Own

About 85–95% of smokers who quit do so on their own. Studies of successful ex-smokers have shown that support from others and regular exercise are two factors that improve the chances of success. On the flip side, the more alcohol one drinks, the less successful one will be at quitting smoking. Some people quit "cold turkey," while others taper off more slowly.

Help from the Pharmacy

Nicotine replacement therapy involves supplying the tobacco user with nicotine from a source other than standard tobacco products. It allows a tobacco user to overcome the psychological and behavioral aspects of a tobacco habit without having to simultaneously endure the physical symptoms of nicotine withdrawal. Nicotine replacements are available in chewing gum and skin patches; both products are available without a prescription. Each piece of gum delivers about as much nicotine as one cigarette; each patch delivers a timed dose of nicotine equal to as much as three-quarters of a pack of cigarettes over a 24-hour period. After a few weeks or months, the reforming tobacco user begins to gradually taper off use of the replacement, avoiding withdrawal symptoms. Some brands of nicotine patches come in several strengths to make it easier to gradually decrease the dosage.

There are drawbacks to nicotine replacement therapy. Many people find it difficult to manage the dosage of nicotine while using the gum. Possible side effects include burning sensations in the mouth and throat, nausea, and vomiting; the patch can cause skin irritation, insomnia, nausea, dry mouth, and nervousness. People who continue to smoke while using a nicotine replacement risk nicotine overdose and possibly heart attack. And some people become hooked on the gum or the patch.

Since nicotine replacement therapy deals only with the physical aspects of addiction, it is usually recommended that users combine it with some type of support group or counseling. Studies indicate that the combination of nicotine replacement therapy and behavioral counseling has twice the success rate of replacement therapy alone.

Help from Your Physician

Two additional forms of nicotine replacement therapy are available with a prescription: a nicotine nasal spray and an oral vapor inhaler. One study found that combining the nicotine patch with the nasal spray doubled the chances of success; the spray works quickly and appears to help smokers overcome sudden urges. The inhaler is similar in appearance to a cigarette, but it delivers nicotine slowly via the lining of the mouth. The antidepressant drug Zyban was recently approved for use in smoking cessation: It increases the success rate among quitters and lessens the weight gain sometimes experienced by smokers who quit. Other antidepressants and anti-anxiety drugs are also currently being tested for use in smoking-cessation programs. Your physician may also have resources to share with you that are unique to your community, such as cessation programs, support groups, or a hotline number.

Group Programs

Formal programs are particularly recommended for people who have tried repeatedly to quit on their own without success. The American Cancer Society, the American Lung Association, and the Seventh-Day Adventist Church all offer well-respected smoking-cessation programs. Your college health center or community hospital may also do so. Some programs now are geared specifically to smokeless tobacco users. Although the effectiveness of programs to help adults quit smoking has been mixed, group programs that use nicotine replacement therapy may have success rates as high as 47%.

Each individual method of quitting smoking may be successful for some people, but a combined approach usually has the highest success rate. Plan carefully how you will quit, to maximize your chance of conquering this powerful addiction.

SOURCES: Blondal, T., et al. 1999. Nicotine nasal spray with nicotine patch for smoking cessation. *British Medical Journal* 318(7179) 285–288. American Cancer Society. 1998. *Quitting Smoking* (retrieved November 22, 1998; http://www.cancer.org/tobacco/quitSmok.html). Nicotine patches: A better way to quit smoking? 1992. *Consumer Reports on Health,* September.

- The overall cost of tobacco use to society is high and includes the cost of both medical care and lost worker productivity.

What Can Be Done?

- There are many avenues individuals and groups can take to act against tobacco use. Nonsmokers can use social pressure and legislative channels to discourage smokers from polluting the air and assert their rights to breathe clean air.
- The EPA's report on environmental tobacco smoke strengthened the call to prohibit smoking in public and in the workplace.

- Tobacco companies have recently aimed marketing programs at narrower segments of the population in which smoking is still popular—minorities, the poor, and young women.

How a Tobacco User Can Quit

- Giving up smoking is a difficult and long-term process. Although most ex-smokers quit on their own, some smokers benefit from stop-smoking programs. OTC and prescription medications can ease withdrawal symptoms, and support groups or counseling can help deal with psychological factors.

You can look forward to a longer and healthier life if you join the 44 million Americans who have quit using tobacco. The steps for quitting described below are discussed in terms of the most popular tobacco product in the United States—cigarettes—but they can be adapted for all forms of tobacco use.

Gather Information

Collect personal smoking information in a detailed journal about your smoking behavior. Use your journal to collect two major types of information: cigarettes smoked and smoking urges. Write down the time you smoke each cigarette of the day, the situation you are in, how you feel, and how strong your craving for the cigarette is, plus any other information that seems relevant. Part of the job is to identify patterns of smoking that are connected with routine situations (for example, the coffee break smoke, the after-dinner cigarette, the tension-reduction cigarette). Use this information to discover the behavior patterns involved in your smoking habit.

Make the Decision to Quit

Choose a date in the near future when you expect to be relatively stress-free and can give quitting the energy and attention it will require. Don't choose a date right before or during finals week, for instance. Consider making quitting a gift: Choose your birthday as your quit date, for example, or make quitting a Father's Day or Mother's Day present. You might also want to coordinate your quit date with a buddy—a fellow tobacco user who wants to quit, or a nonsmoker who wants to give up another bad habit or begin an exercise program. Tell your friends and family when you plan to quit. Ask them to offer encouragement and help hold you to your goal.

Decide what approach to quitting will work best for you. Will you go cold turkey, or will you taper off? Will you use nicotine patches or gum? Will you join a support group or enlist the help of a buddy? Prepare a contract for quitting, as discussed in Chapter 1. Set firm dates and rewards, and sign the contract. Post it in a prominent place.

Prepare to Quit

One of the most important things you can do to prepare to quit is to develop and practice nonsmoking relaxation techniques. Many smokers find that they use cigarettes to help them unwind in tense situations or to relax at other times. If this is true for you, you'll need to find and develop effective substi-

tutes. It takes time to become proficient at relaxation techniques, so begin practicing before your quit date. Refer to the detailed discussion of relaxation techniques in Chapter 2.

Other things you can do to help prepare for quitting include the following:

- Make an appointment to see your physician. Ask about OTC and prescription aids for tobacco cessation and whether one or more might be appropriate for you.

- Make a dentist's appointment to have your teeth cleaned the day after your target quit date.

- Start an easy exercise program, if you're not exercising regularly already. Get in the habit of going to bed and getting up at the same time. Don't let yourself become overworked or fall behind at school or on the job.

- Buy some sugarless gum. Stock your kitchen with low-calorie snacks.

- Clean out your car, and air out your house. Send your clothes out for dry cleaning.

- Throw away all your cigarette-related paraphernalia (ashtrays, lighters, etc.).

- The night before your quit day, get rid of all your cigarettes. Have fun with this—get your friends or family to help you tear them up.

- Make your last few days of smoking inconvenient: Smoke only outdoors and when alone. Don't do anything else while you smoke.

Quitting

Your first few days without cigarettes will probably be the most difficult. It's hard to give up such a strongly ingrained habit, but remember that millions of Americans have done it—and you can too. Plan and rehearse the steps you will take when you experience a powerful craving. Avoid or control situations that you know from your journal are powerfully associated with your smoking (see the table). If your hands feel empty without a cigarette, try holding or fiddling with a small object such as a paper clip or pencil.

Social support can also be a big help. Arrange with a buddy to help you with your weak moments, and call him or her whenever you feel overwhelmed by an urge to smoke. Tell people you've just quit. You may discover many inspiring former

---

TAKE ACTION

1. Interview one or two former tobacco users about their experiences with tobacco and the methods they used to quit. Why did they start smoking or using tobacco, how old were they when they started, and how long did their habit continue? What made them decide to quit? How did they quit? What could a current to-

bacco user learn from their experience of quitting?

2. Make a tour of the public facilities in your community and on your campus, such as movie theaters, auditoriums, business and school offices, and classrooms. What kinds of restrictions on smoking do these

smokers who can encourage you and reassure you that it's possible to quit and lead a happier, healthier life.

Maintaining Nonsmoking

Maintaining nonsmoking over time is the ultimate goal of any stop-smoking program. The lingering smoking urges that remain once you've quit should be carefully tracked and controlled because they can cause relapses if left unattended. Keep track of these urges in your journal to help you deal with them. If certain situations still trigger the urge for a cigarette, change something about the situation to break past associations. If stress or boredom causes strong smoking urges, use a relaxation technique, take a brisk walk, have a stick of gum, or substitute some other activity for smoking.

Don't set yourself up for a relapse. If you allow yourself to get overwhelmed at school or work or to gain weight, it will be easier to convince yourself that now isn't the right time to quit.

This is the right time. Continue to practice time-management and relaxation techniques. Exercise regularly, eat sensibly, and get enough sleep. These habits will not only ensure your success at remaining tobacco-free, but they will also serve you well in stressful times throughout your life.

Watch out for patterns of thinking that can make nonsmoking more difficult. Focus on the positive aspects of not smoking, and give yourself lots of praise—you deserve it. Stick with the schedule of rewards you developed for your contract.

Keep track of the emerging benefits that come from having quit. Items that might appear on your list include improved stamina, an increased sense of pride at having kicked a strong addiction, a sharper sense of taste and smell, no more smoker's cough, and so on. Keep track of the money you're saving by not smoking, and spend it on things you really enjoy. And if you do lapse, be gentle with yourself. Lapses are a normal part of quitting. Forgive yourself, and pick up where you left off.

Strategies for Dealing with High-Risk Smoking Situations

Cues and High-Risk Situations	Suggested Strategies
Awakening in morning	Brush your teeth as soon as you wake up. Stay busy, and try not to think about smoking.
Drinking coffee	Do something else with your hands. Drink tea or another beverage instead.
Eating meals	Eat in a different location. Sit in nonsmoking sections of restaurants. Get up from the table right away after eating, and start another activity. Brush your teeth right after eating.
Driving a car	Have the car cleaned when you quit smoking. Chew sugarless gum or eat a low-calorie snack. Take public transportation or ride your bike.
Socializing with friends who smoke	Suggest nonsmoking events (movies, theatre, shopping). Tell them you've quit and ask them not to smoke around you, offer you cigarettes, or give you cigarettes if you ask for them.
Drinking at a bar, restaurant, or party	Try to take a nonsmoker with you, or associate with nonsmokers. Let friends know you've just quit. Moderate your intake of alcohol (it can weaken your resolve).
Encountering stressful situations	Practice relaxation techniques. Take some deep breaths. Get out of your room or house. Go somewhere that doesn't allow smoking. Take a shower, chew gum, call a friend, or exercise.

SOURCE: Strategies adapted with permission from *Postgraduate Medicine* 90(1), July 1991.

places have? In your opinion, are they appropriate? If you feel more or different restrictions are in order, write a letter to the editor of your school or local newspaper, and state your case. Support it with convincing arguments and appropriate facts.

3.   Plan what you will say or do the next time you want to ask a smoker to stop smoking around you. Draw up a list of statements you might make to a smoker in various situations. You'll increase the effectiveness of your statements if they are courteous and don't threaten the person's dignity. Practice saying these statements in a way that is assertive rather than aggressive or passive. The next time you're in an appropriate situation, use one of your statements. If it doesn't have the desired effect, think about why, and modify it for the next time.

1. **_Critical Thinking_** Examine advertisements for cigarettes and smokeless tobacco products. What markets are they targeting? How do they try to appeal to their audience? How do the advertisers deal with the mandatory warning labels? Write a short essay describing your findings.

2. **_Critical Thinking_** Restrictions on smoking are increasing in our society. Do you think they're fair? Do they infringe on people's rights? Do they go too far or not far enough? Write a brief essay stating your position on smoking restrictions. Be sure to explain your reasoning. What are the most important factors in your decision? Why do you think you have the opinion you do?

3. **_Critical Thinking_** Research the roles the U.S. government plays in tobacco use and sales. Describe these roles and their effects. Do you think the government is acting appropriately? In your opinion, what role should the government have regarding tobacco use and sales?

FOR MORE INFORMATION

Books

American Council on Science and Health. 1997. _Cigarettes: What the Warning Label Doesn't Tell You: A Comprehensive Guide to the Health Consequences of Smoking._ New York: Prometheus Books. _A detailed look at the known health threats of smoking._

Brigham, J. 1998. _Dying to Quit: Why We Smoke and How We Stop._ Washington, D.C.: National Academy Press. _A discussion of the process and nature of nicotine addiction from both the scientific and personal perspectives._

Glantz, S. A. 1998. _The Cigarette Papers._ Berkeley, Calif.: University of California Press. _Surveys 30 years' worth of internal tobacco industry documents, showing that the industry has long known that smoking is addictive and causes disease._

Pringle, P. 1998. _Cornered: Tobacco Companies at the Bar of Justice._ New York: Henry Holt. _A review of the events leading up to the lawsuits against the major tobacco companies._

Self-help books designed to help smokers quit:

Allison, P., and J. Yost. 1999. _Hooked But Not Helpless, Kicking Nicotine Addiction,_ 3rd ed. Portland, Or.: BridgeCity Bks.

American Lung Association. 1998. _7 Steps to a Smoke-Free Life._ New York: Wiley.

Rustin, T. A. 1996. _Quit and Stay Quit: A Personal Program to Stop Smoking._ Center City, Minn.: Hazelden.

Stevic-Rust, L., and A. Maximin. 1996. _The Stop-Smoking Workbook._ Oakland, Calif.: New Harbinger.

Organizations, Hotlines, and Web Sites

Action on Smoking and Health (ASH). An advocacy group that provides statistics, news briefs, and other information.
202-659-4310
http://ash.org

American Cancer Society (ACS). Sponsor of the annual Great American Smokeout; provides information on the dangers of tobacco, as well as tools for prevention and cessation for both smokers and users of spit tobacco.
1599 Clifton Rd., N.E.
Atlanta, GA 30329
800-ACS-2345
http://www.cancer.org

American Lung Association. Provides information on lung diseases, tobacco control, and environmental health.
1740 Broadway
New York, NY 10019-4374
800-LUNG-USA; 212-315-8700
http://www.lungusa.org

CDC's Tobacco Information and Prevention Source (TIPS). Provides research results, educational materials, and tips on how to quit smoking; Web site includes special sections for kids and teens.
800-CDC-1311; 770-488-5701
http://www.cdc.gov/nccdphp/osh

Environmental Protection Agency Indoor Air Quality/ETS. Provides information and links about secondhand smoke.
800-438-4318
http://www.epa.gov/iaq/ets.html

Nicotine Anonymous. A 12-step program for tobacco users.
http://www.nicotine-anonymous.org

Quitnet. Provides interactive tools and questionnaires, support groups, a library, news on tobacco issues, and quitting programs for both smokers and spit tobacco users.
http://www.quitnet.org

Smokescreen Action Network. Sponsored by an advocacy group for tobacco control, a Web site that provides news and information on congressional representatives' voting records on tobacco-related issues and opportunities to send letters.
http://www.Smokescreen.org

Tobacco BBS. A resource center on tobacco and smoking issues that includes news and information, assistance for smokers who want to quit, and links to related sites.
http://www.tobacco.org

Tobacco Control Resource Center and Tobacco Products Liability Project (TPLP). Provides current information about tobacco-related court cases and legislation; based at the Northeastern School of Law.
http://www.tobacco.neu.edu

World Health Organization Tobacco Free Initiative. Promotes the goal of a tobacco-free world.
http://www.who.int/toh

See also the listings for Chapters 9, 15, and 16.

Action on Smoking and Health. 1998. *Poll Shows Smokers Want to Quit* (retrieved November 22, 1998; http://ash.org/oct98/10-21-98.html).

American Cancer Society. 1999. *Cancer Facts and Figures.* Atlanta, Ga.: American Cancer Society.

American Cancer Society. 1998. *Quitting Smokeless Tobacco* (retrieved November 22, 1998; http://www.cancer.org/tobacco/quitDip.html).

American Lung Association. 1998. *Quit Smoking Action Plan* (retrieved September 10, 1998; http://www.lungusa.org/partner/quit/index.html).

American Medical Association. 1998. *Briefing Assessment of the Multi-State Tobacco Settlement Proposal* (retrieved November 19, 1998; http://www.ama-assn.org/advocacy/statemnt/981117.htm).

Ayanian, J. Z., and P. D. Cleary. 1999. Perceived risk of heart disease and cancer among cigarette smokers. *Journal of the American Medical Association* 281: 1019–1021.

Boffetta P., et al. 1998. Multicenter case-control study of exposure to environmental tobacco smoke and lung cancer in Europe. *Journal of the National Cancer Institute* 90(19): 1440–1450.

Brennan, P. A., E. R. Grekin, and S. A. Mednick. 1999. Maternal smoking during pregnancy and adult male criminal outcomes. *Archives of General Psychiatry* 56(3): 215–219.

Caraballo, R., et al. 1998. Racial and ethnic differences in serum cotinine levels of cigarette smokers. *Journal of the American Medical Association* 280: 135–139.

Centers for Disease Control and Prevention. 1999. Preemptive state tobacco-control laws—United States, 1982–1998. *Morbidity and Mortality Weekly Report* 47(51): 1112–1114.

Dejin-Karlsson, E., et al. 1998. Does passive smoking in early pregnancy increase the risk of small-for-gestational-age infants? *American Journal of Public Health* 88: 1523–1527.

Distefan, J. M., et al. 1999. Do movie stars encourage adolescents to start smoking? Evidence from California. *Preventive Medicine* 28(1): 1–11.

Gergen, P. J., et al. 1998. The burden of environmental tobacco smoke exposure on the respiratory health of children 2 months through 5 years of age in the United States. *Pediatrics.* 101(2): E8 (retrieved November 22, 1998; http://www.pediatrics.org/cgi/content/full/101/2/e8).

Goldstein, A. O., R.A. Sobel, and G. R. Newman. 1999. Tobacco and alcohol use in G-rated children's animated films. *Journal of the American Medical Association* 281: 1131–1136.

He, Jiang, et al. 1999. Passive smoking and the risk of coronary heart disease. A meta-analysis of epidemiologic studies. *New England Journal of Medicine* 340(12): 920–926.

Howard, G., et al. 1998. Cigarette smoking and progression of atherosclerosis. *Journal of the American Medical Association* 279(2): 119–124.

Jorenby, D. E., et al. 1999. A controlled trial of sustained-release bupropion, a nicotine patch, or both for smoking cessation. *New England Journal of Medicine* 340(9): 685–691.

Klesges, R. C., et al. 1998. The prospective relationship between smoking and weight in a young, biracial cohort. *Journal of Consulting and Clinical Psychology* 66(6): 987–993.

Kozlowski, L. T., et al. 1999. Filter ventilation and nicotine content of tobacco in cigarettes from Canada, the United Kingdom, and the United States. *Tobacco Control* 7(4): 369.

Kyrklund-Blombert, N. B., and S. Cnattingius. 1998. Preterm birth and maternal smoking. *American Journal of Obstetrics and Gynecology* 179(4): 1051–1055.

Lackmann, G. M., et al. 1999. Metabolites of a tobacco-specific carcinogen in urine from newborns. *Journal of the National Cancer Institute* 91(5): 459–465.

Mascola, M. A., et al. 1998. Exposure of young infants to environmental tobacco smoke: Breast-feeding among smoking mothers. *American Journal of Public Health* 88(6): 893–896.

Minami, J., T. Ishimitsu, and H. Matsuoka. 1999. Effects of smoking cessation on blood pressure and heart rate variability in habitual smokers. *Hypertension* 33(1 Pt 2): 586–590.

National Association of Attorneys General. 1998. *Tobacco Settlement Summary* (retrieved November 20, 1998; http://naag.org/glance.htm).

National Cancer Institute. 1998. *Cigars: Health Effects and Trends.* Smoking and Tobacco Control Monograph No. 9. Washington, D.C.: National Cancer Institute.

Ness, R. B., et al. 1999. Cocaine and tobacco use and the risk of spontaneous abortion. *New England Journal of Medicine* 340(5): 333–339.

Pérez-Stable, E. J., et al. 1998. Nicotine metabolism and intake in black and white smokers. *Journal of the American Medical Association* 280: 152–156.

Public Citizen. 1998. *Blowing Smoke: Big Tobacco's 1998 Congressional Lobbying Expenses Skyrocket* (retrieved November 25, 1998; http://www.citizen.org/tobacco/oct98lobby.htm).

Rubes, J., et al. 1998. Smoking cigarettes is associated with increased sperm disomy in teenage men. *Fertility and Sterility* 70(4): 715–723.

Santo-Tomas, M., et al. 1999. *Debunking the Yuppie Habit: Cigars and Endothelial Function.* Presented at the American College of Cardiology 48th Annual Scientific Session (retrieved March 27, 1999; http://ex2.excerptamedica.com/99acc/abstracts/abs1042-71.html).

Seductive cigars: New ways to addict the next generation. 1998. *Consumer Reports,* May.

U.S. Department of Health and Human Services. 1998. *Tobacco Use Among U.S. Racial/Ethnic Minority Groups: A Report of the Surgeon General.* Washington, D.C.: U.S. Department of Health and Human Services.

U.S. Federal Trade Commission. 1999. *1999 Smokeless Tobacco Report.* Washington, D.C.: Federal Trade Commission.

Walsh, M. M., et al. 1999. Smokeless tobacco cessation intervention for college athletes: Results after 1 year. *American Journal of Public Health* 89(2): 228–234.

Wechsler, H., et al. 1998. Increased levels of cigarette use among college students. A cause for national concern. *Journal of the American Medical Association* 280: 1673–1678.

Windham, G. C., et al. 1999. Cigarette smoking and effects on menstrual function. *Obstetrics and Gynecology* 93(1): 59–65.

Windham, G. C., et al. 1999. Exposure to environmental and mainstream tobacco smoke and risk of spontaneous abortion. *American Journal of Epidemiology* 149(3): 243–247.

World Health Organization. 1998. *Passive Smoking Does Cause Lung Cancer* (retrieved November 28, 1998; http://www.who.int/inf-pr-1998/en/pr98-29.html).

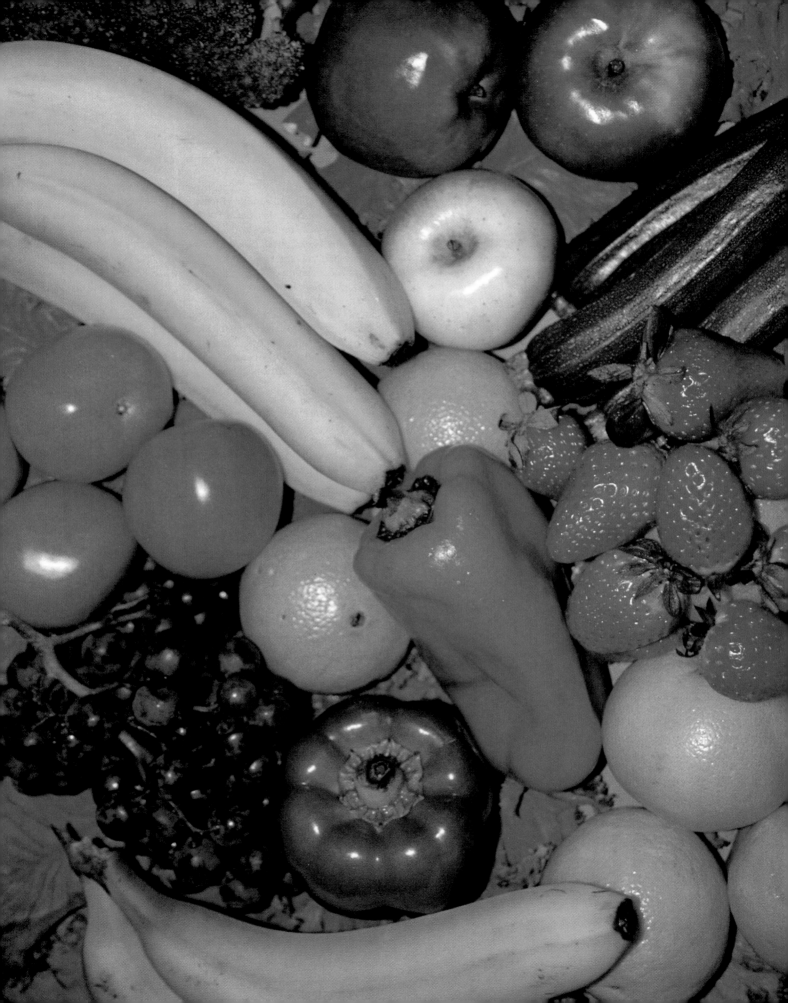

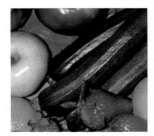

LEARNING OBJECTIVES

After reading this chapter, you should be able to:

- List the essential nutrients, and describe the functions they perform in the body.

- Describe the Dietary Reference Intakes, Food Guide Pyramid, and Dietary Guidelines for Americans.

- Discuss nutritional guidelines for vegetarians and for special population groups.

- Explain how to use food labels to make informed choices about foods.

- Put together a personal nutrition plan based on affordable foods that you enjoy and that will promote wellness, today as well as in the future.

Nutrition Basics

12

TEST YOUR KNOWLEDGE

1. It is recommended that all adults consume one to two servings each of fruits and vegetables every day.
   True or false?

2. Three ounces of chicken or meat, the amount considered to be one serving, is approximately the size of which of the following?
   a. a domino
   b. a deck of cards
   c. a small paperback book

3. Where does most of the sodium in the American diet come from?
   a. It is added during cooking or at the table.
   b. It occurs naturally in foods.
   c. It is found in processed foods such as soups and frozen dinners.

4. The recommended limit for daily fat intake is the equivalent of 10 tablespoons of fat.
   True or false?

5. Which of the following is the best source of fiber?
   a. 1 cup of pinto beans
   b. a baked potato with the skin
   c. 1 cup of raspberries

Answers

1. False. A minimum of five servings per day—two of fruits and three of vegetables—is recommended. The majority of Americans fail to meet this goal; and half of all the vegetables we *do* eat are potatoes—and half of those are french fried.

2. b. Many people underestimate the size of the servings they eat, leading to overconsumption of calories and fat.

3. c. 75% of the sodium Americans consume is from processed foods; 15% is added during cooking or at the table; the remaining 10% occurs naturally in foods.

4. False. No more than 30% of total daily calories should come from fat—the equivalent of 65 grams or 4.5 tablespoons of fat per day in a 2000-calorie diet. This total includes fat found naturally in foods and fat added to foods as butter, salad dressing, and so on.

5. a. All three are good sources of fiber, but pinto beans win the prize with 9 grams. A cup of raspberries has 6 grams; a baked potato has 5 grams.

In your lifetime, you'll spend about 6 years eating—about 70,000 meals and 60 tons of food. What you choose to eat can have profound effects on your health and well-being. Of particular concern is the connection between lifetime nutritional habits and the risk of major chronic diseases, including heart disease, cancer, stroke, and diabetes. Choosing foods that provide adequate amounts of the nutrients you need, while avoiding the substances linked to disease, should be an important part of your daily life. The food choices you make will significantly influence your health—both now and in the future.

Choosing a healthy diet that supports maximum wellness and protects against disease is a two-part project. First, you have to know which nutrients are necessary and in what amounts. Second, you have to translate those requirements into a diet consisting of foods you like to eat that are both available and affordable. Once you have an idea of what constitutes a healthy diet for you, you may want to make adjustments in your current diet to bring it into line with your goals.

This chapter provides the basic principles of **nutrition.** It introduces the six classes of essential nutrients, explaining their role in the functioning of the body. It also provides different sets of guidelines that you can use to design a healthy diet plan. Finally, it offers practical tools and advice to help you apply the guidelines to your own life. Diet is an area of your life in which you have almost total control. Using your knowledge and understanding of nutrition to create a healthy diet plan is a significant step toward wellness.

NUTRITIONAL REQUIREMENTS: COMPONENTS OF A HEALTHY DIET

When you think about your diet, you probably do so in terms of the foods you like to eat—a turkey sandwich and a glass of milk, or a steak and a baked potato. What's important for your health, though, are the nutrients contained in those foods. Your body requires proteins, fats, carbohydrates, vitamins, minerals, and water—about 45 **essential nutrients.** The word *essential* in this context means that you must get these substances from food because your body is unable to manufacture them at all, or at least not fast enough to meet your physiological needs. Plants use energy from the sun to convert chemicals from the air, water, and soil into all the complex chemicals they need. Animals, including humans, must eat foods to obtain the nutrients necessary to keep their bodies growing and functioning properly. Your body obtains these nutrients through the process of **digestion,** in which the foods you eat are broken down into compounds your gastrointestinal tract can absorb and your body can use (Figure 12-1). A diet containing adequate amounts of all essential nutrients is vital because various nutrients provide energy, help build and maintain body tissues, and help regulate body functions.

The energy in foods is expressed as **kilocalories.** One kilocalorie represents the amount of heat it takes to raise the temperature of 1 liter of water 1°C. A person needs about 2000 kilocalories per day to meet his or her energy needs. In common usage, people usually refer to kilocalories as *calories,* which is a much smaller energy unit: 1 kilocalorie contains 1000 calories. We'll use the familiar word *calorie* in this chapter to stand for the larger energy unit.

Three classes of nutrients supply energy: protein, carbohydrates, and fats. Alcohol, though it is not an essential nutrient and has no nutritional value, also supplies energy. Fats provide the most energy, at 9 calories per gram; protein and carbohydrates each provide 4 calories per gram. The high caloric content of fat is one reason experts continually advise against high fat consumption; most of us do not need the extra calories. Alcohol provides 7 calories per gram. And although alcohol has no general nutritional role, alcoholic beverages are a major calorie contributor to the American diet.

But just meeting energy needs is not enough; our bodies require adequate amounts of all the essential nutrients to grow and function properly. Practically all foods contain mixtures of nutrients, although foods are commonly classified according to the predominant nutrient; for example, spaghetti is thought of as a "carbohydrate" food. Let's take a closer look at the function and sources of each class of nutrients.

Proteins—The Basis of Body Structure

Proteins form important parts of the body's main structural components: muscles and bones. Proteins also form important parts of blood, enzymes, some hormones, and cell membranes. As mentioned above, proteins can provide energy for the body (4 calories per gram).

Amino Acids   The building blocks of proteins are called **amino acids.** Twenty common amino acids are found in food; nine of these are essential: histidine, isoleucine, leucine, lysine, methionine, phenylalanine, threonine, tryptophan, and valine. The other 11 amino acids can be produced by the body, given the presence of the needed components supplied by foods.

Complete and Incomplete Proteins   Individual protein sources are considered "complete" if they supply all the essential amino acids in adequate amounts and "incomplete" if they do not. Meat, fish, poultry, eggs, milk, cheese, and other foods from animal sources provide complete proteins. Incomplete proteins, which come from plant sources such as **legumes** and nuts, are good sources of most essential amino acids, but are usually low in one or two. Combining two vegetable proteins, such as wheat and peanuts in a peanut butter sandwich, allows each vegetable protein to make up for the amino acids missing in

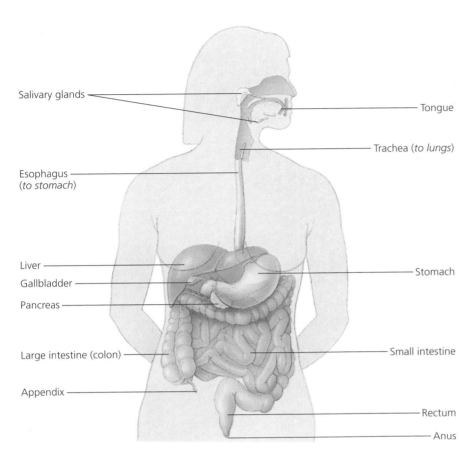

Salivary glands

Tongue

Trachea (*to lungs*)

Esophagus
(*to stomach*)

Liver

Stomach

Gallbladder

Pancreas

Large intestine (colon)

Small intestine

Appendix

Rectum

Anus

Figure 12-1 The digestive system. Food is partially broken down by being chewed and mixed with saliva in the mouth. As food moves through the digestive tract, it is mixed by muscular contractions and broken down by chemicals. After traveling to the stomach via the esophagus, food is broken down further by stomach acids. Most absorption of nutrients occurs in the small intestine, aided by secretions from the pancreas, gallbladder, and intestinal lining. The large intestine reabsorbs excess water; the remaining solid wastes are collected in the rectum and excreted through the anus.

the other protein. The combination yields a complete protein. Your concern with amino acids and complete protein in your diet should focus on what you consume throughout the day, rather that at each meal. It was once believed that vegetarians had to "complement" their proteins at each meal in order to receive the benefit of a complete protein. It is now known, however, that proteins consumed throughout the course of the day can complement each other to form a pool of amino acids the body can draw from to produce the necessary proteins. (Healthy vegetarian diets are discussed later in the chapter.)

Recommended Protein Intake The leading sources of protein in the American diet are (1) beef, steaks, and roasts; (2) hamburger and meatloaf; (3) white bread, rolls, and crackers; (4) milk, and (5) pork. About two-thirds of the protein in the American diet comes from animal sources; therefore, the American diet is rich in amino acids. Most Americans consume more protein than they need each day. Protein consumed beyond what the body needs is synthesized into fat for energy storage or burned for energy requirements. Consuming somewhat above our needs is not harmful, but it does contribute fat to the diet because protein-rich foods are often fat-rich as well. The amount of protein you eat should represent about 10–15% of your total daily calorie intake (Figure 12-2).

Fats—Essential in Small Amounts

Fats, also known as lipids, are the most concentrated source of energy, at 9 calories per gram. The fats stored in your body represent usable energy; they help insulate your body, and they support and cushion your organs. Fats in the diet help your body absorb fat-soluble vitamins, as well as add important flavor and texture to foods.

TERMS

nutrition   The science of food and how the body uses it in health and disease.

essential nutrients   Substances the body must get from foods because it cannot manufacture them at all or fast enough to meet its needs. These nutrients include proteins, fats, carbohydrates, vitamins, minerals, and water.

digestion   The process of breaking down foods in the gastrointestinal tract into compounds the body can absorb.

kilocalorie   A measure of energy content in food; 1 kilocalorie represents the amount of heat needed to raise the temperature of 1 liter of water 1°C; commonly referred to as *calorie*.

protein   An essential nutrient; a compound made of amino acids that contains carbon, hydrogen, oxygen, and nitrogen.

amino acids   The building blocks of proteins.

legumes   Vegetables such as peas and beans that are high in fiber and are also important sources of protein.

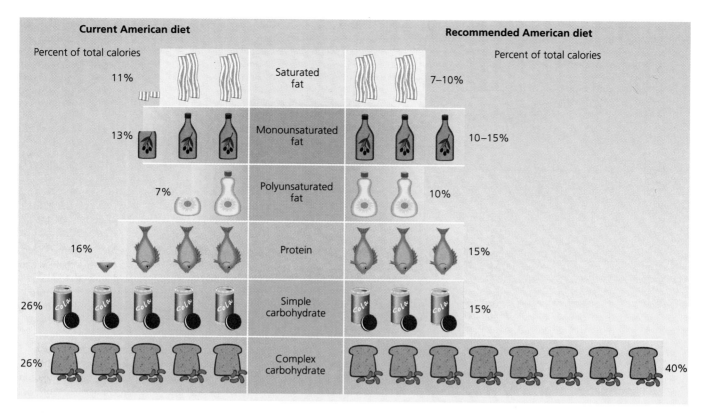

Percent of total calories

Recommended American diet

Percent of total calories

Current %	Category	Recommended %
11%	Saturated fat	7–10%
13%	Monounsaturated fat	10–15%
7%	Polyunsaturated fat	10%
16%	Protein	15%
26%	Simple carbohydrate	15%
26%	Complex carbohydrate	40%

VITAL STATISTICS

Figure 12-2 The current versus the recommended American diet. Health experts recommend that we consume 55% of total daily calories as carbohydrate, 15% as protein, and no more than 30% as fat.

Fats are the major fuel for the body during rest and light activity. Two fats—linoleic acid and alpha-linolenic acid —are essential components of the diet. They are key to the regulation of body functions, such as the maintenance of blood pressure and the progress of a healthy pregnancy.

Types and Sources of Fats Most of the fats in food are in the form of triglycerides, which are composed of a glyceral molecule (an alcohol) plus three fatty acids. A fatty acid is made up of a chain of carbon atoms with oxygen attached at the end and hydrogen atoms attached along the length of the chain. Fatty acids differ in the length of their carbon atom chains and in their degree of saturation (the number of hydrogens attached to the chain). If every available bond from each carbon atom in a fatty acid chain is attached to a hydrogen atom, the fatty acid is said to be **saturated** (Figure 12-3). If not all the available bonds are taken up by hydrogens, the carbon atoms in the chain will form double bonds with each other. Such fatty acids are called unsaturated fats. If there is only one double bond, the fatty acid is called **monounsaturated.** If there are two or more double bonds, the fatty acid is called **polyunsaturated.** The essential fatty

acids, linoleic and alpha-linolenic acids, are both polyunsaturated. The different types of fatty acids have different characteristics and different effects on your health.

Food fats are often composed of both saturated and unsaturated fatty acids; the dominant type of fatty acid determines the fat's characteristics. Food fats containing large amounts of saturated fatty acids are usually solid at room temperature; they are generally found in animal products. The leading sources of saturated fat in the American diet are unprocessed animal flesh (hamburger, steak, roasts), whole milk, cheese, hot dogs, and lunch meats. Food fats containing large amounts of monounsaturated and polyunsaturated fatty acids are usually from plant sources and are liquid at room temperature. Olive, canola, and peanut oils contain mostly monounsaturated fatty acids. Sunflower, corn, and safflower oils contain mostly polyunsaturated fatty acids.

There are notable exceptions to these generalizations. When unsaturated vegetable oils undergo the process of **hydrogenation,** a mixture of saturated and unsaturated fatty acids is produced. Hydrogenation turns many of the double bonds in unsaturated fatty acids into single bonds, increasing the degree of saturation and producing a more solid fat from a liquid oil. Hydrogenation also produces

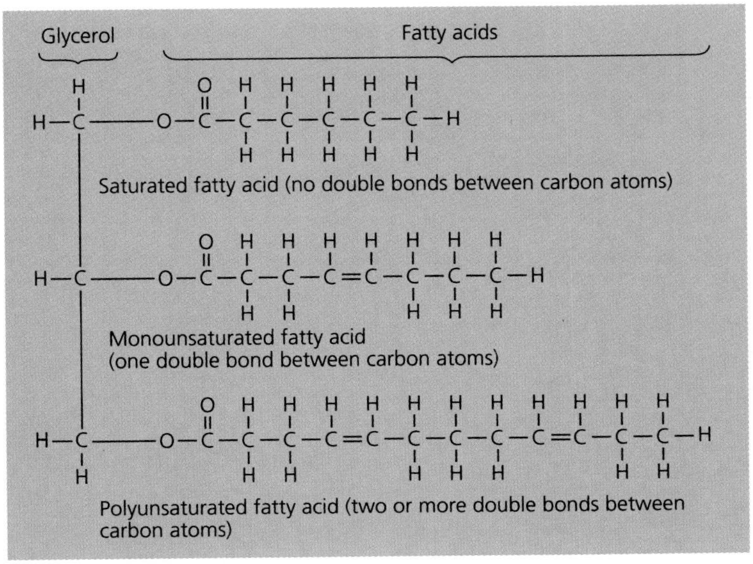

Figure 12-3 Chemical structures of saturated and unsaturated fatty acids. This example of a triglyceride consists of a molecule of glycerol with three fatty acids attached. Fatty acids can differ in the length of their carbon chains and their degree of saturation. SOURCE: Fahey, T. D., P. M. Insel, and W. T. Roth. 1999. *Fit and Well: Core Concepts and Labs in Physical Fitness and Wellness,* 3rd ed. Mountain View, Calif.: Mayfield.

trans fatty acids, unsaturated fatty acids with an atypical shape that affects their behavior during cooking and in the body. Food manufacturers use hydrogenation to increase the stability of an oil so it can be reused for deep frying; to improve the texture of certain foods (to make pastries and pie crusts flakier, for example); to keep oil from separating out of peanut butter; and to extend the shelf life of foods made with oil. Hydrogenation is also used to transform a liquid oil into margarine or vegetable shortening.

Many baked and fried foods are prepared with hydrogenated vegetable oils, so they can be relatively high in saturated and trans fatty acids. Leading sources of trans fats in the American diet are deep-fried fast foods such as french fries and fried chicken (typically fried in vegetable shortening rather than oil); baked and snack foods such as pot pies, cakes, cookies, pastries, doughnuts, and chips; and stick margarine. In general, the more solid a hydrogenated oil is, the more saturated and trans fats it contains; for example, stick margarines typically contain more saturated and trans fats than do tub or squeeze margarines. Small amounts of trans fatty acids are found naturally in meat and milk.

Hydrogenated vegetable oils are not the only plant fats that contain saturated fats. Palm and coconut oils, although derived from plants, are also highly saturated. On the other hand, fish oils, derived from an animal source, are rich in polyunsaturated fats.

Recommended Fat Intake You need only about 1 tablespoon (15 grams) of vegetable oil per day incorporated into your diet to supply the essential fats. The average American diet supplies considerably more than this amount; in fact, fats make up about 33% of our calorie intake. (This is the equivalent of about 75 grams, or 5 tablespoons, of fat per day.) Health experts recommend that we reduce our fat intake to 30%, but not less than 10%, of total daily calories, with less than 10% coming from saturated fat (see Figure 12-2). Among Americans, total fat consumption expressed as a percent of total calories has dropped steadily since 1965. However, some of this decline has been due to an *increase* in total calorie intake rather than a *decrease* in fat intake. Since 1990, total fat consumption in terms of weight (grams) has actually increased for many groups of Americans. The fat content of many common foods is given in Figure 12-4; the box "Setting Goals for Fat, Protein, and Carbohydrate Intake" explains how to set a daily goal for fat consumption.

Fats and Health Different types of fats have very different effects on health. Many studies have examined the effects of dietary fat intake on blood **cholesterol** levels

saturated fat A fat with no carbon-carbon double bonds; solid at room temperature.

monounsaturated fat A fat with one carbon-carbon double bond; liquid at room temperature.

polyunsaturated fat A fat containing two or more carbon-carbon double bonds; liquid at room temperature.

hydrogenation A process by which hydrogens are added to unsaturated fats, increasing the degree of saturation and turning liquid oils into solid fats. Hydrogenation produces a mixture of saturated fatty acids and standard and trans forms of unsaturated fatty acids.

trans fatty acid A type of unsaturated fatty acid produced during the process of hydrogenation; trans fats have an atypical shape that affects their chemical activity.

cholesterol A waxy substance found in the blood and cells and implicated in heart disease.

TERMS

	0–10%	10–30%	30–50%	50–75%	75–100%
Breads, cereals, rice, and pasta	Many dry cereals and breads, rice, pasta, tortillas, pretzels	Plain popcorn, hot cereals, some breads	Granola, buttered popcorn, crackers, biscuits, muffins	Croissants	
Vegetables and fruits	Most fresh, frozen, canned, and dried fruits and vegetables		French fries, onion rings	Potato chips, coconut	Avocado, olives
Milk, yogurt, and cheese	Fat-free milk, yogurt, and cottage cheese	Lowfat cottage cheese and yogurt, lowfat (1%) and reduced fat (2%) milk, buttermilk	Whole milk, regular ice cream	Most cheeses, rich ice cream	Half and half, cream cheese, sour cream, heavy cream
Meat, poultry, fish, dry beans, eggs, nuts	Skinless turkey breast, haddock, cod, most dry beans, egg whites	Skinless white meat chicken, halibut, shrimp, clams, tuna in water, red snapper, trout, lowfat tofu	Beef top round, broiled steak, ham, skinless dark meat poultry, salmon, mackerel, swordfish	Roast beef; ground chuck; pork, lamb, and veal chops; poultry with skin; tuna in oil; regular tofu; eggs	Salami, bacon, hot dogs, spare ribs, most nuts and seeds, peanut butter, egg yolks
Combination foods	Clear soup (bouillon)	Most broth-based soups; vegetarian chili	Hamburger, lasagna, chili with meat, potato salad, vegetable and cheese pizza, macaroni and cheese, enchilada	Cheeseburger; meat pizza; large meat, poultry, or cheese sandwich; taco salad	
Fats, oils, and sweets	Hard candy, chewing gum			Chocolate bars	Butter, margarine, vegetable oil, mayonnaise, salad dressing

Figure 12-4 **Percent of total calories from fat for selected foods.**

and the risk of heart disease. Saturated and trans fatty acids appear to raise blood levels of **low-density lipoprotein (LDL),** or "bad" cholesterol, thereby increasing a person's risk of heart disease. Unsaturated fatty acids, on the other hand, lower LDL. Monounsaturated fatty acids, such as those found in olive and canola oils, may also increase levels of **high-density lipoproteins (HDL),** or "good" cholesterol, providing even greater benefits for heart health. In large amounts, trans fatty acids may lower HDL. Thus, to reduce the risk of heart disease, it is important to substitute unsaturated fats for saturated and trans fats. (See Chapter 15 for more on cholesterol and a heart-healthy diet.)

Most Americans consume more saturated fat than trans fat (11% versus 2–4% of total calories). The best way to reduce saturated fat in your diet is to lower your intake of meat and full-fat dairy products (whole milk, cream, butter, cheese, ice cream). Saturated fats are listed on the nutrition label of prepared foods. Trans fats are not, but you can check for the presence of hydrogenated oils on the ingredient list. If "partially hydrogenated" oils or fats or "vegetable shortening" appears near the top of the list, the product may be high in trans fats.

To lower trans fats, decrease your intake of deep-fried foods and baked goods made with hydrogenated vegetable oils; use liquid oils rather than margarine; and favor tub or squeeze margarines or those labeled low-trans or trans-free over standard stick margarines. (Remember, the softer or more liquid a fat is, the less satu-

rated and trans fat it is likely to contain.) Some trans-free margarines contain plant sterols, compounds that may actually lower cholesterol levels.

Research has indicated that certain forms of polyunsaturated fatty acids—known as **omega-3 fatty acids** and found primarily in fish—may have a particularly positive effect on cardiovascular health. If the endmost double bond of a polyunsaturated fat occurs three carbons from the end of the fatty acid chain, an omega-3 form is produced. (The polyunsaturated fatty acid shown in Figure 12-3 is an omega-3 form.) If the endmost double bond occurs at the sixth carbon atom, an omega-6 form is produced. Most of the polyunsaturated fats currently consumed by Americans are omega-6 forms, primarily from corn oil and soybean oil. However, the consumption of omega-3 fatty acids reduces the tendency of blood to clot, decreases inflammatory responses, raises levels of HDL, and may lower the risk of heart disease in some people. Because of these benefits, nutritionists recommend that Americans increase the proportion of omega-3 polyunsaturated fats in their diet by eating fish two or more times a week. Mackerel, herring, salmon, halibut, sardines, anchovies, tuna, and trout are all good sources of omega-3 fatty acids. Lesser amounts are found in plant sources, including green leafy vegetables and walnut, canola, linseed (flax), and soybean oils.

Dietary fat can affect health in other ways. Diets high in fatty red meat are associated with an increased risk of

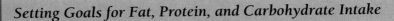

Setting Daily Goals

To meet the recommendations for nutrient intakes, start by setting some overall daily goals.

1. Determine approximately how many calories you consume each day. Depending on your activity level, daily needs range from about 2200 to 3500 calories for men and from about 1600 to 2500 for women.

2. Set percentage goals or limits for your intake of fat, protein, and carbohydrate. Those recommended for the general public are 30% or less of total daily calories from fat, 15% of total daily calories from protein, and 55% of total daily calories from carbohydrate. If your diet already meets these goals, you may want to set more challenging marks, such as raising your daily carbohydrate consumption to 60% of total calories.

3. Change your limits or goals from percentages to grams for easy tracking. A person who eats about 2200 calories per day could calculate her or his goals as follows:

Fat: 2200 calories per day × 30% = 660 calories of fat per day

660 calories ÷ 9 calories per gram = **73 g of fat per day**

Protein: 2200 calories per day × 15% = 330 calories of protein per day

330 calories ÷ 4 calories per gram = **83 g of protein per day**

Carbohydrate: 2200 calories per day × 55% = 1210 calories of carbohydrate per day

1210 calories ÷ 4 calories per gram = **303 g of carbohydrate per day**

(Remember, there are 9 calories per gram of fat and 4 calories per gram of protein and carbohydrate.)

Evaluating an Individual Food Item

You can do the same type of calculations to evaluate a particular food item, to determine whether it is high or low in protein, fat, or carbohydrate. For example, suppose you want to determine how high in fat peanut butter is. First, you need to know the total number of calories and grams of fat it contains. Multiply the grams of fat by 9 (because there are 9 calories in a gram of fat), and then divide that number by the total calories. For a tablespoon of peanut butter (8 grams of fat and 95 calories), you would calculate as follows: 8 × 9 = 72, divided by 95 = 0.76, or 76% of calories from fat. This means peanut butter is relatively high in fat. If your overall daily fat consumption goal is 70 grams of fat, a tablespoon of peanut butter would represent 11% of your daily target.

Of course, you can still eat high-fat foods. But it makes good sense to limit the size of your portions and to balance your intake with lowfat foods. For example, a tablespoon of peanut butter eaten on whole-wheat bread and served with a banana, carrot sticks, and a glass of fat-free milk makes a nutritious lunch—high in protein and carbohydrates, low in fat. Eating three tablespoons of peanut butter on high-fat crackers with potato chips, cookies, and whole milk is a less healthy combination. So while it's important to evaluate individual food items, it is more important to look at them in the context of your overall diet.

Monitoring Your Progress

Depending on your current diet and health needs, you may choose to focus on a particular goal, such as that for fat or protein. For prepared foods, food labels list the number of grams of fat, protein, and carbohydrate; the breakdown for popular fast-food items can be found in Appendix A. For other foods, this information is posted in many grocery stores, published in inexpensive nutrition guides, and available online. By checking these resources, you can keep a running total of the grams of fat, protein, and carbohydrate you eat and determine how close you are to meeting your goals.

---

certain forms of cancer, especially colon cancer. A high-fat diet can also make weight management more difficult. Because fat is a concentrated source of calories (9 calories per gram versus 4 calories per gram for protein and carbohydrate), a high-fat diet is often a high-calorie diet that can lead to weight gain. In addition, there is some evidence that calories from fat are more easily converted to body fat than calories from protein or carbohydrate.

Although more research is needed on the precise effects of different types and amounts of fat on overall health, a

TERMS

low-density lipoprotein (LDL) Blood fat that transports cholesterol to organs and tissues; excess amounts result in the accumulation of deposits on artery walls.

high-density lipoprotein (HDL) Blood fat that helps transport cholesterol out of the arteries, thereby protecting against heart disease.

omega-3 fatty acids Polyunsaturated fatty acids commonly found in fish oils that are beneficial to cardiovascular health; the endmost double bond occurs three carbons from the end of the fatty acid chain.

great deal of evidence points to the fact that most people benefit from lowering their overall fat intake to recommended levels and substituting unsaturated fats for saturated and trans fats.

PERSONAL INSIGHT Do you have emotional attachments to particular kinds of foods or meals, such as those you eat on holidays or at family gatherings? If so, do your attachments make it hard for you to evaluate those foods objectively and admit that some of them may not be good for you?

Carbohydrates—An Ideal Source of Energy

Carbohydrates are needed in the diet primarily to supply energy for body cells. Some cells, such as those found in the brain and other parts of the nervous system and in blood, use only carbohydrates for fuel. During high-intensity exercise, muscles also use primarily carbohydrates for fuel. When we don't eat enough carbohydrates to satisfy the needs of the brain and red blood cells, our bodies synthesize carbohydrates from proteins. In situations of extreme deprivation, when the diet lacks a sufficient amount of both carbohydrates and proteins, the body turns to its own organs and tissues, breaking down proteins in muscles, the heart, kidneys, and other vital organs to supply carbohydrate needs. This rarely occurs, however, because consuming the equivalent of just three or four slices of bread supplies the body's daily need for carbohydrates.

Simple and Complex Carbohydrates Carbohydrates are classified into two groups: simple and complex. Simple carbohydrates contain only one or two sugar units in each molecule; they include sucrose (table sugar), fructose (fruit sugar, honey), maltose (malt sugar), and lactose (milk sugar). Simple carbohydrates provide much of the sweetness in foods and are found naturally in fruits and milk and are added to soft drinks, fruit drinks, candy, and sweet desserts. There is no evidence that any type of simple sugar is more nutritious than others.

Starches and most types of dietary fiber are complex carbohydrates; they consist of chains of many sugar molecules. Starches are found in a variety of plants, especially grains (wheat, rye, rice, oats, barley, millet), legumes, and tubers (potatoes and yams). Most other vegetables contain a mix of starches and simple carbohydrates. Dietary fiber is found in fruits, vegetables, and grains.

Many nutritionists also distinguish between refined (processed) and unrefined carbohydrates. Before they are processed, all grains are **whole grains,** consisting of an inner layer of germ, a middle layer called the endosperm, and an outer layer of bran. During processing, the germ and bran are often removed, leaving just the starchy endosperm. The refinement of whole grains transforms whole-wheat flour to white flour, brown rice to white rice, and so on.

Refined carbohydrates usually retain all the calories of their unrefined counterparts, but they tend to be much lower in fiber, vitamins, minerals, and other beneficial compounds. In general, unrefined carbohydrates tend to take longer to chew and digest than refined ones; they also enter the bloodstream more slowly. This slower digestive pace tends to make people feel full sooner and for a longer period, lessening the chance that they will overeat. It also helps keep blood sugar and insulin levels low, which may decrease the risk of diabetes and heart disease. Whole grains are also high in dietary fiber and so have all the benefits of fiber (see the next section). For all these reasons, whole grains are recommended over those that have been refined. This does not mean that you should never eat refined carbohydrates such as white bread or white rice, simply that whole-wheat bread, brown rice, and other whole grains are healthier choices.

During digestion in the mouth and small intestine, your body breaks down starches and double sugars into single sugar molecules, such as **glucose,** for absorption. Once glucose is in the bloodstream, cells take it up and use it for energy. The liver and muscles also take up glucose to provide carbohydrate storage in the form of the animal starch **glycogen.** Some people have problems metabolizing glucose, a disorder called diabetes mellitus (see Chapter 14 for more on diabetes).

Carbohydrates consumed beyond the body's requirements for carbohydrate and energy are synthesized into fat and stored as such once glycogen reserves are full. Any type of diet where calorie intake exceeds calorie needs can lead to fat storage and weight gain. This is true whether these excess calories come from carbohydrate, protein, fat, or alcohol.

Recommended Carbohydrate Intake On average, Americans consume over 250 grams of carbohydrates per day, well above the minimum of 50–100 grams of essential carbohydrate required by the body. However, health experts recommend that Americans increase their consumption of carbohydrates—particularly complex carbohydrates—to 55% of total daily calories.

Experts also recommend that Americans alter the proportion of simple and complex carbohydrates in the diet, lowering simple carbohydrate intake from 26% to about 15% of total daily calories. To accomplish this change, reduce your intake of foods like candy, sweet desserts, soft drinks, and sweetened fruit drinks, which are high in simple sugars but low in other nutrients. The bulk of the simple carbohydrates in your diet should come from fruits, which are excellent sources of vitamins and minerals, and milk, which is high in protein and calcium. Instead of prepared foods high in added sugars, choose a variety of foods rich in unrefined complex carbohydrates.

Athletes in training can especially benefit from high-carbohydrate diets (60–65% of total daily calories), which enhance the amount of carbohydrates stored in their muscles (as glycogen) and therefore provide more carbohydrate fuel for use during endurance events or long workouts. In addition, carbohydrates consumed during prolonged athletic events can help fuel muscles and extend the availability of the glycogen stored in muscles. Caution is in order, however, because overconsumption of carbohydrates can lead to feelings of fatigue and underconsumption of other nutrients.

Dietary Fiber—A Closer Look

Dietary fiber consists of carbohydrate plant substances that are difficult or impossible for humans to digest. Instead, fiber passes through the intestinal tract and provides bulk for feces in the large intestine, which in turn facilitates elimination. In the large intestine, some types of fiber are broken down by bacteria into acids and gases, which explains why consuming too much fiber can lead to intestinal gas. Because humans cannot digest dietary fiber, fiber is not a source of carbohydrate in the diet; however, the consumption of dietary fiber is necessary for good health.

Types of Dietary Fiber   Nutritionists classify fibers as soluble or insoluble. **Soluble fiber** slows the body's absorption of glucose and binds cholesterol-containing compounds in the intestine, lowering blood cholesterol levels and reducing the risk of cardiovascular disease. **Insoluble fiber** binds water, making the feces bulkier and softer so they pass more quickly and easily through the intestines.

Both kinds of fiber contribute to disease prevention. A diet high in soluble fiber can help people manage diabetes and high blood cholesterol levels. A diet high in insoluble fiber can help prevent a variety of health problems, including constipation, hemorrhoids, and **diverticulitis.** Some studies have linked high-fiber diets with a reduced risk of colon and rectal cancer; more recent evidence suggests that other characteristics of diets rich in fruits, vegetables, and whole grains may be responsible for this reduction in risk (see Chapter 16 for more on cancer and diet).

Sources of Dietary Fiber   All plant foods contain some dietary fiber, but fruits, legumes, oats (especially oat bran), barley, and psyllium (found in some laxatives) are particularly rich in it. Wheat (especially wheat bran), cereals, grains, and vegetables are all good sources of insoluble fiber. However, the processing of packaged foods can remove fiber, so it's important to depend on fresh fruits and vegetables and foods made from whole grains as sources of dietary fiber.

Recommended Intake of Dietary Fiber   Although it is not yet clear precisely how much and what types of fiber are ideal, most experts believe the average American would benefit from an increase in daily fiber intake. Currently, most Americans consume about 16 grams of dietary fiber a day, whereas the recommended daily amount is 20–35 grams of fiber—not from supplements, which should be taken only under medical supervision. However, too much fiber—more than 40–60 grams a day—can cause health problems, such as excessively large stools or the malabsorption of important minerals. In fiber intake, as in all aspects of nutrition, balance and moderation are key principles.

To increase the amount of fiber in your diet, try the following:

- Choose whole-grain bread instead of white bread, brown rice instead of white rice, and whole-wheat pasta instead of regular pasta. Select high-fiber breakfast cereals (those with 5 or more grams of fiber per serving). Look for breads, crackers, and cereals that list a whole grain first in the ingredient list: Whole-wheat flour, whole-grain oats, and whole-grain rice are whole grains; wheat flour is not.

- Eat whole, unpeeled fruits rather than drinking fruit juice. Top cereals, yogurt, and desserts with berries, apple slices, or other fruit.

- Include beans in soups and salads. Prepare salads that combine raw vegetables with pasta, rice, or beans.

- Substitute bean dip for cheese-based or sour cream–based dips or spreads. Use raw vegetables rather than chips for dipping.

TERMS

carbohydrate   An essential nutrient; sugars, starches, and dietary fiber are all carbohydrates.

whole grain   The entire edible portion of a grain such as wheat, rice, or oats, including the germ, endosperm, and bran. During milling or processing, parts of the grain are removed, often leaving just the endosperm.

glucose   A simple sugar that is the body's basic fuel.

glycogen   An animal starch stored in the liver and muscles.

dietary fiber   Carbohydrates and other substances in plants that are difficult or impossible for humans to digest.

soluble fiber   Fiber that dissolves in water or is broken down by bacteria in the large intestine.

insoluble fiber   Fiber that does not dissolve in water and is not broken down by bacteria in the large intestine.

diverticulitis   A digestive disorder in which abnormal pouches form in the walls of the intestine and become inflamed.

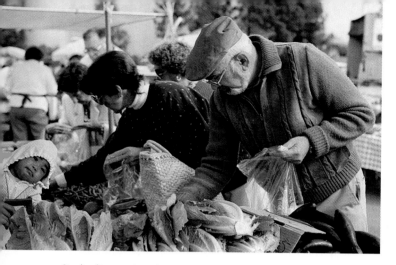

Our bodies require adequate amounts of all essential nutrients—water, proteins, carbohydrates, fats, vitamins, and minerals—in order to grow and function properly. Choosing foods to satisfy these nutritional requirements is an important part of a healthy lifestyle.

Vitamins—Organic Micronutrients

Vitamins are organic (carbon-containing) substances required in very small amounts to promote specific chemical reactions within living cells (Table 12-1). Humans need 13 vitamins. Four are fat-soluble (A, D, E, and K), and nine are water-soluble (C, and the eight B-complex vitamins: thiamin, riboflavin, niacin, vitamin B-6, folate, vitamin B-12, biotin, and pantothenic acid). Solubility affects how a vitamin is absorbed, transported, and stored in the body. The water-soluble vitamins are absorbed directly into the bloodstream, where they travel freely; excess water-soluble vitamins are detected by the kidneys and excreted in urine. Fat-soluble vitamins require a more complex digestive process; they are usually carried in the blood by special proteins and are stored in the body in fat tissues rather than excreted.

Functions of Vitamins　Vitamins help chemical reactions take place. They provide no energy to the body directly but help unleash the energy stored in carbohydrates, proteins, and fats. Vitamins are critical in the production of red blood cells and the maintenance of the nervous, skeletal, and immune systems. Some vitamins also form substances that act as **antioxidants**, which help preserve

healthy cells in the body. Key vitamin antioxidants include vitamin E, vitamin C, and the vitamin A precursor beta-carotene. (The actions of antioxidants will be described in greater detail later in the chapter.)

Sources of Vitamins　The human body does not manufacture most of the vitamins it requires and must obtain them from foods. Vitamins are abundant in fruits, vegetables, and grains. In addition, many processed foods, such as flour and breakfast cereals, are enriched with certain vitamins during the manufacturing process. On the other hand, both vitamins and minerals can be lost or destroyed during the storage and cooking of foods. For tips on minimizing such losses, see the box "Keeping the Nutrient Value in Food."

A few vitamins are made in certain parts of the body: The skin makes vitamin D when it is exposed to sunlight, and intestinal bacteria make vitamin K and possibly biotin. Nonetheless, you still need to obtain vitamin D, vitamin K, and biotin from foods.

Vitamin Deficiencies and Excesses　If your diet lacks sufficient amounts of a particular vitamin, characteristic symptoms of deficiency develop (see Table 12-1.) For example, vitamin A deficiency can cause blindness and vitamin B-6 deficiency can cause seizures. The best known deficiency disease is probably **scurvy,** caused by vitamin C deficiency. In the eighteenth century, it killed many sailors on long ocean voyages, until people realized that eating citrus fruits could prevent it. Even today people develop scurvy; its presence suggests a very poor intake of fruits and vegetables, which are rich sources of vitamin C.

Vitamin deficiency diseases are most often seen in developing countries; they are relatively rare in the United States because vitamins are readily available from our food supply. People suffering from alcoholism and malabsorption disorders probably run the greatest risk of vitamin deficiencies. However, intakes below recommended levels can have adverse effects on health even if they are not low enough to cause a deficiency disease. For example, low intake of folate increases a woman's chance of giving birth to a baby with a neural tube defect (a congenital malformation of the central nervous system).

Extra vitamins in the diet can be harmful, especially when taken as supplements. High doses of vitamin A are toxic and increase the risk of birth defects, for example. Vitamin B-6 can cause irreversible nerve damage when taken in large doses. Megadoses of fat-soluble vitamins are particularly dangerous because the excess will be stored in the body rather than excreted, increasing the risk of toxicity. Even when vitamins are not taken in excess, relying on supplements for an adequate intake of vitamins can be a problem: There are many substances in foods other than vitamins and minerals, and some of these compounds may have important health effects. Later in the chapter we will discuss specific recommendations for vitamin intake

TABLE 12-1	Facts About Vitamins

Vitamin	Important Dietary Sources	Major Functions	Signs of Prolonged Deficiency	Toxic Effects of Megadoses
Fat-Soluble				
Vitamin A	Liver, milk, butter, cheese, and fortified margarine; carrots, spinach, and other orange and deep-green vegetables and fruits	Maintenance of vision, skin, linings of the nose, mouth, digestive and urinary tracts, immune function	Night blindness; dry, scaling skin; increased susceptibility to infection; loss of appetite; anemia; kidney stones	Headache, vomiting and diarrhea, vertigo, double vision, bone abnormalities, liver damage, miscarriage and birth defects
Vitamin D	Fortified milk and margarine, fish liver oils, butter, egg yolks (sunlight on skin also produces vitamin D)	Development and maintenance of bones and teeth, promotion of calcium absorption	Rickets (bone deformities) in children; bone softening, loss, and fractures in adults	Kidney damage, calcium deposits in soft tissues, depression, death
Vitamin E	Vegetable oils, whole grains, nuts and seeds, green leafy vegetables, asparagus, peaches	Protection and maintenance of cellular membranes	Red blood cell breakage and anemia, weakness, neurological problems, muscle cramps	Relatively nontoxic, but may cause excess bleeding or formation of blood clots
Vitamin K	Green leafy vegetables; smaller amounts widespread in other foods	Production of factors essential for blood clotting	Hemorrhaging	Anemia, jaundice
Water-Soluble				
Vitamin C	Peppers, broccoli, spinach, brussels sprouts, citrus fruits, strawberries, tomatoes, potatoes, cabbage, other fruits and vegetables	Maintenance and repair of connective tissue, bones, teeth, and cartilage; promotion of healing; aid in iron absorption	Scurvy, anemia, reduced resistance to infection, loosened teeth, joint pain, poor wound healing, hair loss, poor iron absorption	Urinary stones in some people, acid stomach from ingesting supplements in pill form, nausea, diarrhea, headache, fatigue
Thiamin	Whole-grain and enriched breads and cereals, organ meats, lean pork, nuts, legumes	Conversion of carbohydrates into usable forms of energy, maintenance of appetite and nervous system function	Beriberi (symptoms include muscle wasting, mental confusion, anorexia, enlarged heart, abnormal heart rhythm, nerve changes)	None reported
Riboflavin	Dairy products, enriched breads and cereals, lean meats, poultry, fish, green vegetables	Energy metabolism; maintenance of skin, mucous membranes, and nervous system structures	Cracks at corners of mouth, sore throat, skin rash, hypersensitivity to light, purple tongue	None reported
Niacin	Eggs, poultry, fish, milk, whole grains, nuts, enriched breads and cereals, meats, legumes	Conversion of carbohydrates, fats, and protein into usable forms of energy	Pellagra (symptoms include diarrhea, dermatitis, inflammation of mucous membranes, dementia)	Flushing of the skin, nausea, vomiting, diarrhea, liver dysfunction, glucose intolerance
Vitamin B-6	Eggs, poultry, fish, whole grains, nuts, soybeans, liver, kidney, pork	Protein and neurotransmitter metabolism; red blood cell synthesis	Anemia, convulsions, cracks at corners of mouth, dermatitis, nausea, confusion	Neurological abnormalities and damage
Folate	Green leafy vegetables, yeast, oranges, whole grains, legumes, liver	Amino acid metabolism, synthesis of RNA and DNA, new cell synthesis	Anemia, weakness, fatigue, irritability, shortness of breath, swollen tongue	Masking of vitamin B-12 deficiency
Vitamin B-12	Eggs, milk, meats, other animal foods	Synthesis of red and white blood cells; other metabolic reactions	Anemia, fatigue, nervous system damage, sore tongue	None reported
Biotin	Cereals, yeast, egg yolks, soy flour, liver; widespread in foods	Metabolism of fats, carbohydrates, and proteins	Rash, nausea, vomiting, weight loss, depression, fatigue, hair loss	None reported
Pantothenic acid	Animal foods, whole grains, broccoli, legumes; widespread in foods	Metabolism of fats, carbohydrates, and proteins	Fatigue, numbness and tingling of hands and feet, gastrointestinal disturbances	None reported

SOURCES: Food and Nutrition Board. 1998. *Dietary Reference Intakes for Thiamin, Riboflavin, Niacin, Vitamin B₆, Folate, Vitamin B₁₂, Pantothenic Acid, and Choline.* Washington, D.C.: National Academy Press. National Research Council. 1989. *Recommended Dietary Allowances,* 10th ed. Washington, D.C.: National Academy Press. Copyright © 1989, 1998 by the National Academy of Sciences. Adapted with permission from the National Academy Press, Washington, D.C.; Shils, M. E., et al., eds. 1998. *Modern Nutrition in Health and Disease,* 9th ed. Baltimore: Williams & Wilkins.

1. *Consume or process vegetables immediately after purchasing (or harvesting).* The longer vegetables are kept before they are eaten or processed, the more vitamins are lost.

2. *Store vegetables and fruits properly.* If you can't eat fruits and vegetables immediately after purchasing (or harvesting) but plan to do so within a few days, keep them in the refrigerator. Place them in covered containers or plastic bags to minimize moisture loss. Freezing is the best method for longer-term preservation.

3. *Minimize the preparation and cooking of vegetables and other foods.* The more preparation and cooking of foods that is done before eating, the greater the nutrient loss. To reduce the losses:

- When possible, cook vegetables, like potatoes, in their skins.
- Don't soak and rinse rice before cooking.
- Cook in as little water as possible.
- Don't add baking soda to vegetables to enhance the green color.
- Bake, steam, broil, or microwave vegetables.
- When boiling, use tight-fitting lids to minimize evaporation of water.
- Cook vegetables as little as possible. Develop a taste for a crunchier texture.
- Don't thaw frozen vegetables before cooking.
- Prepare lettuce salads right before eating.

and when a vitamin supplement is advisable. For now, keep in mind that it's best to obtain most of your vitamins from foods rather than supplements.

Minerals—Inorganic Micronutrients

Minerals are inorganic (non–carbon-containing) compounds you need in relatively small amounts to help regulate body functions, aid in the growth and maintenance of body tissues, and help release energy (Table 12-2). There are about 17 essential minerals. The major minerals, those that the body needs in amounts exceeding 100 milligrams, include calcium, phosphorus, magnesium, sodium, potassium, and chloride. The essential trace minerals, those that you need in minute amounts, include copper, fluoride, iodide, iron, selenium, and zinc.

Characteristic symptoms develop if an essential mineral is consumed in a quantity too small or too large for good health. The minerals most commonly lacking in the American diet are iron, calcium, zinc, and magnesium. Focus on good food choices for these nutrients (see Table 12-2). Lean meats are rich in iron and zinc, while lowfat or fat-free dairy products are excellent choices for calcium. Plant foods are good sources of magnesium. Iron-deficiency **anemia** is a problem in many age groups and researchers fear poor calcium intakes are sowing the seeds for future **osteoporosis**, especially in women. See the box "Osteoporosis" on p. 312 to learn more.

TERMS   **minerals**   Inorganic compounds needed in relatively small amounts for regulation, growth, and maintenance of body tissues and functions.

anemia   A deficiency in the oxygen-carrying material in the red blood cells.

osteoporosis   A condition in which the bones become extremely thin and brittle and break easily.

Water—Vital But Often Ignored

Water is the major component in both foods and the human body: You are composed of about 60% water. Your need for other nutrients, in terms of weight, is much less than your need for water. You can live up to 50 days without food, but only a few days without water.

Water is distributed all over the body, among lean and other tissues and in urine and other body fluids. Water is used in the digestion and absorption of food and is the medium in which most of the chemical reactions take place within the body. Some water-based fluids like blood transport substances around the body, while other fluids serve as lubricants or cushions. Water also helps regulate body temperature.

Water is contained in almost all foods, particularly in liquids, fruits, and vegetables. The foods and fluids you consume provide 80–90% of your daily water intake; the remainder is generated through metabolism. You lose water each day in urine, feces, and sweat and through evaporation in your lungs. To maintain a balance between water consumed and water lost, you need to take in about 1 milliliter of water for each calorie you burn—about 2 liters, or 8 cups, of fluid per day—more if you live in a hot climate or engage in vigorous exercise.

Thirst is one of the body's first signs of dehydration that we can actually recognize. However, by the time we are actually thirsty, our cells have been needing fluid for quite some time. A good motto to remember, especially when exercising is: Drink *before* you're thirsty. If the thirst mechanism is faulty, as it may be during illness or vigorous exercise, hormonal mechanisms can help conserve water by reducing the output of urine. Severe dehydration causes weakness and can lead to death.

Other Substances in Food

There are many substances in food that are not essential nutrients but which may influence health.

	Important Dietary Sources	**Major Functions**	**Signs of Prolonged Deficiency**	**Toxic Effects of Megadoses**
TABLE 12-2 *Facts About Selected Minerals*				
Mineral				
Calcium	Milk and milk products, tofu, fortified orange juice and bread, green leafy vegetables, bones in fish	Maintenance of bones and teeth, control of nerve impulses and muscle contraction	Stunted growth in children, bone mineral loss in adults; urinary stones	Constipation, calcium deposits in soft tissues, inhibition of mineral absorption
Fluoride	Fluoride-containing drinking water, tea, marine fish eaten with bones	Maintenance of tooth and bone structure	Higher frequency of tooth decay	Increased bone density, mottling of teeth, impaired kidney function
Iron	Meat, legumes, eggs, enriched flour, dark-green vegetables, dried fruit, liver	Component of hemoglobin, myoglobin, and enzymes	Iron-deficiency anemia, weakness, impaired immune function, gastrointestinal distress	Liver and kidney damage, joint pains, sterility, disruption of cardiac function, death
Iodine	Iodized salt, seafood	Essential part of thyroid hormones, regulation of body metabolism	Goiter (enlarged thyroid), cretinism (birth defect)	Depression of thyroid activity, hyperthyroidism in susceptible people
Magnesium	Widespread in foods and water (except soft water); especially found in grains, legumes, nuts, seeds, green vegetables	Transmission of nerve impulses, energy transfer, activation of many enzymes	Neurological disturbances, cardiovascular problems, kidney disorders, nausea, growth failure in children	Nausea, vomiting, diarrhea, central nervous system depression, coma; death in people with impaired kidney function
Phosphorus	Present in nearly all foods, especially milk, cereal, legumes, meat, poultry, fish	Bone growth and maintenance, energy transfer in cells	Impaired growth, weakness, kidney disorders, cardiorespiratory and nervous system dysfunction	Drop in blood calcium levels, calcium deposits in soft tissues, bone loss
Potassium	Meats, milk, fruits, vegetables, grains, legumes	Nerve function and body water balance	Muscular weakness, nausea, drowsiness, paralysis, confusion, disruption of cardiac rhythm	Cardiac arrest
Selenium	Seafood, meat, eggs, whole grains	Protection of cells from oxidative damage, immune response	Muscle pain and weakness, heart disorders	Hair and nail loss, nausea and vomiting, weakness, irritability
Sodium	Salt, soy sauce, salted foods, tomato juice	Body water balance, acid-base balance, nerve function	Muscle weakness, loss of appetite, nausea, vomiting; sodium deficiency is rarely seen	Edema, hypertension in sensitive people
Zinc	Whole grains, meat, eggs, liver, seafood (especially oysters)	Synthesis of proteins, RNA, and DNA; wound healing; immune response; ability to taste	Growth failure, loss of appetite, impaired taste acuity, skin rash, impaired immune function, poor wound healing	Vomiting, impaired immune function, decline in blood HDL levels, impaired copper absorption

SOURCES: Food and Nutrition Board. 1997. *Dietary Reference Intakes for Calcium, Phosphorus, Magnesium, Vitamin D, and Fluoride.* Washington, D.C.: National Academy Press. National Research Council. 1989. *Recommended Dietary Allowances,* 10th ed. Washington, D.C.: National Academy Press. Copyright © 1989, 1998 by the National Academy of Sciences. Reprinted with permission from National Academy Press, Washington, D.C.; Shils, M. E., et al., eds. 1998. *Modern Nutrition in Health and Disease,* 9th ed. Baltimore: Williams & Wilkins.

Vitamin-like Compounds   Various vitamin-like compounds are necessary to maintain the proper functioning of the body; they include choline, carnitine, inositol, and taurine. A healthy body is able to manufacture them from common building blocks like glucose and amino acids—meaning that although they are also available in foods, they are not essential nutrients. However, infants and people with some diseases may not be able to manufacture

all of these necessary compounds in sufficient amounts, making dietary intake essential. Recommended intakes were recently established for choline, and ongoing research may determine that other of these compounds are essential nutrients for certain population groups.

Antioxidants   When the body uses oxygen or breaks down certain fats or proteins as a normal part of metabo-

Osteoporosis is a condition in which the bones become dangerously thin and fragile over time. It currently afflicts some 25 million Americans, 80% of them women, and results in about 1.5 million bone fractures each year. The incidence of osteoporosis may double in the next 25 years as the population ages.

The bones in your body are continually being broken down and rebuilt in order to adapt to mechanical strain. About 20% of your body's bone mass is replaced each year. In the first few decades of life, bones become thicker and stronger as they are rebuilt. Most of your bone mass (95%) is built by age 18. After bone mass peaks between the ages of 25 and 35, the rate of bone loss exceeds the rate of replacement, and bones become less dense. In osteoporosis, this loss of density becomes so severe that bones become very fragile.

Fractures are the most serious consequence of osteoporosis; up to 25% of all people who suffer a hip fracture die within a year. Other problems associated with osteoporosis are loss of height and a stooped posture caused by vertebral fractures, severe back and hip pain, and breathing problems caused by changes in the shape of the skeleton.

Who Is at Risk?

Women are at greater risk than men for osteoporosis because they have 10–25% less bone in their skeleton. As they lose bone mass with age, women's bones become dangerously thin sooner than men's bones. More men will probably develop osteoporosis in the future as they live into their eighties and nineties. Bone loss accelerates in women during the first 5–10 years after the onset of menopause because of a drop in estrogen production. (Estrogen improves calcium absorption and reduces the amount of calcium the body excretes.)

Other risk factors include a family history of osteoporosis, early menopause (before age 45), abnormal menstruation, a history of anorexia, and a thin, small frame. Thyroid medication, corticosteroid drugs for asthma or arthritis, and certain other medications can also have a negative impact on bone mass. African American women tend to have a *lower* risk of osteoporosis than women from other ethnic groups.

What Can You Do?

To prevent osteoporosis, the best strategy is to build as much bone as possible during your young years and then do everything you can to maintain it as you age. Up to 50% of bone loss is determined by controllable lifestyle factors.

Ensure Adequate Intake of Calcium and Vitamin D Consuming an adequate amount of calcium is important throughout life to build and maintain bone mass. Americans average 600–800 mg of calcium per day, only about half of what is recommended. Milk, yogurt, and calcium-fortified orange juice, bread, and cereals are all good sources. Nutritionists suggest that you obtain calcium from foods first and then take supplements only if needed to make up the difference.

Vitamin D is necessary for bones to absorb calcium; a daily intake of 400–800 IU is recommended by the National Osteoporosis Foundation. Vitamin D can be obtained from foods (milk and fortified cereals, for example) and is manufactured by the skin when exposed to sunlight. Candidates for vitamin D supplements include people who don't eat many foods rich in vitamin D; those who don't expose their face, arms, and hands to the sun (without sunscreen) for 5–15 minutes a few times each week; and people who live north of an imaginary line roughly between Boston and the Oregon–California border (the sun is weaker in northern latitudes). Adequate intake of vitamin K has also been linked to a lower risk of bone fractures (see Table 12-2 for sources of vitamin K).

Exercise Weight-bearing aerobic activities help build and maintain bone mass throughout life, but they must be performed regularly in order to have lasting effects. Strength training is also helpful: It improves bone density, muscle mass, strength, and balance, protecting against both bone loss and falls, a major cause of fractures. Even low-intensity strength training has been shown to improve bone density—even in women in their seventies.

Don't Smoke, and Drink Alcohol Only in Moderation Smoking reduces the body's estrogen levels and is linked to earlier menopause and more rapid postmenopausal bone loss. Alcohol reduces the body's ability to absorb calcium and may interfere with estrogen's bone-protecting effects.

Be Moderate in Your Consumption of Protein, Sodium, and Caffeine A high intake of protein and sodium has been shown to increase calcium loss in the urine and may lead to loss of calcium from the skeleton. Caffeine may also cause small losses of urinary calcium, and experts often recommend that heavy caffeine consumers take special care to include calcium-rich foods in their diet. Adding milk to coffee or tea seems to offset the effects of caffeine on urinary calcium loss.

Manage Depression and Stress Some women with depression experience significant bone loss that may increase their risk of fractures. Researchers haven't identified the mechanism, but it may be linked to increases in the stress hormone cortisol.

After Menopause, Consider Testing and Treatment The National Osteoporosis Foundation recommends bone mineral density testing for all women over age 65 as well as younger postmenopausal women who have a fracture or who have one or more osteoporosis risk factors. Results of bone mineral density testing can be used to gauge an individual's risk of fracture and help determine an appropriate course of action.

Hormone replacement therapy (HRT) combats bone loss as well as menopausal symptoms and heart disease (see Chapters 15 and 19). However, estrogen acts on many tissues in the body, and HRT is not without side effects and risks, including a slight increase in the risk of breast cancer. Compounds called selective estrogen receptor modulators, or SERMs, have been found to act like estrogen on some body tissues but not others. Researchers hope to develop SERMs that have all of estrogen's beneficial effects without the associated risks. Although currently not as effective as HRT in preventing bone loss, SERMs such as raloxifene (Evista) may be a good choice for some women. Other drug treatments include alendronate (Fosamax) and calcitonin (Miacalcin), which slow the resorption of bone by the body, and fluoride, which helps build bone in women who already have osteoporosis.

lism, it gives rise to substances called **free radicals.** Environmental factors like cigarette smoke, exhaust fumes, radiation, excessive sunlight, certain drugs, and stress can increase free radical production. A free radical is a chemically unstable molecule that is missing an electron; it will react with any molecule it encounters from which it can take an electron. In their search for electrons, free radicals react with fats, proteins, and DNA, damaging cell membranes and mutating genes. Because of this, free radicals have been implicated in aging, cancer, cardiovascular disease, and degenerative diseases like arthritis.

Antioxidants found in foods can help protect the body from damage by free radicals in several ways. Some dietary antioxidants prevent or reduce the formation of free radicals; others remove free radicals from the body by reacting with them directly by donating electrons. Antioxidants can also repair some types of free radical damage after it occurs. Some antioxidants, such as vitamin C, vitamin E, and selenium, are also essential nutrients; others, such as carotenoids, found in yellow, orange, and deep-green vegetables, are not. Obtaining a regular intake of these nutrients is vital for maintaining the health of the body. Many fruits and vegetables are rich in antioxidants.

Phytochemicals Antioxidants are a particular type of **phytochemical,** a substance found in plant foods that may help prevent chronic disease. Researchers have just begun to identify and study all the different compounds found in foods, and many preliminary findings are promising. For example, certain substances found in soy foods may help lower cholesterol levels. Sulforaphane, a compound isolated from broccoli and other **cruciferous vegetables,** may render some carcinogenic compounds harmless. Allyl sulfides, a group of chemicals found in garlic and onions, appear to boost the activity of cancer-fighting immune cells. Further research on phytochemicals may extend the role of nutrition to the prevention and treatment of many chronic diseases.

If you want to increase your intake of phytochemicals, it is best to obtain them by eating a variety of fruits and vegetables rather than relying on supplements. Like many vitamins and minerals, isolated phytochemicals may be harmful if taken in high doses. In addition, it is likely that their health benefits are the result of chemical substances working in combination. Phytochemicals are discussed in greater detail in Chapters 15 and 16.

NUTRITIONAL GUIDELINES: PLANNING YOUR DIET

The second part of putting together a healthy food plan—after you've learned about necessary nutrients—is choosing foods that satisfy nutritional requirements and meet your personal criteria. Various tools have been created by scientific and government groups to help people design

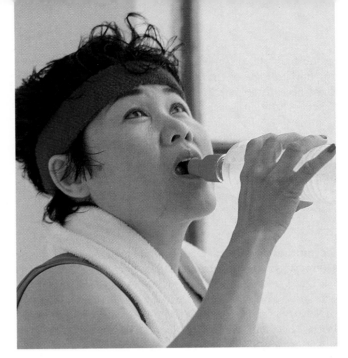

Often overlooked but absolutely crucial to life, water is an essential part of the diet. You need to drink about 8 cups of fluid per day—more if you live in a hot climate or exercise vigorously.

healthy diets. The **Recommended Dietary Allowances (RDAs), Dietary Reference Intakes (DRIs),** and related guidelines are standards for nutrient intake designed to prevent nutritional deficiencies and reduce the risk of chronic disease. The **Food Guide Pyramid** translates these nutrient recommendations into a balanced food-group plan that includes all essential nutrients. To provide further guidance, **Dietary Guidelines for Americans** have been established to address the prevention of diet-related chronic diseases. Together, these tools make up a complete set of resources for dietary planning.

> **PERSONAL INSIGHT**   How have your eating habits changed since you've entered college? Do you feel more comfortable with your current habits or less? Why?

Recommended Dietary Allowances (RDAs) and Dietary Reference Intakes (DRIs)

The Food and Nutrition Board of the National Academy of Sciences establishes the RDAs, DRIs, and related guidelines. The RDAs were developed as standards to prevent nutritional deficiency diseases such as rickets, scurvy, and anemia (see Tables 12-1 and 12-2). First published in 1941, the RDAs have been updated periodically to keep pace with new research findings; the most recent version was published in 1989. RDAs include intake recommendations for individual nutrients in one of three categories: (1) the RDAs themselves, which give specific recommended intakes of nutrients that are well known and well researched; (2) the Estimated Safe and Adequate Daily Dietary Intakes (ESADDIs), which provide a range of values for nutrients about which our knowledge is still sketchy; and (3) Estimated Minimum Requirements, which provide minimum values for three minerals.

Scientific knowledge about nutrition has increased dramatically since the inception of the RDAs, and current research focuses not just on the prevention of nutrient deficiencies but also on the role of nutrients in preventing chronic diseases such as osteoporosis, cancer, and cardiovascular disease. This expanded focus is the basis for the development of a new system of recommendations, the Dietary Reference Intakes. The DRIs, which will eventually replace the RDAs, include standards for both recommended intakes and maximum safe intakes.

- Recommended nutrient intakes can be expressed as three different types of standards—Adequate Intake (AI), Estimated Average Requirement (EAR), and Recommended Dietary Allowance (RDA). The type of standard used for a particular nutrient or age group depends on the amount of scientific information available and the intended use of the standard. Regardless of the type of standard attached to a particular nutrient, the DRI represents the best available estimate of intake for optimal health.

- Maximum intake level guidelines are expressed as the Tolerable Upper Intake Level (UL), the maximum daily intake by a healthy person that is unlikely to cause health problems. Because of lack of

suitable data, ULs have not been established for all nutrients. This does not mean that people can tolerate chronic intakes of these vitamins above recommended levels. Like all chemical agents, nutrients can produce adverse effects if intakes are excessive; when data are limited, extra caution may be warranted. There is no established benefit from consuming nutrients at levels above the AI or RDA.

The DRIs are being issued in stages, and they have not yet been established for all vitamins and minerals. Table 12-3 is an abridged version of the 1989 RDAs; it includes nutrients for which DRIs have not yet been set. Table 12-4 gives recommended intakes for the vitamins and minerals for which DRIs have been set. Table 12-5 lists the upper intake levels for adults; as described earlier, ULs have not been established for all nutrients. (For more on updates and additions to the DRIs, call or visit the Web site of the Food and Nutrition Board; see For More Information at the end of the chapter.)

Should You Take Supplements?   The aim of the RDAs and DRIs is to guide you in meeting your nutritional needs primarily with food, rather than with vitamin and mineral supplements. This goal is important because recommendations have not yet been set for some essential nutrients. Many supplements contain only nutrients with established recommendations, so using them to meet nutrient needs can leave you deficient in other nutrients. Supplements also lack potentially beneficial phytochemicals that are found only in whole foods. Nutrition scientists generally agree that most Americans can obtain most of the vitamins and minerals they need to prevent deficiencies by consuming a varied, nutritionally balanced diet. Ongoing research is examining whether supplements of particular vitamins and minerals should be recommended for their potential disease-fighting properties, as for the antioxidant vitamins C and E.

The question of whether or not to take supplements is a serious one. Some vitamins and minerals are dangerous when ingested in excess, as shown in Tables 12-1 and 12-2. Large doses of particular nutrients can also cause health problems by affecting the absorption of other vitamins and minerals. For all these reasons, you should think carefully about whether or not to take supplements; consider consulting a physician or registered dietitian.

In 1998, the Food and Nutrition Board of the National Academy of Sciences recommended supplements of particular nutrients for the following groups:

- Women who are capable of becoming pregnant should take 400 µg per day of folic acid from fortified foods and/or supplements in addition to folate from a varied diet. Research indicates that this level of folate intake will reduce the risk of neural tube defects. (This defect occurs early in pregnancy, before most women know they are pregnant; therefore,

Category	Age (years) or Condition	Protein (g/kg)[d]	Vitamins Vitamin A (μg RE)[e]	Vitamin E (mg α-TE)[f]	Vitamin K (μg)	Vitamin C (mg)	Minerals Iron (mg)	Zinc (mg)	Iodine (μg)	Selenium (μg)
Infants	0.0–0.5	2.2	375	3	5	30	6	5	40	10
	0.5–1.0	1.6	375	4	10	35	10	5	50	15
Children	1–3	1.2	400	6	15	40	10	10	70	20
	4–6	1.1	500	7	20	45	10	10	90	20
	7–10	1.0	700	7	30	45	10	10	120	30
Males	11–14	1.0	1000	10	45	50	12	15	150	40
	15–18	0.9	1000	10	65	60	12	15	150	50
	19–24	0.8	1000	10	70	60	10	15	150	70
	25–50	0.8	1000	10	80	60	10	15	150	70
	51+	0.8	1000	10	80	60	10	15	150	70
Females	11–14	1.0	800	8	45	50	15	12	150	45
	15–18	0.8	800	8	55	60	15	12	150	50
	19–24	0.8	800	8	60	60	15	12	150	55
	25–50	0.8	800	8	65	60	15	12	150	55
	51+	0.8	800	8	65	60	10	12	150	55
Pregnant		+10g	800	10	65	70	30	15	175	65
Lactating	1st 6 Months	+15g	1300	12	65	95	15	19	200	75
	2nd 6 Months	+12g	1200	11	65	90	15	16	200	75

[a] This table includes RDAs for those nutrients for which DRIs had not yet been established as of June 1999. The allowances, expressed as average daily intakes over time, are intended to provide for individual variations among most healthy people as they live in the United States under usual environmental stresses. Diet should be based on a variety of common foods in order to provide other nutrients for which human requirements have been less well defined.

[b] Estimated Safe and Adequate Daily Dietary Intakes (ESADDIs) for adults: 1.5–3.0 mg copper; 2.0–5.0 mg manganese; 50–200 μg chromium; 75–250 mg molybdenum. (For information on other age groups, see National Research Council. 1989. *Recommended Dietary Allowances*, 10th ed. Washington, D.C.: National Academy Press.)

[c] Estimated Minimum Requirements of healthy adults: 500 mg sodium; 750 mg chloride; 2000 mg potassium. (For information on other age groups, see *Recommended Dietary Allowances*, 10th ed.)

[d] The RDA for protein is expressed as grams of protein per kilogram of body weight. To calculate the RDA, multiply body weight in kilograms (1 kilogram = 2.2 pounds) by the appropriate number from the protein column. For example, a 19-year-old male who weighs 165 pounds would calculate his protein RDA as follows: 165 lb ÷ 2.2 kg/lb = 75 kg × 0.8 g/kg (from table) = 60 g protein per day. For pregnant or lactating women, calculate RDA based on age and then add the appropriate number of additional grams listed in the table.

[e] Retinol equivalents: 1 retinol equivalent = 1 μg retinol or 6 μg ß-carotene.

[f] α-Tocopherol equivalents: 1 mg d-α tocopherol = 1 α-TE.

SOURCE: Reprinted with permission from *Recommended Dietary Allowances*, 10th ed. Copyright © 1989, 1998 by the National Academy of Sciences. Courtesy of the National Academy Press, Washington, D.C.

the recommendation for folate intake applies to all women of reproductive age rather than only to pregnant women.) Since 1998, enriched breads, flours, corn meals, rice, noodles, and other grain products have been fortified with small amounts of folic acid. Folate is found naturally in leafy green vegetables, legumes, citrus fruits and juices, and most berries.

- People over age 50 should consume foods fortified with vitamin B-12, B-12 supplements, or a combination of the two in order to meet the majority of the DRI of 2.4 mg of B-12 daily. Up to 30% of people over 50 may have problems absorbing vitamin B-12; the consumption of supplements and fortified

foods can overcome this problem and help prevent a deficiency.

Supplements may also be recommended in the following cases:

- Women with heavy menstrual flows may need extra iron to compensate for the monthly loss.
- Some vegetarians may need extra calcium, iron, zinc, and vitamin B-12.

Dietary Guidelines for Americans General principles of good nutrition intended to help prevent certain diet-related diseases. **TERMS**

TABLE 12-4 *Dietary Reference Intakes (DRIs): Recommended Levels for Individual Intake*

Life Stage	Group	Calcium (mg/day)	Phosphorus (mg/day)	Magnesium (mg/day)	Vitamin D (µg/day)[a,b]	Fluoride (mg/day)	Thiamin (mg/day)	Riboflavin (mg/day)
Infants	0–5 months	210	100	30	5	0.01	0.2	0.3
	6–11 months	270	275	75	5	0.5	0.3	0.4
Children	1–3 years	500	**460**	**80**	5	0.7	**0.5**	**0.5**
	4–8 years	800	**500**	**130**	5	1	**0.6**	**0.6**
Males	9–13 years	1300	**1250**	**240**	5	2	**0.9**	**0.9**
	14–18 years	1300	**1250**	**410**	5	3	**1.2**	**1.3**
	19–30 years	1000	**700**	**400**	5	4	**1.2**	**1.3**
	31–50 years	1000	**700**	**420**	5	4	**1.2**	**1.3**
	51–70 years	1200	**700**	**420**	10	4	**1.2**	**1.3**
	>70 years	1200	**700**	**420**	15	4	**1.2**	**1.3**
Females	9–13 years	1300	**1250**	**240**	5	2	**0.9**	**0.9**
	14–18 years	1300	**1250**	**360**	5	3	**1.0**	**1.0**
	19–30 years	1000	**700**	**310**	5	3	**1.1**	**1.1**
	31–50 years	1000	**700**	**320**	5	3	**1.1**	**1.1**
	51–70 years	1200	**700**	**320**	10	3	**1.1**	**1.1**
	>70 years	1200	**700**	**320**	15	3	**1.1**	**1.1**
Pregnancy	≤18 years	1300	**1250**	**400**	5	3	**1.4**	**1.4**
	19–30 years	1000	**700**	**350**	5	3	**1.4**	**1.4**
	31–50 years	1000	**700**	**360**	5	3	**1.4**	**1.4**
Lactation	≤18 years	1300	**1250**	**360**	5	3	**1.5**	**1.6**
	19–30 years	1000	**700**	**310**	5	3	**1.5**	**1.6**
	31–50 years	1000	**700**	**320**	5	3	**1.5**	**1.6**

NOTE: This table includes Dietary Reference Intakes for those nutrients for which DRIs had been set through June 1999. The table includes values for the type of DRI standard—Adequate Intake (AI) or Recommended Dietary Allowance (RDA)—that has been established for that particular nutrient and life stage; RDAs are shown in **bold type**.

[a] As cholecalciferol. 1 µg cholecalciferol = 40 IU vitamin D.
[b] In the absence of adequate exposure to sunlight.
[c] As niacin equivalents. 1 mg of niacin = 60 mg of tryptophan.
[d] As dietary folate equivalents (DFE). 1 DFE = 1 µg food folate = 0.6 µg of folic acid (from fortified food or supplement) consumed with food = 0.5 µg of synthetic (supplemental) folic acid taken on an empty stomach.
[e] Although AIs have been set for choline, there are few data to assess whether a dietary supply of choline is needed at all stages of the life cycle, and it may be that the choline requirement can be met by endogenous synthesis at some of these stages.
[f] Since 10–30% of older people may malabsorb food-bound B-12, it is advisable for those older than 50 years to meet their RDA mainly by consuming foods fortified with B-12 or a B-12-containing supplement.
[g] In view of evidence linking folate intake with neural tube defects in the fetus, it is recommended that all women capable of becoming pregnant consume 400 µg of synthetic folic acid from fortified food and/or supplements in addition to intake of food folate from a varied diet.
[h] It is assumed that women will continue consuming 400 µg of folic acid until their pregnancy is confirmed and they enter prenatal care, which ordinarily occurs after the end of the periconceptional period—the critical time for formation of the neural tube.

SOURCES: Food and Nutrition Board. Institute of Medicine. National Academy of Sciences. 1997. *Dietary Reference Intakes for Calcium, Phosphorus, Magnesium, Vitamin D, and Fluoride.* Washington, D.C.: National Academy Press. Food and Nutrition Board. Institute of Medicine. National Academy of Sciences. 1998. *Dietary Reference Intakes for Thiamin, Riboflavin, Niacin, Vitamin B₆, Folate, Vitamin B₁₂, Pantothenic Acid, Biotin, and Choline.* Washington, D.C.: National Academy Press. Copyright © 1998 by the National Academy of Sciences. Reprinted with permission from National Academy Press, Washington, D.C.

- Newborns need a single dose of vitamin K, which must be administered under the direction of a physician.
- People who are unable to consume adequate calories may need a range of vitamins and minerals.
- People who have certain diseases or who take certain medications may need specific vitamin and mineral supplements. Such supplement decisions must be made by a physician because some vitamins and minerals counteract the actions of certain medications.

In deciding whether to take a vitamin and mineral supplement, consider whether you already regularly consume a fortified breakfast cereal. If you do decide to take a supplement, choose a balanced formulation that contains 50–100% of the adult Daily Value for vitamins and

TABLE 12-4

TABLE 12-4 *Dietary Reference Intakes (DRIs)*

Niacin (mg/day)[c]	Vitamin B-6 (mg/day)	Folate (µg/day)[d]	Vitamin B-12 (µg/day)	Pantothenic Acid (mg/day)	Biotin (µg/day)	Choline[e] (mg/day)
2	0.1	65	0.4	1.7	5	125
3	0.3	80	0.5	1.8	6	150
6	0.5	150	0.9	2	8	200
8	0.6	200	1.2	3	12	250
12	1.0	300	1.8	4	20	375
16	1.3	400	2.4	5	25	550
16	1.3	400	2.4	5	30	550
16	1.3	400	2.4	5	30	550
16	1.7	400	2.4[f]	5	30	550
16	1.7	400	2.4[f]	5	30	550
12	1.0	300	1.8	4	20	375
14	1.2	400[g]	2.4	5	25	400
14	1.3	400[g]	2.4	5	30	425
14	1.3	400[g]	2.4	5	30	425
14	1.5	400[g]	2.4[f]	5	30	425
14	1.5	400	2.4[f]	5	30	425
18	1.9	600[h]	2.6	6	30	450
18	1.9	600[h]	2.6	6	30	450
18	1.9	600[h]	2.6	6	30	450
17	2.0	500	2.8	7	35	550
17	2.0	500	2.8	7	35	550
17	2.0	500	2.8	7	35	550

TABLE 12-5 *Tolerable Upper Intake Levels for Adults*

Nutrient	Upper Intake Level
Calcium	2500 mg/day
Phosphorus	4000 mg/day
Magnesium (nonfood sources)	350 mg/day
Vitamin D	50 µg/day
Fluoride	10 mg/day
Niacin	35 mg/day
Vitamin B-6	100 mg/day
Folate	1000 µg/day
Choline	3500 mg/day

This table includes the adult Tolerable Upper Intake Level (UL) standard of the Dietary Reference Intakes (DRIs). For some nutrients, there is insufficient data on which to develop a UL. This does not mean that there is no potential for adverse effects from high intake, and when data about adverse effects are limited, extra caution may be warranted. In healthy individuals, there is no established benefit from nutrient intakes above the RDA or AI.

SOURCES: Food and Nutrition Board. Institute of Medicine. National Academy of Sciences. 1997. *Dietary Reference Intakes for Calcium, Phosphorus, Magnesium, Vitamin D, and Fluoride.* Washington, D.C.: National Academy Press. Food and Nutrition Board. Institute of Medicine. National Academy of Sciences. 1998. *Dietary Reference Intakes for Thiamin, Riboflavin, Niacin, Vitamin B₆, Folate, Vitamin B₁₂, Pantothenic Acid, Biotin, and Choline.* Washington, D.C.: National Academy Press.

minerals. Avoid supplements containing large doses of particular nutrients. See pp. 327–331 for more on choosing and using supplements.

Daily Values Because the RDAs and DRIs are far too cumbersome to use as a basis for food labels, the U.S. Food and Drug Administration developed another set of dietary standards, the **Daily Values.** The Daily Values are based on several different sets of guidelines and include standards for fat, cholesterol, carbohydrate, dietary fiber, and selected vitamins and minerals. On food labels, they are expressed as a percentage of a 2000-calorie diet, an average daily calorie intake for Americans. Using a single set of recommendations—the Daily Values—on food labels helps make nutrition information more accessible to the consumer. Food labels are described in more detail later in the chapter.

The Food Guide Pyramid

The Food Guide Pyramid is a food-group plan developed by the U.S. Department of Agriculture that gives a

Daily Values A simplified version of the RDAs used on food labels; also included are values for nutrients with no RDA per se.

TERMS

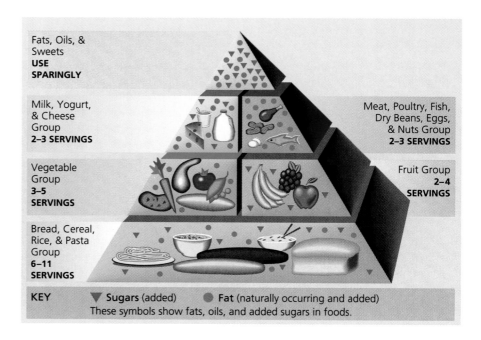

Figure 12-5 The Food Guide Pyramid: a guide to daily food choices. The Pyramid is an outline of what to eat each day—not a rigid prescription, but a general guide that lets you choose a healthful diet that's right for you. It calls for eating a variety of foods to get the nutrients you need and at the same time the right amount of calories to maintain a healthy weight. The Pyramid also focuses on fat because many Americans eat too much fat, especially saturated fat. SOURCE: U.S. Department of Agriculture, Human Nutrition Information Service. 1992. *Food Guide Pyramid.* Home and Garden Bulletin No. 249.

Within the pyramid image:

Fats, Oils, & Sweets
USE SPARINGLY

Milk, Yogurt, & Cheese Group
2–3 SERVINGS

Meat, Poultry, Fish, Dry Beans, Eggs, & Nuts Group
2–3 SERVINGS

Vegetable Group
3–5 SERVINGS

Fruit Group
2–4 SERVINGS

Bread, Cereal, Rice, & Pasta Group
6–11 SERVINGS

KEY ▼ Sugars (added) ● Fat (naturally occurring and added)
These symbols show fats, oils, and added sugars in foods.

recommended number of servings for six different food groups (Figure 12-5). A range of servings is given for each group: The smaller number is for people who consume about 1600 calories a day, the larger number for those who consume about 2800 calories a day. Serving sizes and examples of foods are described below for each group. The fundamental principles of the Food Guide Pyramid are moderation, variety, and balance—a theme echoed throughout this chapter. A diet is balanced if it contains appropriate amounts of each nutrient, and choosing foods from each of the food groups helps ensure that balance.

It is important to choose a variety of foods within each group because different foods have different combinations of nutrients: for example, within the vegetable group, potatoes are high in vitamin C, while spinach is a rich source of vitamin A. Foods also vary in their amount of calories and nutrients, and people who do not need many calories should focus on nutrient-rich foods within each group (foods that are high in nutrients relative to the number of calories they contain). Many foods you eat contain servings from more than one food group.

For more on the basic pyramid and alternative pyramids for special populations such as young children, vegetarians, and people choosing particular ethnic diets, contact the USDA's Food and Nutrition Center (see For More Information at the end of the chapter).

Bread, Cereals, Rice, and Pasta (6–11 Servings)

Foods from this group are usually low in fat and rich in complex carbohydrates, dietary fiber, and many vitamins and minerals, including thiamin, riboflavin, iron, niacin, folate, and zinc. Although 6–11 servings may seem like a

large amount of food, many people eat several servings at a time. A single serving is the equivalent of the following:

- 1 slice of bread or half of a hamburger bun, English muffin, or bagel
- 1 small roll, biscuit, or muffin
- 1 ounce of ready-to-eat cereal
- ½ cup cooked cereal, rice, or pasta
- 5–6 small or 2–3 large crackers

If you are one of the many people who have trouble identifying an ounce of cereal or half a cup of rice, see the strategies in the box "Judging Serving Sizes." Choose foods that are typically made with little fat or sugars (bread, rice, pasta) over those that are high in fat and sugars (croissants, chips, cookies, doughnuts). For maximum nutrition, choose whole-grain breads, high-fiber cereals, whole-wheat pasta, and brown rice.

Vegetables (3–5 Servings)

Vegetables are rich in carbohydrates, dietary fiber, vitamin A, vitamin C, folate, magnesium, and other nutrients. They are also naturally low in fat. A serving of vegetables is equivalent to the following:

- 1 cup raw leafy vegetables
- ½ cup raw or cooked vegetables
- ¾ cup vegetable juice
- ½ cup tomato sauce
- ½ cup cooked dry beans

Good choices from this group include dark-green leafy vegetables such as spinach, chard, and collards; deep-orange and red vegetables such as carrots, winter squash,

Studies have shown that most people underestimate the size of their food portions, in many cases by as much as 50%. If you need to retrain your eye, try using measuring cups and spoons and an inexpensive kitchen scale when you eat at home. With a little practice, you'll learn the difference between 3 and 8 ounces of chicken or meat, and what a half-cup of rice really looks like. For quick estimates, use the following equivalents:

- 1 teaspoon of margarine = the tip of your thumb
- 1 ounce of cheese = your thumb or four dice stacked together

- 3 ounces of chicken or meat = a deck of cards or an audio-cassette tape
- ½ cup of rice or cooked vegetables = an ice cream scoop or one-third of a soda can
- 2 tablespoons of peanut butter = a ping pong ball
- 1 cup of pasta = a woman's fist or a tennis ball
- 1 medium potato = a computer mouse

red bell peppers, and tomatoes; broccoli, cauliflower, and other cruciferous vegetables; peas; green beans; potatoes; and corn. Dry beans (legumes) such as pinto, navy, kidney, and black beans can be counted as servings of vegetables or as alternatives to meat.

Fruits (2–4 Servings)

Like vegetables, fruits are rich in carbohydrates, dietary fiber, and many vitamins, especially vitamin C. The serving sizes used in the Pyramid are as follows:

- 1 medium (apple, banana, peach, orange, pear) or 2 small (apricot, plum) whole fruit(s)
- 1 melon wedge
- ½ cup berries, cherries, or grapes
- ½ grapefruit
- ¼ cup dried fruit
- ½ cup chopped, cooked, canned, or frozen fruit
- ¾ cup fruit juice (100% juice)

Good choices from this group are citrus fruits and juices, melons, pears, apples, bananas, and berries. Choose whole fruits often—they are higher in fiber and often lower in calories than fruit juices. Fruit *juices* typically contain more nutrients than fruit *drinks*. For canned fruits, choose those packed in fruit juice rather than in syrup.

Milk, Yogurt, and Cheese (2–3 Servings)

Foods from this group are high in protein, carbohydrate, calcium, riboflavin, potassium, and zinc. To limit the fat in your diet, it is best to choose servings of lowfat or nonfat items from this group:

- 1 cup milk or yogurt
- 1½ ounces cheese
- 2 ounces processed cheese

Cottage cheese is lower in calcium than most other cheeses, and 1 cup of cottage cheese counts as only half a serving for this food group. Ice cream is also lower in calcium than many other dairy products (½ cup is equivalent to ⅓ serving); in addition, it is high in sugar and fat.

Meat, Poultry, Fish, Dry Beans, Eggs, and Nuts (2–3 Servings)

This group of foods provides protein, niacin, iron, vitamin B-6, zinc, and thiamin, and vitamin B-12 (animal foods only). The Pyramid recommends 2–3 servings each day of foods from this group. The total amount of these servings should be the equivalent of 5–7 ounces of cooked lean meat, poultry, or fish per day. Many people misjudge what makes up a single serving for this food group:

- 2–3 ounces cooked lean meat, poultry, or fish (an average hamburger or a medium chicken breast half is about 3 ounces; 4 slices of bologna, 6 slices of hard salami, or ½ cup of drained canned tuna counts as about 2 ounces)
- The following portions of nonmeat foods are equivalent to 1 ounce of lean meat:

  ½ cup cooked dry beans (if not counted as a vegetable)

  1 egg

  2 tablespoons peanut butter

  ⅓ cup nuts

  ¼ cup seeds

  ½ cup tofu

One egg at breakfast, a cup of pinto beans at lunch, and a hamburger at dinner would add up to the equivalent of 6 ounces of lean meat for the day. To limit your intake of fat and saturated fat, choose lean cuts of meat and skinless poultry, and watch your serving sizes carefully. Nuts and seeds are high in fat, so eat them in moderation. Choose at least one serving of plant proteins every day.

Fats, Oils, and Sweets

The small tip of the Pyramid includes fats, oils, and sweets—foods such as salad dressings, oils, butter, margarine, gravy, mayonnaise, soft drinks, sugar, candy, jellies and jams, syrups, and sweet desserts. Foods from the tip of the Pyramid provide calories but few nutrients; they should not replace foods from the other groups. The total amount of fats, oils, and

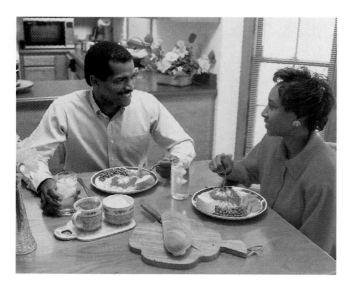

This couple's dinner of spaghetti with marinara sauce, carrots, peas, and bread is high in complex carbohydrates, vitamin A, vitamin C, folate, and dietary fiber.

sweets you consume should be determined by your overall energy needs.

As indicated by the colored triangles and circles in the Pyramid, fats and added sugars are also found within the five major food groups (see Figure 12-5). ("Added sugars" refers to those sugars added to foods in processing or at the table, not the sugars found naturally in fruits and milk.) Foods that come from animals (the meat and milk groups) are naturally higher in fat than foods that come from plants. However, there are many lean meat and low-fat dairy choices available. Fruits, vegetables, and grain products are naturally low in fat, but they can be prepared in ways that make them higher-fat choices—for example, potatoes served as french fries and pasta served as fettucini alfredo. Added sugars in the food groups can be found in foods such as ice cream, sweetened yogurt, canned fruit packed in syrup, and baked goods such as cookies. Reduced-fat versions of foods such as cookies and ice cream are often *very* high in added sugars and just as high in calories as their full-fat versions.

The average American diet currently includes more fat and added sugars than recommended. The Pyramid suggests that Americans limit the fat in their diets to 30% of total calories. You will consume about half this amount if you eat the recommended number of servings from each food group, select the lowest-fat choices, and add no fat during cooking or at the table. Additional fat, up to 30% of total calories, is considered discretionary in that you can decide whether to get it from higher-fat food choices or additions to your foods.

Added sugars are less of a concern to health than fat, but consumption of large amounts of sugars adds empty calories to the diet and can make weight management more difficult. Analysis of the average diet of Americans has revealed that the number of servings from the fruit, dairy, and meat groups is below the recommended ranges, and servings from the grain and vegetable groups are near the bottom of the recommended ranges (Table 12-6). Overconsumption of fat and added sugars leaves fewer calories available for healthier food choices from the five major food groups. For example, the average daily diet among American women includes about 10 teaspoons (40 grams) of added sugars and 5 grams of fat above recommended limits. The 200 calories in these extra sugars and fats could be better used to increase the number of servings from the food groups for which women typically fall short of Pyramid recommendations.

General strategies for controlling intake of fat and added sugars include choosing lower-fat foods within each food group, eating fewer foods that are high in sugar and low in other nutrients, and limiting the amount of fats and sugars added to foods during cooking or at the table.

The Food Guide Pyramid is a general guide to what you should eat every day. By eating a balanced variety of foods from each of the six food groups and including some plant proteins, you can ensure that your daily diet is adequate in all nutrients. A diet using lowfat food choices contains only about 1600 calories but meets all known nutritional needs, except possibly for iron in some women who have heavy menstrual periods. For these women, foods fortified in iron, such as breakfast cereals, can usually make up the deficit.

Dietary Guidelines for Americans

To provide further guidance for choosing a healthy diet, the U.S. Department of Agriculture and the Department of Health and Human Services have issued Dietary Guidelines for Americans, most recently in December of 1995. What follows is a summary of the advice provided by the Dietary Guidelines, with additional comments from other health-related organizations, including the American Heart Association, the National Cancer Institute, the National Academy of Sciences, and the Surgeon General. (Contact the USDA's Food and Nutrition Information Center for more on the development of the 2000 edition of the Dietary Guidelines; see For More Information at the end of the chapter.)

Eat a Variety of Foods To obtain the nutrients and other substances needed for good health, vary the foods you eat. Focus on the Food Guide Pyramid, choosing an appropriate number of servings from each group. Use foods from the base of the Pyramid as the foundation for your meals, and choose a variety of foods from within each group. Everyone, especially adolescent girls and women, should take special care to meet their recommended intakes for calcium and iron.

TABLE 12-6 *Food Guide Pyramid Recommendations Compared with the Average American Diet*

	Recommended Diets at Three Calorie Levels[a]			Average American Diet	
	1600	2200	2800	Women (1600 calories)	Men (2400 calories)
Grain group (servings)	6	9	11	5.7	7.7
Vegetable group (servings)	3	4	5	3.2	4.1
Fruit group (servings)	2	3	4	1.4	1.5
Dairy group (servings)[b]	2–3	2–3	2–3	1.1	1.5
Meat group (ounces)[c]	5	6	7	3.7	6.1
Total fat (grams)[d]	53	73	93	57.9	88.5
Total added sugars (teaspoons)[d,e]	6	12	18	15.9	22.4

[a] The bottom of the recommended range of servings (1600 calories) is about right for many sedentary women and older adults. The middle range (2200 calories) is about right for most children, teenage girls, active women, and many sedentary men. The top of the range (2800 calories) is about right for teenage boys, many active men, and some very active women.
[b] Women who are pregnant or lactating, teenagers, and young adults to age 24 need 3 servings.
[c] The Pyramid recommends 2–3 servings per day, the equivalent of 5–7 ounces of cooked lean meat, poultry, or fish (see p. 319).
[d] Values for total fat and added sugars include fat and added sugars that are in food choices from the five major food groups as well as fat and added sugars from foods in the Fats, Oils, and Sweets group. The total for added sugars does not include sugars that occur naturally in foods such as fruit and milk. The recommended fat totals are based on a limit of 30% of total calories as fat.
[e] A teaspoon of sugar is equivalent to 4 grams (16 calories).

SOURCES: Shaw, A., et al. 1997. *Using the Food Guide Pyramid: A Resource for Nutrition Educators.* Center for Nutrition Policy and Promotion. U.S. Department of Agriculture (retrieved January 8, 1998; http://www.nal.usda.gov/fnic/Fpyr/guide.pdf). U.S. Department of Agriculture. 1997. *Pyramid Servings Data: Results from USDA's 1995 and 1996 Continuing Survey of Food Intakes by Individuals.* Riverdale, Md.: Food Surveys Research Group. U.S. Department of Agriculture (retrieved December 2, 1998; http://www.barc.usda.gov/bhnrc/foodsurvey/home.htm).

Balance the Food You Eat with Physical Activity: Maintain or Improve Your Weight Emphasize balancing food intake with regular physical activity to avoid becoming overweight. Excess body fat increases the risk of diabetes, heart disease, cancer, and other diseases. People who are overweight and have one of these problems should try to lose weight, or at least not gain weight.

Those who are overweight should not try to lose more than ½–1 pound per week; avoid crash diets. Weight loss should be accomplished by increasing physical activity, eating less fat, and controlling portion sizes. If you are sedentary, try to become more active by accumulating 30 minutes or more of moderate physical activity on most or all days of the week. Choose lowfat, low-calorie, nutrient-rich foods—grains, vegetables, fruits, nonfat dairy products, and lean protein sources—rather than fatty foods, sugar and sweets, and alcoholic beverages. Exercise and weight management are discussed in Chapters 13 and 14.

Choose a Diet with Plenty of Grain Products, Vegetables, and Fruits Foods from these food groups provide vitamins, minerals, complex carbohydrates, dietary fiber, and other substances important for good health. They also tend to be low in fat. Five or more servings of fruits and vegetables and six or more servings of grain products will help you reach a daily dietary fiber consumption of 20–35 grams. Emphasize complex, rather than simple, carbohydrates, and eat a variety of foods from each group. The availability of fresh fruits and vegetables varies by season and region of the country, but frozen and canned fruits and vegetables are readily available and are usually as high in nutrients. According to the *Healthy People 2010* report, only about two in five Americans currently meet the Dietary Guidelines' minimum standard for fruit and vegetable intake.

Choose a Diet Low in Fat, Saturated Fat, and Cholesterol Some dietary fat is necessary for good health; good choices are monounsaturated and polyunsaturated fats found in vegetable oils, nuts, and fish. However, many Americans consume high-fat diets that increase their risk of heart disease, certain cancers, and obesity. Limit your overall intake of fat to 30% or less of daily calories, your saturated fat intake to one-third or less of your total daily fat intake (10% or less of total daily calories), and your intake of cholesterol to 300 milligrams per day.

To control your intake of fat and saturated fat, choose lean meat, fish, poultry, and dry beans as protein sources; use nonfat or lowfat milk and milk products; and limit your consumption of high-fat foods. To reduce your intake of trans fats, avoid deep-fried fast foods and other products made with hydrogenated vegetable oils. Refer to the box "Reducing the Fat in Your Diet" for more suggestions.

Although less dangerous for heart health than saturated fat, high cholesterol intake can be a problem for some people. Cholesterol is found only in animal foods. If you want to cut back on your cholesterol intake, follow the Food Guide Pyramid recommendations for

Your overall goal is to limit total fat intake to no more than 30% of total calories. Within that limit, favor unsaturated fats from vegetable oils, nuts, and fish over saturated and trans fats from animal products and foods made with hydrogenated vegetable oils. Limit saturated fat to less than 10% of total calories.

- Be moderate in your consumption of foods high in fat, including fast food, commercially prepared baked goods and desserts, meat, poultry, nuts and seeds, and regular dairy products (see Figure 12-4).

- When you do eat high-fat foods, limit your portion sizes, and balance your intake with foods low in fat.

- Choose lean cuts of meat, and trim any visible fat from meat before and after cooking. Remove skin from poultry before or after cooking.

- Replace whole milk with fat-free or lowfat milk in puddings, soups, and baked products. Substitute plain lowfat yogurt, blender-whipped cottage cheese, or buttermilk in recipes that call for sour cream.

- To reduce saturated fat, use vegetable oil instead of butter or margarine. Use tub or squeeze margarine instead of stick margarine. Look for margarines that are free of trans fats.

- Season vegetables with herbs and spices rather than with sauces, butter, or margarine.

- Try lemon juice on salad, or use a yogurt-based salad dressing instead of mayonnaise or sour cream dressings.

- Steam, boil, or bake vegetables, or stir-fry them in a small amount of vegetable oil.

- Roast, bake, or broil meat, poultry, or fish so that fat drains away as the food cooks.

- Use a nonstick pan for cooking so that added fat will be unnecessary; use a vegetable spray for frying.

- Chill broths from meat or poultry until the fat becomes solid. Spoon off the fat before using the broth.

- Eat a lowfat vegetarian main dish at least once a week.

---

consumption of animal foods; pay particular attention to serving sizes. In addition, limit your intake of foods that are particularly high in cholesterol content, including egg yolks and liver. Food labels provide the cholesterol content of prepared foods.

Choose a Diet Moderate in Sugars   Diets high in simple sugars do not cause hyperactivity or diabetes, but they do promote tooth decay. In addition, some foods that are high in sugar supply calories but few or no nutrients. For people who are very active and have high caloric needs, sugars can be an additional source of energy. However, because eating a nutritious diet and maintaining a healthy body weight are very important, most people should use sugars in moderation; people with low caloric needs should use sugars sparingly.

Moderation here means less than 15% of total calories—about 75 grams (15 teaspoons) of simple sugars per day. To reduce sugar consumption, cut back on items with added sugar, such as baked goods, candies, sweet desserts, sweetened beverages, canned fruits with heavy syrup, and presweetened breakfast cereals.

Choose a Diet Moderate in Salt and Sodium   Sodium is an essential nutrient, but it is required only in small amounts—500 milligrams, or ¼ teaspoon, per day. Most Americans consume 8–12 times this amount. High sodium intake is linked to high blood pressure in some people and may also increase calcium loss, contributing to osteoporosis. It is recommended that you limit sodium intake to no more than 2400 milligrams per day, or about 1¼ teaspoons of salt per day.

Sodium is found primarily in processed and prepared foods; sodium content is provided on food labels. To lower your sodium intake, cut back on salty foods such as lunch meats, salted snack foods, canned soups, regular cheese, many tomato-based products, and many frozen dinners and baked goods. Add less salt during cooking and at the table; use lemon juice, herbs, and spices, rather than salt, to enhance the flavor of food. It usually takes only about a week or two to become accustomed to a lower sodium diet.

If You Drink Alcoholic Beverages, Do So in Moderation   Alcoholic beverages supply calories but few or no nutrients. Current evidence suggests that moderate drinking—no more than one drink daily for women and two drinks for men—is associated with a lower risk of cardiovascular disease in some people. However, higher levels of alcohol intake are associated with an increased risk for many diseases and with higher overall mortality rates. (Refer to Chapter 10 for more on the health risks and benefits of alcohol use.) Adults who drink alcoholic beverages should do so in moderation, with meals, and when consumption does not put themselves or others at risk.

One further recommendation geared primarily for cancer prevention is to use moderation when consuming salt-cured, smoked, and nitrate-cured foods such as bacon and sausage. Curing and smoking of foods helps prevent the growth of certain harmful bacteria. However, nitrates have been associated with an increased risk of colon and other gastrointestinal cancers in some people (see p. 334). The addition of vitamin C and other antioxidants to cured meats decreases the number of carcinogens, but salt-cured, smoked, and nitrate-cured foods should still be consumed in moderation because they are often high in fat, cholesterol, and sodium.

These guidelines do not apply equally to everyone. We vary in our susceptibility to developing high blood cholesterol levels, high blood pressure, obesity, cancer, and the other health problems these guidelines seek to counteract. You should consider your own health status and apply these guidelines appropriately to address current or potential health problems. To determine how your eating habits stack up, take the quiz in the box "How's Your Diet?"

> **PERSONAL INSIGHT** Do you feel good after you eat a healthy meal? Are your good feelings physical or emotional, or both?

The Vegetarian Alternative

Some people choose a diet with one essential difference from the diets we've already described—foods of animal origin (meat, poultry, fish, eggs, milk) are eliminated or restricted. Today, about 12 million Americans follow a vegetarian diet. Most do so because they think foods of plant origin are a more natural way to nourish the body. Some do so for religious, health, ethical, or philosophical reasons. If you choose to be a vegetarian, you can be confident you can meet your nutritional needs by following a few basic rules. (Vegetarian diets for children and pregnant women warrant individual professional guidance.)

Types of Vegetarian Diets   There are various vegetarian styles; the wider the variety of the diet eaten, the easier it is to meet nutritional needs. **Vegans** eat only plant foods. **Lacto-vegetarians** eat plant foods and dairy products. **Lacto-ovo-vegetarians** eat plant foods, dairy products, and eggs. Finally, **partial, semivegetarians,** or **pesco-vegetarians** eat plant foods, dairy products, eggs, and usually a small selection of poultry, fish, and other seafood. Including some animal protein in a diet makes planning much easier, but it is not necessary.

A Food-Group Plan for Vegetarians   A food-group plan has been developed for lacto-vegetarians; it includes 6–11 servings from grains and 2–4 servings from legumes, nuts, and seeds. Add to this 3–5 servings from a vegetable group, 2–4 servings from a fruit group, and 2 or more servings from the milk, yogurt, and cheese group to complete the plan. By following this plan, the lacto-vegetarian should have no problem obtaining an adequate diet. Consuming fruits with most meals is especially helpful, because any vitamin C present will improve iron absorption (the iron in plants is more difficult to absorb than the iron in animal sources).

In contrast to those who eat dairy products, the vegan has to do more planning to obtain all essential nutrients. A vegan must take special care to consume adequate amounts of protein, riboflavin, vitamin D, vitamin B-12, calcium, iron, and zinc; good strategies for obtaining these nutrients include the following:

- Eat proteins from a wide variety of sources, and include a couple of protein sources at each meal. A good rule of thumb is 11 servings of grains and 4 servings of legumes, nuts, and seeds. Soy milk, tofu (soybean curd), and tempeh (a cultured soy product) make important nutrient contributions to this diet plan.

- Eat green leafy vegetables, whole grains, yeast, and legumes to obtain riboflavin.

- Obtain vitamin D by spending 5–15 minutes a day out in the sun, by consuming vitamin D–fortified products like rice milk or soy milk, or by taking a supplement.

- Obtain vitamin B-12 (found only in animal foods) from a supplement or by consuming foods fortified with vitamin B-12, such as special yeast products, soy milk, and breakfast cereals.

- Eat fortified tofu, dark-green leafy vegetables, nuts, tortillas made from lime-processed corn, and fortified orange juice, bread, and soy milk to obtain calcium. Supplements may be necessary.

- Eat whole grains, fortified bread and breakfast cereals, dried fruits, green leafy vegetables, nuts, and legumes to obtain iron. Supplements may be necessary.

- Obtain zinc from whole grains, nuts, and legumes.

It takes a little planning and common sense to put together a good vegetarian diet. If you are a vegetarian or are considering becoming one, devote some extra time and thought to your diet. It's especially important that you eat as wide a variety of foods as possible to ensure that all your nutritional needs are satisfied. Consulting with a registered dietitian will make your planning even easier.

Dietary Challenges for Special Population Groups

The Food Guide Pyramid and Dietary Guidelines for Americans provide a basis that everyone can use to create a healthy diet. However, some population groups face special dietary challenges.

> **vegan**   A vegetarian who eats no animal products at all. **TERMS**
>
> **lacto-vegetarian**   A vegetarian who includes milk and cheese products in the diet.
>
> **lacto-ovo-vegetarian**   A vegetarian who eats no meat, poultry, or fish, but does eat eggs and milk products.
>
> **partial, semivegetarian, or pesco-vegetarian**   A vegetarian who includes eggs, dairy products, and small amounts of poultry and seafood in the diet.

- For each question, circle the plus (+) or minus (−) score(s) that best reflects your diet. If you circle more than one score, average them by adding the scores and dividing by the number of scores you circled.

- For your final score, add your plus scores separately from your minus scores, then subtract your total minus scores from your total plus scores.

- Keep the quiz as incentive. Take it again in a few months to see if your habits have improved.

1. How many times a week do you eat red meat? (Include beef, lamb, pork, veal.)
   - (a) 0   +4
   - (b) 1 or 2   +2
   - (c) 3 or 4   −2
   - (d) 5 or 6   −4
   - (e) More than 6   −5

2. How many ounces of red meat constitute your normal portion? (*Hint:* 3 ounces, cooked, is approximately the size of a deck of cards.)
   - (a) 3 ounces   +2
   - (b) 4 ounces   +1
   - (c) 5 ounces   −2
   - (d) 6 or more ounces   −3

3. What kind of red meat do you usually choose?
   - (a) Loin or round cuts only   +2
   - (b) 80% lean   +1
   - (c) Ribs, T-bone   −4
   - (d) Hot dogs, bacon, bologna   −5

4. How many times a week do you eat seafood? (Omit fried dishes; include shellfish like shrimp and lobster.)
   - (a) 2 or more   +4
   - (b) 1   +2
   - (c) Less than 1   0
   - (d) Never   −3

5. How many ounces of poultry or seafood do you eat for a serving? (Do not count fried items.)
   - (a) 3 ounces   +2
   - (b) 4 ounces   +1
   - (c) 5 ounces   −2
   - (d) 6 or more ounces   −3

6. Do you remove the skin from poultry?
   - (a) Yes   +2
   - (b) Don't eat poultry   0
   - (c) No   −3

7. How many times a week do you eat at least one half-cup serving of legumes? (Include beans like soybeans, navy, kidney, garbanzo, baked beans, lentils.)
   - (a) 3 or more   +4
   - (b) 1 to 2   +2
   - (c) Less than 1   0
   - (d) Never eat legumes   −1

8. What kind of milk do you drink?
   - (a) Skim or 1%   +3
   - (b) Don't drink milk   0
   - (c) 2%   −3
   - (d) Whole   −4

9. What kind of cheese do you usually eat?
   - (a) Fat-free   +2
   - (b) Lowfat (5 grams fat or less per ounce)   +1
   - (c) Don't eat cheese   0
   - (d) Whole-milk cheese   −4

10. How many servings of lowfat, high-calcium foods do you eat daily? (One cup of yogurt or milk, 2 ounces of cheese, or one cup chopped broccoli, kale, or greens count as a serving.)
    - (a) 3 or more   +4
    - (b) 1 or 2   +2
    - (c) 0   −3

11. What kind of bread do you eat most often?
    - (a) 100% whole wheat   +4
    - (b) Whole grain   +2
    - (c) White, "wheat," Italian or French   0
    - (d) Croissant or biscuit   −4

12. Which is part of your most typical breakfast?
    - (a) High-fiber cereal and fruit   +4
    - (b) Bagel or toast   +1
    - (c) Don't eat breakfast   −2
    - (d) Danish, pastry, or doughnut   −3

13. What kind of sauce or topping is usually on the pasta you eat?
    - (a) Vegetables tossed lightly with olive oil   +3
    - (b) Tomato or marinara sauce   +2
    - (c) Meat sauce   −3
    - (d) Alfredo or cream sauce   −4

14. Which would you be most likely to order at a Chinese restaurant?
    - (a) Chicken with steamed vegetables over white rice   +3
    - (b) Cold sesame noodles   −1
    - (c) Twice-fried pork   −4

15. Which would you be most likely to choose as toppings for pizza?
    - (a) Vegetables (e.g., broccoli, peppers)   +3
    - (b) Plain cheese   0
    - (c) Extra cheese   −3
    - (d) Sausage and pepperoni   −4

Women   Women tend to be smaller and weigh less than men, meaning they have lower energy needs and therefore consume fewer calories. Because of this, women have more difficulty getting adequate amounts of all essential nutrients and need to focus on nutrient-dense foods. Two nutrients of special concern are calcium and iron, minerals for which many women fail to meet the RDAs. Low calcium intake may be linked to the development of osteoporosis in later life. The *Healthy People 2010* report sets a goal of increasing from 38% to 90% the proportion of women age 20–49 who meet the dietary recommendation for calcium. Nonfat and lowfat dairy products and fortified cereal, bread, and orange juice are good choices. Iron is also a concern: Menstruating women have higher iron requirements than other groups, and a lack of iron in the diet can lead to iron-deficiency anemia. Lean red

16. What is the most typical snack for you?
    (a) Fresh fruit   +4   (d) Potato chips −3
    (b) Lowfat yogurt   +3   (e) Candy bar   −3
    (c) Pretzels   +1

17. How many half-cup servings of a high vitamin C fruit or vegetable do you eat daily? (Include citrus fruit and juices, kiwi, papaya, strawberries, broccoli, peppers, potatoes, tomatoes.)
    (a) 2 or more +3   (b) 1 +1   (c) None −3

18. How many half-cup servings of a high vitamin A fruit or vegetable do you eat daily? (Include apricots, cantaloupe, mango, broccoli, carrots, greens, spinach, sweet potato, winter squash.)
    (a) 2 or more +3   (b) 1 +1   (c) None −3

19. What kind of salad dressing do you most often choose?
    (a) Fat-free or lowfat   +3
    (b) Lemon juice or herb vinegar   +3
    (c) Olive or canola oil–based   +1
    (d) Creamy or cheese-based   −3

20. What do you usually spread on bread, rolls, or bagels?
    (a) Nothing   +1
    (b) Jam, jelly, or honey   −1
    (c) Light butter or light margarine −2
    (d) Cream cheese   −2
    (e) Margarine   −3
    (f) Butter   −4

21. What spread do you usually choose for sandwiches?
    (a) Nothing   +3   (d) Mayonnaise,
    (b) Mustard   +2   margarine, or
    (c) Light mayonnaise −1   butter   −3

22. Which frozen dessert do you usually choose?
    (a) Don't eat frozen desserts +3
    (b) Fat-free frozen yogurt   +1
    (c) Sorbet or sherbet   +1
    (d) Light ice cream   −2
    (e) Ice cream   −4

23. How many cups of caffeinated beverages (e.g., coffee, tea, or soda) do you usually drink in a typical day?
    (a) None +2   (c) 3 to 4   −1
    (b) 1 to 2 0   (d) 5 or more −4

24. How many total cups of fluid do you drink in a typical day? (Include water, juice, milk.)
    (a) 8 or more +3   (c) 4 or 5   +1
    (b) 6 to 7   +2   (d) Less than 4 −1

25. What kind of cereal do you eat?
    (a) High-fiber cereals such as bran flakes +3
    (b) Low-fiber, low-sugar cereals, such as puffed rice, corn flakes, Corn Chex, or Cheerios.   0
    (c) Sugary, low-fiber cereals, like Frosted Flakes, or fruit-flavored cereals   −2
    (d) Regular (high-fat) granola   −3

26. How many times a week do you eat fried foods?
    (a) never +4   (b) 2 or less 0   (c) 3 or more −3

27. How many times a week do you eat cancer-fighting cruciferous vegetables? (Include broccoli, cauliflower, brussels sprouts, cabbage, kale, bok choy, cooking greens, turnips, rutabaga.)
    (a) 3 or more +4   (b) 1 to 2 +2   (c) Rarely −4

Scoring

65–82: Excellent.
42–64: Very good.
28–41: Good.
27−−16: Fair.
Below −16: Get help!

SOURCE: © 1996, CSPI. Adapted from Nutrition Action Healthletter (1875 Connecticut Ave., N.W., Suite 300, Washington, D.C. 20009-5728. $24 for 10 issues).

meat, green leafy vegetables, and fortified breakfast cereals are good sources of iron. As discussed earlier, all women capable of becoming pregnant should consume adequate folic acid from fortified foods and/or supplements.

Men   Men are seldom thought of as having nutritional deficiencies because they generally have high-calorie diets. However, many men have a diet that does not follow the Food Guide Pyramid but that includes more red meat and fewer fruits, vegetables, and grains than recommended. This dietary pattern is linked to heart disease and some types of cancer. A high intake of calories can lead to weight gain in the long term if a man's activity level decreases as he ages. Men should use the Food Guide Pyramid as a basis for their overall diet and focus on increasing their consumption of fruits, vegetables, and grains to obtain vitamins, minerals, dietary fiber, and phytochemicals.

Children and Teenagers   Young people often simply need to be encouraged to eat. Perhaps the best thing a parent can do for younger children is to provide them with a variety of foods. Add vegetables to casseroles and fruit to cereal; offer fruit and vegetable juices or homemade yogurt or fruit shakes instead of sugary drinks. Allowing children to help prepare meals is another good way to increase overall food consumption and variety. Many children and teenagers enjoy eating at fast-food restaurants;

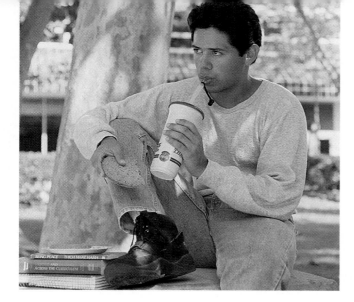

Eating on the run is a common—but not always healthy—habit among college students. After snacking on cookies, this young man should complete his day's diet with a lowfat, nutrient-rich dinner.

they should be encouraged to select the healthiest choices from fast-food menus (see Appendix A) and to complete the day's diet with lowfat, nutrient-rich foods.

College Students   Foods that are convenient for college students are not always the healthiest choices. It is easy for students who eat in buffet-style dining halls to overeat, and the foods offered are not necessarily high in essential nutrients and low in fat. The same is true of meals at fast-food restaurants, another convenient source of quick and inexpensive meals for busy students. Although no food is entirely "bad," consuming a wide variety of foods is critical for a healthy diet. See the box "Eating Strategies for College Students" for tips on making healthy eating convenient and affordable.

Older Adults   As people age, they tend to become less active, so they require fewer calories to maintain their body weight. At the same time, the absorption of nutrients tends to be lower in older adults because of age-related changes in the digestive tract. Thus, they must consume nutrient-dense foods in order to meet their nutritional requirements. As discussed earlier, foods fortified with vitamin B-12 and/or B-12 supplements are recommended for people over age 50. Because constipation is a common problem, consuming foods high in dietary fiber is another important goal. Social and economic factors such as isolation and low income can profoundly influence the eating habits of older Americans. (For more on healthy aging, refer to Chapter 19.)

Athletes   Key dietary concerns for athletes are meeting their increased energy requirements and drinking enough fluids during practice and throughout the day to remain fully hydrated. Endurance athletes may also benefit from increasing the amount of carbohydrate in the diet to 60–65% of total daily calories; this increase should come in the form of complex, rather than simple, carbohydrates. Athletes for whom maintaining low body weight and body fat is important—such as skaters, gymnasts, and wrestlers—should consume adequate nutrients and avoid falling into unhealthy patterns of eating. Eating for exercise is discussed in more detail in Chapter 13; refer to Chapter 14 for information on eating disorders.

People with Special Health Concerns   Many Americans have special health concerns that affect their dietary needs. For example, women who are pregnant or breastfeeding require extra calories, vitamins, and minerals (see Chapter 8). People with diabetes benefit from a well-balanced diet that is low in simple sugars, high in complex carbohydrates, and relatively rich in monounsaturated fats. And people with high blood pressure need to limit their sodium consumption and control their weight. If you have a health problem or concern that may require a special diet, discuss your situation with a physician or registered dietitian (R.D.).

A PERSONAL PLAN: MAKING INFORMED CHOICES ABOUT FOOD

Now that you understand the basis of good nutrition and a healthy diet, you can put together a diet that works for you. Based on your particular nutrition and health status there probably is an ideal diet for you, but there is no single type of diet that provides optimal health for everyone. Many cultural dietary patterns encompass the practices recommended by nutrition experts: eating a variety of foods, maintaining a healthy body weight, and maintaining a physically active lifestyle (see the box "Ethnic Foods," p. 328 for more information).

Focus now on the likely causes of any health problems in your life, and make specific dietary changes to address them. You may also have some specific areas of concern, such as interpreting food labels and dietary supplement labels, avoiding foodborne illnesses and environmental contaminants, and understanding food additives. We turn to these and other topics next.

Reading Food Labels

Consumers can get help in applying the principles of the Food Guide Pyramid and the Dietary Guidelines for Americans from food labels. Since 1994, all processed foods regulated by either the FDA or the USDA have included standardized nutrition information on their labels. Every food label shows serving sizes and the amount of fat, saturated fat, cholesterol, protein, dietary fiber, and

General Guidelines

- Eat slowly, and enjoy your food.

- Eat a colorful, varied diet. The more colorful your diet is, the more varied and rich in fruits and vegetables it will be. Many Americans eat few fruits and vegetables, despite the fact that these foods are typically inexpensive, delicious, rich in nutrients, and low in fat and calories.

- Eat breakfast. You'll have more energy in the morning and be less likely to grab an unhealthy snack later on.

- Choose healthy snacks—fruits, vegetables, grains, and cereals—as often as you can.

- Combine physical activity with healthy eating. You'll feel better and have a much lower risk of many chronic diseases. Even a little exercise is better than none.

Eating in the Dining Hall

- Choose a meal plan that includes breakfast, and don't skip it.

- If menus are posted or distributed, decide what you want to eat before you get in line, and stick to your choices. Consider what you plan to do and eat for the rest of the day before making your choices.

- Ask for large servings of vegetables and small servings of meat and other high-fat main dishes. Build your meals around grains and vegetables.

- Choose leaner poultry, fish, or bean dishes rather than high-fat meats and fried entrees.

- Ask that gravies and sauces to be served on the side; limit your intake.

- Choose broth-based or vegetable soups rather than cream soups.

- Drink nonfat milk, water, mineral water, or 100% fruit juice rather than heavily sweetened fruit drinks or whole milk.

- Choose fruit for dessert rather than pastries, cookies, or cakes.

- Do some research about the foods and preparation methods used in your dining hall or cafeteria. Discuss any food and nutrition suggestions you have with your food service manager.

Eating in Fast-Food Restaurants

- Most fast-food chains can provide a brochure with a nutritional breakdown of the foods on the menu. Ask for it. (See also the information in Appendix A.)

- Order small single burgers with no cheese instead of double burgers with many toppings. If possible, ask for them broiled instead of fried.

- Ask for items to be prepared without mayonnaise, tartar sauce, sour cream, or other high-fat sauces. Ketchup, mustard, and fat-free mayonnaise or sour cream are better choices and are available at many fast-food restaurants.

- Choose whole-grain buns or bread for burgers and sandwiches.

- Choose chicken items made from chicken breast, not processed chicken.

- Order vegetable pizzas.

- At the salad bar, choose a lowfat dressing. Put the dressing on the side and dip your fork into it; don't pour it over your salad. Avoid heavily dressed potato and pasta salads. Don't put croutons and bacon on vegetable salads.

- If you order french fries or onion rings, get the smallest size, and/or share them with a friend.

Eating on the Run

Are you chronically short of time? The following healthy and filling items can be packed for a quick snack or meal: fresh or dried fruit, fruit juices, raw fresh vegetables, plain bagels, bread sticks, fig bars, lowfat cheese sticks or cubes, lowfat crackers or granola bars, nonfat or lowfat yogurt, pretzels, rice or corn cakes, plain popcorn, soup (if you have access to a microwave), or water.

SOURCES: Fahey, T. D., P. M. Insel, and W. T. Roth. 1999. *Fit and Well: Core Concepts and Labs in Physical Fitness and Wellness,* 3rd ed. Mountain View, Calif.: Mayfield. Kleiner, S. M. 1995. Nutrition on the run. *Physician and Sportsmedicine* 23(2): 15–16.

---

sodium in each serving. To make intelligent choices about food, learn to read and understand food labels (see the box "Using Food Labels," p. 329). Research has shown that people who read food labels consume less fat.

Because most meat, poultry, fish, fruits, and vegetables are not packaged, they do not have food labels. You can obtain information on the nutrient content of these items from basic nutrition books, registered dietitians, nutrient analysis computer software, the World Wide Web, and the companies that produce or distribute these foods. Also, supermarkets often have large posters or pamphlets listing the nutrient contents of these foods.

Reading Dietary Supplement Labels

Dietary supplements include vitamins, minerals, amino acids, and herbs and other plant-derived substances. They may come in the form of tablets, capsules, liquids,

There is no one ethnic diet that clearly surpasses all others in providing people with healthful foods. However, every diet has its advantages and disadvantages and, within each cuisine, some foods are better choices. It is in this area of personal choice that individuals can make a difference in their own health. The dietary guidelines described in this chapter can be applied to any ethnic cuisine. For additional guidance, refer to the table below, which lists some of the more and less healthful choices you can make when you eat out at various ethnic restaurants or cook ethnic meals at home.

	Choose Often	**Choose Seldom**
Chinese	Chinese greens Hunan or Szechuan dishes Rice, brown or white Steamed or stir-fry dishes Wonton soup	Crispy duck or beef Egg rolls or fried wontons General Tso's chicken Kung pao or sweet-and-sour dishes Rice, fried
Indian	Chapati (baked, tortilla-like bread) Dal (lentils) Karhi (chickpea soup) Khur (milk and rice dessert) Tandoori, chicken or fish Yogurt-based curry dishes	Bhatura, poori, or paratha (fried breads) Coconut milk–based dishes Ghee (clarified butter) Korma (rich meat dish) Pakoras (fried appetizer) Samosa (fried meat and vegetables in dough)
Italian	Cioppino (seafood stew) Minestrone soup, vegetarian Pasta with marinara sauce Pasta primavera Pasta with red or white clam sauce	Cannelloni, ravioli, or manicotti Fettucine alfredo Fried calamari Garlic bread Veal or eggplant parmigiana
Japanese	Kushiyaki (broiled foods on skewers) Nabemono (boiled dishes) Shabu-shabu (foods in boiling broth) Sushi	Agemono (deep-fried dishes) Sukiyaki Tempura (fried chicken, shrimp, or vegetables) Tonkatsu (fried pork)
Mexican	Beans and rice Burritos, bean or chicken Fajitas, chicken or vegetable Gazpacho Refried beans, nonfat or lowfat Tortillas, steamed	Chiles rellenos Chimichangas, flautas, or quesadillas Enchiladas, beef or cheese Nachos or fried tortillas Refried beans made with lard Taco salad
Thai	Forest salad Larb (chicken salad with mint) Po tak (seafood soup) Yum neua (broiled beef with onions)	Fried fish, duck, or chicken Curries with coconut milk Dishes with peanut sauce Yum koon chaing (sausage with peppers)

SOURCES: The sat fat switch. 1997. *Nutrition Action Healthletter,* January/February. University of Southern Florida Student Health Service. 1997. Ethnic food (http://www.shs.usf.edu/Health/ethnic.html). The best of Asian cuisines. 1993. *University of California at Berkeley Wellness Letter,* January. Eating in ethnic restaurants. 1990. *Runner's World,* January. Reprinted by permission of *Runner's World Magazine.* Copyright © 1990 Rodek Press, Inc. All rights reserved.

or powders. Surveys indicate that over half of American adults use dietary supplements at least occasionally, and sales have more than doubled since 1990, to over $6 billion per year. Although dietary supplements are often thought to be safe and "natural," they do contain powerful, bioactive chemicals that have the potential for harm. About one-quarter of all pharmaceutical drugs are derived from botanical sources—morphine from poppies and digoxin from foxglove, for example. And as described earlier, even essential vitamins and minerals can have toxic effects if consumed in excess.

In the United States, supplements are not considered drugs and are not regulated the way drugs are. Before they are approved by the FDA and put on the market, drugs undergo clinical studies to determine safety, effectiveness, side effects and risks, possible interactions with other substances, and appropriate dosages. The FDA does not authorize or test dietary supplements, and supplements are not required to demonstrate either safety or effectiveness prior to marketing. Although dosage guidelines exist for some of the compounds in dietary supplements, dosages for many are not well established.

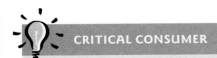

Food labels are designed to help consumers make food choices based on the nutrients that are most important to good health. A food label states how much fat, saturated fat, cholesterol, protein, dietary fiber, and sodium the food contains. In addition to listing nutrient content by weight, the label puts the information in the context of a daily diet of 2000 calories that includes no more than 65 grams of fat (approximately 30% of total calories). For example, if a serving of a particular product has 13 grams of fat, the label will show that the serving represents 20% of the daily fat allowance. If your daily diet contains fewer or more than 2000 calories, you need to adjust these calculations accordingly. Refer to p. 305 for instructions on setting nutrient intake goals.

Food labels contain uniform serving sizes. This means that if you look at different brands of salad dressing, for example, you can compare calories and fat content based on the serving amount. Regulations also require that foods meet strict definitions if their packaging includes the terms "light," "lowfat," or "high-fiber" (see below). Health claims such as "good source of dietary fiber" or "low in saturated fat" on packages are signals that those products can wisely be included in your diet. Overall, the food label is an important tool to help you choose a diet that conforms to the Food Guide Pyramid and the Dietary Guidelines.

Selected Nutrient Claims and What They Mean

Healthy   A food that is low in fat, low in saturated fat, has no more than 360–480 mg of sodium and 60 mg of cholesterol, *and* provides 10% or more of the Daily Value for vitamin A, vitamin C, protein, calcium, iron, or dietary fiber.

Light or lite   One-third fewer calories or 50% less fat than a similar product.

Reduced or fewer   At least 25% less of a nutrient than a similar product; can be applied to fat ("reduced fat"), saturated fat, cholesterol, sodium, and calories.

Extra or added   10% or more of the Daily Value per serving when compared to a similar product.

Good source   10–19% of the Daily Value for a particular nutrient.

High, rich in, or excellent source of   20% or more of the Daily Value for a particular nutrient.

Low calorie   40 calories or less per serving.

High fiber   5 g or more of fiber per serving.

Good source of fiber   2.5–4.9 g of fiber per serving.

Fat-free   Less than 0.5 g of fat per serving.

Lowfat   3 g of fat or less per serving.

Saturated fat-free   Less than 0.5 g of saturated fat and 0.5 g of trans fatty acids per serving.

Low saturated fat   1 g or less of saturated fat per serving and no more than 15% of total calories.

Cholesterol free   Less than 2 mg of cholesterol and 2 g or less of saturated fat per serving.

Low cholesterol   20 mg or less of cholesterol and 2 g or less of saturated fat per serving.

Low sodium   140 mg or less of sodium per serving.

Very low sodium   35 mg or less of sodium per serving.

Lean   Cooked seafood, meat, or poultry with less than 10 g of fat, 4 g of saturated fat, and 95 mg of cholesterol per serving.

Extra lean   Cooked seafood, meat, or poultry with less than 5 g of fat, 2 g of saturated fat, and 95 mg of cholesterol per serving.

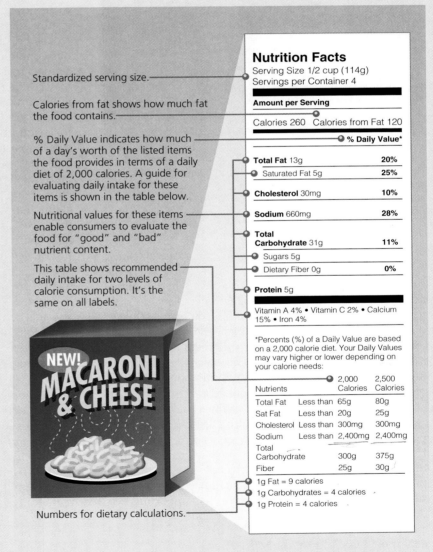

Standardized serving size.

Calories from fat shows how much fat the food contains.

% Daily Value indicates how much of a day's worth of the listed items the food provides in terms of a daily diet of 2,000 calories. A guide for evaluating daily intake for these items is shown in the table below.

Nutritional values for these items enable consumers to evaluate the food for "good" and "bad" nutrient content.

This table shows recommended daily intake for two levels of calorie consumption. It's the same on all labels.

Numbers for dietary calculations.

Nutrition Facts
Serving Size 1/2 cup (114g)
Servings per Container 4

Amount per Serving

Calories 260   Calories from Fat 120

	% Daily Value*
Total Fat 13g	20%
Saturated Fat 5g	25%
Cholesterol 30mg	10%
Sodium 660mg	28%
Total Carbohydrate 31g	11%
Sugars 5g	
Dietary Fiber 0g	0%
Protein 5g	

Vitamin A 4% • Vitamin C 2% • Calcium 15% • Iron 4%

*Percents (%) of a Daily Value are based on a 2,000 calorie diet. Your Daily Values may vary higher or lower depending on your calorie needs:

Nutrients		2,000 Calories	2,500 Calories
Total Fat	Less than	65g	80g
Sat Fat	Less than	20g	25g
Cholesterol	Less than	300mg	300mg
Sodium	Less than	2,400mg	2,400mg
Total Carbohydrate		300g	375g
Fiber		25g	30g

1g Fat = 9 calories
1g Carbohydrates = 4 calories
1g Protein = 4 calories

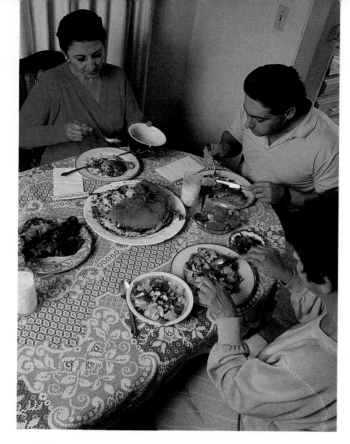
Careful food handling greatly reduces the risk of foodborne illness. Helpful strategies include washing all fruits and vegetables, using separate cutting boards for meat and for foods that will be eaten raw, cooking meat thoroughly, and refrigerating leftovers promptly.

Many ingredients in dietary supplements are classified by the FDA as "generally recognized as safe," but some have been found to be dangerous on their own or to interact with prescription or over-the-counter drugs in dangerous ways. Garlic supplements, for example, can cause bleeding if taken with anticoagulant ("blood thinning") medications. Even products that are generally considered safe can have side effects—St. John's wort, for example, increases the skin's sensitivity to sunlight. If the FDA receives reports of serious reactions or effects, it can then act to restrict the sale or use of a product.

Preliminary studies of the health effects of some compounds in popular dietary supplements are encouraging. However, some supplements are likely far more effective than others, and proof of effectiveness is not required prior to marketing. Supplement manufacturers have to supply only a single scientific report as supporting evidence for any health claims they make about a product—and then only after the product has been introduced and only if the FDA asks for the report.

There are also key differences between how drugs and supplements are manufactured. FDA-approved medications are standardized for potency, and quality control and proof of purity are required. Dietary supple-

ment manufacture is not so closely regulated, and there is no guarantee that a product even contains a given ingredient, let alone in the appropriate amount. The potency of herbal supplements tends to vary widely due to differences in growing and harvesting conditions, preparation methods, and storage. (A 1998 test of 10 brands of St. John's wort supplements found that two had only about 20% of the potency listed on the label and another six had 50–90%; the remaining two were 30–40% more potent than labeled.) Some manufacturers attempt to standardize their products by isolating the compounds believed to be responsible for an herb's action and combining batches to achieve a consistent strength. However, potency is often still highly variable, and when several compounds are thought to be responsible for an herb's effect, often only one is standardized. In addition, herbs can be contaminated or misidentified at any stage from harvest to packaging; the FDA has recalled several products due to the presence of dangerous contaminants, including heavy metals and pharmaceutical drugs.

With increased consumer knowledge and demand, it is likely that both the research base and the manufacturing standards for dietary supplements will improve. In an effort to provide consumers with more reliable and consistent information about supplements, the FDA has developed new labeling regulations. Since March 1999, labels similar to those found on foods have been required for dietary supplements; health claims about supplements are also regulated. See the box "Using Dietary Supplement Labels" for more information.

Finally, it is important to remember that dietary supplements are no substitute for a healthy diet. Supplements do not provide all the known—or yet-to-be-discovered—benefits of whole foods. Supplements should also not be used as a replacement for medical treatment for serious illnesses.

Protecting Yourself Against Foodborne Illness

Many people worry about additives or pesticide residues in their food. However, the greatest threat to the safety of the food supply comes from microorganisms that cause foodborne illnesses. Raw or undercooked animal products, such as chicken, hamburger, and oysters, pose the greatest risk for contamination. The CDC estimates that 6.5–33 million Americans become ill and 9000 die each year as a result of foodborne illness. Your last bout of flu may very well have been a foodborne illness. The symptoms of both are often the same: diarrhea, vomiting, fever, and weakness. Although the effects of foodborne illnesses are usually not serious, some groups, such as children and the elderly, are more at risk for severe complications like rheumatic diseases, seizures, blood poisoning, other ailments, and death.

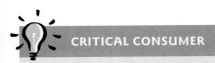
Since 1999, specific types of information have been required on the labels of dietary supplements. In addition to basic information about the product, labels include a "Supplement Facts" panel, modeled after the "Nutrition Facts" panel used on food labels (see the figure). Under the Dietary Supplement Health and Education Act (DSHEA) and food labeling laws, supplement labels can make three types of health-related claims:

- *Nutrient-content claims*, such as "high in calcium," "excellent source of vitamin C," or "high potency." The claims "high in" and "excellent source of" mean the same as they do on food labels. A "high potency" single ingredient supplement must contain 100% of its Daily Value; a "high potency" multi-ingredient product must contain 100% or more of the Daily Value of at least two-thirds of the nutrients present for which Daily Values have been established.

- *Disease claims*, if they have been authorized by the FDA or another authoritative scientific body. The association between adequate calcium intake and lower risk of osteoporosis is an example of an approved disease claim.

- *Structure-function claims*, such as "antioxidants maintain cellular integrity" or "this product enhances energy levels." Because these claims are not reviewed by the FDA, they must carry a disclaimer (see the sample label).

Tips for Choosing and Using Dietary Supplements

- Check with your physician before taking a supplement. Many are not meant for children, elderly people, women who are pregnant or breastfeeding, people with chronic illnesses, or people taking prescription or OTC medications.

- Choose brands made by nationally known food and drug manufacturers or "house brands" from large retail chains. Due to their size and visibility, such sources are likely to have higher manufacturing standards.

- Look for the *USP* or *NF* designation, indicating that the product meets some minimum safety and purity standard developed by the United States Pharmacopeia. (The United States Pharmacopeia develops standards for purity and potency for pharmaceutical drugs and has also set standards for vitamins, minerals, and some herbal products.)

- Follow the cautions, instructions for use, and dosage given on the label.

- If you experience side effects, discontinue use of the product and contact your physician. Report any serious reactions to the FDA's MedWatch monitoring program (800-FDA-1088; http://www.fda.gov/medwatch).

For More Information About Dietary Supplements

Blumenthal, M., ed. 1998. *The Complete German Commission E Monographs: Therapeutic Guide to Herbal Medicines.* Tallahassee, Fla.: Integrative Medicine. (*Herbal products have been studied more thoroughly in Germany; Commission E is the German equivalent of the FDA.*)

Herbal Rx: The promises and the pitfalls. 1999. *Consumer Reports*, March.

O'Hara, M., et al. 1998. A review of 12 commonly used medicinal herbs. *Archives of Family Medicine* 7: 523–536.

Physician's Desk Reference. 1998. *PDR for Herbal Medicines.* Montvale, N.J.: Medical Economics.

Robbers, J. E., and V. E. Tyler. 1998 *Tyler's Herbs of Choice: The Therapeutic Use of Phytomedicinals,* 2nd ed. Binghamton, N.Y.: Haworth Press.

U.S. Pharmacopeia. 1996. *The USP Guide to Vitamins and Minerals.* New York: Avon.

FDA Information About Dietary Supplements (http://Vm.cfsan.fda.gov/~dms/supplmnt.html)

National Institutes of Health Office of Dietary Supplements (http://odp.od.nih.gov/ods)

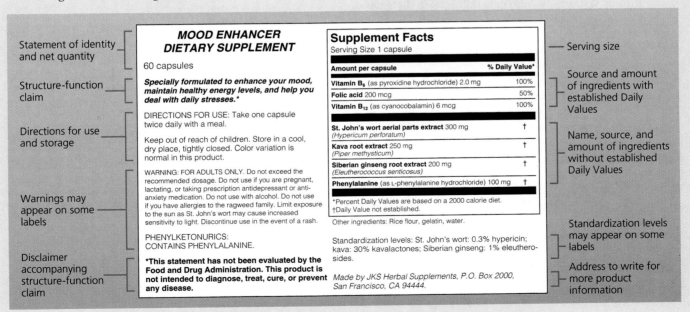

Causes of Foodborne Illnesses Most cases of foodborne illness are caused by **pathogens**, disease-causing microorganisms. Food can be contaminated with pathogens through improper handling; pathogens can grow if food is prepared or stored improperly. *Salmonella* bacteria are responsible for almost 60% of all cases of foodborne illness; they are most often found in eggs, poultry, meat, milk, and inadequately refrigerated and reheated leftovers. The recent identification of an antibiotic-resistant strain of *Salmonella* has raised concerns about a potential increase in serious illness from *Salmonella*.

The bacterium *Staphylococcus aureus* lives mainly in the nasal passages and in skin sores; it causes about 20–40% of all cases of foodborne illness. It is transferred to food when people handle or sneeze or cough over food; ham, egg salad, cheese, seafood, whipped cream, and milk are common sources. Illness from the *Clostridium botulinum* bacterium is rare, but it can be deadly. Botulism results primarily from improperly canned foods, especially meats and vegetables; but *C. botulinum* is found in the soil, so any food grown in the ground may carry it.

The bacterium *Escherichia coli* (typically found in the intestinal tract of humans and other animals) can be dangerous because a certain strain of the bacterium, known as *E. coli* O157:H7, produces a toxin that can cause serious illness. In 1992, a shipment of Jack-in-the-Box hamburgers that were contaminated with *E. coli* and not cooked thoroughly caused hundreds of cases of illness and several deaths. In 1996 in Japan, *E. coli* O157:H7 caused 11 deaths and more than 9500 cases of illness.

There are also deadly strains of *Listeria monocytogenes*, a bacteria that sickens about 1200–1800 Americans a year, causing death in about 20–25% of cases. *Listeria* is particularly dangerous to pregnant women and their fetuses, babies and children, older adults, and people with weakened immune systems. A multistate outbreak in the winter of 1998–1999 sickened more than 70 people, killing 11 adults and causing 5 miscarriages or stillbirths; it was traced to contaminated hot dogs and deli meats produced under many brand names by one manufacturer.

Other organisms that can cause types of foodborne illness include the bacteria *Clostridium perfringens, Campylobacter jejuni, Shigella dysenteriae,* and *Yersinia enterocolitica;* the hepatitis A virus; the parasites *Trichinella spiralis* (found in pork and wild game), *Anisakis* (found in raw fish), *Cyclospora cayetanensis,* and tapeworms; and certain molds.

Preventing and Treating Foodborne Illnesses Because every teaspoon of the soil that our food grows in contains about 2 billion bacteria (only some of them pathogenic), we are always exposed to the possibility of a foodborne illness. You can't tell by taste, smell, or sight whether a food is contaminated. Currently, at least 10% of all ground beef and 25% of all chickens sold in the United States are contaminated with pathogenic bacteria. Some studies have revealed high levels of contamination. In

1998, *Consumer Reports* tested 400 chickens purchased in grocery stores and found that 71% were contaminated with *Campylobacter* and 10% with *Salmonella.*

Although pathogens are usually destroyed during cooking, the U.S. government is taking steps to bring down levels of contamination. New federal regulations require more precise national surveillance; inspectors at meat and poultry processing plants must also use microbiological testing methods, in addition to visual inspections, to check for the presence of pathogens. The number of recalls of potentially contaminated foods has increased under the new system; the 1998 recall of 35 million pounds of hot dogs and lunch meat from one plant due to possible *Listeria* contamination was one of the largest recalls to date. The new tests will not eliminate all contamination, however, and other regulations are designed to help prevent illness from contaminated foods that do make it to consumers. Raw meat and poultry products are now sold with safe handling and cooking instructions, and all packaged, unpasteurized fresh fruit and vegetable juices carry warnings about potential contamination. To decrease your risk of foodborne illness, follow the guidelines in the box "Safe Food Handling."

If you think you may be having a bout of foodborne illness, drink plenty of clear fluids to offset the effects of diarrhea, and rest in bed to speed recovery. To prevent further contamination, wash your hands often and always before handling food until the diarrhea disappears. A fever higher than 102°F, blood in the stool, or dehydration deserves a physician's evaluation, especially if the symptoms persist for more than 2–3 days. In cases of suspected botulism—characterized by symptoms such as double vision, paralysis, dizziness, and vomiting—consult a physician immediately, because the use of an antitoxin may help you recover sooner.

Environmental Contaminants

Contaminants are also present in the food-growing environment, but few of them ever enter the food and water supply in amounts sufficient to cause health problems. Environmental contaminants include various minerals, antibiotics, hormones, pesticides, the industrial chemicals known as **PCBs (polychlorinated biphenyls),** and naturally occurring substances such as cyanogenic glycosides (found in lima beans and the pits of some fruits) and certain molds. Their effects depend on many factors, including concentration, length of exposure, and the age and health status of the person involved. Safety regulations attempt to keep our exposure to environmental contaminants at safe levels, but monitoring is difficult and many substances (such as pesticides) persist in the environment long after being banned from use.

Some people who are concerned about pesticides and other environmental contaminants choose to buy foods that are **certified organic.** To be given such a designation,

- Don't buy food in containers that leak, bulge, or are severely dented. Refrigerated foods should be cold, and frozen foods should be solid.

- Refrigerate perishable items as soon as possible after purchase. Use or freeze fresh meats within 3–5 days and fresh poultry, fish, and ground meat within 1–2 days.

- Thaw frozen food in the refrigerator or in the microwave oven, not on the kitchen counter.

- Thoroughly wash your hands with soapy water for 20 seconds before and after handling food, especially raw meat, fish, poultry, or eggs.

- Make sure counters, cutting boards, dishes, and other equipment are thoroughly cleaned before and after use. If possible, use separate cutting boards for meat and for foods that will be eaten raw, such as fruits and vegetables. Wash dishcloths and kitchen towels frequently.

- Thoroughly rinse and scrub fruits and vegetables with a brush, if possible, or peel off the skin.

- Cook foods thoroughly, especially beef, poultry, fish, pork, and eggs. Cooking kills most microorganisms, as long as an appropriately high temperature is reached. The USDA now recommends that consumers use a food thermometer to verify that hamburgers are cooked to 160°F. When eating out, order red meat cooked "well-done."

- Cook stuffing separately from poultry; or wash poultry thoroughly, stuff immediately before cooking, and transfer the stuffing to a clean bowl immediately after cooking.

- Store foods below 40°F. Do not leave cooked or refrigerated foods, such as meats or salads, at room temperature for more than 2 hours. Use cooked leftovers within 3–4 days.

- Don't eat raw animal products. Use only pasteurized milk and juice.

- According to the USDA, "When in doubt, throw it out."

a food must meet strict growing and production criteria. For produce, these criteria usually include limits on pesticide residues and nonorganic ingredients; meat and poultry are generally considered organic if the animals eat organic feed, are not given antibiotics or hormones, and are allowed to go outside. Different private and state agencies may set standards for organic labels, and the U.S. Department of Agriculture is developing national organic standards.

Foods that are certified organic are not chemical-free, however. They may be contaminated with pesticides used on neighboring lands or on foods transported in the same train or truck. However, they do tend to have lower levels of pesticide residues than conventionally grown crops. In 1998, Consumer's Union tested a thousand pounds of produce and found that the organic samples were less than half as likely as the conventionally grown ones to have traces of pesticides. The organic samples that *were* contaminated tended to have lower levels of less toxic residues than those found on the conventionally grown produce.

There are strict pesticide limits for all foods—organic and conventional—and the debate about the potential health effects of long-term exposure to small amounts of pesticide residues is ongoing. The benefits of a diet rich in fruits and vegetables far outweigh any potential long-term risks of exposure to pesticide residues. Some studies indicate that washing produce in a highly diluted liquid soap solution removes most pesticide residues, but many experts feel that the use of running water is sufficient.

Supporters of organic foods also note that practices associated with organic farming help maintain biodiversity of crops and are less likely to degrade soil, contaminate water, or expose farm workers to dangerous chemicals. Organic foods tend to be more expensive than those grown conventionally, however, and there is no evidence that they contain more nutrients or fewer foodborne pathogens. But some people choose to pay the higher prices for organic foods to support agricultural practices they believe promote a healthier environment.

Adequate nutrition from a varied diet provides a key part of your defense against small doses of contaminants, since a healthy body has a much greater level of resistance to their effects. If you eat a variety of foods in moderation, you will have less chance of suffering negative health consequences from contaminants. The presence of mercury in swordfish may concern you, for example, but it's a health risk only if your diet is dominated by swordfish.

Additives in Food

Today, some 2800 substances are intentionally added to foods for one or more of the following reasons: (1) to maintain or improve nutritional quality, (2) to maintain freshness, (3) to help in processing or preparation, or (4) to alter taste or appearance. Additives make up less than

TERMS

pathogen   A microorganism that causes disease.

polychlorinated biphenyl (PCB)   An industrial chemical used as a insulator in electrical transformers and linked to certain human cancers.

certified organic   A designation applied to foods grown and produced according to strict guidelines limiting the use of pesticides and nonorganic ingredients.

1% of our food. The most widely used are sugar, salt, and corn syrup; these three, plus citric acid, baking soda, vegetable colors, mustard, and pepper, account for 98% by weight of all food additives used in the United States.

Some additives may be of concern for certain people, because either they are consumed in large quantities or they cause some type of allergic reaction. Additives having potential health concerns include the following:

- *Nitrates and nitrites:* Used to protect meats from contamination from the botulism pathogen. Their consumption is associated with the synthesis of cancer-causing agents in the stomach, but the cancer risk appears to be low, except for people with low stomach acid output (such as some elderly people). The use of nitrates or nitrites is allowed in small quantities.

- *BHA and BHT:* Used to help maintain the freshness of foods. Some studies indicate a potential link between BHT and an increased risk of certain cancers. The FDA is reviewing the use of BHT and BHA, but any risk to the diet from these agents is low. Many manufacturers have stopped using BHT and BHA.

- *Sulfites:* Used to keep vegetables from turning brown. They can cause severe allergic reactions in some people. The FDA severely limits the use of sulfites and requires any foods containing sulfites to be clearly labeled.

- *Monosodium glutamate (MSG):* Typically used as a flavor enhancer. MSG may cause some people to experience episodes of high blood pressure and sweating. If you are sensitive to MSG, check food labels when shopping, and ask to have it left out of dishes you order at restaurants.

- *Food irradiation:* Used to prevent the growth of microorganisms, parasites, and insects. Because it alters food, it is regulated like a food additive. Studies indicate that foods exposed to low doses of irradiation are safe to eat and do not undergo significant changes in nutrient composition. However, few companies have marketed irradiated foods because of logistical problems and concerns about consumer response. In 1999, the FDA approved the use of food irradiation for red meat as a means of combatting foodborne pathogens. Under the FDA's proposed rule, irradiated foods would be identified with the international radiation symbol.

Food additives pose no significant health hazard to most people because the levels used are well below any that could produce toxic effects. Eat a variety of foods in moderation. If you have a sensitivity to an additive, check food labels when you shop, and ask questions when you eat out.

Genetically Altered Foods

Genetic engineering involves inserting DNA from one plant, animal, or microorganism into another. A number of genetically engineered products are already widely used, including insulin to treat diabetes and the enzyme chymosin to produce cheese. Food producers have begun working with genetic engineering techniques to introduce genes for qualities such as disease resistance and slow ripening into common food plants like tomatoes, potatoes, and squash.

Potential benefits of genetically altered foods include improved quality, lower price, and less use of pesticides. As with all new technologies, however, there may be unexpected effects. Gene manipulation could elevate levels of naturally occurring toxins and allergens or could permanently change the botanical gene pool. Critics also fear that genes for antibiotic resistance could be transferred from foods to bacteria in the intestine during digestion, thus creating antibiotic-resistant bacteria.

Genetically altered whole foods are not yet widely available, in part due to consumer resistance and concerns over labeling. Under current rules, the FDA requires labeling only when a food's composition is changed significantly or when a known allergen is introduced. For example, soybeans that have peanut genes would have to be labeled because peanuts are a common allergen. Special labeling would be expensive, but many people feel that public acceptance of genetically engineered foods will not occur without strict labeling guidelines.

Overall, the American food supply is very safe, whether you're concerned with additives, pesticides, or bacteria. By preparing foods carefully and avoiding substances to which you are sensitive, you can be confident that the food supply is not causing you harm. By far the greatest dietary risks to your long-term health come from an overconsumption of fat and calories and an underconsumption of fruits, vegetables, and grains.

SUMMARY

- Choosing foods that provide needed nutrients is an important part of daily life. Food choices made during our youth can significantly affect our health in later years.

Nutritional Requirements: Components of a Healthy Diet

- The fuel potential in our diet is expressed in calories.

- To function at its best, the human body requires about 45 essential nutrients in specific proportions. People get the nutrients needed to fuel their bodies and maintain tissues and organ systems from foods; the body cannot synthesize most of them.

- Proteins, made up of amino acids, form muscles and bones and help make up blood, enzymes, hormones, and cell membranes. Foods from animal sources provide complete proteins; plants provide incomplete proteins.

- Fats, a concentrated source of energy, also help insulate the body and cushion the organs; 1 tablespoon of vegetable oil per day supplies the essential fats. Dietary fat intake should be limited to 30% of total daily calories. Unsaturated fats should be favored over saturated and trans fats.

- Carbohydrates supply energy to the brain and other parts of the nervous system as well as to red blood cells. The body needs 50–100 grams of carbohydrates a day, but much more is usually consumed.

- Dietary fiber includes plant substances that are difficult or impossible for humans to digest. Insoluble fiber holds water and increases bulk in the stool. Soluble fiber binds cholesterol-containing compounds in the intestine and slows glucose absorption.

- The 13 vitamins needed in the diet are organic substances that promote specific chemical and cell processes within living tissue. Deficiencies or excesses can cause serious illnesses and even death.

- The approximately 17 minerals needed in the diet are inorganic substances that regulate body functions, aid in the growth and maintenance of body tissues, and help in the release of energy from foods.

- Water is used to digest and absorb food, transport substances around the body, lubricate joints and organs, and regulate body temperature. A lack of water can cause death within a few days.

- Foods contain other substances such as phytochemicals, which may not be essential nutrients but which may protect against chronic diseases.

Nutritional Guidelines: Planning Your Diet

- Recommended Dietary Allowances (RDAs) and Dietary Reference Intakes (DRIs) are recommended intakes for essential nutrients that meet the needs of healthy people.

- The Food Guide Pyramid contains six food groups; choosing foods from each group every day helps ensure the appropriate amounts of necessary nutrients. The fundamental principles of the Food Guide Pyramid are moderation, variety, and balance.

- The Dietary Guidelines for Americans address the prevention of diet-related diseases like cardiovascular disease, cancer, and diabetes. The guidelines advise us to eat a variety of foods; to balance the food we eat with physical activity to maintain or improve our weight; to choose a diet with plenty of grain products, vegetables, and fruits; to choose a diet low in fat, saturated fat, and cholesterol and moderate in sugars and salt; and to drink alcohol only in moderation, or not at all.

- A vegetarian diet can meet human nutritional needs.

- Different population groups may face special dietary challenges. Women need to focus on nutrient-dense foods; men should limit fat intake and increase their consumption of fruits, vegetables, and grains.

A Personal Plan: Making Informed Choices About Food

- No single diet provides wellness for everyone; people should focus on the likely causes of health problems in their lives and make the appropriate dietary changes.

- Almost all foods have labels that show how much fat, cholesterol, protein, fiber, and sodium they contain. Serving sizes are standardized, and health claims are carefully regulated. Dietary supplements also have uniform labels.

- Foodborne illnesses are a greater threat to health than additives and environmental contaminants. Specific precautions in handling and preparing food, especially animal products like chicken and hamburger, can help prevent foodborne illnesses.

- Food additives maintain or improve nutritional quality, maintain freshness, help in processing, and alter taste or appearance.

TAKE ACTION

1. Read the list of ingredients on three or four canned or packaged foods that you enjoy eating. If any ingredients are unfamiliar to you, find out what they are and why they have been used. A nutrition textbook from the library may be a helpful resource.

2. Investigate the nutritional and dietary guidelines that are used to prepare the food served in your school. Are they consistent with what you've learned in this chapter? If not, try to find out more about the guidelines that have been used and why they were chosen.

3. Prepare a flavorful lowfat vegetarian and/or ethnic meal. (Use the suggestions in the chapter, and check your local library for appropriate cookbooks.) How do the foods included in the meal and the preparation methods differ from what you're used to?

If you want to alter your diet, some of the behavior change strategies we have already examined can help you. Here are some suggestions to help you lower your fat consumption, raise your fiber intake, or make other changes in your diet.

Establishing a Baseline

Let's say that you want to do two things to your diet: (1) Cut out all candy while walking between classes or while doing errands in town, and (2) eat more fresh fruits and raw vegetables.

Begin by keeping track of your candy consumption. In your health journal, jot down the time of day and what occurred before and after you ate the candy. On a chart such as the one shown here, keep track of the number of times each day you eat candy. Because you also want to add more fruits and vegetables to your diet, also keep notes on the kinds of foods you've been eating at meals. You can include this information on the same chart, or you can keep two graphs.

Intervention

Once you have established your baseline levels, begin to make some changes in those routines that seem to precede your eating candy. For example, you might find that you have been eating candy from a vending machine that you walk by every day after class. If this is the case, try another route that allows you to avoid the machine. If you find that you usually are hungry at one particular time of day and that you rarely have lunch or a healthful snack with you, try to keep a healthful snack on hand so that you won't be caught off guard and be pushed toward eating candy (which always seems to be available). Putting fresh or dried fruit in a backpack or pocket every morning can help. You can use the same sort of strategy to increase the number of fruits and vegetables in your diet: Specifically, you'll need to shop for these food items *in advance* and prepare them *ahead of time* so that they are readily available.

Revision (If Needed)

You may discover that your initial plan works perfectly, or that it works well for 3 weeks but then loses its effectiveness. Watch out for programs that become stale and lose their strength, and, of course, revise an ineffective program entirely once you have given it a real try. The critical data from your journal can help you decide how to revise your program. Plotting the data on a prominently displayed chart can encourage you to continue.

Social Eating Events

Avoiding an attractive candy vending machine may be a lot easier than cutting back on late-night pizza binges; the former involves only you, while the latter involves you and your friends. It's harder to make adjustments in social eating patterns, but there are some strategies you can try. First, tell your friends that you would prefer to try something new to eat instead of pizza, such as plain popcorn. Being assertive in such matters can be very helpful; you may discover some allies who share your views about the type of food you want to eat. Second, try to cut down on these group activities without eliminating them entirely. Of course, you can try to change or limit the kinds of food you eat at these times, but it's generally very difficult to refrain from joining in once you're actually in the social situation.

Systematic Changes in Other Habits

Many people begin an exercise program or begin to increase their routine activity levels (walks after meals, and so on) at the same time that they try to adjust their diet. While it isn't a good idea to try to make too many significant changes at one time, you may want to experiment with other changes while making adjustments in your eating habits.

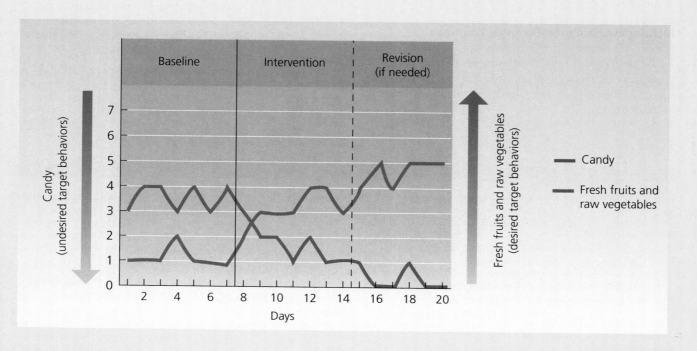

1. In your health journal, keep track of everything you eat and drink for 3–4 days. Calculate the average number of servings from each food group you consume each day. Then see how well your average daily intake meets the guidelines in the Food Guide Pyramid.

2. Put together three sample daily menus that follow the Food Guide Pyramid. Keep the dietary guidelines in mind as you make your food selections from each group. Also, be sure to base your menus on foods you enjoy eating.

3. *Critical Thinking* Analyze patterns of food advertising on television by recording the number and types of ads that appear each hour. If possible, compare the number and types of products advertised during an hour of cartoons or other children's programs, an hour of daytime programs, and an hour of prime-time programs. What patterns do you see? What types of information do the ads present? Are they geared toward different segments of the population? Do they encourage healthy eating?

FOR MORE INFORMATION

For reliable nutrition advice, talk to a faculty member in the nutrition department on your campus, a registered dietitian (R.D.), or your physician. Many large communities have a telephone service called Dial-a-Dietitian. By calling this number, people can receive nutrition information from an R.D. free of charge.

Experts on quackery suggest that you steer clear of anyone who puts forth any of the following false statements:

- Most diseases are caused by faulty nutrition.

- Large doses of vitamins are effective against many diseases.

- Hair analysis can be used to determine a person's nutritional state.

- A computer-scored nutritional deficiency test is a basis for prescribing vitamins.

Any practitioner—licensed or not—who sells vitamins in his or her office should be thoroughly scrutinized.

Books

American Dietetic Association. 1999. *The Essential Guide to Nutrition and the Foods We Eat: Everything You Need to Know About the Foods You Eat.* New York: HarperCollins. *An excellent review of current nutrition information and issues.*

Consumers Guide Editors. 1998. *Complete Book of Vitamins and Minerals.* Revised edition. New York: Signet. *A comprehensive review of vitamins and minerals.*

Havala, S. 1999. *The Complete Idiot's Guide to Being a Vegetarian.* Indianapolis, In.: Macmillan. *Provides information on the health benefits of vegetarian diets and how to plan healthy meals; advice is given for vegetarian diets for special population groups, including children.*

Luke, B. 1998. *Good Bones: The Complete Guide to Building and Maintaining the Healthiest Bones.* Palo Alto, Calif.: Bull Publishing. *Provides practical advice for lifestyle prevention of osteoporosis.*

Wardlaw, G. M. 1999. *Perspectives in Nutrition,* 4th ed. Boston: McGraw-Hill. *An easy-to-understand review of major concepts in nutrition.*

Newsletters

Environmental Nutrition: P.O. Box 420235, Palm Coast, FL 32142; 800-829-5384.

Nutrition Action Health Letter: 1875 Connecticut Ave., N.W., Suite 300, Washington DC 20009-5728; 202-332-9110 (http://www.cspinet.org).

Tufts University Health & Nutrition Letter: P.O. Box 420235, Palm Coast, FL 32142; 800-274-7581.

Organizations, Hotlines, and Web Sites

American Dietetic Association. Provides a wide variety of nutrition-related educational materials.

216 West Jackson Blvd., Suite 800
Chicago, IL 60606
800-366-1655 (For general nutrition information and referrals to registered dietitians.)
900-CALL-AN-RD (For customized answers to nutrition questions.)
http://www.eatright.org

American Medical Association Personal Nutritionist. Includes a brief online nutrition assessment and tips on making healthy dietary changes.

http://www.ama-assn.org/insight/gen_hlth/pernutri/pernutri.htm

Ask the Dietitian. Questions and answers on many topics relating to nutrition.

http://www.dietitian.com

CyberDiet. Provides a variety of resources, including a profile that calculates calorie and nutrient needs and a database that provides nutrition information in food label format.

http://www.CyberDiet.com

FDA Center for Food Safety and Applied Nutrition. Offers information about topics such as food labeling, food additives, dietary supplements, and foodborne illness.

http://vm.cfsan.fda.gov

Food Safety Hotlines. Provide information on safe purchase, handling, cooking, and storage of food.

800-FDA-4010 (FDA)
800-535-4555 (USDA)

Gateway to Government Food Safety Information. Provides access to government resources relating to food safety, including consumer advice and information on specific pathogens.

http://www.foodsafety.gov

International Food Information Council. Provides helpful information on food safety and nutrition for consumers, journalists, and educators.

1100 Connecticut Ave., N.W., Suite 430
Washington, DC 20036
http://ificinfo.health.org

Martindale's "Virtual" Nutrition Center. Provides information and links to many sites, including nutrition dictionaries, recipes, food safety information, and online nutrition calculators.

http://sun2.lib.uci.edu/HSG/Nutrition.html

Meals Online. Provides a database of over 10,000 recipes, searchable by recipe title or ingredient.

http://www.meals.com

Meat and Poultry Hotline. Information from USDA experts on topics such as the proper handling, preparation, storage, and cooking of food.

800-535-4555

National Academies' Food and Nutrition Board. Provides information about the Dietary Reference Intakes and related guidelines.

http://www4.nationalacadamies.org/IOM/IOMHome.nsf/
Pages/Food+and+Nutrition+Board

National Institutes of Health Osteoporosis and Related Bone Diseases—National Resource Center. Provides information about osteoporosis prevention and treatment; includes a special section on men and osteoporosis.

http://www.osteo.org

National Osteoporosis Foundation. Provides up-to-date information on the causes, prevention, detection, and treatment of osteoporosis.

1150 17th Street, N.W., Suite 500
Washington, DC 20036
202-223-2226
http://www.nof.org

Tufts University Nutrition Navigator. Provides descriptions and ratings for many nutrition-related Web pages.

http://navigator.tufts.edu

USDA Food and Nutrition Information Center. Provides a variety of materials relating to the Dietary Guidelines, food labels, Food Guide Pyramid, and many other topics; Web site includes extensive links.

10301 Baltimore Blvd., Room 304
Beltsville, MD 20705
301-504-5719
http://www.nal.usda.gov/fnic

Specific USDA programs include the *Center for Nutrition Policy and Promotion,* which provides information on the Dietary Guidelines and the Food Guide Pyramid (http://www.usda.gov/cnpp); the *Food Safety and Inspection Service,* which provides comsumer resources on food safety and irridiation (http://www.fsis.usda.gov); and the *Agricultural Marketing Service,* which provides information on food standards, including those for organic foods, and has a helpful series of consumer "How to Buy . . ." publications (http://www.ams.usda.gov).

Vegetarian Resource Group. Information and links for vegetarians and people interested in learning more about vegetarian diets.

http://www.vrg.org

You can obtain nutrient breakdowns of individual food items from the following sites:

Nutrition Analysis Tool, University of Illinois, Urbana/Champaign
http://www.ag.uiuc.edu/~food-lab/nat

USDA Food and Nutrition Information Center
http://www.nal.usda.gov/fnic/foodcomp

See also the resources listed in the dietary supplements box on p. 331 and in the For More Information sections in Chapters 13–16.

SELECTED BIBLIOGRAPHY

A fresh look at chicken safety. 1998. *Consumer Reports,* October.

Allison, D. B., et al. 1999. Estimated intakes of trans fatty and other fatty acids in the U.S. population. *Journal of the American Dietetic Association* 99(2): 166–174.

Altekruse, S. F., et al. 1999. *Campylobacter jejuni*—an emerging foodborne pathogen. *Emerging Infectious Diseases* 5(1) (retrieved February 2, 1999; http://www.cdc.gov/ncidod/EID/vol5no1/altekruse.htm).

American Society for Clinical Nutrition/American Institute of Nutrition Task Force. 1996. Position paper on trans fatty acids. *American Journal of Clinical Nutrition* 63: 663–670.

Centers for Disease Control and Prevention. 1999. Incidence of foodborne illnesses: Preliminary data from the Foodborne Disease Active Surveillance Network (Food Net). *Morbidity and Mortality Weekly Report* 48(9): 189–194.

Centers for Disease Control and Prevention. 1999. *Update Multistate Outbreak of Listeriosis* (retrieved February 12, 1999; http://www.cdc.gov/od/oc/media/pressrel/r990114.htm).

Centers for Disease Control and Prevention. 1998. Osteoporosis among estrogen-deficient women—United States, 1988–1994. *Morbidity and Mortality Weekly Report* 47(45): 969–973.

Chatenoud, L., et al. 1998. Whole-grain food intake and cancer risk. *International Journal of Cancer* 77(1): 24–28.

Commission on Dietary Supplement Labels. 1997. *Report of the Commission on Dietary Supplement Labels, November 1997.* Washington, D.C.: U.S. Government Printing Office (Stock No. 017-001-00531-2).

DeMarco, H. M., et al. 1999. Pre-exercise carbohydrate meals: Application of glycemic index. *Medicine and Science in Sports and Exercise* 31(1): 164–170.

Feskanich, D., et al. 1999. Vitamin K intake and hip fractures in women: A prospective study. *American Journal of Clinical Nutrition* 69(1): 74–79.

Food and Nutrition Board. 1998. *Dietary Reference Intakes for Thiamin, Riboflavin, Niacin, Vitamin B$_6$, Folate, Vitamin B$_{12}$, Pantothenic Acid, Biotin, and Choline.* Washington, D.C.: National Academy Press.

Food and Nutrition Board. 1998. *Proposed Definition and Plan for Review of Dietary Antioxidants and Related Compounds.* Washington, D.C.: National Academy Press.

Food and Nutrition Board. 1997. *Dietary Reference Intakes for Calcium, Phosphorus, Magnesium, Vitamin D, and Fluoride.* Washington, D.C.: National Academy Press.

Food Safety and Inspection Service. 1998. *USDA Urges Consumers to Use Food Thermometers When Cooking Ground Beef-patties* (retrieved December 10, 1998; http://www.fsis.usda.gov/OA/news/colorpr.htm).

Ford, E. S., et al. 1999. Diabetes mellitus and serum carotenoids. *American Journal of Epidemiology* 149(2): 168–176.

Greener greens? The truth about organic farming. 1998. *Consumer Reports,* January.

Guide to drug-herb interactions. 1999. *Environmental Nutrition,* January.

Hallikainen, M. A., and M. I. Uusitupa. 1999. Effects of 2 lowfat stanol ester–containing margarines on serum cholesterol concentrations as part of a low-fat diet in hypercholesterolemic subjects. *American Journal of Clinical Nutrition* 69(3): 403–410.

Holman, R. T. 1998. The slow discovery of the importance of omega-3 essential fatty acids in human health. *Journal of Nutrition* 128(2 Suppl): 427S–433S.

Hu, F. B., et al. 1997. Dietary fat intake and the risk of coronary heart disease in women. *New England Journal of Medicine* 337(21): 1491–1499.

Institute of Medicine. 1998. *Ensuring Safe Food from Production to Consumption.* Washington, D.C.: National Academy Press.

Jacobs, D. R., et al. 1999. Is whole grain intake associated with reduced total and cause-specific death rates in older women? The Iowa Women's Health Study. *American Journal of Public Health* 89: 322–329.

Judd, J. T., et al. 1998. Effects of margarine compared with those of butter on blood lipid profiles related to cardiovascular disease risk factors in normolipemic adults fed controlled diets. *American Journal of Clinical Nutrition* 68(4): 768–777.

Kleiner, S. M. 1999. Water: An essential but overlooked nutrient. *Journal of the American Dietetic Association* 99(2): 200–206.

Knekt, P., et al. 1999. Risk of colorectal and other gastro-intestinal cancers after exposure to nitrate, nitrite and N-nitroso compounds. A follow-up study. *International Journal of Cancer* 80(6): 852–856.

Kurtzweil, P. 1998. An FDA guide to dietary supplements. *FDA Consumer,* September/October.

Levinson, W., and D. Altkorn. 1998. Primary prevention of postmenopausal osteoporosis. *Journal of the American Medical Association* 280(21): 1821–1822.

Messina, V. K., and K. I. Burke. 1997. Position of the American Dietetic Association: Vegetarian diets. *Journal of the American Dietetic Association* 97(11): 1317–1321.

Miller, E. R., L. J. Appel, and T. H. Risby. 1998. Effect of dietary patterns on measures of lipid peroxidation: Results from a randomized clinical trial. *Circulation* 98(22): 2390–2395.

Misciagna, G., et al. 1999. Diet, physical activity, and gallstones —a population-based, case-control study in southern Italy. *American Journal of Clinical Nutrition* 69(1): 120–126.

National Osteoporosis Foundation. 1998. *Physician's Guide to Prevention and Treatment of Osteoporosis.* Washington, D.C.: National Osteoporosis Foundation.

Nelson, G. J. 1998. Dietary fat, trans fatty acids, and risk of coronary heart disease. *Nutrition Reviews* 56(8): 250–252.

Nelson, M. E. 1997. *Strong Women Stay Young.* New York: Bantam.

Neuhouser, M. L., A. R. Kristal, and R. E. Patterson. 1999. Use of food nutrition labels is associated with lower fat intake. *Journal of the American Dietetic Association* 99(1): 45–50, 53.

Russell, R. M., H. Rasmussen, and A. H. Lichtenstein. 1999. Modified food guide pyramid for people over seventy years of age. *Journal of Nutrition* 129(3): 751–753.

Salmeró, J., et al. 1997. Dietary fiber, glycemic load, and risk of non-insulin-dependent diabetes mellitus in women. *Journal of the American Medical Association* 277(6): 472–477.

Shaw, A., et al. 1997. *Using the Food Guide Pyramid: A Resource for Nutrition Educators.* USDA Center for Nutrition Policy and Promotion (retrieved January 8, 1998; http://www.nal.usda.gov/fnic/Fpyr/guide.pdf).

Shils, M. E., et al., eds. 1998. *Modern Nutrition in Health and Disease.* Baltimore: Williams & Wilkins.

Slutsker, L., et al. 1997. *Escherichia coli* O157:H7 diarrhea in the United States: Clinical and epidemiologic features. *Annals of Internal Medicine* 126(7): 505–513.

Sundram, K., et al. 1997. Trans (elaidic) fatty acids adversely affect the lipoprotein profile relative to specific fatty acids in humans. *Journal of Nutrition* 127(3): 514S–520S.

Tavelli, S., et al. 1998. Sources of error and nutritional adequacy of the Food Guide Pyramid. *Journal of American College Health* 47(2): 77–82.

U.S. Department of Agriculture. 1999. *Tips for Using the Food Guide Pyramid for Young Children 2 to 6 Years Old.* Program Aid 1647.

U.S. Department of Agriculture. 1997. *Data Tables: Results from USDA's 1994–96 Continuing Survey of Food Intakes by Individuals and 1994–96 Diet and Health Knowledge Survey* (retrieved December 2, 1998; http://www.barc.usda.gov/bhnrc/foodsurvey/home.htm).

U.S. Department of Agriculture. 1995. *Nutrition and Your Health: Dietary Guidelines for Americans,* 4th ed. Home and Garden Bulletin No. 232.

U.S. Department of Agriculture Center for Nutrition Policy and Promotion. 1998. Is total fat consumption really decreasing? *Nutrition Insights,* April.

U.S. Department of Agriculture Food Safety and Inspection Service. 1999. *Listeria monocytogens and Listeriosis* (retrieved February 12, 1999; http://www.fsis.usda.gov/OA/pubs/listeria.htm).

U.S. Department of Agriculture Food Safety and Inspection Service. 1999. *Using the Claim "Certified Organic By . . ." on Meat and Poultry Product Labeling* (retrieved February 12, 1999; http://www.fsis.usda.gov/OA/background/organic.htm).

U.S. Food and Drug Administration. 1998. Irradiation: A safe measure for safer food. *FDA Consumer,* May/June.

U.S. Food and Drug Administration. 1996. *Fact Sheet: Folic Acid Fortification* (retrieved February 21, 1997; http://vm.cfsan.fda.gov/~dms/wh-folic.html).

U.S. Food and Drug Administration Center for Food Safety and Applied Nutrition. 1998. *Foodborne Pathogenic Microorganisms and Natural Toxins Handbook* ("The Bad Bug Book") (retrieved December 10, 1998; http://vm.cfsan.fda.gov/~mow/intro.html).

Uusi-Rasi, K., et al. 1998. Association of physical activity and calcium intake with bone mass and size in healthy women at different ages. *Journal of Bone Mineral Research* 13(1): 133–142.

Van Beneden, C. A., et al. 1999. Multinational outbreak of *Salmonella enterica* serotype Newport infections due to contaminated alfalfa sprouts. *Journal of the American Medical Association* 281(2): 158–162.

Van Loan, M. D. 1998. What makes good bones? Factors affecting bone health. *ACSM Health and Fitness Journal* 2(4): 27–34.

Volpe, S. L. 1998. Butter vs. margarine: What should we eat? *Healthline* 17(4): 6–7.

Wardlaw, G. M. 1999. *Perspectives in Nutrition,* 4th ed. Boston: McGraw-Hill.

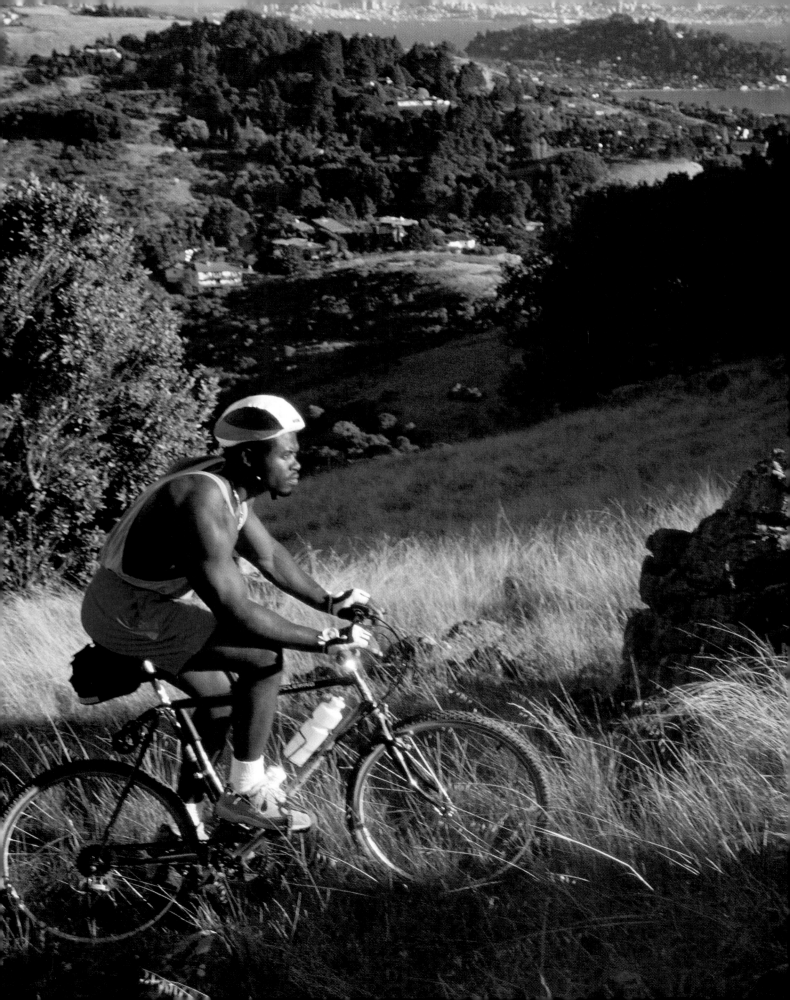

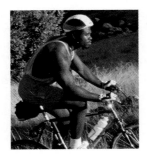

LEARNING OBJECTIVES

After reading this chapter, you should be able to:

- Define physical fitness, and list the health-related components of fitness.

- Explain the wellness benefits of physical activity and exercise.

- Describe how to develop each of the health-related components of fitness.

- Discuss how to choose appropriate exercise equipment, how to eat and drink for exercise, how to assess fitness, and how to prevent and manage injuries.

- Put together a personalized exercise program that you enjoy and that will enable you to achieve your fitness goals.

Exercise for Health and Fitness 13

TEST YOUR KNOWLEDGE

1. About what percentage of home exercise equipment is not being used?
   a. 10
   b. 20
   c. 40

2. To improve your health, you must do high-intensity exercise.
   True or false?

3. The best time to do stretching exercises is after a workout.
   True or false?

4. If you want to lose fat around your middle to have a flat stomach, you should do sit-ups.
   True or false?

5. If you think you've sprained your ankle or hurt a muscle, you should
   a. do nothing until you've seen a physician.
   b. apply heat immediately.
   c. apply ice immediately.

Answers

1. **c.** The 43% of equipment currently gathering dust includes 8% that was *never* used. On average, Americans spend 15 minutes per day exercising and 150 minutes per day watching television.

2. **False.** Even moderate physical activity—walking the dog or doing yard work—has significant health benefits.

3. **True.** Your muscles can stretch farther with a lower risk of injury when they are warm, so it's best to do stretching as part of your cool-down after cardiorespiratory endurance exercise or strength training.

4. **False.** The energy burned by sit-ups comes from fat stores throughout the body, not just from the abdomen, so sit-ups are no better at trimming fat from your stomach than any other calisthenic exercise.

5. **c.** Always ice an acute injury immediately, and continue icing for 10–20 minutes every 2 hours for the next day or two or until the swelling subsides.

Your body is a wonderful moving machine. Your bones, joints, and ligaments provide a support system for movement; your muscles perform the motions of work and play; your heart and lungs nourish your cells as you move through your daily life. But your body is made to work best when it is physically active. It readily adapts to practically any level of activity and exercise: The more you ask of your body—your muscles, bones, heart, lungs—the stronger and more fit they become. The opposite is also true. Left unchallenged, bones lose their density, joints stiffen, muscles become weak, and cellular energy systems begin to degenerate. To be truly healthy, human beings must be active.

The benefits of physical activity are both physical and mental, immediate and far-reaching. Being physically fit makes it easier to do everyday tasks, such as lifting; it provides reserve strength for emergencies; and it helps people to look and feel good. Over the long term, physically fit individuals are less likely to develop heart disease, cancer, high blood pressure, diabetes, and many other degenerative diseases. Their cardiorespiratory systems tend to resemble those of people 10 or more years younger than themselves. As they get older, they may be able to avoid weight gain, muscle and bone loss, fatigue, memory loss, and other problems associated with aging. With a healthy heart, strong muscles, a lean body, and a repertoire of physical skills they can call on for recreation and enjoyment, fit people can maintain their physical and mental well-being throughout their entire lives.

Unfortunately, modern life for most Americans provides few built-in occasions for vigorous activity. Technological advances have made our lives increasingly sedentary: We drive cars, ride escalators, watch television, and push papers around at school and work. According to *Healthy People 2010*, levels of physical activity remain low for all populations of Americans (Table 13-1). In 1996, the U.S. Surgeon General published *Physical Activity and Health,* a report designed to reverse these trends and get Americans moving. The report's conclusions include the following:

- People of all ages, both male and female, benefit from regular physical activity.

- People can obtain significant health benefits by including a moderate amount of physical activity on most, if not all, days of the week. Through a modest increase in daily activity, most Americans can improve their health and quality of life.

- Additional health benefits can be gained through greater amounts of physical activity. People who can maintain a regular regimen of more vigorous or longer-duration activity are likely to obtain even greater benefits.

- Physical activity reduces the risk of premature mortality, improves psychological health, and is important for the health of muscle, bones, and joints.

Are you one of the 60% of Americans who are not regularly active? Or one of the 25% who are not active at all? This chapter will give you the basic information you need to put together a physical fitness program that will work for you. If approached correctly, physical activity can contribute immeasurably to overall wellness, add fun and joy to life, and provide the foundation for a lifetime of fitness.

WHAT IS PHYSICAL FITNESS?

Physical fitness is the ability of the body to adapt to the demands of physical effort—that is, to perform moderate-to-vigorous levels of physical activity without becoming overly tired. Physical fitness has many components, some related to general health and others related more specifically to particular sports or activities. The five components of fitness most important for health are cardiorespiratory endurance, muscular strength, muscular endurance, flexibility, and body composition (proportion of fat to fat-free mass).

Cardiorespiratory Endurance

Cardiorespiratory endurance is the ability to perform prolonged, large-muscle, dynamic exercise at moderate-to-high levels of intensity. It depends on such factors as the ability of the lungs to deliver oxygen from the environment to the bloodstream, the heart's capacity to pump blood, the ability of the nervous system and blood vessels to regulate blood flow, and the capability of the body's chemical systems to use oxygen and process fuels for exercise. When levels of cardiorespiratory fitness are low, the heart has to work very hard during normal daily activities and may not be able to work hard enough to sustain high-intensity physical activity in an emergency. As cardiorespiratory fitness improves, the heart begins to function more efficiently. It doesn't have to work as hard at rest or during low levels of exercise. The heart pumps more blood per heartbeat, resting heart rate slows down, blood volume increases, blood supply to the tissues improves, the body is better able to cool itself, and resting

TERMS **physical fitness** The ability of the body to respond or adapt to the demands and stress of physical effort.

cardiorespiratory endurance The ability of the body to perform prolonged, large-muscle, dynamic exercise at moderate-to-high levels of intensity.

muscular strength The amount of force a muscle can produce with a single maximum effort.

muscular endurance The ability of a muscle or group of muscles to remain contracted or to contract repeatedly for a long period of time.

flexibility The range of motion in a joint or group of joints; flexibility is related to muscle length.

TABLE 13-1	Adults Who Regularly Engage in Physical Activity	
	Moderate Intensity[a]	High Intensity[b]
Overall[c]	20.1%	14.4%
Sex		
Men	21.5	12.9
Women	18.9	15.8
Ethnicity		
White	20.8	15.3
Black	15.2	9.4
Hispanic (Latino)	20.1	11.9
Education		
Less than 12 years	15.6	8.2
12 years	17.8	11.5
13–15 years	22.7	14.9
16 or more years	23.5	21.9
Income		
Less than $10,000	17.6	9.0
$10,000–$19,999	18.7	10.8
$20,000–$34,999	20.3	14.2
$35,000–$49,999	20.9	16.3
$50,000 or more	23.5	20.5
Geographic region		
Northeast	20.2	13.8
North Central	18.2	13.7
South	19.0	13.8
West	24.0	16.8

[a]Adults who engage in moderate-intensity physical activity 5 or more times per week for at least 30 minutes per session.
[b]Adults who engage in high-intensity physical activity 3 or more times per week for at least 20 minutes per session.
[c] The goals set in the *Healthy People 2010* report are 30% for moderate exercise and 25% for vigorous exercise.

SOURCE: U.S. Department of Health and Human Services. 1996. *Physical Activity and Health: A Report of the Surgeon General.* Atlanta, Ga.: U.S. Department of Health and Human Services.

blood pressure decreases. A healthy heart can better withstand the strains of everyday life, the stress of occasional emergencies, and the wear and tear of time. Endurance training also improves the functioning of biochemical systems, particularly in the muscles and liver, thereby enhancing the body's ability to use energy supplied by food.

Cardiorespiratory endurance is considered the most important component of health-related fitness because the functioning of the heart and lungs is so essential to overall wellness. A person simply cannot live very long or very well without a healthy heart. Low levels of cardiorespiratory fitness are linked with heart disease, the leading cause of death in the United States. Cardiorespiratory endurance is developed by activities that involve continu-

ous rhythmic movements of large-muscle groups like those in the legs—for example, walking, jogging, cycling, and aerobic dance.

Muscular Strength

Muscular strength is the amount of force a muscle can produce with a single maximum effort. Strong muscles are important for the smooth and easy performance of everyday activities, such as carrying groceries, lifting boxes, and climbing stairs, as well as for emergency situations. They help keep the skeleton in proper alignment, preventing back and leg pain and providing the support necessary for good posture. Muscular strength has obvious importance in recreational activities. Strong people can hit a tennis ball harder, kick a soccer ball farther, and ride a bicycle uphill more easily.

Muscle tissue is an important element of overall body composition. Greater muscle mass makes possible a higher rate of metabolism and faster energy use. Maintaining strength and muscle mass is vital for healthy aging. Older people tend to lose muscle cells, and many of the remaining muscle cells become nonfunctional because they lose their attachment to the nervous system. Strength training helps maintain muscle mass and function in older people, which greatly enhances their quality of life and prevents life-threatening injuries. Muscular strength can be developed by training with weights or by using the weight of the body for resistance during calisthenic exercises such as push-ups and sit-ups.

Muscular Endurance

Muscular endurance is the ability to sustain a given level of muscle tension—that is, to hold a muscle contraction for a long period of time, or to contract a muscle over and over again. Muscular endurance is important for good posture and for injury prevention. For example, if abdominal and back muscles are not strong enough to hold the spine correctly, the chances of low-back pain and back injury are increased. Muscular endurance helps people cope with the physical demands of everyday life and enhances performance in sports and work. It is also important for most leisure and fitness activities. Like muscular strength, muscular endurance is developed by stressing the muscles with a greater load (weight) than they are used to. The degree to which strength or endurance develops depends on the type and amount of stress that is applied.

Flexibility

Flexibility is the ability to move the joints through their full range of motion. Although range of motion is not a significant factor in everyday activities for most people, inactivity causes the joints to become stiffer with age.

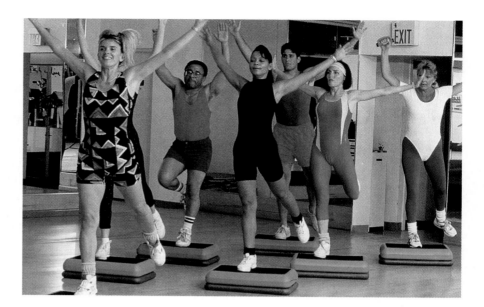

Cardiorespiratory endurance exercise conditions the heart, improves the function of the entire cardiorespiratory system, and has many other health benefits. An effective personal fitness program should be built around an activity like running, walking, biking, swimming, or aerobic dance.

Stiffness often causes older people to assume unnatural body postures, and it can lead to back pain. The majority of Americans experience low-back pain at some time in their lives, often because of stiff joints. Stretching exercises can help ensure a normal range of motion.

Body Composition

Body composition refers to the relative amounts of fat-free mass (muscle, bone, and water) and fat in the body. Healthy body composition involves a high proportion of fat-free mass and an acceptably low level of body fat. A person with excessive body fat is more likely to experience a variety of health problems, including heart disease, high blood pressure, stroke, joint problems, diabetes, gallbladder disease, cancer, and back pain. The best way to lose fat is through a lifestyle that includes a sensible diet and exercise. The best way to add muscle mass is through resistance training such as weight training. (Body composition is discussed in more detail in Chapter 14.)

In addition to these five health-related components of physical fitness, physical fitness for a particular sport or activity might include any or all of the following: coordination, speed, reaction time, agility, balance, and skill. Sport-specific skills are best developed through practice. The skill and coordination needed to play basketball, for example, are developed by playing basketball.

TERMS **body composition** The relative amounts of fat-free mass (muscle, bone, and water) and fat in the body.

cardiovascular disease (CVD) A collective term for diseases of the heart and blood vessels.

THE BENEFITS OF EXERCISE

As mentioned above, the human body is very adaptable. The greater the demands made on it, the more it adjusts to meet the demands. Over time, immediate, short-term adjustments translate into long-term changes and improvements. For example, when breathing and heart rate increase during exercise, the heart gradually develops the ability to pump more blood with each beat. Then, during exercise, it doesn't have to beat as fast to meet the body's demand for oxygen. The goal of regular physical activity is to bring about these kinds of long-term changes and improvements in the body's functioning.

Scientists have been actively studying these effects of exercise and their impact on health for over 40 years. They have found that exercise is one of the most important things you can do to improve your level of wellness (see the box "Benefits of Exercise and Physical Fitness"). Regular exercise increases energy levels, improves emotional and psychological well-being, and boosts the immune system. It prevents heart disease, some types of cancer, stroke, high blood pressure, Type 2 diabetes, obesity, and osteoporosis. At any age, people who exercise are less likely to die from all causes than their sedentary peers.

Improved Cardiorespiratory Functioning

Every time you take a breath, some of the oxygen in the air you take into your lungs is picked up by red blood cells and transported to your heart. From there, this oxygenated blood is pumped by the heart throughout the body to organs and tissues that use it. During exercise, the cardiorespiratory system (heart, lungs, and circulatory system) must work harder to meet the body's increased demand for oxygen. Regular endurance exercise improves

Physical Benefits

- Increased life expectancy.
- Decreased risk of developing and dying from cardiovascular disease.
- Decreased risk of developing and dying from certain cancers, particularly colon cancer.
- Decreased risk of Type 2 diabetes.
- Decreased risk of bone fractures from osteoporosis.
- Improved cardiac function.
- Control of blood pressure levels.
- Improved blood fat levels.
- Improved regulation of blood clotting.
- Improved ability to deliver oxygen to tissues.
- Improved body chemistry.
- Increased protection against the physiological effects of stress.
- Quicker recovery from illness and injury.
- Increased resistance to fatigue.
- Improved posture and body mechanics.
- Strengthened tendons, ligaments, bones, and muscles.
- Increased muscle mass.

- Decreased body fat.
- Decreased risk of injury.
- Reduced risk of low-back pain.
- Improved joint health.
- Decreased postexercise muscle soreness.
- Improved performance in sport, work, and recreational activities.

Psychological Health Benefits

- Tension relief.
- Reduced symptoms of stress.
- Improved sleeping habits.
- Increased energy levels and resistance to mental fatigue.
- Increased opportunities for positive interaction with others.
- Improved appearance.
- Improved self-image.
- Improved quality of life.

SOURCE: Fahey, T. D., P. M. Insel, and W. T. Roth. 1999. *Fit and Well: Core Concepts and Labs in Physical Fitness and Wellness*, 3rd ed. Mountain View, Calif.: Mayfield.

the functioning of the heart and the ability of the cardiorespiratory system to carry oxygen to body tissues. It also reduces the risk of cardiovascular disease.

More Efficient Metabolism

Endurance exercise improves metabolism, the process by which food is converted to energy and tissue is built. This process involves oxygen, nutrients, hormones, and enzymes. A physically fit person is better able to generate energy, to use fats for energy, and to regulate hormones. Physical training may also protect the body's cells from damage from free radicals, which are produced during normal metabolism (see Chapter 12). Training activates antioxidant enzymes that prevent free radical damage and maintain the health of the body's cells.

Improved Body Composition

Healthy body composition means that the body has a high proportion of fat-free mass (primarily composed of muscle) and a relatively small proportion of fat. Too much body fat is linked to a variety of health problems, including heart disease, cancer, and diabetes. Healthy body composition can be difficult to achieve and maintain

because a diet that contains all essential nutrients can be relatively high in calories, especially for someone who is sedentary. Excess calories are stored in the body as fat.

Exercise can improve body composition in several ways. Endurance exercise significantly increases daily calorie expenditure; it can also raise *metabolic rate,* the rate at which the body burns calories, for several hours after an exercise session. Strength training increases muscle mass, thereby tipping the body composition ratio toward fat-free mass and away from fat. It can also help with losing fat because metabolic rate is directly proportional to fat-free mass: The more muscle mass, the higher the metabolic rate. (Metabolism, energy balance, and the role of exercise in improving body composition are discussed in detail in Chapter 14.)

Disease Prevention and Management

Regular physical activity lowers your risk of many chronic, disabling diseases. It can also help people with those diseases improve their health.

Cardiovascular Disease A sedentary lifestyle is one of the six major risk factors for **cardiovascular disease (CVD)** (see Chapter 15). The others are smoking, unhealthy cholesterol levels, high blood pressure, diabetes, and obesity. People who are sedentary have CVD death rates significantly higher than fit individuals. There is a dose-response relationship between exercise and CVD: The benefit of physical activity occurs at moderate levels of activity and increases with increasing levels of activity. Many research studies have shown conclusively that exercise not only affects the risk factors for CVD but also directly interferes with the disease process itself.

BLOOD FAT LEVELS   Endurance exercise has a positive effect on the balance of lipids that circulate in the blood. High concentrations of lipids such as cholesterol and triglycerides are linked to heart disease because they contribute to the formation of fatty deposits on the linings of arteries. When such deposits block an artery, a heart attack or stroke can occur.

Cholesterol is carried in the blood by **lipoproteins,** which are classified according to size and density. Cholesterol carried by low-density lipoproteins (LDLs) tends to stick to the walls of coronary arteries. High-density lipoproteins (HDLs) tend to pick up excess cholesterol in the bloodstream and carry it back to the liver for excretion from the body. High LDL levels and low HDL levels are associated with a high risk of cardiovascular disease. High levels of HDL and low levels of LDL are associated with lower risk.

More information about cholesterol and heart disease is provided in Chapter 15. For our purposes in this chapter, it is important to know only that endurance exercise influences blood lipid, or fat, levels in a positive way, by increasing HDL and decreasing LDL and triglycerides—thereby helping reduce the risk of CVD.

HIGH BLOOD PRESSURE   Regular exercise tends to reduce high blood pressure, a contributing factor in diseases such as coronary heart disease, stroke, kidney failure, and blindness. People who exercise for a longer duration and at a higher intensity receive the greatest benefit, but even moderate exercise can produce significant improvements.

CORONARY HEART DISEASE   Coronary heart disease (CHD) involves blockage of one of the coronary arteries. These blood vessels supply the heart with oxygenated blood, and an obstruction in one of them can cause a heart attack. Exercise directly interferes with the disease process that causes coronary artery blockage. It also minimizes other risk factors—such as obesity, high blood pressure, and blood fat levels—that contribute to CHD.

STROKE   A stroke occurs when a blood vessel leading to the brain is blocked, often through the same disease process that leads to heart attacks. Regular exercise reduces the risk of stroke.

Cancer   Some studies have shown a relationship between increased physical activity and a reduction in a person's risk of all types of cancer, but these findings are not conclusive. There is strong evidence that exercise reduces the risk of colon cancer, and promising data that it reduces the risk of cancer of the breast and reproductive organs in women. Exercise may decrease the risk of colon cancer by speeding the movement of food through the gastrointestinal tract (quickly eliminating potential carcinogens), enhancing immune function, and reducing blood fats. The protective mechanism in the case of reproductive system cancers is less clear, but physical activity during the high school and college years may be particularly important for preventing breast cancer later in life.

Osteoporosis   A special benefit of exercise, especially for women, is protection against osteoporosis, a disease that results in loss of bone density and poor bone strength (see Chapter 12). Weight-bearing exercise, which includes almost everything except swimming, helps build bone during the teens and twenties. Older people with denser bones can better endure the bone loss that occurs with aging. Strength training can increase bone density throughout life. With stronger bones and muscles and better balance, fit people are less likely to experience debilitating falls and bone fractures. (But too much exercise can depress levels of estrogen, which helps maintain bone density, thereby leading to bone loss, even in young women.)

Diabetes   People with diabetes are prone to heart disease, blindness, and severe problems of the nervous and circulatory systems. Recent studies have shown that exercise actually prevents the development of Type 2 diabetes, the most common form. Exercise burns excess sugar and makes cells more sensitive to insulin. Exercise also helps keep body fat at healthy levels. (Obesity is a key risk factor for Type 2 diabetes.) For people who have diabetes, physical activity is an important part of treatment. (See Chapter 14 for more on diabetes.)

Improved Psychological and Emotional Wellness

The joy of a well-hit cross-court backhand, the euphoria of a walk through the park, or the rush of a downhill schuss through deep snow powder provides pleasure that

TERMS   **lipoproteins** Substances in blood, classified according to size, density, and chemical composition, that transport fats.

endorphins Brain chemicals that seem to be involved in modulating pain and producing euphoria.

neurotransmitters Brain chemicals that transmit nerve impulses.

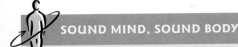
If you've ever gone for a long, brisk walk after a hard day's work, you know how refreshing exercise can be. Exercise can improve mood, stimulate creativity, clarify thinking, relieve anxiety, and provide an outlet for anger or aggression. But why does exercise make you feel good? Does it simply take your mind off your problems? Or does it cause a physical reaction that affects your mental state?

Current research indicates that exercise triggers many physical changes in the body that can alter mood. Scientists are now trying to explain how and why exercise affects the mind. One theory has to do with the physical structure of the brain. The area of the brain responsible for the movement of muscles in the body is near the area responsible for thought and emotion. As muscles work vigorously, the resulting stimulation in the muscle center of the brain may also stimulate the thought and emotion center, producing improvements in mood and cognitive functions.

Other researchers suggest that exercise stimulates the release of **endorphins**, chemicals in the brain that can suppress fatigue, decrease pain, and produce euphoria. The "runner's high" often experienced after running several miles may be due to an increased production of endorphins.

A third area of research focuses on changes in brain activity during and after exercise. One change is an increase in alpha brain wave activity. Alpha waves indicate a highly relaxed state; meditation also induces alpha wave activity. A second change is an alteration in the levels of **neurotransmitters**, brain chemicals that increase alertness and reduce stress.

Higher levels of neurotransmitters such as serotonin may explain how exercise improves mild to moderate cases of depression. Researchers have found that exercise can be as effective as psychotherapy in treating depression, and even more effective when used in conjunction with other therapies. In addition to boosting neurotransmitter activity, exercise provides a distraction from stressful stimuli, enhances self-esteem, and may provide opportunity for positive social interactions.

Another benefit of regular exercise is improved body image. According to a recent study, women who worked out on a regular basis rated their bodies as more attractive and healthy than did sedentary women. Of course, the exercisers may have had particularly attractive bodies, but they weighed an average of 11–12 pounds more than the less active women, suggesting that active women are more comfortable bucking cultural ideals of body shape.

Although most people don't associate exercise with mental skills, physical activity has been shown to have positive effects on cognitive functioning in both the short term and the long term. Exercise improves alertness and memory and can help you perform cognitive tasks at your peak level. Exercise may also help boost creativity. In a study of college students, those who ran regularly or took aerobic dance classes scored significantly higher on standard psychological tests of creativity than sedentary students. Over the long term, exercise can slow and possibly even reverse certain age-related declines in cognitive performance, including slowed reaction time and loss of short-term memory and nonverbal reasoning skills.

The message from this research is that exercise is a critical factor in developing *all* the dimensions of wellness, not just physical health. Even moderate exercise like walking briskly a few times per week can significantly improve your well-being. A lifetime of physical activity can leave you with a healthier body and a sharper, happier, more creative mind.

---

transcends health benefits alone. People who are physically active experience many social, psychological, and emotional benefits. For example:

- *Reduced stress.* In response to stressors, physically fit people experience milder physical responses and less emotional distress than sedentary individuals. Physical activity also provides protection against the effects of stress that have been linked to poor cardiorespiratory health. Psychological stress causes increased secretion of epinephrine and norepinephrine, the so-called fight-or-flight hormones, which are thought to speed the development of atherosclerosis, or hardening of the arteries. Excessive hostility is also associated with a risk of heart disease. Endurance exercise decreases the secretion of hormones triggered by emotional stress. It also can diffuse hostility and alleviate feelings of stress and anxiety by proving an emotional outlet and inducing feelings of relaxation. Regular exercise can also relieve sleeping problems.

- *Reduced anxiety and depression.* Sedentary adults have a much higher risk of feeling fatigue and depression than those who are physically active. Exercise is an effective treatment for people with depression and improves mood in nondepressed people who feel fine or who feel a little bit "down."

- *Improved self-image.* Performing physical activities provides proof of skill and self-control, thus enhancing self-concept. Exercise also helps you look and feel better, boosting self-confidence and body image.

- *Enjoyment.* Exercise is fun! It offers an arena for harmonious interaction with other people, as well as opportunities to strive and excel. Physically fit people can perform everyday tasks—such as climbing stairs and carrying books or groceries—with ease. They have plenty of energy and can lead lives that are full and varied.

For more on the psychological benefits of physical activity, see the box "Exercise and the Mind."

Physical fitness and athletic achievement are not limited to the able-bodied. People with disabilities can also attain high levels of fitness and performance, as shown by the elite athletes who compete in the Paralympics. The premier event for athletes with disabilities, the Paralympics is held in the same year and city as the Olympics. The athletes who participate include people with cerebral palsy, people with visual impairments, paraplegics, quadriplegics, and others. They compete in wheelchair races and wheelchair basketball, tandem cycling, in which a blind cyclist pedals with a sighted athlete, and other events. The performance of these skilled athletes makes it clear that people with disabilities can be active, healthy, and extraordinarily fit.

Paralympians point out that able-bodied athletes and athletes with disabilities have two important things in common: both are striving for excellence, and both can serve as role models. One athlete commented, "I'd like to let kids who have a disability know there is a sports option. The possibilities are endless."

Currently, some 34–43 million Americans are estimated to have chronic, significant disabilities. Some disabilities are the result of injury, such as spinal cord injuries sustained in car crashes. Other disabilities result from illness, such as the blindness that sometimes occurs as a complication of diabetes or the joint stiffness that accompanies arthritis. And some disabilities are present at birth, as in the case of congenital limb deformities or cerebral palsy.

Exercise and physical activity are as important for people with disabilities as for able-bodied individuals—if not *more* important. Being active helps prevent secondary conditions that may result from prolonged inactivity, such as circulatory or muscular problems. It also provides an emotional boost that helps support a positive attitude. Currently, about 10% of peo-ple with disabilities engage in regular vigorous activity and 27% engage in moderate activity.

People with disabilities don't have to be Paralympians to participate in sports and lead an active life. Depending on the nature of the disability, numerous options exist, including tennis, basketball, cycling, swimming, and running. Some fitness centers offer modified aerobics, mild exercise in warm water, and other exercises adapted for people with disabilities.

For those who prefer to get their exercise at home, special aerobic workout videos are available. Most of these videos are produced by hospitals and health associations and are geared to specific disabilities. For example, the Arthritis Foundation produces two videos, at different levels, called "People with Arthritis Can Exercise." There are also workout videos designed especially for individuals with hearing impairments (instructors both speak and sign); for women who have had breast surgery and need to strengthen arm, shoulder, and back muscles; for people who use wheelchairs; and many others. Some types are designed so that both able-bodied people and people with disabilities can participate.

If you want to try one of these videos or participate in some form of adapted physical activity, check with your physician about what's appropriate for you. Remember that no matter what your level of ability or disability, it's possible to make exercise an integral part of your life.

SOURCES: U.S. Department of Health and Human Services. 1996. *Physical Activity and Health: A Report of the Surgeon General.* Atlanta, Ga.: U.S. Department of Health and Human Services. Nemeth, M. 1992. Willing and able. *Maclean's,* 7 September. Silver, M. 1990. All the right moves. *U.S. News & World Report,* 12 December.

Improved Immune Function

Exercise can have either positive or negative effects on the immune system, the physiological processes that protect us from disease. It appears that moderate endurance exercise boosts immune function, while excessive training depresses it. Physically fit people get fewer colds and upper respiratory tract infections than people who are not fit. The immune system—and ways to strengthen it—are discussed further in Chapter 17.

Prevention of Injuries and Low-Back Pain

Increased muscle strength provides protection against injury because it helps people maintain good posture and appropriate body mechanics when carrying out everyday activities like walking, lifting, and carrying. Strong muscles in the abdomen, hips, low back, and legs support the back in proper alignment and help prevent low-back pain, which afflicts over 85% of all Americans at some time in their lives.

Improved Wellness over the Life Span

Although people differ in the maximum levels of fitness they can achieve through exercise, the wellness benefits of exercise are available to everyone (see the box "Fitness and Disability"). Exercising regularly may be the single most important thing you can do now to improve the quality of your life in the future. All the benefits of exercise continue to accrue but gain new importance as the resilience of youth begins to wane. Simply stated, exercising can help you live a longer and healthier life.

DESIGNING YOUR EXERCISE PROGRAM

The best exercise program has two primary characteristics: It promotes your health, and it's fun for you to do. Exercise does not have to be a chore. On the contrary, it can provide some of the most pleasurable moments of your day, once you make it a habit. A little thought and planning will help you achieve these goals.

Physical Activity and Exercise for Health and Fitness

Physical activity can be defined as any movement of the body that is carried out by the muscles and requires energy to produce. Different types of physical activity can be arranged on a continuum based on the amount of energy they require. Quick, easy movements such as standing up or walking down a hallway require little energy or effort; more intense, sustained activities such as cycling 5 miles or running in a race require considerably more.

The term *exercise* is usually used to refer to a subset of physical activity—planned, structured, repetitive movement of the body designed specifically to improve or maintain physical fitness. As described earlier, levels of fitness depend on physiological factors such as the heart's ability to pump blood. To develop fitness, a person must perform a sufficient amount of physical activity to stress the body and cause long-term physiological changes. The precise type and amount of activity required to develop fitness will be discussed in greater detail later in the chapter. For now, just remember that only some types of physical activity—what is commonly referred to as exercise—will develop fitness. This distinction is important for setting goals and developing a program.

Lifestyle Physical Activity for Health Promotion
The Surgeon General's report recommends that all Americans include a moderate amount of physical activity on most, preferably all, days of the week. The report suggests a goal of 150 calories per day, or about 1000 calories per week. Because energy expenditure is a function of both intensity and duration of activity, the same amount of benefit can be obtained in longer sessions of moderate-intensity activities as in shorter sessions of more strenuous activities. Thus, 30 minutes of brisk walking is equivalent to 15 minutes of running (Figure 13-1).

In this lifestyle approach to physical activity, the daily total of activity can be accumulated in multiple short bouts—for example, two 10-minute bicycle rides to and from class and a brisk 15-minute walk to the post office. Everyday tasks at school, work, and home can be structured to contribute to the daily activity total (see the box "Becoming More Active" for suggestions).

By increasing lifestyle physical activity in accordance with the guidelines given in the Surgeon General's report, people can expect to significantly improve their health and well-being. Such a program may not, however, increase physical fitness.

Exercise Programs to Develop Physical Fitness
The Surgeon General's report also summarized the benefits of more formal exercise programs. It concluded that people can obtain even greater health benefits by increasing the duration and intensity of activity. Thus a person who engages in a structured, formal exercise program designed to measurably improve physical fitness will obtain even

Washing and waxing a car for 45–60 minutes
Washing windows or floors for 45–60 minutes
Playing volleyball for 45 minutes
Playing touch football for 30–45 minutes
Gardening for 30–45 minutes
Wheeling self in wheelchair for 30–40 minutes
Walking 1¾ miles in 35 minutes (20 min/mile)
Basketball (shooting baskets) for 30 minutes
Bicycling 5 miles in 30 minutes
Dancing fast (social) for 30 minutes
Pushing a stroller 1½ miles in 30 minutes
Raking leaves for 30 minutes
Walking 2 miles in 30 minutes (15 min/mile)
Water aerobics for 30 minutes
Swimming laps for 20 minutes
Wheelchair basketball for 20 minutes
Basketball (playing a game) for 15–20 minutes
Bicycling 4 miles in 15 minutes
Jumping rope for 15 minutes
Running 1½ miles in 15 minutes (10 min/mile)
Shoveling snow for 15 minutes
Stairwalking for 15 minutes

Less Vigorous, More Time

More Vigorous, Less Time

Figure 13-1   Examples of moderate amounts of physical activity. A moderate amount of physical activity is roughly equivalent to physical activity that uses approximately 150 calories of energy per day, or 1000 calories per week. Some activities can be performed at various intensities; the suggested durations correspond to expected intensity of effort. SOURCE: U.S. Department of Health and Human Services. 1996. *Physical Activity and Health. A Report of the Surgeon General: At-A-Glance.* Washington, D.C.: U.S. Department of Health and Human Services.

greater improvements in quality of life and greater reductions in disease and mortality risk.

How Much Exercise Is Enough?
The Surgeon General's report has generated controversy among researchers. Some experts feel that people get most of the health benefits of a formal exercise program simply by becoming more active over the course of the day. Others feel that the lifestyle approach sets too low an activity goal; they argue that people should exercise long and intensely enough to improve their body's capacity for exercise—that is, to improve physical fitness. More research is needed to resolve this debate, but there is probably truth in both of these positions. Regular physical activity, regardless of intensity, makes you healthier and can help protect you from many chronic diseases. But you obtain even greater benefits when you are physically fit.

Where does this leave you? Most experts agree that some physical activity is better than none, but that more—as long as it does not result in injury or become obsessive—is probably better than some. A physical activity pyramid to guide you in meeting these goals for physical activity is shown in Figure 13-2. If you are sedentary, start at the bottom of the pyramid and gradually increase the amount of

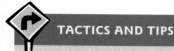

TACTICS AND TIPS   *Becoming More Active*

- Take the stairs instead of the elevator or escalator.
- Walk to the mailbox, post office, store, bank, or library whenever possible.
- Park your car a mile or even just a few blocks from your destination, and walk briskly.
- Do at least one chore every day that requires physical activity: wash the windows or your car, clean your room or house, mow the lawn, rake the leaves.
- Take study or work breaks to avoid sitting for more than 30 minutes at a time. Get up and walk around the library, your office, or your home or dorm; go up and down a flight of stairs.

- Stretch when you stand in line or watch TV.
- When you take public transportation, get off one stop down the line and walk to your destination.
- Go dancing instead of to a movie.
- Walk to visit a neighbor or friend rather than calling him or her on the phone. Go for a walk while you chat.
- Put your remote controls in storage; when you want to change TV or radio stations, get up and do it by hand.
- Seize every opportunity to get up and walk around. Move more and sit less.

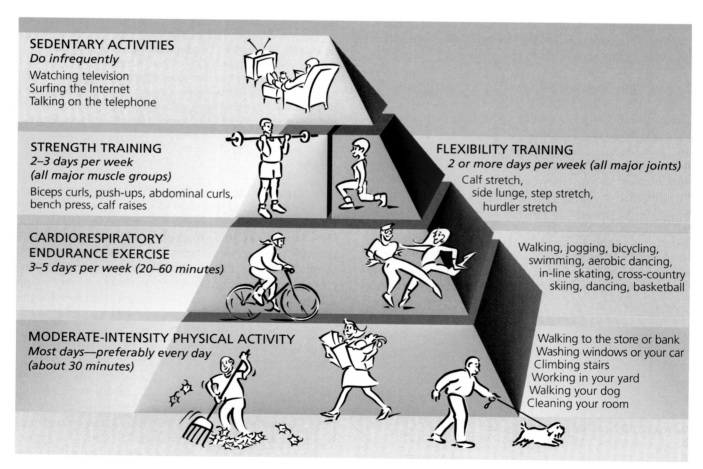

SEDENTARY ACTIVITIES
Do infrequently
Watching television
Surfing the Internet
Talking on the telephone

STRENGTH TRAINING
2–3 days per week
(all major muscle groups)
Biceps curls, push-ups, abdominal curls, bench press, calf raises

FLEXIBILITY TRAINING
2 or more days per week (all major joints)
Calf stretch, side lunge, step stretch, hurdler stretch

CARDIORESPIRATORY ENDURANCE EXERCISE
3–5 days per week (20–60 minutes)

Walking, jogging, bicycling, swimming, aerobic dancing, in-line skating, cross-country skiing, dancing, basketball

MODERATE-INTENSITY PHYSICAL ACTIVITY
Most days—preferably every day
(about 30 minutes)

Walking to the store or bank
Washing windows or your car
Climbing stairs
Working in your yard
Walking your dog
Cleaning your room

Figure 13-2   Physical activity pyramid.   Similar to the Food Guide Pyramid, this physical activity pyramid is designed to help people become more active. If you are currently sedentary, begin at the bottom of the pyramid and gradually increase the amount of moderate-intensity physical activity in your life. If you are already moderately active, begin a formal exercise program that includes cardiorespiratory endurance exercise, flexibility training, and strength training to help you develop all the health-related components of fitness.

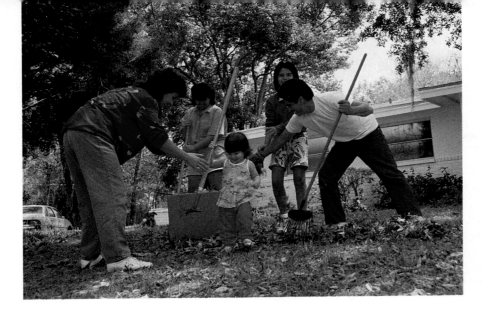

The Surgeon General recommends that all Americans accumulate at least 30 minutes of moderate-intensity activity on most days of the week. Yard work is one of many household chores that can contribute to your daily total of physical activity.

moderate-intensity physical activity in your daily life. You don't have to exercise vigorously, but you should experience a moderate increase in your heart and breathing rates; appropriate activities include walking, climbing stairs, doing yard work, and washing your car. As described earlier, your activity time can be broken up into small blocks over the course of a day.

For even greater benefits, move up to the next two levels of the pyramid, which illustrate parts of a formal exercise program. The American College of Sports Medicine has established guidelines for creating an exercise program that includes **cardiorespiratory endurance (aerobic) exercise**, strength training, and flexibility training (Table 13-2). Such a program will develop all the health-related components of physical fitness. The following sections of this chapter will show you how to develop a personalized exercise program that is fun and that will enable you to enjoy all the physical and psychological benefits of physical fitness.

First Steps

Are you thinking about starting a formal exercise program? A little planning can help make it a success.

Medical Clearance   Previously inactive men over 40 and women over 50 should get a medical examination before beginning an exercise program. Diabetes, asthma, heart disease, and extreme obesity are conditions that may call for a modified program. If you have an increased risk of heart disease because of smoking, high blood pressure, or obesity, have a physical checkup, including an **electrocardiogram (ECG or EKG),** before beginning an exercise program. This checkup will help ensure that your program will be a benefit to your health, rather than a potential hazard.

Basic Principles of Physical Training   As discussed earlier, fitness has many components; each has value and

requires specific exercises. Lifting weights develops muscle strength, for example, but it does not do much to condition heart and lungs. Running is excellent for increasing cardiorespiratory capacity, but it contributes little to upper-body strength. Different sports and activities call for different skills; and to become proficient in them, you have to practice the specific movements they require. Therefore, to develop all the fitness components, you must participate in a variety of activities.

Your body adapts to the demands of exercise by improving its functioning. When the amount of exercise, also called **overload**, is progressively increased, fitness continues to improve. The amount of overload is very important. Too little exercise will have no effect on fitness; too much may cause injury. The amount of exercise needed depends on your current level of fitness, your fitness goals, and the fitness components being developed. A novice, for example, might experience fitness benefits from jogging a mile in 10 minutes, but this level of exercise would cause no physical adaptations in a trained distance runner.

The amount of overload needed to maintain or improve a particular level of fitness is determined in terms of three dimensions:

1. *Frequency, or how often.* Optimum exercise frequency, expressed in number of days per week,

| TABLE 13-2 | *Exercise Recommendations for Healthy Adults* |

Exercise to Develop and Maintain Cardiorespiratory Endurance and Body Composition

Mode of activity	Any activity that uses large-muscle groups, can be maintained continuously, and is rhythmical and aerobic in nature; for example, walking-hiking, running-jogging, cycling-bicycling, cross-country skiing, group exercise (aerobic dance), rope skipping, rowing, stairclimbing, swimming, skating, and endurance game activities.
Frequency of training	3–5 days per week.
Intensity of training	55/65–90% of maximum heart rate or 40/50–85% of maximum oxygen uptake reserve. The lower intensity values (55–64% of maximum heart rate and 40–49% of maximum oxygen uptake reserve) are most applicable to individuals who are quite unfit.
Duration of training	20–60 total minutes of continuous or intermittent (in sessions lasting 10 or more minutes) aerobic activity. Duration is dependent on the intensity of activity; thus, lower-intensity activity should be conducted over a longer period of time (30 minutes or more). Lower-to-moderate-intensity activity of longer duration is recommended for the nonathletic adult.

Exercise to Develop and Maintain Muscular Strength and Endurance, Flexibility, and Body Composition

Resistance training	One set of 8–10 exercises that condition the major muscle groups should be performed 2–3 days per week. Most people should complete 8–12 repetitions of each exercise; for older and more frail people (approximately 50–60 years of age and above), 10–15 repetitions with a lighter weight may be more appropriate. Multiple-set regimens may provide greater benefits if time allows.
Flexibility training	Stretches for the major muscle groups should be performed a minimum of 2–3 days per week; at least four repetitions, held for 10–30 seconds, should be completed.

SOURCES: American College of Sports Medicine. 1998. ACSM position stand: The recommended quantity and quality of exercise for developing and maintaining cardiorespiratory and muscular fitness, and flexibility in healthy adults. *Medicine and Science in Sports and Exercise* 30(6): 975–991.

varies with the component being developed and your goals. A frequency of 3–5 days per week is recommended for cardiorespiratory endurance exercise, 2–3 days per week for strength training, and 2 or more days per week for stretching.

2. *Intensity, or how hard.* Fitness benefits occur when you exercise harder than your normal level of activity. To develop cardiorespiratory endurance, you must raise your heart rate above normal; to develop muscular strength, you must lift a heavier weight than normal; to develop flexibility, you must stretch your muscles beyond their normal length. A gradual increase in intensity is recommended to avoid injury.

3. *Duration, how long.* If fitness benefits are to occur, exercise sessions must last for an extended period of time. Depending on the component being developed and your intensity level, a duration of 20–60 minutes is usually recommended.

Each of these dimensions of overload will be described as it applies to the health-related components of fitness.

Selecting Activities   If you have been inactive, you should begin slowly by gradually increasing the amount of moderate physical activity in your life (the bottom of

the activity pyramid). Once your body has adjusted to your new level of activity, you will be ready to choose additional activities for your exercise program.

Consider your choices carefully. First, be sure the activities you choose contribute to your overall wellness. Choose activities that make sense for you. Are you competitive? If so, try racquetball, basketball, or squash. Do you prefer to exercise alone? Then consider cross-country skiing or road running. Have you been sedentary? A walking program may be a good place to start.

If you think you may have trouble sticking with an exercise program, find a structured activity that you can do with a buddy or a group. If you don't have any favorite sports or activities, try something new. Take a physical education class, join a health club, or sign up for jazz dancing. You're sure to find an activity that's both enjoyable and good for you.

Be realistic about the constraints presented by some sports, such as accessibility, expense, and time. For example, if you have to travel for hours to get to a ski area, skiing may not be a good choice for your regular exercise program. If you don't have large blocks of time available, you may have trouble squeezing in eighteen holes of golf. And if you've never played tennis, it will probably take you a fair amount of time to reach a reasonable skill level; you may be better off with a program of walking or jogging to get good workouts while you're improving your tennis game.

A general fitness program that supports an active lifestyle and promotes good health should contain the following components: cardiorespiratory endurance exercises, muscular strength and endurance exercises, flexibility exercises, and training in specific skills.

> **PERSONAL INSIGHT**   Do you exercise because you like it or because you think you should? Is there any form of exercise that you do just for the love of it?

Cardiorespiratory Endurance Exercises

Exercises that condition your heart and lungs should have a central role in your fitness program. The best exercises for developing cardiorespiratory endurance are those that stress a large portion of the body's muscle mass for a prolonged period of time. These include walking, jogging, running, swimming, bicycling, and aerobic dancing. Many popular sports and recreational activities such as racquetball, tennis, basketball, and soccer are also good if the skill level and intensity of the game are sufficient to provide a vigorous workout.

Frequency   The optimal workout schedule for endurance training is 3–5 days per week. Beginners should start with 3 and work up to 5 days. Training more than 5 days a week often leads to injury for recreational athletes. While you do get health benefits from exercising very vigorously only 1–2 days per week, you risk injury because your body never gets a chance to adapt fully to regular exercise training.

Intensity   The most misunderstood aspect of conditioning, even among experienced athletes, is training intensity. Intensity is the crucial factor in attaining a significant training effect—that is, in increasing the body's cardiorespiratory capacity. A primary purpose of endurance training is to increase **maximal oxygen consumption (MOC)**. MOC represents the maximum ability of the cells to use oxygen and is considered the best measure of cardiorespiratory capacity. Intensity of training is the crucial factor in improving MOC.

However, it's not true that the harder you work, the better it is for you. Working too hard can cause injury, just as not working hard enough provides less benefit. One of the easiest ways to determine exactly how intensely you should work involves measuring your heart rate. It is not necessary or desirable to exercise at your maximum heart rate—the fastest heart rate possible before exhaustion sets in—in order to improve your cardiorespiratory capacity.

Beneficial effects occur at lower heart rates with a much lower risk of injury. **Target heart rate** is the rate at which you should exercise to obtain cardiorespiratory benefits. To find out how you can determine the intensity at which you should exercise, refer to the box "Determining Your Target Heart Rate," p. 354.

After you begin your fitness program, you may improve quickly because the body adapts readily to new exercises at first; the rate of improvement may slow after the first month or so. The more fit you become, the harder you will have to work to improve. By monitoring your heart rate, you will always know if you are working hard enough to improve, not hard enough, or too hard. For most people, a fitness program involves attaining an acceptable level of fitness and then maintaining that level. There is no need to keep working indefinitely to improve; doing so only increases the chance of injury. After you have reached the level you want, you can maintain fitness by exercising at the same intensity at least 3 nonconsecutive days per week.

Duration   A total duration of 20–60 minutes is recommended; exercise can take place in a single session or in multiple bouts lasting 10 or more minutes. The total duration of exercise depends on its intensity. To improve cardiorespiratory endurance during a low- to moderate-intensity activity such as walking or slow swimming, you should exercise for 45–60 minutes. For high-intensity exercise performed at the top of your target heart rate zone, a duration of 20 minutes is sufficient. It is usually best to start off with less-vigorous activities and only gradually increase intensity.

You can use these three dimensions of cardiorespiratory endurance training—frequency, intensity, and duration—to develop a fitness program that strengthens your heart and lungs and provides all the benefits described earlier in this chapter. Build your program around at least 20 minutes of endurance exercise at your target heart rate three to five times a week. Then add exercises that develop the other components of fitness.

The Warm-Up and Cool-Down   It is always important to warm up before you exercise and to cool down afterward. Warming up enhances your performance and decreases your chances of injury. Your muscles work better when their temperature is elevated slightly above resting level. Warming up helps your body's physiology gradually

> **maximal oxygen consumption (MOC)**   The body's maximum ability to transport and use oxygen.
>
> **target heart rate**   The heart rate at which exercise yields cardiorespiratory benefits.

TERMS

Your target heart rate is the rate at which you should exercise to experience cardiorespiratory benefits. Your target heart rate is based on your maximum heart rate, which can be estimated from your age. (If you are a serious athlete or face possible cardiovascular risks from exercise, you may want to have your maximum heart rate determined more accurately through a treadmill test in a physician's office, hospital, or sports medicine laboratory.) Your target heart rate is actually a range; the lower value corresponds to moderate-intensity exercise, while the higher value is associated with high-intensity activities. Target heart rates are shown in the accompanying table.

You can monitor the intensity of your workouts by measuring your pulse either at your wrist or at one of your carotid arteries, located on either side of your Adam's apple. Your pulse rate drops rapidly after exercise, so begin counting immediately after you have finished exercising. You will obtain the most accurate results by counting beats for 15 seconds and then multiplying by 4 to get your heart rate in beats per minute (bpm). The 15-second counts corresponding to each target heart rate range are also shown in the table at the right.

Age (years)	Target Heart Rate Range (bpm)*	15-Second Count (beats)*
20–24	127–182	32–46
25–29	124–176	31–44
30–34	121–171	30–43
35–39	118–167	30–42
40–44	114–162	29–41
45–49	111–158	28–40
50–54	108–153	27–38
55–59	105–149	26–37
60–64	101–144	25–36
65+	97–140	24–35

*Target heart rates lower than those shown here are appropriate for individuals who are quite unfit. Ranges are based on the following formula: Target heart rate = 0.65 to 0.90 of maximum heart rate, assuming maximum heart rate = 220 – age.

progress from rest to exercise. Blood needs to be redirected to active muscles, and your heart needs time to adapt to the increased demands of exercise. A warm-up helps spread **synovial fluid** throughout the joints, which helps protect joint surfaces from wear and tear. (It's like warming up a car to spread oil through the engine parts before shifting into gear.)

A warm-up session should include low-intensity movements similar to those in the activity that will follow. Examples of low-intensity movements are hitting forehands and backhands before a tennis game and running a 12-minute mile before progressing to an 8-minute one. Some experts also recommend warm-up stretching exercises for flexibility after the general warm-up and before intense activity.

Cooling down after exercise is important to restore the body's circulation to its normal resting condition. When you are at rest, a relatively small percentage of your total blood volume is directed to muscles, but during exercise, as much as 85% of the heart's output is directed to them. During recovery from exercise, it is important to continue exercising at a low level to provide a smooth transition to the resting state. Cooling down helps regulate the return of blood to your heart.

Developing Muscular Strength and Endurance

Any program designed to promote health should include exercises that develop muscular strength and endurance. Your ability to maintain correct posture and move efficiently depends in part on adequate muscle fitness. Strengthening exercises also increase muscle tone, which improves the appearance of your body. A lean, healthy-looking body is certainly one of the goals and one of the benefits of an overall fitness program.

Types of Strength Training Exercises   Muscular strength and endurance can be developed in many ways, from weight training to calisthenics. Common exercises such as sit-ups, push-ups, pull-ups, and wall-sitting (leaning against a wall in a seated position and supporting yourself with your leg muscles) maintain the muscular strength of most people if they practice them several times a week. To condition and tone your whole body, choose exercises that work the major muscles of the shoulders, chest, back, arms, abdomen, and legs.

To increase strength, you must do **resistance exercise**—exercises in which your muscles must exert force against a significant amount of resistance. Resistance can be provided by weights, exercise machines, or your own body weight. **Isometric exercises** involve applying force without movement, such as when you contract your abdominal muscles. This static type of exercise is valuable

TERMS   **synovial fluid**   Fluid found within many joints that provides lubrication and nutrition to the cells of the joint surface.

resistance exercise   Exercise that forces muscles to contract against increased resistance; also called *strength training*.

isometric exercise   The application of force without movement; also called *static exercise*.

isotonic exercise   The application of force with movement.

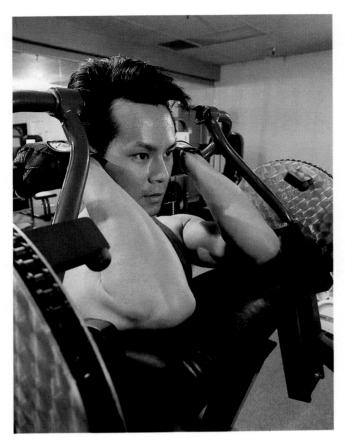

Building muscular strength is an important component of a fitness program. Weight training is just one way to increase strength, improve muscle tone, and enhance the overall appearance of the body.

for toning and strengthening muscles. Isometrics can be practiced anywhere and do not require any equipment. For maximum strength gains, hold an isometric contraction maximally for 6 seconds; do 5–10 repetitions. Don't hold your breath—that can restrict blood flow to your heart and brain. Within a few weeks, you will notice the effect of this exercise. Isometrics are particularly useful when recovering from an injury.

Isotonic exercises involve applying force with movement, as, for example, in weight training exercises such as the bench press. These are the most popular type of exercises for increasing muscle strength and seem to be most valuable for developing strength that can be transferred to other forms of physical activity. They include exercises using barbells, dumbbells, weight machines, and the body's own weight, as in push-ups or sit-ups.

Choosing Equipment Weight machines are preferred by many people because they are safe, convenient, and easy to use. You just set the resistance (usually by placing a pin in the weight stack), sit down at the machine, and start working. Machines make it easy to isolate and work specific muscles. Free weights require more care, balance,

and coordination to use, but they strengthen your body in ways that are more adaptable to real life. For free weights, you need to use a spotter, someone who stands by to assist in case you lose control over a weight (see the box "Safe Weight Training," p. 356).

Choosing Exercises A complete weight training program works all the major muscle groups: neck, upper back, shoulders, arms, chest, abdomen, lower back, thighs, buttocks, and calves. It usually takes about 8–10 different exercises to get a complete workout. If you are also training for a particular activity, include exercises to strengthen the muscles important for optimal performance and the muscles most likely to be injured.

Intensity and Duration The amount of weight (resistance) you lift in weight training exercises is equivalent to intensity in cardiorespiratory endurance training; the number of repetitions of each exercise is equivalent to duration. In order to improve fitness, you must do enough repetitions of each exercise to temporarily fatigue your muscles. The number of repetitions needed to cause fatigue depends on the amount of resistance: The heavier the weight, the fewer repetitions to reach fatigue. In general, a heavy weight and a low number of repetitions (1–5) build strength, while a light weight and a high number of repetitions (20–25) build endurance. For a general fitness program to build both strength and endurance, try to do 8–12 repetitions of each exercise; a few exercises, such as abdominal crunches and calf raises, may require more. (For people who are 50–60 years of age and older, 10–15 repetitions of each exercise using a lighter weight is recommended.)

Begin with a weight that you can lift fairly easily, and do 8–12 repetitions of each exercise. As you progress, add weight when you can do more than 12 repetitions of an exercise. By gradually increasing resistance over a period of weeks, you will increase your muscle strength and endurance without causing injury.

For developing strength and endurance for general fitness, a single set (group) of each exercise is sufficient, provided you use enough resistance (weight) to fatigue your muscles. Doing more than 1 set of each exercise may increase strength development, and most serious weight trainers do at least 3 sets of each exercise. If you do perform more than 1 set of an exercise, rest long enough between sets to allow your muscles to recover.

As with cardiorespiratory endurance exercise, you should warm up before every weight training session and cool down afterward.

Frequency You should train with weights 2–3 days per week. Allow your muscles a day of rest between workouts to avoid soreness and injury. If you enjoy weight training and would like to train more often, try working different muscle groups on alternate days. Refer to the box

General Strategies

- Lift weights from a stabilized body position. Protect your back from dangerous positions. Don't twist your body while lifting.

- Don't lift beyond the limits of your strength.

- Be aware of what's going on around you so that you don't bump into someone or get too close to a moving weight stack.

- Don't use defective equipment; report any equipment problems immediately.

- Don't hold your breath while doing weight training exercises. Exhale when exerting the greatest force, and inhale when moving the weight into position. (Holding your breath causes a decrease in blood returning to the heart and can make you become dizzy and faint.)

- Rest between lifts.

- Always warm up before training and cool down afterward.

Free Weights

- Use spotters to avoid injury. A spotter can help you if you cannot complete a lift or if the weight tilts.

- Secure weight plates to barbells with a collar to prevent them from sliding off.

- Keep weights as close to your body as possible. Do most of your lifting with your legs; keep your hips and buttocks tucked in.

- Lift weights smoothly and slowly; don't bounce or jerk them. Control the weight through the entire range of motion.

- When holding barbells and dumbbells, wrap your thumbs around the bar when gripping it.

Weight Machines

- Stay away from moving parts of the machine that could pinch your skin.

- Adjust each machine for your body so that you don't have to work in an awkward position.

- Beware of broken bolts, frayed cables, broken chains, or loose cushions that can give way and cause serious injury.

- Make sure the machines are clean. Carry a towel with you, and place it on the machine where you will sit or lie down.

A CLOSER LOOK   *A Sample Weight Training Program for General Fitness*

Guidelines

Type of activity: 8–10 weight training exercises that focus on major muscle groups

Frequency: 2–3 days per week

Resistance: Weights heavy enough to cause muscle fatigue when performed for the selected number of repetitions

Repetitions: 8–12 of each exercise (10–15 with a lower weight for people over age 50–60)

Sets: 1 (Doing more than 1 set per exercise may result in faster and greater strength gains.)

Sample Program

1. Warm-up (5–10 minutes)

2. Weight training exercises (see table at right)

3. Cool-down (5–10 minutes)

Exercise	Resistance (lb)	Repetitions	Sets
Bench press	60	10	1
Overhead press	40	10	1
Lat pulls	40	10	1
Lateral raises	5	10	1
Biceps curls	25	10	1
Squats	30	10	1
Toe raises	25	15	1
Abdominal curls	—	30	1
Spine extensions	—	10	1
Neck flexion	—	10	1

"A Sample Weight Training Program for General Fitness" for suggestions on beginning a program.

Gender Differences in Muscle Size and Strength Men are generally stronger than women because they typically have larger bodies overall and larger muscles. But when the amount of muscle tissue is taken into account, men are only 1–2% stronger than women in the upper body and about equal to women in the lower body. (Men have a larger proportion of muscle tissue in the upper body, so it's easier for them to build upper-body strength than it is for women.) This disparity is probably due in large part to androgens, naturally occurring male hormones that are responsible for the development of secondary sex characteristics (facial hair, deep voice, and so on; see Chapter 5). Androgens also promote the growth of muscle tissue, and androgen levels are about 6–10 times higher in men than in women.

However, both men and women can increase strength through resistance training. Men tend to build larger, stronger, more shapely muscles. Women tend to lose inches, increase strength, and develop greater muscle definition. (Because of their lower levels of androgens, women do not develop large muscles from moderate strength training.) The lifetime wellness benefits of strength training are available to everyone.

A Caution About Supplements No nutritional supplement or drug will change a weak, untrained person into a strong, fit person. Those changes require regular training that stresses the body and causes physiological adaptations. Supplements or drugs that promise quick, large gains in strength usually don't work and are often either dangerous or expensive, or both. The long-term effects of many supplements have not been studied. Use your critical thinking skills to evaluate claims made about supplements, and stay with the proven method of a steady, progressive fitness program to build strength.

About 2.4% of male college students and 0.4% of female college students report having used **anabolic steroids,** the drugs most often taken in an effort to build strength and power. Steroids have dangerous side effects, including the disruption of the body's hormone system. In men, they can cause testicular atrophy. In women and children, steroid use can have masculinizing effects, including hair growth on the face and body, deepening of the voice, and baldness. Steroids can also harm the immune system and the liver, and they increase the risk of coronary heart disease. Anabolic steroids are not a safe way to increase strength.

Flexibility Exercises

Although flexibility, or stretching, exercises are perhaps the most neglected part of fitness programs, they are extremely important. They are necessary for maintaining the normal range of motion in the major joints of the body. Some exercises, such as running, can actually decrease flexibility because they require only a partial range of motion. A good stretching program includes exercises for all the major muscle groups and joints of the body: neck, shoulders, back, hips, thighs, hamstrings, and calves. A sequence of appropriate stretching exercises is given in the box "Exercises for Flexibility," on pp. 358–359.

Proper Stretching Technique Stretching should be performed statically. "Bouncing" (known as ballistic stretching) is dangerous and counterproductive. Stretching can either be active or passive. In active stretching, a muscle is stretched by a contraction of opposing muscles. In passive stretching, an outside force or resistance provided by yourself, a partner, gravity, or a weight helps your joints move through their range of motion. You can achieve a greater range of motion and a more intense stretch using passive stretching, but there is a greater risk of injury. The safest and most convenient technique may be active static stretching with a passive assist. For example, you might do a seated stretch of your calf muscles both by contracting the muscles on the top of your shin and by grabbing your feet and pulling them toward you.

Intensity and Duration For each exercise, stretch to the point of tightness in the muscle, and hold the position for 10–30 seconds. Rest for 30–60 seconds, then repeat, trying to stretch a bit farther. Relax and breathe easily as you stretch. You should feel a pleasant, mild stretch as you let the muscles relax; stretching should not be painful. Do at least 4 repetitions of each exercise. A complete flexibility workout usually takes about 20–30 minutes.

Increase your intensity gradually over time. Improved flexibility takes many months to develop. There are large individual differences in joint flexibility. Don't feel you have to compete with others during stretching workouts.

Frequency Do stretching exercises a minimum of 2–3 days per week. You can set apart a special time for these exercises, or do them before or after cardiorespiratory endurance exercise or strength training. You may develop more flexibility if you do them after exercise, during your cool-down, because your muscles are warmer then and can be stretched farther.

Training in Specific Skills

The final component in your fitness program is learning the skills required for the sports or activities in which you choose to participate. Taking the time and effort to acquire competence means that instead of feeling ridiculous, becoming frustrated, and giving up in despair, you achieve a sense of mastery and add a new physical activity to your repertoire.

The first step in learning a new skill is getting help. Sports like tennis, golf, sailing, and skiing require mastery of basic movements and techniques, so instruction from a qualified teacher can save you hours of frustration and increase your enjoyment of the sport. Skill is also important in conditioning activities such as jogging, swimming, and cycling. Even if you learned a sport as a child, additional instruction now can help you refine your

anabolic steroids Synthetic male hormones used to increase **TERMS** muscle size and strength.

The exercises shown here work all the major joints of the body and have a minimum risk of injury. Perform each one on both sides of your body. Hold each stretch for 10–30 seconds; do at least 4 repetitions.

1. Head Turns and Tilts

Turn your head to the side, and hold the stretch. Tilt your head to the side, and hold the stretch.

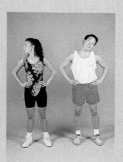

2. Towel Stretch

Roll up a towel and grasp it with both hands, palms down. With your arms straight, slowly lift it back over your head as far as possible. The closer together your hands are, the greater the stretch.

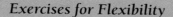

3. Across-the-Body Stretch

Keep your back straight, cross your left arm in front of your body, and grasp it with your right hand. Stretch your arm, shoulders, and back by gently pulling your arm as close to your body as possible.

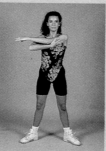

4. Upper Back Stretch

Stand with your feet shoulder-width apart, knees slightly bent, and pelvis tucked under. Clasp your hands in front of your body, and press your palms forward.

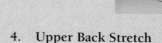
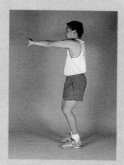

5. Lateral Stretch

Stand with your feet shoulder-width apart, knees slightly bent, and pelvis tucked under. Raise one arm over your head, and bend sideways from the waist. Support your trunk by placing the hand or forearm of your other arm on your thigh or hip for support. Be sure you bend directly sideways, and don't move your body below the waist.

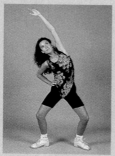

6. Step Stretch

Step forward and flex your forward knee, keeping your knee directly above your ankle. Stretch your other leg back so that it's parallel to the floor. Press your hips forward and down to stretch. Your arms can be at your sides, on top of your knee, or on the ground for balance.

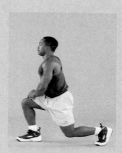

7. Side Lunge

Stand in a wide straddle, with your legs turned out from your hip joints and your hands on your thighs. Lunge to one side by bending one knee and keeping the other leg straight. Keep your knee directly over your ankle; do not bend it more than 90 degrees.

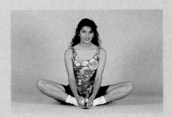

8. Sole Stretch

Sit with the soles of your feet together. Push your knees toward the floor using your hands or forearms.

9. Trunk Rotation

Sit with your right leg straight, left leg bent and crossed over the right knee, and left hand on the floor next to your left hip. Turn your trunk as far as possible to the left by pushing against your left leg with your right forearm or elbow. Keep your left foot on the floor.

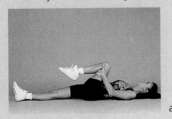

10. Modified Hurdler Stretch

Sit with your right leg straight and your left leg tucked close to your body. Reach toward your right foot as far as possible.

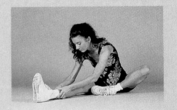

11. Alternate Leg Stretcher

Lie flat on your back with both legs straight. (a) Grasp your left leg behind the thigh, and pull in to your chest. (b) Hold this position, then extend your left leg toward the ceiling. (c) Hold this position, then bring your left knee back to your chest, and pull your toes toward your shin with your left hand. Stretch the back of the leg by attempting to straighten your knee.

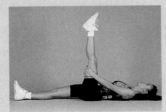

12. Lower Leg Stretch

Stand with one foot about 1–2 feet in front of the other, with both feet pointing forward. (a) Keeping your back leg straight, lunge forward by bending your front knee and pushing your rear heel backward. Hold this position. (b) Then pull your back foot in slightly, and bend your back knee. Shift your weight to your back leg and hold.

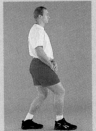

SOURCE: Fahey, T. D., P. M. Insel, and W. T. Roth. 1999. *Fit and Well: Core Concepts and Labs in Physical Fitness and Wellness*, 3rd ed. Mountain View, Calif.: Mayfield.

TABLE 13-3　*A Summary of Sports and Fitness Activities*

This table classifies sports and activities as high (H), moderate (M), or low (L) in terms of their ability to develop each of the five components of physical fitness: cardiorespiratory endurance (CRE), muscular strength (MS), muscular endurance (ME), flexibility (F), and body composition (BC). The skill level needed to obtain fitness benefits is noted: Low (L) means little or no skill is required to obtain fitness benefits; moderate (M) means average skill is needed to obtain fitness benefits; and high (H) means much skill is required to obtain fitness benefits. The fitness prerequisite, or conditioning needs of a beginner, is also noted: Low (L) means no fitness prerequisite is required, moderate (M) means some preconditioning is required, and high (H) means substantial fitness is required. The last two columns list the calorie cost of each activity when performed moderately and vigorously. To determine how many calories you burn, multiply the value in the appropriate column by your body weight and then by the number of minutes you exercise. Work up to using 300 or more calories per workout.

Sports and Activities	Components					Skill Level	Fitness Prerequisite	Approximate Calorie Cost (cal/lb/min)	
	CRE	MS*	ME*	F*	BC			Moderate	Vigorous
Aerobic dance	H	M	H	H	H	L	L	.046	.062
Backpacking	H	M	H	M	H	L	M	.032	.078
Badminton, skilled, singles	H	M	M	M	H	M	M	—	.071
Ballet (floor combinations)	M	M	H	H	M	M	L	—	.058
Ballroom dancing	M	L	M	L	M	M	L	.034	.049
Baseball (pitcher and catcher)	M	M	H	M	M	H	M	.039	—
Basketball, half court	H	M	H	M	H	M	M	.045	.071
Bicycling	H	M	H	M	H	M	L	.049	.071
Bowling	L	L	L	L	L	L	L	—	—
Calisthenic circuit training	H	M	H	M	H	L	L	—	.060
Canoeing and kayaking (flat water)	M	M	H	M	M	M	M	.045	—
Cheerleading	M	M	M	M	M	M	L	.033	.049
Fencing	M	M	H	H	M	M	L	.032	.078
Field hockey	H	M	H	M	H	M	M	.052	.078
Folk and square dancing	M	L	M	L	M	L	L	.039	.049
Football, touch	M	M	M	M	M	M	M	.049	.078
Frisbee, ultimate	H	M	H	M	H	M	M	.049	.078
Golf (riding cart)	L	L	L	M	L	L	L	—	—
Handball, skilled, singles	H	M	H	M	H	M	M	—	.078
Hiking	H	M	H	L	H	L	M	.051	.073
Hockey, ice and roller	H	M	H	M	H	M	M	.052	.078
Horseback riding	M	M	M	L	M	M	M	.052	.065
Interval circuit training	H	H	H	M	H	L	L	—	.062
Jogging and running	H	M	H	L	H	L	L	.060	.104

*Ratings are for the muscle groups involved.

technique, get over stumbling blocks, and relearn skills that you may have learned incorrectly.

Putting It All Together

Now that you know the basic components of a fitness program, you can put them all together in a program that works for you. Remember to include the following:

- *Cardiorespiratory endurance exercise:* Do at least 20 minutes of aerobic exercise at your target heart rate three to five times a week.

- *Muscular strength and endurance:* Work the major muscle groups (1 set of 8–10 exercises) two to three times a week.

- *Flexibility exercise:* Do stretches at least two to three times a week.

- *Skill training:* Incorporate some or all of your aerobic or strengthening exercise into an enjoyable sport or physical activity.

A summary of the fitness benefits of a variety of activities is provided in Table 13-3 to help you plan your program.

There are as many different adequate fitness programs as there are different individuals. Consider these examples:

Maggie is a person whose life revolves around sports. She's been on volleyball teams, softball teams, and swim

TABLE 13-3   A Summary of Sports and Fitness Activities

Sports and Activities	Components					Skill Level	Fitness Prerequisite	Approximate Calorie Cost (cal/lb/min)	
	CRE	MS*	ME*	F*	BC			Moderate	Vigorous
Judo	M	H	H	M	M	M	L	.049	.090
Karate	H	M	H	H	H	L	M	.049	.090
Lacrosse	H	M	H	M	H	H	M	.052	.078
Modern dance (moving combinations)	M	M	H	H	M	L	L	—	.058
Orienteering	H	M	H	L	H	L	M	.049	.078
Outdoor fitness trails	H	M	H	M	H	L	L	—	.060
Popular dancing	M	L	M	M	M	M	L	—	.049
Racquetball, skilled, singles	H	M	M	M	H	M	M	.049	.078
Rock climbing	M	H	H	H	M	H	M	.033	.033
Rope skipping	H	M	H	L	H	M	M	.071	.095
Rowing	H	H	H	H	H	L	L	.032	.097
Rugby	H	M	H	M	H	M	M	.052	.097
Sailing	L	L	M	L	L	M	L	—	—
Skating, ice, roller, and in-line	M	M	H	M	M	H	M	.049	.095
Skiing, alpine	M	H	H	M	M	H	M	.039	.078
Skiing, cross-country	H	M	H	M	H	M	M	.049	.104
Soccer	H	M	H	M	H	M	M	.052	.097
Squash, skilled, singles	H	M	M	M	H	M	M	.049	.078
Stretching	L	L	L	H	L	L	L	—	—
Surfing (including swimming)	M	M	M	M	M	H	M	—	.078
Swimming	H	M	H	M	H	M	L	.032	.088
Synchronized swimming	M	M	H	H	M	H	M	.032	.052
Table tennis	M	L	M	M	M	M	L	—	.045
Tennis, skilled, singles	H	M	M	M	H	M	M	—	.071
Volleyball	M	L	M	M	M	M	M	—	.065
Walking	H	L	M	L	H	L	L	.029	.048
Water polo	H	M	H	M	H	H	M	—	.078
Water skiing	M	M	H	M	M	H	M	.039	.055
Weight training	L	H	H	H	M	L	L	—	—
Wrestling	H	H	H	H	H	H	H	.065	.094
Yoga	L	L	M	H	L	H	L	—	—

*Ratings are for the muscle groups involved.

SOURCE: Kusinitz, I., and M. Fine. 1995. *Your Guide to Getting Fit,* 3rd ed. Mountain View, Calif.: Mayfield.

teams, and now she's on her college varsity soccer team. She follows a rigorous exercise regimen established by her soccer coach. Soccer practice is from four to six afternoons a week. It begins with warm-ups, drills, and practice in specific skills, and it ends with a scrimmage and then a jog around the soccer field. Games are every Saturday. Maggie likes team sports, but she also enjoys exercising alone, so she goes on long bicycle rides whenever she can fit them in. She can't imagine what it would be like not to be physically active every day.

Janine is a young mother of twins. Her life is so busy caring for them that she hardly has time to comb her hair, much less spend a lot of time exercising. To keep in shape, she joined a health club with a weight room, exercise classes, and child care. Every Monday, Wednesday, and Friday morning, she takes the twins to the club and attends the 7:00 "wake-up" low-impact aerobics class. The instructor leads the class through warm-ups; a 20-minute aerobic workout; exercises for the arms, abdomen, buttocks, and legs; stretches; and a relaxation exercise. Janine is exhilarated and ready for the rest of the day before 9:00 A.M.

Tom is an engineering student with a lot of studying to do and an active social life as well. For exercise, he plays tennis. He likes to head for the courts around 6:00 P.M., when most people are eating dinner. He warms up for 10 minutes by practicing his forehand and backhand against a backboard, and then plays a hard, fast game with his regular partner

CRITICAL CONSUMER   *Choosing Exercise Footwear*

Footwear is perhaps the most important item of equipment for almost any activity. Shoes protect and support your feet and improve your traction. When you jump or run, you place as much as six times more force on your feet than when you stand still. Shoes can help cushion against the stress that this additional force places on your lower legs, thereby preventing injuries. Some athletic shoes are also designed to help prevent ankle rollover, another common source of injury.

Shoe Terminology

Understanding the structural features of athletic shoes can help you make sound choices.

Outsole: The bottom of the shoe that touches the ground and provides traction. The shape and composition of an outsole depend on the activity for which the shoe is designed.

Insole: The insert or sock lining that the foot rests on inside the shoe, usually contoured to fit the foot and containing cushioning and arch and heel support.

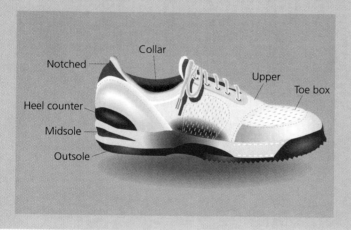

Midsole: The layer of shock-absorbing material located between the insole and the outsole; typically composed of polyurethane, ethyl vinyl acetate (EVA), rubber, or another cushioning material. For improved durability, some shoe midsoles include encapsulated air or gel.

Collar: The opening of the shoe where the foot goes in.

Upper: The top part of the shoe, usually made of nylon, canvas, or leather.

Toe box: The front part of the upper, which surrounds the toes.

Heel counter: The stiff cup in the back of the inside of the shoe that provides support and stability.

Notched heel: Some shoes have raised heel padding to support the Achilles tendon.

Stabilizers: Bars or strips of rubber, polyurethane, or nylon near the heel or forefoot area of some shoes; they provide additional stability.

Wedge: The thick portion of the midsole that makes the heel higher than the ball of the foot in some shoes.

General Guidelines

When choosing athletic shoes, first consider the activity you've chosen for your exercise program. Shoes appropriate for different activities have very different characteristics. For example, running shoes typically have highly cushioned midsoles, rubber outsoles with elevated heels, and a great deal of flexibility in the forefoot. The heels of walking shoes tend to be lower, less padded, and more beveled than those designed for running. For aerobic dance, shoes must be flexible in the forefoot and have straight, nonflared heels to allow for safe and easy lateral movements. Court shoes also provide substantial support for lateral movements; they typically have outsoles made from white rubber that will not damage court surfaces.

---

for 45 minutes to an hour. After he walks back to his room, he does some stretching exercises while his muscles are still warm. Then he showers and gets ready for dinner. Twice a week he works out at the gym, with particular attention to keeping his arms strong and his elbows limber. On Saturday nights, he goes dancing with his girlfriend.

Each of these people has worked an adequate or more-than-adequate fitness program into their busy daily routine. How can you find the time to include exercise in your life?

PERSONAL INSIGHT   In our society, boys and men tend to be more active in sports and physical activities than girls and women. Why do you think that is? How do you feel about it?

GETTING STARTED AND STAYING ON TRACK

Once you have a program that fulfills your basic fitness needs and suits your personal tastes, adhering to a few basic principles will help you improve at the fastest rate, have more fun, and minimize the risk of injury. These principles include buying appropriate equipment, eating and drinking properly, and managing your program so it becomes an integral part of your life.

Selecting Equipment and Facilities

When you're sure of the activities you're going to do, buy the best equipment you can afford. Good equipment will enhance your enjoyment and decrease your risk of injury. Appropriate safety equipment is particularly important.

Also consider the location and intensity of your workouts. If you plan to walk or run on trails, you should choose shoes with water-resistant, highly durable uppers and more outsole traction. If you work out intensely or have a relatively high body weight, you'll need thick, firm midsoles to avoid bottoming-out the cushioning system of your shoes.

Foot type is another important consideration. If your feet tend to roll inward excessively, you may need shoes with additional stability features on the inner side of the shoe to counteract this movement. If your feet tend to roll outward excessively, you may need highly flexible and cushioned shoes that promote foot motion. For aerobic dancers with feet that tend to roll inward or outward, mid-cut to high-cut shoes may be more appropriate than low-cut aerobic shoes or cross-trainers (shoes designed to be worn for several different activities). Compared with men, women have narrower feet overall and narrower heels relative to the forefoot. Most women will get a better fit if they choose shoes that are specifically designed for women's feet rather than those that are down-sized versions of men's shoes.

For successful shoe shopping, keep the following strategies in mind:

- Shop at an athletic shoe or specialty store that has personnel trained to fit athletic shoes and a large selection of styles and sizes.

- Shop late in the day or, ideally, following a workout. Your foot size increases over the course of the day and as a result of exercise.

- Wear socks like those you plan to wear during exercise. If you have an old pair of athletic shoes, bring them with you. The wear pattern on your old shoes can help you select a pair with extra support or cushioning in the places you need it the most.

- Ask for help. Trained salespeople know which shoes are designed for your foot type and your level of activity. They can also help fit your shoes properly.

- Don't insist on buying shoes in what you consider to be your typical shoe size. Sizes vary from shoe to shoe. In addition, foot sizes change over time, and many people have one foot that is larger or wider than the other. Try several sizes in several widths, if necessary. Don't buy shoes that are too small.

- Try on both shoes, and wear them around for 10 or more minutes. Try walking on a noncarpeted surface. Approximate the movements of your activity: walk, jog, run, jump, and so on.

- Check the fit and style carefully:

  Is the toe box roomy enough? Your toes will spread out when your foot hits the ground or you push off. There should be at least one thumb's width of space from the longest toe to the end of the toe box.

  Do the shoes have enough cushioning? Do your feet feel supported when you bounce up and down? Try bouncing on your toes and on your heels.

  Do your heels fit snugly into the shoe? Do they stay put when you walk, or do they rise up?

  Are the arches of your feet right on top of the shoes' arch supports?

  Do the shoes feel stable when you twist and turn on the balls of your feet? Try twisting from side to side while standing on one foot.

  Do you feel any pressure points?

- If the shoes are not comfortable in the store, don't buy them. Don't expect athletic shoes to stretch over time in order to fit your feet properly.

Before you invest in a new piece of equipment, investigate it. Is it worth the money? Does it produce the results its proponents claim for it? Is it safe? Does it fit properly, and is it in good working order? Does it provide a genuine workout? Will you really use it regularly? Ask the experts (coaches, physical educators, and sports instructors) for their opinion. Better yet, educate yourself. Every sport, from running to volleyball, has its own magazine. A little effort to educate yourself will be well rewarded. Footwear is probably the most important piece of equipment for almost any activity; refer to the box "Choosing Exercise Footwear" for shopping strategies.

Are you thinking of becoming a member of a health club or fitness center? Be sure to choose one that has the right programs and equipment available at the times you will use them. The facility should be clean and well-maintained, the staff well-trained and helpful. Ask for a short-term trial membership before committing to a long-term contract. Be wary of promotion gimmicks and high-pressure sales tactics. Find out whether the club belongs to the Association of Physical Fitness Centers or the International Racquet Sports Association. These trade associations have established standards to help protect consumer health, safety, and rights. Find a facility that you feel comfortable with and that meets your needs.

Eating and Drinking for Exercise

Most people do not need to change their eating habits when they begin a fitness program. Many athletes and other physically active people are lured into buying aggressively advertised vitamins, minerals, and protein supplements. But in almost every case, a well-balanced diet contains all the energy and nutrients needed to sustain an exercise program (see Chapter 12 for more information).

A balanced diet is also the key to improving your body composition when you begin to exercise more. One of the promises of a fitness program is a decrease in body fat and an increase in muscular body mass. As mentioned earlier, the control of body fat is determined by the balance of energy in the body. If more calories are consumed than are expended through metabolism and exercise, then fat increases. If the reverse is true, fat is lost. The best way to control body fat is to follow a diet containing adequate but not excessive calories and to exercise.

One of the most important principles to follow when exercising is to drink enough water. Your body depends on water to sustain many chemical reactions and to maintain correct body temperature. Sweating during exercise depletes the body's water supply and can lead to dehydration if fluids are not replaced. Serious dehydration can cause reduced blood volume, accelerated heart rate, elevated body temperature, muscle cramps, heat stroke, and other serious problems. Drinking water before and during exercise is important to prevent dehydration and enhance athletic performance.

Thirst alone is not a good indication of how much you need to drink, because thirst is quickly depressed by drinking even small amounts of water. Most of the weight lost immediately after exercise is from the loss of fluids. If you rely on thirst, it can take 24 hours or more to replace these fluids. Ideally, you should restore your body fluids before you exercise vigorously again. As a rule of thumb, try to drink about 8 ounces of water (more in hot weather) for every 30 minutes of heavy exercise. Bring a water bottle with you when you exercise so you can replace your fluids while they're being depleted. Water, preferably cold, and commercial sports drinks are the best fluid replacements. Sports drinks are good because they also supply energy and electrolytes, such as sodium and potassium. You don't need to take salt pills—your body is very efficient at sparing electrolytes during exercise.

Managing Your Fitness Program

How can you tell when you're in shape? When do you stop improving and start maintaining? How can you stay motivated? If your program is going to become an integral part of your life, and if the principles behind it are going to serve you well in the years ahead, these are very important questions.

Consistency: The Key to Physical Improvement
It is important to be able to recognize when you have achieved the level of fitness that is adequate for you. This level will vary, of course, depending on your goals, the intensity of your program, and your natural ability. Your body gets into shape by adapting to increasing levels of physical stress. If you don't push yourself by increasing the intensity of your workout—by adding weight or running a little faster or a little longer—no change will occur in your body.

But if you subject your body to overly severe stress, it will break down and become distressed, or injured. Overdoing exercise is just as bad as not exercising hard enough. No one can become fit overnight. Your body needs time to adapt to increasingly higher levels of stress. The process of improving fitness involves a countless number of stresses and adaptations. If you feel extremely sore and tired the day after exercising, then you have worked too hard. Injury will slow you down just as much as a missed workout.

Consistency is the key to getting into shape without injury. Steady fitness improvement comes when you overload your body consistently over a long period of time. The best way to ensure consistency is by keeping a training journal in which you record the details of your workouts: how far you ran, how much weight you lifted, how many laps you swam, and so on. This record will help you evaluate your progress and plan your workout sessions intelligently. Don't increase your exercise volume by more than 5–10% per week.

Assessing Your Fitness
When are you "in shape"? It depends. One person may be out of shape running a mile in 5 minutes; another may be in shape running a mile in 12 minutes. As mentioned earlier, your ultimate level of fitness depends on your goals, your program, and your natural ability. The important thing is to set goals that make sense for you.

If you are interested in finding out exactly how fit you are before you begin a program, the best approach is to get an assessment from a modern sports medicine laboratory. Such laboratories can be found in university physical education departments and medical centers. Here you will receive an accurate profile of your capacity to exercise. Typically, your endurance will be measured on a treadmill or bicycle, your body fat will be estimated, and your strength and flexibility will be tested. This evaluation will reveal whether your physical condition is consistent with good health, and the staff members at the laboratory can suggest an exercise program that will be appropriate for your level of fitness. To assess your own approximate level of cardiorespiratory endurance, take the test in the box "The 1.5-Mile Run-Walk Test."

Preventing and Managing Athletic Injuries
Although annoying, most injuries are neither serious nor permanent. However, an injury that is not cared for properly can escalate into a chronic problem. It is important to learn how to deal with injuries so they don't derail your fitness program.

Some injuries require medical attention. Consult a physician for head and eye injuries, possible ligament

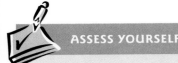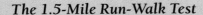
You can obtain a general rating of your cardiorespiratory fitness by taking the 1.5-mile run-walk test. Don't attempt this test unless you have completed at least 6 weeks of some type of conditioning activity. Also, if you are over age 35 or have questions about your health, check with your physician before taking this test.

You'll need a stopwatch, clock, or watch with a second hand, and a running track or course that is flat and provides measurements of up to 1.5 miles. You may want to practice pacing yourself prior to taking the test to avoid going too fast at the start and becoming fatigued before you finish. Allow yourself a day or two to recover from your practice run before taking the test.

Warm up before taking the test with some walking, easy jogging, and stretching exercises. The idea is to cover the distance as fast as possible, at a pace that is comfortable for you. You can run or walk the entire distance, or use some combination of running and walking. If possible, monitor your own pace, or have someone call out your time at various intervals to help you determine whether your pace is correct. When you have completed the test, refer to the table for your cardiorespiratory fitness rating. Be sure to cool down by walking or jogging slowly for about 5 minutes.

Standards for the 1.5-Mile Run-Walk Test (minutes:seconds)

	Superior	Excellent	Good	Fair	Poor	Very Poor
Women						
Age: 18–29	11:00 or less	11:15–12:45	13:00–14:15	14:30–15:45	16:00–17:30	17:45 or more
30–39	11:45 or less	12:00–13:30	13:45–15:15	15:30–16:30	16:45–18:45	19:00 or more
40–49	12:45 or less	13:00–14:30	14:45–16:30	16:45–18:30	18:45–20:45	21:00 or more
50–59	14:15 or less	14:30–16:30	16:45–18:30	18:45–20:30	20:45–23:00	23:15 or more
60 and over	14:00 or less	14:15–17:15	17:30–20:15	20:30–22:45	23:00–24:45	25:00 or more
Men						
Age: 18–29	9:15 or less	9:30–10:30	10:45–11:45	12:00–12:45	13:00–14:00	14:15 or more
30–39	9:45 or less	10:00–11:00	11:15–12:15	12:30–13:30	13:45–14:45	15:00 or more
40–49	10:00 or less	10:15–11:45	12:00–13:00	13:15–14:15	14:30–16:00	16:15 or more
50–59	10:45 or less	11:00–12:45	13:00–14:15	14:30–15:45	16:00–17:45	18:00 or more
60 and over	11:15 or less	11:30–13:45	14:00–15:45	16:00–17:45	18:00–20:45	21:00 or more

SOURCES: Formula for maximal oxygen consumption taken from McArdle, W. D., F. I. Katch, and V. L. Katch. 1991. *Exercise Physiology: Energy, Nutrition, and Human Performance.* Philadelphia: Lea & Febiger, pp. 225–226. Ratings based on norms from the Cooper Institute for Aerobics Research, Dallas, Texas. *The Physical Fitness Specialist Manual,* revised 1993. Used with permission.

injuries, broken bones, and internal disorders such as chest pain, fainting, and intolerance to heat. Also seek medical attention for apparently minor injuries that do not get better within a reasonable amount of time.

For minor cuts and scrapes, stop the bleeding and clean the wound with soap and water. Treat soft tissue injuries (muscles and joints) with the R-I-C-E principle: rest, ice, compression, elevation. Use ice for 48 hours after the injury or until all swelling is gone. (Because of the danger of frostbite, don't leave ice on one spot for more than 20 minutes at a time.) Elevate the affected part of the body above the level of the heart, and compress it with an elastic bandage to minimize swelling. Take care not to wrap the bandage too tightly; it can cut off circulation. Nonprescription medication that decreases inflammation, such as aspirin, ibuprofen, or naproxen sodium, is also helpful in treating soft tissue injuries.

Do not use heat on an injury initially because heat draws blood to the area and increases swelling. After the swelling has subsided (usually about 24–48 hours after the injury occurred), apply heat to speed up the healing process. Heat helps relieve pain, relax muscles, and reduce stiffness.

After a minor athletic injury, gradually reintroduce the stress of the activity until you are capable of returning to full intensity. Before returning to full exercise participation, you should have a full range of motion in your joints, normal strength and balance among your muscles, normal coordinated patterns of movement, with no injury-compensation movements, such as limping, and little or no pain.

To prevent injuries in the future, follow a few basic guidelines:

1. Stay in condition; haphazard exercise programs invite injury.

2. Warm up thoroughly before exercise.

3. Use proper body mechanics when lifting objects or executing sports skills.

4. Don't exercise when you're ill or overtrained (extreme fatigue due to overexercising).

5. Use the proper equipment.

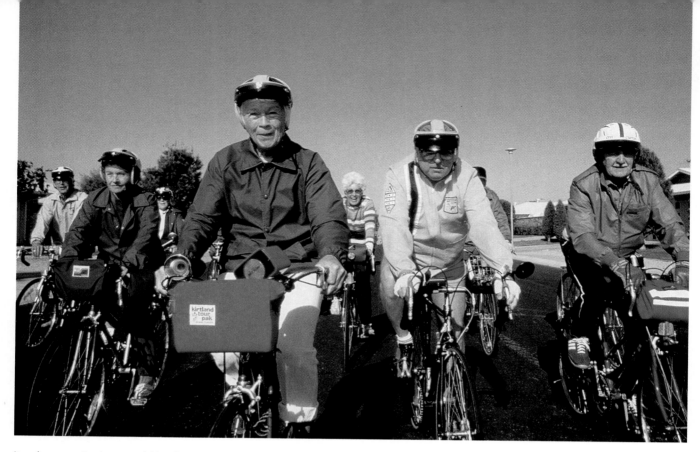

It makes sense to choose activities that will add enjoyment to your life for years to come. In this group of older people, we can see the rewards of a lifetime of fitness and smart exercise habits.

6. Don't return to your normal exercise program until athletic injuries have healed.

Professional athletes appear to recover quickly from their injuries because they treat them promptly and correctly. You can keep your fitness program on track by doing the same.

Staying with Your Program Once you have attained your desired level of fitness, you can maintain it by exercising regularly at a consistent intensity, three to five times a week. You must work at the intensity that brought you to your desired fitness level. If you don't, your body will become less fit because less is expected of it. In general, if you exercise at the same intensity over a long period, your fitness will level out and can be maintained easily.

What if you run out of steam? Although good health is an important *reason* to exercise, it's a poor *motivator* for consistent adherence to an exercise program. A variety of specific suggestions for staying with your program are given in the box "Maintaining Your Exercise Program" and in the Behavior Change Strategy at the end of the chapter. It's a good idea to have a meaningful goal, any-

thing from fitting into the same-size jeans you used to wear to successfully skiing down a new slope.

Varying your program is another key strategy. Some people alternate two or more activities—swimming and jogging, for example—to improve a particular component of fitness. The practice, called **cross-training**, can help prevent boredom and overuse injuries. Explore many exercise options. Consider competitive sports at the recreational level: swimming, running, racquetball, volleyball, golf, and so on. Find out how you can participate in an activity you've never done before: canoeing, hang gliding, windsurfing, backpacking. Try new activities, especially ones that you will be able to do for the rest of your life. Get maps of the recreational or wilderness areas near you, and go exploring. Fill a canteen, pack a good lunch, and take along a wildflower or bird book. Every step you take will bring you closer to your ultimate goal—fitness and wellness that last a lifetime.

PERSONAL INSIGHT Was exercise part of your family life when you were growing up? How much do your parents exercise? Do you think you're influenced by their attitudes and habits? How will you motivate your own children to exercise?

TERMS **cross-training** Participating in two or more activities to develop a particular component of fitness.

- *Set realistic goals.* Unrealistically high goals will only discourage you.

- *Sign a contract.* Also, keep records of your activities, and track your progress.

- *Start slowly, and increase your intensity and duration gradually.* Overzealous exercising can result in discouraging discomforts and injuries. Your program is meant to last a lifetime. The important first step is to break your established pattern of inactivity.

- *Make your program fun.* Participate in a variety of different activities that you enjoy. Vary the routes you take walking, running, or biking.

- *Exercise with a friend.* The social side of exercise is an important factor for many regular exercisers.

- *Focus on the positive.* Concentrate on the improvements you obtain from your program, how good you feel during and after exercise.

- *Revisit and revise.* If your program turns out to be unrealistic, revise it. Expect to make many adjustments in your program along the way.

- *Expect fluctuation.* On some days, your progress will be excellent, while on others, you'll barely be able to drag yourself through your scheduled activities.

- *Expect lapses.* Don't let them discourage you or make you feel guilty. Instead, feel a renewed commitment to your exercise program.

- *Reward yourself.* Give yourself frequent rewards for sticking with your program.

- *Renew your attitude.* If you notice you're slacking off, try to list the negative thoughts and behaviors that are causing noncompliance. Devise a strategy to decrease the frequency of negative thoughts and behaviors. Make changes in your program plan and reward system to help renew your enthusiasm and commitment.

- *Review your goals.* Visualize what it will be like to reach them, and keep these pictures in your mind as an incentive to stick to your program.

SOURCE: Fahey, T. D., P. M. Insel, and W. T. Roth. 1999. *Fit and Well: Core Concepts and Labs in Physical Fitness and Wellness,* 3rd ed. Mountain View, Calif.: Mayfield.

SUMMARY

What Is Physical Fitness?

- The five components of physical fitness most important to health are cardiorespiratory endurance, muscular strength, muscular endurance, flexibility, and body composition.

- Elements of fitness for a specific activity might include coordination, speed, reaction time, agility, balance, and skill.

The Benefits of Exercise

- Exercise improves the functioning of the heart and the ability of the cardiorespiratory system to carry oxygen to the body's tissues. A fit heart does not have to work as hard in daily life and can meet emergency needs.

- Exercise increases the efficiency of the body's metabolism and improves body composition.

- Exercise lowers the risk of cardiovascular disease by improving blood fat levels, reducing high blood pressure, and interfering with the disease process that causes coronary artery blockage.

- Exercise reduces the risk of cancer, osteoporosis, and diabetes. It improves immune function and helps prevent injuries and low-back pain.

- Exercise can improve psychological health by reducing stress, anxiety, and depression; enhancing self-image; and providing opportunities for enjoyable social interaction.

Designing Your Exercise Program

- Everyone should accumulate at least 30 minutes per day of moderate endurance-type physical activity. Additional health and fitness benefits can be achieved through longer or more vigorous activity.

- The body adapts to the demands of exercise by improving its functioning. The amount of overload is expressed in terms of frequency, intensity, and duration of exercise.

- Cardiorespiratory endurance exercises stress a large portion of the body's muscle mass. Endurance exercise should be performed 3–5 days per week for a total of 20–60 minutes per day. Intensity can be evaluated by measuring the heart rate.

- Warming up before exercising and cooling down afterward improve your performance and decrease your chances of injury.

- Exercises that develop muscular strength and endurance involve exerting force against a significant resistance. A strength training program for general fitness typically involves 1 set of 8–12 repetitions of 8–10 exercises, 2–3 days per week.

Although most people recognize the importance of incorporating exercise into their lives, many find it difficult to do. No single strategy will work for everyone, but the general steps outlined here should help you create an exercise program that fits your goals, preferences, and lifestyle. A carefully designed contract and program plan can help you convert your vague wishes into a detailed plan of action. And the strategies for program compliance outlined here and in Chapter 1 can help you enjoy and stick with your program for the rest of your life.

Step 1: Set Goals

Setting specific goals to accomplish by exercising is an important first step in a successful fitness program because it establishes the direction you want to take. Your goals might be specifically related to health, such as lowering your blood pressure and risk of heart disease, or they might relate to other aspects of your life, such as improving your tennis game or the fit of your clothes. If you can decide why you're starting to exercise, it can help you keep going.

Think carefully about your reasons for incorporating exercise into your life, and then fill in the goals portion of the Personal Fitness Contract.

Step 2: Select Activities

As discussed in the chapter, the success of your fitness program depends on the consistency of your involvement. Select activities that encourage your commitment: The right program will be its own incentive to continue; poor activity choices provide obstacles and can turn exercise into a chore.

When choosing activities for your fitness program, consider the following:

- Is this activity fun? Will it hold my interest over time?
- Will this activity help me reach the goals I have set?
- Will my current fitness and skill level enable me to participate fully in this activity?
- Can I easily fit this activity into my daily schedule? Are there any special requirements (facilities, partners, equipment, etc.) that I must plan for?
- Can I afford any special costs required for equipment or facilities?
- (If you have special exercise needs due to a particular health problem.) Does this activity conform to my special

health needs? Will it enhance my ability to cope with my specific health problem?

Refer to Table 13-3, which summarizes the fitness benefits and other characteristics of many activities. Using the guidelines listed above, select a number of sports and activities. Fill in the Program Plan portion of the Fitness Contract, using Table 13-3 to include the fitness components your choices will develop and the intensity, duration, and frequency standard you intend to meet for each activity. Does your program meet the criteria of a complete fitness program discussed in the chapter?

Step 3: Make a Commitment

Complete your Fitness Contract and Program Plan by signing your contract and having it witnessed and signed by someone who can help make you accountable for your progress. By completing a written contract, you will make a firm commitment and will be more likely to follow through until you meet your goals.

Step 4: Begin and Maintain Your Program

Start out slowly to allow your body time to adjust. Be realistic and patient—meeting your goals will take time. The following guidelines may help you to start and stick with your program:

- Set aside regular periods for exercise. Choose times that fit in best with your schedule, and stick to them. Allow an adequate amount of time for warm-up, cool-down, and a shower.
- Take advantage of any opportunity for exercise that presents itself (for example, walk to class, take the stairs instead of the elevator).
- Do what you can to avoid boredom. Do stretching exercises or jumping jacks to music, or watch the evening news while riding your stationary bicycle.
- Exercise with a group that shares your goals and general level of competence.
- Vary the program. Change your activities periodically. Alter your route or distance if biking or jogging. Change racquetball partners, or find a new volleyball court.
- Establish minigoals or a point system, and work rewards into your program. Until you reach your main goals, a system of self-rewards will help you stick with your program. Rewards should be things you enjoy and that are easily obtainable.

- A good stretching program includes exercises for all the major muscle groups and joints of the body. Do a series of active, static stretches (possibly with a passive assist) 2 or more days per week. Hold each stretch for 10–30 seconds; do at least 4 repetitions.
- Learning the skills required for specific sports or activities helps people achieve a sense of mastery and adds new activities to their exercise programs.

Getting Started and Staying on Track

- Equipment and facilities should be chosen carefully to enhance enjoyment and prevent injuries.
- A well-balanced diet contains all the energy and nutrients needed to sustain a fitness program. When exercising, it's important to remember to drink enough water.

Personal Fitness Contract

I, _____, am contracting with myself to follow an exercise program to work at the following goals.

Fitness Goals
(Note as many as appropriate)

1. _____
2. _____
3. _____
4. _____
5. _____

Program Plan

Activities	Components (Check ✔)					Intensity	Duration	Frequency (Check ✔)						
	CRE	MS	ME	F	BC			M	Tu	W	Th	F	Sa	Su
1. _____														
2. _____														
3. _____														
4. _____														
5. _____														

I will begin my program on _____.

I agree to maintain a record of my activity, assess my progress periodically, and, if necessary, revise my goals.

Signed _____ Date _____

Witness _____

Note: You should conduct activities for achieving CRE goals at your target heart rate.

Step 5: Record and Assess Your Progress

Keeping a record that notes the daily results of your program will help remind you of your ongoing commitment to your program and give you a sense of accomplishment. Create daily and weekly program logs that you can use to track your progress. Record the activity type, frequency, and duration. Keep your log handy, and fill it in immediately after each exercise session. Post it in a visible place to remind you of your activity schedule and provide incentive for improvement.

SOURCE: Adapted from Kusinitz, I., and M. Fine. 1995. *Your Guide to Getting Fit,* 3rd ed. Mountain View, Calif.: Mayfield.

- Subjecting the body to severe stress will cause injury. Consistency leads to steady improvement.
- The ultimate level of fitness depends on the goals, the program, and natural ability.
- Rest, ice, compression, and elevation (R-I-C-E) are the appropriate treatments for muscle and joint injuries. Heat can be used after swelling has subsided.
- A desired level of fitness can be maintained by exercising three to five times a week at a consistent intensity.
- Strategies for maintaining an exercise program over the long term include having meaningful goals, varying the program, and trying new activities.

1. Go to your school's physical education office and ask for a comprehensive listing of all the exercise and fitness facilities available on your campus. Visit the facilities you haven't yet seen, and investigate the activities that are done there. If there are sports or activities you'd like to try, consider doing so.

2. Investigate the fitness clubs in your community. How do they compare with each other? How do they measure up in terms of the guidelines provided in this chapter?

1. In your health journal, list the positive behaviors and attitudes that help you avoid a sedentary lifestyle and stay fit. How can you strengthen these behaviors and attitudes? Then list the negative behaviors and attitudes that block a physically active lifestyle. Which ones can you change? How can you change them?

2. Habit helps us conserve energy as we go through our daily lives, but it also blinds us to areas we could change. Make a list of ten ways you can incorporate more

physical activity into your life by changing a habit, such as walking instead of riding the bus, taking the stairs in a certain building instead of the elevator, and so on.

3. *Critical Thinking* Study the ads for fitness products and clubs on television, in popular magazines, and in your local newspaper. What markets are they targeting? How do they try to appeal to their audience? What other messages are they sending? Write a short essay describing your findings.

Books

American College of Sports Medicine. 1998. *ACSM Fitness Book,* 2nd ed. Champaign, Ill.: Human Kinetics. *A brief, easy-to-use guide to creating a successful fitness program.*

Fahey, T. 2000. *Basic Weight Training for Men and Women,* 4th ed. Mountain View, Calif.: Mayfield. *A practical guide to developing training programs tailored to individual needs.*

Fahey, T., P. Insel, and W. Roth. 1999. *Fit and Well: Core Concepts and Labs in Physical Fitness and Wellness,* 3rd ed. Mountain View, Calif.: Mayfield. *A comprehensive guide to developing a complete fitness program.*

Nieman, D. C. 1999. *Exercise Testing and Prescription: A Health-Related Approach,* 4th ed. Mountain View, Calif.: Mayfield. *A comprehensive discussion of the effects of exercise and exercise testing and prescription.*

U.S. Department of Health and Human Services. 1996. *Physical Activity and Health: A Report of the Surgeon General.* Atlanta, Ga.: Department of Health and Human Services. (Also available online: http://www.cdc.gov/nccdphp/sgr/sgr.htm) *Provides a summary of the evidence for the benefits of physical activity as well as recommendations for activity and exercise.*

Williams, M. H. 1998. *The Ergogenics Edge: Pushing the Limits of Sports Performance.* Champaign, Ill.: Human Kinetics. *An excellent review of the scientific basis of substances and techniques used to improve athletic performance.*

Organizations, Hotlines, and Web Sites

Aerobics and Fitness Association of America/Your Body. Provides information on exercise, including how to choose an instructor, class, or facility; how to begin a walking program; and how to maintain an exercise program while traveling.
  http://www.afaa.com/your_body/yourbody.html

American College of Sports Medicine. Provides brochures, publications, and audio- and videotapes on the positive effects of exercise.
  P.O. Box 1440
  Indianapolis, IN 46206
  317-637-9200
  http://www.acsm.org

American Council on Exercise. Promotes exercise and fitness for all Americans; the Web site features fact sheets on many consumer topics, including choosing shoes, cross-training, steroids, and getting started on an exercise program.
  5820 Oberlin Dr., Suite 102
  San Diego, CA 92121
  800-529-8227 (Consumer Fitness Hotline)
  http://www.acefitness.org

American Heart Association: Just Move. Provides practical advice for people of all fitness levels plus an online fitness diary.
  http://www.justmove.org

American Medical Association/Personal Trainer. Includes a fitness assessment and guidelines for creating a safe, effective program for developing the health-related components of fitness.
  http://www.ama-assn.org/insight/gen_hlth/trainer

Disabled Sports USA. Provides sport and recreation services to people with physical or mobility disorders.
  http://www.nas.com/~dsusa

Fitness Management Magazine's Fitness World. Includes current issues of the magazine, information about exercise books and videos, news highlights related to exercise, and answers to frequently asked questions.
  http://www.fitnessworld.com

Physical Activity and Health Network. Provides resources and links on the relationship between activity and health.

http://www.pitt.edu/~pahnet

Worldguide Health and Fitness Forum. Provides information on anatomy, cardiorespiratory endurance exercise, strength training, nutrition, and sports medicine.

http://www.worldguide.com/Fitness/hf.html

Information on many specific sports, activities, and fitness issues is available on the Web; use the following sites that provide many links or use a search engine to locate appropriate sites (see Appendix C).

FitnessLink

http://www.fitnesslink.com

Fitness Partner Connection Jumpsite

http://www.primusweb.com/fitnesspartner

Medicine and Sports Related Links

http://www.mspweb.com

NetSweat: The Internet's Fitness Resource

http://www.netsweat.com

Yahoo! Recreation and Sports

http://dir.yahoo.com/recreation/sports

See also the listings for Chapters 12, 14, and 15.

SELECTED BIBLIOGRAPHY

American College of Sports Medicine. 1998. ACSM position stand: The recommended quantity and quality of exercise for developing and maintaining cardiorespiratory and muscular fitness, and flexibility in healthy adults. *Medicine and Science in Sports and Exercise* 30(6): 975–991.

Andersen, R. E., et al. 1999. Effects of lifestyle activity vs. structured aerobic exercise in obese women. *Journal of the American Medical Association* 281: 335–340.

Artal, M. 1998. Exercise against depression. *Physician and Sportsmedicine* 26(10).

Brooks, G. A., T. D. Fahey, and T. P. White. 2000. *Exercise Physiology: Human Bioenergetics and its Applications,* 3rd ed. Mountain View, Calif.: Mayfield.

Centers for Disease Control and Prevention. 1997. Youth risk behavior surveillance: National College Health Risk Behavior Survey. *Morbidity and Mortality Weekly Report Surveillance Summary* 46(SS-6).

Cullinen, K., and M. Caldwell. 1998. Weight training increases fat-free mass and strength in untrained young women. *Journal of the American Dietetic Association* 98(4): 414–418.

Dengel, D. R., et al. 1998. The independent and combined effects of weight loss and aerobic exercise on blood pressure and oral glucose tolerance in older men. *American Journal of Hypertension* 11(12): 1405–1412.

DiLorenzo, T. M., et al. 1999. Long-term effects of aerobic exercise on psychological outcomes. *Preventive Medicine* 28(1): 75–85.

Dunn, A. L., et al. 1999. Comparison of lifestyle and structured interventions to increase physical activity and cardiorespiratory fitness. *Journal of the American Medical Association* 281: 327–334.

Erikssen, G., et al. 1998. Changes in physical fitness and changes in mortality. *Lancet* 352: 759–762.

Exercise Special Report: Workouts that work. 1999. *Consumer Reports,* February.

Fahey, T., P. Insel, and W. Roth. 1999. *Fit and Well: Core Concepts and Labs in Physical Fitness and Wellness,* 3rd ed. Mountain View, Calif.: Mayfield.

Feigenbaum, M. S., and M. L. Pollock. 1997. Strength training: Rationale for current guidelines for adult fitness programs. *Physician and Sportsmedicine* 25(2): 44–49.

Folsom, A. R., et al. 1997. Physical activity and incidence of coronary heart disease in middle-aged women and men. *Medicine and Science in Sports and Exercise* 29: 901–909.

Jetta, A. M., et al. 1999. Exercise—it's never too late: The strong-for-life program. *American Journal of Public Health* 89(1): 66–72.

Katz, W. A. 1998. Exercise for osteoporosis. *Physician and Sportsmedicine* 26(2).

Kushi, L. H., et al. 1997. Physical activity and mortality in postmenopausal women. *Journal of the American Medical Association* 277(16): 1287–1292.

Lee, I. M., and R. S. Paffenbarger. 1998. Physical activity and stroke incidence: The Harvard Alumni Health Study. *Stroke* 29: 2049–2054.

McMurray, R. G., et al. 1998. Is physical activity or aerobic power more influential on reducing cardiovascular disease risk factors? *Medicine and Science in Sports and Exercise* 30(10): 1521–1529.

National Institute on Drug Abuse. 1998. *NIDA Infofax: Anabolic Steroids* (retrieved November 30, 1998; http://www.nida.nih.gov/infofax/steroids.html).

Nieman, D. C. and B. K. Pedersen. 1999. Exercise and immune function. Recent developments. *Sports Medicine* 27(2): 73–80.

Nieman, D. C. 1999. *Exercise Testing and Prescription: A Health-Related Approach,* 4th ed. Mountain View, Calif.: Mayfield.

Nieman, D. C. 1998. The human body: Designed for action. *ACSM's Health and Fitness Journal* 2(3): 30–34.

Perna, F. M., et al. 1999. Cognitive-behavioral intervention effects on mood and cortisol during exercise training. *Annals of Behavioral Medicine* 20(2): 92–98.

Rippe, J. M., and S. Hess. 1998. The role of physical activity in the prevention and management of obesity. *Journal of the American Dietetic Association* 98(10 Suppl 2): S31–S38.

Shephard, R. J., and G. J. Balady. 1999. Exercise as cardiovascular therapy. *Circulation* 99(7): 963–972.

Stanford, B. 1998. Weight training basics. Part 1: Choosing the best options. *Physician and Sportsmedicine* 26(2).

Ten reasons why warming up is important. 1999. *ACSM's Health and Fitness Journal* 3(1): 52.

van Praag, H., G. Kempermann, and F. H. Gage. 1999. Running increases cell proliferation and neurogenesis in the adult mouse dentate gyrus. *Nature Neuroscience* 2(3): 266–270.

Villeneuve, P. J., et al. 1998. Physical activity, physical fitness, and risk of dying. *Epidemiology* 9(6): 626–631.

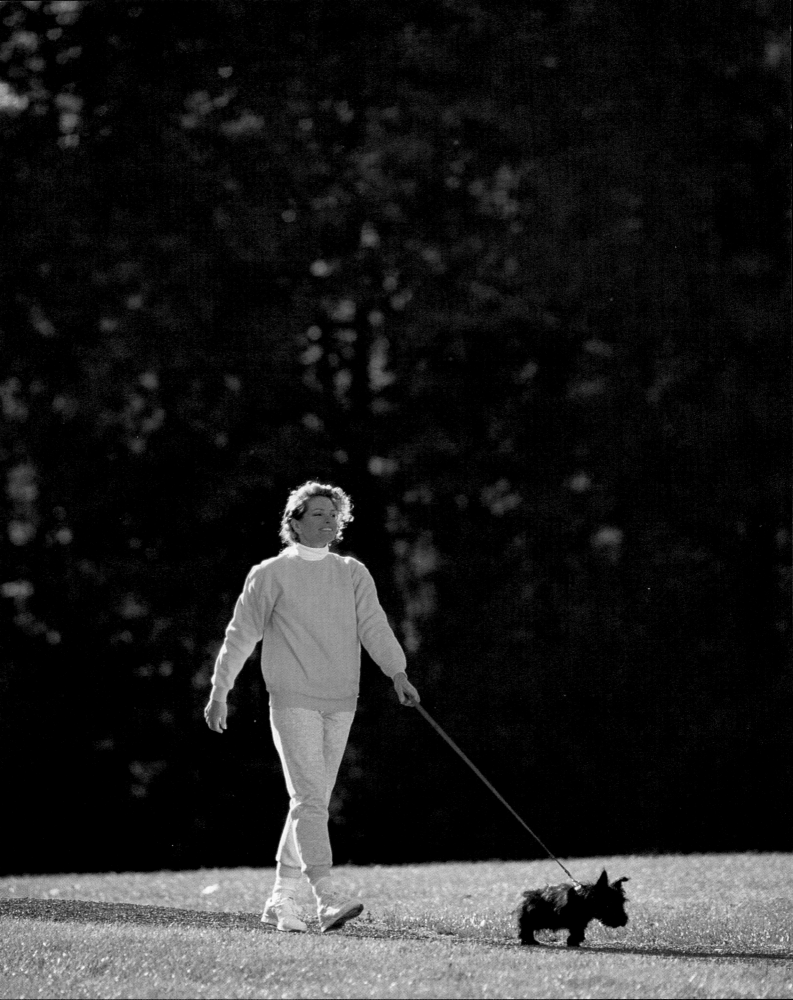

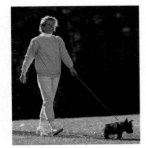

LEARNING OBJECTIVES

After reading this chapter, you should be able to:

- Explain the health risks associated with obesity.

- Discuss different methods for assessing body weight and body composition.

- Explain factors that may contribute to a weight problem, including genetic, environmental, and personal considerations.

- Describe lifestyle factors that contribute to weight gain and loss, including the role of diet, exercise, and emotional factors.

- Identify and describe the symptoms of eating disorders and the health risks associated with them.

- Design a personal plan for successfully managing body weight.

Weight Management

14

TEST YOUR KNOWLEDGE

1. Short-term restrictive diets are effective for long-term weight management.
   True or false?

2. About what percentage of participants in commercial weight-loss programs maintain a substantial proportion of their weight loss in the long term?
   a. 10%
   b. 20%
   c. 40%

3. The consumption of low-calorie sweeteners has helped Americans control their weight.
   True or false?

4. If Barbie were a full-size human being, her measurements would be
   a. 38-26-36
   b. 38-18-33
   c. 33-23-33

5. Approximately how many female high school and college students have either anorexia or bulimia?
   a. 1 in 250
   b. 1 in 100
   c. 1 in 30

Answers

1. *False.* The most effective strategies for long-term weight management are regular exercise and a moderate diet.

2. *a.* About 40% of participants actually gain back more than they lose during the program. Regular exercise is the strongest predictor of weight-loss maintenance.

3. *False.* Since the introduction of low-calorie sweeteners, both total calorie intake and total sugar intake have increased, as has the proportion of Americans who are overweight.

4. *b.* The measurements in answer c correspond to the average fashion model, who is 5 inches taller and 30 pounds lighter than the average American woman.

5. *c.* About 2–4% of female students suffer from bulimia or anorexia, and many more occasionally engage in behaviors associated with anorexia or bulimia.

Achieving and maintaining a healthy body weight is a serious public health challenge in the United States and a source of distress for many Americans. Millions struggle to lose weight, while others fall into dangerous eating patterns such as binge eating or self-starvation. At any given time, more than one-third of the American public is dieting. Research shows that many girls start dieting during adolescence, and the rate of dieting among female college students can reach 60% or more.

Despite widespread dieting, Americans are getting fatter. Under standards published by the National Institutes of Health in 1998, 55% of American adults are overweight; of these, 22% are obese (Table 14-1). Lifestyle changes are at the root of this increase. The Centers for Disease Control and Prevention estimates that while the fat intake of Americans (as a percentage of total calories) has declined during the past decade, total calorie intake has increased. People are also less active during the day. More are working in white-collar and service professions rather than jobs involving physical activity; increased access to home computers and cable television may also be contributing to a more sedentary lifestyle.

Although not completely understood, managing body weight is not a mysterious process. The "secret" is balancing calories consumed with calories expended in daily activities—in other words, eating a moderate, lowfat diet and exercising regularly. Unfortunately, this simple formula is not as exciting as the latest fad diet or "scientific breakthrough" that promises slimness without effort. The American public is assaulted year after year by a steady stream of diet books, dietary supplements, commercial weight-loss programs, and medical procedures for weight loss. Many people fail in their efforts to manage their weight because they emphasize short-term weight loss rather than permanent changes in lifestyle. Successful management of body weight requires the long-term coordination of many aspects of a wellness lifestyle, including proper nutrition, adequate physical activity, and stress management.

This chapter explores the factors that contribute to a weight problem, takes a closer look at weight management through lifestyle, and suggests specific strategies for permanent weight loss. This information is designed to provide the tools necessary for integrating effective weight management into a wellness lifestyle.

BASIC CONCEPTS OF WEIGHT MANAGEMENT

How many times have you or one of your friends said, "I'm too fat. I need to lose weight"? If you are like most people, you are concerned about what you weigh and whether or not you are too fat. But how do you decide if you are overweight? At what point does being overweight present a health risk? And just how much should you weigh?

Body Composition, Overweight, and Obesity

The human body can be divided into fat-free mass and body fat. Fat-free mass is all the body's nonfat tissues: bone, water, muscle, connective and organ tissues, and teeth. Body fat includes both essential and nonessential body fat. **Essential fat** includes lipids incorporated into the nerves and organs. These fat deposits, crucial for normal body functioning, make up about 3% of total body weight in men and 12% in women. (The larger percentage in women is due to fat deposits in the breasts, uterus, and other sites specific to females.) **Nonessential (storage) fat** exists primarily within fat cells, often located just below the skin and around major organs. The amount of storage fat varies from individual to individual based on many factors, including gender, age, heredity, metabolism, diet, and activity level. When we talk about wanting to "lose weight," most of us are referring to storage fat.

How much body fat should you have? In the past, many people relied on height-weight charts to answer this question. Based on insurance company statistics, these list a range of body weights associated with lowest mortality. People whose weight falls above the range recommended for their gender, age, and height are considered **overweight**. Although easy to use, height-weight charts can be highly inaccurate for some people, and they provide only an indirect measure of fatness. (Methods for assessing body weight and body composition are discussed later in this chapter.)

The most important consideration in looking at body composition is not total weight but the proportion of the body's total weight that is fat—the **percent body fat.** For example, two women may both be 5 feet, 5 inches tall and weigh 130 pounds. But one woman, an endurance runner, may have only 15% of her body mass as fat, while the second, sedentary woman could have 32% body fat. While neither woman is overweight by most standards, the second woman is overfat. Most sources agree that women should have 8–30% body fat, while men should have 5–20% body fat (Table 14-2). Since most people use the word "overweight" to describe the condition of

TERMS **essential fat** The fat in the body necessary for normal body functioning.

nonessential (storage) fat Extra fat or fat reserves stored in the body.

overweight Body weight that falls above the range associated with minimum mortality.

percent body fat The percentage of total body weight that is composed of fat.

obesity The condition of having an excess of nonessential body fat; weighing 20% or more over recommended weight, having a body mass index of 30 or greater, or having a percent body fat greater than 25% for men and 33% for women.

TABLE 14-1	The Prevalence of Obesity: Populations of Special Concern		
Group		Estimated Prevalence of Obesity*	Healthy People 2010 Target
Children (age 6–11)		11%	5%
Adolescents (age 12–19)		10	5
Adults (age 20–74)		22	15
Men		20	15
Women		25	15
Low-income people		26	15
Black women		37	15
Mexican American women		33	15

*Children and adolescents are classified as obese if they have a BMI at or above the appropriate 95th percentile for body mass index (BMI); adults are classified as obese if they have a BMI of 30 or above.

SOURCE: U.S. Department of Health and Human Services. 1998. *Healthy People 2010 Objectives: Draft for Public Comment.* Washington, D.C.: U.S. Government Printing Office.

TABLE 14-2	Percent Body Fat Classifications	
Percent Body Fat		
Males	Females	Classification
Less than 5%	Less than 8%	Excessively lean
5–11%	8–19%	Lean
12–20%	20–30%	Acceptable
21–25%	31–33%	Borderline obese
More than 25%	More than 33%	Obese

These represent approximate standards for body composition; the healthy range varies, depending on health status and risk factors for disease. For example, a man with high blood pressure and high cholesterol levels might want to reduce his percentage of body fat, even if it is within the acceptable range for the general population.

having too much body fat, we'll use it in this chapter, although "overfat" is actually a more accurate word.

Obesity is usually defined as excess storage fat beyond what is considered normal and healthy for a person's size, gender, age, and body type. Typically, obesity means being 20% or more over the desirable weight. According to this definition, a man is obese if his body fat exceeds 20% of his total body mass, and a woman is obese at over 30% body fat. On the flip side, levels of body fat below 8% for women and 5% for men can lead to health problems.

Energy Balance

The key to keeping a healthy ratio of fat to lean body mass is maintaining an energy balance (Figure 14-1, p. 376). You take in energy (calories) from the food you eat. Your body uses energy (calories) to maintain vital body functions (resting metabolism), to digest food, and to fuel physical activity. When energy in equals energy out, you maintain your current weight. To change your weight and body composition, you must tip the energy balance equation in a particular direction. If you take in more calories daily than your body burns, the excess calories will be stored as fat, and you will gain weight over time. If you eat fewer calories than you burn each day, you will lose some of that storage fat, and probably lose weight.

The two parts of the energy balance equation over which you have the most control are the energy you take in as food and the energy you burn during physical activity. To lose weight and body fat, you can increase the amount of energy you burn by increasing your level of physical activity and/or decrease the amount of energy you take in by consuming fewer calories. Specific strategies for altering energy balance are discussed later in the chapter.

Weight Management and Wellness

The amount of fat in the body—and its location—can have profound effects on health.

The Health Risks of Excess Body Fat   Obese people have an overall mortality rate almost twice that of non-obese people. They are more than three times as likely to develop diabetes (see the box "Diabetes" for more information). Obesity is associated with unhealthy cholesterol levels and impaired heart function. It is estimated that if all Americans had a healthy body composition, the incidence of coronary heart disease (CHD) would drop by 25%. Other health risks associated with obesity include hypertension, many kinds of cancer, impaired immune function, gallbladder and kidney diseases, and bone and joint disorders. These risks from obesity increase with its severity, and they are much more likely to occur in people who are more than twice their desirable body weight.

The effects of obesity on health were further clarified by the Nurses' Health Study, in which Harvard researchers have followed more than 120,000 women since 1976. It found that even mildly to moderately overweight women had an 80% increased risk of developing CHD compared to leaner women. This study also confirmed that to reduce the risk of dying prematurely of any cause, maintaining a desirable body weight is important.

The distribution of body fat is also an important indicator of future health. People who tend to gain weight in the abdominal area ("apples") have a risk of CHD, high

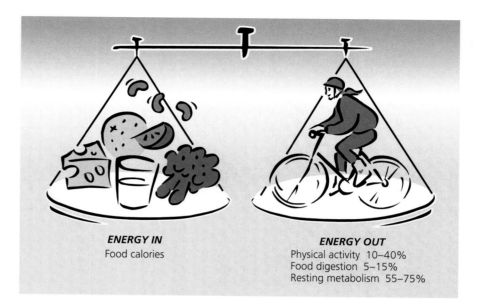

Figure 14-1 The energy balance equation. In order to maintain your current weight, you must burn up as many calories as you take in as food each day.

ENERGY IN
Food calories

ENERGY OUT
Physical activity 10–40%
Food digestion 5–15%
Resting metabolism 55–75%

blood pressure, diabetes, and stroke twice as high as those who tend to gain weight in the hip area ("pears"). The reason for this increased risk is not entirely clear, but it appears that fat in the abdomen is more easily mobilized and sent into the bloodstream, increasing disease-related blood fat levels.

In addition to risking physical health, obesity can impair psychological health. Being perceived as fat can be the source of ridicule, ostracism, and sometimes discrimination from others; it can contribute to psychological problems such as depression and low self-esteem. For some, the stigma associated with obesity can give rise to a negative body image, body dissatisfaction, and eating disorders (discussed later in the chapter).

Is It Possible to Be Too Lean? Health experts have generally viewed very low levels of body fat as a threat to wellness. Extremely lean people may experience muscle wasting and fatigue; they are also more likely to suffer from a dangerous eating disorder. For women, an extremely low percentage of body fat is associated with **amenorrhea,** the absence of menstruation, and a loss of bone mass.

Body Image The collective picture of the body as seen through the mind's eye, **body image** consists of perceptions, images, thoughts, attitudes, and emotions. A nega-

tive body image is characterized by dissatisfaction with the body in general or some part of the body in particular. Recent surveys indicate that more than 40% of Americans, many of whom are not actually overweight, are unhappy with their body weight or with some aspect of their appearance.

This dissatisfaction can cause significant psychological distress. A person can become preoccupied by a perceived defect in appearance, thereby damaging self-esteem and interfering with relationships. Adolescents and adults who have a negative body image are more likely to diet restrictively, eat compulsively, or develop some other form of disturbed eating. Losing weight does not necessarily improve body image. And even if it does, if the individual regains the weight, he or she will likely experience a return of body dissatisfaction and the accompanying psychological distress. On the other hand, improvements in body image may occur in the absence of weight loss. Many experts now believe that body image issues must be dealt with as part of treating obesity and eating disorders. See pp. 393–397 for more information on body image and eating disorders.

Wellness for Life A healthy body composition is vital for wellness throughout life. Strong scientific evidence suggests that controlling your weight will increase your life span; reduce your risk of heart disease, cancer, diabetes, and back and joint pain; increase your energy level; and improve your self-esteem.

TERMS **amenorrhea** The absence of menstruation.

body image The mental representation a person holds about his or her body at any given moment in time, consisting of perceptions, images, thoughts, attitudes, and emotions about the body.

PERSONAL INSIGHT What do you think when you see someone who is especially thin or heavy? Do you associate particular personality traits with different body types? Where do you think your ideas come from?

Diabetes mellitus is a disease that causes a disruption of normal metabolism. The pancreas, a long, thin organ located behind the stomach, normally secretes the hormone insulin, which stimulates cells to take up glucose to produce energy. In a person with diabetes, this process is disrupted, causing a buildup of glucose in the bloodstream. Over the long term, diabetes is associated with kidney failure, nerve damage, circulation problems, retinal damage and blindness, and increased rates of heart attack, stroke, and hypertension. The rate of diabetes has increased steadily over the past 40 years, and it is currently the seventh leading cause of death in the United States.

Types of Diabetes

Approximately 16 million Americans—nearly 6% of the population—have one of two major forms of diabetes. About 5–10% of people with diabetes have the more serious form, known as Type 1 diabetes. In this type of diabetes, the pancreas produces little or no insulin, so daily doses of insulin are required. (Without insulin, a person with Type 1 can lapse into a coma.) Type 1 diabetes usually strikes before age 30.

The remaining 15 million Americans with diabetes have Type 2 diabetes. This condition can develop slowly, and about half of affected individuals are unaware of their condition. In Type 2 diabetes, the pancreas doesn't produce enough insulin, the cells don't respond to the hormone, or both. This condition is usually diagnosed in people over age 40, although it is becoming more common at earlier ages. About one-third of people with Type 2 diabetes must take insulin; others may take medications that increase insulin production or stimulate cells to take up glucose.

A third type of diabetes occurs in about 2–3% of women during pregnancy. So-called *gestational diabetes* usually disappears after pregnancy, but more than half of women who experience it eventually develop Type 2 diabetes.

The major factors involved in the development of diabetes are age, obesity, physical inactivity, a family history of diabetes, and lifestyle. Excess body fat reduces cell sensitivity to insulin, and it is a major risk factor for Type 2 diabetes. Ethnic background also plays a role. African Americans and people of Hispanic background are 55% more likely than non-Hispanic whites to develop Type 2 diabetes; over 20% of Hispanics over age 65 have diabetes. Native Americans also have a higher-than-average incidence of diabetes.

Treatment

There is no cure for diabetes, but it can be successfully managed. Treatment involves keeping blood sugar levels within safe limits through diet, exercise, and, if necessary, medication. Blood sugar levels can be monitored using a home test. Recent research indicates that close monitoring and control of glucose levels can significantly reduce the rate of serious complications among people with diabetes. Nearly 90% of people with Type 2 diabetes are overweight when diagnosed, and an important step in treatment is to lose weight. Even a small amount of weight loss can be beneficial. People with diabetes should eat regular meals with an emphasis on complex carbohydrates and ample dietary fiber; a dietitian can help design a healthy eating plan. Regular exercise and a healthy diet are often sufficient to control Type 2 diabetes.

Prevention

Recent studies have shown that exercise can help prevent the development of Type 2 diabetes, a benefit especially important in individuals with one or more risk factors for the disease. Exercise burns excess sugar and makes cells more sensitive to insulin. Exercise also helps keep body fat at healthy levels.

Eating a healthy diet to help control body fat is perhaps the most important dietary recommendation for the prevention of diabetes. However, there is some evidence that the composition of the diet may also be important. In a long-term study of over 65,000 nurses, a diet low in fiber and high in sugar and refined carbohydrates was found to increase risk for Type 2 diabetes. The foods most closely linked to higher diabetes risk were regular (nondiet) cola beverages, white bread, white rice, french fries, and potatoes; consumption of cereal fibers such as those found in cold breakfast cereals was associated with lower risk. (See Chapter 12 for more information on different types of carbohydrates and specific strategies for increasing fiber intake.)

Warning Signs and Testing

A wellness lifestyle that includes a healthy diet and regular exercise is the best strategy for preventing diabetes. If you do develop diabetes, the best way to avoid complications is to recognize the symptoms and get early diagnosis and treatment. Be alert for the following warning signs:

- Frequent urination
- Extreme hunger or thirst
- Unexplained weight loss
- Extreme fatigue
- Blurred vision
- Frequent infections, especially of the bladder, gums, skin, or vagina
- Cuts and bruises that are slow to heal
- Tingling or numbness in the hands and feet
- Generalized itching, with no rash

Type 2 diabetes is often asymptomatic in the early stages, and major health organizations now recommend routine screening for people over age 45 and anyone younger who is at high risk, including anyone who is obese. (The Web site for the American Diabetes Association, listed in the For More Information section at the end of the chapter, includes an interactive diabetes risk assessment.) Screening involves a blood test to check glucose levels after either a period of fasting or the administration of a set dose of glucose. If you are concerned about your risk for diabetes, talk with your physician about being tested.

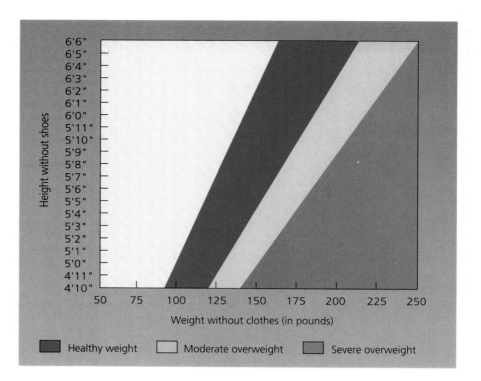

Figure 14-2 Suggested weights for adults. Weights are grouped in ranges because people of the same height may have equal amounts of body fat but different amounts of muscle and bone. The higher weights in each range apply to people with more muscle and bone, such as many men. Although weights are presented in ranges, gaining weight over time, even within the same range, is not healthy. SOURCE: Adapted from U.S. Department of Agriculture. Agricultural Research Service. Dietary Guidelines Committee. 1995. *Report of the Dietary Guidelines Advisory Committee on the Dietary Guidelines for Americans.* Springfield, Va.: National Technical Information Service, pp. 23–24.

Assessing Your Body Composition

Body weight, percent body fat, and the distribution of body fat can be measured and evaluated by a variety of means. The results of these assessments can help you determine whether you could improve your health by making changes in your body composition.

Assessing Body Weight Body weight is only an indirect indicator of body composition, but it is easy to measure.

HEIGHT-WEIGHT CHARTS The morning weighing ritual on the bathroom scale cannot reveal whether a fluctuation in weight is due to a change in muscle, body water, or fat and cannot differentiate between overweight and overfat. Despite these limitations, height and weight recommendations are published as part of the Dietary Guidelines for Americans (Figure 14-2).

BODY MASS INDEX Although also based on the concept that a person's weight should be proportional to height, **body mass index (BMI)** is a more accurate assessment method than height-weight charts. In 1998, new federal

BMI guidelines were released by the National Heart, Lung, and Blood Institute (NHLBI), a division of the National Institutes of Health. Under these guidelines, a person with a BMI of 25 or above is classified as overweight and a person with a BMI of 30 or above is considered obese. BMI is calculated by dividing your weight in kilograms by the square of your height in meters; a shortcut calculation method is given in the box "Calculate and Rate Your Body Mass Index (BMI)."

In classifying the health risks associated with overweight and obesity, the new NHLBI guidelines also consider body fat distribution (as indicated by waist circumference) and other disease risk factors. As described earlier, excess fat in the abdomen is of greater concern than excess fat in other areas. At a given level of overweight, people with a large waist circumference and/or additional disease risk factors are at greater risk for health problems. For example, a man with a BMI of 27, a waist circumference above 40 inches, and high blood pressure is at greater risk for health problems than another man who has a BMI of 27 but has a smaller waist and no other risk factors. Thus, optimal BMI for good health depends on many factors; if your BMI is 25 or above, consult a physician for help in determining a healthy BMI for you.

Determining Percent Body Fat There are several different methods for assessing body composition and determining percent body fat. Refer to Table 14-2 for body composition ratings based on percent body fat.

TERMS **body mass index (BMI)** A measure of relative body weight that takes height into account and is highly correlated with more direct measures of body fat; calculated by dividing total body weight (in kilograms) by the square of height (in meters).

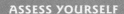
Calculate your BMI using the following formula:

$$BMI = \frac{703 \times \text{body weight (lb)}}{\text{height (in)}^2}$$

For example, if you are 5 feet, 6 inches tall (66 inches) and weigh 150 pounds, you would calculate your BMI as follows:

$$BMI = \frac{703 \times 150}{66 \times 66} = 24$$

Refer to the table below for the appropriate rating of your BMI. For additional information about the health risks associated with your BMI value, measure your waist. Take measurements at your smallest waist circumference or, if you don't have a natural waist, at the level of your navel. Find the disease risk rating that applies to your BMI and waist measurement in the table.

Body Mass Index (BMI) Classifications

Classification	BMI (kg/m^2)	Obesity Class	Disease Risk Relative to Normal Weight and Waist Circumference[a]	
			Men ≤40 in (102 cm) Women ≤35 in (88 cm)	>40 in (102 cm) >35 in (88 cm)
Underweight[b]	Less than 18.5		—	—
Normal[c]	18.5–24.9		—	—
Overweight	25.0–29.9		Increased	High
Obesity	30.0–34.9	I	High	Very high
	35.0–39.9	II	Very high	Very high
Extreme obesity	40.0 and higher	III	Extremely high	Extremely high

[a]Disease risk for type 2 diabetes, hypertension, and cardiovascular disease. The waist circumference cutoff points for increased risk are 40 inches (102 cm) for men and 35 inches (88 cm) for women.
[b]Research suggests that a low BMI can be healthy in some cases, as long as it is not the result of smoking, an eating disorder, or an underlying disease process.
[c]Increased waist circumference can also be a marker for increased risk even in persons of normal weight.

SOURCE: Adapted from National Heart, Lung, and Blood Institute. 1998. *Clinical Guidelines on the Identification, Evaluation, and Treatment of Overweight and Obesity in Adults: The Evidence Report.* Bethesda, Md.: National Institutes of Health.

HYDROSTATIC (UNDERWATER) WEIGHING   One of the most accurate techniques is hydrostatic weighing. In this method, a person is submerged and weighed under water. Percent body fat can be calculated from body density. Muscle has a higher density and fat a lower density than water, so people with more fat tend to float and weigh less under water, while lean people tend to sink and weigh relatively more under water.

SKINFOLD MEASUREMENTS   The skinfold thickness technique measures the thickness of fat under the skin. A technician grasps a fold of skin at a predetermined location and measures it using an instrument called a caliper. Measurements are taken at several sites and plugged into formulas that predict body fat percentages.

ELECTRICAL IMPEDANCE ANALYSIS   In this method, electrodes are attached to the body and a harmless electrical current is transmitted from electrode to electrode. The electrical conduction through the body favors the path of the fat-free tissues over the fat tissues. A computer can calculate fat percentages from current measurements.

SCANNING PROCEDURES   High-tech scanning procedures are highly accurate means of assessing body composition, but they require expensive equipment. These procedures include computed tomography (CT), magnetic resonance imaging (MRI), dual-energy X ray absorptiometry, and dual-photon absorptiometry.

Assessing Fat Distribution   Two simple methods of assessing body fat distribution are waist measurement and waist-to-hip ratio calculation. In the first method, you measure your waist circumference; in the second, you divide your waist measurement by your hip measurement. Waist measurements over 40 inches (102 cm) for men and 35 inches (88 cm) for women and waist-to-hip ratios above 0.94 for men and 0.82 for women are associated with a significantly increased risk of disease.

What Is the Right Weight for You?

For most of us, our body weight and percentage of body fat fall somewhere below the levels associated with significant health risks. For us, these assessment tests do not

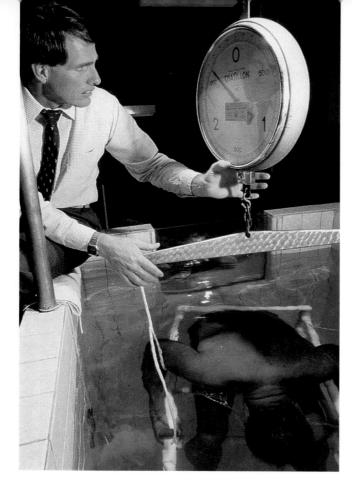

This man is being submerged as part of a hydrostatic weighing procedure, one of several methods for measuring the percentage of body weight that is fat. A very high or very low percentage of body fat is associated with health problems.

really answer the question: How much should I weigh? Height-weight charts, body composition analyses, and BMI and waist-to-hip ratio measurements can best serve as general guides or estimates for body weight. They cannot account for individual genetic or ethnic differences that cause variations from "average" population weights but that may still be healthy.

Perhaps it's time for a radical idea: To answer the question of what you "should" weigh, let your lifestyle be your guide. Don't focus on a particular weight as your goal. Instead, focus on living a lifestyle that includes eating moderate amounts of healthful foods, getting plenty of exercise, thinking positively, and learning to cope with stress. Then let the pounds fall where they may. For most people, the result will be close to the recommended weight ranges discussed earlier. For some, their weight will be somewhat higher than societal standards—but right for them. By letting a healthy lifestyle determine your weight, you can avoid developing unhealthy patterns of eating and a negative body image.

FACTORS CONTRIBUTING TO WEIGHT PROBLEMS

Although the picture is far from complete, we know that physical factors, as well as psychological, cultural, and social factors, play a significant role in determining body weight. In particular, heredity and metabolism have been linked to a tendency toward obesity.

Genetic Factors Versus Environmental Factors

Both genetic and environmental factors influence the development of obesity. Genes influence body size and shape, body fat distribution, and metabolic rate. Genetic factors also affect the ease with which weight is gained as a result of overeating and where on the body extra weight is added. If both parents are overweight, their children are twice as likely to be overweight as children who have only one overweight parent. In studies that compared adoptees and their biological parents, the weights of the adoptees were found to be more like those of the biological parents than the adoptive parents, again indicating a strong genetic link.

In studies of mice, scientists located a gene (named *ob*) that appears to influence appetite and the development of obesity. The gene produces a hormonelike protein called leptin that is secreted by the body's fat cells and carried to the brain. Leptin seems to let the brain know how big or small the body's fat stores are, and the brain can regulate appetite and metabolic rate accordingly. Mice with a defective or missing *ob* gene overate and gained weight. But when injected with leptin, the obese mice ate less, had higher metabolic rates, and lost weight. Even mice of normal weight lost weight when injected with leptin.

Could leptin "cure" obesity in humans? As encouraging as this finding is, obesity in humans is likely to turn out to be more complicated than a one-gene phenomenon. Many obese people have been found to have normal or higher-than-normal levels of leptin in their bloodstream; researchers hypothesize that they may have faulty leptin receptors in their brains. Other recently identified chemicals that may also be significant in controlling appetite include orexin, cortisol, gluconlike peptide-1 (GLP-1), neuropeptide Y (NPY), and peptide YY. However, additional studies will be needed before a treatment can be developed based on any of these findings.

All this research points to a genetic component in the determination of body weight. However, hereditary influences must be balanced against the contribution of environmental factors. Not all children of obese parents become obese, and normal-weight parents also have overweight children. The incidence of obesity is rising in the United States, but not in all parts of the world. In a study comparing men born and raised in Ireland with their biological brothers who lived in the United States, the American men were found to weigh, on average, 6% more than their Irish brothers. Environmental factors like diet and exercise are probably responsible for this difference in weight. Thus, the *tendency* to develop obesity may be inherited, but the expression of this tendency is affected by environmental influences.

The message you should take from this research is that genes are not destiny. It is true that some people have a harder time losing weight and maintaining weight loss than others. However, with increased exercise and attention to diet, even those with a genetic tendency toward obesity can maintain a healthy body weight. And regardless of genetic factors, lifestyle choices remain the cornerstone of successful weight management.

Metabolism and Energy Balance

Metabolism is the sum of all the vital processes by which food energy and nutrients are made available to and used by the body. The largest component of metabolism, **resting metabolic rate (RMR),** is the energy required to maintain vital body functions, including respiration, heart rate, body temperature, and blood pressure, while the body is at rest. As shown in Figure 14-1, RMR accounts for 55–75% of daily energy expenditure. The energy required to digest food accounts for an additional 5–15% of daily energy expenditure. The remaining 10–40% is expended during physical activity.

Both heredity and behavior affect metabolic rate. Men, who have a higher proportion of muscle mass than women, have a higher RMR (muscle tissue is more metabolically active than fat). Also, some individuals inherit a higher or lower RMR than others. A higher RMR means that a person burns more calories while at rest and can therefore take in more calories without gaining weight.

Weight loss or gain also affects metabolic rate. When a person loses weight, both RMR and the energy required to perform physical tasks decrease. The body thus "defends" its original weight by conserving energy and making it easier to regain lost pounds. For example, a man who formerly weighed 165 pounds but who now weighs 150 pounds must eat about 15% fewer calories to maintain his new, lower weight than a man who has weighed 150 pounds throughout his adult life. The reverse occurs when weight is gained; RMR increases, pushing weight back down toward its original level. The message from this research is that although weight loss can be achieved and maintained, it requires ongoing commitment.

Exercise has a positive effect on metabolism. When people exercise, they increase their RMR—the number of calories their bodies burn at rest. They also increase their muscle mass, which is associated with a higher metabolic rate. The exercise itself also burns calories, raising total energy expenditure. The higher the energy expenditure, the more the person can eat without gaining weight. (The role of exercise in weight management is discussed in greater detail later in the chapter.)

The Fat Cell Theory

According to the fat cell theory, the quantity of fat stored in the body is the result of the number and size of fat cells in the body. People who have an above-average number of fat cells or particularly large fat cells may have been born with them or may have developed them at certain critical times because of overeating. As the theory goes, having more or larger fat cells creates a biological pressure to keep these cells full. It is unclear whether the number of fat cells can be decreased if weight is kept off for an extended period. More research is needed to determine the relevance of the fat cell theory to the development and maintenance of obesity in humans.

Weight Cycling

It has been hypothesized that repeated dieting resulting in cycles of weight loss and weight gain ("yo-yo dieting") is harmful both to weight management and to overall health. Researchers proposed that cycling increases the body's efficiency at extracting and storing calories from food, making weight loss increasingly difficult with each successive diet. Although some studies have found support for this idea, most have not; and current thinking is that weight cycling probably does not result in increased efficiency. Concerns have also been raised that weight cycling may alter body fat distribution, increase the preference for dietary fat, raise the risk of gallbladder disease and death from CVD, and lead to disordered patterns of eating. Again, however, research results have been mixed. More studies are needed to clarify the relationship between weight cycling, weight management, and disease mortality. On balance, when the substantial health benefits of even modest weight loss are compared with the uncertain potential adverse health consequences of losing weight or weight cycling, the benefits of losing weight clearly exceed the potential risks.

The Restrained Eating Theory

According to the restrained eating theory, restrictive dieting can cause excessive hunger and feelings of deprivation, possibly leading to binge eating. Attempts to restrain food intake may contribute to confusion about internal hunger cues and increase susceptibility to external cues (the sight of food, for example). As hunger or fatigue

resting metabolic rate (RMR) The energy required to maintain vital body functions, including respiration, heart rate, body temperature, and blood pressure, while the body is at rest. **TERMS**

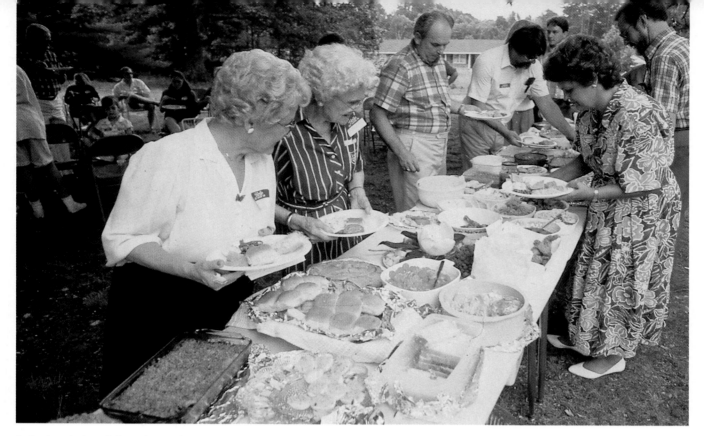

Eating is so intimately bound up with the social fabric of life that people trying to change their diets often meet unexpected obstacles and difficulties. High-fat foods are an integral part of this family reunion, not easily avoided even by those very concerned with their fat intake.

increases, or if confronted with cues in the environment, a person's restraint may falter. For many restrained eaters, once they violate their self-imposed diet rules, they simply give up and overeat or even binge. This overeating is usually followed by feelings of guilt, shame, and self-blame. Binge eating may contribute to the development of obesity in some people.

Although restrictive dieting can trigger inappropriate eating, binge eating is not always caused by dieting. Other triggers include particular emotions, situations, or physical states. To learn more about your eating habits, take the quiz in the box "What Triggers Your Eating?"

Psychological, Social, and Cultural Factors

Many people have learned to use food as a means of coping with stress and negative emotions. Eating can provide a powerful distraction from difficult feelings—loneliness, anger, boredom, anxiety, shame, sadness, inadequacy. It can be used to combat low moods, low energy levels, and low self-esteem. When food and eating become the primary means of regulating emotions, binge eating or other disturbed eating patterns can develop.

Obesity is strongly associated with socioeconomic status. The prevalence of obesity goes down as income level goes up. More women are obese at lower income levels than men, but men are somewhat more obese at higher levels. These differences may reflect the greater sensitivity and concern for a slim physical appearance among upper-income women, as well as greater access to information about nutrition and to lowfat and low-calorie foods. It may also reflect the greater acceptance of obesity among certain ethnic groups, as well as different cultural values related to food choices.

In some families and cultures, food is used as a symbol of love and caring. It is an integral part of social gatherings and celebrations. In such cases, it may be difficult to change established eating patterns because they are linked to cultural and family values.

ADOPTING A HEALTHY LIFESTYLE FOR SUCCESSFUL WEIGHT MANAGEMENT

When all the research has been assessed, it is clear that most weight problems are lifestyle problems. Even though more and more young people are developing weight problems, most arrive at early adulthood with the advantage of having a "normal" body weight—neither too fat nor too thin. In fact, many young adults get away with terrible eating and exercise habits and don't develop a weight problem. But as the rapid growth of adolescence

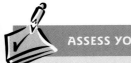

Hunger isn't the only reason people eat. Efforts to maintain a healthy body weight can be sabotaged by eating related to other factors, including emotions, environment, and patterns of thinking. This quiz is designed to provide you with a score for five factors that describe many people's eating habits. This information will put you in a better position to manage your eating behavior and control your weight. Circle the number that indicates to what degree each situation is likely to make you start eating.

	Very Unlikely								Very Likely	

Social

1. Arguing or having a conflict with someone. 1 2 3 4 5 6 7 8 9 10
2. Being with others when they are eating. 1 2 3 4 5 6 7 8 9 10
3. Being urged to eat by someone else. 1 2 3 4 5 6 7 8 9 10
4. Feeling inadequate around others. 1 2 3 4 5 6 7 8 9 10

Emotional

5. Feeling bad, such as being anxious or depressed. 1 2 3 4 5 6 7 8 9 10
6. Feeling good, happy, or relaxed. 1 2 3 4 5 6 7 8 9 10
7. Feeling bored or having time on my hands. 1 2 3 4 5 6 7 8 9 10
8. Feeling stressed or excited. 1 2 3 4 5 6 7 8 9 10

Situational

9. Seeing an advertisement for food or eating. 1 2 3 4 5 6 7 8 9 10
10. Passing by a bakery, cookie shop, or other enticement to eat. 1 2 3 4 5 6 7 8 9 10
11. Being involved in a party, celebration, or special occasion. 1 2 3 4 5 6 7 8 9 10
12. Eating out. 1 2 3 4 5 6 7 8 9 10

Thinking

13. Making excuses to myself about why it's OK to eat. 1 2 3 4 5 6 7 8 9 10
14. Berating myself for being fat or unable to control my eating. 1 2 3 4 5 6 7 8 9 10
15. Worrying about others or about difficulties I'm having. 1 2 3 4 5 6 7 8 9 10
16. Thinking about how things should or shouldn't be. 1 2 3 4 5 6 7 8 9 10

Physiological

17. Experiencing pain or physical discomfort. 1 2 3 4 5 6 7 8 9 10
18. Experiencing trembling, headache, or light-headedness associated with no eating or too much caffeine. 1 2 3 4 5 6 7 8 9 10
19. Experiencing fatigue or feeling overtired. 1 2 3 4 5 6 7 8 9 10
20. Experiencing hunger pangs or urges to eat, even though I've eaten recently. 1 2 3 4 5 6 7 8 9 10

Scoring

Total your scores for each category, and enter them below. Then rank the scores by marking the highest score 1, next highest score 2, and so on. Focus on the highest-ranked categories first, but any score above 24 is high and indicates that you need to work on that category.

Category	Total Score	Rank Order
Social (Items 1–4)	_____	_____
Emotional (Items 5–8)	_____	_____
Situational (Items 9–12)	_____	_____
Thinking (Items 13–16)	_____	_____
Physiological (Items 17–20)	_____	_____

What Your Score Means

Social   A high score here means you are very susceptible to the influence of others. Work on better ways to communicate more assertively, handle conflict, and manage anger. Challenge your beliefs about the need to be polite and the obligations you feel you must fulfill.

Emotional   A high score here means you need to develop effective ways to cope with emotions. Work on developing skills in stress management, time management, and communication. Practicing positive but realistic self-talk can help you handle small daily upsets.

Situational   A high score here means you are especially susceptible to external influences. Try to avoid external cues and respond differently to those you cannot avoid. Control your environment by changing the way you buy, store, cook, and serve food. Anticipate potential problems, and have a plan for handling them.

Thinking   A high score here means that the way you think—how you talk to yourself, the beliefs you hold, your memories, and your expectations—have a powerful influence on your eating habits. Try to be less self-critical, less perfectionistic, and more flexible in your ideas about the way things ought to be. Recognize when you're making excuses or rationalizations that allow you to eat.

Physiological   A high score here means that the way you eat, what you eat, or medications you are taking may be affecting your eating behavior. You may be eating to reduce physical arousal or deal with physical discomfort. Try eating three meals a day, supplemented with regular snacks if needed. Avoid too much caffeine. If any medication you're taking produces adverse physical reactions, switch to an alternative, if possible. If your medications may be affecting your hormone levels, discuss possible alternatives with your physician.

SOURCE: Adapted from Nash, J. D. 1997. *The New Maximize Your Body Potential.* Palo Alto, Calif.: Bull Publishing. Reprinted with permission from Bull Publishing Company.

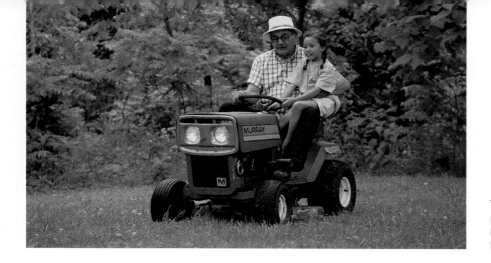

The typical American lifestyle does not lead naturally to healthy weight management. Labor-saving devices such as lawn mowers help reinforce our sedentary habits.

slows and family and career obligations increase, maintaining a healthy weight becomes a greater challenge. A good time to develop a lifestyle for successful weight management is during early adulthood, when healthy behavior patterns have a better chance of taking a firm hold.

Permanent weight loss is not something you start and stop. You need to adopt healthy behaviors that you can maintain throughout your life. Lifestyle factors that are critical for successful long-term weight management include eating habits, level of physical activity, an ability to think positively and manage your emotions effectively, and the coping strategies you use to deal with the stresses and challenges in your life.

Diet and Eating Habits

In contrast to "dieting," which involves some form of food restriction, "diet" refers to your daily food choices. Everyone has a diet, but not everyone is dieting. You need to develop a diet that you enjoy and that enables you to maintain a healthy body composition.

Total Calories   To maintain your current weight, the total number of calories you eat must equal the number you burn (refer to the energy balance equation in Figure 14-1). To lose weight, you must decrease your calorie intake and/or increase the number of calories you burn. According to the CDC, the average calorie intake by Americans has increased by 100–300 calories per day over the past decade. Levels of physical activity did not increase during this period, so the net result was a substantial increase in the number of Americans who are obese. To calculate your daily calorie needs, complete the calculations in the box "How Many Calories Do You Need?"

The best approach for weight loss is probably combining an increase in physical activity with moderate calorie restriction. Don't go on a "crash diet." You need to consume enough food to meet your need for essential nutrients. Also, to maintain weight loss, you will probably have to maintain some degree of the calorie restriction you used to lose the weight. Therefore, it is important that

you adopt a level of food intake that you can live with over the long term.

Portion Sizes   Overconsumption of total calories is closely tied with portion sizes. Most of us significantly underestimate the amount of food we eat. Limiting portion sizes to those recommended in the Food Guide Pyramid is critical for weight management. For many people, concentrating on portion sizes is also a much easier method of monitoring and managing total food intake than counting calories. (Refer to Chapter 12 for more on appropriate portion sizes.)

Fat Calories   Although some fat is needed in the diet to provide essential nutrients, you should avoid overeating fatty foods. There is some evidence that fat calories are more easily converted to body fat than calories from protein or carbohydrate. Limiting fat in the diet can also help you limit your total calories. As described in Chapter 12, fat should supply no more than 30% of your average total daily calories, which translates into no more than 66 grams of fat in a 2000-calorie diet each day. Foods rich in fat include oils, margarine, butter, cream, and lard, which are almost pure fat; meat and processed foods, which contain a great deal of "hidden" fat; and nuts, seeds, and avocados, which are plant sources of fats.

Some people are better fat burners than others; that is, they burn more of the fat they take in as calories and therefore have less fat to store. Low fat burners convert more dietary fat to stored body fat. This tendency to hoard fat calories may be an important part of the genetic tendency toward obesity. For low fat burners, restricting fat calories to a level even below 30% may be helpful in weight management.

As Chapter 12 made clear, moving toward a diet strong in complex carbohydrates and fresh fruits and vegetables, and away from a reliance on meat and processed foods, is an effective approach to reducing fat consumption. Watch out for processed foods labeled "fat-free" or "reduced fat," as they may be high in calories (see the box "Evaluating Fat and Sugar Substitutes" on p. 386). In addition,

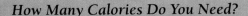

Use the following steps to estimate your total daily energy needs.

1. Add a zero to the end of your present weight.

2. If you are a woman, add your weight again to that number to get your estimated resting metabolic rate (RMR). If you are a man, add twice your weight to the number from step 1.

3. Multiply the number obtained in step 2 by 30% (0.3) to obtain an estimate of the calories you need for your daily activities.

4. Add your RMR value from step 2 and your daily activity number from step 3 to obtain an estimate of the number of calories you need to maintain your current weight.

Example: A woman who weighs 140 pounds.

1. 140, add a 0 = 1400

2. 1400 + 140 = 1540 calories for RMR.

3. 1540 × 30% = 462 calories for daily activities.

4. 1540 + 462 = 2002 calories to maintain current weight.

To estimate the number of calories you would need to maintain a lower weight, repeat the four steps using your target weight instead of your current weight. Remember, these numbers are only estimates. Your actual daily calorie needs depend on your age, level of activity, body composition, and other factors.

---

researchers have found that many Americans compensate for a lower-fat diet by consuming more calories overall.

Complex Carbohydrates   It has long been the fashion among dieters to cut back on bread, pasta, and potatoes to control weight. But complex carbohydrates from these sources, as well as from vegetables, legumes, and whole grains, are precisely the nutrients that can help you achieve and maintain a healthy body weight. They help provide a feeling of satiety, or fullness, that can keep you from overeating. Carbohydrates should make up about 55–65% of your total daily calories. Avoid high-fat toppings and sauces, however; try plain yogurt instead of sour cream on your baked potato and tomato-based sauces rather than cream sauces on your pasta.

Simple Sugars and Refined Carbohydrates   Foods high in added simple sugars provide calories but few nutrients. There is also some evidence that foods high in sugar and/or refined carbohydrates may trigger overeating in some people by affecting the rate of glucose absorption and the levels of hormones that influence appetite. Choose fresh fruits and whole grains instead of foods high in added sugars and refined carbohydrates.

Protein   The typical American consumes more than an adequate amount of protein. Special dietary supplements that provide extra protein are unnecessary for most people, and protein not needed by the body for growth and tissue repair will be stored as fat. Foods high in protein are often also high in fat. Stick to the recommended protein intake of 10–15% of total daily calories.

Periodically, new diet books hit the market proclaiming a "scientific breakthrough" involving a high-protein, low-carbohydrate diet. Such diets also typically involve significant calorie restriction, which is what actually causes any weight loss that occurs. A high-protein, low-carbohydrate diet does not conform to the Dietary Guidelines for Americans and is difficult to maintain. Most authorities recommend diets high in complex carbohydrates and moderate in protein consumption.

Eating Habits   Equally important to weight management is eating small, frequent meals—three or more a day plus snacks—on a dependable, regular schedule. Skipping meals leads to excessive hunger, feelings of deprivation, and increased vulnerability to binge eating or snacking on high-calorie, high-fat, or sugary foods. A regular pattern of eating, along with some personal "decision rules" governing food choices, is a way of thinking about and then internalizing the many details that go into a healthy, low-fat diet. Decision rules governing breakfast might be these, for example: Choose a sugar-free, high-fiber cereal with nonfat milk most of the time; once in a while (no more than once a week), have a hard-boiled egg; save pancakes and waffles for special occasions.

Decreeing some foods "off limits" generally sets up a rule to be broken. The better principle is "everything in moderation." If a particular food becomes troublesome, it might be placed off limits temporarily until control over it is regained. The ultimate goal for achieving a healthy diet that ensures successful weight management is to eat in moderation; no foods need to be entirely off limits, though some should be eaten judiciously. Making the healthier choice more often than not is the essence of moderation.

Physical Activity and Exercise

Regular physical activity is another important lifestyle factor in weight management. Physical activity and exercise burn calories and keep the metabolism geared to using food for energy instead of storing it as fat. See the box "Exercise and Weight Management" for more information on how physical activity affects metabolism.

As described in Chapter 13, the first step in becoming more active is to incorporate more physical activity into your daily life. Accumulate 30 minutes or more of moderate-intensity physical activity—walking, gardening,

For successful weight management, some people find it helpful to limit their intake of foods high in fat and simple sugars. Foods made with fat and sugar substitutes are often promoted for weight loss. But just what are fat and sugar substitutes? And can they really contribute to weight management?

Fat Substitutes

A variety of substances are used to replace fats in processed foods and other products. Some contribute calories, protein, fiber, and/or other nutrients, while others do not. Fat replacers can be classified into three general categories:

• *Carbohydrate-based fat replacers* include starch, fibers, gums, cellulose, polydextrose, and fruit purees. They are the oldest and most widely used form of fat replacer and are found in dairy and meat products, baked goods, salad dressing, and many other prepared foods. Newer types such as Oatrim, Z-trim, and Nu-trim are made from types of dietary fiber that may actually lower cholesterol levels. Carbohydrate-based fat replacers contribute 0–4 calories per gram.

• *Protein-based fat replacers* are typically made from milk, egg whites, soy, or whey; trade names include Simplesse, Dairy-lo, and Supro. They are used in cheese, sour cream, mayonnaise, margarine spreads, frozen desserts, salad dressing, and baked goods. Protein-based fat replacers typically contribute 1–4 calories per gram.

• *Fat-based fat replacers* include glycerides, olestra, and other special types of fatty acids. Some of these compounds are not absorbed well by the body and so provide fewer calories per gram (5 calories compared with the standard 9 for fats); others are impossible for the body to digest and so contribute no calories at all. Olestra, marketed under the trade name Olean and used in fried snack foods, is an example of the latter type of compound. Concerns have been raised about the safety of olestra because it reduces the absorption of fat-soluble nutrients and certain antioxidants and because it causes gastrointestinal distress in some people.

Nonnutritive Sweeteners

Sugar substitutes are often referred to as nonnutritive sweeteners because they provide no calories or essential nutrients. By 1999, four types of nonnutritive sweeteners had been approved for use in the United States: acesulfame-K (Sunett), aspartame (NutraSweet, Equal, NatraTaste), saccharin (Sweet 'N Low), and sucralose (Splenda). They are used in beverages, desserts, baked goods, yogurt, chewing gum, and products such as toothpaste, mouthwash, and cough syrup. Other nonnutritive sweeteners currently under review include alitame, cyclamate, neotame, and stevia.

Fat and Sugar Substitutes in Weight Management

Whether fat and sugar substitutes help you achieve and maintain a healthy weight depends on your lifestyle—your overall eating and activity habits. When evaluating foods containing fat and sugar substitutes, consider these issues:

• *Is the food lower in calories or just lower in fat?* Reduced-fat foods often contain extra sugar to improve the taste and texture lost when fat is removed, so such foods may be as high or even higher in total calories than their fattier counterparts. Limiting fat intake is an important goal for weight management, but so is controlling total calories.

• *Are you choosing foods with fat and/or sugar substitutes* instead of *foods you typically eat or* in addition to *foods you typically eat?* If you consume low-fat, no-sugar-added ice cream instead of regular ice cream, you may save calories. But if you add such ice cream to your daily diet simply because it is lower in fat and sugar, your overall calorie consumption—and your weight—may increase.

• *How many foods containing fat and sugar substitutes do you consume each day?* Although the FDA has given at least provisional approval to all the fat and sugar substitutes currently available, health concerns about some of these products linger. One way to limit any potential adverse effects is to read labels and monitor how much of each product you consume. Remember that fat and sugar substitutes are found in a wide variety of products.

• *Is an even healthier choice available?* Many of the foods containing fat and sugar substitutes are low-nutrient snack foods. Although substituting a lower-fat or lower-sugar version of the same food may be beneficial, fruits, vegetables, and whole grains are healthier snack choices.

housework, and so on—on most, or preferably all, days of the week. Take advantage of routine opportunities to be more active; in the long term, even a small increase in activity level can help maintain your current weight or help you lose a moderate amount of weight (Table 14-3). In fact, research suggests that fidgeting—stretching, squirming, standing up, and so on—may help prevent weight gain after overeating in some people.

Once you become more active every day, consider beginning a formal exercise program that includes cardiorespiratory endurance exercise, resistance training, and stretching exercises. Moderate cardiorespiratory endurance exercise, sustained for 45 minutes to 1 hour, can help trim body fat permanently. Strength training helps increase fat-free mass, which results in more calorie burning even outside of exercise periods. See Chapter 13 for advice on creating a complete fitness program.

The message about exercise is that regular exercise, maintained throughout life, makes weight management easier. The sooner you establish good habits, the better. The key to success is making exercise an integral part of the lifestyle you can enjoy now and will enjoy in the future. Chapter 13 contains many suggestions for becoming a more active, physically fit person.

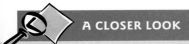

Exercise is a crucial component of a weight-management program. In order to achieve long-term success, you must be able to stick with your program for a lifetime. Cutting food intake in order to lose weight is a difficult strategy to maintain; increasing your physical activity is a much better approach. A 45-minute exercise session burns a significant number of calories—in addition to its many other health benefits. And exercise has weight-management benefits beyond the increased energy expenditure that occurs during each exercise session.

Both strength training and cardiorespiratory endurance exercise can raise your metabolic rate. Strength training builds muscle mass, and more muscle translates into a higher metabolic rate. It can also help you maintain your muscle mass during a period of weight loss, helping you avoid the significant drop in RMR associated with weight loss.

Endurance exercise increases the rate at which your body uses calories after your exercise session is over. One study found that a 30-minute session of endurance exercise increased RMR by an extra 150 calories over the 12-hour period following the workout. The number of excess calories burned during the recovery period can equal up to 50% of the calories burned during the exercise itself. That's like getting the weight-management benefits of an extra 15 minutes of walking, jogging, or stair climbing.

Refer to Chapter 13 for information on setting up an exercise program to achieve fitness and help you develop and maintain a healthy body weight.

SOURCES: Fahey, T. D. 1995. Exercise burns more calories. *Healthline,* March. Ask the experts. 1994. *University of California at Berkeley Wellness Letter,* November.

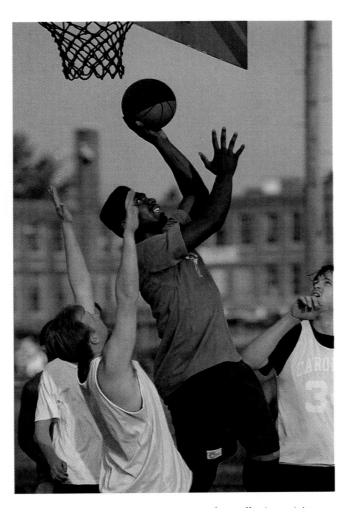

Physical activity is an essential component of any effective weight-management plan. Playing basketball is just one of innumerable activities that can help you keep in shape.

TABLE 14-3 *Energy Costs of Selected Physical Activities**

To determine how many calories you burn when you engage in a particular activity, multiply the calorie multiplier given below by your body weight (in pounds) and then by the number of minutes you exercise.

Activity	Cal/lb/ min	×	Body Weight	×	Min	=	Total Calories
Cycling (13 mph)	.071		_____		_____		_____
Digging	.062		_____		_____		_____
Driving a car	.020		_____		_____		_____
Housework	.029		_____		_____		_____
Painting a house	.034		_____		_____		_____
Shoveling snow	.052		_____		_____		_____
Sitting quietly	.009		_____		_____		_____
Sleeping and resting	.008		_____		_____		_____
Standing quietly	.012		_____		_____		_____
Typing or writing	.013		_____		_____		_____
Walking briskly (4.5 mph)	.048		_____		_____		_____

*See Chapter 13 for the energy costs of fitness activities.

SOURCE: Adapted from Kusinitz, I., and M. Fine. 1995. *Your Guide to Getting Fit,* 3rd ed. Mountain View, Calif.: Mayfield.

Thinking and Emotions

What goes on in your head is another factor in a healthy lifestyle and successful weight management. The way you think about yourself and your world influences, and is influenced by, how you feel and how you act. Certain kinds of thinking produce negative emotions, which can undermine a healthy lifestyle.

Research on people who have a weight problem indicates that low self-esteem and the negative emotions that accompany it are significant problems. This often results in part from mentally comparing the actual self to an internally held picture of the "ideal self." The greater the discrepancy, the larger the impact on self-esteem and the more likely the presence of negative emotions.

Often our internalized "ideal self" is the result of having adopted perfectionistic goals and beliefs about how we and others "should" be. Examples of such beliefs are: "If I don't do things perfectly, I'm a failure" and "It's terrible if I'm not thin." These irrational beliefs may actually cause stress and emotional disturbance. The remedy is to challenge such beliefs and replace them with more realistic ones.

The beliefs and attitudes you hold give rise to self-talk, an internal dialogue you carry on with yourself about events that happen to and around you. Positive self-talk includes leading yourself through the steps of a job and then praising yourself when it's successfully completed. Negative self-talk takes the form of self-deprecating remarks, self-blame, and angry and guilt-producing comments. Negative self-talk can undermine efforts at self-control and lead to feelings of anxiety and depression (see Chapter 3).

Your beliefs and attitude influence how you interpret what happens to you and what you can expect in the future, as well as how you feel and react. A healthy lifestyle is supported by having realistic beliefs and goals and by engaging in positive self-talk and problem-solving efforts.

> **PERSONAL INSIGHT** Do you sometimes overeat? If so, are you more likely to overeat in certain situations, at certain times of the day, or with particular people? Do you overeat when you're in a certain frame of mind?

Coping Strategies

Adequate and appropriate coping strategies for dealing with the stresses and challenges of life are another lifestyle factor in weight management. One strategy that some people adopt for coping is eating. (Others use drugs, alcohol, smoking, spending, gambling, and so on, to cope.) When boredom occurs, eating can provide entertainment. Food may be used to alleviate loneliness or as a pickup for fatigue. Eating provides distraction from difficult problems and is a means of punishing the self or others for real or imagined transgressions.

People with a healthy lifestyle have more effective ways to get their needs met. Having learned to communicate assertively and to manage interpersonal conflict effectively, they don't shrink from problems or overreact. The person with a healthy lifestyle knows how to create and maintain relationships with others and has a solid network of friends and loved ones. Food is used appropriately—to fuel life's activities and gain personal satisfaction, not to manage stress.

The healthy lifestyle that naturally and easily results in a reasonable body weight is one characterized by good nutrition, adequate exercise, positive thinking and emotions, and effective coping strategies and behavior patterns. You can make positive changes in your lifestyle to promote permanent weight control; see the box "Strategies for Managing Your Weight" for ideas.

APPROACHES TO OVERCOMING A WEIGHT PROBLEM

What should you do if you are overweight? There are several options available to you.

Doing It Yourself

Research indicates that people are far more successful than was previously thought at losing weight and keeping it off. One study found that about 64% of the subjects achieved long-term success without joining a formal program or getting special help. Supporting these findings, a U.S. Public Health Service survey indicated that about 50% of the general public succeed with long-term weight management.

Other researchers investigated the characteristics that distinguished those who lost at least 20% of their body weight and maintained this loss for 2 years or more. Although some had used diet alone to lose weight, some had used exercise alone, and others had used a combination of diet and exercise, virtually all maintained their success by making exercise a permanent part of their lifestyle. They also kept tabs on their weight and habits. In addition, they learned to develop their own diet, exercise, and maintenance plans, and they became more involved in and excited by activities other than eating—such as careers, projects, and special interests. Long-term success depends on maintaining the lifestyle changes that helped you lose the weight in the first place (see the box "Strategies of Successful Weight Managers").

If you need to lose weight, focus on adopting the healthy lifestyle described throughout this book. The "right" weight for you will naturally evolve, and you won't

You need to adopt a weight-management plan that will last a lifetime. Look through the following list of strategies, and adopt those that will be most useful for you.

- When shopping for food, make a list and stick to it. Don't shop when you're hungry. Avoid aisles that contain problem foods.

- When serving food, use a small food scale to measure out portions before putting them on your plate.

- Serve meals on small plates and in small bowls to help you eat smaller portions without feeling deprived.

- Eat three meals a day; replace impulse snacking with planned, healthy snacks. Drink plenty of water to help fill you up.

- Eat only in specifically designated spots. Remove food from other areas of your house or apartment.

- When you eat, just eat—don't do anything else, such as read or watch TV.

- Eat more slowly. Pay attention to every bite and enjoy your food. Try putting your fork or spoon down between bites.

- For problem foods, try eating small amounts under controlled conditions. Go out for a scoop of ice cream, for example, rather than buying half a gallon for your freezer.

- If you cook a large meal for friends, send leftovers home with your guests.

- When you eat out, choose a restaurant where you can make healthy food choices. Ask the waiter or waitress not to put bread and butter on the table before the meal; request that sauces and salad dressings be served on the side.

- If you're eating at a friend's, eat a little and leave the rest. Don't eat to be polite; if someone offers you food you don't want, thank the person and decline firmly. To turn down dessert or second helpings, try "No thank you, I've had enough" or "It's delicious, but I'm full."

- Develop strategies for handling stress—go for a walk or use a relaxation technique. Practice positive self-talk.

- Increase your level of daily physical activity. If you have been sedentary for a long time or are seriously overweight, increase your level of physical activity slowly. Start by walking 10 minutes at a time, and work toward 30 minutes of moderate physical activity per day.

- Begin a formal exercise program that includes cardiorespiratory endurance exercise, resistance training, and stretching (see Chapter 13).

- Tell family members and friends that you're making some changes in your eating and exercise habits. Ask them to be supportive.

SOURCES: Nash, J. D. 1997. *The New Maximize Your Body Potential.* Palo Alto, Calif.: Bull Publishing. Ferguson, J. M., and C. Ferguson. 1997. *Habits Not Diets: The Secret to Lifetime Weight Control,* 3rd ed. Palo Alto, Calif.: Bull Publishing. Reprinted with permission from Bull Publishing Company.

---

have to diet. However, if you must diet, do so in combination with exercise, and avoid very-low-calorie diets. Don't try to lose more than 0.5–1 pound per week. Realize that most low-calorie diets cause a rapid loss of body water at first. When this phase passes, weight loss declines. As a result, dieters are often misled into believing that their efforts are not working. They then give up, not realizing that smaller losses later in the diet are actually better than the initial big losses, because later loss is mostly fat loss, whereas initial loss was primarily fluid.

For more tips on losing weight on your own, refer to the Behavior Change Strategy at the end of the chapter.

Diet Books

Many people who try to lose weight by themselves fall prey to one or more of the dozens of diet books on the market. Although a very few of these do contain useful advice and tips for motivation, most make empty promises. Some guidelines for evaluating and choosing a diet book are as follows:

1. Reject books that advocate an unbalanced way of eating. These include books advocating a high-carbohydrate-only diet or those advocating low-carbohydrate, high-protein diets.

2. Reject books that claim to be based on a "scientific breakthrough" or to have the "secret" to success.

3. Reject books that use gimmicks, like combining foods in special ways to achieve weight loss, rotating levels of calories, or purporting that a weight problem is due to food allergies, food sensitivities, yeast infections, or hormone imbalances.

4. Reject books that promise quick weight loss or that limit the selection of foods.

5. Accept books that advocate a balanced approach to diet plus exercise and sound nutrition advice.

A recent crop of popular books has advocated diets high in protein, low in carbohydrate, and relatively high in fat. The American College of Sports Medicine, the American Dietetic Association, the Cooper Institute for Aerobics Research, and the Women's Sports Foundation released a joint statement saying that such diets are not a good weight-loss strategy, will not improve athletic performance, and can be harmful in some cases. The only reason such plans help some people lose weight is that the diets they advocate provide so few calories; but as

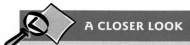

Studies of weight-loss programs have consistently shown that most people gain back lost weight within a fairly short period of time. But what about those people who *do* succeed in losing weight and keeping it off? Why are they successful? What can "yo-yo dieters" learn from their experiences? Researchers recently set out to answer these questions with the National Weight Control Registry (NWCR), a large-scale study of people who have dropped an average of 60 pounds and kept it off for 5 years. The average body mass index of NWCR participants fell from 35 to 24, bringing it into the healthy range (see p. 379). Findings from the NWCR study include the following:

- About half of the NWCR participants joined formal weight-loss programs; the remainder lost weight on their own. Fewer than 5% used any type of prescription medication.

- In order to maintain weight loss, participants made permanent changes in both their diet and their exercise habits. They incorporated the strategies they used to lose the weight into their daily routines.

- Common dietary strategies included restricting certain foods, cutting portion sizes, and monitoring calories or fat grams. (Other studies of successful weight managers have shown that increasing intake of vegetables, fruits, and dietary fiber is also helpful.) Participants did not skip meals, and they ate out an average of three times per week.

- NWCR participants expended lots of energy in physical activity—an average of 2700 calories per week, the equivalent of walking 28 miles. This is well above the Surgeon General's minimum physical activity recommendation of 1000 calories per week. Popular activities among participants included walking, cycling, aerobic dance, and stair climbing.

- Nearly all participants reported improvements in energy level, mobility, mood, self-confidence, and physical health. They felt that the results of their lifestyle changes were well worth the effort.

People who have struggled with their weight should take heart from the NWCR. Most of the successful weight managers who participated in the study had tried unsuccessfully to lose weight in the past, and many of them had been overweight since childhood. The message from the NWCR is that weight management is possible but that it requires lifetime commitment and effort.

SOURCES: Weight loss: The secrets of success. 1998. *Harvard Women's Health Watch*, January. Klem, M. L., et al. 1997. A descriptive study of individuals successful at long-term maintenance of substantial weight loss. *American Journal of Clinical Nutrition* 66(2): 239–246.

with all such plans, they are difficult to maintain over any period of time. (See the January 1998 issue of *Consumer Reports* and the January 1999 issue of *Environmental Nutrition* for reviews of many top-selling diet books.)

Dietary Supplements

Using commercially available supplements for modified fasting can be dangerous, especially if they are the sole source of nutrition, because there is no medical monitoring by a physician. Such approaches include powders used to make shakes that substitute for some or all of the daily food intake, as well as food bars. Many provide fewer than 800 calories a day.

Although the products available today are much improved over the liquid-protein supplements that contributed to many dieters' deaths during the 1970s, only careful medical evaluation and monitoring can significantly reduce the risk of such an approach. Furthermore, dietary supplements teach reliance on patented products, not on sound, lifelong eating habits. And although weight loss can be rapid, muscle tends to be lost too, and the lost weight is often regained.

Nonprescription Diet Pills and Diet Aids

A large number of over-the-counter (OTC) diet aids are available to those seeking a "magic pill" to do away with

extra pounds. Many of these products promote such gimmicks as exotic-sounding herbs, grapefruit juice extract, and amino acids, none of which has been proven to affect appetite or weight loss.

The most common ingredient in OTC diet aids is *phenylpropanolamine hydrochloride (PPA)*, which acts as a mild stimulant and suppresses the desire to eat. The results of studies on the effectiveness of PPA are contradictory. A recent study found that while PPA was effective in suppressing appetite, the average weight loss of people taking it over a 6-week period was only 2 pounds greater than for those receiving a placebo. Without a conscious effort to reduce calorie intake, increase physical activity, and change eating behavior, such weight loss is unlikely to be maintained. And there is concern over the safety of PPA. Some reports suggest it can cause dizziness, headaches, rapid pulse, palpitations, sleeplessness, and hypertension. The use of PPA is not approved by the FDA for periods longer than 12 weeks.

The second most common ingredient of diet aids sold in drug stores is fiber. Manufacturers claim these products work by "swelling in the stomach and absorbing liquids" to provide a feeling of fullness. In fact, dietary fiber acts as a bulking agent in the large intestine, not in the stomach. The FDA has found no data to warrant classifying any type of fiber as an aid in weight control or as an appetite suppressant. And most of these products provide a mere 1–3 grams of fiber per day, which does not

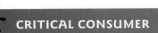

In 1999, the Partnership for Healthy Weight Management, a coalition of government and private organizations, issued guidelines for weight-loss programs. Any commercial plan or program you consider should provide the following:

• A description of the central components of the program (diet, exercise, behavior modification, and so on) and information about staff credentials and training.

• Information about the risks associated with overweight and obesity and the benefits of modest weight loss.

• Information about the risks, side effects, and potential complications associated with the product or program.

• An itemized list of all costs of the plan, including membership fees and any special meals or supplements. Costs that are nonrefundable should be clearly identified.

• If possible, information about outcomes of the program— how much weight clients lose on average and how much weight they keep off over time—that enable people to make informed choices among weight-loss products and services.

The guidelines also recommend that any program documentation include a statement to the effect that many people who lose weight are likely to find it difficult to keep off and that they can improve their chances by adopting a lifelong commitment to frequent and regular physical activity and healthy eating in accordance with the Dietary Guidelines for Americans.

SOURCE: Partnership for Healthy Weight Management (http://www.consumer.gov/weightloss).

contribute much toward the recommended daily intake of 20–35 grams.

There are many other types of dietary supplements and over-the-counter products marketed for weight loss. Use your critical thinking skills and the resources given in the discussion of dietary supplements in Chapter 12 to evaluate these types of products. The bottom line on nonprescription diet aids is: *Caveat emptor*—let the buyer beware. There is no quick and easy way to lose weight. The most effective approach is developing healthy diet and exercise habits and making them part of your lifestyle.

Commercial, Group, and Medical Programs

A variety of options are available if you want help, support, or advice about managing your weight. Different types of programs may work for different people, but a little research can help you locate a program that suits your needs and preferences. Many commercial weight-loss programs include counseling sessions, nutrition education, exercise planning, and behavior modification training. They can be expensive, though, and some require purchasing special foods or supplements. If you are considering a commercial program, use the tips in the box "How to Evaluate Commercial Weight-Loss Programs."

Maintenance is an especially important feature of any program. Studies indicate that only about 10–15% of program participants maintain their weight loss—the rest gain back all or more than they had lost. One study of participants found that regular exercise was the best predictor of maintaining weight loss, while frequent television viewing was the best predictor of weight gain. This finding reinforces the idea that successful weight management requires long-term lifestyle changes.

Self-help groups that focus on weight management can provide support and encouragement. Your physician or a registered dietitian can also help you put together a successful weight-management program. Many R.D.s can be found in private practice or conducting weight-management programs through hospitals or clinics. For cases of severe obesity, consult a physician.

Prescription Drugs

A number of prescription drugs are designed to facilitate weight loss and treat obesity. Currently available drugs include the following:

• Phentermine (Ionamin), an amphetamine-like stimulant that suppresses appetite. It can produce dependence and is recommended for only short-term use.

• Sibutramine (Meridia), which affects appetite by increasing levels of serotonin and norepinephrine. Sibutramine may trigger increases in blood pressure and heart rate and must be used with caution.

• Orlistat (Xenical), which lowers calorie consumption by blocking fat absorption in the intestines; it prevents about 30% of the fat in food from being digested. Similar to the fat substitute olestra, orlistat reduces the absorption of fat-soluble vitamins and antioxidants; it can also cause cramping, diarrhea, and other gastrointestinal problems if users do not follow a low-fat diet.

Other drugs under study include leptin, cholecystokinin boosters, and neuropeptide Y inhibitors.

Studies have generally found that these drugs produce modest weight loss—a 5–15% weight reduction. They do not eliminate the need to exercise and reduce food intake. Unfortunately, most people regain the weight they've lost if they stop taking the drugs. Most researchers agree that what is truly needed is an effective medication that can be taken safely for many years. Weight management is a lifelong project.

As with all drugs, there are risks and side effects. In 1997, the FDA asked that two other prescription weight-loss drugs, fenfluramine (Pondimin) and dexfenfluramine (Redux), be removed from the market after their use was linked to potentially life-threatening heart valve problems. The scope and extent of these problems is still under investigation, but it appears that people who took these drugs over a long period or at high dosages are at greatest risk. Because heart valve problems may not cause symptoms, the FDA recommends that anyone who has taken either of these drugs be examined by a physician.

Clearly, prescription weight-loss drugs are not for people who want to lose a few pounds to wear a smaller size of jeans. The latest federal guidelines advise people to try lifestyle modification for at least 6 months before trying drug therapy. Prescription drugs are recommended—in conjunction with lifestyle changes—only in certain cases: for people who have been unable to lose weight with non-drug options and who have a BMI over 30 (or over 27 if two or more additional risk factors such as diabetes and high blood pressure are present). For severely obese people who have been unable to lose weight by other methods, prescription drugs may provide a good option. Even modest weight loss provides significant health benefits for obese individuals.

Surgery

For people who are 100% or more overweight, obesity is considered a serious medical condition, and surgical intervention may be necessary as a treatment of last resort. Generally, this involves a *gastric resection,* in which a portion of the small intestine is bypassed to decrease the body's ability to absorb nutrients. This procedure can produce major weight loss, but it is associated with serious side effects, including frequent diarrhea, possible liver damage, and various nutritional deficiencies. Lifetime medical management is also necessary.

An alternative procedure is *gastroplasty,* or stomach stapling. During this operation, the stomach is reduced in size by using surgical staples to close off a portion. The reduced capacity of the stomach decreases the amount of food that can be consumed at any one time, and the patient feels full more quickly after eating a small meal. Unfortunately, it is also possible for the patient to overeat and burst a staple, resulting in a medical emergency.

Recently, *liposuction* has become popular for removing localized fat deposits. This cosmetic procedure should not be considered a viable approach to overall weight loss. In addition to being a medically serious operation, it is associated with considerable pain and discomfort, bruising, swelling, discoloration, the risk of infection, and possible unexpected contour changes. Furthermore, it takes from 6 months to a year to see satisfactory results from a liposuction procedure.

Psychological Help

Many people can lose weight just by increasing their physical activity level and moderately restricting total calories, especially fat calories. When concern about body weight and shape have developed into an eating disorder, the help of a professional is recommended. In choosing a therapist, be sure to ask about credentials and experience (see Chapter 3). The therapist should have experience working with body image issues, eating disorders, addictions, and abuse issues. Your physician may be able to provide a referral.

Choosing a Weight-Reduction Approach

No single approach to weight reduction is appropriate for all individuals, and no one type of program stands above all others. After eliminating those approaches that are dangerous or fraudulent, you will have a number of options. The challenge is to find the one that's best for you.

The first step is to decide how serious your weight problem is. If you are less than 20% overweight, you might consider a self-directed approach—cutting back on fat calories and increasing exercise on your own—or reconsidering whether in fact you need to lose weight. Be sure you are pursuing a reasonable weight, given your family history and lifestyle.

If you are 20–40% overweight, you might consider joining a self-help group, one of the commercial weight-loss programs, a behavioral program led by a health professional, or a work site program. More serious degrees of overweight, 40–100%, may require a more aggressive approach. Consider getting private counseling, joining a hospital-based program, participating in a medically supervised very-low-calorie diet with a maintenance program, or going to a residential program.

If you are 100% or more overweight, or have 100 pounds or more to lose, a medically supervised very-low-calorie diet should be your first choice. With appropriate pretreatment assessment, open-ended treatment that includes a maintenance program, and the help of a professional staff that includes dietitians, physicians, and psychologists, such an approach has been found to be quite effective for about 65% of those who participate. If this approach fails, the most drastic (but often successful) treatment is surgery. Discuss this alternative with your physician.

Once you narrow your options, consider your own needs and preferences. You may prefer a group program to individual care. You may need supervised exercise, or you may be able to exercise on your own. Choosing a program that fits your lifestyle will increase your chances of success.

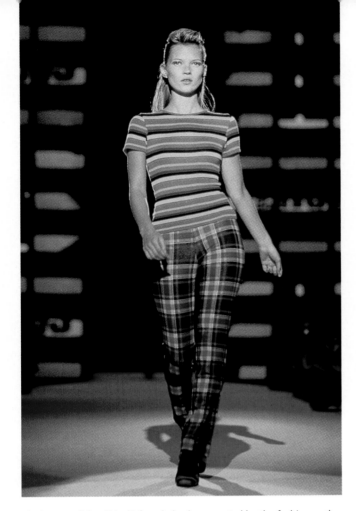

The image of the "ideal" female body promoted by the fashion and fitness industries doesn't reflect the wide range of body shapes and sizes that are associated with good health. An overconcern with body image can contribute to low self-esteem and the development of eating disorders.

Hazards and Rewards in the Search for the "Perfect" Body

The American focus on attaining a perfect body has prompted a flood of weight-loss programs, fad diets, health clubs, exercise equipment, appetite-reducing drugs, and books on diet, nutrition, and fitness. Presumably, with the right combination of programs, exercise, and eating plans, one can attain the promised rewards of a healthier, slimmer, fitter, more aesthetically appealing body.

Dieting is part of the American way of life. Data from two large national surveys indicate that about 24% of men and 40% of women are currently dieting. The rates are even higher among young people. A national survey found that 61% of adolescent girls and 28% of adolescent boys had dieted during the previous year. Another study found that up to 15% of girls and 3% of boys were "chronic dieters"—that is, they reported that they always dieted or had been on a diet more than 10 times in the past year. Chronic dieting among teenagers can lead to

retarded physical growth, menstrual irregularities, and to the development of eating disorders.

During adolescence, both boys and girls become sensitive about their size and physical appearance. Studies have consistently shown a high prevalence of dissatisfaction with body weight or shape among male and female teenagers. The cultural pressure to be thin, especially for female adolescents, coupled with the social stigma of obesity, may well predispose weight-conscious youths to dieting, abnormal eating patterns, and eating disorders (see the box "Gender, Ethnicity, and Body Image").

Setting unrealistic weight-loss goals in response to cultural ideals of attractiveness can set people up for failure and psychological distress. Dieters may suffer from depression, persistent irritability, an inability to concentrate, sleep disturbances, and preoccupation with food and weight. When they fail to attain their goal of thinness, they may feel they're weak or suffer from a character flaw. Such ideas can undermine their chances of developing a truly healthy lifestyle, one that will enable them to maintain a reasonable body weight easily and naturally.

Realistic weight-loss goals are much more achievable and can have very beneficial effects. For an obese person, losing as few as 10 pounds can reduce blood pressure as much as antihypertensive medication. Participants in behavioral weight-loss programs often experience improvement in mood after losing as few as 10 pounds.

Obesity is a serious health risk, but weight management needs to take place in a positive and realistic atmosphere. The hazards of excessive dieting and overconcern about body weight need to be countered by a change in attitude about what constitutes the perfect body and a reasonable body weight. The current ideal of ultrathin must change. A reasonable body weight should take into account a person's weight history, social circumstances, metabolic profile, and psychological well-being.

> **PERSONAL INSIGHT** How do you feel about your body weight, shape, and size? Do you have strong feelings about what an ideal male and female body should look like? Where do you think you've learned these ideals?

EATING DISORDERS

Problems with body weight and weight control are not limited to excessive body fat. A growing number of people, especially adolescent girls and young women, experience **eating disorders**, characterized by severe disturbances in

eating disorder A serious disturbance in eating patterns or eating-related behavior, characterized by a negative body image and concerns about body weight or body fat. **TERMS**

The image of the "perfect woman" seems to be everywhere, from television shows to magazine covers to fashion advertisements. The mass media expose us to this single "right" look relentlessly, and the beauty and fitness industries promise to help us attain it. For American women, success is still too often equated with how we look rather than who we are.

The incidence of dieting, eating disorders, and obesity are all higher among girls and women than boys and men. According to one study, 61% of adolescent girls have dieted in the past year, compared with 28% of adolescent boys. Only 30% of eighth-grade girls are content with their bodies, while 70% of their male classmates expressed satisfaction with their looks. This critical evaluation of their bodies happens at the same time as a drop in overall self-esteem among teenage girls. Some girls and women come to feel that they can't be successful or worthwhile people unless they look like the underweight models shown in the media. Many become slaves to the mirror and bathroom scale, which robs energy from more important pursuits and may lead to eating disorders. Indeed, women are 20 times more likely than men to have anorexia nervosa or bulimia nervosa.

The thin, toned look as a feminine ideal is just a fashion and is not shared by all American women. The African American community is much more accepting of larger, more voluptuous body shapes than white Americans have been. In many traditional African societies, full-figured women's bodies are seen as symbols of health, prosperity, and fertility. African American teenage girls have a much more positive body image than white girls. Two-thirds of black teenage girls in one survey defined beauty as "the right attitude," while white girls were much more preoccupied with weight and body shape. (Take the quiz below to assess your body image.) African American women are less likely to suffer from eating disorders than their Latina, Native American, or white counterparts. However, black women have higher rates of obesity than women of other ethnic backgrounds. Nearly 50% of African American women are more than 20% over their ideal body weight, and black women as a group have a low level of physical fitness. (Some studies indicate that black women on average have lower resting metabolic rates than white women.)

How does socioeconomic status fit into this picture? Obesity is more common among Americans of lower income, regardless of ethnicity; poor women are twice as likely as more affluent women to be overweight. One theory is that people with lower incomes must eat a less expensive diet that is also higher in fat. Lowfat food and fresh fruits and vegetables are often unavailable in poor communities, and places for physical activity may be limited. Minority women in middle and upper income brackets tend to be thinner than poor minority women. They also have rates of eating disorders that approach those of white women. The relationship between ethnicity, income, and rates of overweight and eating disorders is obviously a complex one.

For women (or men) of any cultural or ethnic background, a sensible approach to body image is focusing on good physical and psychological health, not a number on a scale. When you see idealized standards presented by the beauty and fitness industries, realize that one of their goals is to increase your dissatisfaction with yourself so you will buy their products. Most of all, put your concerns about your physical appearance in perspective. Remember, your worth as a human being is not a function of how you look.

How's Your Body Image?

	Never	Some-times	Often	Always
1. I dislike seeing myself in mirrors.	0	1	2	3
2. When I shop for clothing, I am more aware of my weight problem, and consequently I find shopping for clothes somewhat unpleasant.	0	1	2	3
3. I'm ashamed to be seen in public.	0	1	2	3
4. I prefer to avoid engaging in sports or public exercise because of my appearance.	0	1	2	3
5. I feel somewhat embarrassed about my body in the presence of someone of the other sex.	0	1	2	3
6. I think my body is ugly.	0	1	2	3
7. I feel that other people must think my body is unattractive.	0	1	2	3
8. I feel that my family or friends may be embarrassed to be seen with me.	0	1	2	3
9. I find myself comparing myself with other people to see if they are heavier than I am.	0	1	2	3
10. I find it difficult to enjoy activities because I am self-conscious about my physical appearance.	0	1	2	3
11. Feeling guilty about my weight problem preoccupies most of my thinking.	0	1	2	3
12. My thoughts about my body and physical appearance are negative and self-critical.	0	1	2	3

Now, add up the number of points you have circled in each column: _____   0 + _____ + _____ + _____

Score Interpretation

The lowest possible score is 0, and this indicates a positive body image. The highest possible score is 36, and this indicates an unhealthy body image. A score higher than 14 suggests a need to develop a healthier body image.

SOURCE: Nash, J. D. 1997. *The New Maximize Your Body Potential*. Palo Alto, Calif.: Bull Publishing. Reprinted with permission from Bull Publishing Company.

eating patterns and eating-related behaviors. The major eating disorders are anorexia nervosa, bulimia nervosa, and binge-eating disorder. **Anorexia nervosa** is characterized by a refusal to maintain a minimally normal body weight. **Bulimia nervosa** is characterized by repeated episodes of binge eating followed by compensatory behaviors such as self-induced vomiting, the misuse of laxatives or diuretics, fasting, or excessive exercise. **Binge-eating disorder** is characterized by binge eating without any compensatory behaviors. Eating disorders are associated with depression, anxiety, low self-esteem, and increased health risks, including, in some cases, increased risk of premature death.

Eating disorders are more prevalent in developed countries than in developing ones. At any given time, about 0.5–1.0% of Americans suffer from anorexia and 3.0% have bulimia. Binge-eating disorder may affect 25–45% of people who join formal weight-reduction programs.

In the United States, eating disorders affect far more women than men: Of the 1 million Americans who develop anorexia or bulimia each year, 90% are female. Eating disorders appear to be more prevalent among people of middle and upper-middle socioeconomic status. Preliminary research findings suggest that eating disorders are equally common among white females and Latinas, more common among Native American females, and less common among African American and Asian American females. Among minority groups, females most at risk for eating disorders are those who are younger, heavier, and better educated, and who identify with middle-class values.

Factors in Developing an Eating Disorder

Many factors are probably involved in the development of an eating disorder. Although many widely different explanations have been proposed, they share one central feature: a dissatisfaction with body image and body weight. Such dissatisfaction is created by distorted thinking, including perfectionistic beliefs, unreasonable demands for self-control, and excessive self-criticism.

Dissatisfaction with body weight leads to dysfunctional attitudes about eating, such as fear of fat and preoccupation with food, and problematic eating behaviors, including excessive dieting, constant calorie counting, and frequent weighing. If a significant family dysfunction—such as a rigid or overprotective parent or a family in which there is hostility, abuse, or lack of cohesion—is added to body dissatisfaction, an eating disorder is a likely outcome.

A person with a sensitive temperament, or someone who has been taught to care for the needs of others before her or his own needs, may have a higher risk of developing an eating disorder. This is especially true if the person has not learned how to express and deal with difficult emotions. Comparing oneself negatively with others can damage self-esteem and increase vulnerability. Young people who fail to develop a firm sense of self or who see themselves as lacking control over their lives are also at high risk for eating disorders.

Eating disorders can also be described as an obsession with weight and an addiction to abnormal eating behavior. A person with an eating disorder experiences obsessive, anxiety-producing thinking, revolving around the fear of gaining weight. The abnormal eating behavior—starvation, **purging,** or binge eating—reduces anxiety by producing numbness and alleviating emotional pain. Thus, an eating disorder is a means of coping with stress and relieving tension. A person who has an eating disorder often lacks an adequate repertoire of skills for dealing with stress.

Anorexia Nervosa

A person suffering from anorexia nervosa does not eat enough food to maintain a reasonable body weight. Anorexia affects 1–3 million Americans, 95% of them female. Although it can occur later, anorexia typically develops between the ages of 12 and 18.

Characteristics of Anorexia Nervosa People suffering from anorexia have an intense fear of gaining weight or becoming fat. Their body image is distorted, so that even when emaciated, they think they are fat. They may engage in compulsive behaviors or rituals that help keep them from eating, though some may also binge and purge. They commonly use vigorous and prolonged physical activity to reduce body weight as well. Although they may express a great interest in food, even taking over the cooking responsibilities for the rest of the family, their own diet becomes more and more extreme. People with anorexia often hide or hoard food without eating it.

Anorexic people are typically introverted, emotionally reserved, and socially insecure. They are often "model

---

TERMS

anorexia nervosa An eating disorder characterized by a refusal to maintain body weight at a minimally healthy level and an intense fear of gaining weight or becoming fat; self-starvation.

bulimia nervosa An eating disorder characterized by recurrent episodes of binge eating and purging: overeating and then using compensatory behaviors such as vomiting and excessive exercise to prevent weight gain.

binge-eating disorder An eating disorder characterized by binge eating and a lack of control over eating behavior in general.

purging The use of vomiting, laxatives, excessive exercise, restrictive dieting, enemas, diuretics, or diet pills to compensate for food that has been eaten and that the person fears will produce weight gain.

children" who rarely complain and are anxious to please others and win their approval. Although school performance is typically above average, they are often critical of themselves and not satisfied with their accomplishments. For people with anorexia nervosa, their entire sense of self-esteem may be tied up in their evaluation of their body shape and weight.

Health Risks of Anorexia Nervosa   Because of extreme weight loss, females with anorexia often stop menstruating, become intolerant of cold, and develop low blood pressure and heart rate. They develop dry skin that is often covered by fine body hair like that of an infant. Their hands and feet may swell and take on a blue color.

Anorexia nervosa has been linked to a variety of medical complications, including disorders of the cardiovascular, gastrointestinal, and endocrine systems. When body fat is virtually gone and muscles are severely wasted, the body turns to its own organs in a desperate search for protein. Death can occur from heart failure caused by electrolyte imbalances. As many as 18% of patients with anorexia nervosa die of complications related to the disorder. Depression is also a serious risk, and about half the fatalities relating to anorexia are suicides.

Bulimia Nervosa

A person suffering from bulimia nervosa engages in recurrent episodes of binge eating followed by purging. Bulimia is often difficult to recognize because sufferers conceal their eating habits and usually maintain a normal weight, although they may experience weight fluctuations of 10–15 pounds. Although bulimia usually begins in adolescence or young adulthood, it has recently begun to emerge at increasingly younger (11–12 years) and older (40–60 years) ages.

Characteristics of Bulimia Nervosa   During a binge, a bulimic person may rapidly consume anywhere from 1,000–60,000 calories. This is followed by an attempt to get rid of the food by purging, usually by vomiting or using laxatives or diuretics. During a binge, they feel as though they have lost control and cannot stop or limit how much they eat. Some binge and purge only occasionally, while others do so many times every day.

In public, people suffering from bulimia may appear to eat normally, but they are rarely comfortable around food. Binges usually occur in secret and can become nightmarish—ravaging the kitchen for food, going from one grocery store to another to buy food, or even stealing food. During the binge, all feelings are blocked out, and food acts as an anesthetic. Afterward, they feel physically drained and emotionally spent. They usually feel deeply ashamed and disgusted with both themselves and their behavior and terrified that they will gain weight from what they've eaten.

Major life changes such as leaving for college, getting married, having a baby, or losing a job can trigger a binge-purge cycle. At such times, stress is high and the person may have no good outlet for emotional conflict or tension. As with anorexia, bulimia sufferers are often insecure and depend on others for approval and self-esteem. They may hide difficult emotions such as anger and disappointment from themselves and others. Binge eating and purging becomes a way of dealing with feelings.

Health Risks of Bulimia Nervosa   The binge-purge cycle of bulimia places a tremendous strain on the body and can have serious health effects. Contact with vomited stomach acids erodes tooth enamel. Bulimic people often develop tooth decay because they binge on foods that contain large amounts of simple sugars. Repeated vomiting or the use of laxatives, in combination with deficient calorie intake, can damage the liver and kidneys and cause cardiac arrhythmia. Chronic hoarseness and esophageal tearing with bleeding may also result from vomiting. More rarely, binge eating can lead to rupture of the stomach. Although many bulimic women maintain normal weight, even small amounts of weight loss to a lower-than-normal weight can cause menstrual problems. And although less often associated with suicide or premature death than anorexia, bulimia is associated with increased depression, excessive preoccupation with food and body image, and sometimes disturbances in cognitive functioning.

Binge-Eating Disorder

Binge-eating disorder is characterized by uncontrollable eating, usually followed by feelings of guilt and shame with weight gain. Common eating patterns are eating more rapidly than normal, eating until uncomfortably full, eating when not hungry, and preferring to eat alone. Binge eaters may eat large amounts of food throughout the day, with no planned mealtimes. Many people with binge-eating disorder mistakenly see rigid dieting as the only solution to their problem. However, rigid dieting usually causes feelings of deprivation and a return to overeating.

Compulsive overeaters rarely eat because of hunger. Instead, food is used as a means of coping with stress, conflict, and other difficult emotions or to provide solace and entertainment. People who do not have the resources to deal effectively with stress may be more vulnerable to binge-eating disorder. Inappropriate overeating often begins during childhood. In some families, eating may be used as an activity to fill otherwise empty time. Parents may reward children with food for good behavior or withhold food as a means of punishment, thereby creating distorted feelings about the use of food.

Binge eaters are almost always obese, so they face all the health risks associated with obesity. In addition, binge eaters may have higher rates of depression and anxiety. To

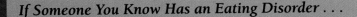
- Educate yourself about eating disorders and their risks and about treatment resources in your community. (See the For More Information section at the end of this chapter for suggestions.)

- Write down specific ways the person's eating problem is affecting you or others in the household. Call a house meeting to talk about how others are affected by the problem and how to take action.

- Consider consulting a professional about the best way to approach the situation. Obtain information about how and where your friend can get help. Attend a local support group.

- Arrange to speak privately with the person, along with other friends or family members. Let one person lead the group and do most of the talking. Discuss specific incidents and the consequences of disordered eating.

- If you are going to speak with your friend, write down ahead of time what your concerns are and what you would like to say. Expect that the person you are concerned about will deny there is a problem, minimize it, or become angry with you. Remain calm and nonjudgmental, and continue to express your concern.

- Avoid giving simplistic advice about eating habits. Gently encourage your friend to eat properly.

- Take time to listen to your friend, and express your support and understanding. Encourage honest communication. Emphasize your friend's good characteristics, and compliment all her or his successes.

- Help maintain the person's sense of dignity by encouraging personal responsibility and decision making. Be patient and realistic; recovery is a long process. Continue to love and support your friend.

- If the situation is an emergency—if the person has fainted or attempted suicide, for example—take immediate action. Call 911 for help.

- If you feel very upset about the situation, seek professional help. Remember, you are not to blame for another person's eating disorder.

overcome binge eating, a person must learn to put food and eating into proper perspective and develop other ways of coping with stress and painful emotions.

Treating Eating Disorders

The treatment of eating disorders must address both problematic eating behaviors and the misuse of food to manage stress and emotions. Anorexia nervosa treatment first involves averting a medical crisis by restoring adequate body weight; then the psychological aspects of the disorder can be addressed. The treatment of bulimia nervosa or binge-eating disorder involves first stabilizing the eating patterns, then identifying and changing the patterns of thinking that lead to disordered eating. Concurrent problems, such as depression or anxiety, must also be addressed. In 1996, the antidepressant Prozac became the first medication approved by the FDA for the treatment of bulimia.

Treatment usually involves a combination of psychotherapy and medical management. The therapy may be carried out individually or in a group; sessions involving the entire family may be recommended. A support or self-help group can be a useful adjunct to such treatment. Medical professionals, including physicians, dentists, gynecologists, and registered dietitians, can evaluate and manage the physical damage caused by the disorder. If a patient is severely depressed or emaciated, hospitalization may be necessary. Depending on the severity of the disorder, treatment may last from a few months to several years.

Friends and family members often want to know what they can do to help someone with an eating disorder. For suggestions, see the box "If Someone You Know Has an Eating Disorder. . . ."

Today's Challenge

Eating disorders can be seen as the logical extension of the concern with weight that pervades American society. Although most people don't succumb to irrational or distorted ideas about their bodies, many do become obsessed with dieting. The challenge facing Americans today is achieving a healthy body weight without excessive dieting—by adopting and maintaining sensible eating habits, an active lifestyle, realistic and positive attitudes and emotions, and creative ways of handling stress.

SUMMARY

Basic Concepts of Weight Management

- Body composition is the relative amounts of fat-free mass and fat in the body. *Overweight* and *obesity* are often used interchangeably; they refer to body weight or the percentage of body fat that exceeds what is associated with good health.

- The key to weight management is maintaining a balance of calories in (food) and calories out (resting metabolism, food digestion, and physical activity).

- Too much or too little body fat is linked to health problems. Obesity is a risk factor for premature death, cardiovascular disease, cancer, diabetes, and other disorders. The distribution of fat throughout the body is also a significant factor.

- An inaccurate or negative body image is very common and is associated with psychological distress.

- Body weight provides an indirect measure of body composition; it can be assessed using height-weight charts and body mass index (BMI).

- Percent body fat can be determined through a variety of methods, including hydrostatic weighing and skinfold measurements. The health risks of body fat distribution can be assessed using waist measurements or the waist-to-hip ratio.

Factors Contributing to Weight Problems

- Although genetic factors help determine a person's weight, the influence of heredity can be overcome with attention to diet and physical activity.

- Resting metabolic rate (RMR) is partly determined by heredity, gender, and lifestyle; it can be increased through exercise and an increase in muscle mass.

- Other possible factors in weight problems are having excess or large fat cells, engaging in restrictive dieting, and using food to express or deal with emotions. Certain cultural patterns of food use may also contribute.

Adopting a Healthy Lifestyle for Successful Weight Management

- Nutritional guidelines for weight management include consuming a moderate number of calories; limiting portion sizes and the intake of fat, simple sugars, refined carbohydrates, and protein to recommended levels; increasing the intake of complex carbohydrates; and developing an eating schedule and decision rules for food choices.

- Activity guidelines for weight management emphasize daily physical activity and regular sessions of cardiorespiratory endurance exercise and strength training.

- Weight management requires rejecting irrational, perfectionistic beliefs and developing positive, realistic self-talk and self-esteem.

- A repertoire of appropriate techniques for handling stress and other emotional and physical challenges prevents the misuse of food as a coping mechanism.

Approaches to Overcoming a Weight Problem

- People can be successful at long-term weight loss on their own, usually through a combination of diet and exercise.

- Diet books, OTC diet aids, diet supplements, and commercial weight-loss programs should be assessed for safety and efficacy.

- Professional help is needed in cases of severe obesity; medical treatments include prescription drugs, surgery, and psychological therapy.

- The high rate of dieting in the United States is due in part to unrealistic cultural ideals of thinness. Modest weight loss can benefit health.

Eating Disorders

- Eating disorders can have serious physical and psychological consequences. Dissatisfaction with weight and shape are common to all eating disorders.

- Anorexia nervosa is characterized by self-starvation, increased physical activity, distorted body image, and an intense fear of gaining weight. It is potentially fatal.

- Bulimia nervosa is characterized by recurrent episodes of uncontrolled binge eating and frequent purging, either by self-induced vomiting or the use of laxatives or diuretics.

- Binge-eating disorder involves binge eating without compensatory purging. It is most common among obese dieters.

- Although eating disorders are extreme conditions, many Americans are obsessed with weight and dieting. The challenge is to maintain normal body weight without excessive dieting—by balancing a healthy diet with exercise.

TAKE ACTION

1. Interview some people who have successfully lost weight and kept it off. What were their strategies and techniques? Do you think their approach would work for others?

2. Find out what percentage of your body weight is fat by taking one of the tests described in this chapter at your campus health clinic, sports medicine clinic, or health club. If you have too high or too low a proportion of body fat, consider taking steps to change it.

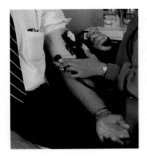

LEARNING OBJECTIVES

After reading this chapter, you should be able to:

- List the major components of the cardiovascular system, and describe how blood is pumped and circulated throughout the body.

- Describe the controllable and uncontrollable risk factors associated with cardiovascular disease.

- Discuss the major forms of cardiovascular disease and how they develop.

- List the steps you can take to lower your personal risk of developing cardiovascular disease.

Cardiovascular Health

15

TEST YOUR KNOWLEDGE

1. Reducing the amount of cholesterol you eat is the most important dietary change you can make to improve your blood cholesterol levels.
   True or false?

2. Women are about as likely to die of cardiovascular disease as they are to die of breast cancer.
   True or false?

3. Which of the following behaviors lowers the risk of heart disease?
   a. exercising regularly
   b. eating a high-fiber diet
   c. managing stress and anger

4. Which of the following is a possible sign of a heart attack?
   a. chest pain that spreads to the shoulders and arms
   b. uncomfortable pressure or fullness in the chest lasting more than a few minutes
   c. chest discomfort with nausea

5. Which of the following foods would be a good choice for promoting heart health?
   a. kidney beans
   b. oat bran
   c. olive oil

Answers

1. **False.** Limiting your intake of saturated and trans fats, which promote the production of cholesterol by the liver, is the key dietary change for improving blood cholesterol levels; dietary cholesterol has much less of an effect on blood cholesterol.

2. **False.** Cardiovascular disease kills far more. Among American women, about 1 in 2 deaths is due to cardiovascular disease and about 1 in 27 is due to breast cancer.

3. **All three.** Everyone has the ability to significantly reduce the risk of heart disease through lifestyle choices.

4. **All three.** Quick recognition of symptoms and early treatment can greatly reduce the severity of a heart attack and increase the chances of survival.

5. **All three.** These foods all contain substances that improve cholesterol levels; kidney beans and oat bran are high in fiber, and olive oil is rich in monounsaturated fatty acids.

Cardiovascular disease (CVD) is the leading cause of death in the United States, claiming one life every 33 seconds. Nearly half of all Americans alive today will die from CVD. Though we typically think of CVD as primarily affecting men and older adults, heart attack is the number-one killer of American women, and 45% of heart attacks occur in people under age 65. But not all the news is bad. In the past 50 years, lifestyle changes and medical advances have led to significant progress in the fight against CVD.

Much of the incidence of CVD is due to the American way of life. Too many Americans eat a high-fat diet, are overweight and sedentary, smoke cigarettes, manage stress ineffectively, have uncontrolled high blood pressure or high cholesterol levels, and don't know the signs of CVD. Not all the risk factors for CVD are controllable—some people have an inherited tendency toward high blood pressure, for example. But many factors can be changed, treated, or modified, and you have the power to significantly reduce your risk.

Exactly what is CVD, and how does it do its damage? More important, what steps can you take now to make sure you keep your heart healthy throughout your life? This chapter will provide some answers to these questions.

THE CARDIOVASCULAR SYSTEM

The cardiovascular system consists of the heart and blood vessels (veins, arteries, and capillaries); together, they pump and circulate blood throughout the body. A person weighing 150 pounds has about 5 quarts of blood, which is circulated about once every minute.

The heart is a four-chambered, fist-size muscle located just beneath the ribs under the left breast (Figure 15-1). Its role is to pump oxygen-poor blood to the lungs and oxygenated (oxygen-rich) blood to the rest of the body. Blood actually travels through two separate circulatory systems: The right side of the heart pumps blood to and from the lungs in what is called **pulmonary circulation,** and the left side pumps blood through the rest of the body in **systemic circulation.**

Used, oxygen-poor blood enters the right upper chamber, or **atrium,** of the heart through the **vena cava,** the largest vein in the body (Figure 15-2). Valves prevent the blood from flowing the wrong way. As the right atrium fills, it contracts and pumps blood into the right lower chamber, or **ventricle,** which, when it contracts, pumps blood through the pulmonary artery into the lungs. There, blood picks up oxygen and discards carbon dioxide. Cleaned, oxygenated blood then flows through the pulmonary veins into the left atrium. As this chamber fills, it contracts and pumps blood into the powerful left ventricle, which pumps it through the **aorta,** the body's largest artery, to be fed into the rest of the body's blood

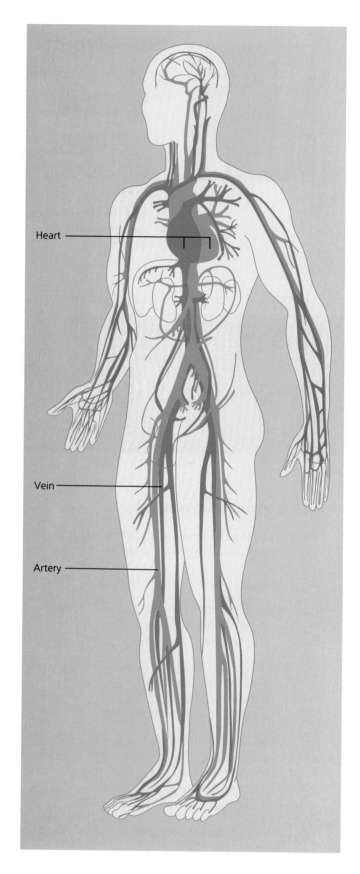

Heart

Vein

Artery

Figure 15-1   The cardiovascular system.

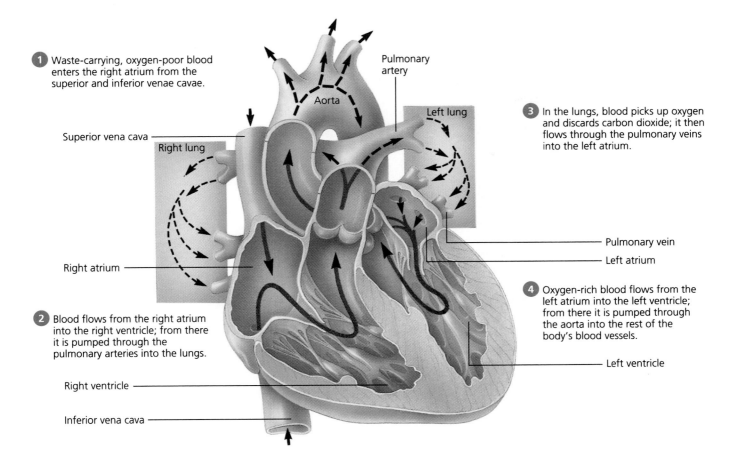

1 Waste-carrying, oxygen-poor blood enters the right atrium from the superior and inferior venae cavae.

Pulmonary artery

Aorta

Left lung

3 In the lungs, blood picks up oxygen and discards carbon dioxide; it then flows through the pulmonary veins into the left atrium.

Superior vena cava

Right lung

Pulmonary vein

Left atrium

Right atrium

4 Oxygen-rich blood flows from the left atrium into the left ventricle; from there it is pumped through the aorta into the rest of the body's blood vessels.

2 Blood flows from the right atrium into the right ventricle; from there it is pumped through the pulmonary arteries into the lungs.

Left ventricle

Right ventricle

Inferior vena cava

Figure 15-2   Circulation in the heart.

vessels. The period of the heart's contraction is called **systole;** the period of relaxation is called **diastole.**

The heartbeat—the split-second sequence of contractions of the heart's four chambers—is controlled by electrical impulses. These signals originate in a bundle of specialized cells in the right atrium called the pacemaker. Unless it is speeded up or slowed down by the brain in response to such stimuli as danger or exhaustion, the heart produces electrical impulses at a steady rate.

Blood vessels are classified by size and function. **Veins** carry blood to the heart; **arteries** carry blood away from the heart. Veins have thin walls, but arteries have thick elastic walls that enable them to expand and relax with the volume of the blood being pumped through them. After leaving the heart, the aorta branches into smaller and smaller vessels. Two vital arteries, called the **coronary arteries,** branch off the aorta to carry blood back to the heart tissues themselves (Figure 15-3, p. 406).

The smallest arteries branch still further into **capillaries,** tiny vessels only one cell thick. The capillaries deliver oxygen and nutrient-rich blood to the tissues and receive oxygen-poor, waste-carrying blood. From the capillaries, this blood empties into small veins and then into larger veins that return it to the heart. From there the cycle is repeated.

TERMS

cardiovascular disease (CVD)   The collective term for various forms of diseases of the heart and blood vessels.

pulmonary circulation   The part of the circulatory system governed by the right side of the heart; the circulation of blood between the heart and the lungs.

systemic circulation   The part of the circulatory system governed by the left side of the heart; the circulation of blood between the heart and the rest of the body.

atria   The two upper chambers of the heart in which blood collects before passing to the ventricles; also called *auricles.*

vena cava   The large vein through which blood is returned to the right atrium of the heart.

ventricles   The two lower chambers of the heart from which blood flows through arteries to the lungs and other parts of the body.

aorta   The large artery that receives blood from the left ventricle and distributes it to the body.

systole   Contraction of the heart.

diastole   Relaxation of the heart.

veins   Vessels that carry blood to the heart.

arteries   Vessels that carry blood away from the heart.

coronary arteries   Two arteries branching from the aorta that provide blood to the heart muscle.

capillaries   Very small blood vessels that distribute blood to all parts of the body.

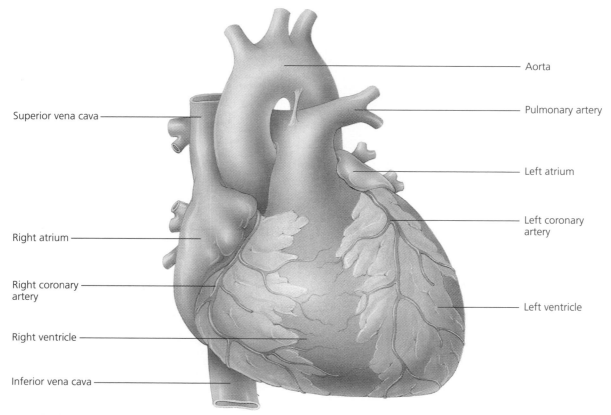

Superior vena cava

Right atrium

Right coronary artery

Right ventricle

Inferior vena cava

Aorta

Pulmonary artery

Left atrium

Left coronary artery

Left ventricle

Figure 15-3   Blood supply to the heart.

RISK FACTORS FOR CARDIOVASCULAR DISEASE

Researchers have identified a variety of factors associated with an increased risk of developing cardiovascular disease. They are grouped into two categories: major risk factors and contributing risk factors. Some major risk factors, such as diet, exercise habits, and use of tobacco, are linked to controllable aspects of lifestyle and can therefore be changed. Others, such as age, sex, and heredity, are beyond an individual's control.

Major Risk Factors That Can Be Changed

The American Heart Association (AHA) has identified six major risk factors for CVD that can be changed: tobacco use, high blood pressure, unhealthy blood cholesterol levels, physical inactivity, obesity, and diabetes.

Tobacco Use   Nearly 1 in 5 deaths from CVD are attributable to smoking. People who smoke a pack of cigarettes a day have twice the risk of heart attack that nonsmokers have; smoking two or more packs a day triples the risk. And when smokers do have heart attacks, they are two to four times more likely than nonsmokers to die from them. Women who smoke and use oral contraceptives are up to 39 times more likely to have a heart attack and up to 22 times more likely to have a stroke than women who don't smoke and take the pill.

Smoking harms the cardiovascular system and raises risk for CVD in several ways. Nicotine, a central nervous system stimulant, increases blood pressure and heart rate; the carbon monoxide in cigarette smoke displaces oxygen in the blood, reducing the amount of oxygen available to the heart and other parts of the body. Smoking damages the linings of arteries, and it contributes to unhealthy blood fat levels by reducing levels of high-density lipoproteins (HDL), "good cholesterol," and raising levels of triglycerides and low-density lipoproteins (LDL), "bad cholesterol." It causes the **platelets** in the blood to become sticky and cluster, promoting clotting. Smoking also permanently accelerates the rate at which fatty deposits are laid down in arteries.

You don't have to smoke to be affected. The risk of death from coronary heart disease increases up to 30% among those exposed to environmental tobacco smoke (ETS) at home or at work. Researchers estimate that 50,000 nonsmokers die from CVD each year as a result of exposure to ETS.

High Blood Pressure   High blood pressure, or **hypertension,** is a risk factor for many forms of CVD but is also

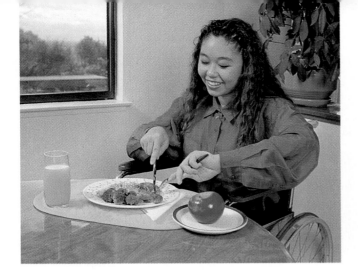

A diet high in fiber and low in fat and saturated fat can help lower levels of total cholesterol and LDL. This young woman is enjoying a healthy dinner of baked chicken, broccoli, rice, fruit, and juice.

considered a disease itself. High blood pressure occurs when too much force or pressure is exerted against the walls of the arteries. If your blood pressure is high, your heart has to work harder to push the blood forward. Over time, a strained heart weakens and tends to enlarge, which weakens it further. Increased blood pressure also scars and hardens arteries, making them less elastic. Heart attacks, strokes, **atherosclerosis,** and kidney failure can result.

Hypertension usually has no early warning signs, so it's important to have your blood pressure tested at least once every two years (more often if you have CVD risk factors). If yours is consistently high, your physician can help you lower it through diet, weight management, exercise, and, if necessary, medication. (High blood pressure and atherosclerosis are discussed later in the chapter.)

Cholesterol Cholesterol is a fatty, waxlike substance that circulates through the bloodstream and is an important component of cell membranes, sex hormones, vitamin D, the fluid that coats the lungs, and the protective sheaths around nerves. Adequate cholesterol is essential for the proper functioning of the body. However, excess cholesterol can clog arteries and increase the risk of cardiovascular disease.

Our bodies obtain cholesterol in two ways: from the liver, which manufactures it, and from the foods we eat. Cholesterol levels vary depending on diet, age, sex, heredity, and other factors.

GOOD VERSUS BAD CHOLESTEROL   Cholesterol is carried in the blood in protein-lipid packages called lipoproteins. Lipoproteins can be thought of as one-way shuttles that transport cholesterol to and from the liver through the circulatory system (Figure 15-4, p. 408). **Low-density lipoproteins (LDLs)** shuttle cholesterol from the liver to the organs and tissues that require it. LDL is known as "bad" cholesterol because if there is more than the body

can use, the excess is deposited in the blood vessels. When it accumulates, it can block arteries and cause heart attacks and strokes. **High-density lipoproteins (HDLs),** or "good" cholesterol, shuttle unused cholesterol back to the liver for recycling.

RECOMMENDED BLOOD CHOLESTEROL LEVELS   The risk for CVD increases with increasing blood cholesterol levels The first step in managing your cholesterol is to be tested. The National Cholesterol Education Program (NCEP) recommends testing at least once every 5 years for all adults, beginning at age 20, or at least every 3 years for people with a family history of heart disease. General cholesterol guidelines are given in Table 15-1, p. 409. A total cholesterol level below 200 mg/dl (milligrams per deciliter) is considered desirable and indicates a relatively low risk of CVD; high levels over 240 mg/dl carry approximately double the CVD risk of desirable levels. An estimated 98 million American adults—over half the adult population—have total cholesterol levels of 200 mg/dl or higher.

Laboratory blood tests can measure your LDL and HDL levels. In general, high LDL levels and low HDL levels are associated with a high risk for CVD; low levels of LDL and high levels of HDL are associated with lower risk. HDL is especially important because a high HDL level seems to offer protection from CVD even in cases where total cholesterol is high. On the other hand, low total cholesterol may be associated with high CVD risk if HDL is also very low. For this reason, some experts use the ratio of total cholesterol to HDL to evaluate CVD risk (see Table 15-1).

BENEFITS OF CONTROLLING CHOLESTEROL   Experts calculate that people can cut their heart attack risk by 2% for every 1% that they reduce their total blood cholesterol levels. People who lower their total cholesterol from 250 to 200 mg/dl, for example, reduce their risk of heart attack by 40%. In addition, studies indicate that lowering total blood cholesterol levels not only reduces the

---

TERMS

platelets Microscopic disk-shaped cell fragments in the blood that disintegrate on contact with foreign objects and release chemicals that are necessary for the formation of blood clots.

hypertension Sustained abnormally high blood pressure.

atherosclerosis A form of CVD in which the inner layers of artery walls are made thick and irregular by plaque deposits; arteries become narrow and blood supply is reduced.

low-density lipoproteins (LDL) Blood fat that transports cholesterol from the liver to organs and tissues; excess is deposited on artery walls, where it can eventually block the flow of blood to the heart and brain; "bad" cholesterol.

high-density lipoprotein (HDL) Blood fat that helps transport cholesterol out of the arteries and thus protects against heart diseases; "good" cholesterol.

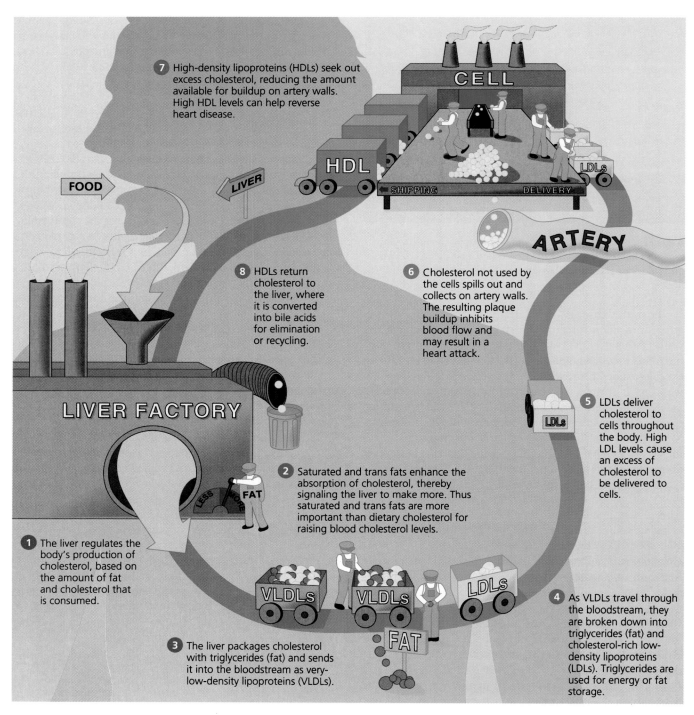

Figure 15-4   Travels with cholesterol.

likelihood that arteries will become clogged, it can also reverse deposits on artery walls, thereby actually helping clean out diseased arteries.

How can you improve your cholesterol levels? Important dietary changes include cutting total fat intake, substituting unsaturated for saturated and trans fats, and increasing soluble fiber intake. Decreasing your intake of saturated and trans fats is particularly important because they promote the production and excretion of cholesterol by the liver. You can raise your HDL levels by exercising regularly and, if you smoke, kicking the habit. These and other lifestyle changes for lowering cholesterol and promoting heart health are discussed in greater detail later in this chapter.

TABLE 15-1	*Cholesterol Guidelines*[a]
Total blood cholesterol	
Less than 200 mg/dl	Desirable[b]
200–239 mg/dl	Borderline high
240 mg/dl or more	High
LDL cholesterol	
Less than 130 mg/dl	Desirable[b]
130–159 mg/dl	Borderline high
160 mg/dl or more	High
HDL cholesterol	
More than 45 mg/dl	Desirable[b]
35–45 mg/dl	Borderline low
Less than 35 mg/dl	Low
Cholesterol ratio (total ÷ HDL)[c]	
4.5	Average
3.5 or less	Optimal

[a]These guidelines are based on large-scale studies of middle-aged Americans; younger people should strive for somewhat lower levels. For example, for those age 19 and under, the desirable level for total blood cholesterol is below 170 mg/dl.
[b]For adults without known heart disease.
[c]Higher ratios indicate higher risk.

SOURCES: American Heart Association. National Cholesterol Education Program.

Physical Inactivity   An estimated 35–50 million Americans are so sedentary that they are at high risk for developing CVD. Exercise is thought to be the closest thing we have to a "magic bullet" against heart disease. It lowers CVD risk by helping decrease blood pressure, increase HDL levels, maintain desirable weight, and prevent or control diabetes. One recent study found that women who accumulated at least 3 hours of brisk walking each week cut their risk of heart attack and stroke by more than half. A minimum of 30 minutes per day of moderate physical activity is recommended; more intense or longer duration exercise has even greater health benefits. Refer to Chapter 13 for more on the benefits of physical activity and guidelines for creating an exercise program.

PERSONAL INSIGHT   What sort of health habits did your family have when you were growing up? Did members of your family exercise? Smoke? What kind of diet did they eat? How do your current habits compare? In what ways have your family's habits affected your current lifestyle?

Obesity   A person whose body weight is more than 30% above the recommended level is at higher risk for heart disease and stroke, even if no other risk factors are present. Excess weight increases the strain on the heart by contributing to high blood pressure and high cholesterol. It can also lead to diabetes, another CVD risk factor (see below). As discussed in Chapter 14, distribution of body fat is also significant: Fat that collects in the torso is more dangerous than fat that collects around the hips. A sensible diet and regular exercise are the best ways to achieve and maintain a healthy body weight. For someone who is overweight, even modest weight reduction can reduce CVD risk by lowering blood pressure, improving cholesterol levels, and reducing diabetes risk.

Diabetes   As described in Chapter 14, diabetes is a disorder characterized by elevated blood glucose levels due to either insufficient supply or action of insulin. People with diabetes are at increased risk for CVD, partially because the disease affects cholesterol levels. Careful control of glucose levels is beneficial, but even people whose diabetes is under control face an increased risk of CVD. For that reason, careful management of other CVD risk factors is critical for people with diabetes.

Contributing Risk Factors That Can Be Changed

Various other factors that can be changed have been identified as contributing to CVD risk, including triglyceride levels and psychological and social factors.

Triglyceride Levels   Like cholesterol, triglycerides are blood fats that can be obtained from the diet and manufactured by the body. Studies have shown that high triglyceride levels are a reliable predictor of heart disease, especially if associated with other risk factors, such as low HDL levels, obesity, and diabetes. Elevated triglyceride levels are especially dangerous for women and for people who smoke.

Much of the picture regarding triglycerides remains unclear, however. Studies have yet to show whether lowering triglyceride levels through lifestyle changes or medication will actually decrease heart disease. Elevated triglyceride levels are most often seen in people with other lipid abnormalities such as high total cholesterol and low HDL. The lifestyle modifications that help lower cholesterol also help decrease triglycerides, making it difficult to identify any potential independent benefit of lowering triglyceride levels.

Physicians often recommend that people with other risk factors for CVD have their total triglyceride level measured. If it is high (400 mg/dl or more), steps should be taken to bring levels down into the healthy range (below 150–200 mg/dl). The best ways to reduce triglycerides seem to be weight loss, regular exercise, and a diet that is high in fiber and low in simple and refined carbohydrates, and that favors unsaturated over saturated fats. (Simple carbohydrates are those found in non-diet soda, candy, and other desserts; sources of refined carbohydrates include white rice and anything made with white flour, such as white bread and pasta.) Being moderate in the use of alcohol is also important because alcohol elevates triglyceride levels.

Psychological and Social Factors Many of the psychological and social factors that influence other areas of wellness are also important risk factors for CVD.

- *Stress.* Excessive stress can strain the heart and blood vessels over time and contribute to CVD. A full-blown stress response causes blood pressure to rise; blood platelets become more likely to cluster, possibly enhancing the formation of artery-clogging clots. People sometimes also adopt unhealthy habits such as smoking or overeating as a means of dealing with severe stress.

- *Chronic hostility and anger.* Certain traits in the hard-driving "Type A" personality—hostility, cynicism, and anger—are associated with increased risk of heart disease. Men prone to anger have two to three times the heart attack risk of calmer men. For more information on this connection, see the box "Hostility and CVD."

- *Suppressing psychological distress.* Consistently suppressing anger and other negative emotions may also be hazardous to a healthy heart. People who hide psychological distress appear to have higher rates of heart disease than people who experience similar distress but share it with others. People with so-called "Type D" personalities tend to be pessimistic, negative, and unhappy and to suppress these feelings. Researchers are not yet certain why the Type D trait is dangerous. It may have physical effects, or it may lead to social isolation and poor communication with physicians.

- *Depression and anxiety.* Both mild and severe depression are linked to an increased risk of CVD. In one study, people with low self-esteem, low motivation, and feelings of despair and hopelessness had a 70% greater risk of heart attack than those who were not depressed. Researchers have also found a strong association between anxiety disorders and an increased risk of death from heart disease, particularly sudden death from heart attack. Both depression and anxiety have physical effects, including irregular heart rhythms, that have short- and long-term effects on the cardiovascular system. Despite the fact that these disorders are more common in women, most studies on the links among depression, anxiety, and CVD have been carried out on men. For more on inequities in research, see the box "Closing the Gender Gap in Health Research," p. 412.

- *Social isolation.* People with little social support are at higher risk of dying from CVD than people with close ties to others. A strong social support network is a major antidote to stress. Friends and family members can also promote and support a healthy lifestyle.

- *Low socioeconomic status.* Low socioeconomic status and low educational attainment also increase risk for CVD. These associations are probably due to a variety of factors, including lifestyle and access to health care.

> **PERSONAL INSIGHT** Would you characterize yourself as a hostile or cynical person? If not, do you know anyone you would characterize that way? What do you think causes a person to have this type of personality?

Major Risk Factors That Can't Be Changed

A number of major risk factors for CVD cannot be changed: heredity, aging, being male, and ethnicity.

Heredity The tendency to develop CVD seems to be inherited. If your father or mother has had heart or blood vessel disease, you have a greater risk of developing CVD yourself. High cholesterol levels, abnormal blood-clotting problems, diabetes, and obesity are other CVD risk factors that have genetic links. But it's important to remember that people who inherit a tendency for CVD are not destined to develop it. They may, however, have to work harder than other people to prevent CVD.

Aging The risk of heart attack increases dramatically after age 65. About 70% of all heart attack victims are age 65 or older, and more than four out of five who suffer fatal heart attacks are over 65. For people over 55, the incidence of stroke more than doubles in each successive decade. However, many people in their thirties and forties, especially men, have heart attacks.

Being Male Although CVD is the leading killer of both men and women in the United States, men face a greater risk of heart attack than women, especially earlier in life. Until age 55, men also have a greater risk of hypertension than women. The incidence of stroke is about 19% higher for males than females. Estrogen production, which is highest during the childbearing years, may offer premenopausal women some protection against CVD (see the box "Women and CVD," p. 413). By age 75, the gender gap nearly disappears.

Ethnicity Death rates from heart disease vary among ethnic groups in the United States, with African Americans having much higher rates of hypertension, heart disease, and stroke than other groups (see the box "African Americans and CVD," p. 414).

Puerto Rican Americans, Cuban Americans, and Mexican Americans are also more likely to suffer from high blood pressure and angina (a warning sign of heart disease) than non-Hispanic white Americans. These differences may be due in part to differences in education,

Current research indicates that people who have a persistently hostile outlook, a quick temper, and a mistrusting, cynical attitude toward life are more likely to develop heart disease than those with a calmer, more trusting attitude. The link between chronic hostility and the heart is most likely to be found in the physiological mechanism of the stress response (see Chapter 2). People who are prone to chronic hostility experience the stress response more intensely and frequently than more relaxed individuals. When they encounter the irritations of daily life, their blood pressure increases much more. They also seem to have trouble shutting down the stress response. Less hostile people tend to calm down much more quickly, taking the stress off their bodies—especially their hearts.

Are You Hostile?

Assess your hostility quotient by checking any of the following statements that are true for you:

_____ 1. Stuck in a long line at the express checkout in the grocery store, I often count the number of items the people in front of me have to see if anyone is over the limit.

_____ 2. I am often irritated by people's incompetence.

_____ 3. If a cashier gives me the wrong change, I assume he or she is probably trying to cheat me.

_____ 4. I've been so angry at someone that I've thrown things or slammed a door.

_____ 5. If someone is late, I plan the angry words I'm going to say.

_____ 6. I tend to remember irritating incidents and get mad all over again.

_____ 7. If someone cuts me off in traffic, I honk, flash my lights, pound the steering wheel, or shout.

_____ 8. Little annoyances have a way of adding up during the day, leaving me frustrated and impatient.

_____ 9. If the person who cuts my hair trims off more than I want, I fume about it for days afterward.

_____ 10. When I get into an argument, I feel my jaw clench and my pulse and breathing rate climb.

_____ 11. If someone mistreats me, I look for an opportunity to pay them back, just for the principle of it.

_____ 12. I get annoyed at little things my spouse or significant other does that get under my skin.

Add up the number of items you checked. A score of 3 or less indicates a generally cool head. A score between 4 and 8 indicates that your level of hostility could be raising your risk of heart disease. A score of 9 or more indicates a hot head—a level of cynicism, anger, and aggression high enough to endanger both heart health and interpersonal relationships.

Managing Your Anger

If you are one of the 20% of Americans who meet the criteria for hot-headedness, take time out to develop calmer responses to life's little annoyances. Keep a log of your hostile responses to people and situations. Familiarize yourself with the patterns of thinking that lead to hostile feelings, and try to head them off before they develop into full-blown anger. If you feel your anger starting to build, ask yourself the following questions:

1. *Is this really important enough to get angry about?* For example, is having to wait an extra 5 minutes for a late bus so important that you should stew about it for the entire 15-minute ride?

2. *Am I really justified in getting angry?* Is the person in front of you really driving slowly, or are you trying to speed?

3. *Is getting angry going to make any real difference in this situation?* Will slamming the door really help your friend find the concert tickets he misplaced?

If you answer "yes" to all three questions, then you should calmly but assertively ask for what you want. A "no" to any question means that you should try to defuse your anger. Reason with yourself, distract your mind with another activity, or try one of the techniques for meditation or deep breathing described in Chapter 2. Your heart—and the people around you—will benefit from your calmer, more positive outlook.

SOURCE: Adapted from Williams, R. B., and V. Williams. 1993. *Anger Kills.* Copyright © 1993 by R. B. Williams, M.D., and V. Williams, Ph.D. By permission of Times Books, a division of Random House, Inc.

---

income, and other socioeconomic factors. Asian Americans historically have had far lower rates of CVD than white Americans. However, cholesterol levels among Asian Americans appear to be rising, presumably because of the adoption of a high-fat American diet.

Possible Risk Factors Currently Being Studied

In recent years, a number of other possible risk factors for cardiovascular disease have been identified. These include homocysteine, specific types of cholesterol, infectious agents, inflammation, and others.

Homocysteine   High levels of homocysteine, an amino acid circulating in the blood, are associated with an increased risk of CVD. Researchers are not yet certain, however, whether it is a direct cause of CVD or simply a marker for some other risk factor. In laboratory studies, homocysteine appears to damage the lining of blood vessels, resulting in inflammation and the development of fatty deposits in artery walls. These changes can lead to the formation of clots and blockages in arteries, which in turn can cause heart attacks and strokes.

Homocysteine levels tend to be higher in men than in women and are particularly high in people who have

Traditionally, medical research has not focused on the prevention and treatment of health problems in women, except in areas of reproductive health. It was assumed that the same approaches that work for men would work for women. As a result of these biases, men have been much more frequently recruited for medical research studies, as well as being the researchers in charge of these studies. As recently as 1989, only 15% of the National Institutes of Health (NIH) resources went to women's health issues.

In the last few years, some major attempts have been made to close this gender gap. In 1990, the Office of Research on Women's Health was established at the NIH. That office has set up the largest clinical trial ever launched in this country: the 15-year, $625 million Women's Health Initiative. Researchers hope to enroll more than 160,000 women in the study, which will look at the relationships among lifestyle, health, risk factors, and disease. It will focus on strategies to prevent diseases common to women, such as heart disease, cancer, and osteoporosis. The study also includes many groups who have been all but ignored in past scientific investigations, like postmenopausal women and women of color. Some specific areas being investigated by the Women's Health Initiative include whether a low-fat diet reduces the risk of breast, colon, and rectal cancers; the effects of calcium and vitamin D supplements

on osteoporosis risk; and the risks and benefits of hormone replacement therapy.

One major study preceded the Women's Health Initiative and is still ongoing: the Nurses' Health Study, inaugurated in 1976. Some 120,000 women between the ages of 30 and 55 fill out extensive questionnaires on their health and lifestyle every 2 years. The study has produced more than 100 reports so far. Among the findings to date are that regular exercise benefits health, that abdominal fat increases CVD risk, that drinking alcohol increases the risk of breast cancer, that suntanning increases the risk of skin cancer, and that oral contraceptives are not linked to an increased risk of CVD.

In addition to these landmark studies, the medical establishment is becoming more aware of the need to include women in research investigations. Women are becoming physicians and researchers in almost the same numbers as men these days, and they may be more sensitive to gender issues in health research. Although we still have a long way to go, the gender gap is definitely closing.

SOURCES: Advances in women's health. 1999. *Harvard Women's Health Watch*, March. Lessons from the nurses. 1997. *Harvard Women's Health-Watch*, May. National Center for Health Statistics. 1996. *Health, United States, 1995*. Hyattsville, Md.: Public Health Service.

chronic illnesses such as cancer and in otherwise healthy people who have diets deficient in vitamin B-12, vitamin B-6, and folic acid. Increasing your intake of fruits, vegetables, and other foods rich in these vitamins brings homocysteine levels down; supplements may also be used. It has yet to be shown, however, if decreasing homocysteine levels will actually reduce CVD risk.

Lipoprotein(a) A high level of a specific type of LDL called lipoprotein(a), or Lp(a), has been identified as a possible independent risk factor for CHD. Lp(a) levels have a strong genetic component and are difficult to treat. Preliminary research indicates that hormone replacement therapy in postmenopausal women, a diet rich in omega-3 fatty acids, and treatment for lowering elevated LDL levels may help reduce the associated risk.

LDL Particle Size Recent research has shown that LDL particles differ in size and density and that the concentrations of different particles vary among individuals. LDL cholesterol profiles can be divided into three general types: people with pattern A have mostly large, buoyant LDL particles; people with pattern B have mostly small, dense LDL particles; and people with pattern C have a mixture of particle types. Small, dense LDL particles pose a greater CVD risk than larger particles; thus, people with LDL pattern B are at greater risk for CVD. At this time, testing to identify LDL particle size is expensive and not

widely available, and further research is needed before routine screening and treatment for LDL pattern B can be recommended. Exercise and a low-fat diet may help lower CVD risk in people with LDL pattern B.

Infectious Agents Several infectious agents have been identified as possible culprits in the development of CVD. *Chlamydia pneumoniae*, a common cause of flu-like respiratory infections, has been found in sections of clogged, damaged arteries but not in sections of healthy arteries. In one study, evidence of infection with *C. pneumoniae* was found in 90% of patients who had recently had a heart attack but in only 25% of healthy control subjects. Research in animals indicates that *C. pneumoniae* infection can damage arteries. Studies are underway to determine if antibiotic treatment for heart attack victims who show evidence of *C. pneumoniae* infection will reduce the risk of a second heart attack.

Other infectious agents may also play a role in CVD. *Cytomegalovirus,* a common type of herpes virus, is linked to the recurrence of blockages in patients who have been treated for CHD. The bacteria that cause gingivitis (gum disease) and *Helicobacter pylori,* the bacterium that causes the majority of peptic ulcers, have also been implicated in the development of heart disease.

Inflammation and C-Reactive Protein Recent research suggests that inflammation plays a key role in the devel-

Cardiovascular disease has traditionally been thought of as a "man's disease." It is true that men have a higher incidence of cardiovascular problems than women, especially before age 50. Until recently, this has been the justification for carrying out almost all CVD research on men. But heart disease is the leading cause of death among women, and more women actually die of CVD than men, though they tend to do so at older ages. Polls indicate that women vastly underestimate their risk of dying of a heart attack and overestimate their risk of dying of breast cancer. In reality, nearly 1 in 2 women dies of CVD, while 1 in 27 dies of breast cancer.

Risk factors for CVD are generally similar for both sexes. But there are important gender differences in how and when CVD develops, is diagnosed, and is treated.

Premenopausal Women: Protected by Estrogen

One important protective factor is unique to women—estrogen. It has long been observed that women seem to avoid heart disease until after menopause. The hormone estrogen, produced naturally by women's bodies until menopause or surgical removal of the ovaries, improves blood fat concentrations by increasing HDL levels and decreasing LDL levels. After menopause, when estrogen levels drop, rates of heart disease among women rapidly increase. Some women choose hormone replacement therapy (HRT) to keep estrogen levels high after menopause. Most studies have shown that HRT cuts CVD risk substantially. However, one recent study showed that women who already have heart disease might actually have more serious health problems during the first year of HRT than women with heart disease who are not on HRT. These findings are controversial, though, and do not apply to women with no history of CVD. Although more research is needed, many experts feel that for the majority of postmenopausal women, the benefits of HRT outweigh the risks. (HRT is discussed further in Chapter 19.)

There is one special caution for premenopausal women: The combination of smoking and using oral contraceptives makes a woman up to 39 times more likely to have a heart attack than a woman who doesn't both smoke and use birth control pills.

Postmenopausal Women: At Risk

Heart attack is the leading killer of women in the United States, and women are more likely than men to die within 1 year following a heart attack. Why are heart attacks more deadly for women? One answer is that women tend to develop heart disease at older ages, when they are more likely to have other health problems that complicate treatment. In addition, recent studies have shown that women tend to have more severe heart attacks than men. Because of physiological differences, some common diagnostic tests are less accurate for women (false positives on ECGs are common). Women also tend to have smaller hearts and arteries, possibly making surgery both more difficult and less successful.

The mortality difference cannot entirely be explained by age and anatomy, however. It also appears that medical personnel evaluate and treat women less aggressively than men. One study of emergency room treatment of heart attack patients found that women had to wait longer than men did—by about 23 minutes—before receiving clot-dissolving drugs. Women may complain less about their pain, or they may describe somewhat different symptoms than male heart attack victims. Some physicians may not immediately consider heart attack when dealing with a female patient. An older woman's health problems may be easier to dismiss than those of a man in the "prime" of his life. In another study, a heart condition causing periodic episodes of rapid heartbeat was twice as likely to be misdiagnosed as anxiety or stress in female patients than in male patients—again indicating gender bias.

Researchers are now focusing more attention on the health problems of women, and more accurate diagnostic techniques may soon be in use. In the meantime, women with chest pain or other symptoms should be persistent in seeking diagnosis and effective treatment.

---

opment of CVD. When an artery is injured by smoking, cholesterol, infectious agents, or other factors, the body's response produces inflammation. A substance called C-reactive protein is released into the bloodstream during the inflammatory response, and studies suggest that high levels of C-reactive protein indicate a substantially elevated risk of heart attack and stroke. Testing levels of C-reactive protein may someday be an important way to assess CVD risk. Aspirin, which reduces both clotting and inflammation, is often recommended for people at high risk for heart attacks and strokes.

Fibrinogen Fibrinogen is a protein that is essential for the formation of blood clots. High levels of fibrinogen are linked to increased risk for coronary heart disease and stroke. Hormone replacement therapy and quitting smoking both help lower fibrinogen levels.

Blood Viscosity and Iron High blood viscosity (thickness) may increase the risk of CVD; excess iron stores have also been linked to higher risk, especially for men and postmenopausal women (iron stores are usually lower in younger women because of menstrual blood loss). Regular blood donation, which reduces iron stores and blood viscosity, is associated with lower CVD risk in men. Drinking five or more glasses of water a day may also reduce risk be reducing blood viscosity. On the flip side, high consumption of heme iron—found in meat, fish, and poultry—is associated with an increased risk of heart attack. Men and postmenopausal women should consult a physician before taking iron supplements.

Syndrome X Researchers have found that certain CVD risk factors are often found in a cluster. As a group, these risk factors—high blood pressure, high triglycerides, low

Although cardiovascular disease is the leading cause of death for all Americans, African Americans are far more likely to experience CVD than white Americans. Black men are nearly 50% more likely to die from a heart attack than white men, and death from stroke is five times more common among African Americans than in other Americans. Hypertension, which is both a disease in and of itself and a risk factor for other forms of CVD, is twice as common in blacks. What accounts for these higher rates of CVD among African Americans? Contributing factors can be grouped into three areas: biological/genetic factors, low income and discrimination, and lifestyle factors.

Biological/Genetic Risk Factors

A number of genetic factors may contribute to CVD in African Americans, including heightened sensitivities to lead and salt, which can lead to high blood pressure. Heredity may also play a role in higher cholesterol levels among blacks. And sickle-cell disease, a genetic disorder that occurs mainly in blacks, can lead to impaired blood flow and heart failure.

Researchers have also found that African Americans respond to stress differently: As part of the fight-or-flight reaction, nitric oxide signals blood vessels to dilate (open up) to allow increased blood flow to muscles. Compared to whites, African Americans are not as sensitive to nitric oxide, so their blood vessels don't dilate as readily. And poor dilation is a key characteristic of hypertension.

Low Income and Discrimination

Another factor in the high incidence of CVD among African Americans is low income. One-third live below the official poverty line. Economic deprivation usually means reduced access to adequate health care and health insurance. Associated with low income are poorer educational opportunities, which often mean less information about preventive health measures, such as diet and stress management.

Discrimination may also play a role in CVD among blacks. Research has shown that many physicians and hospitals treat the medical problems of African Americans differently than those of whites. Discrimination, along with low income and other forms of deprivation, may also increase stress, which is linked with hypertension and CVD.

Lifestyle Factors

Lifestyle factors may be the key in explaining high CVD rates among African Americans. A recent large-scale study determined that birthplace, not ethnicity, is the key indicator of CVD risk among African Americans. The study found that among New Yorkers born in the Northeast, blacks and whites have nearly identical risk for CVD. But black New Yorkers who were born in the South have a sharply higher risk, and black New Yorkers born in the Caribbean have a significantly lower risk. Researchers speculate that some risk factors for CVD, including smoking and a high-fat diet, may be more common in the South. When combined with urban stress, these factors create a lifestyle that is far from heart-healthy. And people with low incomes, who are disproportionately African American, tend to smoke more, use more salt, and exercise less than those with higher incomes. In addition, half of black women and one-third of black men are significantly overweight.

All Americans are advised to have their blood pressure checked regularly, exercise, eat a healthy diet, manage stress, and avoid smoking. These general preventive strategies may be particularly critical for African Americans. In addition, recent research has identified several specific dietary factors that may be of special importance for blacks. Studies have found that diets high in potassium and calcium improve blood pressure in African Americans. Fruits, vegetables, grains, and nuts are rich in potassium; dairy products are high in calcium.

SOURCES: Morris, R. C., et al . 1999. Normotensive salt sensitivity: Effects of race and dietary potassium. *Hypertension* 33(1): 18–23. Cardillo, C., et al. 1998. Racial differences in nitric-oxide mediated vasodilator response to mental stress in the forearm circulation. *Hypertension* 31(6): 1235–1239. Fang, J., S. Madhaven, and M. H. Alderman. 1996. The association between birthplace and mortality from cardiovascular causes among black and white residents of New York City. *New England Journal of Medicine* 335(21): 1545–1551.

HDL cholesterol, abdominal obesity, and glucose intolerance—are called syndrome X. The underlying causes are not well understood, but syndrome X is thought to have a genetic basis. A treatment plan that addresses all the risk factors together may be the best strategy for people with syndrome X.

MAJOR FORMS OF CARDIOVASCULAR DISEASE

Collectively, the various forms of CVD kill more Americans than the next four leading causes of death combined (Figure 15-5). The financial burden of CVD, including the costs of medical treatments and lost productivity, exceeds $280 billion annually.

The main forms of CVD are hypertension, atherosclerosis, heart disease and heart attack, stroke, congestive heart failure, congenital heart disease, and rheumatic heart disease. Many forms are interrelated and have elements in common; we treat them separately here for the sake of clarity.

Hypertension

Blood pressure, the force exerted by the blood on blood vessel walls, is created by the pumping action of the heart. When the heart contracts (systole), blood pressure in-

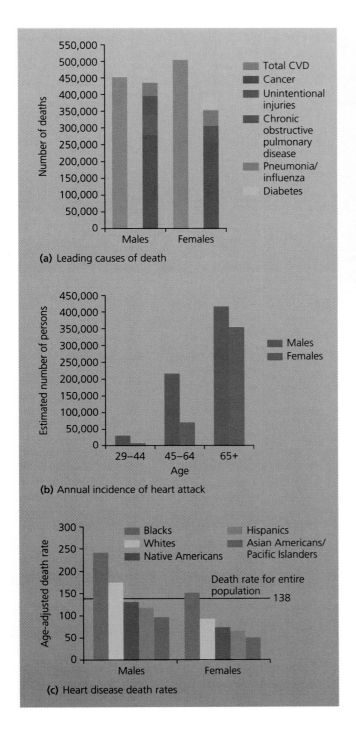

(a) Leading causes of death

(b) Annual incidence of heart attack

Death rate for entire population 138

(c) Heart disease death rates

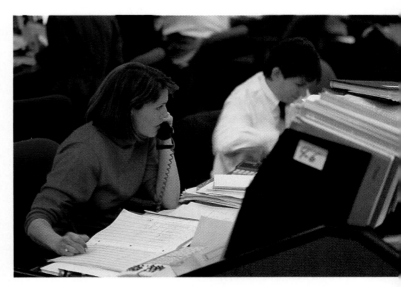

Before age 65, women are less susceptible to cardiovascular disease than men. Even though this woman has to cope with the same on-the-job stresses as men in her profession, she is less likely to have a heart attack in middle age than they are.

VITAL STATISTICS

Figure 15-5 A statistical look at cardiovascular disease in the United States. (a) The leading causes of death. CVD causes more deaths than the next four causes combined. (b) Estimated numbers of Americans who have a heart attack each year. Among heart attack victims under age 65, men significantly outnumber women; after age 65, women start to catch up. (c) Heart disease death rates by gender and ethnicity. SOURCES: American Heart Association. 1999. *Heart and Stroke Facts Statistical Update.* National Center for Health Statistics. 1998. *Health, United States, 1998.* Hyattsville, Md.: U.S. Public Health Service, DHHS Pub. No. (PHS) 98-1232.

creases; when the heart relaxes (diastole), pressure decreases. Many factors affect blood pressure; for example, excitement or exercise causes the heart to pump more blood into the arteries, resulting in a rise in blood pressure. Short periods of high blood pressure are normal, but blood pressure that is continually at an abnormally high level is known as hypertension.

Blood pressure is measured with a stethoscope and an instrument called a sphygmomanometer. It is expressed as two numbers—for example, 120 over 80—and measured in millimeters of mercury. The first and larger number is the systolic blood pressure; the second is the diastolic blood pressure. Average blood pressure readings for young adults in good physical condition are 110–120 systolic over 70–80 diastolic. High blood pressure in adults is defined as equal to or greater than 140 over 90 (Table 15-2).

High blood pressure results from either an increased output of blood by the heart, often as a result of overweight, or because of increased resistance to blood flow in the arteries. The latter condition can be caused by atherosclerosis, discussed in the next section, or by constriction of smooth muscle surrounding the arteries. When a person has high blood pressure, the heart must work harder than normal to force blood through the arteries, thereby straining both the heart and arteries.

High blood pressure is often called a "silent killer," because it usually has no symptoms. A person may have high blood pressure for years without realizing it. But during that time, it damages vital organs and increases the risk of heart attack, congestive heart failure, stroke,

TABLE 15-2 *Blood Pressure Classification for Healthy Adults*

Category[a]	Systolic (mm Hg)		Diastolic (mm Hg)	Recommended Follow-Up
Optimal[b]	below 120	and	below 80	Recheck in 2 years
Normal	below 130	and	below 85	Recheck in 2 years
High-normal	130–139	or	85–89	Recheck in 1 year
Hypertension[c]				
Stage 1	140–159	or	90–99	Confirm within 2 months
Stage 2	160–179	or	100–109	Physician evaluation within 1 month
Stage 3	180 and above	or	110 and above	Immediate physician evaluation

[a]When systolic and diastolic pressure fall into different categories, the higher category should be used to classify blood pressure status.
[b]Optimal blood pressure with respect to cardiovascular risk is below 120/80 mm Hg; however, unusually low readings should be evaluated.
[c]Based on the average of two or more readings taken at different physician visits.

SOURCE: *The Sixth Report of the Joint National Committee on Prevention, Detection, Evaluation, and Treatment of High Blood Pressure.* 1997. Bethesda, Md.: National Heart, Lung, and Blood Institute. National Institutes of Health (NIH Publication No. 98-4080).

kidney failure, and blindness. In about 90% of people with high blood pressure, the cause is unknown. So-called primary hypertension is probably due to a mixture of genetic and environmental factors, including obesity, stress, excessive alcohol intake, inactivity, and a high-fat, high-salt diet. In the remaining 10% of cases, the condition is caused by an underlying illness and is referred to as secondary hypertension.

Hypertension is common, occurring in about 1 in 4 adults. Its incidence rises dramatically with increasing age; however, it can occur among children and young adults, and women sometimes develop hypertension during pregnancy (blood pressure usually returns to normal after the baby is born).

Primary hypertension cannot be cured, but it can be controlled. The key to avoiding the complications of hypertension is to have your blood pressure checked regularly and to follow your physician's advice about lifestyle changes and medication. Unfortunately, of the estimated 50 million Americans with hypertension, only about one-third of them have it under control.

People with mild hypertension can frequently lower their blood pressure through lifestyle changes, including quitting smoking, exercising regularly, and improving diet. Controlling total calorie intake is important for achieving and maintaining a healthy body weight. Increasing intake of fruits, vegetables, and whole grains is recommended because these foods are rich in potassium and fiber, both of which may reduce blood pressure. Moderate sodium restriction can also be helpful. About half of all people with hypertension are "salt-sensitive," meaning that their blood pressure will decrease significantly when salt intake is restricted. Salt restriction has less impact on those who are not salt-sensitive, but it may still be beneficial. Most experts feel that restricting sodium intake to about 2400 mg per day is a good strategy for all people—whether they have hyper-

tension or not. For people with severe hypertension, drug therapy is usually needed in addition to lifestyle changes.

Atherosclerosis

Atherosclerosis is a slow, progressive hardening and narrowing of the arteries that can begin in childhood. Arteries become narrowed by deposits of fat, cholesterol, and other substances. As these deposits, called **plaques,** accumulate on artery walls, the arteries lose their elasticity and their ability to expand and contract, restricting blood flow. Once narrowed by a plaque, an artery is vulnerable to blockage by blood clots (Figure 15-6).

If the heart, brain, and/or other organs are deprived of blood, and thus the vital oxygen it carries, the effects of atherosclerosis can be deadly. Coronary arteries, which supply the heart with blood, are particularly susceptible to plaque buildup, a condition called **coronary heart disease (CHD),** or *coronary artery disease.* The blockage of a coronary artery causes a heart attack. If a cerebral artery (leading to the brain) is blocked, the result is a stroke.

The main risk factors for atherosclerosis are cigarette smoking, physical inactivity, high levels of blood cholesterol, and high blood pressure.

Heart Disease and Heart Attacks

Every year, about 1.1 million Americans have a heart attack (see Figure 15-5). Although a **heart attack** may come without warning, it is the end result of a long-term disease process. The most common form of heart disease is coronary artery disease caused by atherosclerosis. When one of the coronary arteries, the arteries that branch off the aorta and supply blood directly to the heart muscle, becomes blocked by a blood clot, a heart attack results. A heart attack caused by a clot is called a **coronary throm-**

Blood lipids (cholesterol)   Artery-lining cells   Platelets   Fibrous cap   Fatty core

Plaque buildup begins when excess fat particles (lipids) collect beneath cells lining the artery that have been damaged by smoking, high blood pressure, or other causes.

Platelets, components of one of the body's protective mechanisms, collect at the damaged area and cause a cap of cells to form, isolating the plaque within the artery wall.

The narrowed artery is now vulnerable to blockage by clots that can form if the cap breaks and the fatty core of the plaque combines again with platelets and other clot-producing factors in the blood.

Figure 15-6 Stages of plaque development.

bosis, a **coronary occlusion**, or a **myocardial infarction (MI)**. In myocardial infarction, part of the heart muscle (myocardium) may die from lack of oxygen. If an MI is not fatal, the heart muscle may partially repair itself.

Angina   Arteries narrowed by disease may still be open enough to deliver blood to the heart. At times, however—primarily during emotional excitement, stress, or physical exertion—the heart requires more oxygen than narrowed arteries can accommodate. When the need for oxygen exceeds the supply, chest pain, called **angina pectoris,** may occur. Angina pain is felt as an extreme tightness in the chest and heavy pressure behind the breastbone or in the shoulder, neck, arm, hand, or back. This pain, although not actually a heart attack, is a warning that the load on the heart must be reduced. Angina may be controlled in a number of ways (with drugs or surgical procedures), but its course is unpredictable. Over a period of months or years, the narrowing may go on to full blockage and a heart attack.

Arrhythmia   The pumping of the heart is controlled by electrical impulses that maintain a regular heartbeat of 60–100 beats per minute. If this electrical conduction system is disrupted, the heart may beat too quickly, too slowly, or in an irregular fashion, a condition known as **arrythmia.** Arrythmia can cause symptoms ranging from imperceptible to severe, and it can even cause sudden death. Abnormal heart rhythms can often be controlled by medications or a pacemaker to deliver electrical stimulation to the heart.

Helping a Heart Attack Victim   Most people who die from a heart attack do so within 2 hours from the time they experience the first symptoms. Unfortunately, half of all heart attack victims wait more than 2 hours before getting help. Recognizing the signals and responding immediately by getting to the nearest hospital or clinic with 24-hour emergency cardiac facilities is critical (see the box "What to Do in Case of a Heart Attack or Stroke").

If the person loses consciousness, emergency **cardiopulmonary resuscitation (CPR)** should be initiated by a qualified person. Damage to the heart muscle increases with time. If the victim gets to the emergency room quickly enough, a clot-dissolving agent can be injected to dissolve a clot in the coronary artery. These relatively new "clot-busting" drugs, such as streptokinase, urokinase, and tissue plasminogen activator (TPA), are being used successfully to treat not only heart attacks but also some types of stroke. The sooner these drugs are used, the more effective they are.

Detecting and Treating Heart Disease   Physicians have a variety of diagnostic tools to evaluate the condition of the heart and the arteries. To determine whether a person

TERMS

plaque A deposit of fatty (and other) substances on the inner wall of the arteries.

coronary heart disease (CHD) Heart disease caused by hardening of the arteries that supply oxygen to the heart muscle; also called *coronary artery disease.*

heart attack Damage to, or death of, heart muscle, sometimes resulting in a failure of the heart to deliver enough blood to the body.

coronary thrombosis A clot in a coronary artery, often causing sudden death.

coronary occlusion Partial or total obstruction of a coronary artery, as by a clot; usually resulting in myocardial infarction.

myocardial infarction (MI) A heart attack in which the heart muscle is damaged by a lack of blood supply.

angina pectoris A condition in which the heart muscle does not receive enough blood, causing severe pain in the chest and often in the left arm and shoulder.

arrhythmia A change in the normal pattern of the heartbeat.

cardiopulmonary resuscitation (CPR) A technique involving mouth-to-mouth breathing and chest compression to keep oxygen flowing to the brain.

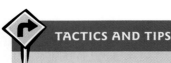
Know the Signals of a Heart Attack

- Uncomfortable pressure, fullness, squeezing, or pain in the center of the chest lasting more than a few minutes.
- Pain spreading to the shoulders, neck, or arms.
- Chest discomfort with lightheadedness, fainting, sweating, nausea, or shortness of breath.

Know the Signals of a Stroke

- Sudden weakness or numbness of the face, arm, or leg, especially on one side of the body.
- Sudden confusion or trouble speaking or understanding.
- Sudden trouble seeing in one or both eyes.
- Sudden trouble walking, dizziness, or loss of balance or coordination.
- Sudden, severe headache with no known cause.

Know What Emergency Action to Take

- *If you have symptoms:* Not all the signals listed above will occur in every heart attack or stroke, and some symptoms may come and go. If you experience one or more of these signs, don't wait. Call your emergency medical service immediately. If you can get to a hospital much faster by going yourself and not waiting for an ambulance, have someone drive you there. If you have heart attack symptoms, chew and swallow one adult aspirin tablet (325 mg).

- *If you are with someone who is having symptoms:* Take action—even if the person denies there is something wrong. Call the emergency medical services or get to the nearest hospital emergency room that offers 24-hour emergency cardiac care. Give CPR if it's necessary and you are properly trained.

SOURCE: American Heart Association (http://www.americanheart.org). © 1998 American Heart Association, Inc. All rights reserved. Used with permission.

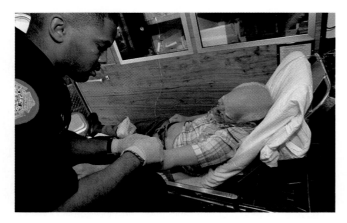

Many heart attack victims aren't sure they've had an attack and wait too long—2 hours or more—before getting help. Prompt attention from a paramedic greatly improves this man's chance of survival.

is at risk of a heart attack, the physician orders a stress or exercise test, in which the patient runs on a treadmill while being monitored for heart rhythm abnormalities with an **electrocardiogram (ECG or EKG).** Certain characteristic changes in the heart's electrical activity while under stress can reveal particular heart problems, such as restricted blood flow to the heart muscle.

Other tools enable the physician to visualize the patient's heart and arteries. **Magnetic resonance imaging (MRI)** uses powerful magnets to look inside the heart. **Radionuclide imaging** involves injecting radioactive markers into the bloodstream. The markers are taken up by the heart in areas where there is adequate blood flow. Sensitive cameras can then be used to determine if the

heart is adequately supplied with blood and its chambers are functioning properly. Other tests involve threading a catheter through arteries and into the heart. Dye is injected through the catheter; X rays are used to trace the liquid's flow. The resulting pictures, called **angiograms,** reveal the presence of any obstructions. A newer test uses a catheter tipped with a tiny ultrasound transducer. The transducer sends out a beam of sound waves that bounce off the tissue of the arteries and create pictures of the artery walls.

Various treatments, ranging from changes in diet to major surgery, are available if a problem is detected. Along with a lowfat diet, regular exercise, and smoking cessation, one frequent nonsurgical recommendation for people at high risk for CVD is to take half an aspirin tablet a day. Aspirin has an anticlotting effect, discouraging platelets in the blood from sticking to arterial plaques and forming clots; it also reduces inflammation. Prescription drugs can help control heart rate, dilate arteries, lower blood pressure, and reduce the strain on the heart—raising both quality and quantity of life in heart patients.

A common surgical procedure for treating heart disease is **balloon angioplasty.** This technique involves threading a catheter with an inflatable balloon tip through the artery until it reaches the area of blockage. The balloon is then inflated, flattening the fatty plaque and widening the arterial opening. However, repeat clogging of the artery, known as *re-stenosis,* is common.

New variations on this technique are being tried to decrease the occurrence and severity of restenosis. Surgeons have put lasers, rotating blades, drill bits, and even miniature ultrasound "jackhammers" on the tips of catheters and threaded them into blocked arteries, where

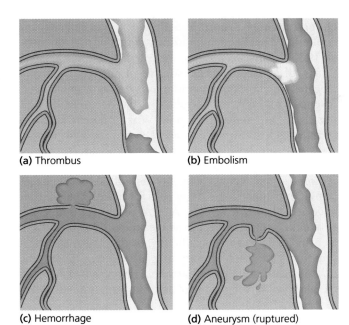

(a) Thrombus

(b) Embolism

(c) Hemorrhage

(d) Aneurysm (ruptured)

Figure 15-7   Causes of stroke.   Five out of six strokes are caused by blood clots, either (a) a thrombus or (b) an embolism. A hemorrhagic stroke (c) is more serious and occurs when a blood vessel in the brain bursts. When an aneurysm ruptures (d), a stroke results.

Types of Strokes   There are three major types of stroke. The most common is the *thrombotic stroke,* caused by a blood clot, or **thrombus,** that forms in one of the cerebral arteries (Figure 15-7). This condition, called **cerebral thrombosis,** is likely to occur when the cerebral arteries become narrowed or damaged by atherosclerosis. If a cerebral artery is clogged with plaque, the formation of clots is more likely. The risk of stroke is much higher in people with hypertension than in those with normal blood pressure, since high blood pressure accelerates the process of atherosclerosis.

A second type of stroke, an *embolic stroke,* occurs when a wandering blood clot, or **embolus,** is carried in the bloodstream and becomes wedged in one of the cerebral arteries. This event is called a **cerebral embolism.**

The third type of stroke, a *hemorrhagic stroke,* is the least common but most severe type of stroke. It occurs when a blood vessel in the brain bursts, spilling blood into the surrounding tissue and causing damage to it. When a **cerebral hemorrhage** occurs, cells normally nourished by the artery are deprived of blood and cannot

they vaporize, shave, drill, or pulverize plaques. To keep arteries open following angioplasty, many surgeons also permanently implant coronary stents—flexible, stainless steel tubes that remain in place as a framework to prop the artery open and prevent restenosis.

Every year, **coronary bypass surgery** is performed on nearly 400,000 men and women, about half of whom are under age 65. Surgeons remove a healthy blood vessel, usually a vein from one of the patient's legs, and graft it to one or more coronary arteries to bypass a blockage. A heart-lung machine maintains circulation during the surgery.

Whatever treatment is used, the person with heart disease is also advised to make behavior and lifestyle changes, such as changing the diet to improve blood cholesterol levels and quitting smoking. Otherwise, the arteries simply become clogged again, and the same problems recur a few years later.

Stroke

For brain cells to function as they should, they must have a continuous and ample supply of oxygen-rich blood. If brain cells are deprived of blood for more than a few minutes, they die. A **stroke,** also called a *cerebrovascular accident (CVA),* occurs when the blood supply to the brain is cut off. Stroke is particularly serious because brain cells, unlike those of other organs, cannot regenerate.

TERMS

electrocardiogram (ECG or EKG)   A test to detect abnormalities by measuring the electrical activity in the heart.

magnetic resonance imaging (MRI)   A computerized imaging technique that uses a strong magnetic field and radio frequency signals to examine a thin cross section of the body; also known as *nuclear magnetic resonance imaging* (NMR).

radionuclide imaging   An imaging technique that uses radioisotopes and a scanning camera to produce a pictorial representation of the radioisotope markers taken up in a particular organ, such as the heart.

angiogram   A picture of the arterial system taken after injecting a dye that is opaque to X rays; also called *arteriogram.*

balloon angioplasty   A technique in which a catheter with a balloon on the tip is inserted into an artery; the balloon is then inflated at the point of obstruction in the artery, pressing the plaque against the artery wall to improve blood supply; also known as *percutaneous transluminal coronary angioplasty* (PTCA).

coronary bypass surgery   Surgery in which a vein is grafted from a point above to a point below an obstruction in a coronary artery, improving the blood supply to the heart.

stroke   An impeded blood supply to some part of the brain resulting in the destruction of brain cells; also called *cerebrovascular accident.*

thrombus   A blood clot that forms in a blood vessel and remains attached there.

cerebral thrombosis   A clot in a vessel that supplies blood to the brain.

embolus   A blood clot that breaks off from its place of origin in a blood vessel and travels through the bloodstream.

cerebral embolism   Blockage of a blood vessel in the brain, caused by blood clots or other material carried in the blood from other parts of the body.

cerebral hemorrhage   Bleeding in or near the brain.

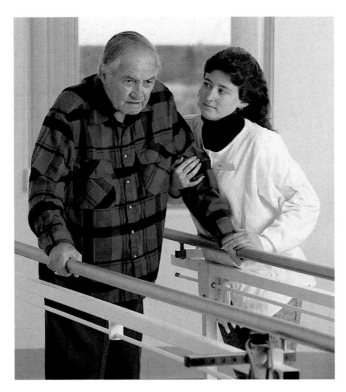

Rehabilitation after a stroke can be a long and arduous process. Complete recovery eludes many stroke victims.

Detecting and Treating Stroke   Death rates from stroke have declined significantly over the past decades. In 1950, nearly 90% of victims died; today, about two-thirds of stroke victims survive. Effective treatment requires the prompt recognition of symptoms and correct diagnosis of the type of stroke that has occurred. Signals of a stroke are listed in the box "What to Do in Case of a Heart Attack or Stroke" on p. 418. Anyone who experiences one or more of these signs should obtain emergency medical help immediately.

Some stroke victims have a **transient ischemic attack (TIA),** or ministroke, days, weeks, or months before they have a full-blown stroke. A TIA produces temporary strokelike symptoms, such as weakness or numbness in an arm or a leg, speech difficulty, or dizziness, but these symptoms are brief, often lasting just a few minutes, and do not cause permanent damage. However, TIAs should be taken as warning signs of a stroke, and anyone with a suspected TIA should get immediate medical help.

Until recently, there was very little that could be done to treat strokes. But now they should be thought of as "brain attacks" and treated with the same urgency as heart attacks. A person with stroke symptoms should be rushed to the hospital. A **computed tomography (CT)** scan, which uses a computer to construct an image of the brain from X rays, can assess brain damage and determine the type of stroke. Newer diagnostic techniques using MRI and ultrasound are becoming increasingly available and should improve the speed and accuracy of stroke diagnosis.

If tests reveal that a stroke is caused by a blood clot—and if help is sought within a few hours of the onset of symptoms—the person can be treated with the same kind of clot-dissolving drugs that are used to treat coronary artery blockages. If the clot is dissolved quickly enough, brain damage is minimized and symptoms may disappear. (The longer the brain goes without oxygen, the greater the risk of permanent damage.) Drugs that help protect healthy brain cells from the effects of stroke are currently being tested. People who have had TIAs or who are at high risk for stroke due to narrowing of the carotid arteries may undergo a procedure called *carotid endarterectomy,* in which plaque is surgically removed.

If tests reveal that a stroke was caused by a cerebral hemorrhage, drugs may be prescribed to lower the blood pressure, which will usually be high. Careful diagnosis is crucial, because administering clot-dissolving drugs to a person suffering a hemorrhagic stroke would cause more bleeding and potentially more brain damage.

If detection and treatment of stroke come too late, rehabilitation is the only treatment. Although damaged or destroyed brain tissue cannot regenerate, nerve cells in the brain can make new pathways, and some functions can be taken over by other parts of the brain. Some spontaneous recovery starts immediately after a stroke and continues for a few months.

Rehabilitation consists of various types of therapy:

function. People who suffer from both atherosclerosis and high blood pressure are more likely to suffer a cerebral hemorrhage than are those who have only one condition or neither. About two in ten strokes is caused by a brain hemorrhage rather than a blood clot.

Bleeding of an artery in the brain may also be caused by a head injury or by the bursting of an **aneurysm,** a blood-filled pocket that bulges out from a weak spot in an artery wall. Aneurysms in the brain may remain stable and never break. But when they do, the result is a stroke.

The Effects of a Stroke   The interruption of the blood supply to any area of the brain prevents the nerve cells there from functioning—in some cases, causing death. Of the 600,000 Americans who have strokes each year, nearly one-third die within a year. Those who survive usually have some lasting disability. Which parts of the body are affected depends on the area of the brain affected (Figure 15-8). Nerve cells control sensation and most of our body movements, and a stroke may cause paralysis, walking disability, speech impairment, or memory loss. The severity of the stroke and its long-term effects depend on which brain cells have been injured, how widespread the damage is, how effectively the body can restore the blood supply, and how rapidly other areas of the brain can take over.

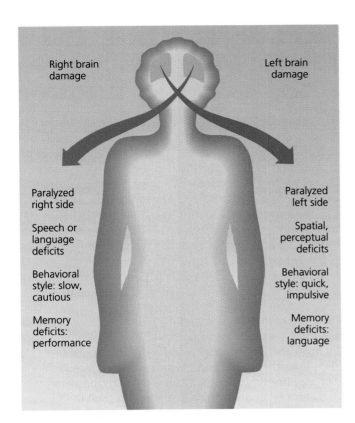

Figure 15-8 Damage caused by strokes. SOURCE: American Heart Association. 1993. *Heart and Stroke Facts.*

physical therapy, which helps strengthen muscles and improve balance and coordination; speech and language therapy, which helps those whose speech has been damaged; and occupational therapy, which helps improve hand-eye coordination and everyday living skills. Progress varies from person to person and can be unpredictable. Some people recover completely in a matter of days or weeks, but most stroke victims who survive must adapt to a lifelong disability.

Congestive Heart Failure

A number of conditions—high blood pressure, heart attack, atherosclerosis, rheumatic fever, birth defects—can damage the heart's pumping mechanism. When the heart cannot maintain its regular pumping rate and force, fluids begin to back up. When extra fluid seeps through capillary walls, edema (swelling) results, usually in the legs and ankles, but sometimes in other parts of the body as well. Fluid can collect in the lungs and interfere with breathing, particularly when a person is lying down. This condition is called **pulmonary edema,** and the entire process is known as **congestive heart failure.**

Congestive heart failure can be controlled. Treatment includes reducing the workload on the heart, modifying salt intake, and using drugs that help the body eliminate excess fluid. Drugs used to treat congestive heart failure include digitalis, which increases the pumping action of the heart; diuretics, which help the body eliminate excess salt and water; and vasodilators, which expand the blood vessels, decrease the pressure, and allow blood to flow more easily, which in turn makes the heart's work easier.

Heart Disease in Children

Although most cardiovascular disease occurs in adults—and usually in middle-aged or older adults at that—it can occur in children, usually as congenital heart disease or as a result of rheumatic fever.

Congenital Heart Disease About 32,000 children born each year in the United States have a defect or malformation of the heart or major blood vessels. These conditions are collectively referred to as **congenital heart disease,** and they cause about 5000 deaths a year.

The most common congenital defects are holes in the wall that divides the chambers of the heart. With these defects the heart produces a distinctive sound, making diagnosis relatively simple. Another defect is *coarctation of the aorta,* a narrowing, or constriction, of the aorta. Heart failure may result unless the constricted area is repaired by surgery.

Most of the common congenital defects can now be accurately diagnosed and treated with medication or surgery. Important in saving lives is early recognition that the newborn who has a bluish appearance or respiratory difficulty or who fails to thrive may be suffering from congenital heart disease.

Rheumatic Heart Disease Worldwide, a leading cause of heart trouble is **rheumatic fever,** a consequence of certain types of untreated streptococcal throat infections

TERMS

aneurysm A sac formed by a distention or dilation of the artery wall.

transient ischemic attack (TIA) A small stroke; usually a temporary interruption of blood supply to the brain, causing numbness or difficulty with speech.

computed tomography (CT) The use of computerized X-ray images to create a cross-sectional depiction (scan) of tissue density.

pulmonary edema The accumulation of fluid in the lungs.

congestive heart failure A condition resulting from the heart's inability to pump out all the blood that returns to it; blood backs up in the veins leading to the heart, causing an accumulation of fluid in various parts of the body.

congenital heart disease A defect or malformation of the heart or its major blood vessels, present at birth.

rheumatic fever A disease, mainly of children, characterized by fever, inflammation, and pain in the joints; often damages the heart muscle.

(group A ß-hemolytic). Rheumatic fever can damage the heart muscle and heart valves. Many of the approximately 70,000 operations on heart valves performed annually are related to rheumatic heart disease (RHD), and about 5000 Americans die each year from RHD.

Symptoms of strep throat are the sudden onset of a sore throat, painful swallowing, fever, swollen glands, headache, nausea, and vomiting. Careful laboratory diagnosis is important because strep throat is treated with antibiotics, which are not useful in the treatment of far more common viral sore throats. Symptoms of rheumatic fever are generally vague, but in children they include weight loss or a failure to gain weight, fever, poor appetite, repeated nosebleeds, jerky body movements, fatigue, weakness, and pain in the arms, legs, or abdomen. Rheumatic fever can be prevented by treating strep throat, when it occurs, with antibiotics.

PROTECTING YOURSELF AGAINST CARDIOVASCULAR DISEASE

There are several important steps you can take now to lower your risk of developing CVD in the future.

Eat Heart-Healthy

For most Americans, changing to a heart-healthy diet involves cutting total fat intake, substituting unsaturated fats for saturated and trans fats, and increasing fiber. Such changes can lower a person's blood levels of total cholesterol, LDL cholesterol, and triglycerides. A moderate amount of alcohol may also be beneficial for some people.

Decreased Fat and Cholesterol Intake The NCEP recommends that all Americans over the age of 2 adopt a diet in which total fat consumption is no more than 30% of total daily calories. No more than one-third of those fat calories should come from saturated fat, which is found in animal products, palm and coconut oil, and hydrogenated vegetable oils; the latter is also high in trans fats. Saturated and trans fats influence the production and excretion of cholesterol by the liver, so decreasing saturated and trans fat intake is the most important dietary change you can make to control your cholesterol (see the Behavior Change Strategy at the end of the chapter).

One-third or more of your fat calories should come from monounsaturated fats, such as olive or canola oil; consuming these oils may raise levels of beneficial HDL. Up to one-third of your fat calories should come from polyunsaturated fats; these can lower your total cholesterol level, although they may also reduce HDL slightly. By controlling your intake of total fat as well as trans and saturated fats, you can reduce your risk of cardiovascular disease.

Animal products contain cholesterol as well as saturated fat. The NCEP and AHA recommend that you limit dietary cholesterol intake to no more than 300 mg per day. However, recent studies have called into question the assumed association between dietary cholesterol and blood cholesterol. But because total fat and saturated fat are known to adversely affect blood fat levels, it is better to limit your intake of whole milk, cheese, meat, butter, and other animal products that are high in cholesterol as well as total and saturated fat. Vegetable products do not contain cholesterol. The total fat and cholesterol content of packaged foods is provided on the food label. Unfortunately, the trans fat content of foods is not currently listed on food labels; but many experts have recommended that this information be added in the future. As described in Chapter 12, you can check for the presence of trans fats by checking the list of ingredients for hydrogenated or partially hydrogenated vegetable oils.

Refer to Chapter 12 for a more complete discussion of the different types of dietary fats and their health effects.

Increased Fiber Intake Soluble fiber traps the bile acids the liver needs to manufacture cholesterol and carries them to the large intestine, where they are excreted. It also slows the production of proteins that promote blood clotting. Insoluble fiber may interfere with the absorption of dietary fat and may also help you cut total food intake because foods rich in insoluble fiber tend to be filling. Studies have shown that heart attack risk decreases by nearly 20% for each 10-gram increase in total dietary fiber intake. To obtain the recommended 20–35 grams of dietary fiber per day, choose a diet rich in whole grains, fruits, and vegetables. Good sources of fiber include oatmeal, some breakfast cereals, barley, legumes, and most fruits and vegetables.

Alcohol As described in Chapter 10, a moderate use of alcohol has been shown to increase HDL cholesterol, thereby improving heart health. Moderate alcohol use also appears to reduce the risk of stroke, possibly by dampening the inflammatory response or by affecting blood-clotting factors. ("Moderate" means no more than one drink per day for women or two drinks per day for men.) Excessive alcohol consumption, however, can lead to an increased risk of a variety of serious health problems, including hypertension, stroke, some cancers, liver disease, alcohol dependence, and injuries. For this reason, public health authorities have been unwilling to recommend alcohol use to the general public as a means of improving heart health. If you do drink, do so moderately, with food, and at times when drinking will not put you or others at risk. Refer to Chapter 10 for more on the dangers and potential benefits of moderate drinking.

Other Dietary Factors Researchers have identified other dietary factors that may affect CVD risk:

- *Omega-3 fatty acids.* Found in fish, shellfish, and some plant foods (nuts and canola, soybean, and flaxseed oils), omega-fatty acids may reduce plaque formation. Many experts recommend eating fish two or three times a week; fish oil capsules may be appropriate for some people who won't eat fish, but they add fat and calories to the diet and may raise LDL levels.

- *Vitamin E.* The antioxidant vitamin E—found in nuts, vegetable oils, wheat germ, margarine, avocados, and leafy green vegetables—may help prevent CVD by inhibiting the buildup of fatty plaques on artery walls. Many experts now recommend that people increase their intake of foods high in vitamin E.

- *Plant sterols.* Sterol compounds found in plants reduce the absorption of cholesterol in the body and may help lower LDL levels. Some new types of trans-free margarines also contain plant sterols.

- *Folic acid, vitamin B-6, and vitamin B-12.* These vitamins affect CVD risk by lowering homocysteine levels. See Chapter 12 for a list of foods rich in these vitamins and information on supplements.

- *Salt.* As described earlier, excessive salt consumption raises blood pressure in salt-sensitive people and is not recommended for anyone. Follow the Dietary Guidelines' recommendation of consuming no more than 2400 mg of sodium per day: limit your intake of processed and fast foods, choose low-sodium products, and eat plenty of naturally low-sodium foods such as fruits and vegetables.

- *Potassium and calcium.* Studies indicate that diets rich in potassium and calcium are helpful in preventing and treating hypertension; they may also decrease the risk of stroke. The best way to ensure adequate intake of these minerals is to consume the recommended number of servings of fruits, vegetables, and low-fat or nonfat dairy products. The same dietary changes that limit sodium intake usually also increase intake of potassium and calcium.

- *Soy protein.* Replacing some animal proteins with soy protein may lower LDL cholesterol. Soy-based foods include tofu and tempeh.

DASH A dietary plan that reflects many of the suggestions described here was released as part of a 1997 study called Dietary Approaches to Stop Hypertension, or DASH. The DASH study found that a diet low in fat and high in fruits, vegetables, and low-fat dairy products reduces blood pressure. (It also follows the recommendations for lowering one's risk of heart disease, cancer, and osteoporosis.) The DASH diet plan is as follows:

- 7–8 servings per day of grains and grain products
- 4–5 servings per day of vegetables
- 4–5 servings per day of fruits
- 2–3 servings per day of low-fat or nonfat dairy products

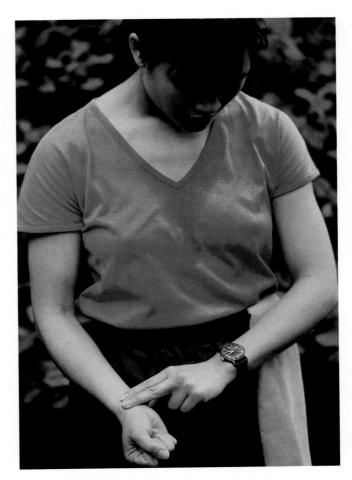

One of the primary benefits of endurance exercise is its conditioning effect on the heart and lungs. A lifetime of sensible exercise habits offers protection against cardiovascular disease later in life.

- 2 or fewer servings per day of meats, poultry, and fish
- 4–5 servings per *week* of nuts, seeds, and legumes
- 2–3 servings per day of added fats, oils, and salad dressings
- 5 servings per *week* of snacks and sweets

Before you act on new dietary advice, remember not to seize on one particular food as a cure-all for CVD (see the box "Evaluating Health News"). The fight against CVD will not be won by any single dietary change; success depends on the collective effects of your entire diet. Eat a varied, moderate diet rich in fruits, vegetables, and whole grains—the DASH diet provides a good model. And use your common sense. For example, substituting olive oil or canola oil for butter is a helpful change because it lowers saturated fat intake. But adding a new oil to your diet—without subtracting fat elsewhere—will add calories and fat and not be nearly as beneficial.

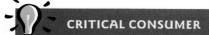
Health-related research is now described in popular newspapers and magazines rather than just medical journals, meaning that more and more people have access to the information. Greater access is certainly a plus, but news reports of research studies may oversimplify both the results and what those results mean to the average person. Researchers do not set out to mislead people, but they must often strike a balance between reporting promising preliminary findings to the public, thereby allowing people to act on them, and waiting 10–20 years until long-term studies confirm (or disprove) a particular theory.

All this can leave you in a difficult position. You cannot become an expert on all subjects, capable of effectively evaluating all the available health news. However, the following questions can help you better assess the health advice that appears in the popular media:

1. *Is the report based on research or on an anecdote?* Information or advice based on one or more carefully designed research studies has more validity than one person's experiences.

2. *What is the source of the information?* A study published in a respected peer-reviewed journal has been examined by editors and other researchers in the field, people who are in a position to evaluate the merits of a study and its results. Research presented at medical meetings should be considered very preliminary because the results have not yet undergone a thorough pre-publication review. It is also wise to ask who funded a study to determine whether there is any potential for bias. Information from government agencies and national research organizations is usually considered fairly reliable.

3. *How big was the study?* A study that involves many subjects is more likely to yield reliable results than a study involving only a few people. Another indication that a finding is meaningful is if several different studies yield the same results.

4. *Who were the subjects involved in the study?* Research findings are more likely to apply to you if you share important characteristics with the subjects of the study. For example, the results of a study on men over age 50 who smoke may not be particularly meaningful for a 30-year-old nonsmoking woman. Even less applicable are studies done in test tubes or on animals. Such research should be considered very preliminary in terms of its applicability to humans. Promising results from laboratory or animal research frequently cannot be replicated in human study subjects.

5. *What kind of study was it?* Epidemiological studies involve observation or interviews in order to trace the relationship among lifestyle, physical characteristics, and diseases. While epidemiological studies can suggest links, they cannot establish cause-and-effect relationships. Clinical or interventional studies or trials involve testing the effects of different treatments on groups of people who have similar lifestyles and characteristics. They are more likely to provide conclusive evidence of a cause-and-effect relationship. The best interventional studies share the following characteristics:

- *Controlled.* A group of people who receive the treatment is compared with a matched group who do not receive the treatment.

- *Randomized.* The treatment and control groups are selected randomly.

- *Double-blind.* Researchers and participants are unaware of who is receiving the treatment.

- *Multicenter.* The experiment is performed at more than one institution.

Some studies have characteristics of both epidemiological and interventional studies.

6. *What do the statistics really say?* First, are the results described as "statistically significant"? If a study is large and well designed, its results can be deemed statistically significant, meaning there is less than a 5% chance that the findings resulted from chance. Second, are the results stated in terms of relative or absolute risk? Many findings are reported in terms of relative risk—how a particular treatment or condition affects a person's disease risk. Consider the following examples of relative risk:

- According to some estimates, taking estrogen without progesterone can increase a postmenopausal woman's risk of dying from endometrial cancer by 233%.

- Giving AZT to HIV-infected pregnant women reduces prenatal transmission of HIV by 66%.

The first of these two findings seems far more dramatic than the second—until one also considers absolute risk, the actual risk of the illness in the population being considered. The absolute risk of endometrial cancer is 0.3%; a 233% increase based on the effects of estrogen raises it to 1%, a change of 0.7%. Without treatment, about 25% of infants born to HIV-infected women will be infected with HIV; with treatment, the absolute risk drops to about 8%, a change of 17%. Because the absolute risk of an HIV-infected mother passing the virus to her infant is so much greater than a woman's risk of developing endometrial cancer (25% compared with 0.3%), a smaller change in relative risk translates into a much greater change in absolute risk.

7. *Is new health advice being offered?* If the media report new guidelines for health behavior or medical treatment, examine the source. Government agencies and national research foundations usually consider a great deal of evidence before offering health advice. Above all, use common sense, and check with your physician before making a major change in your health habits based on news reports.

SOURCES: Medicine and the media. 1999. Harvard Women's Health Watch, February. Medical hype: How to read between the lines. 1998. *Consumer Reports on Health,* October. Making sense of health research. 1998. *Healthline,* May. Yet another study—should you pay attention? 1998. *Tufts University Health and Nutrition Letter,* September.

Exercise Regularly

You can significantly reduce your risk with a moderate amount of physical activity. Follow the guidelines for physical activity and exercise described in Chapter 13. Begin by accumulating at least 30 minutes of moderate-intensity physical activity each day. Activities like brisk walking, gardening, and stair climbing are appropriate. Increasing the duration or intensity of exercise can provide even greater health benefits. The next step, then, is to begin a formal exercise program that develops cardio-respiratory endurance and other components of fitness. There is no need to exercise too intensely, however, because very intense exercise provides little added benefit in terms of CVD prevention, although it can improve your strength, endurance, and athletic performance.

Avoid Tobacco

Remember: The number-one risk factor for CVD that you can control is smoking. If you smoke, quit. If you don't, don't start. The majority of people who start don't believe they will become hooked, but most do. If you live or work with people who smoke, encourage them to quit—for their sake and yours. Regular exposure to ETS in social settings, at home, or at work raises your risk of CVD. If you find yourself breathing in smoke, take steps to prevent or stop this exposure.

Until recently, many experts believed that 5 or more years after quitting smoking, a former smoker's CVD risk would drop to about that of a person who had never smoked. However, new research indicates that the rate of plaque formation in arteries is significantly greater in former smokers than in those who have never smoked. What seems to matter most for CVD risk is the total amount of smoking over a lifetime rather than whether a person is currently smoking. The same study also showed that people exposed to environmental tobacco smoke have a significantly higher rate of plaque formation than nonsmokers who are not exposed to ETS.

The bottom line? Quitting smoking is highly beneficial. But abstaining from cigarette smoking and avoiding ETS throughout your entire life is even better.

Know and Manage Your Blood Pressure

Currently, only about 30% of Americans with hypertension have their blood pressure under control; the *Healthy People 2010* report sets the goal of increasing this number to 50%. If you have no CVD risk factors, have your blood pressure measured at least once every two years; yearly tests are recommended if you have other risk factors. Self-administered blood pressure tests in pharmacies and other public places may be misleading and are no substitute for a test performed by a trained professional. If your blood pressure is high, follow your physician's advice on how to lower it. For those with severe hypertension, a vast array of antihypertensive medications are available.

Know and Manage Your Cholesterol Levels

Have your blood cholesterol levels measured if you've never had it done. Finger-prick tests at health fairs and other public places are generally fairly accurate, especially if they're offered by a hospital or other reputable health group. When you know your "number," follow these guidelines from the National Cholesterol Education Program (NCEP):

- *Total cholesterol below 200 mg/dl.* If your HDL is 35 mg/dl or higher and you have no other risk factors for CVD, your risk of a heart attack is relatively low. It is still a good idea to maintain a healthy lifestyle, including eating a lowfat diet, getting regular exercise, maintaining a healthy body weight, and not smoking. Get another test within 5 years.

If your HDL level is less than 35 mg/dl, you should have your LDL level measured and evaluated. Maintain a healthy lifestyle, and follow your physician's advice for controlling your risk factors and having your cholesterol levels rechecked.

- *Total cholesterol between 200 and 239 mg/dl.* If your HDL is 35 mg/dl or higher and you have fewer than two other risk factors for CVD, you may or may not be at increased risk. However, you should take steps to reduce your cholesterol by modifying your diet, increasing your physical activity, and making other positive lifestyle changes. Work with your physician to control other CVD risk factors, and have your cholesterol levels rechecked in 1–2 years.

If your HDL level is less than 35 mg/dl or you have two or more other risk factors for CVD, you may have about twice the risk of people whose levels are less than 200. You should have your LDL level checked and evaluated. To reduce your risk, modify your diet, increase your physical activity, and work with your physician to control your other risk factors. Your physician will determine how frequently you should have your cholesterol levels rechecked.

- *Total cholesterol 240 mg/dl or more.* Your risk of heart disease may be substantially higher than average. Your physician should order a more detailed cholesterol analysis and recommend therapy based on the results. Adopt a heart-healthy lifestyle immediately, including a cholesterol-improving diet and regular exercise. Follow your physician's advice for controlling other CVD risk factors, and have your cholesterol levels rechecked as recommended.

There is some disagreement among experts about the benefits of cholesterol testing and treatment for certain groups of Americans, especially young and older adults.

Of 212 clinical studies that evaluated the effect of religious commitment on health and well-being of Americans, 75% found a positive effect, according to research presented at the American Association for the Advancement of Science 1996 annual meeting. The report, sponsored by the National Institute for Health Care Research, found that religion was beneficial for both physical and psychological problems—including depression, hypertension, and heart disease—as well as overall quality of life.

The critical factor, says author Dale Matthews, M.D., of Georgetown University School of Medicine, seems to be the intensity of religious commitment: In general, those who had the greatest involvement with their church and the strongest devotion were the healthiest. For example, in one study of heart surgery patients, the death rate within 6 months of surgery was 5% for regular churchgoers, compared to a national average of 9%, and 0% for those who considered themselves "deeply religious." Overall, the report found these and other effects to be unrelated to a particular denomination.

The mechanism behind religion's apparent health benefits is still unclear, but Dr. Matthews speculates that the church provides a strong community that keeps people from becoming isolated and acts as a safety net when they are ill. Studies have consistently shown that social isolation contributes to poor health. In addition, people who are religious may have a healthier lifestyle than the general population and be less inclined to smoke and drink excessive amounts of alcohol. Research has also found that the act of worship promotes relaxation, which itself confers other health benefits. And, of course, there is the possibility that all of this is outside the realm of medical science.

"I think religion *is* good for your health," Dr. Matthews says. "But we still need to do more research to understand how this works and whether there is a healing mechanism separate from the social one."

SOURCE: Religion: Good for the body as well as the soul? 1996. *Healthnews* 2(5): 5.

However, the lifestyle recommendations for controlling cholesterol, such as regular exercise and a moderate diet, are highly recommended for everyone because of their beneficial effects both on heart health and overall wellness. If cholesterol levels remain less than optimal despite efforts at lifestyle changes, medications may be prescribed.

Develop Effective Ways to Handle Stress and Anger

To reduce the psychological and social risk factors for CVD, develop effective strategies for handling the stress in your life. Shore up your social support network, and try some of the techniques described in Chapter 2 for managing stress (see also the box "Religion and Wellness"). If anger and hostility are problems for you, try some of the tips on p. 411 for defusing your anger.

Manage Other Risk Factors and Medical Conditions

Know your CVD risk factors—take the quiz in the box "Are You at Risk for CVD?"—and follow your physician's advice for testing, lifestyle modification, and any drug treatments. If you are a postmenopausal woman, discuss the health risks and benefits of hormone replacement therapy with your physician.

If you are at high risk for CVD, consult a physician about taking small doses of aspirin. As described earlier, aspirin reduces inflammation and the blood's tendency to clot, thereby reducing the risk of CVD for some people. The recommended prescription use of aspirin for treating CVD was recently updated by the FDA. Low doses (50–325 mg) are recommended for men and women to treat TIA, stroke, angina, heart attack, and certain other cardiovascular problems. Because of possible side effects, including gastrointestinal bleeding and increased risk for certain types of strokes, the FDA cautions people to consult with their physician before taking aspirin regularly.

PERSONAL INSIGHT Have you taken any steps to lower your chances of developing CVD later in life? If you haven't, why haven't you? When do you think you will?

SUMMARY

The Cardiovascular System

- The cardiovascular system pumps and circulates blood throughout the body. The heart pumps blood to the lungs via the pulmonary artery and to the body via the aorta.

- The exchange of nutrients and waste products takes place between the capillaries and the tissues.

Risk Factors for Cardiovascular Disease

- The six major risk factors that can be changed are smoking, high blood pressure, unhealthy cholesterol levels, inactivity, obesity, and diabetes.

- Effects of smoking include lower HDL levels, increased blood pressure and heart rate, accelerated plaque formation, and increased risk of blood clots.

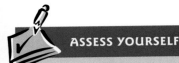

Your chances of suffering an early heart attack or stroke depend on a variety of factors, many of which are under your control. The best time to identify your risk factors and change your behavior to lower your risk is when you are young. You can significantly affect your future health and quality of life if you adopt healthy behaviors. To help identify your risk factors, circle the response for each risk category that best describes you:

1. Gender
   - 0 Female.
   - 2 Male.

2. Heredity
   - 0 Neither parent suffered a heart attack or stroke before age 60.
   - 3 One parent suffered a heart attack or stroke before age 60.
   - 7 Both parents suffered a heart attack or stroke before age 60.

3. Smoking
   - 0 Never smoked.
   - 3 Quit more than 2 years ago and lifetime smoking is less than 5 pack-years.*
   - 6 Quit less than 2 years ago and/or lifetime smoking is greater than 5 pack-years.*
   - 8 Smoke less than $1/2$ pack per day.
   - 13 Smoke more than $1/2$ pack per day.
   - 15 Smoke more than 1 pack per day.

4. Environmental Tobacco Smoke
   - 0 Do not live or work with smokers.
   - 2 Exposed to ETS at work.
   - 3 Live with a smoker.
   - 4 Both live and work with smokers.

5. Blood Pressure

   The average of the last three readings:
   - 0 130/80 or below.
   - 1 131/81–140/85.
   - 5 141/86–150/90.
   - 9 151/91–170/100.
   - 13 Above 170/100.

6. Total Cholesterol

   The average of the last three readings:
   - 0 Lower than 190.
   - 1 190–210.
   - 2 Don't know.
   - 3 211–240.
   - 4 241–270.
   - 5 271–300.
   - 6 Over 300.

7. HDL Cholesterol

   The average of the last three readings:
   - 0 Over 65 mg/dl.
   - 1 55–65.
   - 2 Don't know HDL.
   - 3 45–54.
   - 5 35–44.
   - 7 25–34.
   - 12 Lower than 25.

8. Exercise
   - 0 Aerobic exercise three times a week.
   - 1 Aerobic exercise once or twice a week.
   - 2 Occasional exercise less than once a week.
   - 7 Rarely exercise.

9. Diabetes
   - 0 No personal or family history.
   - 2 One parent with diabetes.
   - 6 Two parents with diabetes.
   - 9 Non–insulin-dependent diabetes.
   - 13 Insulin-dependent diabetes.

10. Weight
   - 0 Near ideal weight.
   - 1 6 pounds or less above ideal weight.
   - 3 7–19 pounds above ideal weight.
   - 5 20–40 pounds above ideal weight.
   - 7 More than 40 pounds above ideal weight.

11. Stress
   - 0 Relaxed most of the time.
   - 1 Occasional stress and anger.
   - 2 Frequently stressed and angry.
   - 3 Usually stressed and angry.

Scoring

Total your risk factor points. Refer to the list below to get an approximate rating of your risk of suffering an early heart attack or stroke.

Score	Estimated Risk
Less than 20	Low risk
20–29	Moderate risk
30–45	High risk
Over 45	Extremely high risk

*Pack-years can be calculated by multiplying the number of packs you smoked per day by the number of years you smoked. For example, if you smoked a pack and a half a day for 5 years, you would have smoked the equivalent of 1.5 × 5 = 7.5 pack-years.

The American Heart Association recommends that no more than 10% of the calories in your diet come from saturated fat. Foods from animals that have the highest amounts of saturated fat include beef, veal, lamb, pork, lard, poultry skin and fat, butter, cream, whole milk, cheese, and other dairy products made from whole milk. Most plant foods are low in saturated fat, but there are a few exceptions: coconut and palm oils, cocoa butter, and hydrogenated vegetable oils.

Monitor Your Current Diet

To see how your diet measures up, monitor yourself for a week, keeping track of everything you eat in your health journal. Information about the calorie and fat content of the foods you eat is available on many food labels, in books and on the World Wide Web (see Chapter 12). You can use Appendix A in this text to look up nutritional information for many fast-food items.

At the end of the week, enter the calories and grams of saturated fat for each of the foods you've eaten. For foods that contain saturated fat, compute the percentage of calories from saturated fat: Multiply grams of saturated fat by 9 and divide the product by the total calories in the food. (Remember, all types of fat contain 9 calories per gram.) Repeat the calculations for each day (based on total grams of saturated fat and total calorie intake) and for the week. How close do the daily and weekly percentages you've calculated come to the goal of 10% or fewer calories from saturated fat?

Making Heart-Healthy Changes

If your diet includes more than your fair share of saturated fat, you can take steps to reduce it. Set an overall limit on saturated fat based on the total calories you typically consume. For example, if your daily diet contains about 2000 calories, no more than 200 calories (10% of 2000) should come from saturated fat. (This corresponds to about 20 grams of saturated fat per day.) Then try keeping a running daily total of saturated fat intake, and manage your food choices accordingly. For example, if your lunch includes a fatty hamburger, you can choose a dinner low in saturated fat and still stay within the daily limit you've set for yourself.

Take a close look at your food record. What are the leading sources of saturated fat in your diet? Do you choose many foods high in saturated fat, or is it your portion sizes that are causing problems? Do you usually go for hamburgers, hot dogs, steaks, and chips? Choose lean meat, chicken, or fish instead. Do you have a salami and cheese on rye for lunch? Try turkey for a change. Is ice cream your downfall? Fruit and yogurt are delicious alternatives (see the table for more substitution ideas). When you do choose foods that are rich in saturated fats, watch your portion sizes carefully (see Chapter 12). Choose cuts of meat that have the least amount of visible fat, and trim off what you see. Choose only lean ground beef, and drain the fat after cooking. Remove the skin from poultry.

If there is a lot of saturated fat in your diet, you may have to change some of your habits for a while. You may have to avoid fast-food restaurants or skip going for pizza at night with your friends. Put your best effort into finding appealing, satisfying, and enjoyable activities as substitutes, such as trying out restaurants that serve lowfat dishes. If you can recruit some friends to join you in your campaign, it will be easier to stick with it.

Remember, cardiovascular disease often starts when people are in their teens or early twenties. By making a conscious effort to establish a healthy diet and cut down on saturated fat now, you'll be doing yourself a favor that will give you benefits for your whole life.

- High LDL and low HDL cholesterol levels contribute to clogged arteries and increase the risk of CVD.

- Physical inactivity, obesity, and diabetes are interrelated and are associated with high blood pressure and unhealthy cholesterol levels.

- Contributing risk factors that can be changed include high triglyceride levels and psychological and social factors such as high levels of stress, a hostile personality, lack of social support, and low income.

- Risk factors for CVD that can't be changed include being over 65, being male, being African American, and having a family history of CVD.

- Possible risk factors under study include homocysteine, lipoprotein(a), LDL particle size, infectious agents, and inflammation.

Major Forms of Cardiovascular Disease

- Hypertension occurs when blood pressure exceeds normal limits most of the time. It weakens the heart, scars and hardens arteries, and can damage the eyes and kidneys.

- Atherosclerosis is a progressive hardening and narrowing of arteries that can lead to restricted blood flow and even complete blockage. Plaques form from deposits of fat, cholesterol, and other substances.

- Heart attacks are usually the result of a long-term disease process. Warning signs of a heart attack include angina pectoris and arrhythmia.

- A stroke occurs when the blood supply to the brain is cut off by a blood clot or hemorrhage. A transient ischemic attack (TIA) is a warning sign of stroke.

- Congestive heart failure occurs when the heart's pumping action becomes less efficient and fluid collects in the lungs or in other parts of the body.

- Heart disease in children is usually the result of rheumatic fever or a congenital defect in the heart or major blood vessels.

Switch from	Switch to
Meat, poultry, seafood	
Hamburger, meatloaf	Ground turkey breast, veggie burger
T-bone, rib eye, prime rib, etc.	Round steak, sirloin
Pork chops, ribs	Pork tenderloin
Regular hot dog, bologna, sausage, etc.	Fat-free or lowfat hot dog, bologna, sausage, etc.
Poultry with skin	Skinless poultry
Fried chicken or fish	Broiled, grilled, or roasted chicken or fish
Chicken thigh, wing	Chicken breast, drumstick
Dairy products	
Whole or reduced fat (2%) milk	lowfat (1%) or fat-free milk
Regular cheese	Reduced-fat or lowfat cheese
Regular ice cream	Lowfat or fat-free ice cream or frozen yogurt
Regular cream cheese	Light or fat-free cream cheese
Sweets and desserts	
Cheesecake, cheese danish, croissant, cinnamon roll, brownie, pie, regular or gourmet ice cream, fudge brownie sundae, doughnut, pound cake	Fruit or *small* serving of a lowfat sweet (muffin, cake, cookie, pie, pastry, ice cream, frozen yogurt, sherbet, sorbet, etc.)
Snacks	
Chocolate bar, sandwich crackers, ice cream, Bugles, popcorn popped in coconut oil	Fruits, vegetables, whole-grain crackers, "light" popcorn, pretzels, baked potato chips, corn chips, rice cakes
Condiments	
Butter or margarine, sour cream	Whipped light butter, lower-fat tub margarine, fat-free or low-fat sour cream

SOURCE: Table copyright © 1997, Center for Science in the Public Interest. Adapted from *Nutrition Action Healthletter* (1875 Connecticut Ave., N.W., Suite 300, Washington, DC 20009-5728. $24 for 10 issues).

Protecting Yourself Against Cardiovascular Disease

- Dietary changes that can protect against CVD include decreasing your intake of fat, saturated fat, trans fat, and cholesterol; increasing your intake of fiber; and drinking alcohol in moderation.

- CVD risk can also be reduced by engaging in regular exercise, not smoking cigarettes and avoiding environmental tobacco smoke, knowing and managing your blood pressure and cholesterol levels, developing effective ways of handling stress and anger, and managing other risk factors and medical conditions.

TAKE ACTION

1. The CPR courses given by the American Red Cross and other groups provide invaluable training that may help you save a life some day. Anyone can take these courses and become qualified to perform CPR. Investigate CPR courses in your community, and sign up to take one.

2. Do some research into your family medical history. Is there cardiovascular disease in your family, as indicated by premature deaths from heart attack, stroke, or congestive heart failure? Such a history is a risk factor for you. Keep that in mind as you consider whether you need to make lifestyle changes to avoid CVD.

1. If the hostility quiz in the box "Hostility and CVD" indicates that you may have a hostile personality, examine your thoughts and behavior more carefully. In your health journal, keep track of your cynical thoughts, angry feelings, and aggressive acts. For each entry, include the time, place, and cause of your cynical thoughts; what thoughts actually went through your head; the emotions you felt; and any actions you took. Review your journal at the end of a week to learn more about the frequency and kinds of situations that trigger these thoughts and behaviors.

2. *Critical Thinking* How much responsibility does an individual have for his or her health? Do people have an obligation to take care of themselves as best they can to help avoid becoming a burden on their family and on society? Do people have a right to choose whatever lifestyle they want—no matter how unhealthy? In your health journal, write an essay describing your opinion about individual responsibility for good health. Be sure to explain your reasoning.

FOR MORE INFORMATION

Books

American Heart Association. 1998. *American Heart Association Guide to Heart Attack Treatment, Recovery, and Prevention.* New York: Times Books. *A clear discussion of CVD—who is at risk, what the warning signs are, what treatments are available, and what lifestyle changes are recommended.*

American Heart Association and American Cancer Society. 1999. *Living Well, Staying Well: The Ultimate Guide to Help Prevent Heart Disease and Cancer.* New York: Times Books. *Provides practical, easy-to-follow guidelines to help you reduce your risk of developing CVD and cancer.*

Carlson, K. J., S. A. Eisenstat, and T. Ziporyn. 1997. *The Women's Concise Guide to a Healthier Heart.* Boston: Harvard University Press. *A guide to the causes, prevention, and treatment of CVD in women.*

Kwiterovich, P. O. 1998. *The Johns Hopkins Complete Guide to Preventing and Reversing Heart Disease.* Rocklin, Calif.: Prima. *A clear explanation of CVD risk factors and how to modify them.*

Ornish, D. 1998. *Love and Survival: The Scientific Basis for the Healing Power of Intimacy.* New York: HarperCollins. *Written by a researcher known for using diet, exercise, and stress management to treat heart disease, this book focuses on the role of intimacy in promoting good health.*

Williams, V., and R. Williams. 1998. *Lifeskills.* New York: Times Books. *An exploration of why relationships are essential for physical health, with practical tips for improving your interactions with others; written by the authors of* Anger Kills, *which focuses on why hostility is dangerous to heart health.*

Organizations and Web Sites

American Heart Association. Provides information on hundreds of topics relating to the prevention and control of cardiovascular disease; sponsors a general Web site as well as several sites focusing on specific topics.
7272 Greenville Ave.
Dallas, TX 75231
800-AHA-USA1 (general information)
888-MY-HEART (women's health information)
800-553-6321 (Stroke Connection)
http://www.americanheart.org (general information)
http://www.deliciousdecisions.org (dietary advice)
http://www.justmove.org (fitness advice)
http://women.americanheart.org (women and CVD)

Cardiology Compass. An index and links to cardiovascular information on the Internet.
http://www.cardiologycompass.com

Dietary Approaches to Stop Hypertension (DASH). Provides information about the design, diets, and results of the DASH study, including tips on how to follow the DASH diet at home.
http://dash.bwh.harvard.edu

Franklin Institute Science Museum/The Heart: An On-Line Exploration. An online museum exhibit containing information on the structure and function of the heart, how to monitor your heart's health, and how to maintain a healthy heart.
http://www.fi.edu/biosci/heart.html

Heart Disease Prevention System. Provides educational materials on improving lifestyle for heart health, including information on smoking cessation, low-fat diets, and exercise.
http://www.fammed.wisc.edu/research/heart

HeartInfo—Heart Information Network. Provides information for heart patients and others interested in learning how to identify and reduce their risk factors for heart disease; includes links to many related sites.
http://www.heartinfo.org

HeartPoint. Presents news, information, and tips relating to heart health.
http://www.heartpoint.com

National Heart, Lung, and Blood Institute. Provides information on a variety of topics relating to cardiovascular health and disease, including cholesterol, smoking, obesity, and hypertension; Web site has special fact sheets covering women and heart disease.
P.O. Box 30105
Bethesda, MD 20824
800-575-WELL
http://www.nhlbi.nih.gov/nhlbi/nhlbi.htm
http://rover.nhlbi.nih.gov/chd

National Stroke Association. Provides information and referrals for stroke victims and their families; the Web site has a stroke risk assessment.
96 Inverness Drive East, Suite I
Englewood, CO 80112
800-STROKES
http://www.stroke.org

See also the listings for Chapters 2 and 12–14.

SELECTED BIBLIOGRAPHY

American Heart Association. 1999. *1999 Heart and Stroke Statistical Update.* Dallas, Tex.: American Heart Association.

American Heart Association. 1998. *Risk Factors and Coronary Heart Disease: AHA Scientific Position* (retrieved January 22, 1999; http://www.americanheart.org/ Heart_and_Stroke_A_Z_Guide/riskfact.html).

Bots, M. L., et al. 1999. Homocysteine and short-term risks of myocardial infarction and stroke in the elderly. *Archives of Internal Medicine* 159: 38–44.

Caplan, L. R. 1998. Stroke treatment: Promising but still struggling. *Journal of the American Medical Association* 279(16): 1304–1306.

Carney, R., et al. 1998. New CAD risk factors: Interesting, but how useful? *Patient Care* 32(11): 134–165.

Cooper, R. S., C. N. Rotimi, and R. Ward. 1999. The puzzle of hypertension in African-Americans. *Scientific American* 280(2): 56–63.

Dunn, M. I., et al. 1998. Cause or coincidence: *C. pneumoniae* and CAD. *Patient Care* 32(13): 89–96.

Eckel, R. H., and R. M. Krauss. 1998. Obesity as a major risk factor for coronary heart disease. *Circulation* 97(21): 2099–2100.

Ford, D. E., et al. 1998. Depression is a risk factor for coronary artery disease in men. *Archives of Internal Medicine* 158: 1422–1426.

Gorelick, P. B., et al. 1999. Prevention of a first stroke. *Journal of the American Medical Association* 281: 1112–1120.

Gotto, A. M., Jr. 1998. Impact of multiple risk factors on coronary artery disease: Beyond total cholesterol. *American Journal of Cardiology* 82(9A): 1Q–2Q.

Henkel, J. 1999. Keeping cholesterol under control. *FDA Consumer,* January.

Howard, G., et al. 1998. Cigarette smoking and progression of atherosclerosis. *Journal of the American Medical Association* 337(21): 1491–1499.

Hulley, S., et al. 1998. Randomized trial of estrogen plus progestin for secondary prevention of CHD in postmenopausal women. *Journal of the American Medical Association* 280: 605–613.

Kaplan, N. 1998. *Clinical Hypertension.* Baltimore: Williams & Wilkins.

Klipstein-Grobusch, K., et al. 1999. Dietary iron and risk of myocardial infarction in the Rotterndam Study. *American Journal of Epidemiology* 149(5): 421–428.

Knox, S. S., et al. 1998. Hostility, social support, and coronary heart disease in the NHLBI Family Heart Study. *American Journal of Cardiology* 82(10): 1192–1196.

Koenig, W., et al. 1999. C-reactive protein, a marker of inflammation, predicts future risk of coronary heart disease in initially healthy middle-aged men. *Circulation* 99(2): 237–242.

Lee, I., and R. S. Paffenbarger. 1998. Physical activity and stroke incidence. *Stroke* 29: 2049–2054.

Lloyd-Jones, D. M., et al. 1999. Lifetime risk of developing coronary heart disease. *Lancet* 353(9147): 89–92.

Lowe, L. P., et al. 1998. Impact of major CVD risk factors, particularly in combination, on 22-year mortality in women and men. *Archives of Internal Medicine* 158: 2007–2014.

Malinow, M. R., A. G. Bostom, and R. M. Krauss. 1999. Homocyst(e)ine, diet and cardiovascular diseases: A statement from the Nutrition Committee, American Heart Association. *Circulation* 99(1): 178–182.

Maron, D., et al. 1998. Current strategies for the primary prevention of CAD. *Patient Care* 32(19): 19–38.

Marrugat, J., et al. 1998. Mortality differences between men and women following first myocardial infarction. *Journal of the American Medical Association* 280: 1405–1409.

O'Connor, R. E., P. McGraw, and L. Edelsohn. 1999. Thrombolytic therapy for acute ischemic stroke. *Annals of Emergency Medicine* 33(1): 9–14.

Ornish, D., et al. 1998. Intensive lifestyle changes for reversal of coronary heart disease. *Journal of the American Medical Association* 280: 2001–2007.

Pickering, T. G. 1999. Advances in the treatment of hypertension. *Journal of the American Medical Association* 281: 114–116.

Prescription labels for aspirin will address heart disease. 1999. *FDA Consumer,* January.

Rexrode, K. M. 1998. Abdominal adiposity and coronary heart disease in women. *Journal of the American Medical Association* 280(21): 1843–1848.

Ross, R. 1999. Atherosclerosis—an inflammatory disease. *New England Journal of Medicine* 340(2): 115–126.

Salonen, J. T., et al. 1998. Donation of blood is associated with reduced risk of myocardial infarction. *American Journal of Epidemiology* 148(5): 445–451.

Schauer, J., et al. 1998. Atherosclerotic vascular disease prevention: Advances in risk factor management. *Family Practice Recertification* 20(10): 13–35.

Strong, J. P., et al. 1999. Prevalence and extent of atherosclerosis in adolescents and young adults. *Journal of the American Medical Association* 281: 727–735.

Suarez, E. C., et al. 1998. Neuroendocrine, cardiovascular, and emotional responses of hostile men: The role of interpersonal challenge. *Psychosomatic Medicine* 60(1): 78–88.

Svetkey, L. P., et al. 1999. Effects of dietary patterns on blood pressure. *Archives of Internal Medicine* 159: 285–293.

Vaccarino, V., et al. 1998. Sex differences in mortality after myocardial infarction. *Archives of Internal Medicine* 158: 2054–2062.

Wamala, S. P., et al. 1999. Potential explanations for the educational gradient in coronary heart disease. *American Journal of Public Health* 89(3): 315–321.

Wannamethee, S. G., et al. 1998. Hypertension, serum insulin, obesity, and the metabolic syndrome. *Journal of Human Hypertension* 12(11): 735–741.

Watkins, L. L., and P. Grossman. 1999. Association of depressive symptoms with reduced baroreflex cardiac control in coronary artery disease. *American Heart Journal* 137(3): 453–457.

What you should know about cholesterol. 1999. *Journal of the American Medical Association* 281(2): 113.

Winkleby, M. A., et al. 1998. Ethnic and socioeconomic differences in cardiovascular disease risk factors. *Journal of the American Medical Association* 280(4): 356–362.

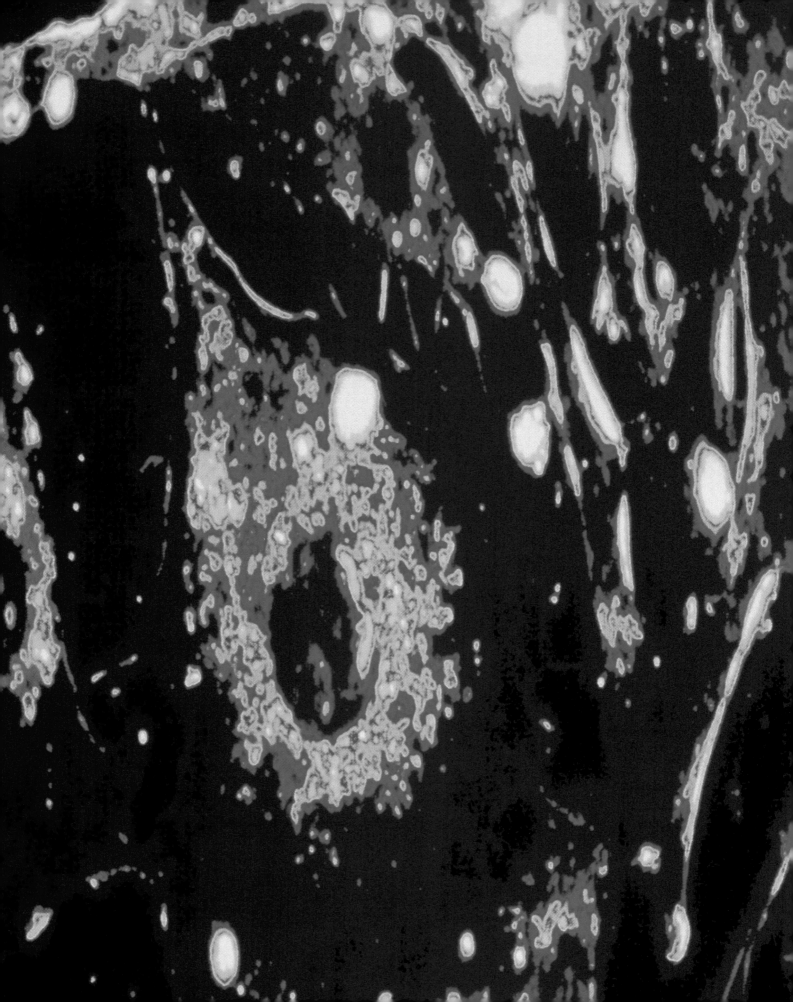

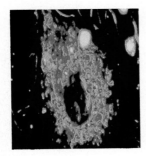

LEARNING OBJECTIVES

After reading this chapter, you should be able to:

- Explain what cancer is and how it spreads.

- List and describe common cancers—their risk factors, signs and symptoms, treatments, and approaches to prevention.

- Discuss some of the causes of cancer and how they can be avoided or minimized.

- Describe how cancer can be detected, diagnosed, and treated.

- List specific actions you can take to lower your risk of cancer.

Cancer

16

TEST YOUR KNOWLEDGE

1. Which type of cancer kills the most women each year?
   - a. breast cancer
   - b. lung cancer
   - c. ovarian cancer

2. What is the most common cancer in men under age 30?
   - a. skin cancer
   - b. oral cancer
   - c. testicular cancer

3. The use of condoms during sexual intercourse can prevent cancer in women.
   True or false?

4. Using a sunscreen with an SPF rating of 15 means that you
   - a. can stay in the sun for 15 minutes without getting burned.
   - b. can stay in the sun 15 times longer without getting burned than if you didn't use it.
   - c. are protected against the full range of ultraviolet (UV) radiation.

5. If you test positive for a cancer-related gene, it means that you'll definitely develop cancer at some point in your life?
   True or false?

Answers

1. *b.* There are more cases of breast cancer each year, but lung cancer kills more women. Smoking is the primary risk factor for lung cancer.

2. *c.* Although rare, testicular cancer is the most common cancer in men under age 30. All men should perform regular self-exams to aid in its detection.

3. *True.* The primary cause of cervical cancer is infection with human papillo-mavirus (HPV), a sexually transmitted pathogen. The use of condoms helps prevent HPV infection.

4. *b.* Choose a sunscreen that has an SPF rating of 15 or higher and that protects against both UVA and UVB rays. Apply it generously; most people use less than half the recommended amount.

5. *False.* Testing positive for a cancer-related gene may indicate higher risk, but it doesn't guarantee cancer will develop just as a negative test doesn't guarantee you'll remain cancer-free. A healthy lifestyle is the best protection against cancer.

*C*ancer is a word derived from the Greek for crab, *karki-nos*. The early Greek physicians who first described cancerous tumors had no notion of their cause or true nature, but they were struck by the resemblance of some invasive tumors to crabs: a hard mass with clawlike extensions and an aggressive nature. Today, though we know a great deal about cancer, the old metaphor still has power; cancer has maintained its reputation as an alien presence in the body, capable of causing pain and great harm. Cancer causes more than 550,000 deaths in the United States each year, and it is the second most common cause of death, after heart disease.

While medical science struggles to find cures for the various cancers that plague us, evidence indicates that more than half of all cancers in the United States could be prevented by simple changes in lifestyle. Tobacco use is responsible for about one-third of all cancer deaths (Table 16-1). Diet and exercise habits, including their effect on obesity, account for another large proportion of cancer deaths. Although cancer is primarily a disease of older adults, your behavior now will determine your cancer risk in the future. Experts estimate that through changes in lifestyle, most Americans can cut their lifetime cancer risk in half.

WHAT IS CANCER?

Cancer is the abnormal, uncontrolled growth of cells, which if left untreated, can ultimately cause death.

Benign Versus Malignant Tumors

Most cancers take the form of tumors, although not all tumors are cancerous. A tumor is simply a mass of tissue that serves no physiological purpose. It can be benign, like a wart, or malignant, like most lung cancers. The term **malignant tumor** (or *neoplasm*) is synonymous with cancer.

Benign tumors are made up of cells similar to the surrounding normal cells and are enclosed in a membrane that prevents them from penetrating neighboring tissues. They are dangerous only if their physical presence interferes with body functions. A benign brain tumor, for example, can cause death if it blocks the blood supply to the brain.

A malignant tumor, or cancer, is capable of invading surrounding structures, including blood vessels, the **lymphatic system,** and nerves. It can also spread to distant sites via the blood and lymphatic circulation, thereby producing invasive tumors in almost any part of the body. A few cancers, like leukemia, cancer of the blood, do not produce a mass and therefore are not properly called tumors. But since leukemia cells do have the fundamental property of rapid, uncontrolled growth, they are still malignant and therefore cancers.

VITAL STATISTICS

TABLE 16-1   *Causes of Cancer*

Risk Factor	Percentage of All Cancer Deaths Linked to Risk Factor
Tobacco	30
Diet and obesity	30
Sedentary lifestyle	5
Family history of cancer	5
Occupational factors	5
Viruses and other biological agents	5
Alcohol	3
Environmental pollution	2
Ultraviolet radiation	2

SOURCE: Harvard Center for Cancer Prevention. 1996. *Harvard Report on Cancer Prevention. Vol. 1: Causes of Human Cancer.*

Every case of cancer begins as a change in a cell that allows it to grow and divide when it should not. Normally (in adults), cells divide and grow at a rate just sufficient to replace dying cells. When you cut your finger, for example, the cells around the wound divide more rapidly to heal the wound. When the wound is healed, the rate of cell growth and division returns to normal. In contrast, a malignant cell divides without regard for normal control mechanisms and gradually produces a mass of abnormal cells, or a tumor. It takes about a billion cells to make a mass the size of a pea, so a single tumor cell must go through many divisions, often taking years, before the tumor grows to a noticeable size.

Eventually a tumor produces a sign or symptom that is determined by its location in the body. In the breast, for example, a tumor may be felt as a lump and diagnosed as cancer by an X ray or **biopsy.** In less accessible locations, like the lung, ovary, or intestine, a tumor may be noticed only after considerable growth has taken place and may then be detected only by an indirect symptom—for instance, a persistent cough or unexplained bleeding or pain. In the case of leukemia, there is no lump, but the changes in the blood will eventually be noticed as increasing fatigue, infection, or abnormal bleeding.

How Cancer Spreads: Metastasis

Metastasis, the spreading of cancer cells, occurs because cancer cells do not stick to each other as strongly as normal cells do and therefore may not remain at the site of

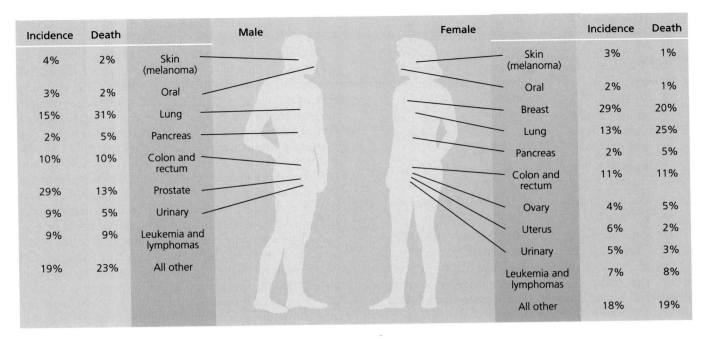

Incidence	Death	Male	Female	Incidence	Death
4%	2%	Skin (melanoma)	Skin (melanoma)	3%	1%
3%	2%	Oral	Oral	2%	1%
15%	31%	Lung	Breast	29%	20%
2%	5%	Pancreas	Lung	13%	25%
10%	10%	Colon and rectum	Pancreas	2%	5%
29%	13%	Prostate	Colon and rectum	11%	11%
9%	5%	Urinary	Ovary	4%	5%
9%	9%	Leukemia and lymphomas	Uterus	6%	2%
19%	23%	All other	Urinary	5%	3%
			Leukemia and lymphomas	7%	8%
			All other	18%	19%

VITAL STATISTICS

Figure 16-1   Cancer incidence and deaths by site and sex.   The Incidence column indicates what percentage of all cancers occurred in each site; the Death column indicates what percentage of all cancer deaths were attributed to each type.   SOURCE: American Cancer Society, 1999. *Cancer Facts and Figures, 1999.* Atlanta, Ga.: American Cancer Society.

the *primary tumor,* the original location. They break away and can pass through the lining of lymph or blood vessels to invade nearby tissue. They can also drift to distant parts of the body, where they establish new colonies of cancer cells. This traveling and seeding process is called metastasizing, and the new tumors are called *secondary tumors,* or *metastases.*

Traveling cancer cells can follow two courses. They can produce secondary tumors in the lymph nodes and be carried through the lymph system to form secondary sites elsewhere, or they can invade blood vessels and circulate through the vessels to colonize other organs. This ability of cancer cells to metastasize makes early cancer detection critical. To control the cancer and prevent death, every cancerous cell must be removed. Once cancer cells enter either the lymphatic system or the bloodstream, it is extremely difficult to stop their spread to other organs of the body. In fact, counting the number of lymph nodes that contain cancer cells is one of the principal methods of predicting the outcome of the disease; the probability of a cure is much greater when the lymph nodes do not contain cancer cells.

Types of Cancer

The behavior of tumors arising in different body organs is characteristic of the tissue of origin. (Figure 16-1 shows the major cancer sites and the incidence of each type.) Because each cancer begins as a single (altered) cell with a specific function in the body, the cancer will retain some of the properties of the normal cell for a time. For instance, cancer of the thyroid gland may produce too much thyroid hormone and cause hyperthyroidism as well as cancer. Usually, however, cancer cells lose their resemblance to normal tissue as they continue to divide, becoming groups of rogue cells with increasingly unpredictable behavior.

Malignant tumors are classified according to the types of cells that give rise to them:

TERMS

cancer   Abnormal, uncontrolled cellular growth.

malignant tumor   A tumor that is cancerous and capable of spreading.

benign tumor   A tumor that is not cancerous.

lymphatic system   A system of vessels that returns proteins, lipids, and other substances from fluid in the tissues to the circulatory system.

biopsy   The removal and examination of a small piece of body tissue; a needle biopsy uses a needle to remove a small sample; some biopsies require surgery.

metastasis   The spread of cancer cells from one part of the body to another.

- **Carcinomas** arise from **epithelia,** tissues that cover external body surfaces, line internal tubes and cavities, and form the secreting portion of glands. They are the most common type of cancers; major sites include the skin, breast, uterus, prostate, lungs, and gastrointestinal tract.
- **Sarcomas** arise from connective and fibrous tissues like muscle, bone, cartilage, and the membranes covering muscles and fat.
- **Lymphomas** are cancers of the lymph nodes, part of the body's infection-fighting system.
- **Leukemias** are cancers of the blood-forming cells, which reside chiefly in the **bone marrow.**

There is a great deal of variation in how easily different cancers can be detected and how well they respond to treatment. For example, certain types of skin cancer are easily detected, grow slowly, and are very easy to remove; virtually all of the 1 million cases that occur each year in the United States are cured. Cancer of the pancreas, on the other hand, is very difficult to detect or treat, and very few patients survive the disease. In general, it is very difficult for an **oncologist** to predict how a specific tumor will behave because every tumor arises from a unique set of changes in a single cell.

The Incidence of Cancer

Each year, about 1.2 million people in the United States are diagnosed with cancer. More than half will be cured, but about 40% will eventually die as a result of their cancer. These grim statistics exclude more than 1 million cases of the curable types of skin cancer. At current U.S. rates, about 1 in 2 men and 1 in 3 women will develop cancer at some point in their lives.

Are cancer deaths increasing in the United States? Until 1991, the answer was yes, largely due to a wave of lethal lung cancers among men caused by smoking. In 1991, the death rate stopped increasing and began to fall slowly; it has dropped 3% since 1990. This is a very promising trend, as it suggests that efforts at prevention, early detection, and improved therapy are all bearing fruit. Experts estimate that if these trends continue, we may see a decline in death rates of as much as 15–50% over the next 20 years.

Could more people be saved from cancer? The American Cancer Society (ACS) estimates that 90% of skin cancer could be prevented by protecting the skin from the rays of the sun and 87% of lung cancer could be prevented by avoiding exposure to tobacco smoke. Thousands of cases of colon, breast, and uterine cancer could be prevented by improving the diet and controlling body weight. Regular screenings and self-examinations have the potential to save an additional 100,000 lives per year. Although cancer may seem like a mysterious disease, there are many concrete strategies you can adopt to reduce your risk.

> **PERSONAL INSIGHT** Has anyone in your family had cancer or died of cancer? If so, how was it handled? What were you told about it? How do you think it has affected you?

COMMON CANCERS

A discussion of all types of cancer is beyond the scope of this book. In this section we look at some of the most common cancers and their causes, prevention, and treatment.

Lung Cancer

Lung cancer is the most common cause of cancer death in the United States; it is responsible for about 160,000 deaths each year. For over 40 years, breast cancer was the major cause of cancer death in women, but since 1987, lung cancer has surpassed breast cancer as a killer of women.

Risk Factors The chief risk factor for lung cancer is tobacco smoke, which accounts for 87% of cancers. (Other negative effects of tobacco smoke on the lungs were discussed in detail in Chapter 11.) When smoking is combined with exposure to other environmental **carcinogens,** such as asbestos particles, the risk of cancer can be multiplied by a factor of 10 or more.

The smoker is not the only one at risk. In 1993, the U.S. Environmental Protection Agency (EPA) classified environmental tobacco smoke (ETS) as a human carcinogen. Long-term exposure to ETS increases risk for lung

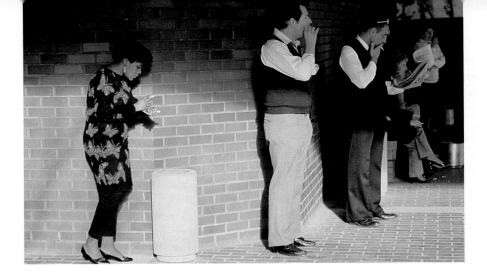

Smoking is responsible for about 30% of all cancer deaths. The benefits of quitting are substantial: Lung cancer risk decreases significantly after one smoke-free year and drops to half that of continuing smokers after 10 smoke-free years.

cancer. Secondhand smoke, the smoke from the burning end of the cigarette, has significantly higher concentrations of the toxic and carcinogenic compounds found in mainstream smoke. It is estimated that ETS causes about 3000 lung cancer deaths each year.

Detection and Treatment Lung cancer is difficult to detect at an early stage and hard to cure even when detected early. Symptoms of lung cancer do not usually appear until the disease has advanced to the invasive stage. Signals such as a persistent cough, chest pain, or recurring bronchitis may be the first indication of a tumor's presence. A diagnosis can usually be made by chest X ray or by studying the cells in sputum. Because almost all lung cancers arise from the cells that line the bronchi, tumors can sometimes be visualized by fiber-optic bronchoscopy, a test in which a flexible lighted tube is inserted into the windpipe and the surfaces of the lung passages are directly inspected.

Treatment for lung cancer depends on the type and stage of the cancer. If caught early, localized cancers can be treated with surgery. But because only about 15% of lung cancers are detected before they spread, radiation and **chemotherapy** are often used in addition to surgery. For cases detected early, 50% of patients are alive 5 years after diagnosis; but overall, the survival rate is only 14%. Phototherapy and gene therapy are being studied in the hope of improving these statistics. In addition, one form of lung cancer, known as small-cell lung cancer and accounting for about 20% of cases, can be treated fairly successfully with chemotherapy—alone or in combination with radiation. A large percentage of cases respond with **remission,** which in some cases lasts for years.

Colon and Rectal Cancer

Another common cancer in the United States is colon and rectal cancer (also called colorectal cancer). It is the second leading cause of cancer death, after lung cancer, for men and women combined.

Risk Factors Age is a key risk factor for colon and rectal cancer, with more than 70% of cases diagnosed in people age 65 and older. Heredity also plays a role: Many cancers arise from preexisting **polyps,** small growths on the wall of the colon that may gradually develop into malignancies. The tendency to form colon polyps appears to be determined by specific genes, and 15–30% of colon cancers may be due to inherited gene mutations. Chronic inflammation of the colon as a result of disorders such as ulcerative colitis also increases the risk of colon cancer.

Lifestyle is also a risk factor for colon and rectal cancer. Regular physical activity appears to reduce a person's risk, while obesity increases risk. A diet rich in red meat is thought to increase risk, although it is unclear whether fat or some other component of meat is the culprit. A diet rich in fruits, vegetables, and whole grains is associated with lower risk. However, a 1999 finding from the ongoing Nurses' Health Study contradicted the longstanding view that dietary fiber prevents colon cancer. Further investigation of different types and sources of fiber and other properties of plant-based diets may help clarify the relationship between diet and colon cancer. Recent studies have suggested a protective role for folic acid and calcium; in contrast, high intake of simple sugars may increase risk. A plant-based, high-fiber diet is still recommended because it is associated with a lower risk of cancer overall and also helps prevent heart disease, hypertension, and diabetes.

Other lifestyle factors that may increase the risk of colon and rectal cancer include excessive alcohol consumption and smoking. Hormone replacement therapy may reduce risk in postmenopausal women. In addition, research indicates that regular use of nonsteroidal anti-inflammatory drugs such as aspirin and ibuprofen decreases the risk for developing colon cancer and other cancers of the digestive tract.

Detection and Treatment If identified early, precancerous polyps and early-stage cancers can be removed before they become malignant or spread. Because polyps may bleed as they progress, the standard warning signs of colon cancer are bleeding from the rectum or a change in bowel habits. Regular screening tests are recommended beginning at age 50 (earlier for people with a family history of the disease). A stool blood test, performed every year, can detect small amounts of blood in the stool long before obvious bleeding would be noticed. More involved screening tests are recommended at 5- or 10-year intervals. In sigmoidoscopy or colonoscopy, a flexible fiberoptic device is inserted through the rectum; part or all of the colon can be examined, and polyps can be biopsied or even removed without major surgery.

Surgery is the primary treatment for colon and rectal cancer. Radiation and chemotherapy may be used before surgery to shrink a tumor or after surgery to destroy any remaining cancerous cells. The survival rate is 91% for colon and rectal cancers detected early and 61% overall.

Breast Cancer

Breast cancer is the most common cancer in women and causes almost as many deaths in women as lung cancer. In men, breast cancer occurs only rarely. In the United States, about one woman in nine will develop breast cancer during her lifetime. The incidence of breast cancer increased during the 1980s but now appears to have leveled off; each year, about 175,000 American women are diagnosed with breast cancer. Although mortality rates declined during the early 1990s, about 44,000 women die from breast cancer each year.

Less than 1% of breast cancer cases occur in women under age 30, but a woman's risk doubles every 5 years between the ages of 30 and 45 and then increases more slowly, by 10–15% every 5 years after age 45. More than 75% of breast cancers are diagnosed in women over 50.

Risk Factors   There is a strong genetic factor in breast cancer. A woman who has two close relatives with breast cancer is four to six times more likely to develop the disease than a woman who has no close relatives with it. However, even though genetic factors are important, only about 15% of cancers occur in women with a family history of breast cancer. (Genetic factors in breast cancer are discussed later in the chapter.)

Other risk factors include early onset of menstruation, late onset of menopause, having no children or having a first child after age 30, current use of hormone replacement therapy, obesity, and alcohol use. The unifying factor for many of these risk factors may be the female sex hormone estrogen, which circulates in a woman's body in high concentrations between puberty and menopause. Fat cells also produce estrogen, and estrogen levels are higher in obese women. Alcohol can interfere with estrogen metabolism in the liver and increases estrogen levels in the blood. Estrogen promotes the growth of cells in responsive sites, including the breast and the uterus, so

any factor that increases estrogen exposure may raise breast cancer risk. In addition, pregnancy and breastfeeding trigger changes in breast cells that make them less susceptible to cancerous changes.

Breast cancer has been called a "disease of civilization" because incidence is high in industrialized Western countries but remains low in developing non-Western countries. Differences in diet and exercise habits have been proposed to explain this pattern, but the connections are still being investigated. Recent studies indicate that a high-fat diet alone may not increase the risk of breast cancer but that the type of fat consumed may be important. Monounsaturated fats have been linked with reduced risk, while certain types of polyunsaturated fats may increase risk. Dietary fiber may also have a protective effect. Regular exercise is extremely important: A study of more than 25,000 women found that those who exercised regularly had a 37% lower risk of breast cancer than those who did not exercise. Vigorous exercise may reduce estrogen levels in the blood, and physical activity of all intensities helps control body weight. Both obesity and significant weight gain during adulthood are linked to increased risk of breast cancer.

Although some of the risk factors for breast cancer—such as heredity and some hormonal factors—cannot be changed, important lifestyle risk factors are under the control of the individual. Eating a low-fat, high-fiber diet, exercising regularly, limiting alcohol intake, and maintaining a healthy body weight can minimize the chance of developing breast cancer, even for women at risk from family history or other factors.

Early Detection   A cure is most likely if breast cancer is detected early, so regular screening is a good investment, even for younger women. The ACS advises a three-part personal program for the early detection of breast cancer:

1. Monthly breast self-examination (BSE) for all women over age 20 (see the box "Breast Self-Examination" on p. 440).

2. A clinical breast exam by a physician every 3 years for women between 20 and 39 and every year for women 40 and older.

3. **Mammograms** (low-dose breast X rays) every year for most women over 40. (Individual risk factors must be considered in determining the frequency of mammograms, and the value of mammograms for women in their forties is an area of debate.)

Treatment   If a lump is detected, it may be scanned by **ultrasonography** and biopsied to see if it is cancerous. The biopsy may be done either by needle in the physician's office or surgically. In 90% of cases, the lump is found to be a cyst or other harmless growth, and no further treatment is needed. If the lump does contain cancer cells, a variety of surgeries may be called for, ranging from a lumpectomy (removal of the lump and surrounding tissue) to a mastectomy (removal of the breast). To determine whether the cancer has spread, lymph nodes from the armpit may be removed and examined. If cancer cells are found, tumor cells remaining in the body can often be slowed or killed by additional therapy, such as radiation, chemotherapy, or both.

The chance of survival in cases of breast cancer varies, depending both on the nature of the tumor and whether it has metastasized. If the tumor is discovered early, before it has spread to the adjacent lymph nodes, the patient has about a 97% chance of surviving more than 5 years. The survival rate for all stages is 84% at 5 years, 69% at 10 years, and 57% at 15 years.

New Strategies for Treatment and Prevention A number of new drugs have recently been developed for the treatment or prevention of breast cancer. A family of drugs called selective estrogen-receptor modulators, or SERMs, act like estrogen in some tissues of the body but block estrogen's effects in others. One SERM, tamoxifen, has long been used in breast cancer treatment because it blocks the action of estrogen in breast tissue. In 1998, the FDA approved the use of tamoxifen to reduce the risk of breast cancer in healthy women who are at high risk for the disease. A large-scale study found that tamoxifen reduced the risk of breast cancer by about 45% among high-risk women. However, the drug has serious potential side effects, including increased risk for blood clots and uterine cancer, and its long-term effects are unknown. Another SERM currently being tested as a potential preventive agent is raloxifene, a drug used to treat osteoporosis that has fewer side effects than tamoxifen. Although still controversial, the use of SERMs in the prevention of breast cancer is a major breakthrough.

A new therapy for advanced breast cancer is Herceptin (trastuzumab), a monoclonal antibody. Antibodies, discussed in Chapter 17, are proteins produced by the immune system that recognize and bind to foreign substances such as bacteria; monoclonal antibodies are a special type of antibody that are produced in the laboratory and designed to bind to a specific cancer-related target. About 30% of metastatic breast cancer tumors produce excess amounts of a growth-promoting protein called HER2. Herceptin binds to the excess HER2, thus blocking its action and slowing tumor growth. Herceptin is used alone or in combination with Taxol (paclitaxel), a drug that interferes with cell division.

Another new treatment approach under investigation targets *angiogenesis*, the process by which new blood vessels are recruited to nourish cancer cells. These new blood vessels are necessary for the continued growth of a tumor, so blocking this process may halt the growth and spread of tumors. Clinical trials of anti-angiogenesis agents are just beginning, however, so it will be some time before any such drugs are available.

Prostate Cancer

The prostate gland is situated at the base of the bladder in men. It produces seminal fluid; if enlarged, it can block the flow of urine. Prostate cancer is the most common cancer in men and, after lung and colon cancer, the cause of the most deaths. About 180,000 new cases are diagnosed each year, and about 37,000 American men die from the disease each year.

Risk Factors Age is the strongest predictor of risk, with about 75% of cases of prostate cancer diagnosed in men over age 65. Inherited genetic predisposition may be responsible for about 5–10% of cases, and men with a family history of the disease should be particularly vigilant about screening. For reasons not well understood, African American men have the highest rate of prostate cancer of any group in the world; both genetic and lifestyle factors may be involved. Diets high in calories and animal fats and low in plant foods have also been implicated as possible culprits in the development of prostate cancer. Compounds in soy foods and tomatoes are being investigated for their possible protective effects.

Detection Warning signs of prostate cancer include changes in urinary frequency, weak or interrupted urine flow, painful urination, and blood in the urine. Screening tests for early detection are recommended annually for men age 50 and over—earlier for African Americans and those with a strong family history of the disease. Most cases of prostate cancer are first detected during a digital rectal exam. A physician can feel the prostate gland through the rectum and determine if it is enlarged or if lumps are present.

The **PSA blood test**, which measures the amount of prostate-specific antigen (PSA) in the blood, can also be used to help diagnose prostate cancer. An elevated level or a rapid increase in PSA can signal trouble. A single measurement of PSA can help catch early prostate cancer,

TERMS

mammography Low-dose X rays of the breasts used to check for early signs of breast cancer.

ultrasonography An imaging method in which sound waves are bounced off body structures to create an image on a TV monitor; also called *ultrasound*.

PSA blood test A diagnostic test for prostate cancer that measures blood levels of prostate-specific antigen (PSA).

By regularly examining your own breasts, you are likely to notice any changes that occur. The best time for breast self-examination (BSE) is about a week after your period ends, when your breasts are not tender or swollen. If you are not having regular periods, do BSE on the same day every month.

1. Lie down with a pillow under your right shoulder and place your right arm behind your head.

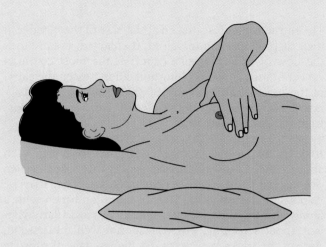

2. Use the finger pads of the three middle fingers on your left hand to feel for lumps in the right breast.

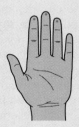

3. Press firmly enough to know how your breast feels. A firm ridge in the lower curve of each breast is normal. If you're not sure how hard to press, talk with your health care professional.

4. Move around the breast in a circular (a), up-and-down line (b), or wedge pattern (c). Be sure to do it the same way every time, check the entire breast area, and remember how your breast feels from month to month.

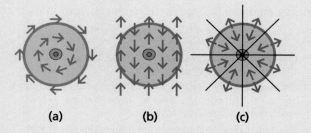

(a)   (b)   (c)

5. Repeat the exam on your left breast, using the finger pads of the right hand. (Move the pillow to under your left shoulder.)

6. If you find any changes, see your health care professional right away.

7. Repeat the examination of both breasts while standing, with your one arm behind your head. The upright position makes it easier to check the upper and outer part of the breasts (toward your armpit). This is where about half of breast cancers are found. You may want to do the standing part of the BSE while you are in the shower. Some breast changes can be felt more easily when your skin is wet and soapy.

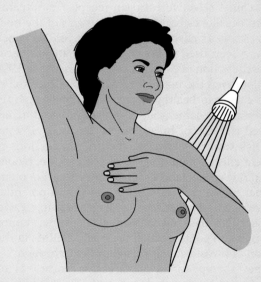

For added safety, you can check your breasts for any dimpling of the skin, changes in the nipple, redness, or swelling while standing in front of a mirror right after your BSE each month.

SOURCE: *How to Do Breast Self-Examination.* © 1999 American Cancer Society, Inc. Reprinted by the permission of the American Cancer Society, Inc.

but it also registers benign conditions (more than half of men over 50 have benign prostate disease). Researchers are looking for ways to make the PSA test more sensitive. One strategy is to repeat the test over time to chart a rate of change. A newer approach involves measuring the percentage of PSA that is free-floating in the blood. PSA made by cancer cells is more likely to circulate bound to other proteins, while PSA from healthy prostate cells is more likely to be unbound. Thus, a low proportion of so-called free PSA indicates greater risk, while a high proportion of free PSA is associated with lower risk.

Ultrasound is used increasingly as a follow-up, to detect lumps too small to be felt and to determine their size, shape, and properties. A needle biopsy of suspicious lumps can be performed relatively painlessly, and whether the biopsied cells are malignant or benign can be determined by examining them under a microscope.

Treatment   Treatments vary based on the stage of the cancer and the age of the patient. A small, slow-growing tumor in an older man may be treated with "watchful waiting" because he is more likely to die from another cause before his cancer becomes life threatening. More aggressive treatment would be indicated for younger men or those with more advanced cancers. Treatment usually involves radical prostatectomy, in which the prostate is removed surgically. While radical surgery has an excellent cure rate, it is major surgery and often results in **incontinence** and **impotence.**

A less-invasive alternative involves surgical implantation of radioactive seeds. Radiation from the seeds destroys the tumor and much of the normal prostate tissue but leaves surrounding tissue relatively untouched. Although there is little risk of incontinence or impotence, this procedure is relatively new and its effectiveness for different stages of cancer is still being evaluated.

Alternative or additional treatments include external radiation, hormones, and anticancer drugs. Survival rates for all stages of this cancer have improved steadily since 1940; the 5-year survival rate is currently about 93%.

Cancers of the Female Reproductive Tract

Because the uterus, cervix, and ovaries are subject to similar hormonal influences, the cancers of these organs can be discussed as a group.

Cervical Cancer   Cervical cancer is at least in part a sexually transmitted disease. Probably more than 80% of cervical cancer stems from infection by the human papillomavirus (HPV), which is transmitted during unprotected sex (see the box "Microbes That Cause Cancer," p. 442). Unlike most cancers, which occur most often after the age of 60, cancer of the cervix occurs frequently in women in their thirties or even twenties. Cancer at this age is especially devastating to women and their families.

The principal risk factors for cervical cancer are many sex partners (because of the risk of HPV transmission), cigarette smoking, and low socioeconomic status.

Screening for the changes in cervical cells that precede cancer is done chiefly by means of the **Pap test.** During a pelvic exam, loose cells are scraped from the cervix, spread on a slide, stained for easier viewing, and examined under a microscope to see whether they are normal in size and shape. If cells are abnormal, a condition commonly referred to as *cervical dysplasia,* the Pap test is repeated at intervals. Sometimes cervical cells spontaneously return to normal, but in about one-third of cases, the cellular changes progress toward malignancy. If this happens, the abnormal cells must be removed, either surgically or by destroying them with a cryoscopic (ultracold) probe or localized laser treatment. When the abnormal cells are in a precancerous state, the small patch of dangerous cells can be completely removed.

Without timely surgery, the malignant patch of cells goes on to invade the wall of the cervix and spreads to adjacent lymph nodes and to the uterus. At this stage, chemotherapy may be used with radiation to kill the fast-growing cancer cells, but chances for a complete cure are lower. Even when a cure can be achieved, it often means surgical removal of the uterus.

Because the Pap test is highly effective, all sexually active women, and women between the ages of 18 and 65, should be tested. Although screening can clearly save lives, *Healthy People 2010* reports lower-than-average rates of Pap testing for certain groups, including women of low socioeconomic status and women with less than a high school education. Mortality rates for cervical cancer are twice as high for black women as for white women.

Uterine or Endometrial Cancer   Cancer of the lining of the uterus, or **endometrium,** most often occurs after the age of 55. The risk factors are similar to those for breast cancer: prolonged exposure to estrogen, early onset of menstruation, late menopause, never having been pregnant, and other medical conditions, including obesity. The use of oral contraceptives, which combine estrogen and progestin, appears to provide protection.

Endometrial cancer is usually detectable by pelvic examination. It is treated surgically, commonly by hysterectomy, or removal of the uterus; radiation treatment and chemotherapy may be used in addition to surgery. When the tumor is detected at an early stage, about 96% of patients are alive and disease-free 5 years later. When

incontinence   The inability to control the flow of urine.

impotence   The inability to have an erection or ejaculate; an inability to perform sexual intercourse.

Pap test   A scraping of cells from the cervix for examination under a microscope to detect cancer.

endometrium   The layers of tissue lining the uterus.

TERMS

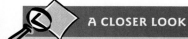

It has long been suspected that microbes, including viruses, bacteria, and parasites, might cause cancer. However, only during the past 20 years have investigators been able to prove this. It is now estimated that about 15% of the world's cancers are caused by microorganisms, although the percentage is much lower in developed countries like the United States.

Viruses seem to play the most important role in cancers caused by microbes. The Epstein-Barr virus is best known for causing mononucleosis, but it is also suspected of contributing to Hodgkin's disease (a lymphoma), cancer of the pharynx, and some stomach cancers. Certain types of human papillomavirus (HPV) are thought to be responsible for 70–80% of cervical cancers worldwide. Hepatitis viruses B and C together cause as many as 80% of the world's liver cancers. HPV and hepatitis are of special concern to college students because they are often transmitted sexually; they are discussed in greater detail below.

So far, only one bacterium, *Helicobacter pylori,* has been linked to cancer. *H. pylori* is believed to cause more than half of the 22,000 cases of stomach cancer that occur in the United States each year. At the beginning of the twentieth century, stomach cancer was the leading cause of cancer death among Americans; researchers now believe that improvements in sanitation that have lowered rates of *H. pylori* infection may be responsible for the huge drop in the number of cases of stomach cancer.

Let's take a closer look at two cancers caused by common microbes.

HPV and Cervical Cancer

The human papillomaviruses are a large group of related viruses that cause both common warts and genital warts. These viruses have the ability to cause cells to divide and grow without the normal control mechanisms. A great deal of data now indicate that infection of cervical cells by certain types of HPV is the critical event in the development of cervical cancer. The initial infection begins when the virus is introduced into the cervix, usually by an infected sex partner. Not surprisingly, cervical cancer is associated with multiple sex partners and is extremely

rare in women who have not had heterosexual intercourse. The regular use of condoms can reduce the risk of transmitting both HPV and other infectious agents that may be important in cervical cancer, including HIV. (Genital warts and other STDs are discussed in Chapter 18.)

Because only a very small percentage of HPV-infected women ever get cervical cancer, other factors must be involved. The most important cofactors seem to be smoking and infection with genital herpes. Both smoking and herpes infection can cause cancerous changes in cells in the laboratory, and they can speed and intensify the cancerous changes begun by HPV.

Hepatitis B and C and Liver Cancer

Hepatitis B is spread mainly though sexual intercourse, though it can also be passed through contact with any body fluid or with contaminated needles. Hepatitis C is most commonly acquired through blood transfusions or injecting drug use, but it, too, can be spread sexually. Most people who develop hepatitis will recover. However, up to 10% of people with hepatitis B and 85% of people with hepatitis C become chronic carriers of the virus. Hepatitis carriers are at high risk for a number of health problems, including liver cancer. The best way to avoid liver cancer is to avoid contracting hepatitis B or C: Limit the number of sex partners you have, practice safer sex, and if you are an injecting drug user, don't share needles. A vaccine for hepatitis B is available. (See Chapters 17 and 18 for more on hepatitis.)

The immune system helps control the damage done by pathogenic microorganisms (see Chapter 17). Normal cellular immunity probably plays the most important role in controlling the initial infection and in preventing progression from infection to malignancy and cancer. Chemicals that suppress elements of the immune system, such as substances in tobacco, are associated with an increase in cancer. Stress, poor nutrition, and frequent infections are additional factors that can interfere with optimal immune functioning; these all appear to be secondary risk factors in microbe-related cancers.

---

the disease has spread beyond the uterus, the 5-year survival rate is only 66%.

Ovarian Cancer   Although ovarian cancer is rare compared with cervical or uterine cancer, it causes more deaths than the other two combined. It cannot be detected by Pap tests or any other simple screening method and is often diagnosed only late in its development, when surgery and other therapies are unlikely to be successful. The risk factors are similar to those for breast and endometrial cancer: increasing age (most ovarian cancer occurs after age 60), never having been pregnant, a family history of breast or ovarian cancer, and specific genetic mutations. A high number of ovulations appears to increase the chance that a cancer-causing genetic muta-

tion will occur, so anything that lowers the number of lifetime ovulation cycles—pregnancy, breastfeeding, or use of oral contraceptives—reduces a woman's risk of ovarian cancer.

There are often no warning signs of developing ovarian cancer. Therefore, women at high risk, because of family history or because they harbor a mutant gene, should have thorough pelvic exams at regular intervals, as recommended by their physician. Pelvic exams may include the use of ultrasound to view the ovaries. A blood test for a tumor marker called CA-125 may assist with diagnosis but is not yet recommended for routine screening.

Ovarian cancer is treated by surgical removal of both ovaries, the fallopian tubes, and the uterus. Radiation and chemotherapy are sometimes used in addition to surgery.

When the tumor is localized to the ovary, the survival rate after 5 years is 95%. But for all stages, the survival rate is only 50%, reflecting the difficulty of early detection.

Other Female Reproductive Tract Cancers During 1938–1971, millions of women were given a synthetic hormone called DES (diethylstilbestrol), which was thought to help prevent miscarriage. It was later discovered that daughters born to these women (DES daughters) have an increased risk, about 1 in 1000, of a vaginal or cervical cancer called clear cell cancer. This cancer is extremely rare in unexposed women. DES daughters may also have an anatomically abnormal reproductive tract and have problems with fertility or miscarriage. Though this is primarily a health threat for daughters, there is also some risk to DES sons, who may have an increased risk of abnormalities of the reproductive tract, including undescended testicles, a risk factor for testicular cancer.

If you suspect you may be a DES daughter or son, you should ask your mother if she took any medications while pregnant, and, if possible, review her medical records for that time. A DES daughter should find a physician who is familiar with the problems of DES exposure; more frequent and more thorough pelvic exams may be recommended. A recent animal study suggested the possibility of an increased third-generation cancer risk from DES, but further research is needed to determine if the finding applies to DES granddaughters.

Skin Cancer

Skin cancer is the most common cancer of all when cases of the highly curable forms are included in the count. (Usually these forms are not included, precisely because they are easily treated.) Of the more than 1 million cases of skin cancer diagnosed each year, 44,000 are the most serious type, **melanoma.** Treatments are usually simple and successful when the cancers are caught early.

Risk Factors Almost all cases of skin cancer can be traced to excessive exposure to **ultraviolet (UV) radiation** from the sun, including longer wavelength ultraviolet A (UVA) and shorter wavelength ultraviolet B (UVB) radiation. UVB radiation causes sunburns and can damage the eyes and the immune system. UVA is less likely to cause an immediate sunburn, but by damaging connective tissue, it leads to premature aging of the skin, giving it a wrinkled, leathery appearance. (Tanning lamps and tanning-salon beds emit mostly UVA radiation.) Both UVA and UVB radiation have been linked to the development of skin cancer, and the NIH's National Toxicology Program has declared both solar and artificial sources of UV radiation to be known human carcinogens.

Both severe, acute sun reactions (sunburns) and chronic low-level sun reactions (suntans) can lead to skin cancer. People with fair skin have less natural protection

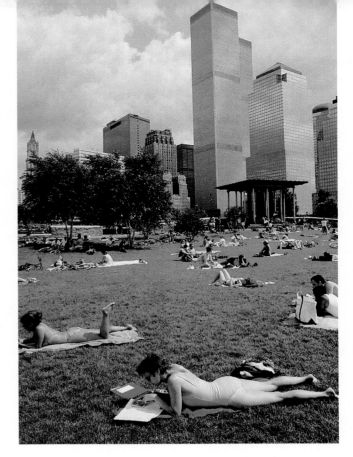

Cumulative exposure to sunlight, beginning in childhood, increases the risk of skin cancer later in life. Blistering sunburns are particularly dangerous, but tanning also poses a hazard. Sunscreens help protect the skin from the sun's radiation.

against skin damage from the sun and a higher risk of developing skin cancer; people with naturally dark skin have a considerable degree of protection (see the box "What's Your UV Risk?"). Whites are about 20 times more likely than African Americans to develop melanoma. Severe sunburns in childhood have been linked to a greatly increased risk of skin cancer in later life, so children in particular should be protected. Because of damage to the ozone layer of the atmosphere (discussed in Chapter 24), there is a chance that we may all be exposed to increasing amounts of UV radiation in the future. Take time now to understand the risks of excessive sun exposure, because the precautions suggested here will become increasingly critical if the ozone shield continues to thin.

melanoma A malignant tumor of the skin that arises from pigmented cells, usually a mole.

ultraviolet (UV) radiation Light rays of a specific wavelength emitted by the sun; most UV rays are blocked by the ozone layer in the upper atmosphere. Exposure to ultraviolet A (UVA) and/or ultraviolet B (UVB) rays is linked to the development of skin cancer.

TERMS

Your risk of skin cancer from the ultraviolet radiation in sunlight depends on several factors. Take the quiz below to see how sensitive you are. The higher your UV-risk score, the greater your risk of skin cancer—and the greater your need to take precautions against too much sun.

Score 1 point for each true statement:

_____ 1. I have blond or red hair.

_____ 2. I have light-colored eyes (blue, gray, green).

_____ 3. I freckle easily.

_____ 4. I have many moles.

_____ 5. I had two or more blistering sunburns as a child.

_____ 6. I spent lots of time in a tropical climate as a child.

_____ 7. I have a family history of skin cancer.

_____ 8. I work outdoors.

_____ 9. I spend a lot of time in outdoor activities.

_____ 10. I like to spend as much time in the sun as I can.

_____ 11. I sometimes go to a tanning parlor or use a sunlamp.

_____ Total score

Score	Risk of skin cancer from UV radiation
0	Low
1–3	Moderate
4–7	High
8–11	Very high

SOURCE: Adapted from Shear, N. 1996. What's your UV-risk score? *Consumer Reports on Health*, June. Copyright © 1996 by Consumers Union of U.S., Inc., Yonkers, N.Y. 10703–1057. Reprinted by permission from *Consumer Reports on Health*. No photocopying or reproduction permitted. To order a subscription, call 1-800-234-1645.

Other risk factors for skin cancer include having many moles, particularly large ones, and a family history of the disease. Skin cancer may also be caused by exposure to coal tar, pitch, creosote, arsenic, and radioactive materials; but compared to sunlight, these agents account for only a small proportion of cases.

Types of Skin Cancer   There are three main types of skin cancer, named for the types of skin cell from which they develop. **Basal cell** and **squamous cell carcinomas** together account for about 95% of the skin cancers diagnosed each year. They are usually found in chronically sun-exposed areas, such as the face, neck, hands, and arms. They usually appear as pale, waxlike, pearly nodules, or red, scaly, sharply outlined patches. These cancers are often painless, although they may bleed, crust, and form an open sore on the skin.

Melanoma is by far the most dangerous skin cancer because it spreads so rapidly. Since 1973, the incidence of melanoma has increased by about 4% per year. It is the most common cancer among women age 25-29 years. It can occur anywhere on the body, but the most common sites are the back, chest, abdomen, and lower legs. A melanoma usu-

ally appears at the site of a preexisting mole. The mole may begin to enlarge, become mottled or varied in color (colors can include blue, pink, and white), or develop an irregular surface or irregular borders. Tissue invaded by melanoma may also itch, burn, or bleed easily.

Prevention   One of the major steps you can take to protect yourself against all forms of skin cancer is to avoid lifelong overexposure to sunlight. Blistering, peeling sunburns from unprotected sun exposure are particularly dangerous, but suntans—whether from sunlight or tanning lamps—also increase your risk of developing skin cancer later in life. People of every age, including babies and children, need to be protected from the sun with **sunscreens** and protective clothing. For a closer look at sunlight and skin cancer, see the box "Protecting Your Skin from the Sun."

Detection and Treatment   The only sure way to avoid a serious outcome from skin cancer is to make sure it is recognized and diagnosed early. In most successfully treated cases, patients themselves bring a melanoma or other skin cancer to their physician's attention. Make it a habit to examine your skin regularly. Most of the spots, freckles, moles, and blemishes on your body are normal; you were born with some of them, and others appear and disappear throughout your life. But if you notice an unusual growth, discoloration, sore that does not heal, or mole that undergoes a sudden or progressive change, see your physician or a dermatologist immediately.

The characteristics that may signal that a skin lesion is a melanoma—asymmetry, border irregularity, color change, and a diameter greater than ¼ inch—are illus-

TERMS   **basal cell carcinoma**   Cancer of the deepest layers of the skin.

squamous cell carcinoma   Cancer of the surface layers of the skin.

sunscreen   A substance used to protect the skin from UV rays; usually applied as an ointment or a cream.

With proper clothing and the use of sunscreens, you can lead an active outdoor life *and* protect your skin against most sun-induced damage.

Clothing

- Wear long-sleeved shirts and long pants made of tightly woven fabric. Thin, white shirts or wet clothing will not protect you sufficiently.
- Wear a wide-brimmed hat to protect your ears and face.
- Wear UV-blocking sunglasses to protect your eyes. A dark color does not imply UV protection; check the label.

Sunscreen

- Use a sunscreen and lip balm with a sun protection factor (SPF) of 15 or higher. (An SPF rating refers to the amount of time you can stay out in the sun before you burn, compared to using no sunscreen; for example, a product with an SPF of 15 would allow you to remain in the sun without burning 15 times longer, on average, than if you didn't apply sunscreen.) If you're fair-skinned or will be outdoors for long hours, use a sunscreen with a high SPF 30+.
- Choose a "broad-spectrum" sunscreen that protects against both UVA and UVB radiation. The SPF rating of a sunscreen currently applies only to UVB, but a number of ingredients, including avobenzone (Parsol 1789), benzophenone, oxybenzone, titanium dioxide, and zinc oxide, are effective at blocking most UVA radiation. Use a water-resistant sunscreen if you swim or sweat quite a bit.
- Apply sunscreen 30 minutes before exposure to allow it time to penetrate the skin; shake it before applying.
- Reapply sunscreen frequently and generously to all sun-exposed areas. Most people use less than half as much as they would need to attain the full SPF rating. One ounce of sunscreen—one-fourth of a 4-ounce container—is about enough to cover an average-size adult in a swimsuit.

- If you're taking medication, ask your physician or pharmacist about possible reactions to sunlight or interactions with sunscreens. If you're using sunscreen and an insect repellent containing DEET, use extra sunscreen (DEET decreases sunscreen effectiveness).
- Don't let sunscreens give you a false sense of security. The effectiveness of sunscreens in preventing skin cancer has not been firmly established, so even if you wear sunscreen and don't burn, sun exposure may increase your cancer risk. For people at greatest risk—those with fair skin and the tendency to develop many moles—avoiding sun exposure may be the safest strategy.

Time of Day and Location

- Avoid sun exposure between 10 A.M. and 4 P.M., when the sun's rays are most intense. Clouds allow as much as 80% of UV rays to reach your skin. Stay in the shade when you can, and use an umbrella at the beach.
- Consult the day's UV Index, which predicts UV levels on a 0–10+ scale, to get a sense of the amount of sun protection you'll need; take special care on days with a rating of 5 or above. UV Index ratings are available in local newspapers, from the weather bureau, or from certain Web sites (see For More Information at the end of the chapter).
- UV rays can penetrate at least 3 feet in water, so swimmers should wear water-resistant sunscreen.
- Locations near the equator or at high altitudes have more intense sunlight, so stronger sunscreens should be used and applied often.
- Snow reflects the sun's rays, so don't forget to apply sunscreen before skiing and other snow activities. Sand and water also reflect the sun's rays, so you still need to apply a sunscreen if you are under a beach umbrella. Concrete and white-painted surfaces are also highly reflective.

---

trated in Figure 16-2. In addition, if someone in your family has had numerous skin cancers or melanomas, you may want to consult a dermatologist for a complete skin examination and discussion of your particular risk.

If you do have an unusual skin lesion, your physician will examine it and possibly perform a biopsy. If the lesion is cancerous, it is usually removed surgically, a procedure that can almost always be performed in the physician's office using a local anesthetic. Occasionally, other forms of treatment may be used. Even for melanoma, the outlook after removal in the early stages is good, with a 5-year survival rate of 96% if the tumor is localized but only 59% if the cancer has spread to adjacent lymph

nodes. Since prevention requires a minimum of time and attention, it pays to be alert.

Oral Cancer

Oral cancer—cancers of the lip, tongue, mouth, and throat—can be traced principally to cigarette, cigar, or pipe smoking, the use of spit tobacco, and the excess use of alcohol. These risk factors work together to multiply a person's risk of oral cancer. The incidence of oral cancer is twice as great in men as in women and most frequent in men over 40. Some prominent sufferers of oral cancer have included Sigmund Freud and Fidel Castro, both

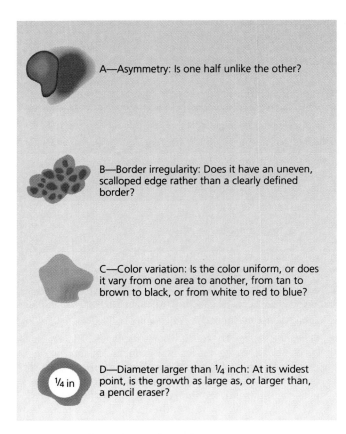

A—Asymmetry: Is one half unlike the other?

B—Border irregularity: Does it have an uneven, scalloped edge rather than a clearly defined border?

C—Color variation: Is the color uniform, or does it vary from one area to another, from tan to brown to black, or from white to red to blue?

D—Diameter larger than ¼ inch: At its widest point, is the growth as large as, or larger than, a pencil eraser?

¼ in

Figure 16-2   The ABCD test for melanoma.

notorious cigar smokers. Sports figures who have cultivated a taste for spit tobacco are now also increasingly being diagnosed with oral cancer. Among long-term snuff users, the excess risk of cancers of the cheek, tongue, and gum is nearly fiftyfold (see Chapter 11 for more on cigars and spit tobacco).

Oral cancers do have the virtue of being fairly easy to detect, but they are often hard to cure. The primary methods of treatment are surgery and radiation. The 5-year survival rates vary from 91% for lip cancer to 26% for throat cancer; the overall survival rate is about 53%.

Testicular Cancer

Testicular cancer is relatively rare, accounting for only 1% of cancer in men (about 7400 cases per year), but it is the most common cancer in men age 20–35. It is much more common among white Americans than Latinos, Asian Americans, or African Americans. Men with undescended testicles are at increased risk for testicular cancer, and for this reason the condition should be corrected in early childhood. Men whose mothers took DES during pregnancy have an increased risk of undescended testicles and other genital anomalies. For this reason, they may have a higher risk of testicular cancer.

Self-examination helps in the early detection of testicular cancer (see the box "Testicle Self-Examination"). Tumors are treated by surgical removal of the testicle and, if the tumor has spread, by chemotherapy. The 5-year survival rate for testicular cancer is over 90%.

Other Cancers

There are about 55,000 new cases of bladder cancer each year in the United States. Bladder cancer is more than twice as common in men as in women, and smoking is the key risk factor. People living in urban areas, and workers exposed to dye, rubber, or leather, are also at increased risk. The first symptoms are likely to be blood in the urine and/or increased frequency of urination. These symptoms should motivate a quick trip to your physician for a thorough exam, because the survival rate for early-stage bladder cancer is 95%.

Pancreatic cancer is the fifth leading cancer killer, with about 29,000 deaths in the United States each year. Pancreatic cancer is both hard to detect and almost always fatal. The major environmental risk factor is, again, smoking. In addition, obesity and a diet high in fat are associated with higher rates of pancreatic cancer. The disease often has a "silent" course, and by the time symptoms occur, the disease is usually far advanced. Very little is known about how to prevent pancreatic cancer, but better diagnostic imaging techniques may eventually allow for earlier detection.

Leukemias, cancers of the blood-forming tissues, are characterized by the abnormal production of immature white blood cells. The rapid growth of these cells displaces red blood cell precursors and can lead to anemia. Because malignant white cells no longer fight infection, the immune system also loses its ability to defend against infectious agents. There are about 30,000 new cases of leukemia each year, and about 22,000 deaths. Risk factors for leukemia have not been clearly established, but certain chemicals and viruses may play a role.

Lymphomas, cancers of the lymph system, are closely related to leukemias; they include Hodgkin's disease and non-Hodgkin's lymphoma. Treatments have been greatly improved, and many patients can lead normal lives for many years. Since the 1970s, the 5-year survival rate for Hodgkin's disease has increased from 40% to over 80%.

THE CAUSES OF CANCER

Although scientists do not know everything about what causes cancer, they have identified genetic, environmental, and lifestyle factors. (For information on possible factors involved in cancer incidence, see the box "Can Poverty Cause Cancer?" on p. 448.) There are usually several steps in the transformation of a normal cell into a cancer cell, and in many cases, different factors may work together in the development of cancer.

Increase your chances of early cancer detection by performing a monthly testicle self-exam. It's important that you know what your own testicles feel like normally so that you'll recognize any changes. The best time to perform the examination is after a warm shower or bath, when the scrotum is relaxed.

- First, stand in front of a mirror and look for any swelling on the scrotum.

- Next, examine each testicle. With your thumb on top of the testicle and two fingers underneath, gently roll the testicle to check for lumps or areas of particular firmness. A normal testicle is smooth, oval, and uniformly firm to the touch. Don't worry if your testicles differ slightly in size; this is common. And don't mistake the epididymis, the sperm-carrying tube at the rear of the testicle, for an abnormality.

- If you find any hard lumps or nodules, or if there has been any change in the shape, size, or texture of the testi-

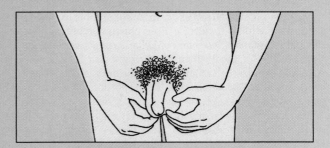

cles, consult a physician. These signs may not indicate a malignancy, but only your physician can make a diagnosis.

SOURCES: Testicular Self-Exam (TSE). 1997. *Cancer Smart* 3(3): 11. American Cancer Society. 1990. *For Men Only: Testicular Cancer and How to Do TSE (a Self-Exam)*. New York: American Cancer Society.

The Role of DNA

Almost daily, the mass media report on some new link between heredity and cancer. But how exactly do genes influence cancer? And what do these links mean for you and your risk of developing particular cancers?

DNA Basics   The nucleus of each cell in your body contains 23 pairs of **chromosomes,** which are made up of tightly packed coils of **DNA** (deoxyribonucleic acid). DNA consists of two long strands wound around each other in a spiral structure, like a twisted ladder; scientists refer to this spiral as a double helix. The rungs of the ladder are made from four different nucleotide bases: adenine, thymine, cytosine, and guanine, or A, T, C, and G. The arrangement of nucleotide bases along the double helix constitutes the genetic code. You can think of this code as a set of instructions for building, operating, and repairing your body.

A **gene** is a smaller unit of DNA made up of a specific sequence of nucleotide bases. Each chromosome contains thousands of genes; you have about 100,000 genes in all. Each of your genes controls the production of a particular protein. The makeup of each protein—which amino acids it contains, and in what sequence—is determined by its precise sequence of A, T, C, and G. Proteins build cells and make them work: They serve both as the structural material for your body and as the regulators of all chemical reactions and metabolic processes. By making different proteins at different times, genes can act as switches to alter the ways a cell works.

Except for sperm and egg cells, every cell in your body contains two copies of each gene, one on each of a pair of chromosomes. You inherit one copy of each gene from

your mother and one from your father. Every cell contains a copy of the complete DNA sequence with all the genes. What makes the cells in your body different from one another in both structure and function—one a nerve cell and one a muscle cell, for example—is not which genes they contain, but which genes are "turned on," or expressed. Some genes are active and producing proteins all the time; others are expressed very seldomly.

Cells reproduce by dividing in two, and your body makes billions of new cells every day. When a cell divides, the DNA replicates itself so that each new cell has a complete set of chromosomes. Through the proteins for which they code, some genes are responsible for controlling the rate of cell division, and some types of cells divide much more rapidly than others. Genes that control the rate of cell division often play a critical role in the development of cancer.

As part of a worldwide initiative known as the Human Genome Project, scientists are mapping the entire DNA sequence—some 6 billion nucleotide bases. This map of the chromosomes should greatly increase our knowledge of how genes function in health and disease.

chromosomes   The threadlike bodies in a cell nucleus that contain molecules of DNA; most human cells contain 23 pairs of chromosomes.

DNA   Deoxyribonucleic acid, a chemical substance that carries genetic information.

gene   A section of a chromosome that contains the nucleotide base sequence for making a particular protein; the basic unit of heredity.

TERMS

Americans with low incomes are more susceptible to cancer and are also more likely to die of it, even if their condition and treatment are similar to those of more affluent cancer victims. As former National Cancer Institute director Samuel Broder has stated, "Poverty is a carcinogen." Why does cancer afflict the economically disadvantaged so disproportionately? A primary factor is lifestyle: People of low socioeconomic status are more likely to smoke, abuse alcohol, and eat high-fat foods—all of which have been associated with cancer. These unhealthy behaviors usually begin early: One study found that 63% of teenagers of parents with low incomes engage in two or more of five cancer-related behaviors: smoking, inactivity, an inadequate intake of fruits and vegetables, excessive fat consumption, and alcohol use. The rates of these behaviors among adolescents of more affluent parents are significantly lower.

Another reason is lack of knowledge and information. Studies have found that low-income people are less exposed to information about cancer, less aware of its early warning signs, and less likely to seek medical care when they have such symptoms. A third reason may be an inability to respond to health information and health needs. Many low-income people know they should eat nutritious foods and get regular checkups, but they still may not be able to afford such foods and may not have transportation or access to health care facilities.

In fact, lifestyle differences account for only about 13% of the gap in death rates between Americans with high and low incomes. Many of the cancer-related threats that people with low incomes face are difficult or impossible to avoid. They may be forced to live and work in unsafe or unhealthy environments. They may have jobs, for example, in which they come into daily contact with carcinogenic chemicals, and they may not have been trained in handling them properly. They face similar risks in their homes and schools, where they may be exposed to asbestos or other carcinogens every day.

But even poor health habits and dangerous living and working conditions don't completely explain the high cancer mortal-ity rates among the economically disadvantaged. One study of cancer patients found that chemotherapy was less effective on the tumors of the poorer patients. They had a lower rate of cancer remission than wealthier patients, even when the latter had more extensive disease. One possible explanation for these statistics is the high levels of stress associated with poverty. Stress can impair the immune system, the body's first line of defense against cancer, and experiments with animals have shown that a stressful environment can enhance the growth of a variety of tumors. The link between poverty, stress, and cancer mortality in humans has not been proven, but studies have shown a link between stress and other illnesses.

What can be done about reducing the rate of cancer and cancer mortality in low-income populations? Educating people about prevention is clearly important, and elementary schools and high schools are places where people can be reached in time to encourage healthy habits and prevent bad habits before they begin. However, people from lower socioeconomic groups tend to have a high rate of school dropout. Furthermore, most people have a difficult time worrying about a disease they might get in 10 or 20 years when their immediate concern is survival.

For these reasons, some medical scientists look to policymakers for solutions. They maintain that living and working conditions in the inner cities must be improved and that access to quality health care must be assured for all Americans. Then, even without new miracle drugs or medical breakthroughs, the United States will see a real decrease in cancer rates in low-income populations.

SOURCES: Institute of Medicine. 1999. *The Unequal Burden of Cancer.* Washington, D.C.: National Academy Press. Lantz, P. M., et al. 1998. Socioeconomic factors, health behaviors, and mortality. *Journal of the American Medical Association* 279: 1703–1708. Grabmeier, J. 1992. Poverty can cause cancer. *USA Today,* July.

DNA Mutations and Cancer   A mutation is any change in the normal sequence of nucleotide bases in a gene. Like a typographical error, it may involve a deletion or a substitution of a certain base—for example, CAA may become CA or CTA. Some mutations are inherited: If the egg or sperm cell that produces a child contains a mutation, so will every one of the child's 30 trillion cells. Environmental agents can also produce mutational damage; these **mutagens** include radiation, certain viruses, and chemical substances in the air we breath. (When a mutagen also causes cancer, it is called a carcinogen.) Some mutations are the result of copying errors that occur when DNA replicates itself as part of cell division.

A mutated gene no longer contains the proper code for producing its protein. Since a cell has two copies of each gene, it can sometimes get by with only one functioning version. In this case, the mutation may have no effect on health. However, if both copies of a gene are damaged, or if the cell needs two normal copies to function properly, then the cell will cease to behave normally.

It usually takes several mutational changes before a normal cell takes on the properties of a cancer cell. Genes in which mutations are associated with the conversion of a normal cell into a cancer cell are known as **oncogenes.** In their undamaged form, many oncogenes play a role in controlling or restricting cell growth; they are called **suppressor genes.** Mutational damage to suppressor genes releases the brake on growth and leads to rapid and uncontrolled cell division—a precondition for the development of cancer.

A good example of how a series of mutational changes can produce cancer is provided by the p53 gene, located on chromosome 17. In its normal form, the protein that is coded for by this gene actually helps prevent cancer: If a cell's DNA is damaged, the p53 protein can either kill the cell outright, or stop it from replicating until the damaged DNA is repaired. For example, if a skin cell's DNA is mutated by exposure to sunlight, the p53 protein activates the cell's "suicide" machinery. By thus preventing the replication of damaged DNA, the p53 protein keeps cells from progressing toward cancer. However, if the p53 gene itself undergoes a mutation, these controls are lost, and the cell can become cancerous. In fact, the damaged version of p53 can actually promote cell division and the spread of cancer.

A damaged p53 gene can be inherited, but carcinogenic damage or DNA copying errors are more common causes of p53 mutations. The carcinogen benzo(a)pyrene, found in tobacco smoke, causes a particular mutation in p53 that is linked to many cases of lung cancer. Other agents contribute to cancer by interfering with the p53 protein after it is produced. For example, human papillomavirus, the infectious agent linked to cervical cancer, destroys the p53 protein. Researchers believe that damage to the p53 gene and protein may be involved, directly and indirectly, in as many as 50–60% of all cancers.

Hereditary Cancer Risks   As we've described, one way to obtain a mutated oncogene is to inherit it. For example, as many as 25% of all Americans have inherited an alteration in one or both copies of a suppressor gene vital for controlling the growth of colon cells. As these people age, they tend to form colon polyps, which can progress to cancer. Another example is BRCA1 (breast cancer gene 1): Women who inherit a damaged copy of this suppressor gene face a significantly increased risk of breast and ovarian cancer.

It is important to remember, however, that most cancers are not linked to heredity; mutational damage usually occurs after birth. For example, only about 5–10% of breast cancer cases can be traced to inherited copies of a damaged BRCA1 gene. In addition, lifestyle is important even for those who have inherited a damaged suppressor gene: A diet high in calcium or folic acid may help keep colon polyps from becoming cancerous.

Testing and identification of hereditary cancer risks can be helpful for some people, especially if it leads to increased attention to controllable risk factors and better medical screening. For more on hereditary cancer risks and the issues involved in genetic testing, see the box "Genetic Testing for Breast Cancer," p. 450.

Cancer Promoters   Substances known as cancer promoters make up another important piece of the cancer puzzle. Carcinogenic agents like UV radiation that cause mutational changes in the DNA of oncogenes are known as "initiators" of cancer. Cancer "promoters," on the other hand, don't directly produce DNA mutations. Instead, they accelerate the growth of cells without damaging or permanently altering their DNA. However, a faster growth rate means less time for a cell to repair DNA damage caused by initiators, so errors are more likely to be passed on. Estrogen, which stimulates cellular growth in the female reproductive organs, is an example of a cancer promoter.

Colon cancer provides a good example of how the combination of initiators and promoters contributes to the development of cancer. Colon cells may divide more rapidly if the diet is high in red meat. Under these circumstances of growth promotion, a cell with a preexisting mutation in an oncogene has an increased chance of progressing toward cancer. Increasing intake of fruits, vegetables, and calcium may reverse this effect and slow the growth of cells that line the colon, thereby decreasing the possibility that cancer develops.

Although much still needs to be learned about the role of genetics in cancer, it's clear that minimizing mutation damage to our DNA will lower our risk of many cancers. Unfortunately, a great many substances produce cancer-causing mutations, and we can't escape them all. By identifying the important carcinogens and understanding how they produce their effects, we can help keep our DNA intact and avoid activating "sleeping" oncogenes. The careful study of oncogenes should also lead to more precise methods of assessing cancer risk, and to new methods of diagnosis and treatment.

Dietary Factors

Diet is one of the most important factors in cancer prevention, but it is also one of the most complex and controversial. Diets high in meat, fast food, refined grains, and simple sugars and low in fruits and vegetables are associated with a higher risk of cancer than are plant-based diets rich in whole grains, fruits, and vegetables. The picture becomes less clear, however, when researchers attempt to identify the particular constituents of foods that affect cancer risk. The foods you eat contain many biologically active compounds, and your food choices affect your cancer risk by both exposing you to potentially dangerous compounds and depriving you of potentially protective ones. For example, snacking on a doughnut instead of an apple means that you consume more fat and simple sugars *and* less fiber and fewer vitamins.

TERMS

mutagen   Any environmental factor that can cause mutation, such as radiation and atmospheric chemicals.

oncogene   A gene involved in the transformation of a normal cell into a cancer cell.

suppressor gene   A type of oncogene that normally functions to restrain cellular growth.

Linda's mother, sister, and grandmother all developed breast cancer at around age 40. Now Linda is wondering if she should be tested for mutations in the so-called breast cancer gene, BRCA1. She is not alone. Recent discoveries of disease-related genes are opening up a host of issues related to genetic testing and associated legal, financial, and ethical concerns. Tests for hereditary mutations in breast cancer genes are now commercially available, but who should be tested?

Researchers identified BRCA1 in 1994. About 1 in 800 women in the general population carries a mutant copy of BRCA1, but in certain groups, most notably women of Ashkenazi (Eastern European) Jewish descent, as many as 1 in 100 may carry an altered gene. Defects in this gene cause breast cancer in as many as 50–60% of affected women; they also increase the risk of ovarian cancer and, in men, prostate cancer. Women with an altered BRCA1 gene tend to develop breast cancer at younger ages than other women, and the cancers that develop appear to be more malignant. The situation is complex, however, because hundreds of different mutations of BRCA1 have been identified, and not all of them carry the same risks. Additional genes influencing risk have been identified—BRCA2 in 1995, TSG101 in 1997—and others will no doubt be found in the future.

Genetic analysis of DNA from a blood sample can identify mutant copies of BRCA1. The tests can be expensive, however, ranging from $200 to more than $2000. (Searching for a mutation on a large gene is a bit like looking for a single typo in a novel.) Good news from a genetic test is reassuring, but it doesn't guarantee freedom from disease. Only about 5–10% of all cases of breast cancer occur among women who inherit an altered version of BRCA1. And a woman with a family history of breast cancer must still be monitored closely, even if she carries a normal version of BRCA1; the cancer-causing genetic defect in her family could be located on another gene.

What about women who test positive for an altered copy of the gene? Options include close monitoring, drug treatment with a SERM such as tamoxifen, and surgical removal of currently healthy breasts or ovaries. None of these strategies completely eliminates risk, and they may expose a woman to a dangerous or drastic treatment that is actually unnecessary. And those who test positive can face problems in addition to an uncertain medical future. Some health insurers use the results of a genetic test to justify canceling coverage; some people have lost their jobs when identified as a "genetic risk." Recent federal legislation should protect patients in group health insurance plans from losing their coverage because of the results of genetic tests, but the law does not apply to everyone, nor does it deal with life and disability insurance or employment issues. Further legislation is pending, but "genetic discrimination" could become a major problem as more and more disease-related genes are identified.

In one recent study, only 43% of women at risk for the BRCA1 mutation decided to take the test when it was offered. Those who decided against it cited genetic discrimination as a major reason. There is no simple answer to the question of who should undergo genetic testing for disease-related genes. If you think you are at high risk for a genetic abnormality because of your family or ethnic background, consider genetic counseling. A counselor can help you consider all the issues related to testing, and can guide you into making the decision that is right for you.

Research into particular food components can help guide you in making dietary choices, but keep in mind that the overall quality of your diet is most important.

Let's take a look at some of the dietary factors that may affect cancer risk.

Dietary Fat and Meat   In general, diets high in fat and meat have been associated with higher rates of certain cancers, including those of the colon and prostate. Dietary fat may promote colon cancer by stimulating the production of bile acids, which are necessary to break down and digest material in the colon. Once produced, these bile acids remove layers of cells from the intestinal epithelium, which in turn are replaced by new cells. Newly formed and rapidly growing cells are particularly susceptible to carcinogens. Although the mechanism is unclear, diets high in animal fats and low in plant fats may also increase the risk of aggressive forms of prostate cancer, possibly by affecting hormone levels.

As is the case for heart disease, certain types of fats may be riskier than others. Some studies suggest that diets favoring omega-6 polyunsaturated fats over the omega-3 forms commonly found in fish may be associated with a higher risk of certain cancers, while monounsaturated fats may have a protective effect (see Chapter 12 for more on different types of fatty acids). Particular fatty acids found in meat or nonfat constituents of meat such as iron may also help explain the association between meat and cancer. In addition, curing, smoking, and grilling and other cooking methods utilizing a direct flame or high temperatures may produce carcinogenic compounds such as polycyclic aromatic hydrocarbons.

Alcohol   Alcohol is associated with an increased incidence of several cancers. An average alcohol intake of three drinks per day is associated with a doubling in the risk of breast cancer. Alcohol and tobacco interact as risk factors for oral cancer, and heavy users of both alcohol and tobacco have a risk for oral cancer up to 15 times greater than that of people who don't drink or smoke.

Fiber   Determining the effects of fiber intake on cancer risk is complicated by the fact that fiber is found in foods that also contain many other potential anticancer agents—fruits, vegetables, and whole grains. Various potential cancer-fighting actions have been proposed for

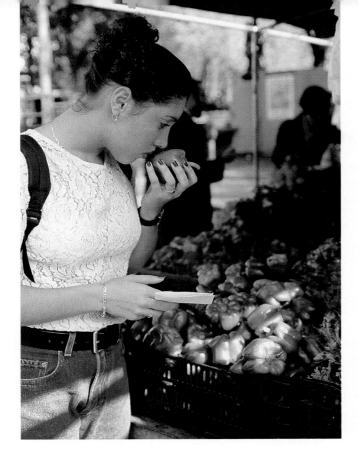

Your food choices significantly affect your risk of cancer. By consuming the recommended 5–9 servings of fruits and vegetables per day, this young woman ensures that her diet is high in fiber and rich in cancer-fighting phytochemicals.

fiber: It may dilute and speed carcinogens through the colon, giving them less of an opportunity to act on cells; it may bind bile acids that promote the development of colon cancer; and it may decrease estrogen levels and thus reduce the risk of female reproductive cancers. None of these actions has been firmly established; and, as described earlier, a 1999 study found no association between total fiber intake and colon cancer risk. Further study is needed to clarify the relationship between fiber intake and cancer risk, and experts still recommend a high-fiber diet for its overall positive effect on health.

Fruits and Vegetables   A massive number of epidemiological studies provides evidence that high consumption of fruits and vegetables reduces the risk of many cancers. Exactly which constituents of fruits and vegetables are responsible for this reduction in risk is less certain. Researchers have identified many mechanisms by which food components may act against cancer: Some may prevent carcinogens from forming in the first place or block them from reaching or acting on target cells. Others boost enzymes that detoxify carcinogens and render them harmless. Still other anticancer agents act on cells that have already been exposed to carcinogens, slowing the development of cancer, or starving cancer cells of oxygen and nutrients by cutting off their blood supply.

Some essential nutrients act as **anticarcinogens**. For example, vitamin C, vitamin E, selenium, and the **carotenoids** (vitamin A precursors) may help block the initiation of cancer by acting as **antioxidants**. As described in Chapter 12, antioxidants prevent **free radicals** from damaging DNA. Vitamin C may also block the conversion of nitrates (food preservatives) into cancer-causing agents. Folic acid may inhibit the transformation of normal cells into malignant cells and strengthen immune function. Calcium inhibits the growth of cells in the colon and may slow the spread of potentially cancerous cells.

Many other anticancer agents in the diet fall under the broader heading of **phytochemicals**, substances in plants that help protect against chronic diseases. One of the first to be identified was **sulforaphane**, a potent anticarcinogen found in broccoli. Sulforaphane induces the cells of the liver and kidney to produce higher levels of protective enzymes, which then neutralize dietary carcinogens. Most fruits and vegetables contain beneficial phytochemicals, and researchers are just beginning to identify them. Some of the most promising are listed in Table 16-2.

To increase your intake of these potential cancer fighters, eat a wide variety of fruits, vegetables, legumes, and grains. Don't try to rely on supplements. Many of these compounds are not yet available in supplement form, and optimal intakes have not been determined. Like many vitamins and minerals, isolated phytochemicals may be harmful if taken in high doses. In addition, it is likely that the anticancer effects of many foods are the result of many chemical substances working in combination. Some practical suggestions for maximizing your intake of anticancer agents are included in the box "A Dietary Defense Against Cancer" and in the Behavior Change Strategy at the end of the chapter.

TERMS

anticarcinogen   An agent that destroys or otherwise blocks the action of carcinogens.

carotenoid   Any of a group of yellow-to-red plant pigments that can be converted to vitamin A by the liver; many act as antioxidants or have other anticancer effects. The carotenoids include beta-carotene, lutein, lycopene, and zeaxanthin.

antioxidant   A substance that can lessen the breakdown of food or body constituents; actions include binding oxygen and donating electrons to free radicals.

free radicals   Electron-seeking compounds that can react with fats, proteins, and DNA, damaging cell membranes and mutating genes in their search for electrons; produced through chemical reactions in the body and by exposure to environmental factors such as sunlight and tobacco smoke.

phytochemical   A naturally occurring substance found in plant foods that may help prevent chronic diseases such as cancer and heart disease; *phyto* means plant.

sulforaphane   A compound found in cruciferous vegetables that can turn on the body's detoxifying enzyme system.

	TABLE 16-2	*Selected Phytochemicals and Their Potential Anticancer Effects*

Compound	Potential Anticancer Effects	Dietary Sources
Allyl sulfides	Increase levels of enzymes that break down potential carcinogens; boost activity of cancer-fighting immune cells	Garlic, onions, leeks, shallots, chives
Capsaicin	Neutralizes the effect of nitrosamines; may block carcinogens in cigarette smoke from acting on cells	Chili peppers (hotter peppers contain more capsaicin)
Carotenoids	Act as antioxidants; reduce levels of cancer-promoting enzymes; inhibit spread of cancer cells	Orange or deep yellow, red or pink, and dark green vegetables and some fruits
Flavonoids	Act as antioxidants; block access of carcinogens to cells; suppress malignant changes in cells; prevent cancer cells from multiplying	Citrus fruits (oranges, lemons, limes), onions, apples, berries, eggplant
Isothiocyanates	Boost production of cancer-fighting enzymes; suppress tumor growth; block effects of estrogen on cell growth	Cruciferous vegetables (broccoli, cabbage, bok choy, cauliflower, kale, brussels sprouts, collards)
Monoterpenes	Help detoxify carcinogens; inhibit spread of cancer cells	Citrus fruits, cherries
Phytic acid	Binds iron, which may prevent iron from creating cell-damaging free radicals	Whole grains, legumes
Phytoestrogens (isoflavones; lignans)	Block effects of estrogen on cell growth; lower blood levels of estrogen; inhibit angiogenesis	Soy foods; whole grains, flax seeds, nuts
Polyphenols	Increase antioxidant activity; prevent cancer cells from multiplying; help speed excretion of carcinogens from the body	Green, oolong, and black teas (Note: drinking tea that is burning hot may *increase* cancer risk)
Resveratrol	Acts as an antioxidant; suppresses tumor growth	Grapes, red wine, peanuts

Inactivity and Obesity

Several common types of cancer are associated with an inactive lifestyle, and research has shown a relationship between increased physical activity and a reduction in cancer risk. There is good evidence that exercise reduces the risk of colon cancer, perhaps by speeding the movement of food through the digestive tract, strengthening immune function, and decreasing blood fat levels. When young girls get adequate exercise, they tend to gain weight more slowly, menstruation begins later, and their risk of breast and ovarian cancers is reduced.

In addition, exercise is important because it helps prevent obesity, an independent risk factor for cancer. A high percentage of body fat appears to increase the risk of cancers of the prostate, breast, female reproductive tract, and kidney and possibly the colon and gallbladder. Obesity may affect hormone levels in the blood, slow the transit time of food through the colon, change the way the body metabolizes fat, and generally promote cell growth. All of these actions have the potential to increase cancer risk.

In the United States, about 150,000 cancer deaths per year appear to be due to a combination of dietary habits and a sedentary lifestyle. One expert estimates that if we were all to exercise for 20 minutes each day and make the dietary changes discussed in this chapter, about 40,000 cancer deaths could be prevented each year.

PERSONAL INSIGHT   Although many people are aware that certain behaviors help prevent cancer, such as using a sunscreen and modifying the diet, a large percentage of them don't act on their knowledge. Do you follow through with behavior changes when you learn that certain things you do increase your risk of cancer? If so, how do you make the changes? If not, why do you think you don't?

Carcinogens in the Environment

Some carcinogens occur naturally in the environment, like the sun's UV rays. Others are manufactured or synthetic substances that show up occasionally in the general environment but more often in the work environments of specific industries.

Ingested Chemicals   The food industry uses preservatives and other additives to prevent food from becoming spoiled or stale (see Chapter 12). Some of these compounds are antioxidants and may actually decrease any cancer-causing properties the food might have. Other compounds, like the nitrates and nitrites found in processed meat, are potentially more dangerous.

Nitrates and nitrites are added to foods like beer and ale, ham, bacon, hot dogs, and lunch meats. The nitrates inhibit the growth of bacteria, which could otherwise cause food poisoning. They also preserve the pink color of the meat, which has no bearing on taste but looks more appetizing to many people. While nitrates and nitrites are not themselves carcinogenic, they can combine with dietary substances in the stomach and be converted to **nitrosamines,** which are highly potent carcinogens. Foods cured with nitrites, as well as those cured by salt or smoke, have been linked to esophageal and stomach cancer, and they should be eaten only in modest amounts.

Environmental and Industrial Pollution   Pollutants in urban air have long been suspected of contributing to the incidence of lung cancer. Fossil fuels and their combustion products, such as complex hydrocarbons, have been of special concern, and most gas stations are now required to provide special nozzles to reduce the amount of gasoline vapor released when you fill your tank. The effect of air pollutants has been difficult to study because of the overwhelmingly greater influence of smoking on lung cancer rates. Urban air pollution appears to have a measurable but limited role in causing lung cancer. (Chapter 24 has more information on the health effects of air pollution.)

The best available data indicate that less than 2% of cancer deaths are caused by general environmental pollution, such as substances in our air and water. Exposure to carcinogenic materials in the workplace is a more serious problem. Occupational exposure to specific carcinogens may account for up to 5% of cancer deaths. Some of the more important workplace carcinogens are listed in Table 16-3, p. 454. With increasing industry and government regulations, we can anticipate that the industrial sources

of cancer risk will continue to diminish, at least in the United States. By contrast, in the former Soviet Union and Eastern European countries, where environmental concerns were sacrificed to industrial productivity for decades, cancer rates from industrial pollution continue to climb.

Radiation   All sources of radiation are potentially carcinogenic, including medical X rays, radioactive substances (radioisotopes), and UV rays from the sun. Striking examples of the effects of radiation can be seen in the survivors of the atomic bombings of Hiroshima and Nagasaki in 1945, and in residents of the area surrounding the Chernobyl nuclear reactor that blew up in 1986. In Japan, new cancers, especially leukemias, are still occurring over 50 years after the bombings. In Belarus, Russia, and Ukraine, the areas most affected by the radioactive debris from Chernobyl, rates of thyroid cancer in children are as much as 30 times higher than before the explosion. Researchers have also found that people living near Chernobyl suffered genetic damage that is being passed on to their children.

The continuing cancer cases in survivors of Hiroshima, Nagasaki, and Chernobyl are a warning to us that any unnecessary exposure to ionizing radiation should be avoided. Most physicians and dentists are quite aware of the risk of radiation, and successful efforts have been made to reduce the amount of radiation needed for mammograms, dental X rays, and other necessary medical X rays.

Another source of environmental radiation is radon gas. Radon is a radioactive decomposition product of radium, which is found in small quantities in some rocks and soils. Because radon is inhaled with the air we breathe, it comes into intimate contact with the cells of the lungs, where its radiation can produce mutations.

nitrosamine   A carcinogen made in the stomach from nitrates and nitrites.

TERMS

Chemical/ Physical Agent	Cancer Type	Exposure of General Population	Examples of Workers Frequently Exposed or Exposure Sources
Arsenic	Lung, skin	Rare	Insecticide and herbicide sprayers; tanners; oil refinery workers
Asbestos	Lung	Uncommon	Brake-lining, shipyard, insulation and demolition workers
Benzene	Leukemia	Common	Painters; distillers and petrochemical workers; dye users; furniture finishers; rubber workers
Diesel exhaust	Lung	Common	Railroad and bus-garage workers; truck operators; miners
Human-made mineral fibers	Lung	Uncommon	Wall and pipe insulation; duct wrapping
Hair dyes	Bladder	Uncommon	Hairdressers and barbers (inadequate evidence for customers)
Ionizing radiation	Bone marrow, several others	Common	Nuclear materials; medical products and procedures
Radon	Lung	Uncommon	Mines; underground structures
Soot	Skin	Uncommon	Chimney sweeps and cleaners; bricklayers; insulators; firefighters; heating-unit service workers

SOURCE: Trichopoulos, D., F. P. Li, and D. J. Hunter. 1996. What causes cancer? *Scientific American,* September. Copyright © 1996 by Scientific American, Inc. All rights reserved. Reprinted with permission.

Radon and smoking together create a more-than-additive risk of lung cancer. Fortunately, in most of our homes and classrooms, radon is rapidly dissipated into the atmosphere, and very low levels of radon do not appear to increase cancer risk. But in certain kinds of enclosed spaces, such as mines, some basements, and airtight houses built of brick or stone, it can rise to dangerous levels (see Chapter 24).

Sunlight is a very important source of radiation, but because its rays penetrate only a millimeter or so into the skin, it could be considered a "surface" carcinogen. Most cases of skin cancer are the relatively benign and highly curable basal cell carcinomas, but a substantial minority are the potentially deadly malignant melanomas. As discussed earlier, all types of skin cancer are increased by early and excessive exposure to the sun, and severe sunburn early in childhood appears to carry with it an added risk of melanoma later in life.

DETECTING, DIAGNOSING, AND TREATING CANCER

Early cancer detection often depends on our willingness to be aware of changes in our own body and to make sure we keep up with recommended diagnostic tests. Although treatment success varies with individual cancers, cure rates have increased—sometimes dramatically—in this century.

Detecting Cancer

Unlike those of some other diseases, early signs of cancer are usually not apparent to anyone but the person who has them. Even pain is not a reliable guide to early detection, because the initial stages of cancer may be painless. Self-monitoring is the first line of defense, and the American Cancer Society recommends that you watch for the seven major warning signs shown in Figure 16-3. Remember them by the acronym CAUTION.

Although none of the warning signs is a sure indication of cancer, the appearance of any one should send you to see your physician. By being aware yourself of the risk factors in your own life, including the cancer history of your immediate family and your own past history, you can often bring a problem to the attention of a physician long before it would have been detected at a routine physical.

In addition to self-monitoring, the ACS recommends a routine cancer checkup every 3 years for people age 20–39 and every year for people age 40 and over, as well as specific screening tests for certain cancers, including those of the breast, colon, and prostate (Table 16-4).

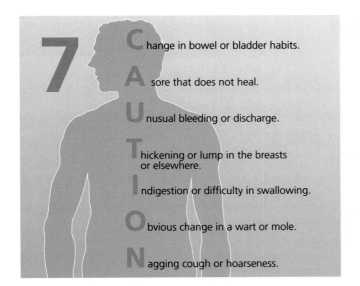

7

C hange in bowel or bladder habits.

A sore that does not heal.

U nusual bleeding or discharge.

T hickening or lump in the breasts or elsewhere.

I ndigestion or difficulty in swallowing.

O bvious change in a wart or mole.

N agging cough or hoarseness.

Figure 16-3   The seven major warning signs of cancer.

Diagnosing Cancer

Detection of a cancer by physical examination is only the beginning. Methods for determining the exact location, type, and degree of malignancy of a cancer continue to improve. Knowledge of the exact location and size of a tumor is necessary for precise and effective surgery or radiation therapy. This is especially true in cases where the tumor may be hard to reach, as in the brain.

A biopsy or exploratory surgery may be performed to identify a cancer's *stage*—a designation based on a tumor's size, location, and spread that helps determine appropriate treatment. New diagnostic imaging techniques have replaced exploratory surgery for some patients. In **magnetic resonance imaging (MRI),** a huge electromagnet is used to detect hidden tumors by mapping, on a computer screen, the vibrations of different atoms in the body. **Computed tomography (CT)** scanning uses X rays to examine the brain and other parts of the body. The process allows the construction of cross sections, which show a tumor's shape and location more accurately than is possible with conventional X rays. For patients undergoing radiation therapy, CT scanning enables the therapist to pinpoint the tumor more precisely, thereby providing more accurate radiation dosage while sparing normal tissue.

Ultrasonography has also been used increasingly in the past few years to view tumors. It has several advantages: It can be used in the physician's office, it is less expensive than other imaging methods, and it is completely safe. Prostate ultrasound (a rectal probe using ultrasonic waves to produce an image of the prostate gland) is currently being investigated for its ability to increase the early detection of small, hidden tumors that would be missed by a digital rectal exam.

Treating Cancer

The ideal cancer therapy would kill or remove all cancerous cells while leaving normal tissue untouched. Sometimes this is almost possible, as when a surgeon removes a small superficial tumor of the skin. Usually the tumor is less accessible, and some combination of surgery, radiation therapy, and chemotherapy must be applied instead. Some patients choose to combine conventional therapies with "alternative" treatments (see the box "Avoiding Cancer Quackery," p. 457).

Surgery   For most cancers, surgery is the most useful therapy. In many cases, the organ containing the tumor is not essential for life and can be partially or completely removed. This is true especially for localized breast, prostate, or testicular cancer, where the surgical removal of one breast, the prostate gland, or one testicle may give a long-lasting cure. Surgery is less effective when the tumor involves cells of the immune system, which are widely distributed throughout the body, or when the cancer has already metastasized. In such cases, surgery must be combined with other techniques.

Chemotherapy   Chemotherapy, or the use of cell-killing drugs to destroy rapidly growing cancer cells, has been in use since the 1940s. Many of these drugs work by interfering with DNA synthesis and replication in rapidly dividing cells. Normal cells, which usually grow slowly, are not destroyed by these drugs. However, some normal tissues such as intestinal, hair, and blood-forming cells are always growing, and damage to these tissues produces the unpleasant side effects of chemotherapy, including nausea, vomiting, diarrhea, and hair loss.

Chemotherapy drugs are often used in combinations or with surgery. Recently, in a procedure called **induction chemotherapy,** physicians have begun to use chemotherapy before surgery, both to shrink the tumor and to kill any existing small metastases as soon as possible.

Radiation   In cancer radiation therapy, a beam of X rays or gamma rays is directed at the tumor, and the tumor cells are killed. Occasionally, when an organ is small enough, radioactive seeds are surgically placed inside the cancerous organ to destroy the tumor, and then removed

magnetic resonance imaging (MRI)   A computerized imaging technique that uses a strong magnetic field and radio frequency signals to examine a thin cross section of the body; also known as *nuclear magnetic resonance imaging (NMR).*

computed tomography (CT)   The use of computerized X ray images to create a cross-sectional depiction of tissue density.

induction chemotherapy   The use of chemotherapy prior to surgery to shrink a cancerous tumor and prevent metastasis; sometimes eliminates the need for radical surgery.

TERMS

TABLE 16-4

Tests Recommended by the American Cancer Society for the Early Detection of Cancer in Asymptomatic People

Site	Recommendation
Breast	Women age 20–39 should have a clinical breast exam (CBE) performed by a health care professional every 3 years and should perform monthly breast self-examination. Women 40 and older should have an annual mammogram, an annual CBE performed by a health care professional, and should perform monthly breast self-examination. The CBE should be conducted close to the scheduled mammogram.
Colon and rectum	Men and women age 50 or older should follow *one* of the following examination schedules: (1) a fecal occult blood test every year and a flexible sigmoidoscopy every 5 years; (2) a colonoscopy every 10 years, or (3) a double-contrast barium enema every 5–10 years. A digital rectal exam should be done at the same time as sigmoidoscopy, colonoscopy, or double-contrast barium enema. People who are at a moderate or high risk for colorectal cancer should talk with a doctor about a different testing schedule.
Prostate	Both the prostate-specific antigen (PSA) blood test and the digital rectal examination should be offered annually, beginning at age 50, to men who have a life expectancy of at least 10 years and to younger men who are at high risk. Men in high risk groups, such as those with a strong familial predisposition (two or more affected first-degree relatives) or African Americans, may begin at a younger age (45 years).
Uterus	*Cervix:* All women who are or have been sexually active or who are 18 and older should have an annual Pap test and pelvic examination. After three or more consecutive satisfactory examinations with normal findings, the Pap test may be performed less frequently. Discuss the matter with your physician. *Endometrium:* Women at high risk for cancer of the uterus should have a sample of endometrial tissue examined when menopause begins.

SOURCE: American Cancer Society. 1999. *Cancer Facts and Figures, 1999.* Atlanta, Ga.: American Cancer Society. Reprinted by the permission of the American Cancer Society, Inc.

later if necessary. Radiation destroys both normal and cancerous cells. But because it can be precisely directed at the tumor, it is usually less toxic for the patient than either surgery or chemotherapy, and it can often be performed on an outpatient basis. Radiation may be used as an exclusive treatment or in combination with surgery and/or chemotherapy.

New and Experimental Techniques   With greater understanding of cellular functions and the genes involved in cancer, a great many new and exciting possibilities have opened up for cancer therapy. Although it is impossible to predict which of these new approaches will be most successful, researchers hope that cancer therapy overall will become increasingly safe and effective.

- *Bone marrow transplants.* In cancers of the blood-forming cells or lymph cells, a patient's own bone marrow may be eliminated by radiation or chemo- therapy to rid the body of cancer cells. Bone marrow can then be restored by transplanting healthy bone marrow cells from a compatible donor. This technique is increasingly being applied to cancers that do not originate in the bone marrow, especially breast cancer.

- *Biological therapies.* Biological therapies are based on enhancing the immune system's reaction to a tumor. Techniques include cancer vaccines, genetic modification of the body's immune cells, and the use of genetically engineered **cytokines,** which enhance immune cell function. Melanomas seem particularly susceptible to these biological approaches.

- *Protease inhibitors.* To spread, cancer cells must activate a set of enzymes known as proteases, which enable them to dissolve the substances between cells and then migrate through normal tissues. **Protease inhibitors** are being developed to interfere with actions of specific proteases, thereby blocking cancer cells' ability to invade normal tissue and metastasize.

- *Anti-angiogenesis drugs.* To obtain nutrients, cancer cells signal the body to produce new blood vessels, a process called angiogenesis. Drugs that block angiogenesis could keep tumors from growing.

- *Telomerase inhibitors.* Normal human cells die after a limited number of divisions; cancer cells do not, in part because of the enzyme telomerase. Researchers hope to develop drugs to block the enzyme.

TERMS   **cytokine**   A chemical messenger produced by a variety of cell types that helps regulate many cell functions; immune system cells release cytokines that help amplify and coordinate the immune response.

protease inhibitor   A drug that inhibits the action of any of the protein-splitting enzymes known as proteases. Because some proteases facilitate metastasis, protease inhibitors are being developed for cancer therapy.

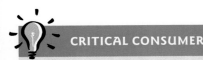
Sometimes conventional treatments for cancer are simply not enough. A patient may be told that there is little conventional therapy can do, other than providing medication to ease pain. Even when therapy is available, it may be painful and even intolerable to some people. Not surprisingly, many cancer patients look for alternatives. These may be therapies within the bounds of legitimate medical practice that have not yet proven themselves in clinical trials. Or, at the other extreme, alternative therapies may be scientifically unsound and dangerous, as well as expensive.

The National Cancer Institute suggests that patients and their families consider the following questions when making decisions about cancer treatment:

- *Has the treatment been evaluated in clinical trials?* Advances in cancer treatment are made through carefully monitored clinical trials. If a patient wants to try a new therapy, participation in a clinical trial may be a treatment option. (See For More Information at the end of the chapter for more on clinical trials.)

- *Do the practitioners of an approach claim that the medical community is trying to keep their cure from the public?* No one genuinely committed to finding better ways to treat a disease would knowingly keep an effective treatment a secret or try to suppress such a treatment.

- *Does the treatment rely on nutritional or diet therapy as its main focus?* Although diet can be a key risk factor in the development of cancer, there is no evidence that diet alone can get rid of cancerous cells in the body.

- *Do those who endorse the treatment claim that it is harmless and painless and that it produces no unpleasant side effects?* Reputable researchers are working to develop less toxic cancer therapies, but because effective treatments for cancer must be very powerful, they frequently have unpleasant side effects.

- *Does the treatment have a "secret formula" that only a small group of practitioners can use?* Scientists who believe they have developed an effective treatment routinely publish their results in reputable journals so they can be evaluated by other researchers.

Many patients who try an alternative treatment do so in combination with conventional medical care. Alternative therapies may thus meet a different need than those used by the medical establishment. Only patients and their families can decide what they want from a particular treatment.

SOURCES: Aulas, J. 1996. Alternative cancer treatments. *Scientific American,* September. National Cancer Institute.

Living with Cancer

Earlier in this century, a diagnosis of cancer was almost equivalent to a death sentence. Gradually, however, survival has become the norm, and there are, in fact, 7.5 million cancer survivors in the United States today. However, for these people, the fear of cancer never completely disappears, and there is always the risk of a recurrence.

Cancer survivors may suffer economic prejudice from insurers, who can refuse to issue or renew health coverage. This sort of problem can be devastating to a cancer survivor who may be struggling both psychologically and financially to restore a normal existence. Several states have passed legislation to prevent this kind of discrimination, but it still exists.

Psychological support is an important factor during treatment for cancer (see the box "Coping with Cancer"). For some patients, family and friends plus a caring physician or nurse provide all the support that is necessary. But often, health care providers are busy or aloof, and family members and friends are just as fearful about the outcome as the patient. For many people, an organized support group can help provide needed social and psychological support. There is even some evidence that cancer patients may live longer when they become part of a professionally led support group (see the box "Support Groups and Cancer Survival"). The possibility that psychological health can enhance cancer survival is controversial, but

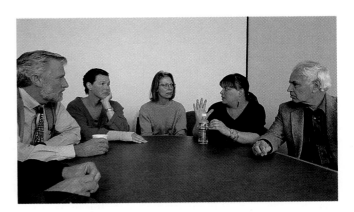

Social support can play a crucial role in cancer treatment for these patients. Studies indicate that support group participants have lower levels of anxiety and depression, manage pain more successfully, and possibly even live longer than cancer patients who are not in support groups.

no one doubts that support groups can promote emotional wellness in both patients and their families.

PREVENTING CANCER

Your lifestyle choices can radically lower your cancer risks, so you *can* take a very practical approach to cancer prevention (Figure 16-4, p. 460).

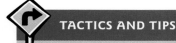
Visiting a Cancer Patient

- Before you visit, call ahead to ask if it's a good time. Surprise visits are often not welcome. Don't overstay your welcome.

- Be a good listener. Allow the person to express all his or her feelings, and don't discount fears or minimize the seriousness of the situation. Let the patient decide whether the two of you talk about the illness. It's human to want to laugh and talk about other things sometimes.

- Ask "What can I get you?" or "How can I help?" instead of saying "Let me know if I can help." Make specific offers: to clean the bathroom, go grocery shopping, do laundry, or give caregivers a break.

- Refrain from offering advice. You may have heard about the latest treatment or hottest physician, but unless you are asked for suggestions, keep them to yourself.

- If you want to take food, ask about dietary restrictions ahead of time. Use a disposable container so the person doesn't have to worry about returning it.

- Don't be put off if your first visit gets a lukewarm reception. Many cancer victims are on an emotional roller coaster, and their feelings and needs will change over time.

If You Are the Patient

- Remember that cancer doesn't always mean death. Many cancers are curable or controllable for long periods, and survivors may return to a normal, healthy life. Hope and optimism can be important elements in cancer survival.

- Don't feel guilty if you can't keep a positive attitude all the time. Having cancer is difficult, and low moods will occur no matter how good you are at coping. But if they become frequent or severe, seek help.

- Use any strategies that have helped you solve problems and manage your emotions in the past. Some people respond to information gathering, talking with others, and prayer or meditation.

- Find a physician you trust and can communicate well with. Ask questions, and insist on being a partner in your treatment.

- Confide your worries to someone close to you. Don't bottle up your feelings to "spare" your loved ones. Ask someone you trust to accompany you on visits to your physician and treatment sessions.

- Explore groups that can help you get through this difficult time. There are many support groups for people who have cancer or who have survived it.

SOURCES: Life with cancer: How to provide support. 1996. *Women's Health Advocate.* September. Holland, J. C. 1996. Cancer's psychological challenges. *Scientific American,* September.

Avoiding Tobacco

Smoking is responsible for 80–90% of all lung cancers and for about 30% of all cancer deaths. People who smoke two or more packs of cigarettes a day have lung cancer mortality rates 15–25 times greater than those of nonsmokers. The carcinogenic chemicals in smoke are transported throughout the body in the bloodstream, making smoking a carcinogen for many forms of cancer other than lung cancer. ETS is dangerous to nonsmokers. If you smoke, stop. If you don't smoke, avoid breathing the smoke from other people's cigarettes.

The use of spit tobacco, highly habit-forming because of its nicotine content, is also dangerous because it increases the risk of cancers of the mouth, larynx, throat, and esophagus. Refer to Chapter 11 for tips on breaking the tobacco habit.

Controlling Diet and Weight

Based on hundreds of studies, the National Cancer Institute estimates that about one-third of all cancers are in some way linked to what we eat. Choose a lowfat, plant-based diet containing a wide variety of fruits, vegetables, and whole grains rich in phytochemicals. See the specific suggestions in the Behavior Change Strategy at the end of this chapter.

Drink alcohol only in moderation, if at all. Oral cancer and cancers of the larynx, throat, esophagus, and liver occur more frequently among heavy drinkers of alcohol. The risk is even higher among heavy drinkers who smoke.

The risk of several cancers increases for obese people. Maintaining a healthy weight through a moderate diet and regular exercise lowers the risk. Chapters 12 and 14 provide strategies for improving your diet and maintaining a healthy body weight.

Regular Exercise

Regular exercise is linked to lower rates of colon and other cancers. It also helps control weight. Refer to Chapter 13 for advice on setting up a lifelong program of regular exercise.

Protecting Skin from the Sun

Almost all cases of nonmelanoma skin cancer are considered to be sun-related, and sun exposure is a major factor

Stanford University psychiatrist Dr. David Spiegel and his colleagues carried out a 3-year study on women with advanced breast cancer to determine how participation in a support group would affect their psychological health. Women in the experimental group not only received standard medical care, they also participated in weekly group therapy sessions. In the support group, women shared their fears, planned means of coping with the threat of death, grieved over the loss of group members, learned to control their pain with self-hypnosis, and looked for ways to live more fully in the time they had left.

At the conclusion of the study, researchers found that women in the study had, indeed, been helped by the support group. They were less anxious and depressed and were better able to control their pain than women in the control group, who received only standard medical treatment. The real surprise came several years later when Dr. Spiegel reexamined the data from this study. He found that the women who participated in the support group also lived on average more than twice as long from the start of the study than women in the control group.

How might support groups improve the survival as well as the psychological health of participants? Researchers have hypothesized several ways in which psychosocial support could be translated into changes in physical health:

- Social support may affect behavior, making patients in a

support group more likely to engage in healthy behaviors such as eating well, exercising regularly, and getting plenty of sleep.

- Cancer patients who benefit from group support might interact more effectively with their physicians, eliciting more vigorous medical treatment.

- Support groups may buffer people against stress, cushioning the body from the effects of the stress response.

- Social support may be particularly helpful in reducing the negative effects of stress on the immune system: A strong immune system may enable the body to fight cancer more effectively.

Additional research should help clarify how support groups benefit cancer patients. In the meantime, this study can serve as a reminder of the powerful effects social support has on our physical and emotional well-being, whether we are coping with a life-threatening illness or the challenges of everyday life.

SOURCES: Spiegel, D., et al. 1998. Effects of psychosocial treatment in prolonging cancer survival may be mediated by neuroimmune pathways. *Annals of the New York Academy of Sciences* 840: 674–683. Spiegel, D. 1993. *Living Beyond Limits: New Hope and Help for Facing Life-Threatening Illness.* New York: Random House.

in the development of melanoma as well. Wear protective clothing when you're out in the sun, and use a sunscreen with an SPF rating of 15 or higher. Don't go to tanning salons; they do not provide "safe tans."

Avoiding Environmental and Occupational Carcinogens

Most medical X rays are adjusted to deliver the lowest dose of radiation possible without sacrificing image quality. Radiation from radon may pose a threat in some homes; remedial steps should be taken if tests indicate high levels of radon. A number of industrial agents that some people are exposed to on the job are associated with cancer, including nickel, chromate, asbestos, and vinyl chloride. Try to avoid occupational exposure to carcinogens, and don't smoke; the cancer risks of many of these agents increase greatly when combined with smoking.

Recommended Screening Tests

Your first line of defense against cancer involves the lifestyle changes described above that help you avoid cancer-causing agents. Your second line of defense involves having any cancers that do develop discovered as quickly as possible through regular self-exams and medical screening tests. Stay alert for the signs and symptoms that could indicate cancer (see Figure 16-3), and follow the

American Cancer Society screening guidelines listed in Table 16-4. Both lifestyle changes and a program of early detection are important to your long-term health.

SUMMARY

What Is Cancer?

- A malignant tumor can invade surrounding structures and spread to distant sites via the blood and lymphatic system, producing additional tumors.

- A malignant cell divides without regard for normal growth. As tumors grow, they produce signs or symptoms that are determined by their location in the body.

- One in two men and one in three women will develop cancer, but more than half will be cured.

Common Cancers

- Lung cancer kills more people than any other type of cancer. Tobacco smoke is the primary cause.

- Colon and rectal cancer is linked to age, heredity, obesity, and a diet rich in red meat and low in fruits and vegetables. Most colon cancers arise from preexisting polyps.

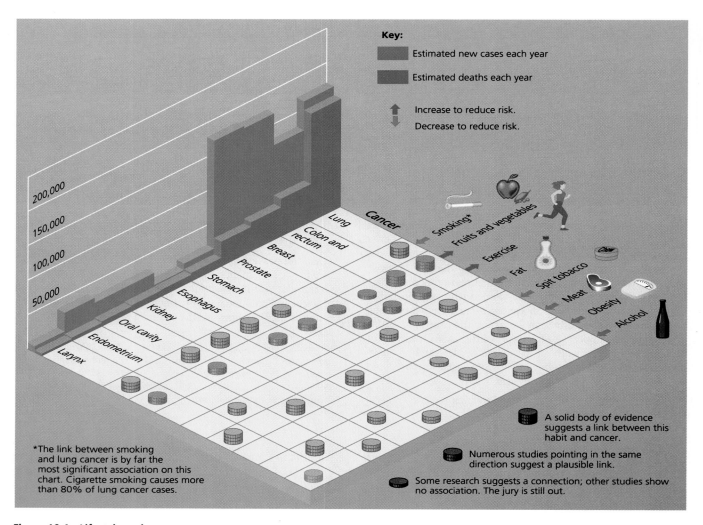

Figure 16-4 Lifestyle and cancer. SOURCE: Beating the odds: Best bets for cancer prevention. 1996. *Tufts University Health and Nutrition Letter,* December. Reprinted with permission. American Cancer Society. 1999. *Cancer Facts and Figures, 1999.* New York: American Cancer Society.

- Breast cancer affects about one in nine women in the United States. Although there is a genetic component to breast cancer, diet and hormones are also risk factors.

- Prostate cancer is chiefly a disease of aging; diet and lifestyle probably are factors in its occurrence. Early detection is possible through rectal examinations, PSA blood tests, and sometimes ultrasound.

- Cancers of the female reproductive tract include cervical, uterine, and ovarian cancer. The Pap test is an effective screening test for cervical cancer.

- Abnormal cellular changes in the epidermis, often a result of exposure to the sun, cause skin cancer, as does chronic exposure to certain chemicals. Skin cancers occur as basal cell carcinoma, squamous cell carcinoma, and melanoma.

- Oral cancer is caused primarily by smoking, excess alcohol consumption, and use of spit tobacco. Oral cancers are easy to detect, but often hard to treat.

- Testicular cancer can be detected early through self-examination. Bladder cancer, often associated with smoking, has a high survival rate if detected at an early stage. Pancreatic cancer is hard to detect and usually fatal.

The Causes of Cancer

- Mutational damage to a cell's DNA can lead to rapid and uncontrolled growth of cells; mutagens include radiation, viral infection, and chemical substances in food and air.

- The genetic basis of some cancers appears to be related to suppressor genes, which normally limit cell growth; people can inherit altered suppressor genes.

When we think of the health benefits of fruits, vegetables, grains, and legumes, we usually focus on the fact that they are high in fiber and low in fat. These properties are important for cancer prevention, but researchers are discovering a new reason to eat more of these foods: phytochemicals. There is a previously undiscovered world of natural chemicals in edible plants that help the body avoid cancer by slowing, stopping, and even reversing the process of cancer.

You don't have to make radical changes in order to increase the amount of phytochemicals in your diet. Begin by monitoring your diet for 1–2 weeks in your health journal. Note both the health-protecting and cancer-promoting foods you eat. Then look for ways to incorporate more plant foods into your diet.

Phase I: Additions

- Add fresh vegetables to omelets, potato dishes, tuna salad, and pasta sauces. Try broccoli or cauliflower florets, mushrooms, sauteed onions and garlic, peas, carrots, or zucchini.

- Use fresh or frozen fruit as a topping for hot or cold cereal, pancakes, and desserts.

- Get creative with sandwiches; lettuce and tomato are just the beginning. Add slices of cucumber or zucchini, bean sprouts, spinach, carrot slivers, or snow peas.

- Add more veggies at the salad bar. Try fresh spinach, red cabbage, squash, cauliflower, broccoli, peas, mushrooms, onions, or peppers.

Phase II: Substitutions

- Instead of snacking on chips or candy, keep fruits or vegetables on hand. Try apples, oranges, bananas, grapes, peaches, carrot and celery sticks, and cherry tomatoes. You can buy prewashed and cut vegetables in the produce section of many grocery stores.

- Choose fruit-filled cookies, such as fig bars.

- Use salsa as a dip for chips and veggies, instead of creamy dips.

- Drink fruit or vegetable juices instead of soda.

- Choose whole-grain breakfast cereals, breads, and crackers instead of processed products.

Phase III: New Recipes

- Try one or two vegetarian meals each week. Some good choices are pasta with tomato-vegetable sauce, baked potato topped with sauteed vegetables, and beans and rice.

- Look for quick-fixing grain side dishes at the supermarket. Try something new, like rice pilaf, couscous, or tabbouleh.

- Experiment with soy products like tofu, soy milk, and roasted soybeans.

- Plan meals around grain products, beans, and vegetables. Treat meat and dairy products as side dishes or condiments.

A diet rich in phytochemicals goes beyond cancer prevention; it will help you manage your weight and avoid other chronic diseases like heart disease, stroke, and diabetes. Try making these changes over the course of a few months, to optimize your wellness and improve your chances for a cancer-free future.

- Cancer-promoting dietary factors include meat, certain types of fats, and alcohol. Certain methods of food preparation may also increase cancer risk.

- Diets high in fruits and vegetables are linked to a lower risk of cancer. Protective elements include vitamin C, vitamin E, and other antioxidants and sulforaphane and other phytochemicals.

- Some carcinogens occur naturally in the environment; others are manufactured substances. Occupational exposure is a risk for some workers.

- All sources of radiation are potentially carcinogenic, including X rays, radioisotopes, radon gas, and the UV rays of the sun.

Detecting, Diagnosing, and Treating Cancer

- Self-monitoring is essential to early cancer detection; the appearance of any early signs necessitates a visit to a physician. The signs can be remembered by using the acronym CAUTION. Regular screening tests are also important.

- Methods of cancer diagnosis include magnetic resonance imaging, computed tomography, and ultrasound.

- Treatment methods usually consist of some combination of surgery, chemotherapy, and radiation. Bone marrow transplants, protease inhibitors, biological therapies, and drugs that inhibit angiogenesis or telomerase also hold promise as effective treatments.

Preventing Cancer

- Strategies for preventing cancer include avoiding tobacco; eating a varied, moderate diet and controlling weight; exercising regularly; protecting skin from the sun; avoiding exposure to environmental and occupational carcinogens; and getting recommended cancer screening tests.

1. Look through the foods listed in Table 16-2 and the Behavior Change Strategy and choose four or five that you don't typically eat. During the next week, make a point of trying each of the foods you've chosen.

2. Devise a plan for incorporating regular self-examinations for cancer (breast self-examination or testicle self-examination) into your life. What strategies will help you remember to do your monthly exam? How can you keep yourself motivated?

3. Interview your parents or grandparents about your family medical history. Are there any cases of cancer in your family, and has anyone died of cancer? Do you see any patterns?

1. In your health journal, list the positive behaviors that help you avoid cancer. How can you strengthen these behaviors? Also list the behaviors that tend to increase your risk, and plan ways to change them.

2. *Critical Thinking* Smoking is responsible for 85–90% of all lung cancers. Are tobacco companies in any way responsible for the high number of deaths from lung cancer each year? Or is each person entirely responsible for his or her own behavior and health? In your health journal, write a brief essay outlining your position on this issue. Then write a brief essay that supports the opposite viewpoint.

3. Make a list of risk factors for cancer over which you have no control, including heredity and personal history. Do these risk factors increase your risk for any cancers? If so, make a list of behaviors you can adopt that will lower your risk.

4. *Critical Thinking* Should people who inherit a genetic defect that increases their risk of cancer pay higher insurance premiums? Should companies be able to deny them employment or health, life, or disability insurance? Should people be held responsible for risk factors like heredity that they cannot control, or only for risk factors they can control, such as smoking? What about risk factors like obesity that are due to a combination of heredity and lifestyle? Write an essay explaining your position.

Books and Newsletters

American Cancer Society and American Heart Association. 1999. *Living Well, Staying Well.* New York: Random House. *A practical guide to reducing cancer risk.*

American Institute for Cancer Research. 1999. *Stopping Cancer Before It Starts.* New York: Golden Books. *Suggests research-based changes in diet and lifestyle to help prevent cancer.*

McKinnell, R. G., et al. 1998. *The Biological Basis of Cancer.* Cambridge: Cambridge University Press. *A thorough review of the causes of cancer.*

Murphy, G. P., ed. 1999. *American Cancer Society's Informed Decisions: The Complete Book of Cancer Diagnosis, Treatment, and Recovery.* New York: Viking. *Provides information to help a patient deal with cancer.*

Scientific American. 1997. *What You Need to Know About Cancer.* New York: Freeman. *A broad survey of cancer, from the molecular details of the causes and spread of cancer to new methods of treatment.*

Scientific American Cancer Outlook. A quarterly newsletter covering a variety of cancer topics (800-996-7522).

Organizations, Hotlines, and Web Sites

American Academy of Dermatology. Provides information on skin cancer prevention.

888-462-DERM
http://www.aad.org

American Cancer Society. Provides a wide range of free materials on the prevention and treatment of cancer.

1599 Clifton Rd., N.E.
Atlanta, GA 30329
800-ACS-2345
http://www.cancer.org

American Institute for Cancer Research. Provides information on lifestyle and cancer prevention, especially nutrition.

1759 R Street, N.W.
Washington, DC 20009
800-843-8114
http://www.aicr.org

Cancer Guide: Steve Dunn's Cancer Information Page. Links to many good cancer resources on the Internet and advice about how to make best use of information.

http://www.cancerguide.org

Cancer News. Provides links to news and information on many types of cancer.

http://www.cancernews.com

Clinical Trials. Information about clinical trials for new cancer treatments can be accessed at the following sites:

http://cancertrials.nci.nih.gov
http://www.centerwatch.com

Dole 5-A-Day/Nutrition Education. Provides resources for parents, children, and educators, including extensive nutrition information about fruits and vegetables.

http://www.dole5aday.com

EPA/UV Index. Information about the UV Index and the effects of sun exposure, with links to sites with daily UV Index ratings for cities in the United States and other countries.

http://www.epa.gov/ozone/uvindex/uvover.html

National Cancer Institute. Provides information on treatment options, screening, and clinical trials and on the national "5 Day for Better Health Program" that promotes greater consumption of fruits and vegetables.

9000 Rockville Pike
Bethesda, MD 20892

800-4-CANCER; 800-624-2511 (Cancer Fax)
http://www.nci.nih.gov
http://cancernet.nci.nih.gov
http://www.dcpc.nci.nih.gov/5ADay

New York Online Access to Health (NOAH)/Cancer. Provides information about cancer—causes, symptoms, types, treatments, clinical trials—and links to related sites.

http://www.noah.cuny.edu/cancer/cancer.html

Oncolink/The University of Pennsylvania Cancer Center Resources. Contains information on different types of cancer and answers to frequently asked questions.

http://www.oncolink.upenn.edu

See also the listings in Chapters 10–14.

SELECTED BIBLIOGRAPHY

American Cancer Society. 1999. *Cancer Facts and Figures, 1999.* Atlanta, Ga.: American Cancer Society.

American Institute for Cancer Research. 1999. *The Obesity Factor* (retrieved January 27, 1999; http://www.aicr.org/nl62ar4.htm).

Baron, J. A., et al. 1999. Calcium supplements for the prevention of colorectal adenomas. *New England Journal of Medicine* 340(2): 101–107.

Berger, D. H., et al. 1999. Mutational activation of K-ras in non-neoplastic exocrine pancreatic lesions in relation to cigarette smoking status. *Cancer* 85(2): 326–332.

Cummings, J. H., and S. A. Bingham. 1998. Diet and the prevention of cancer. *British Medical Journal* 317: 1636–1640.

deLorgeril, M., et al. 1998. Mediterranean dietary pattern in a randomized trial: Prolonged survival and possible reduced cancer rate. *Archives of Internal Medicine* 158(11): 1181–1187.

DES Action. 1999. *Health Risks and Care for DES Daughters* (retrieved January 29, 1999; http://www.desaction.org/daughter.html).

Disease-fighting foods? 1999. *Consumer Reports on Health,* March.

Fuchs, C. S., et al. 1999. Dietary fiber and the risk of colorectal cancer and adenoma in women. *New England Journal of Medicine* 340(3): 169–170.

Giovannucci, E., et al. 1998. Multivitamin use, folate, and colon cancer in women in the Nurses' Health Study. *Annals of Internal Medicine* 129(7): 517–524.

Hanson, K. M., and J. D. Simon. 1998. Epidermal *trans*-urocanic acid and the UV-A-induced photoaging of the skin. *Science* 95(18): 10576–10578.

Hartmann, L. C., et al. 1999. Efficacy of bilateral prophylactic mastectomy in women with a family history of breast cancer. *New England Journal of Medicine* 340(2): 77–84.

Henkel, J. 1998. Prostate cancer: No one answer for testing or treatment. *FDA Consumer,* September/October.

Hirose, K., et al. 1999. Effect of body size on breast-cancer risk among Japanese women. *International Journal of Cancer* 80(3): 349–355.

Holt, P. R., et al. 1998. Modulation of abnormal colonic epithelial cell proliferation and differentiation by low-fat dairy foods. *Journal of the American Medical Association* 280: 1074–1079.

Jumaan, A. O., et al. 1999. Beta-carotene intake and risk of postmenopausal breast cancer. *Epidemiology* 10(1): 49–53.

Kolonel, L. N., A. M. Nomura, and R. V. Cooney. 1999. Dietary fat and prostate cancer: Current status. *Journal of the National Cancer Institute* 91(5): 414–428.

National Cancer Institute. 1999. *Clinical Announcement: Concurrent Chemoradiation for Cervical Cancer* (retrieved April 8, 1999; http://cancertrials.nci.nih.gov/NCI_CANCER_TRIALS/zones/TrialInfo/News/cervcan/clinann.html).

Newbold, R. R., et al. 1998. Increased tumors but uncompromised fertility in the female descendants of mice exposed developmentally to diethylstilbestrol. *Carcinogenesis* 19(9): 1655–1663.

Oriel, K. A., E. M. Hartenbach, and P. L. Remington. 1999. Trends in United States ovarian cancer mortality, 1979–1995. *Obstetrics and Gynecology* 93(1): 30–33.

Osborne, C. K. 1998. Drug therapy: Tamoxifen in the treatment of breast cancer. *New England Journal of Medicine* 339(22): 1609–1618.

Palefsky, J. M., et al. 1999. Cervicovaginal HPV infection in HIV-positive and high-risk HIV-negative women. *Journal of the National Cancer Institute* 91(3): 226–236.

Pegram, M. D., et al. 1998. Phase II study of HER2/neu monoclonal antibody in patients with metastatic breast cancer. *Journal of Clinical Oncology* 16(8): 2659–2671.

Rigel, D. S., E. G. Rigel, and A. C. Rigel. 1999. Effects of altitude and latitude on ambient UVB radiation. *Journal of the American Academy of Dermatology* 40(1): 114–116.

Shephard, R. J., and P. N. Shek. 1998. Associations between physical activity and susceptibility to cancer: Possible mechanisms. *Sports Medicine* 26(5): 293–315.

Slattery, M. L., et al. 1998. Eating patterns and risk of colon cancer. *American Journal of Epidemiology* 148(1): 4–16.

Turner, M. 1998. Sun safety: Avoiding noonday sun, wearing protective clothing, and the use of sunscreen. *Journal of the National Cancer Institute* 90(24): 1854–1855.

Zhang, Y., et al. 1999. Alcohol consumption and risk of breast cancer: The Framingham Study revisited. *American Journal of Epidemiology* 149(2): 93–101.

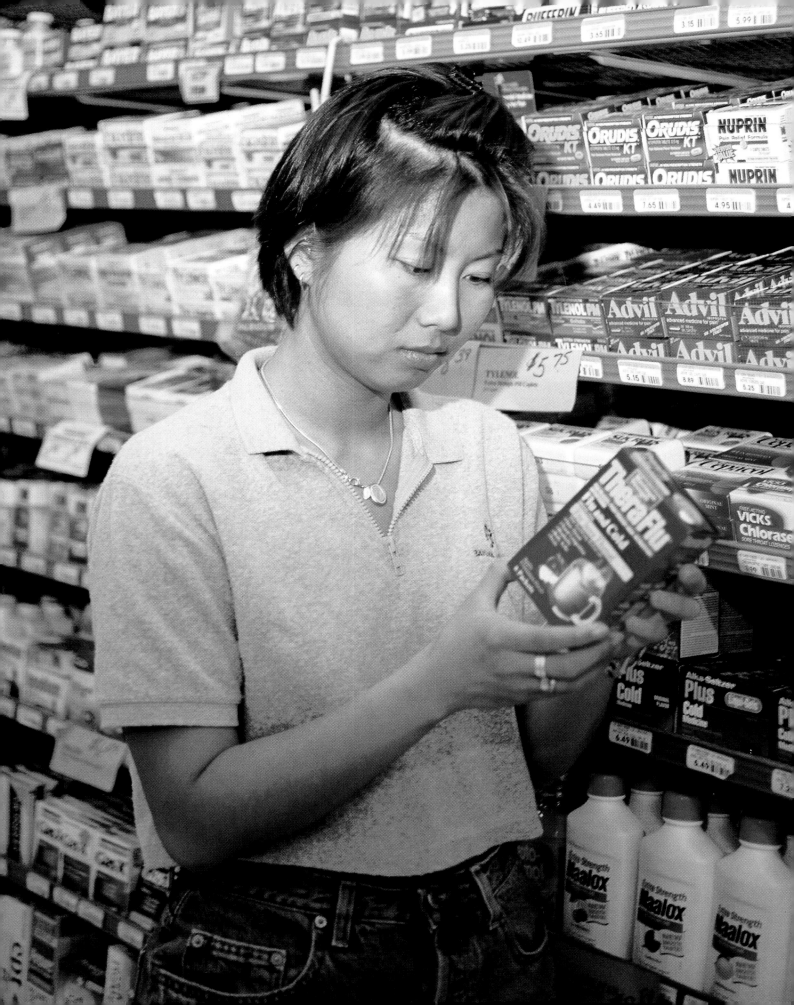

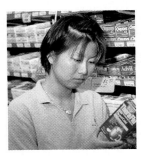

LEARNING OBJECTIVES

After reading this chapter, you should be able to:

- Describe the step-by-step process by which infectious diseases are transmitted.
- List the body's physical and chemical barriers to infection.
- Explain how the immune system responds to an invading micro-organism.
- List the major types of pathogens, and describe the common diseases they cause.
- Discuss steps you can take to prevent infections and strengthen your immune system.

Immunity and Infection

17

TEST YOUR KNOWLEDGE

1. A person with an infectious disease is not contagious unless he or she exhibits symptoms.
   True or false?

2. Which of the following is helpful in treating a cold?
   a. antibiotics
   b. antihistamines
   c. decongestants

3. When taking a prescription antibiotic, you should stop taking the medicine as soon as your infection clears up.
   True or false?

4. If you have ever injected illegal drugs, even if it was only once and many years ago, you are at risk for hepatitis.
   True or false?

5. You can lower your chances of getting sick by
   a. washing your hands frequently
   b. obtaining all recommended immunizations
   c. getting adequate sleep

Answers

1. *False.* A person can be contagious before exhibiting any symptoms and may cease to be contagious before symptoms disappear.

2. *c.* Although 60% of Americans believe that antibiotics are useful for viral infections like colds and the flu, antibiotics are actually effective only against bacteria. Antihistamines are most effective against allergies, not colds.

3. *False.* More than 50% of people fail to take all their medication, leading to relapses and the development of antibi-otic-resistant bacteria.

4. *True.* About 80% of current injecting drug users are infected with hepatitis C virus (HCV), and many people acquire HCV from very limited injecting drug use. The CDC recommends testing for anyone who ever injected drugs.

5. *All three.* Frequent hand washing prevents the transmission of many disease-causing agents. Immunizations prime the body to tackle an invading organism; adequate sleep helps support a healthy immune system.

Most of the time, we go about our daily lives thinking of the world as a place inhabited by beings more or less like ourselves. We seldom think of the countless, unseen microscopic organisms that live around, on, and in us. Although most microbes are beneficial, many of them can cause human disease. But the constant vigilance of our immune system keeps them at bay and our bodies intact and healthy.

Even without these "invaders," our bodies have a tendency to develop problems and diseases. The natural aging process of the human body is a prime example of the second law of thermodynamics: that all things have a tendency toward disorder or disintegration. The immune system works to keep the body from being overwhelmed not just by external invaders that cause **infections,** but also by internal changes, such as cancer.

Most people don't pay much attention to these internal skirmishes unless they become sick and find themselves deprived of their usual feelings of well-being. But many people today are more knowledgeable about the complexities of immunity because they have heard about, or had experience with, HIV infection, which directly attacks the immune system. This chapter provides information that will help you understand immunity, infection, and how you can keep yourself well in a world of disease-causing microorganisms.

THE CHAIN OF INFECTION

Infectious diseases are transmitted from one person to another through a series of steps—a chain of infection (Figure 17-1). New infections can be prevented by interfering with any of the steps in this process.

Links in the Chain

The chain of infection has six major links: the pathogen, its reservoir, a portal of exit, a means of transmission, a portal of entry, and a new host.

TERMS   **infection** A disease caused by an invading microorganism.

pathogen An organism that causes disease.

toxin A poisonous substance produced by a microorganism.

host An organism infected by a pathogen.

vector An insect, rodent, or other organism that carries and transmits a pathogen.

lymphatic system A system of vessels and organs that picks up excess fluid, proteins, lipids, and other substances from the tissues; filters out pathogens and other waste products; and returns the cleansed fluid to the general circulation.

systemic infection An infection spread by the blood or lymphatic system to large portions of the body.

Pathogen   The infectious disease cycle begins with a **pathogen,** a microorganism that causes disease. HIV, the virus that causes AIDS, and the tuberculosis bacterium are examples of pathogens. Many pathogens cause illness because they produce **toxins** that harm human tissue; others do so by directly invading body cells.

Reservoir   The pathogen has a natural environment in which it typically resides. This so-called reservoir can be a person, an animal, or an environmental component like soil or water. A person who is the reservoir for a pathogen may be ill or may be an asymptomatic carrier who, although having no symptoms, is capable of spreading infection.

Portal of Exit   To transmit infection, the pathogen must leave the reservoir through some portal of exit. In the case of a human reservoir, portals of exit include saliva (for mumps, for example), the mucous membranes (for many sexually transmitted diseases), blood (for HIV and hepatitis), feces (for intestinal infections), and nose and throat discharges (for colds and influenza).

Means of Transmission   Transmission can occur directly or indirectly. In direct transmission, the pathogen is passed from one person to another without an intermediate component. Direct transmission usually requires fairly close association with an infected **host,** but not necessarily physical contact. For example, sneezing and coughing can discharge infectious particles into the air, where they can be inhaled by someone nearby. Many common respiratory infections are passed directly: A person with a cold blows her nose and gets some infectious droplets on her hands; she then shakes hands with someone, who later touches his nose and passes the pathogen into his own body. Many intestinal infections are also transmitted hand-to-hand; the initial contamination may result from a failure to wash hands after using the toilet or changing a diaper. Other means of direct transmission include sexual contact and contact with blood.

Transmission can also occur indirectly. Animals or insects such as rats, ticks, and mosquitoes can serve as **vectors,** carrying the pathogen from one host to another. Pathogens can also be transmitted via contaminated soil, food, or water or from inanimate objects, such as eating utensils, doorknobs, and handkerchiefs. Some pathogens float in the air for long periods, suspended on tiny particles of dust or droplets that can travel long distances before they are inhaled and cause infection.

Portal of Entry   To infect a new host, a pathogen must have a portal of entry into the body. Pathogens can enter in one of three general ways:

1. Penetration of the skin or direct contact.
2. Inhalation through the mouth or nose.
3. Ingestion of contaminated food or water.

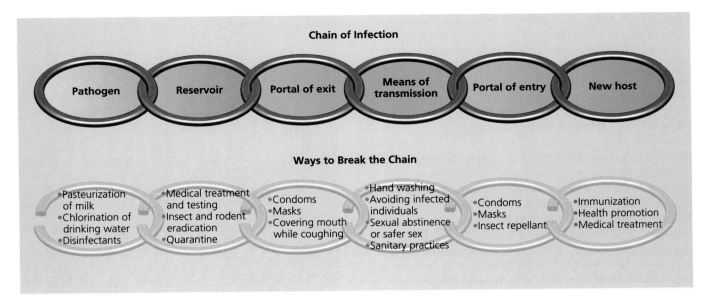

Figure 17-1 **The chain of infection.** Any break in the chain of infection can prevent disease.

Pathogens that enter the skin or mucous membranes can cause a local infection of the tissue, or they may penetrate into the bloodstream or **lymphatic system,** thereby causing a more extensive **systemic infection.** Agents that cause STDs usually enter the body through the mucous membranes lining the urethra (in males) or the cervix (in females). Organisms that are transmitted via respiratory secretions may cause upper respiratory infections or pneumonia, or they may enter the bloodstream and cause systemic infection. Most respiratory infections, however, are contracted through direct contact, from hand to hand and then to mouth or nose, rather than through the inhalation of airborne droplets. Foodborne and waterborne organisms enter the mouth and travel to the location that will best support their reproduction. They may attack the cells of the small intestine or the colon, causing diarrhea and other symptoms, or they may enter the bloodstream via the digestive system and travel to other parts of the body.

The New Host   Once in the new host, a variety of factors determine whether the pathogen will be able to establish itself and cause infection. People with a strong immune system or resistance to a particular pathogen will be less likely to become ill than people with poor immunity (the concept of immunity will be discussed later in the chapter). The number of pathogens that enter the new host is also important; the body's defenses may be able to overcome a few bacteria, for example, but may be overwhelmed by thousands. If conditions are right, the pathogen will multiply and produce disease in the new host. In such a case, the new host may become a reservoir from which a new chain of infection can be started.

Breaking the Chain

Interruption of the chain of infection at any point can prevent disease. Strategies for breaking the chain include a mix of public health measures and individual action. For example, a pathogen's reservoir can be isolated or destroyed, as when a sick individual is placed under quarantine or when insects or animals carrying pathogens are killed. Public sanitation practices, such as sewage treatment and the chlorination of drinking water, can also kill pathogens. Transmission can be disrupted through strategies like hand washing and the use of facemasks. Immunization or the treatment of infected hosts can stop the pathogen from multiplying, producing a serious disease, and being passed on to a new host. Some methods of breaking the chain of infection are given in Figure 17-1.

PERSONAL INSIGHT   How do you feel when you get sick? Do you feel "weak"? Guilty? Angry? Are you impatient to get back on your feet, or do you want to prolong the time you can legitimately be excused from your normal obligations? When you were sick as a child, was it unpleasant, or did it have certain pleasant aspects, such as getting extra attention or staying home from school? How have your childhood experiences affected your current feelings?

THE BODY'S DEFENSE SYSTEM

Our bodies have very effective ways of protecting themselves against invasion by foreign organisms, especially pathogens. The body's first line of defense is a formidable array of physical and chemical barriers. When these barriers are breached, the body's immune system comes into play. Together, these defenses provide an effective response to nearly all the challenges and invasions our bodies will ever experience.

Physical and Chemical Barriers

The skin, the body's largest organ, prevents many microorganisms from entering the body. Although many bacterial and fungal organisms live on the surface of the skin, very few can penetrate it except through a cut or break. Wherever there is an opening in the body, or an area without skin, other barriers exist. The mouth, the main entry to the gastrointestinal system, is lined with mucous membranes, which contain cells designed to prevent the passage of unwanted organisms and particles. Body openings and the fluids that cover them (for example, tears, saliva,

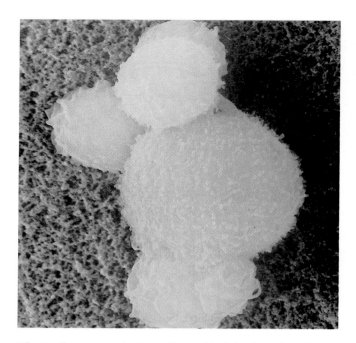

Killer T cells can recognize the antigens of both foreign cells and mutated body cells. In this electron micrograph magnified 2300 times, four killer T cells are in the process of attacking a cancer cell.

and vaginal secretions) are rich in antibodies (discussed in detail later in the chapter) and in **enzymes** that break down and destroy many microorganisms.

The respiratory tract is lined not only with mucous membranes but also with cells having hairlike protrusions called **cilia**. The cilia sweep foreign matter up and out of the respiratory tract. Particles that are not caught by this mechanism may be expelled from the system by a cough. If the ciliated cells are damaged or destroyed, as they are by smoking, a cough is the body's only way of ridding the airways of foreign particles. This is one reason smokers generally have a chronic cough—to compensate for damaged airways.

The Immune System

Once the body has been invaded by a foreign organism, an elaborate system of responses is activated. The immune system operates through a remarkable information network involving billions of cellular defenders who rush to protect the body when a threat arises. We discuss here two of the body's responses: the inflammatory response and the immune response. But before we cover these specific defenses, we'll briefly describe the defenders themselves and the mechanisms by which they work.

Immunological Defenders The immune response is carried out by different types of white blood cells, all of which are continuously being produced in the bone marrow. **Neutrophils**, one type of white blood cell, travel in the bloodstream to areas of invasion, attacking and ingesting pathogens. **Macrophages,** or "big eaters," take up stations in tissues and act as scavengers, devouring pathogens and worn-out cells. **Natural killer cells** directly destroy virus-infected cells and cells that have turned cancerous. **Lymphocytes,** of which there are several types, are white blood cells that travel in both the bloodstream and the lymphatic system. At various places in the lymphatic system there are lymph nodes (or glands), where macrophages congregate and filter bacteria and other substances from the lymph (Figure 17-2). When these nodes are actively involved in fighting an invasion of microorganisms, they fill with cells; physicians use the location of swollen lymph nodes as a clue to the location and cause of an infection.

The two main types of lymphocytes are known as **T cells** and **B cells.** T cells are further differentiated into **helper T cells, killer T cells,** and **suppressor T cells.** B cells are lymphocytes that produce **antibodies.** The first time T cells and B cells encounter a specific invader, some of them are reserved as **memory T and B cells,** enabling the body to mount a rapid response should the same invader appear again in the future. These cells and cell products—macrophages, natural killer cells, T cells, B cells and antibodies, and memory cells—are the primary players in the body's immune response.

The immune system is built on a remarkable feature of these defenders: the ability to distinguish foreign cells from the body's own cells. Because lymphocytes are capable of great destruction, it is essential that they not attack the body itself. When they do, they cause **autoimmune diseases,** such as lupus and rheumatoid arthritis.

How do lymphocytes know when they have encountered foreign substances? All the cells of an individual's body display markers on their surfaces—tiny molecular shapes—that identify them as "self" to lymphocytes that encounter them. Invading microorganisms also display markers on their surface; lymphocytes identify these as foreign, or "nonself." Nonself markers that trigger the immune response are known as **antigens.**

Antibodies have complementary surface markers that work with antigens like a lock and key (Figure 17-3). When an antigen appears in the body, it eventually encounters an antibody with a complementary pattern; the antibody locks onto the antigen, triggering a series of events designed to destroy the invading pathogen. The truly astonishing thing is that the body does not synthesize the appropriate antibody lock after it comes into contact with the antigen key. Rather, antibodies already exist for millions, if not billions, of possible antigens.

The Inflammatory Response When the body has been injured or infected, one of the body's responses is the inflammatory response. Special cells in the area of invasion or injury release **histamine** and other substances that cause blood vessels to dilate and fluid to flow out of capillaries into the injured tissue. This produces increased

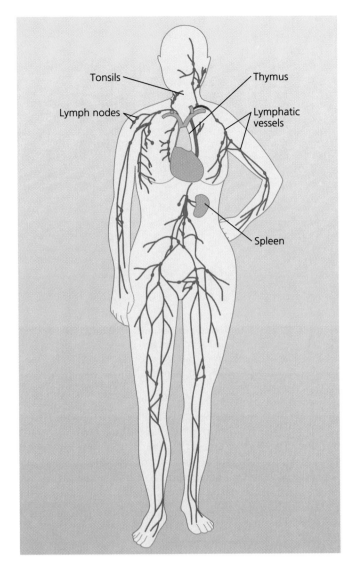

Figure 17-2 The lymphatic system. The lymphatic system consists of a network of vessels and organs, including the spleen, lymph nodes, thymus, and tonsils. The vessels pick up excess fluid and proteins, lipids, and other particles from body tissues. These pass through the lymph nodes, where lymphocytes and macrophages help clear the fluid (lymph) of debris and bacteria and other pathogens. The cleansed lymph is then returned to the bloodstream. The lymphatic organs are production centers for infection-fighting cells and sites for some immune responses.

heat, swelling, and redness in the affected area. White blood cells, including neutrophils and macrophages, are drawn to the area and attack the invaders—in many cases, destroying them. At the site of infection there may be pus, a collection of dead white blood cells and debris resulting from the encounter.

The Immune Response Another bodily reaction to invasion is the immune response (Figure 17-4). For conve-

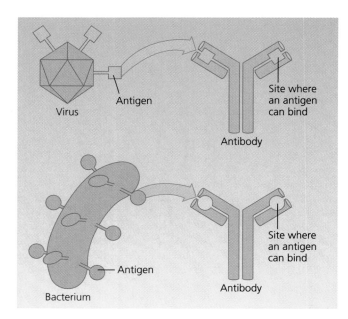

Figure 17-3 The binding of antigen and antibody. The binding sites on the tips of Y-shaped antibodies are specific to a single kind of antigen. When an antibody encounters a corresponding antigen, the two bind together in a kind of lock-and-key fit.

nience, we can think of this response as having four phases: (1) recognition of the invading pathogen, (2) amplification of defenses, (3) attack, and (4) slowdown. In each phase, crucial actions occur that are designed to destroy the invader and restore the body to health.

- *Phase 1.* Macrophages are drawn to the site of the injury and consume the foreign cells; they then provide

TERMS

cytokine A chemical messenger produced by a variety of cell types that helps regulate many cell functions; immune system cells release cytokines that help amplify and coordinate the immune response.

interleukin A cytokine that alerts immune system cells to the presence of foreign organisms and stimulates them into action.

interferon A cytokine that binds to cell membranes, increasing their resistance to many viruses; also stimulates the activities of macrophages and natural killer cells.

immunity Mechanisms that defend the body against infection; specific defenses against specific pathogens.

acquired immunity The body's ability to mobilize the cellular "memory" of an attack by a pathogen to throw off subsequent attacks; acquired through vaccination as well as the normal immune response.

incubation The period when bacteria or viruses are actively multiplying inside the body's cells; usually a period without symptoms of illness.

prodromal period The stage of an infection, following incubation, during which initial symptoms begin to appear but the host does not feel ill; a highly contagious period.

information about the pathogen by displaying its antigen on their surfaces. Helper T cells "read" this information and rush to respond.

- *Phase 2.* Helper T cells multiply rapidly and trigger the production of killer T cells and B cells in the spleen and lymph nodes. **Cytokines,** chemical messengers secreted by lymphocytes, help regulate and coordinate the immune response. **Interleukins** and **interferons** are two examples of cytokines. They stimulate increased production of T cells, B cells, and antibodies; promote the activities of natural killer cells; produce fever; and have special antipathogenic properties themselves.

- *Phase 3.* Killer T cells strike at foreign cells and body cells that have been invaded and infected, identifying them by the antigens displayed on the cell surfaces. Puncturing the cell membrane, they sacrifice body cells in order to destroy the foreign organism within. This type of action is known as a *cell-mediated immune response,* because the attack is carried out by cells. Killer T cells also trigger an amplified inflammatory response and recruit more macrophages to help clean up the site.

B cells work in a different way. Stimulated to multiply by helper T cells, they produce large quantities of antibody molecules, which are released in the bloodstream and tissues. Antibodies are Y-shaped protein molecules that bind to antigen-bearing targets and mark them for destruction by macrophages. This type of response is known as an *antibody-mediated immune response.* Antibodies work against bacteria and against viruses and other substances when they are in the body but outside cells. They do not work against infected body cells or viruses that are replicating inside cells.

- *Phase 4.* The last phase of the immune response is a slowdown of activity. Suppressor T cells regulate the levels of lymphocytes in the body and control their activities. When the danger is over, suppressor T cells halt the immune response and restore stability, or homeostasis. Dead cells, killed pathogens, and other debris that result from the immune response are scavenged by certain types of white blood cells; filtered out of circulation by the liver, spleen, and kidneys; and excreted from the body. (The box "HIV: The Immune System Under Siege," p. 472, explains how the body's response to pathogens is disrupted by HIV.)

Immunity In many infections, survival confers **immunity;** that is, an infected person will never get the same illness again. This is because some of the lymphocytes created during the amplification phase of the immune response are reserved as memory T and B cells. They continue to circulate in the blood and lymphatic system for years or even for the rest of the person's life. If the same antigen enters the body again, the memory T and B cells recognize and destroy it before it can cause illness. This

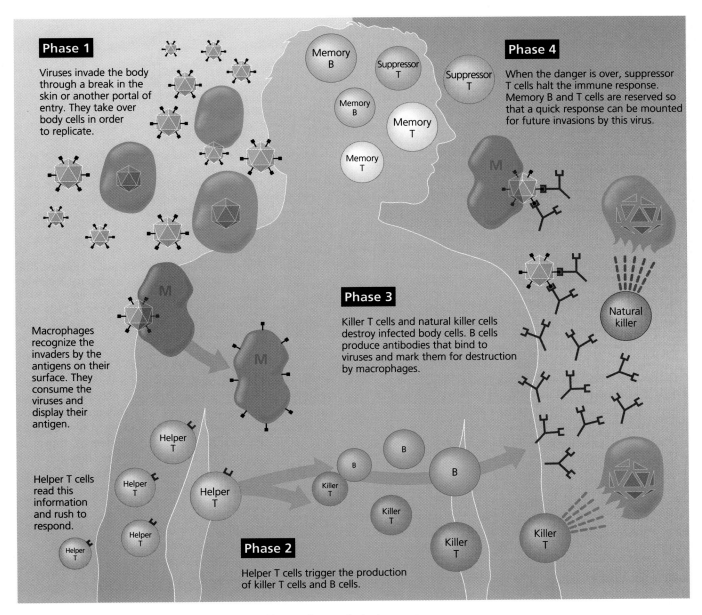

Phase 1

Viruses invade the body through a break in the skin or another portal of entry. They take over body cells in order to replicate.

Macrophages recognize the invaders by the antigens on their surface. They consume the viruses and display their antigen.

Helper T cells read this information and rush to respond.

Phase 2

Helper T cells trigger the production of killer T cells and B cells.

Phase 3

Killer T cells and natural killer cells destroy infected body cells. B cells produce antibodies that bind to viruses and mark them for destruction by macrophages.

Phase 4

When the danger is over, suppressor T cells halt the immune response. Memory B and T cells are reserved so that a quick response can be mounted for future invasions by this virus.

Figure 17-4 The immune response.   Once invaded by a pathogen, the body mounts a complex series of reactions to eliminate the invader. Pictured here are the principal elements of the immune response to a virus; not shown are the many types of cytokines that help coordinate the actions of different types of defenders.

subsequent response takes only a day or two, whereas the original response lasted several days, during which time the individual suffered the symptoms of illness. The ability of memory lymphocytes to remember previous infections is known as **acquired immunity.**

Symptoms and Contagion The immune system is operating at the cellular level within your body all the time, maintaining its vigilance when you're well and fighting invaders when you're sick. How does it all feel to you, the host and playing field for these activities? How

do your symptoms relate to the course of the infection and the immune response?

During **incubation,** when viruses are multiplying in the body or when bacteria are actively multiplying before the immune system has gathered momentum, you may not have any symptoms of the illness, but you may be contagious. During the second and third phases of the immune response, you may still be unaware of the infection, or you may "feel a cold coming on." Symptoms first appear during the **prodromal period,** which follows incubation. If the infected host has prior immunity, the

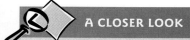
Different viruses attack different types of body cells. The human immunodeficiency virus (HIV) targets helper T cells, also called CD4 T cells after the CD4 protein on their surface. HIV binds to the surface of a CD4 T cell and inserts its own genetic material into the cell. It takes over the reproductive machinery of the cell and uses it to churn out new copies of the virus that can infect even more cells. Infected CD4 T cells are eventually destroyed, and the immune system begins to weaken.

People infected with HIV become susceptible to many secondary infections that people with a healthy, intact immune system have no problem overcoming. It is these **opportunistic infections** that cause most of the serious illnesses and deaths in people with HIV infection. Although T-cell immunity is severely affected by HIV infection, B-cell production of antibodies continues, and the body remains protected against many common diseases. The infections that most often prove deadly for people with HIV seldom occur in people with a healthy immune system.

B cells do produce antibodies to HIV, but unfortunately these antibodies do not protect against the spread of the virus. HIV antibodies are the basis for most of the tests for HIV infection (see Chapter 18). For other diseases, a blood test that reveals an antibody to a particular pathogen may indicate protective immunity—that is, the body would be protected from the organism. In the case of HIV, the presence of the antibody indicates an active case of the disease.

The only situation in which an HIV antibody could be present in the body without indicating ongoing infection is if the antibodies themselves are from another source. For example, HIV antibodies can pass through the placenta of an infected mother to the fetus, regardless of whether the virus itself has been transmitted. In fact, most babies born to infected mothers have HIV antibodies in their blood at birth and would test HIV-positive if given an HIV antibody test. Additional tests that screen for the presence of the virus itself must be done to determine whether a baby with HIV antibodies is actually infected.

infection may be eradicated during the incubation period or prodromal period. In this case, although you may have felt you were coming down with a cold, for example, it does not develop into a full-blown illness.

Many of the symptoms of an illness are actually due to the immune response of the body rather than to the actions or products of the invading organism. For example, fever is thought to be caused by the release and activation of certain cytokines in macrophages and other cells during the immune response. Cytokines travel in the bloodstream to the brain, where they cause the body's thermostat to be "reset" to a higher level. The resulting elevated temperature is thought to help the body in its fight against pathogens by enhancing immune responses. (During an illness, it is necessary to lower a fever only if it is uncomfortably high [over 101.5°F] or if it occurs in an infant who is at risk for seizures from fever.)

Similarly, you get a runny nose when your lymphocytes destroy infected mucosal cells, leading to increased mucus production. You get a sore throat when your lymphocytes destroy infected throat cells, and the malaise and fatigue of the flu may be caused by interferons.

You are contagious when there are active microbes replicating in your body and they can gain access to another person. This may be before a vigorous immune response has occurred, so at times you may be contagious before experiencing any symptoms. This means that you can transmit an illness without knowing you're infected or catch an illness from someone who doesn't appear to be sick. On the other hand, your symptoms may continue after the pathogens have been mostly destroyed, when you are no longer infectious.

PERSONAL INSIGHT   How do you feel when you hear that someone has HIV infection? Herpes? Chicken pox? Bronchitis? If you feel differently about each case, what is the basis for the difference?

Immunization

The ability of the immune system to remember previously encountered organisms and retain its strength against them is the basis for immunization. When a person is immunized against a disease, the immune system is "primed" with an antigen similar to the pathogenic organism but not as dangerous. The body responds by producing antibodies to the organism, which prevent serious infection when and if the person is exposed to the disease itself. These preparations used to manipulate the immune system are known as **vaccines.** (Immunizations available in the United States are listed in Table 17-1.)

Vaccines can be made in several ways. In some cases, microbes are cultured in the laboratory in a way that weakens (attenuates) them. These "live, attenuated" organisms are used in vaccines against such diseases as

TERMS   **opportunistic infection**   An infection caused when organisms take the opportunity presented by a primary (initial) infection to multiply and cause a secondary infection.

vaccine   A preparation of killed or weakened pathogens injected or taken orally, thereby arousing the body's acquired immunity to produce specific antibodies.

TABLE 17-1 — Immunizations Available in the United States

Vaccine	People for Whom Immunization Is Recommended
Diphtheria	All children; adults need boosters every 10 years
H. influenzae type b (Hib)	All children (protects against meningitis)
Hepatitis A	Injecting drug users, men who have sex with men, and others at risk
Hepatitis B	All children; adults at risk, including health care workers, household contacts and sex partners of infected people, injecting drug users, and people with STDs
Influenza	Annual vaccination for adults age 65 and older; nursing home residents; anyone with heart, lung, endocrine, or other chronic disorders (including asthma and diabetes) and others at high risk; women who will be in the second or third trimester of pregnancy during the influenza season; anyone over 6 months of age who wishes to reduce their risk for influenza
Lyme disease	Adults over 15 with frequent or prolonged exposure to ticks in areas where Lyme disease is common
Measles	All children; unvaccinated adults born after 1956 who are not immune (those who received only one dose or were vaccinated between 1963 and 1967 may need revaccination)
Mumps	All children; unvaccinated adults born after 1956 who are not immune
Pertussis (whooping cough)	All children
Pneumococcal poly-saccharide	Adults age 65 and older; anyone with chronic heart or lung disease or with no functional spleen; others at high risk, including Alaskan Natives and certain American Indian groups
Polio	All children; adults at risk, including certain laboratory and health care workers and unvaccinated parents of children receiving the vaccine
Rabies	Anyone at risk from a bite, scratch, or mucous membrane exposure to a potentially rabid animal or from any direct contact with a bat (unless the person can be certain that exposure did not occur); people who work with animals may need preexposure immunization
Rotavirus	Children under age 1 (as determined by parent/guaradian and health care provider)
Rubella (German measles)	All children; unvaccinated adults who are not immune, especially women
Tetanus (lockjaw)	All children; adults need boosters every 10 years (sooner if more than 5 years has elapsed since the previous booster and the individual has a contaminated wound)
Varicella (chicken pox)	Children over age 12 months; unvaccinated adults who have not had varicella, especially health care workers and others at high risk for exposure

For international travelers, the CDC recommends that all standard childhood immunizations be up to date and that additional vaccines such as hepatitis A and influenza be considered. Travelers to areas where certain diseases are common may need others, including vaccines for yellow fever, typhoid fever, meningococcal meningitis, and Japanese or tickborne encephalitis; a one-time polio booster may also be given. Further information about immunization is available from the CDC's National Immunization Program (800-CDC-SHOT; http://www.cdc.gov/nip) and the CDC's Travel Information (877-394-8747; http://www.cdc.gov/travel).

SOURCES: Centers for Disease Control and Prevention. 1999. Recommended childhood immunization schedule. *Morbidity and Mortality Weekly Report* 48(1): 12–16. Centers for Disease Control and Prevention. 1998. *Summary or Adolescent/Adult Immunization Recommendations* (retrieved February 2, 1999; http://www.cdc.gov/nip/schedule/adult/Adult-sched-8x11.pdf). Centers for Disease Control and Prevention. 1999. Availability of Lyme disease vaccine. *Morbidity and Mortality Weekly Report* 48(2): 35–36, 43. Centers for Disease Control and Prevention. 1999. Human rabies prevention—Recommendations of the Advisory Committee on Immunization Practices. *MMWR Recommendations and Reports* 48(RR-1).

measles, mumps, and rubella (German measles). In other cases, when it is not possible to breed attenuated organisms, vaccines are made from pathogens that have been killed in the laboratory but that still retain their ability to stimulate the production of antibodies. Vaccines composed of "killed" viruses are used against influenza viruses, among others. A third type of vaccine has been developed to protect against tetanus. This disease is caused by a bacterium that thrives in deep puncture

wounds and produces a deadly toxin. The vaccine is made from a "toxoid" that resembles the toxin—that is, lymphocytes recognize it as being the same—but that does not produce the same effects.

Vaccines confer what is known as *active immunity*— that is, the vaccinated person produces his or her own antibodies to the microorganism. Another type of injection confers *passive immunity*. In this case, a person exposed to a disease is injected with the antibodies them-

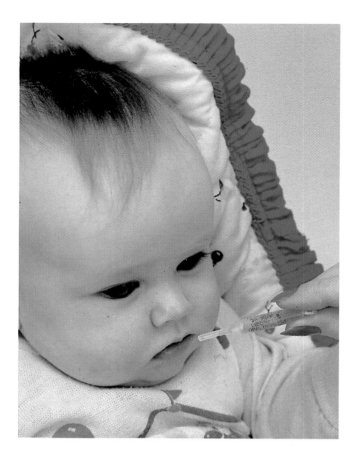

Before polio vaccines were developed by Jonas Salk and Albert Sabin in the 1950s, many people, especially children, were paralyzed or killed by this viral infection. This 1-year-old is being given oral polio vaccine as part of the standard series of childhood immunizations.

selves, produced by other human beings or animals who have recovered from the disease. Injections of **gamma globulin**—a product made from the blood plasma of many individuals, containing all the antibodies they have ever made—are sometimes given to people exposed to a disease against which they have not been immunized. Such injections create a rapid but temporary immunity and are useful against certain viruses, such as hepatitis A. Gamma globulin is also sometimes used to treat antibody deficiency syndromes.

Allergy: The Body's Defense System Gone Haywire

You probably know someone with an **allergy**, or perhaps you have one yourself. Allergic reactions are a response of the immune system, but in this case the response is hypersensitive, inappropriate, annoying, and sometimes even life-threatening. Allergic reactions occur when the body recognizes a relatively harmless substance, such as dust, pollen, or animal hair, as a dangerous antigen and mounts an immune response to it. The hypersensitivity that results in an allergic reaction involves an excess of one or more antibodies belonging to a broad class known as immunoglobulin E, or IgE. IgE antibodies tend to be found in the soft tissues surrounding blood vessels in the lungs, sinuses, skin, and other areas. When activated by the presence of a particular allergen, IgE signals for the release of large quantities of histamine.

Histamine has many effects, including increasing the inflammatory response and stimulating mucus production. The precise symptoms depend on what part of the body is affected. In the nose, histamine causes flushing, congestion, and sneezing; in the eyes, it can produce itching, tearing, and inflammation; in the skin, it can cause redness, swelling, and itching; and in the lungs, it can cause the muscles surrounding air passages to contract, making breathing difficult. In some people, an **allergen**, a substance that triggers an allergy, can cause an asthma attack (see the box "Asthma"). The most serious, but rare, kind of allergic reaction involves a release of histamine throughout the body, causing a life-threatening loss of blood pressure known as anaphylactic shock.

Many allergens can provoke an allergic reaction in a sensitive individual, including animal dander, dust mites (microscopic insects found in the home), pollen, molds, insect stings, medications, and certain foods. The most effective treatment for an allergy is total avoidance of the allergen, but often this is impossible. Over-the-counter antihistamines and decongestants may bring relief but often cause drowsiness. Prescription medications include newer, nonsedating antihistamines and steroid sprays that reduce inflammation. In some cases, a course of desensitizing injections ("allergy shots") may be given.

THE TROUBLEMAKERS: PATHOGENS AND DISEASE

Now that we've discussed the intricate system that protects us from disease, let's consider some pathogens, the disease-producing organisms that live within us and around us. When they succeed in gaining entry to body tissue, they can cause illness and sometimes death to the unfortunate host. Worldwide, infectious diseases are responsible for more than 13 million deaths each year (Table 17-2). Pathogenic organisms include bacteria, viruses, fungi, protozoa, and parasitic worms.

More than 17 million Americans have asthma, including more than 5 million children and teenagers. The symptoms of asthma—wheezing, tightness in the chest, and shortness of breath—may be mild and occur only occasionally, or they may be severe and occur daily. Asthma can be disabling and even fatal if not controlled. Asthma is caused by both inflammation of the airways and a spasm of the muscles surrounding the airways. The spasm causes constriction, and the inflammation causes the airway linings to swell and secrete extra mucus, which further obstructs the passages. The inflammation can become chronic, making airways even more sensitive to triggers of attacks. The tendency to develop asthma may be hereditary.

An asthma attack begins when something sets off a spasm in the bronchial tubes. Usually it's an allergic reaction to an inhaled allergen, most commonly dust mites, mold, animal dander, or pollen. Anything that irritates or overtaxes the bronchial airways can also trigger spasms: exercise, cold air, environmental pollutants, tobacco smoke, infection, emotional stress, or even a hearty laugh. In female asthmatics, who make up about 60% of adults with asthma, hormonal changes that occur as menstruation starts may increase vulnerability to attacks.

Inhaling a muscle-relaxing medication from a bronchodilator can relieve an asthma attack immediately by opening the bronchial tubes. Inhaled anti-inflammatory drugs are designed to treat the underlying inflammation. Both types of treatments may be needed to get asthma under control. Asthmatics can monitor their condition by self-testing their "peak air flow" several times a day (a drop in peak air flow can signal an upcoming attack). As with allergies, it's also a good idea to avoid allergens when possible.

The incidence of asthma is increasing throughout the world, for reasons not completely understood. Since 1980, the number of Americans with asthma has more than doubled; and despite better treatment options, the death rate has also increased. Particularly affected are people over 65, children, African Americans, Latinos, and people living in inner cities. A combination of factors may well be responsible for this increased incidence, including greater exposure to indoor air pollutants due to poorer ventilation, higher levels of outdoor air pollution, and better diagnosis of asthma cases. In addition, the combination of cockroach allergy and exposure to the insects has been shown to be an important cause of asthma-related illness among children in inner-city areas.

SOURCES: Centers for Disease Control and Prevention. 1998. Forecasted state-specific estimates of self-reported asthma prevalence—United States, 1998. *Morbidity and Mortality Weekly Report* 47(47): 1022–1025. Treating the real causes of asthma attacks. 1992. *Consumer Reports on Health*, October.

Bacteria

Among the microorganisms that exist everywhere in the environment are single-celled organisms called **bacteria.** Essential for life as we know it, bacteria break down dead organic matter, allowing it to be restructured for use by other organisms so that life can go on. They also perform a similar task in our intestines, helping digest food for better absorption by the body. (A large portion of human feces consists of bacteria.) These "friendly" bacteria cause disease only if the integrity of the bowel is compromised, as when an appendix ruptures. "Unfriendly" bacteria in the intestines, such as those that cause foodborne illness, disrupt the normal harmony by invading the cells that line the intestine or by producing toxins that cause damage.

If we view the entire digestive tract as a long hollow tube beginning in the mouth and moving down the esophagus, stomach, small and large intestine to the anus, we see that even though bacteria reside inside the intestine, they are not really a part of the body. Underneath the skin, within the bloodstream, tissues, and organs, the body is devoid of bacteria, or "sterile." Bacteria found in these areas are almost always pathogenic. It is here that the immune system keeps up its constant surveillance, seeking out and destroying any invaders.

Bacteria can cause infection almost anywhere in or on the body. They can cause meningitis, an infection of the

VITAL STATISTICS

TABLE 17-2	*Top Infectious Diseases Worldwide*

Disease	Approximate Number of Deaths per Year
Pneumonia	3,452,000
HIV/AIDS	2,285,000
Diarrheal diseases	2,219,000
Tuberculosis	1,498,000
Malaria	1,110,000
Measles	888,000
Tetanus	410,000
Pertussis (whooping cough)	346,000
Syphilis	159,000
Meningitis	143,000

In addition, many of the 609,000 deaths from liver cancer each year can be traced to viral hepatitis. Overall, infectious diseases kill more than 13 million people each year, representing nearly 25% of all deaths.

SOURCE: World Health Organization. 1999. *The World Health Report 1999: Making a Difference.* Geneva: World Health Organization.

spinal fluid and tissue surrounding the brain; conjunctivitis, infection of the layer of cells surrounding the eyes; pharyngitis, or sore throat; bronchitis, infection of the airways (bronchi); pneumonia, infection of the lung itself;

gastroenteritis, infection of the gastrointestinal tract; cellulitis, infection of the soft tissues; osteomyelitis, infection of the bones; and so on, for every tissue and organ.

To diagnose a bacterial infection, a sample must be taken from a diseased patient, grown on a special medium, then viewed through a microscope. A special stain called a Gram stain is used to help visualize bacteria, which are classified according to their shape and how they stain. Organisms are "gram-positive" if they stain dark blue and "gram-negative" if they appear light red. The major shapes are cocci (spheres), bacilli (rods), and spirochetes (long spirals).

Gram-Positive Bacteria

The bacterium that often inflames the tonsils and throat is the **streptococcus**, a gram-positive coccus (sphere) that often grows in chains. This same microbe often causes skin infections such as impetigo and erysipelas. A particularly virulent type of the bacterium responsible for strep throat can cause local destruction of tissue (giving it the name "flesh-eating strep") or a dangerous systemic illness. Other species of streptococci are implicated in pneumonia and endocarditis (infection of the heart lining and valves). A streplike organism known as enterococcus ("sphere from the gut") is a major cause of hospital-acquired infections.

Another gram-positive coccus is **staphylococcus**, which appears in small clusters under the microscope. Its name means "cluster of grapes." These bacteria may reside on the skin or in the nasal passages even in healthy individuals, but can cause many diseases, including boils and other skin infections. A species of these bacteria, *Staphylococcus aureus,* is responsible for toxic shock syndrome (TSS). The bacteria produce a deadly toxin that causes shock (potentially life-threatening low blood pressure), high fever, a peeling skin rash, and inflammation of several organ systems. TSS was first diagnosed in women using highly absorbent tampons, which appear to allow the growth of staphylococci. The disease has since been found in women not using tampons and in men as well.

Gram-Negative Bacteria

Gram-negative bacteria are more commonly **bacilli** (rod-shaped). Many types of gram-negative rods inhabit human intestines but generally are not present in the mouth or on the skin of healthy people. These organisms most often cause disease when there is a breakdown in the normal immune system or when the integrity of the intestinal tract is breached. The vagina normally contains gram-negative bacteria, but if these bacteria travel up the urethra to the bladder, they can cause urinary tract infections.

Gram-negative *Legionella* cause about 15,000 cases of severe pneumonia in the United States each year. Most are isolated cases, but it was an outbreak at a 1976 American Legion convention that led to the bacteria's identification. *Legionella* flourish in moist environments like cooling towers and plumbing systems. A 1999 outbreak in the Netherlands that sickened over 200 people and killed over 20 was tentatively traced to a whirlpool spa at a flower show; it was the largest outbreak to date.

Spirochete Infections

Spirochetes, spiral-shaped bacteria, are very difficult to grow in culture. As a result, researchers have had difficulty in understanding their life cycle as well as in diagnosing infections caused by these pathogens. The sexually transmitted disease syphilis is caused by the spirochete *Treponema pallidum;* syphilis and other STDs are described in detail in Chapter 18.

A different spirochete, *Borrelia burgdorferi,* causes the illness known as Lyme disease. The spirochete is transmitted by the deer tick *Ixodes,* which makes its home on deer and mice, except in California, where the culprit is the closely related black-legged tick, which also lives on wood rats. Ticks acquire the spirochete by ingesting the blood of an infected animal; then they may transmit the microbe to their next host. Lyme disease has been reported throughout the United States and is most common in the northeast and mid-Atlantic states and in Wisconsin and Minnesota; in some areas, up to 75% of deer ticks carry the spirochete.

Symptoms of Lyme disease vary from person to person; they typically occur in three stages. In the first stage, an expanding red rash develops from the area of the tick bite, usually about 2 weeks after the bite occurs; some people develop flulike symptoms as well. The second stage occurs weeks to months later in about 10–20% of untreated patients. Symptoms may involve the nervous and cardiovascular systems and can include impaired motor coordination, partial facial paralysis, and heart rhythm abnormalities. These symptoms usually disappear within a few weeks. The third stage, which occurs in about half of untreated people, can occur years after the tick bite and usually consists of chronic or recurring arthritis (an inflammation of the joints), almost always

TERMS

streptococcus   A spherical bacterium that causes infections such as strep throat, which can lead to serious cardiac damage.

staphylococcus   A spherical, clustered bacterium found on skin and in the nose, that can cause infection if allowed to multiply in food and then be ingested.

bacillus   A rod-shaped bacterium.

spirochete   A spiral-shaped bacterium that causes various infections, including syphilis and Lyme disease.

tuberculosis (TB)   A bacterial disease that almost always infects the lungs.

mycoplasma   A small bacterium that causes pneumonia and sore throat.

chlamydia   A bacterium that causes a type of pneumonia, certain STDs, and possibly heart disease.

rickettsia   A bacterium that can reproduce only inside living cells, transmitted by ticks, fleas, and lice; causes Rocky Mountain spotted fever.

If you live in an area where Lyme disease is prevalent and spend time in the woods or even in your yard—especially between May and September—take these steps:

1. Wear light-colored, long-sleeved, long-legged clothing outdoors. Tuck pant legs into socks or boots and then tape the area so ticks can't crawl under clothing. Wear closed shoes and a hat to protect your feet and scalp.

2. After an outing, thoroughly check your entire body, clothes, and gear. Also check children and pets. Look for both adult ticks and the immature nymphs (see the illustration). Nymphs, which are about the size of a pinhead, are responsible for up to 90% of all cases of Lyme disease. A nymph will feed on you for 2–3 days, an adult tick for up to a week. The sooner you remove it, the better your chance of avoiding infection. Recent studies reveal that if the tick is on you for less than 24 hours, you will probably not develop the disease.

3. Use an insect repellent containing DEET (short for N, N-diethyltoluamide) on your skin and a spray containing the insecticide permethrin on your clothing. (DEET has caused

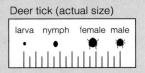

Deer tick (actual size)

larva   nymph   female   male

allergic reactions in some children and should be used with caution.)

4. Remove a tick with fine-tipped tweezers; always carry a pair with you when outdoors. (It is almost impossible to remove a small tick with your fingers.) Exert a slow, steady pull. Don't twist the tick.

5. Put the tick in a small jar containing alcohol (carry one with you if you're out hiking) so you can take it to your physician or health department for identification.

SOURCES: National Center for Infectious Diseases (http://www.cdc.gov/ncidod). Lyme disease: Hard to catch. 1995. *University of California at Berkeley Wellness Letter,* August. © 1995 Health Letter Associates. Used with permission.

---

affecting the knees. Lyme disease can also cause fetal damage or death at any stage of pregnancy. A vaccine is available for adults at high risk, but it is not 100% effective against the disease, so precautions are still needed (see the box "Protecting Yourself Against Lyme Disease").

Other Bacteria   A multitude of organisms are not easily categorized by Gram staining. **Tuberculosis (TB)** is caused by a rod-shaped bacterium that requires a special stain. TB is spread via the respiratory route through prolonged contact with someone who has the disease in its active form. Symptoms include coughing, fatigue, night sweats, weight loss, and fever.

About 10–15 million Americans have been infected with, and therefore continue to carry, the tuberculosis bacterium. However, only about 10% of them will actually come down with the disease. Although their skin tests for TB antibodies register positive, the immune system of the majority prevents the disease from becoming active. In the United States, active TB is most common among people infected with HIV, recent immigrants, and those who live in inner cities. Most strains of tuberculosis respond to antibiotics, but only over a long course of treatment lasting at least 6 months. Failure to complete treatment can lead to relapse and the development of strains of antibiotic-resistant bacteria. Worldwide, about one-third of all people are infected with TB, and TB kills about 1.5 million people each year.

Mycoplasma is a bacterium with an incomplete cell wall. It will not grow on the usual laboratory culture media, so special techniques are required to culture it.

Mycoplasmas are the most common cause of pneumonia in young adults and may also cause ear infections and sore throats. **Chlamydias** are bacteria similar to mycoplasmas; they are implicated as the cause of pneumonia, STDs, and possibly heart disease (see Chapter 15). Sexually transmitted chlamydia is the most common bacterial infection in the United States (see Chapter 18). **Rickettsias** are the agents of Rocky Mountain spotted fever and typhus and are transmitted by ticks, fleas, and lice.

Antibiotic Treatments   The body's immune system can fight off many, if not most, bacterial infections. However, while the body musters its defenses, some bacteria can cause a great deal of damage: Inflammation, caused by the gathering of white blood cells, may lead to scarring and permanently damaged tissues. To help the body deal with these infections, science and medicine have made a considerable contribution: antibiotics.

Antibiotics are both naturally occurring and synthetic substances having the ability to kill bacteria. Most antibiotics work in a similar fashion: They interrupt the production of new bacteria by damaging some part of their reproductive cycle or by causing faulty parts of new bacteria to be made. Penicillins inhibit the formation of the cell wall when bacteria divide to form new cells. Other antibiotics inhibit the production of certain necessary proteins by the bacteria, and still others interfere directly with the reading of genetic material (DNA) during the process of bacterial reproduction.

When antibiotics inhibit a specific bacterial strain's growth, these bacteria are said to be "sensitive." Unfor-

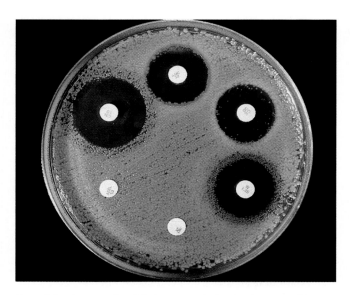

One of the dangers of antibiotic overuse is the development of bacteria resistant to drugs. Cultures of *E. coli* (a bacterium normally present in the human intestine) in this laboratory dish are sensitive to four different types of antibiotics, as indicated by the wide circles where no bacteria are growing, but they are resistant to two other types, which have no effect on their growth.

tunately, antibiotic-resistant strains (types) of many common bacteria have developed, including strains of gonorrhea (an STD), salmonellosis (a foodborne illness), and tuberculosis. A bacterium can become resistant from a chance genetic mutation or through the transfer of genetic material from one bacterium to another. In any given population of bacteria, a few are always resistant. When exposed to antibiotics, these resistant bacteria can grow and flourish, while the antibiotic-sensitive bacteria die off. Eventually, an entire colony of bacteria can become resistant to one or more antibiotics. The more often bacteria encounter antibiotics, the more likely they are to develop resistance. Antibiotic resistance is a major factor contributing to the recent rise in problematic infectious

diseases (see the box "Emerging Infectious Diseases").

You can help prevent the development of antibiotic-resistant strains of bacteria by using antibiotics properly:

- Don't expect to take an antibiotic every time you get sick. They are mainly helpful for bacterial infections; against viruses, they are ineffective.

- Use antibiotics as directed, and finish the full course of medication even if you begin to feel better. This helps ensure that all targeted bacteria are killed off.

- Never take an antibiotic without a prescription. If you take an antibiotic for a viral infection, take the wrong one, or take an insufficient dose, your illness will not improve, and you'll give bacteria the opportunity to develop resistance.

Viruses

Visible only with an electron (high-magnification) microscope, **viruses,** the smallest of the pathogens, are on the borderline between living and nonliving matter. Viruses lack all the enzymes essential to energy production and protein synthesis in normal animal cells, and they cannot grow or reproduce by themselves. Viruses are **parasites;** they use what they need for growth and reproduction from the cells they invade. Once a virus is inside the host cell, it sheds its protein covering and its genetic material takes control of the cell and manufactures more viruses like itself (Figure 17-5). The normal functioning of the host cell is thereby disrupted.

Different viruses affect different kinds of cells, and the seriousness of the disease they cause depends greatly on which kind of cell is affected. The viruses that cause colds, for example, attack upper respiratory tract cells, which are constantly cast off and replaced. The disease is therefore mild. Poliovirus, in contrast, attacks nerve cells that cannot be replaced, and the consequences, such as paralysis, are severe. HIV infection, a viral illness that destroys immune system cells, can destroy the body's ability to fight infectious diseases (see Chapter 18 for more on HIV/AIDS).

Common Viral Illnesses   Illnesses caused by viruses are the most common forms of **contagious disease.** They include most of the minor ailments that cause short-lived illness and are rarely precisely diagnosed. Among these are the common cold, a variety of brief and undiagnosed respiratory infections, **influenza,** gastrointestinal upsets that cause diarrhea, and assorted aches and pains. More serious are the diseases that occur mainly in childhood and frequently cause a severe rash, such as measles, chicken pox, and mumps. Smallpox, which used to be the most severe of these diseases, has now been eliminated, thanks to a worldwide vaccination program carried out by the World Health Organization (WHO) in the 1960s and 1970s.

TERMS   **virus**   The smallest pathogenic organism; cannot grow or reproduce by themselves.

parasite   An organism that derives nutrients from a living host.

contagious disease   A disease that can be transmitted from one person to another; most are viral diseases, such as the common cold and flu.

influenza   A usually mild viral disease, highly infective and adaptable; the form changes so easily that every year new strains arise, making treatment difficult; commonly known as the flu.

herpesvirus   A family of viruses responsible for cold sores, chicken pox, and the STD known as herpes.

Epstein-Barr virus (EBV)   A herpesvirus that causes infectious mononucleosis.

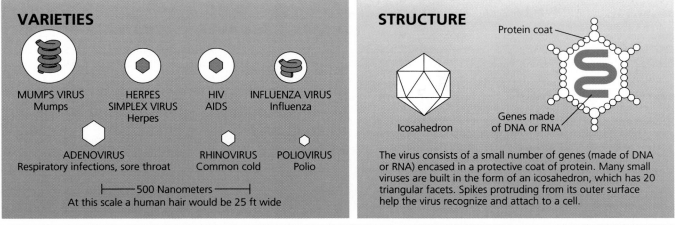

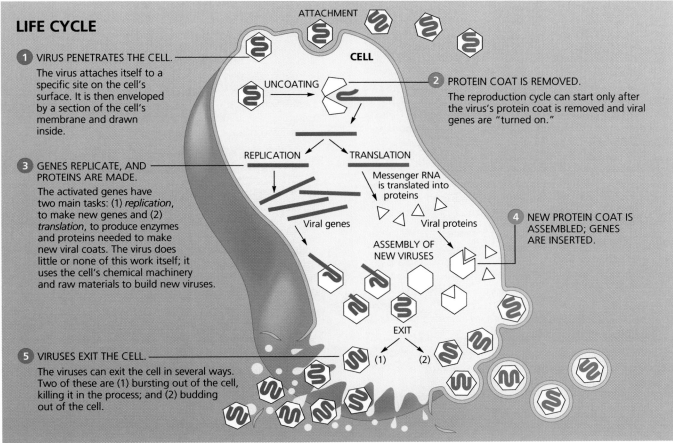

Figure 17-5 **Viruses: varieties, structure, and life cycle.**

The **herpesviruses** are a large and important group of viruses. Once infected, the host is never free of the virus. The virus lies latent within certain cells and becomes active periodically, producing symptoms. Herpesviruses are particularly dangerous for people with a depressed immune system, as in the case of HIV infection. The family of herpesviruses includes the following:

• Herpes simplex types 1 and 2, which cause cold sores

and the STD known as herpes (see Chapter 18).

• Varicella-zoster, which causes chicken pox and shingles.

• Cytomegalovirus (CMV), which causes severe infections of the lungs, brain, colon, and eyes in people with a suppressed immune system.

• **Epstein-Barr virus (EBV),** which causes infectious mononucleosis. Mono, as it is commonly called, is

"Mad cow disease," "flesh-eating bacteria," "Ebola outbreaks"—are they media monsters or cause for alarm? Although the chances of the average American contracting an exotic infectious disease are very slim, emerging infections are a concern to public health officials and represent a challenge to all nations in the future. The CDC defines emerging infectious diseases as diseases of infectious origin whose incidence in humans has increased within the past two decades or threatens to increase in the near future. They include both known diseases that have experienced a resurgence, such as tuberculosis and cholera, and diseases that were previously unknown or confined to specific areas, such as Ebola. Known diseases can reappear or spread when pathogens become resistant to drugs or when public health measures break down. New diseases can appear when genetic mutations occur or when humans are exposed to new reservoirs or vectors of pathogens.

Some of the emerging infections that concern scientists include the following:

- *Escherichia coli O157:H7.* This potentially deadly strain of *E. coli,* transmitted in contaminated food, can cause bloody diarrhea and kidney damage. The first major outbreak occurred in 1993, when over 600 people became ill and four children died after eating contaminated and undercooked fast-food hamburgers. Additional outbreaks have been linked to lettuce, alfalfa sprouts, and unpasteurized juice. In 1998, more than 25 children became ill after swimming in the same public pool; health officials suspect fecal contamination of the water by a sick child as the source of the bacteria.

- *Hantavirus.* Since first being recognized in 1993, over 500 cases of hantavirus pulmonary syndrome (HPS) have been reported in the United States and South America. HPS is caused by the rodent-borne Sin Nombre virus (SNV) and is spread primarily through airborne viral particles from rodent urine, droppings, or saliva. It is characterized by a dangerous fluid buildup in the lungs and is fatal in about 45% of cases.

- *Necrotizing fascitis.* The "flesh-eating bacteria" that cause necrotizing fascitis are a virulent strain of streptococci that also cause scarlet fever, toxic shock syndrome, and the lethal type of pneumonia that killed Muppets creator Jim Henson in 1990. The bacteria break down tissue and damage blood vessels at the site of a wound, sometimes leading to gangrene, shock, and, in about 20% of cases, death. The disease is rare (about 500–1500 cases per year in the United States).

- *Mad cow disease.* By 1999, more than 35 Britons had died of a new variant of a rare, incurable brain affliction called Creutzfeldt-Jakob disease (CJD). Researchers suspect that this new variant of CJD is caused by people eating beef from cows infected with bovine spongiform encephalopathy (BSE), commonly called mad cow disease. Both BSE and CJD are characterized by spongelike holes in the brain, leading to loss of coordination, dementia, and death. CJD may be caused by a newly recognized type of transmissible agent called a prion. No cases have been reported in the United States.

- *Ebola.* So far, outbreaks of the often fatal Ebola hemorrhagic fever (EHF) in humans have occurred only in Africa. The Ebola virus is transmitted by direct contact with infected blood or other body secretions, and many cases of EHF have been linked to unsanitary conditions in medical facilities. Because symptoms appear quickly and 75% of victims die, usually within a few days, the virus tends not to spread widely (unlike HIV or hepatitis, which can infect a person for years before any symptoms appear).

- *Influenza A(H5NI).* By January 1998, 6 of 18 people in Hong Kong infected with this unusual strain of influenza had died. Local authorities contained the outbreak quickly by tracing its source to infected chickens, ducks, and geese and then ordering the slaughter of all domestic poultry. Although small, the outbreak raised the specter of the influenza **pandemic** that killed more than 20 million people in 1918. A strain like A(H5N1) is so unique that few, if any, people have immunity from past exposure; had it mutated into a form that more easily infects humans, influenza A(H5N1) could conceivably have killed as many as 30% of the world's people.

- *Common infectious diseases on the rise.* Diseases that were once under control in many parts of the world but are now increasing and spreading include cholera, malaria, tuberculosis, yellow fever, hepatitis, and many STDs. People with lowered immunity, such as those undergoing cancer treatments and those infected with HIV, are particularly susceptible to these infections.

spread by close contact and usually affects children and young adults, causing a sore throat, fever, and fatigue.

Some herpes viruses have been linked to the development of certain forms of cancer, and new forms continue to be discovered.

Hepatitis (inflammation of the liver) is usually caused by one of the three most common hepatitis viruses. Hepatitis A virus (HAV) causes the mildest form of the disease and is usually transmitted by food or water contaminated by sewage or an infected person. Hepatitis B virus (HBV) is usually transmitted sexually; it is discussed in detail in Chapter 18. Hepatitis C virus (HCV) can also be transmitted sexually, but it more commonly passes through direct contact with infected blood via injecting drug use or, prior to the development of screening tests, blood transfusions. HBV and, to a lesser extent, HCV, can also be passed from a pregnant woman to her child. Although there are effective vaccines for hepatitis A and B, there are up to 500,000 new cases of hepatitis in the United States each year.

Symptoms of acute hepatitis infection can include fatigue, jaundice, abdominal pain, loss of appetite, nausea, and diarrhea. Most people recover from hepatitis A

What's behind this rising tide of infectious diseases? Contributing factors, unfortunately, are complex and interrelated. They include the following:

• *Drug resistance.* New or increasing drug resistance has been found in organisms that cause malaria, gonorrhea, influenza, AIDS, and pneumococcal, staphylococcal, and enterococcal infections. A new multidrug-resistant strain of tuberculosis is now **endemic** in New York. Infections caused by drug-resistant organisms prolong illness, and—if not treated in time with more expensive drugs—they can cause death. Some bacterial strains now appear to be resistant to all available antibiotics; unless new drugs are developed or these strains contained, some diseases may become untreatable as they were in the pre-antibiotic era. The cost of drug resistance is increasing and approaches $30 billion per year.

• *Poverty.* More than 1 billion people live in extreme poverty, and half of the world's population has no regular access to essential drugs. Population growth, urbanization, overcrowding, and migration (including the movement of refugees) also contribute to the spread of infectious diseases.

• *The breakdown of public health measures.* A poor public health infrastructure is often associated with poverty and social upheaval, but problems occur even in industrial countries. In 1993, the Milwaukee municipal water supply was contaminated with the intestinal parasite *Cryptosporidium.* Over 400,000 people had prolonged diarrhea and about 4400 were hospitalized; this was the largest outbreak of waterborne illness in U.S. history. During 1990–1995, a breakdown in programs for childhood vaccination in Russia led to over 50,000 cases of diphtheria.

• *Environmental changes.* Changes in land use—deforestation, the damming of rivers, the spread of ranching and farming—alter the distribution of disease vectors and bring people in contact with new pathogens. A shift in rainfall patterns caused by global warming may allow mosquito-borne diseases to spread from the tropics into temperate zones. Isolated cases of malaria in New York and New Jersey have already occurred in years that were particularly hot and humid. Heavy rainfall and the associated rise in rodent and mosquito populations is linked to an outbreak of hantavirus in the Four Corners area of the western United States and to a recent **epidemic** of Rift Valley Fever in eastern Africa.

• *Travel and commerce.* More than 500 million travelers cross national borders each year, and international tourism and trade open the world to infectious agents. Cholera was reintroduced into the Western Hemisphere after almost a century-long absence when, in 1991, a Chinese freighter discharged bilge water along the Peruvian coast. The bilge water from Asian seas contained billions of cholera-carrying algae, and the infection spread rapidly through contaminated seafood and unchlorinated drinking water. Since that time, millons of Latin Americans have fallen ill and thousands have died.

• *Mass food production and distribution.* Food travels long distances to our table, and microbes are transmitted along with it. Mass production of food increases the likelihood that a chance contamination can lead to mass illness. A 1996 *E.coli* outbreak in Japan that sickened more than 6000 children is thought to have originated in a facility that prepared more than 40,000 school lunches daily. A 22-state U.S. outbreak of listeriosis in 1998–1999 was traced to hot dogs and deli meats produced under many brand names by one manufacturer.

• *Human behavior.* Changes in patterns of human behavior also have an impact on the spread of infectious diseases. The widespread use of IV drugs rapidly transmits HIV infection and hepatitis. Changes in sexual behavior over the past 30 years have led to a proliferation of new and old STDs. The use of day-care facilities for children has led to increases in the incidence of infections caused by *E. coli,* hepatitis A, *Cryptosporidium,* and other pathogens. Many of these illnesses are carried home and spread to other family members.

Public health officials are very much aware of the problem of emerging infections, and international efforts at monitoring, preventing, and controlling their spread are under way. These efforts require worldwide coordination because microbes do not respect national borders; only a global response can make the world a safer and healthier place for everyone.

SOURCES: Centers for Disease Control and Prevention. 1998. Preventing emerging infectious diseases: A strategy for the 21st century. *MMWR Recommendations and Reports* 47(RR-15). World Health Organization. 1998. *Emerging and Re-Emerging Infectious Diseases* (retrieved February 2, 1999; http://www.who.int/inf-fs/en/fact097.html). National Center for Infectious Diseases (http://www.cdc.gov/ncidod).

within a month or so. However, about 5–10% of people infected with HBV and 85–90% of people infected with HCV become chronic carriers of the virus, capable of infecting others for the rest of their lives. Some chronic carriers remain asymptomatic, while others slowly develop chronic liver disease, cirrhosis of the liver, or liver cancer. An estimated 4 million Americans are chronic carriers of HCV and another million carry HBV: worldwide, more than 500 million people may be chronic carriers of hepatitis. Each year in the United States, HCV is responsible for up to 10,000 deaths and HBV up to 6000 deaths, and these numbers are

expected to climb as more people infected in the 1970s and 1980s develop problems. HCV infection is already the most frequent reason for liver transplants among U.S.

TERMS

pandemic A disease epidemic that is unusually severe or widespread; often used to refer to worldwide epidemics affecting a large proportion of the population.

endemic Persistent and relatively widespread in a given population.

epidemic The occurrence in a particular community or region of more than the expected number of cases of a particular disease.

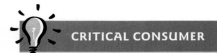
Unfortunately, there is no cure for the common cold. But there are some practical things you can do to avoid catching a cold, and to relieve the symptoms of any colds you do catch.

Prevention

Colds are usually spread by hand-to-hand contact with another person or with objects such as doorknobs and telephones, which an infected person may have handled. The best way to avoid transmission is to wash your hands frequently with warm water and soap. Cold viruses can also be transmitted in very small airborne particles produced by a cough or a sneeze, but this requires very close contact and is relatively rare. Keeping your immune system strong is another good prevention strategy (see the guidelines provided later in the chapter).

Home Treatments

- Get some extra rest. It isn't usually necessary to stay home in bed, but you will need to slow down a little from your usual routine to give your body a chance to fight the infection.

- Drink plenty of liquids to prevent dehydration. Hot liquids such as herbal tea and clear chicken soup will soothe a sore throat and loosen secretions; gargling with a glass of slightly salty water may also help. Avoid alcoholic beverages when you have a cold.

- Hot showers or the use of a humidifier can help eliminate nasal stuffiness and soothe inflamed membranes.

Over-the-Counter Treatments

Avoid multisymptom cold remedies. Because these products include drugs to treat symptoms you may not even have, you risk suffering from side effects from medications you don't need. It's better to treat each symptom separately:

- *Analgesics*—aspirin, acetaminophen (Tylenol), ibuprofen (Advil or Motrin), and naproxen sodium (Aleve)—all help lower fever and relieve muscle aches. Use of aspirin is associated with an increased risk of a serious condition called Reye's syndrome in children; for this reason, aspirin should not be given to children.

- *Decongestants* shrink nasal blood vessels, relieving swelling and congestion. However, they may dry out mucous membranes in the throat and make a sore throat worse.

- *Cough medicines* may be helpful when your cough is non-productive (not bringing up mucus) or if it disrupts your sleep or work. Expectorants make coughs more productive by increasing the volume of mucus and decreasing its thickness, thereby helping remove irritants from the respiratory airways. Suppressants (antitussives) reduce the frequency of coughing.

- *Antihistamines* decrease nasal secretions caused by the effects of histamine, so they are much more useful in treating allergies than colds. *Caution:* Many antihistamines can make you drowsy.

Antibiotics will not help a cold unless a bacterial infection such as strep throat is also present, and overuse of antibiotics leads to the development of drug resistance. *Healthy People 2010* estimates that 15 million courses of antibiotics are inappropriately prescribed for colds each year. The jury is still out on whether other remedies, including zinc gluconate lozenges, echinacea, and vitamin C, will relieve symptoms or shorten the duration of a cold. Researchers are also studying antiviral drugs that target the most common types of cold viruses.

Sometimes a cold leads to a more serious complication, such as bronchitis, pneumonia, or strep throat. If a fever of 102°F or higher persists, or if cold symptoms don't get better after 2 weeks, see your physician.

---

adults; and it is thought to be a major factor in the 70% increase in U.S. liver cancer rates since the 1970s.

The extent of HCV infection among Americans has only recently been recognized, and most infected people are unaware of their condition. To ensure proper monitoring, treatment, and prevention, testing for HCV may be recommended for the following individuals:

- People who ever injected illegal drugs, including those who injected once or a few times many years ago.

- People who received a blood transfusion or a donated organ prior to July 1992 or have been notified they received blood from a donor infected with HCV.

- People who received clotting factor prior to 1987 or have been on long-term dialysis.

- People with high-risk sexual behavior, multiple

partners, and/or sexually transmitted diseases.

- People who had body piercing, tattoos, or acupuncture involving unsterile equipment.

Routine testing may be recommended for children born to women infected with HCV and health care workers and others who may be exposed to infected blood. A home test for HCV infection was approved in 1999.

Another serious viral infection is **poliomyelitis,** or polio, which attacks muscle-controlling nerves. In some cases, polio leads to permanent paralysis. Fortunately, there is an effective vaccine for polio and the disease is now rare in the Western Hemisphere. WHO hopes to completely eradicate polio within the next few years.

Certain viruses can also cause cell proliferation. The human disease resulting from this property is warts, which is usually very mild but can become extremely

TABLE 17-3	*What's Causing My Symptoms?*			
Symptom	**Influenza**	**Common Cold**	**Allergy**	**Sinus Infection**
Headache	Always	Occasionally	Occasionally	Always
Muscle aches	Always (severe)	Usually (mild)	Rarely	Rarely
Fatigue, weakness	Always (severe; sudden onset; may last several weeks)	Usually (mild)	Rarely	Rarely
Fever	Always (high, typically 102–104°F; sudden onset; lasts 3–4 days)	Occasionally (mild)	Never	Occasionally
Cough	Usually (often severe)	Occasionally	Occasionally	Usually
Runny, stuffy nose	Occasionally	Usually	Usually	Always (stuffy)
Nasal discharge	Occasionally	Usually (thick; clear to yellowish green)	Usually (watery; clear)	Always (thick; yellowish green)
Sneezing	Rarely	Occasionally	Usually	Rarely
Sore throat	Rarely	Usually	Occasionally	Rarely
Itchy eyes, nose, throat	Rarely	Rarely	Usually	Never

SOURCE: Is that really the flu? 1997. *Consumer Reports on Health,* October.

severe if the resistance of the infected person breaks down. There are many members of the human wart virus family, and some of them are responsible for cervical cancer in women (see Chapter 16). Another virus, called HTLV-1 and related to HIV, causes a rare leukemia in adults (T-cell leukemia). As our knowledge of the molecular biology of cancer increases, other tumors may turn out to be caused by viruses, but most human cancers are thought to be caused by other factors.

Certain viruses have also been implicated as causes of *chronic fatigue syndrome* (CFS), a disorder characterized by severe chronic fatigue, impaired memory or concentration, and physical symptoms such as persistent sore throat or muscle pain. However, CFS has not been linked to any single infectious agent; other possible causes include abnormalities in immunity, hormone levels, and the regulation of blood pressure and heart rate.

Treating Viral Illnesses Although most viruses cannot be treated medically, there are a few antiviral drugs. These drugs work by interfering with some part of the viral life cycle; for example, they may prevent a virus from entering body cells. Herpes can be treated with acyclovir, an antiviral medication that helps alleviate symptoms and decrease the length of each recurrence. However, it cannot eradicate the latent virus. HIV infection can be treated with AZT (zidovudine), Crixivan (indinavir), or other antivirals that inhibit the virus and slow its progress (see Chapter 18). Influenza antivirals are also available; they help prevent the virus from gaining a foothold in the body

and may relieve the duration and severity of illness in people who take them after they already feel sick.

Most other viral diseases must simply run their course. OTC cold remedies and pain relievers treat symptoms, not their viral cause (see the box "Preventing and Treating the Common Cold"). Sometimes it's difficult to determine whether your symptoms are due to a virus (as for colds, flu, and some sinus infections), a bacterium (as for other sinus infections), or an allergy, but this information is important for appropriate treatment (Table 17-3).

Fungi, Protozoa, and Parasitic Worms

A **fungus** is a primitive plant. Fungi may be multicellular (like molds) or unicellular (like yeasts). Mushrooms and the molds that form on bread and cheese are all examples of fungi. Only about 50 fungi out of many thousands of species cause disease in humans, and these diseases are usually restricted to the skin, mucous membranes, and lungs. Some fungal diseases are extremely difficult to treat. To defend themselves against treatments, some fungi form spores, which are an especially resistant dormant stage of the organism.

Candida albicans is a common fungus found naturally in the vagina of most women. In normal amounts, it

poliomyelitis A disease of the nervous system, sometimes crippling; vaccines now prevent most cases of polio. **TERMS**

fungus A mold, mushroom, or yeast; fungal diseases include yeast infections, athlete's foot, and ringworm.

DIMENSIONS OF DIVERSITY *Women and Autoimmune Diseases*

Although the immune systems of men and women are essentially the same, women have much higher rates of many autoimmune diseases. The reason is somewhat of a mystery. One clue may come from pregnancy: In order to conceive and carry a baby to term, a woman's body must temporarily suppress its immune response so it doesn't attack the sperm or the fetus. Another factor seems to be related to estrogen. Estrogen receptors have been found on suppressor T cells, pointing to a possible link between the glands controlling immunity and those controlling sex hormones. Women also appear to have somewhat enhanced immunity compared to men, a factor that could be linked to both longer life spans and higher rates of autoimmune disorders.

Systemic lupus erythematosus is an autoimmune disease in which the immune system attacks the body's normal tissue, causing inflammation of the joints, blood vessels, heart, lungs, brain, and kidneys. Its symptoms include painful swollen joints, a rash on the nose and cheeks, sensitivity to sunlight, chest pain, fatigue, and dizziness. There are about 1.4–2 million Americans with lupus, 80% of them women; the disorder is especially common among Native American and African American women. Lupus usually begins before menopause and may flare up during pregnancy; for some women, symptoms also increase in severity during menstruation or with the use of oral contraceptives. A link between these exacerbating factors is

increased levels of estrogen, but this connection is not well understood. Researchers have also identified genetic mutations that may be associated with lupus.

In rheumatoid arthritis, the body's immune system attacks the membranes lining the joints, causing pain and swelling. Among the estimated 1% of American adults with rheumatoid arthritis, women outnumber men 3 to 1. The causes of the disease are not well understood. Researchers have hypothesized that an as-yet-unidentified virus may stimulate the immune system and trigger the disease. When the disease is present in younger women, symptoms often improve during pregnancy, when estrogen levels are higher, the opposite of what is seen in the case of lupus. Therefore, although estrogen levels may play a role in these disorders, its effects appear to be influenced by many other factors.

Other autoimmune disorders more common among women than men include multiple sclerosis, a neurological disease caused by the destruction of the protective coating around nerves; scleroderma, a connective tissue disease characterized by thickening, hardening, and tightening of the skin; and Graves' disease, characterized by an increase in the production of thyroid hormone, which affects metabolism and many body systems. Continued scientific investigation will help pinpoint the causes and triggers of autoimmune disorders and explain their higher incidence among women.

---

causes no problems, but when excessive growth occurs, the result is itching and discomfort, commonly known as a yeast infection. Factors that increase the growth of *C. albicans* include the use of antibiotics, clothing that keeps the vaginal area excessively warm and moist, pregnancy, oral contraceptive use, and certain diseases, include diabetes and HIV infection. The most common symptom is usually a thick white or yellowish discharge. Treatment consists of OTC antifungal creams and suppositories or prescription oral antifungal medication. Women should not self-treat unless they are certain from a past medical

diagnosis that they have a yeast infection. (Misdiagnosis could mean that a different and more severe infection goes untreated.) *C. albicans* overgrowth can occur in other areas of the body, especially in the mouth in infants (a condition known as thrush).

Other common fungal conditions affect the skin, including athlete's foot, jock itch, and ringworm, a disease of the scalp. These three mild conditions are usually easy to cure and rarely cause major problems.

Fungi can also cause systemic diseases that are severe, life-threatening, and extremely difficult to treat, including histoplasmosis and coccidioidomycosis. Histoplasmosis causes pulmonary and sometimes systemic disease and is most common in the Mississippi and Ohio River Valleys. Coccidioidomycosis is also known as "valley fever" because it is most frequently seen in the San Joaquin Valley of California. Fungal infections can be especially deadly in people with an impaired immune system.

Another group of pathogens are **protozoa,** microscopic single-celled animals, which are associated with such tropical diseases as **malaria, African sleeping sickness,** and **amoebic dysentery.** Many protozoa-based diseases are recurrent. The pathogen remains in the body, alternating between activity and inactivity. Hundreds of millions of Asians, Africans, and South Americans suffer from protozoal infections. The most common protozoal

TERMS **protozoan** A microscopic single-celled animal that often produces recurrent, cyclical attacks of disease.

malaria A severe, recurrent, mosquito-borne protozoal disease.

African sleeping sickness A severe, recurrent, insect-borne protozoal disease characterized by lethargy and fatigue.

amoebic dysentery A protozoal infection of the intestines.

parasitic worm A pathogen that causes intestinal and other infections; includes tapeworms, hookworms, pinworms, and flukes.

anti-inflammatory medication A drug such as aspirin, ibuprofen, and corticosteroids that is often used to treat autoimmune diseases.

disease in the United States is trichomoniasis, a relatively mild vaginal infection (see Chapter 18). Another protozoal disease, which can be contracted by drinking untreated water even in pristine wilderness areas, is giardiasis, characterized by diarrhea, nausea, and abdominal cramps.

Finally, the **parasitic worms** are the largest organisms that can enter the body to cause infection. The tapeworm, for example, can grow to a length of several feet. Worms, including such intestinal parasites as the tapeworm, hookworm, and pinworm cause a great variety of relatively mild infections. Smaller worms known as flukes infect such organs as the liver and lungs and, in large numbers, can be deadly. Generally speaking, worm infections originate from contaminated food or drink and can be controlled by careful attention to hygiene.

Other Immune Disorders: Cancer and Autoimmune Diseases

The immune system has evolved to protect the body from invasion by foreign microorganisms. Sometimes, as in the case of cancer, the body comes under attack by its own cells. As explained in Chapter 16, cancer cells cease to cooperate normally with the rest of the body and multiply uncontrollably. The immune system can often detect cells that have recently become cancerous and then destroy them just as it would a foreign microorganism. But if the immune system breaks down, as it may when people get older, when they have certain immune disorders (including HIV infection), or when they are receiving chemotherapy for other diseases, the cancer cells may multiply out of control before the immune system recognizes the danger. By the time the immune system gears up to destroy the cancerous cells, it may be too late.

Another immune disorder occurs when the body confuses its own cells with foreign organisms. As described earlier, the immune system must recognize many thousands of antigens as foreign and then be able to recognize the same antigens again and again. Our own tissue cells also are antigenic; that is, they would be recognized by another person's immune system as foreign. A delicate balance must be maintained to ensure that one's immune system recognizes only truly foreign antigens as enemies; erroneous recognition of one's own cells as foreign produces havoc.

This is exactly what happens in what are known as autoimmune diseases. In this type of malady, the immune system seems to be a bit too sensitive and begins to misapprehend itself as "nonself." Rheumatoid arthritis and systemic lupus erythematosus are examples of autoimmune diseases. For reasons not well understood, these conditions are much more common in women than men (see the box "Women and Autoimmune Disease").

Autoimmune diseases and a number of similar disorders are treated with drugs called **anti-inflammatory medications,** which counteract some of the immune effects. Steroids such as prednisone have a more powerful effect on the immune system and cause the immune response to diminish to the point where the patient can actually have an immune deficiency and become susceptible to a number of serious diseases.

GIVING YOURSELF A FIGHTING CHANCE: HOW TO SUPPORT YOUR IMMUNE SYSTEM

Pathogens pose a formidable threat to wellness, but you can take many steps to prevent them from getting control of your body and compromising your health. Public health measures protect people from many diseases that are transmitted via water, food, or insects. A clean water supply and adequate sewage treatment help control typhoid fever and cholera, for example; and mosquito eradication programs control malaria and encephalitis. Proper food inspection and preparation prevent illness caused by foodborne pathogens. These include the parasitic roundworm *Trichina spiralis,* which causes trichinosis and is found in some uncooked meat, especially pork; the *Salmonella* bacterium, which is often found in chicken; and *E. coli* O157:H7, a potentially deadly strain of *E. coli* that has been traced to improperly cooked meat and unpasteurized juice. In response to recent outbreaks of foodborne illness, the USDA is developing a new, more stringent inspection program. For more on this program and on how to prevent foodborne illness at home, see Chapter 12.

But what can you do as an individual to strengthen your immune system to help prevent infection? The most important thing you can do is to take good care of your body, with adequate nutrition, exercise, rest, and moderation in lifestyle. Medical science has not come up with anything that can improve upon the millions of years of evolution that have culminated in your immune system. Of course, once infection has begun, some diseases can be fought with the aid of antibiotics and antiviral drugs. But these medications are not helpful in *preventing* infection, except in circumstances where normal immunity is breached, such as in surgery.

Scientists have discovered, however, that even the strongest immune system (as measured by the number of helper T cells) fluctuates throughout a person's life. You are most susceptible to disease at the extremes of life—when first born, before you have developed active immunity against most pathogens, and in old age, when the immune system, like the rest of the body, starts to deteriorate. You can't avoid being young or old, but you can make sure you get appropriate vaccinations to help the immune system in case of invasion by specific pathogens (see Table 17-1).

One factor that is known to influence the immune response and that can also be affected by lifestyle and attitudes is stress. Research has shown that the actual num-

Many people believe that stress makes them more vulnerable to illness. Studies have shown that rates of illness are higher for weeks or even months in people who have experienced the severe emotional trauma of divorce or the death of a loved one. Can more commonplace anxieties and stresses also cause measurable changes in the immune system? And can common stress-management techniques actually boost the immune system?

Psychologist Janice Kiecolt-Glaser and immunologist Ronald Glaser, both of Ohio State University, conducted some of the first studies suggesting that poor emotional health suppresses the body's ability to fight disease. They studied how well medical students taking final exams could mount an immune response to a hepatitis vaccination. Compared to students who received the vaccine under unstressed conditions, the stressed students showed much weaker immune responses as measured by levels of natural killer cells and other blood components.

Additional research suggests that long-term anxiety, depression, and stress also affect a person's susceptibility to disease. Researchers studying caregivers of patients with Alzheimer's disease found that stressed caregivers had much higher blood levels of the stress hormone epinephrine and much lower levels of some types of T cells than a comparable group of less stressed caregivers. Lower T cell levels make people more vulnerable to illness, and the stressed caregivers reported three times more days of illness than the control group.

Mary Banks Jasnoski of the George Washington University is studying the opposite side of the relationship between stress and immunity—whether therapies that induce positive emotions can boost immune functioning. She has shown that relaxation and imagery of a powerfully functioning immune system increases T-cell levels for people with "high absorption ability." (High absorbers, who make up about 20% of the general population, have the ability to concentrate intently and respond intensively to experiences and imagination.) Jasnoski is currently studying the effects of relaxation and imagery on levels of antibodies, cytokines, and T cells.

In seeking to explain these effects, researchers are looking at the connections between emotions, stress, hormones, and immunity. Some hormones, such as cortisol, have been found to impair the ability of immune cells to multiply and function. Others, such as prolactin, seem to give immune cells a boost. By matching stress levels and hormonal changes to the ups and downs of immune function, researchers hope to gain a better grasp of the shifting chemistry of mind and immunity.

SOURCES: Mills, P. J., et al. 1999. Vulnerable caregivers of patients with Alzheimer's disease have a deficit in circulating CD62L\-T lymphocytes. *Psychosomatic Medicine* 61: 168–174. Mind-body meld may boost immunity. 1994. *Journal of the National Cancer Institute* 86(4): 256–258. Jaret, P. 1992. Mind over malady. *Health,* November/December.

ber of helper T cells rises and falls inversely with stress; that is, the higher the stress, the lower the T-cell count (see the box "Immunity and Stress"). As described in Chapter 2, stress encompasses many variables, ranging from emotional stressors, such as anger, anxiety, depression, and grief, to physical stressors, such as poor nutrition, sleep deprivation, overexertion, and substance abuse. Developing effective ways of coping with stress can improve many of the dimensions of wellness. A 1999 study of people with asthma or rheumatoid arthritis found that spending just 20 minutes a day during a three-day period writing down thoughts and feelings about particularly stressful events helped reduce symptoms by up to 30%—and the improvements were still evident four months later.

In addition to managing the stress in your life and getting all your immunizations, you can help your body defend itself against disease by following the guidelines in the box "How to Keep Yourself Well." As is the case with all your body systems, your immune system works best when you support it with a healthy lifestyle.

PERSONAL INSIGHT   Have you ever noticed a connection between high levels of stress in your life and a tendency to get sick? Do you feel that the two are linked?

SUMMARY

The Chain of Infection

- The step-by-step process by which infections are transmitted from one person to another includes the pathogen, its reservoir, a portal of exit, a means of transmission, a portal of entry, and a new host.

- Infection can be prevented by breaking the chain at any point. Strategies include public health measures such as treatment of drinking water and individual action such as hand washing.

The Body's Defense System

- Physical and chemical barriers to microorganisms include skin, mucous membranes, and the cilia lining the respiratory tract.

- The immune response is carried out by white blood cells that are continuously produced in the bone marrow. These include neutrophils, macrophages, natural killer cells, and lymphocytes.

- B cells are lymphocytes that produce antibodies. T cells consist of helper T cells, killer T cells, and suppressor T cells.

- Eat a balanced diet, and maintain a healthy weight. Consume a variety of lowfat foods to obtain the recommended amount of nutrients every day (see Chapter 12).

- Get enough sleep, 6–8 hours every night. Sleep is extremely important in helping the body replenish itself. Adequate sleep allows the proper production and performance of all immune system cells and functions. Insufficient sleep predisposes you to a great number of illnesses and more severe infections.

- Exercise (but not while you're sick). Moderate endurance exercise is an excellent way to reduce stress and strengthen the body, thereby preventing infection. However, exercising vigorously while you are sick may actually decrease your immunity and can prolong the infection, probably by facilitating the replication of the viruses.

- Don't smoke, and drink alcohol only in moderation. Smoking decreases the levels of some immune cells and heavy and long-term drinking interferes with the normal functioning of the immune system.

- Wash your hands frequently. Remove your rings, and rub all surfaces of your hands with lather for at least 10–20 seconds; rinse thoroughly. Antibacterial soaps may reduce the risk of infection, but some experts are concerned that widespread use of antibacterial products may contribute to the development of drug-resistant bacteria. The most important thing is to wash your hands well and often. (One study found that although 94% of adults claim they wash their hands after using a public restroom, only about 68% actually do.)

- Avoid contact with people who are contagious with infectious diseases transmitted via the respiratory route, such as influenza, chicken pox, and tuberculosis.

- Don't eat raw meats, poultry, seafood, eggs, or milk; don't drink water from streams or lakes near campsites.

- Avoid contact with ticks, rodents, and other disease carriers.

- To protect yourself against diseases such as hepatitis and HIV infection, practice safer sex (see Chapter 18) and don't inject drugs.

- Get all appropriate immunizations.

- If you do become ill, allow yourself time to recover. Be courteous to others by washing your hands frequently and covering your nose and mouth when you sneeze or cough.

- Lymphocytes recognize the antigens of invading organisms as foreign. When a foreign organism appears in the body, the appropriate antibody locks onto the antigen and sets off the immune response.

- The inflammatory response occurs when cells in the area of invasion or injury release histamines and other substances that cause blood vessels to dilate and fluid to flow out of capillaries.

- The immune response has four stages: recognition of the invading pathogen; rapid replication of killer T cells and B cells; attack by killer T cells and macrophages; suppression of the immune response.

- Immunization is based on the body's ability to remember previously encountered organisms and retain its strength against them. Vaccines are preparations made of antigens similar to a pathogen but not as dangerous.

- Allergic reactions occur when the immune system responds to harmless substances as if they were dangerous antigens.

The Troublemakers: Pathogens and Disease

- Bacteria are single-celled organisms; some cause disease in humans, including streptococcus, staphylococcus, and the bacteria that cause syphilis, Lyme disease, tuberculosis, and chlamydia.

- Most antibiotics work by interrupting the production of new bacteria. Bacteria can become resistant to antibiotics, which do not work against viruses.

- Viruses cannot grow or reproduce themselves; different viruses cause HIV infection, polio, hepatitis, herpes, warts, measles, mumps, influenza, the common cold, and other diseases.

- Other diseases are caused by certain types of fungi, protozoa, and parasitic worms.

- The immune system often detects malignant cells and destroys them as if they were pathogens.

- Autoimmune diseases occur when the body identifies its own cells as foreign.

Giving Yourself a Fighting Chance: How to Support Your Immune System

- Public health measures protect people from pathogens carried by water, food, and insects.

- The immune system needs little help other than adequate nutrition and rest, a moderate lifestyle, and protection from excessive stress. Vaccinations also help protect against disease.

1. Find out from your parents or your health records which immunizations you have had, including when you last had a tetanus shot. Are your immunizations up to date? If they aren't, or if you're not sure, check with your school health center about what they recommend.

2. Go to your local pharmacy and examine the cold and cough remedies. Exactly which symptoms does each one claim to alleviate, and with what active ingredient? If possible, ask the pharmacist which ones he or she recommends for various symptoms.

JOURNAL ENTRY

1. In your health journal, list the positive behaviors that help you avoid or resist infection. Consider how you can strengthen those behaviors. Then list the behaviors that tend to block your positive behaviors and put you at risk for contracting an infection. Consider which of these you can change.

2. Monitor yourself the next time you feel a cold coming on. Write down the symptoms, how they felt, the time and date of their occurrence, what you were doing, how you were feeling emotionally, and what you did in response to the symptoms. Keep the record until the cold is gone, noting how long it takes to run its course. Is there an association between your emotional state and how you experienced the symptoms? Between your emotional state and the length of the cold? Does taking medication (decongestant, cough syrup, etc.) make a difference in the symptoms or the duration of the cold?

3. *Critical Thinking* Does the government have the right to quarantine people who have serious infectious diseases such as tuberculosis or measles? Which should take precedence—concerns about public safety, or the rights of individuals? Are there aspects of an illness, such as the seriousness of the illness or the mode of transmission, that should be considered in making this decision? Write an essay outlining your position on this issue; describe what circumstances, if any, you feel would warrant quarantining an infectious person.

FOR MORE INFORMATION

Books

Biddle, W. 1996. *A Field Guide to Germs.* New York: Anchor Books. *An entertaining and informative look at many different kinds of pathogens.*

Farrell, J. 1998. *Invisible Enemies: Stories of Infectious Diseases.* New York: Farrar, Straus & Giroux. *A brief, easy-to-read introduction to infectious diseases, with coverage of tuberculosis, AIDS, cholera, malaria, and others.*

Garrett, L. 1995. *The Coming Plague: Newly Emerging Diseases in a World Out of Balance.* New York: Penguin. *Traces the emergence of new and drug-resistant microbes over the past 50 years, including conditions that promote their spread.*

Oldstone, M. B. A. 1998. *Viruses, Plagues, and History.* New York: Oxford. *An introduction to epidemic diseases and their impact on human history.*

Ryan, F. 1997. *Virus X: Tracking the New Killer Plagues Out of the Present and Into the Future.* Boston: Little, Brown. *Describes the relationship between pathogens and their hosts and the human activities that foster emerging infections.*

Task Force on Allergic Disorders. 1999. *The Allergy Report.* Milwaukee, Wisc.: American Academy of Allergy, Asthma, and Immunology. *Provides treatment recommendations for physicians and patients.*

Organizations, Hotlines, and Web Sites

Alliance for the Prudent Use of Antibiotics. Provides information on antibiotics and their proper usage as well as tips for avoiding infections.

　http://www.healthsci.tufts.edu/apua/apua.html

American Academy of Allergy, Asthma, and Immunology. Provides information and publications; pollen counts are available from the hotline and Web site.

　611 E. Wells St.
　Milwaukee, WI 53202
　800-9-POLLEN; 877-9-ACHOO
　http://www.aaaai.org

American College of Allergy, Asthma, and Immunology. Provides information for patients and physicians; Web site includes an extensive glossary of terms related to allergies and asthma.

　85 W. Algonquin Rd., Suite 550
　Arlington Heights, IL 60005
　847-427-1200
　http://allergy.mcg.edu

Bugs in the News! Provides information about microbiology—allergies, antibodies, antibiotics, mad cow disease, and more—in easy-to-understand language.

　http://falcon.cc.ukans.edu/~jbrown/bugs.html

Cells Alive! Includes micrographs of immune cells and pathogens at work.

> http://www.cellsalive.com

CDC National Center for Infectious Diseases. Provides extensive information on a wide variety of infectious diseases, including emerging infections.

> 404-332-4555; 888-CDC-FAXX
>
> http://www.cdc.gov/ncidod

CDC National Immunization Program. Information and answers to frequently asked questions about immunizations.

> 800-CDC-SHOT
>
> http://www.cdc.gov/nip
>
> 877-394-8747 (international travel information)
>
> http://www.cdc.gov/travel

Lung Facts/National Jewish Medical and Research Center. Provides information about allergies, asthma, chronic bronchitis, and other lung-related problems.

> 800-552-LUNG
>
> http://www.NationalJewish.org

Lyme Disease Foundation. Provides strategies for the prevention and treatment of Lyme disease and other tickborne infections.

> 800-886-LYME (24-hour recorded information)
>
> http://www.lyme.org

National Foundation for Infectious Diseases. Provides information about a variety of diseases and disease issues.

> http://www.nfid.org

National Institute of Allergy and Infectious Diseases. Sponsors research and publishes newsletters and journals; Web site includes fact sheets about many topics relating to allergies and infectious diseases, including tuberculosis and STDs.

> 31 Center Dr., MSC 2520
>
> Bethesda, MD 20892-2520
>
> 301-496-5717
>
> http://www.niaid.nih.gov

Outbreak. Provides information and links about emerging infectious diseases, including facts about current epidemics and background information on key diseases.

> http://www.outbreak.org

World Health Organization/Disease Information. Provides fact sheets about many emerging and tropical diseases as well as information about current outbreaks.

> http://www.who.int/whosis

See also the listings in Chapter 12 (food safety), Chapter 18, and Appendix B.

SELECTED BIBLIOGRAPHY

American Autoimmune Related Diseases Association. 1999. *Autoimmune Diseases in Women* (retrieved February 4, 1999; http://www.aarda.org/women.html).

Armstrong, G. L., L. A. Conn, and R. W. Pinner. 1999. Trends in infectious disease mortality in the United States during the 20th century. *Journal of the American Medical Association* 281: 61–66.

Beyer, W. E., et al. 1999. Protection against influenza after annually repeated vaccination: A meta-analysis of serologic and field studies. *Archives of Internal Medicine* 159(2): 182–188.

CDC Special Pathogens Branch. 1999. *Fact Sheet: Ebola Hemorrhagic Fever* (retrieved February 4, 1999; http://www.cdc.gov/ncidod/dvrd/spb/mnpages/dispages/ebola.htm).

Centers for Disease Control and Prevention. 1999. Achievements in public health, 1900–1999. Impact of vaccines universally recommended for children. *Morbidity and Mortality Weekly Report* 48(12): 243–248.

Centers for Disease Control and Prevention. 1999. *Hantavirus Pulmonary Syndrome Case Information* (retrieved February 3, 1999; http://www.cdc.gov/ncidod/diseases/hanta/hps/noframes/whatsnew.htm).

Centers for Disease Control and Prevention. 1998. Preventing emerging infectious diseases: A strategy for the 21st century. *MMWR Recommendations and Reports* 47(RR-15).

Centers for Disease Control and Prevention. 1998. Recommendations for prevention and control of hepatitis C virus (HCV) infection and HCV-related chronic disease. *MMWR Recommendations and Reports* 47(RR-19).

Christie, G. L., et al. 1999. Asthma, wheezy bronchitis, and atopy across two generations. *American Journal of Respiratory and Critical Care Medicine* 159(1):125–129.

Dhabhar, F. S., and B. S. McEwen. 1999. Enhancing versus suppressive effects of stress hormones on skin immune function. *Proceedings of the National Academy of Sciences* 96(3): 1059–1064.

El-Serag, H. B., and A. C. Mason. 1999. Rising incidence of hepatocellular carcinoma in the United States. *New England Journal of Medicine* 340(10): 745–750.

Gadsby, P. 1999. Fear of flu. *Discover,* January.

Georgia Division of Public Health. 1998. *Press Release: 26 Children Confirmed with E. Coli O157:H7* (retrieved February 4, 1999; http://www.ph.dhr.state.ga.us/news/ecolicobb.htm).

Henkel, J. 1999. Hepatitis C. *FDA Consumer,* March/April.

Is it just a cold? What to do about a cold or flu. 1999. *Consumer Reports,* January.

Laver, W. G., N. Bischofberger, and R. G. Webster. 1999. Disarming flu viruses. *Scientific American* 280(1): 78–87.

Levy, S. B. 1998. The challenge of antibiotic resistance. *Scientific American* 279(3).

McMurry, L. M., M. Oethinger, and S. B. Levy. 1998. Triclosan targets lipid syntheseis. *Nature* 394: 531–532.

National Center for Infectious Diseases. 1998. *Lyme Disease* (retrieved February 2, 1999; http://www.cdc.gov/ncidod/diseases/lyme/lyme.htm).

Rotun, S. S., et al. 1999. *Staphylococcus aureus* with reduced susceptibility to vancomycin isolated from a patient with fatal bacteremia. *Emerging Infectious Diseases* (retrieved February 5, 1999; http://www.cdc.gov/ncidod/ EID/vol5no1/rotun.htm).

UK Creutzfeldt-Jakob Disease Surveillance Unit. 1999. *CJD Statistics* (retrieved April 12, 1999; http://www.cjd.ed.ac.uk/figures.htm).

Vitek, C. R., and M. Wharton. 1998. Diphtheria in the former Soviet Union: Reemergence of a pandemic disease. *Emerging Infectious Diseases* (retrieved February 2, 1999; http://www.cdc.gov/ncidod/EID/vol4no4/vitek.htm).

World Health Organization. 1998. *Hepatitis C: 170 Million Infected Worldwide and Still No Vaccine* (retrieved September 3, 1998; http://www.who.org/inf-pr-1998/en/pr98-36.html).

World Health Organization. 1998. *Fact Sheet: Influenza A(H5N1)* (retrieved February 4, 1999; http://www.who.int/inf-fs/en/fact188.htm).

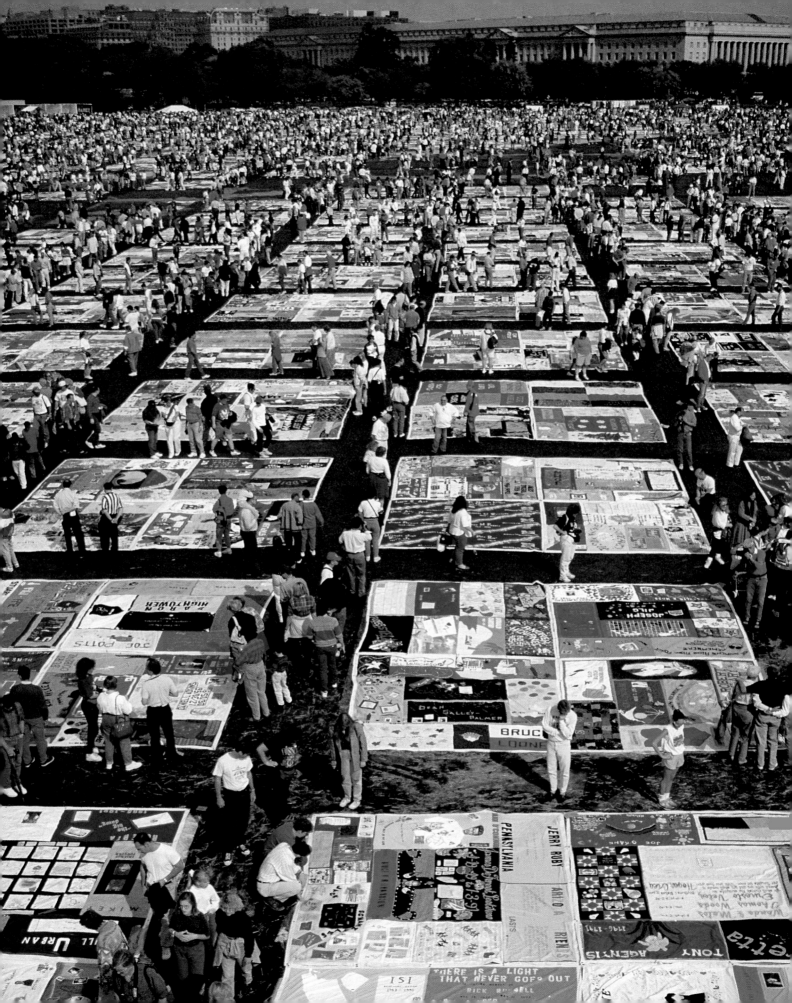

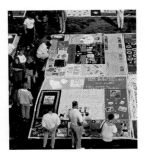

LEARNING OBJECTIVES

After reading this chapter, you should be able to:

- Explain how HIV infection affects the body and how it is transmitted, diagnosed, and treated.
- Discuss the symptoms, risks, and treatments for the other major STDs.
- List strategies for protecting yourself from STDs.

Sexually Transmitted Diseases

18

TEST YOUR KNOWLEDGE

1. If you have a sexually transmitted disease (STD), you will know it.
   True or false?

2. STDs can cause infertility in women.
   True or false?

3. About how many American adults are infected with HIV, the virus that causes AIDS?
   a. 1 in 30
   b. 1 in 300
   c. 1 in 3000

4. A man with an STD is more likely to transmit the infection to a female partner than vice versa.
   True or false?

5. The new and very effective drugs for HIV infection are successfully controlling the HIV/AIDS epidemic in the United States.
   True or false?

6. Douching after intercourse helps decrease the risk of STDs.
   True or false?

Answers

1. *False.* Many people with STDs have no symptoms and do not know they are infected; however, they can still pass an infection to their partners.

2. *True.* Untreated STDs, especially gonorrhea and chlamydia, are the leading cause of infertility in young women.

3. *b.* Worldwide, the figure is 1 in 100. In the United States, about 1 in 160 males and 1 in 800 females over age 12 is infected with HIV.

4. *True.* For many STDs, infected men are at least twice as likely as infected women to transmit an STD to their partner. And many STDs are more physically damaging to women than to men.

5. *False.* New drug treatments have reduced AIDS deaths, but the number of new infections among Americans is holding steady at about 40,000 per year. Anyone who is HIV-positive, even if on effective combination drug therapy, can transmit HIV.

6. *False.* Douching can actually increase a woman's chance of getting pelvic inflammatory disease.

Acquired immunodeficiency syndrome (AIDS) is a leading cause of death in many parts of the world. Most of the more than 33 million people around the world who are infected with **human immunodeficiency virus (HIV)**, the virus that causes AIDS, will likely die within the next 10 years. Although the death rate from AIDS in the United States began to decline in 1996, more than 400,000 of the 700,000 Americans who had been diagnosed with AIDS by 1999 had died from the disease, and it remains a major killer of Americans.

Although recent public education campaigns have focused primarily on HIV infection, all the **sexually transmitted diseases (STDs)**—gonorrhea, genital warts, chlamydia, herpes, syphilis, and others—continue to have a high incidence among Americans. The United States has the highest rate of STDs of any developed nation. Worldwide, nearly 300 million people are affected by STDs each year.

STDs are a particularly insidious group of diseases because a person can be infected, and be able to transmit the disease to others, yet not look or feel sick. The cost of unprotected sex may not become apparent for many years. Then a person may find that an undiagnosed STD has led to infertility, contributed to the development of cancer, or caused a birth defect in a child. In the case of HIV infection, the immune system becomes weakened and can no longer provide protection from disease.

It is important that everyone have a clear understanding of what STDs are, how they are transmitted, and—most importantly—how they can be prevented. The crucial message is that they *can* be prevented. And many can also be cured if they are treated early and properly. This chapter is designed to provide information about healthy, safer sexual behavior and to help you understand what you can do to reduce the further spread of these diseases.

PERSONAL INSIGHT How would you feel if your partner told you he or she exposed you to an STD? How would you feel if you contracted an STD?

TERMS

acquired immunodeficiency syndrome (AIDS) A generally fatal, incurable, sexually transmitted viral disease.

human immunodeficiency virus (HIV) The virus that causes HIV infection and AIDS.

sexually transmitted disease (STD) A disease that can be transmitted by sexual contact; some STDs can also be transmitted by other means.

HIV infection A chronic, progressive disease that damages the immune system.

CD4 T cell A type of white blood cell that helps coordinate the activity of the immune system; the primary target for HIV infection. A decrease in the number of these cells correlates with the risk and severity of HIV-related illness.

THE MAJOR STDS

In general, seven different STDs pose major health threats: HIV/AIDS, hepatitis, syphilis, chlamydia, gonorrhea, herpes, and genital warts. These diseases are considered major because they are serious in themselves, cause serious complications if left untreated, and/or pose risks to a fetus or newborn. In addition, pelvic inflammatory disease (PID) is a common complication of gonorrhea and chlamydia and merits discussion as a separate disease.

HIV Infection and AIDS

HIV infection is one of the most serious and challenging problems facing the United States and the world today. It is soon expected to surpass the influenza epidemic of 1918 that killed 20 million people. Despite the intense efforts of health professionals all around the world, HIV infection continues to spread, and a cure is yet to be found.

By 1999, an estimated 650,000–900,000 Americans were believed to be living with HIV—about 1 in 160 males and 1 in 800 females over age 12 (Figure 18-1). Although the death rate from AIDS among Americans has declined, new infections are holding steady at about 40,000 per year, meaning the number of Americans living with HIV infection is growing.

Worldwide, it is estimated that more than 50 million people have been infected since the epidemic began and more than 15 million have died (see the box "HIV Infection Around the World," on p. 494). Eleven people are infected every minute, and half of these new infections are in people age 15–24.

What Is HIV Infection? **HIV infection** is a chronic disease that progressively damages the body's immune system, making an otherwise healthy person less able to resist a variety of infections and disorders. Under normal conditions, when a virus or other pathogen enters the body, it is targeted and destroyed by the immune system. But the human immunodeficiency virus (HIV) attacks the immune system itself, invading and taking over **CD4 T cells,** monocytes, and macrophages, which are essential elements of the body's defense system (see Chapter 17). HIV enters a human cell and converts its own genetic material, RNA, into DNA. It then inserts this DNA into the chromosomes of the host cell. The viral DNA takes over the CD4 cell, causing it to produce new copies of HIV; it also makes the CD4 cell incapable of performing its immune functions.

Immediately following infection with HIV, billions of infectious particles are produced every day. For a time, the immune system keeps pace, also producing billions of new cells. Unlike the virus, however, the immune system cannot make new cells indefinitely; as long as the virus keeps replicating, it wins in the end. The destruction of

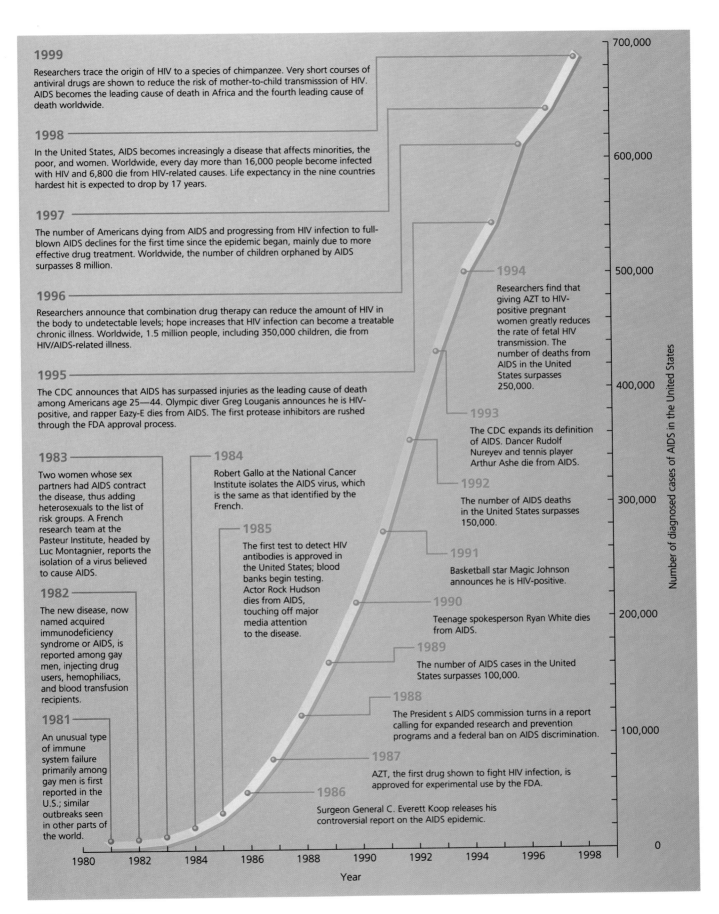

1999

Researchers trace the origin of HIV to a species of chimpanzee. Very short courses of antiviral drugs are shown to reduce the risk of mother-to-child transmisssion of HIV. AIDS becomes the leading cause of death in Africa and the fourth leading cause of death worldwide.

1998

In the United States, AIDS becomes increasingly a disease that affects minorities, the poor, and women. Worldwide, every day more than 16,000 people become infected with HIV and 6,800 die from HIV-related causes. Life expectancy in the nine countries hardest hit is expected to drop by 17 years.

1997

The number of Americans dying from AIDS and progressing from HIV infection to full-blown AIDS declines for the first time since the epidemic began, mainly due to more effective drug treatment. Worldwide, the number of children orphaned by AIDS surpasses 8 million.

1996

Researchers announce that combination drug therapy can reduce the amount of HIV in the body to undetectable levels; hope increases that HIV infection can become a treatable chronic illness. Worldwide, 1.5 million people, including 350,000 children, die from HIV/AIDS-related illness.

1995

The CDC announces that AIDS has surpassed injuries as the leading cause of death among Americans age 25—44. Olympic diver Greg Louganis announces he is HIV-positive, and rapper Eazy-E dies from AIDS. The first protease inhibitors are rushed through the FDA approval process.

1983

Two women whose sex partners had AIDS contract the disease, thus adding heterosexuals to the list of risk groups. A French research team at the Pasteur Institute, headed by Luc Montagnier, reports the isolation of a virus believed to cause AIDS.

1982

The new disease, now named acquired immunodeficiency syndrome or AIDS, is reported among gay men, injecting drug users, hemophiliacs, and blood transfusion recipients.

1981

An unusual type of immune system failure primarily among gay men is first reported in the U.S.; similar outbreaks seen in other parts of the world.

1984

Robert Gallo at the National Cancer Institute isolates the AIDS virus, which is the same as that identified by the French.

1985

The first test to detect HIV antibodies is approved in the United States; blood banks begin testing. Actor Rock Hudson dies from AIDS, touching off major media attention to the disease.

1986

Surgeon General C. Everett Koop releases his controversial report on the AIDS epidemic.

1987

AZT, the first drug shown to fight HIV infection, is approved for experimental use by the FDA.

1988

The President s AIDS commission turns in a report calling for expanded research and prevention programs and a federal ban on AIDS discrimination.

1989

The number of AIDS cases in the United States surpasses 100,000.

1990

Teenage spokesperson Ryan White dies from AIDS.

1991

Basketball star Magic Johnson announces he is HIV-positive.

1992

The number of AIDS deaths in the United States surpasses 150,000.

1993

The CDC expands its definition of AIDS. Dancer Rudolf Nureyev and tennis player Arthur Ashe die from AIDS.

1994

Researchers find that giving AZT to HIV-positive pregnant women greatly reduces the rate of fetal HIV transmission. The number of deaths from AIDS in the United States surpasses 250,000.

Year

Number of diagnosed cases of AIDS in the United States

VITAL STATISTICS

Figure 18-1   AIDS milestones.

Although first detected among heterosexuals in Africa, AIDS captured world attention in the early 1980s as a disease occurring primarily among homosexual men in the United States and Europe. Since then, AIDS has spread around the world. Over 50 million people worldwide have been infected with HIV since the epidemic began, and more than 14 million have died. In the next decade, the number of people who have been infected is expected to grow to 60–110 million.

The vast majority of cases—95%—have occurred in developing countries, where heterosexual contact is the primary means of transmission, responsible for 75–85% of all adult infections. In the developed world, HIV is increasingly becoming a disease that disproportionately affects the poor and ethnic minorities, especially women, youth, and children. Worldwide, women are the fastest-growing group of newly infected people, and nearly half the new cases of HIV infection in 1998 occurred in women. In addition, an estimated 1.2 million children are living with HIV infection and about 8 million children are AIDS orphans. It is estimated that the number of AIDS orphans will reach 40 million by 2010.

Currently, more than 22 million of those infected with HIV are in Africa, where AIDS has become the leading cause of death. Sub-Saharan Africa remains the hardest hit of all areas of the world; in some countries, 20–30% of adults carry the virus, and overall life expectancy has begun to decline dramatically. However, because the epidemic started about 10 years later in Asia than in Africa, experts expect an explosion of new cases in Asia, where already more than 6 million people are infected. And because Asia accounts for more than 50% of the world's population, the pool of people at risk is much larger than in Africa. HIV is also spreading rapidly in Eastern Europe, where injecting drug use and commercial sex are increasing.

Efforts to combat AIDS are complicated by political, economic, and cultural barriers in many parts of the world. Education and prevention programs are often hampered by resistance from social and religious institutions and by the taboo on openly discussing sexual issues. Condoms are unfamiliar in many countries, and women in many societies do not have sufficient control over their lives to demand that men use condoms during sex. Prevention approaches that have had success include STD treatment and education, public education campaigns about safer sex, and syringe exchange programs for injecting drug users. International efforts are under way to make condoms more available by lowering their price and to develop effective antiviral creams and spermicides that women can use without the knowledge of their partners. In countries such as Thailand and Uganda, where governments have worked hard to prevent the spread of HIV through education and other public health measures, rates of new infection have declined substantially.

In developed nations such as the United States, new drugs are reversing AIDS symptoms and lowering viral levels dramatically for some patients. But these drugs are almost entirely unavailable in the developing world. Ultimately what is needed is an effective vaccine. But until a vaccine or low-cost cure is developed, efforts must continue to focus on widespread educational campaigns and prevention through behavior change.

SOURCES: Joint United National Programme on HIV/AIDS. 1998. *AIDS Epidemic Update: December 1998* (retrieved February 6, 1999; http://www. unaids.org/highband/document/epidemio/wadr98e.pdf); Centers for Disease Control and Prevention. 1998. *The HIV/AIDS Epidemic in the United States, 1997–1998* (retrieved February 6, 1999; http://www.cdc.gov/ nchstp/hiv_aids/pubs/facts/hivrepfs.htm).

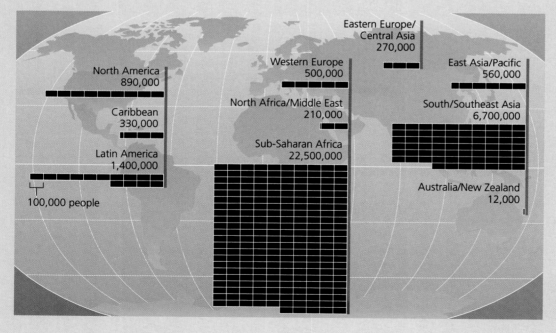

Approximate number of people with HIV/AIDS at the beginning of 1999.

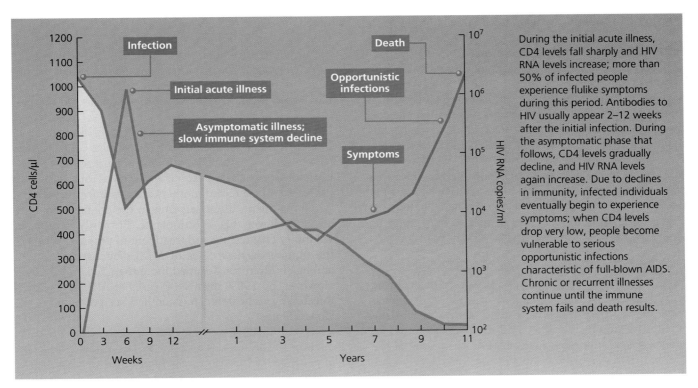

During the initial acute illness, CD4 levels fall sharply and HIV RNA levels increase; more than 50% of infected people experience flulike symptoms during this period. Antibodies to HIV usually appear 2–12 weeks after the initial infection. During the asymptomatic phase that follows, CD4 levels gradually decline, and HIV RNA levels again increase. Due to declines in immunity, infected individuals eventually begin to experience symptoms; when CD4 levels drop very low, people become vulnerable to serious opportunistic infections characteristic of full-blown AIDS. Chronic or recurrent illnesses continue until the immune system fails and death results.

Figure 18-2   The general pattern of HIV infection.   The shaded area under the curve represents the amount of CD4 cells in the blood, a marker for the status of the immune system. The line shows the amount of HIV RNA in the blood. If successful drug therapy is initiated, especially early in the infection, HIV RNA can drop to undetectable levels and CD4 cell levels can rise to normal. However, research thus far indicates that a cure is not achieved because some viable virus remains hidden in cells.   SOURCE: Adapted from Fauci, A. S., et al. 1996. Immunopathogenic mechanisms of HIV infection. *Annals of Internal Medicine* 124: 654–663. Reprinted with permission of the publisher.

the immune system is signaled by the loss of CD4 T cells (Figure 18-2). As the number of CD4 cells declines, an infected person may begin to experience mild to moderately severe symptoms. A person is diagnosed with full-blown AIDS when he or she develops one of the conditions defined as a marker for AIDS or when the number of CD4 cells in the blood drops below a certain level (200/μl). People with AIDS are vulnerable to a number of serious, often fatal, secondary, or opportunistic, infections.

The **asymptomatic** period of HIV—the time between the initial viral infection and the onset of disease symptoms—may range from 2 to 20 years. In adults, the average is 11 years. More than 50% of infected people experience flulike symptoms shortly after the initial infection, but most remain generally healthy for years. During this time, however, the virus is progressively infecting and destroying the cells of the immune system. People infected with HIV can pass the virus to others—even if they have no symptoms, and even if they do not know they have been infected. In the early days and weeks of infection, the most commonly used test for HIV remains negative. An infected individual may feel fine, but viral levels are often high at this stage. These asymptomatic individuals,

unaware that they are infected but with high viral levels, are responsible for much of the spread of HIV.

Transmitting the Virus   HIV lives only within cells and body fluids, not outside the body. It is transmitted by blood and blood products, semen, vaginal and cervical secretions, and breast milk. It cannot live in air, in water, or on objects or surfaces such as toilet seats, eating utensils, or telephones. The three main routes of HIV transmission are: (1) from specific kinds of sexual contact, (2) from direct exposure to infected blood, and (3) from an HIV-infected woman to her fetus during pregnancy or childbirth or to her infant during breastfeeding.

SEXUAL CONTACT   Of the different types of sexual contact, HIV is more likely to be transmitted by unprotected anal or vaginal intercourse than by other sexual activities. Oral-genital contact carries some risk of transmission, although less than anal or vaginal intercourse. HIV can be

asymptomatic   Showing no signs or symptoms of a disease.   TERMS transmitted through tiny tears in the fragile lining of the vagina, cervix, penis, anus, and mouth and through direct infection of cells in some of these areas.

The presence of lesions, blisters, or inflammation from other STDs in the genital, anal, or oral areas makes it two to five times easier for the virus to be passed. In addition, any trauma or irritation of tissues, such as might occur from rough or unwanted intercourse, the overuse of spermicides, or the use of enemas prior to anal intercourse, increases the risk. The risk of HIV transmission during oral sex increases if a person has poor oral hygiene, oral sores, or has brushed or flossed just before or after oral sex. During vaginal intercourse, male-to-female transmission is more likely to occur than female-to-male transmission. HIV has been found in preejaculatory fluid, so transmission can occur before ejaculation.

DIRECT CONTACT WITH INFECTED BLOOD   Direct contact with the blood of an infected person is the second major route of HIV transmission. Needles used to inject drugs (including heroin, cocaine, and anabolic steroids) are routinely contaminated by the blood of the user. If needles are shared, small amounts of one person's blood are directly injected into another person's bloodstream. HIV may be transmitted through subcutaneous and intramuscular injection as well, from needles or blades used in acupuncture, tattooing, ritual scarring, and piercing of the earlobes, nose, lip, nipple, navel, or other body part.

HIV has been transmitted in blood and blood products used in the medical treatment of injuries, serious illnesses, and **hemophilia,** resulting in about 12,000 cases of AIDS. The blood supply in all licensed blood banks and plasma centers in the United States is now screened for HIV. The odds are less than 1 in 600,000 that a unit of HIV-infected donated blood will fail to be detected with today's testing methods, and new genetic tests will further reduce the risk.

A small number of health care workers have acquired HIV on the job; most of these cases involve needle sticks, in which a health care worker is accidentally stuck with a needle used on an infected patient. The only reported cases of possible transmission *to* patients are those of six patients of a Florida dentist and one patient of a French orthopedic surgeon. A method of transmission was never determined with certainty in the first case; in the second, an injury to the hand of the surgeon during an operation may have exposed the patient to infected blood. In general, the risk of infection is far greater for health care workers than it is for patients because they are much more likely to be exposed to infected body fluids.

What about contact with other body fluids? Trace amounts of HIV have been found in the saliva and tears of some infected people. However, researchers believe that these fluids do not carry enough of the virus to infect another person. (In the rare cases of HIV infection linked to deep kissing or biting, the virus is thought to have been transmitted in blood from oral sores rather than in saliva.) HIV has been found in urine and feces, and contact with the urine or feces of an infected person may carry some risk. Contact with an infected person's sweat is not believed to carry any risk. There is absolutely no evidence that the virus can be spread by insects such as mosquitoes.

MOTHER-TO-CHILD TRANSMISSION   The final major route of HIV transmission is mother-to-child, also called *vertical transmission,* which can occur during pregnancy, childbirth, or breastfeeding. About 25–30% of infants born to untreated HIV-infected mothers are also infected with the virus; treatment, discussed later in the chapter, can substantially lower this infection rate. Primarily because of voluntary HIV testing and treatment of pregnant women, the number of new cases of AIDS diagnosed each year among children has declined more than 50% since 1994. However, by 1999, over 8400 cases of AIDS in children infected by vertical transmission had been reported in the United States.

NOT THROUGH CASUAL CONTACT   A person is not at risk of getting HIV infection by being in the same classroom, dining room, or even household with someone who is infected. Before this was generally known, many people with HIV infection, including children, were the targets of ostracism, hysteria, and outright violence. Today, it is an acknowledged responsibility of everyone to treat people with HIV infection with respect and compassion, regardless of their age or how they became infected.

Populations of Special Concern for HIV Infection

Among Americans with AIDS, the most common means of exposure to HIV has been sexual activity between men; injecting drug use (IDU) and heterosexual contact are the next most common (Figure 18-3). Changes in the sexual behavior of homosexual men and the screening of all donated blood have slowed the rate of infection from these sources, and HIV in the United States is increasingly becoming a disease that disproportionately affects minorities, women, children, and the poor.

The rate of HIV infection is eight times higher in African Americans than it is in whites, and the rate among Hispanics is twice that of whites. African American and Hispanic women account for nearly 80% of new HIV cases among women in the United States. In 1998, about 80% of children reported with AIDS were African American or Hispanic. While a large majority of HIV infection among whites in the United States is due to sexual contact between men, among minorities, IDU contributes to about half of cases. Of young women with AIDS, more than half were infected through heterosexual contact, often with an injecting drug user.

AIDS incidence and deaths have declined since 1996 among all groups of Americans, but these declines have been smaller among women and minorities compared to

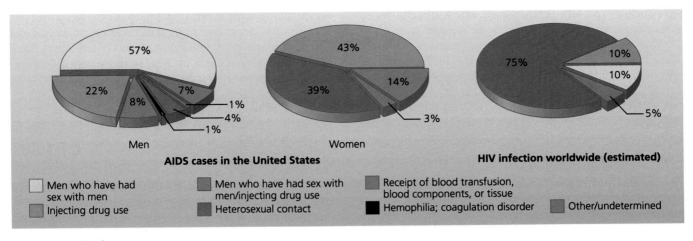

VITAL STATISTICS

Figure 18-3   Routes of HIV transmission among adults.   SOURCES: Centers for Disease Control and Prevention. 1999. *HIV/AIDS Surveillance Report* 10(2). Joint United Nations Programme on HIV/AIDS (UNAIDS). 1998. *AIDS Epidemic Update: December 1998* (retrieved February 6, 1999; http://www.unaids.org/highband/document/epidemio/wadr98e.pdf).

other groups. Between 1985 and 1998, the proportion of new U.S. AIDS cases reported each year in women increased from 7% to 22%. Women with HIV infection or AIDS often face tremendous challenges when they are ill because they may be caring for family members—children and spouses—who may also be infected and ill. Many women are also dealing with substance-abuse problems in themselves or in family members. In addition, there is some evidence that women may actually become sicker at lower viral loads compared to men.

About 90% of all cases of HIV infection in children are the result of transmission from infected mothers. HIV-infected children rarely appear ill at birth, but they begin to develop health problems over the first months and years of life. About 20% of infected children become very ill and progress to AIDS or death by age 4; the remaining 80% develop problems more slowly. In the United States, new treatments to reduce vertical transmission are in use, and the number of new cases of HIV infection in children has declined significantly. The situation worldwide is bleak, however: In 1997, fewer than 1 in 20 children born to HIV-positive women in the United States became infected with HIV; in developing countries, the average was about 1 in 3. The major reasons for this disparity are the lack of HIV testing and treatment in developing countries and breastfeeding practices. In developing countries, infants often acquire HIV through breastfeeding, whereas in the United States, HIV-infected mothers generally do not breastfeed their infants.

Also of concern are younger homosexual men. Although the overall transmission rates of HIV infection have dropped substantially among gay men in general, the reductions are not as great for men under 30. Surveys indicate that younger gay and bisexual men are much more likely to engage in unsafe sexual activity, especially unprotected receptive anal intercourse, than older men.

These patterns of HIV infection reflect complex social, economic, and behavioral factors. Reducing the rates of HIV transmission and AIDS death in minorities, women, and other groups at risk will require dealing with the difficult problems of drug abuse, poverty, and discrimination. HIV prevention programs must be tailored to meet the special needs of minority communities.

Symptoms of HIV Infection   Within a few days or weeks of infection with HIV, some 40–90% of people will develop symptoms of acute HIV infection. These can include fever, fatigue, rashes, headache, swollen lymph nodes, body aches, night sweats, sore throat, nausea, and diarrhea. Because the symptoms of acute HIV infection are similar to those of many common viral illnesses, the condition often goes undiagnosed, even if an infected individual sees a physician.

Diagnosis of HIV at this very early stage of infection, although uncommon, is extremely beneficial. Immediate treatment may help preserve immune function, slow the progress of the disease, and reduce transmission of HIV to others. For these reasons, it is critical for people who have engaged in behavior that places them at risk for HIV infection and who then experience symptoms of acute HIV infection to immediately inform their physician of their risk status. Standard tests for HIV will usually be negative in the very early stages of infection, so specialized

hemophilia   A hereditary blood disease in which blood fails   **TERMS** to clot and abnormal bleeding occurs, requiring transfusions of blood products with a specific factor to aid coagulation.

tests such as the **HIV RNA assay,** which directly measures the amount of virus in the body, must be used.

Other than the initial flulike symptoms associated with acute HIV infection, most people in the first months or years of HIV infection have few if any symptoms. As the immune system weakens, however, a variety of symptoms can develop—persistent swollen lymph nodes; lumps, rashes, sores, or other growths on or under the skin or on the mucous membranes of the eyes, mouth, anus, or nasal passages; persistent yeast infections; unexplained weight loss; fever and drenching night sweats; dry cough and shortness of breath; persistent diarrhea; easy bruising and unexplained bleeding; profound fatigue; memory loss; the loss of a sense of balance; tremors or seizures; changes in vision, hearing, taste, or smell; difficulty in swallowing; changes in mood and other psychological symptoms; and persistent or recurrent pain. Obviously, many of these symptoms can also occur with a variety of other illnesses.

Because the immune system is weakened, people with HIV infection are highly susceptible to infections, both common and uncommon (Table 18-1). The infection most often seen among people with HIV is *Pneumocystis carinii* **pneumonia,** a protozoal infection. **Kaposi's sarcoma,** a rare form of cancer, is common in HIV-infected men. Women with HIV infection often have frequent and difficult-to-treat vaginal yeast infections.

Cases of tuberculosis (TB) are also increasingly being reported in people with HIV, and the Centers for Disease Control and Prevention recommends TB testing for anyone with HIV infection. In Africa, drug-resistant strains of TB are now the most deadly infection among people with AIDS.

Diagnosing HIV Infection   Early diagnosis of HIV infection is important to minimize the impact of the disease. The most commonly used screening blood test for HIV is the **HIV antibody test.** This test consists of an initial screening called an **ELISA** test, and a more specific confirmation test called the **Western blot.** These tests determine whether a person has **antibodies** to HIV circulating in the bloodstream, a sign that the virus is present in the body (see the box "Getting an HIV Test"). Because antibodies may not appear in the blood for weeks or months after infection, the standard HIV antibody tests will be negative immediately following exposure. If recent infection with HIV is suspected, a special blood test such as the HIV RNA assay must be used.

If a person is diagnosed as **HIV-positive,** the next step is to determine the current severity of the disease in order to plan appropriate treatment. The status of the immune system can be gauged by taking CD4 T-cell measurements every few months. The infection itself can be monitored by tracking the amount of virus in the body (the "viral load") through the HIV RNA assay. Keeping track of viral load changes helps physicians evaluate the effects of treatment and can also help predict the likeli-

hood of long-term survival in a person infected with HIV.

Although rates vary from state to state, surveys indicate that about 40% of adults in the United States have been tested for HIV. About 20% of those tested had the test for personal or health reasons. The majority were tested to obtain insurance or enter the military or for reasons related to employment.

Diagnosing AIDS   As mentioned earlier, AIDS is the most severe form of HIV infection. The CDC's criteria for a diagnosis of AIDS reflect the stage of HIV infection at which a person's immune system becomes dangerously compromised. Since January 1993, a diagnosis of AIDS has been made if a person is HIV-positive and either has developed an infection defined as an AIDS indicator or has a severely damaged immune system (as measured by CD4 T-cell counts).

Reporting   All diagnosed cases of AIDS must be reported to public health authorities. Before effective treatments for HIV infection were available, officials could use AIDS statistics to track the epidemic because nearly everyone with HIV eventually developed AIDS within a fairly predictable time frame. However, the advent of more effective treatments has lengthened the time between infection and the onset of full-blown AIDS for many patients, making it more difficult to track the U.S. epidemic based on AIDS statistics alone. For this reason, the CDC recommended in 1999 that states require reporting of both HIV infection and full-blown AIDS.

Despite efforts to safeguard confidentiality and prohibit discrimination, mandatory reporting of HIV infection remains a controversial issue. If people believe they are risking their jobs, friends, or social acceptability, they may be less likely to be tested. At the same time, it is essential that enough information be disclosed through reporting to monitor the epidemic. The CDC recommends that states continue to provide opportunities for people to be tested anonymously; home HIV tests also allow anonymous testing.

Treatment   Although there is no known cure for HIV infection, medications can significantly alter the course of the disease and extend life. The drop in the number of U.S. AIDS deaths that has occurred since 1996 is in large part due to the increasing use of combinations of new drugs. Researchers hope that HIV infection will become a chronic disease that can be managed with medication.

Antiviral Drugs   Antiviral drugs in current use to combat HIV fall into two major categories. The first type are **reverse transcriptase inhibitors,** which include the widely used drug zidovudine (AZT). These drugs work by inhibiting the enzyme reverse transcriptase, which is used by HIV to integrate its genetic material into human cells (Figure 18-4, p. 501). The second class of antivirals are

TABLE 18-1 Infections or Disorders Commonly Associated with HIV/AIDS

Condition	Symptoms
Pneumocystis carinii pneumonia	Shortness of breath, persistent dry cough, sharp chest pains, difficulty breathing
Kaposi's sarcoma	Purple or brownish lesions that resemble bruises but are painless and do not heal
Tuberculosis (TB)	Fever, night sweats, fatigue, cough, weight loss
AIDS dementia	Sensory disturbances; impaired memory and judgment; loss of cognitive, social, or occupational abilities
Lymphadenopathy syndrome	Persistent swollen glands in the absence of other illness
Cytomegalovirus (CMV) retinitis	Blurred vision, visual impairment, "floaters" (vision partially blocked by shapes that seem to float), blindness
Mycobacterium avium complex	High fever, night sweats, weakness
Cryptosporidiosis	Severe diarrhea, abdominal cramping, weight loss, vomiting, loss of appetite
Invasive cervical cancer	Bleeding from the vagina between menstrual periods or after menopause, dull backache, general poor health

protease inhibitors; these target the enzyme HIV protease, which is used by the virus to create a protein coat for each new copy of the virus. Treatment with combinations of drugs, referred to as highly active antiretroviral therapy, or HAART, can reduce HIV in the blood to undetectable levels in some people. However, research indicates that latent virus is still present in the body and that HIV-infected men on HAART carry potentially transmissable HIV in their semen.

A major development in HIV treatment in the last few years has been the very early use of antiviral therapy. At one time, antiviral medications were "saved" for the later stages of immune dysfunction; but now, multiple drugs are being used much earlier in the course of the infection—to help decrease damage to the immune system and to help reduce the development of drug resistance.

Antiviral medications are even being used in some cases in an attempt to prevent infection in people who have been exposed to the virus. The CDC currently recommends that health care workers who have significant exposure to HIV-infected blood or body fluids via a needle stick or other mishap consider starting antiviral medication as soon as possible (preferably within a few hours of exposure) to decrease the risk of infection. Some experts feel that in certain situations people who have had nonoccupational exposure to HIV—such as unprotected high-risk sex or needle sharing with an HIV-positive individual—should also have the option of this type of post-exposure treatment. This approach is controversial for many reasons and its effectiveness is unknown; it is not currently recommended in most cases.

Researchers are working to develop new antiviral drugs that will attack different parts of the HIV replication process. An important step in developing new treatment came in 1996, when researchers discovered that people who carry a particular genetic mutation are resistant to HIV infection. One receptor on the cell wall of CD4 cells that HIV uses as a doorway to enter and infect a cell is called CCR-5. People with one type of mutation in one

TERMS

HIV RNA assay A test used to determine the amount of HIV in the blood (the "viral load").

***Pneumocystis carinii* pneumonia** A protozoal infection that is common in people infected with HIV.

Kaposi's sarcoma A form of cancer characterized by purple or brownish lesions that are generally painless and occur anywhere on the skin; usually appears in men infected with HIV.

HIV antibody test A blood test to determine whether a person has been infected by HIV; becomes positive within weeks or months of exposure.

ELISA (enzyme-linked immunosorbent assay) A blood test that detects the presence of antibodies to HIV.

Western blot A blood test that detects the presence of HIV antibodies; a more accurate and more expensive test, and used to confirm positive results from an ELISA test.

antibody A protein produced in the blood in response to a foreign substance to which it binds.

HIV-positive A diagnosis resulting from the presence of HIV in the bloodstream; also referred to as seropositive.

reverse transcriptase inhibitor An antiviral drug used to treat HIV infection that works by inhibiting reverse transcriptase, the enzyme that converts viral RNA to DNA.

protease inhibitor A drug that inhibits the action of any of the protein-splitting enzymes known as proteases. Protease inhibitors have been developed to block the action of HIV protease and thus prevent the replication of HIV.

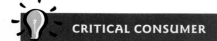

Getting an early diagnosis of HIV infection is more important than ever, but many people with HIV do not know they are infected. Anyone who has engaged in any of the following activities is potentially at risk and should consider being tested:

- You have had unprotected sex (vaginal, anal, or oral) with more than one partner or with a partner who was not in a mutually monogamous relationship with you.

- You have used or shared needles, syringes, or other paraphernalia for injecting drugs (including steroids).

- You received a transfusion of blood or blood products prior to 1985.

- You have been diagnosed with an STD.

Testing Options

If you decide to get an HIV test, either you can visit a physician or health clinic or you can take a home test. A big advantage to having the test performed by a physician or clinician is that you will get one-on-one counseling about the test, your results, and ways to avoid future infection or spreading the disease. If you have good reason to think you may test positive, it is probably best to be tested by a physician or clinic, where follow-up counseling and medical care will be intensive. The home test is a good alternative for people at low risk who just want to be sure. The advantages of the home test are that it can be done privately and anonymously, and it may be attractive to people who would not otherwise get tested.

Physician or Clinic Testing

Your physician, student health clinic, Planned Parenthood, public health department, or local AIDS association can arrange your HIV test. It usually costs $50–$100, but public clinics often charge little or nothing. The test itself is fairly simple. The procedure will be explained to you, then a sample of blood will be drawn and sent to a laboratory for analysis for the presence of antibodies to HIV. If the first stage of testing, the ELISA test, proves positive, it is followed by a confirmatory test, the Western blot. You'll be asked to phone or come in personally to get your results, which should include appropriate counseling. (Some clinics now also offer "rapid tests" that yield results within about 10–30 minutes; positive results must still be confirmed with the standard antibody tests and may require an additional week or two.) If you test negative, you need to know how to stay uninfected. If you test positive, you'll need to know what your medical options are; what the psychological, social,

and financial repercussions might be; and how to avoid spreading the disease.

Alternative tests may be used in some circumstances. The Orasure test uses oral fluid, which is collected by placing a treated cotton pad in the mouth for several minutes. Urine tests are also available. Oral fluid and urine tests may be helpful for people who avoid blood tests because of fear of needles.

Before you get an HIV test, be sure you understand what will be done with the results. Results from confidential tests may still become part of your medical record and/or reported (with your name or some other identifier) to state and federal public health agencies. If you decide you want to be tested anonymously—in which case the results will not be reported to anyone but yourself—check with your physician or counselor about how to obtain an anonymous test or use a home test.

Home Testing

Home test kits for HIV are now available; they cost about $40. (Take care to avoid testing kits that are not FDA-approved; many such unapproved kits are being sold over the Internet.) To use a home test, you prick a finger with a supplied lancet, blot a few drops of blood onto blotting paper, and mail it to the company's laboratory. There the sample is tested for HIV by the same methods used for samples collected by physicians. In about a week, you call a toll-free number to find out your results. Anyone testing positive is routed to a trained counselor, who can provide emotional and medical support.

The results of home test kits are completely anonymous. Your blood sample is assigned an identification number, and you never give your name or address. Even if you test positive and receive counseling, your conversation will be anonymous.

Understanding the Results

A negative test result means that no antibodies were found in your sample. However, it usually takes at least a month (and possibly as long as 6 months in some people) after exposure to HIV for antibodies to appear, a process called **seroconversion.** Therefore, an infected person may get a false-negative result. If you think you've been exposed to HIV, get a test immediately; if it's negative but your risk of infection is high, ask about obtaining an HIV RNA assay, which allows very early diagnosis.

A positive result means that you are infected. It is important to seek medical care and counseling immediately. Rapid progress is being made in treating HIV, and treatments are potentially much more successful when begun early.

copy of the CCR-5 gene have half as many cellular doorways for HIV as people with two normal genes, so the virus spreads more slowly in them. People with mutations in both copies of the gene are completely lacking in doorways and appear highly resistant to HIV infection. Lacking CCR-5 receptors does not appear to harm health in any way, so researchers hope to develop a drug that will mimic its effect. (On the flip side, researchers have found

another CCR-5 gene mutation that actually *increases* the number of cellular doorways for HIV and thus increases the risk of infection and the rate of spread of the virus).

Studies indicate that about 1 in 5 white Americans has one copy of the protective CCR-5 gene defect and 1 in 100 has two copies. The protective gene defect is much less common in African Americans and almost never occurs in Native Americans or Asian Americans, although

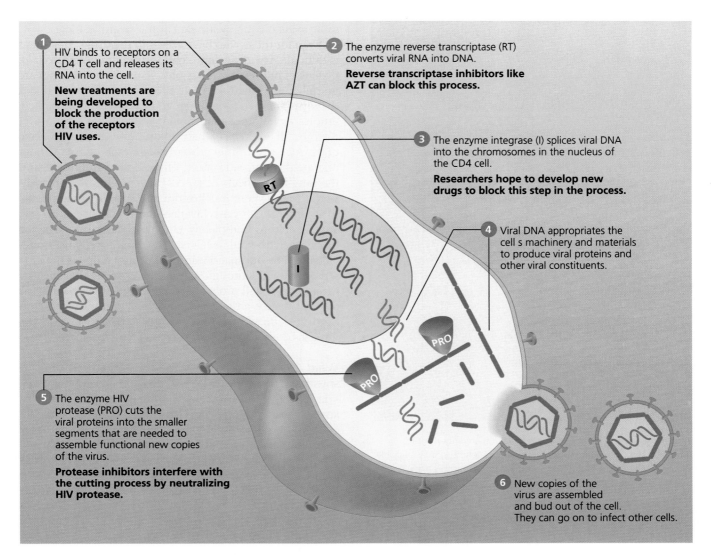

① HIV binds to receptors on a CD4 T cell and releases its RNA into the cell.

New treatments are being developed to block the production of the receptors HIV uses.

② The enzyme reverse transcriptase (RT) converts viral RNA into DNA.

Reverse transcriptase inhibitors like AZT can block this process.

③ The enzyme integrase (I) splices viral DNA into the chromosomes in the nucleus of the CD4 cell.

Researchers hope to develop new drugs to block this step in the process.

④ Viral DNA appropriates the cell's machinery and materials to produce viral proteins and other viral constituents.

⑤ The enzyme HIV protease (PRO) cuts the viral proteins into the smaller segments that are needed to assemble functional new copies of the virus.

Protease inhibitors interfere with the cutting process by neutralizing HIV protease.

⑥ New copies of the virus are assembled and bud out of the cell. They can go on to infect other cells.

Figure 18-4 The life cycle of HIV: How antiviral drugs work. Different classes of drugs block the replication of HIV at different points in the virus's life cycle. SOURCES: Dickinson, G., et al. 1998. The latest recommendations for antiretroviral therapy. *Patient Care,* 15 August. Disrupting the assembly line. 1996. *Newsweek,* 2 December.

these groups may have other protective gene mutations. The CCR-5 gene defect that promotes infection also appears more common among white Americans.

Many new antiviral drugs for HIV/AIDS are being developed. For updates, contact one of the agencies or Web sites listed in For More Information at the end of the chapter.

TREATMENTS FOR OPPORTUNISTIC INFECTIONS   In addition to antiviral drugs, most patients with low CD4 T-cell counts also take a variety of antibiotics to help prevent opportunistic infections such as *Pneumocystis carinii* pneumonia and tuberculosis. A person with advanced HIV infection may need to take 20 or more pills every day. All these medications have potential side effects, which can become severe when so many drugs are used in combination.

HIV AND PREGNANCY   Early stage HIV infection does not appear to significantly affect a woman's chance of becoming pregnant. Without treatment, about 25% of infants born to HIV-infected women are themselves infected with the virus. But treatment with antiviral drugs during pregnancy, labor, and early infancy has been shown to decrease a child's chance of contracting HIV by at least 65%; a cesarean delivery may decrease the risk even further. Because treatment can make such a dramatic difference in the health of the baby, HIV testing is strongly

seroconversion   The appearance of antibodies to HIV in the blood of an infected person; usually occurs 1–6 months after infection.   **TERMS**

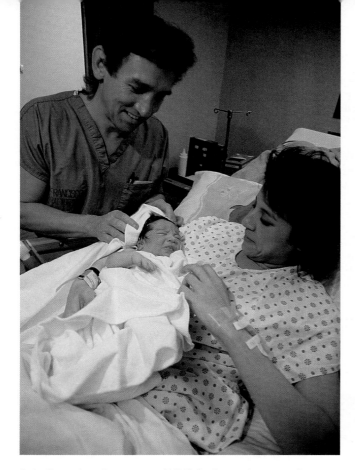

Early diagnosis and treatment of HIV infection are important for everyone, but particularly so for pregnant women. Currently available treatments can significantly increase the chance that this baby, born to an HIV-infected mother, will be free of the virus.

recommended for all pregnant women. HIV-infected women are usually advised not to breastfeed, because this has been shown to transmit HIV.

Testing and the use of antiviral drugs by pregnant HIV-positive women has had a dramatic effect in the United States: The number of new cases of HIV infection in children has declined by more than 60% since 1992. Unfortunately, long-term combination antiviral therapy is very expensive and is out of reach for most of the world's HIV-positive women. Recent studies indicate that very short courses of antiviral drugs given around the time of birth can also reduce vertical transmission, and health authorities are working with drug companies to provide less expensive treatment regimens that will meet the needs of women in developing nations.

TREATMENT CHALLENGES   The cost of treatment for HIV continues to be an area of major concern. Promising drug combinations can cost $10,000–$15,000 annually; for someone with full-blown AIDS, treatment may cost $20,000 or more per year. These costs are tremendous even for a relatively wealthy country like the United States. But 95% of people with HIV infection live in developing countries, where these treatments are unlikely to be available to anyone except the wealthiest few.

Even for those who have access to the drugs, treatment is difficult. The drug combinations require people to take dozens of pills every day at precise times. If the drugs are not taken on schedule, their effectiveness is reduced and the virus is much more likely to develop drug resistance. Studies have found that missing or delaying even 5% of the prescribed doses of medication causes the success rate of HAART to decline substantially. Some people cannot tolerate the toxic side effects of these powerful drugs, and the long-term effects of HAART are not known. In addition, the drugs are much more effective for some people than others. Currently available antiviral drugs do not appear able to completely eliminate the virus from the body, even if viral levels in the blood become undetectable. The optimal duration of drug therapy is not currently known, although many scientists feel that lifelong drug therapy will probably be necessary. It is also unclear to what degree a damaged immune system can rebound from the effects of long-term HIV infection even if the virus is brought under control with antiviral medication.

What About a Vaccine?   The best hope for preventing the spread of HIV worldwide rests with the development of a safe, effective, and inexpensive vaccine. Many different approaches to the development of an AIDS vaccine are currently under investigation, and human trials have begun on several vaccines. No vaccine is likely to be ready for widespread use within the next 5 years. The virus's ability to mutate, and the fact that many different strains of HIV exist, pose major challenges to scientists working on a vaccine.

Prevention   Although AIDS is currently incurable, it is preventable. You can protect yourself by avoiding behaviors that may bring you into contact with HIV. This means making careful choices about sexual activity and not sharing needles if you inject drugs.

MAKE CAREFUL CHOICES ABOUT SEXUAL ACTIVITY   In a sexual relationship, the current and past behaviors of you and your partner determine the amount of risk involved. If you are uninfected and in a mutually monogamous relationship with another uninfected person, you are not at risk for HIV. Of course, it is often hard to know for sure whether your partner is completely faithful and is truly uninfected. Having a series of monogamous relationships is not a safe prevention strategy.

For anyone not involved in a long-term, mutually monogamous relationship, abstinence from any sexual activity that involves the exchange of body fluids is the only sure way to prevent HIV infection (Figure 18-5). Safer sex includes many activities that carry virtually no risk of HIV infection, like hugging, massaging, closed-lip kissing, rubbing clothed bodies together, kissing your partner's skin, and mutual masturbation.

High Risk

Unprotected anal sex is the riskiest sexual behavior, especially for the receptive partner.

Unprotected vaginal intercourse is the next riskiest, especially for women, who are much more likely to be infected by an infected male partner than vice versa.

Oral sex is probably considerably less risky than anal and vaginal intercourse.

Sharing of sex toys can be risky because they can carry blood, semen, or vaginal fluid.

Use of a condom reduces risk considerably but not completely for any type of intercourse. Anal sex with a condom is riskier than vaginal sex with a condom; oral sex with a condom is less risky, especially if the man does not ejaculate.

Hand-genital contact and deep kissing are less risky but could still theoretically transmit HIV; the presence of cuts or sores increases risk.

Sex with only one uninfected and totally faithful partner is without risk, but effective only if both partners are uninfected and completely monogamous.

Activities that don't involve the exchange of body fluids carry no risk: hugging, massage, closed-mouth kissing, masturbation, phone sex, and fantasy.

Abstinence is completely without risk. For many people, it can be an effective and reasonable method of avoiding HIV infection and other STDs during certain periods of life.

No Risk

Figure 18-5   What's risky and what's not: The approximate relative risk of HIV transmission of various sexual activities. Safer sex strategies that reduce the risk of HIV infection will also help protect you against other STDs. The main point to remember is that any activity that involves contact with blood, semen, or vaginal fluid can transmit HIV.

Anal and vaginal intercourse are the sexual activities associated with the highest risk of HIV infection. If you have intercourse, always use a latex condom. Condoms are not perfect, and they do not provide risk-free sex; however, used properly, a latex condom provides a high level of protection against HIV. In one study of 124 couples that had one infected partner and that used condoms consistently, none of the uninfected partners acquired the virus during the 20-month study period. Condoms should also be worn during oral sex. Some experts also suggest the use of latex squares and dental dams, rubber devices that can be used as barriers during oral-genital or oral-anal sexual contact.

Limiting the number of partners you have—particularly those who have engaged in risky sexual behaviors in the past—can also lower your risk of exposure to HIV. Take the time to talk with a potential new partner about HIV and safer sex. Talking about sex may seem embarrassing and uncomfortable, but good communication is critical for your health. Asking a partner about past sexual experiences can also be helpful, but you cannot always depend on that information. Recent surveys of HIV-positive people found that 40–50% failed to reveal their HIV status to sexual partners; of these, nearly two-thirds failed to always use a condom. Take precautions with every partner. Don't agree to have intercourse or give up precautions as a way to show your love or commit-

ment to a relationship. Your specific sexual practices can be just as important as the number of partners you have.

Removing alcohol and other drugs from sexual activity is another crucial component of safer sex. The use of alcohol and mood-altering drugs may lower inhibitions and affect judgment, making you more likely to engage in unsafe sex. The use of drugs is also associated with sexual activity with multiple partners.

Remember, you can't tell if someone is infected by looking at him or her. Researchers believe that HIV has been in the United States since the mid- to late 1970s; anyone who has engaged in an unsafe behavior since that time is potentially at risk for HIV infection. Consider in advance what you will say and do in particular situations. Be assertive, and negotiate for safer sex practices.

Surveys of college students indicate that the majority of students are not engaging in safer sex. Although most students know that condom use can protect against HIV infection, this knowledge is often not translated into action. Many students also report a willingness to lie about past sexual activity in order to obtain sex. In addition, many students believe their risk of contracting HIV depends on "who they are" rather than on their sexual behavior. These attitudes and behaviors place college students at continued high risk for contracting HIV.

If you are sexually active, take responsibility for undergoing testing for HIV and other STDs at least once a

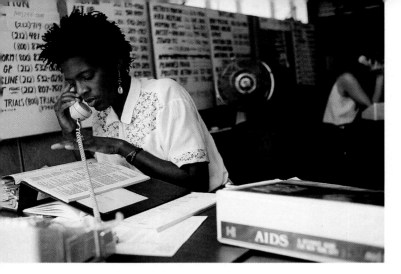

Accurate, confidential answers to personal questions are available from local and national STD hotlines. Separate AIDS hotlines, such as the one shown here, provide referrals, information, and updates on the success of the latest treatments for HIV infection and AIDS.

year—more often if you have a new sexual partner or multiple partners. Remember that having any other STD makes you much more likely to acquire HIV infection. Prompt detection and treatment of other STDs can help decrease your risk of HIV infection.

DON'T SHARE DRUG NEEDLES   People who inject drugs should avoid sharing needles, syringes, or anything that might have blood on it. Any injectable drug, legal or illegal, can be associated with HIV transmission. Needles can be decontaminated with a solution of bleach and water, but it is not a foolproof procedure and HIV can survive in a syringe for a month or longer. (Boiling needles and syringes does not necessarily destroy HIV either.) If you are an injecting drug user, your best protection against HIV is to obtain treatment and refrain from using drugs. (See Chapter 9 for more information about drug abuse.)

PARTICIPATE IN AN HIV EDUCATION PROGRAM   Many schools and colleges have peer education programs about preventing the transmission of HIV. These programs give you a chance to practice communicating with potential sex partners and negotiating safer sex, to engage in role

playing to build self-confidence, and to learn how to use condoms. Studies show that educational programs in which students learn from their peers and then try out what they've learned through role playing are more likely to result in real behavior change.

Many young people still believe that they are invulnerable to most kinds of harm and persist in thinking of themselves as not being at risk for HIV. The attitude of "It won't happen to me" is pervasive among high school and college students and is a major stumbling block to HIV/AIDS prevention. Until there is a vaccine and a cure, HIV infection will remain one of the biggest challenges of this generation. Education and individual responsibility can lead the way to controlling this devastating epidemic (see the box "Preventing HIV Infection and Other STDs").

Chlamydia

Chlamydia trachomatis causes **chlamydia,** the most prevalent bacterial STD in the United States. About 3 million new cases occur each year, down from a high of about 4 million; the drop is likely due to increased screening and treatment. An estimated 5–10% of all sexually active American women are infected with chlamydia; rates among men are similar. The highest rates of infection occur in single people between ages 18 and 24. About 20–40% of people who are diagnosed with gonorrhea also have chlamydia. *C. trachomatis* can be transmitted by oral sex as well as by other forms of sexual intercourse.

Both men and women are susceptible to chlamydia, but as with most STDs, women bear the greater burden because of possible complications and consequences of the disease. In most women, chlamydia produces no early symptoms. If left untreated, it can lead to pelvic inflammatory disease (PID), a serious infection involving the oviducts (fallopian tubes) and uterus. PID, discussed later in this chapter, is a leading cause of infertility, and even an infection that produces no symptoms can cause significant scarring of the oviducts. Chlamydia also greatly increases a woman's risk for ectopic (tubal) pregnancy. Because rates of infection are high and most women with chlamydia have no symptoms, many physicians screen sexually active women at the time of their routine pelvic exam; for young sexually active women, some experts recommend screening every 6 months.

Chlamydia can also lead to infertility in men, although not as often as in women. In men under age 35, chlamydia is the most common cause of **epididymitis,** inflammation of the sperm-carrying ducts. And up to half of all cases of **urethritis,** inflammation of the urethra, in men are caused by chlamydia. Despite these statistics, many infected men have no symptoms. And although equally likely to be infected, men are much less likely than women to be screened routinely for chlamydia.

Infants of infected mothers can acquire the infection through contact with the pathogen in the birth canal dur-

For those who don't have a long-term monogamous relationship with an uninfected partner, abstinence is the only truly safe option. Individuals should remember that it's OK to say no to sex and drugs.

Safer sexual activities that allow close person-to-person contact with almost no risk of contracting STDs or HIV include fantasy, hugging, massage, rubbing clothed bodies together, self-stimulation by both partners, and kissing with lips closed.

If you choose to be sexually active, talk with potential partners about HIV, safer sex, and the use of condoms before you begin a sexual relationship. The following behaviors will help lower your risk of exposure to HIV during sexual activities:

- Limit the number of partners. Avoid sexual contact with people who have HIV or an STD or who have engaged in risky behaviors in the past, including unprotected sex and injecting drug use.

- Use latex condoms during every act of intercourse and oral sex. Even if your partner claims to have been tested for HIV and STDs, there is no guarantee that he or she is uninfected. Many STDs are not easy to diagnose in their asymptomatic stage, which can last for years; and asymptomatic individuals can still infect others. No matter what your partner says, you have no guarantee that you will not contract an STD during any sexual encounter. If you choose to have intercourse, your best protection is to *always* use a condom. They do not provide perfect protection, but they greatly reduce your risk of contracting an infection.

- Use condoms properly to obtain maximum protection (refer to the instructions for condom use in Chapter 6). Use a water-based lubricant; don't use oil-based lubricants such as petroleum jelly or baby oil or any vaginal product containing mineral or vegetable oil. Unroll condoms gently to avoid tearing them, and smooth out any air bubbles.

- Avoid sexual contact that could cause cuts or tears in the skin or tissue.

- Get periodic screening tests for STDs and HIV. Young women need yearly pelvic exams and Pap tests.

- Get vaccinated for hepatitis B. Take advantage of this safe and effective vaccine.

- Get prompt treatment for any STDs you contract.

- Don't drink or use drugs in sexual situations. Mood-altering drugs can affect your judgment and make you more likely to engage in risky behaviors. Having sex when intoxicated is associated with a significantly increased risk of STDs.

If you inject drugs of any kind, don't share needles, syringes, or anything that might have blood on it. Decontaminate needles and syringes with household bleach and water.

If you are at risk for HIV infection, don't donate blood, sperm, or body organs. Don't have unprotected sex or share needles or syringes. Get tested for HIV soon, and get treated. HIV-infected people who get early treatment generally feel better and live longer than those who delay.

---

ing delivery. Every year, over 150,000 newborns suffer from eye infections and pneumonia as a result of untreated maternal chlamydial infections.

Symptoms In men, chlamydia symptoms include painful urination, a slight watery discharge from the penis, and sometimes pain around the testicles. Although most women with chlamydia are asymptomatic, some notice increased vaginal discharge, burning with urination, pain or bleeding with intercourse, and lower abdominal pain. Less common symptoms in both men and women include arthritis, conjunctivitis, and rectal inflammation and pain (in people who become infected during receptive anal intercourse). Symptoms in both men and women can begin within 5 days of infection. However, most people experience few or no symptoms, increasing the likelihood that they will inadvertently spread the infection to their partners.

Diagnosis Chlamydia is typically diagnosed through laboratory tests. Specimens are usually obtained by collecting a urine sample or a small amount of fluid from the urethra or cervix with a swab. The lab test may involve growing the organism in culture, special dyes to detect bacterial proteins, or a process that quickly copies and detects genetic material from the bacteria. Testing pregnant women and treating those with chlamydia is a highly effective way to prevent infection of newborns.

Treatment Once chlamydia has been diagnosed, the infected person and his or her partner(s) are given antibiotics—usually doxycycline, erythromycin, or a newer drug, azithromycin, which can cure infection in one dose. Chlamydia is an expensive disease, with costs running higher than $2 billion annually in the United States. And for an individual, the physical and emotional costs—damaged reproductive organs, infertility, or an infected infant—can be devastating.

Gonorrhea

In the United States, an estimated 650,000 new cases of **gonorrhea** are diagnosed every year. The highest incidence is among 15–24-year-olds. Like chlamydia, untreated gonorrhea can cause PID in women and urethritis and epididymitis in men. It can also cause arthritis and rashes, and it occasionally involves internal organs. An infant passing through the birth canal of an infected mother may contract **gonococcal conjunctivitis**, an infection in the eyes that can cause blindness if not treated. In most states, all newborn babies are routinely treated with antimicrobial eyedrops to prevent infection.

Gonorrhea is caused by the bacterium *Neisseria gonorrhoeae,* which flourishes in mucous membranes, including the moist linings of the mouth, throat, vagina, cervix, urethra, and anal canal. The microbe cannot thrive outside the warm, moist environment of the human body and dies within moments of exposure to light and air. Consequently, gonorrhea cannot be contracted from toilet seats, towels, or other objects.

Symptoms   In males, the incubation period for gonorrhea is brief, generally 2–7 days. The first symptoms are due to urethritis, which causes urinary discomfort and a thick, yellowish-white or yellowish-green discharge from the penis. The lips of the urethral opening may become inflamed and swollen. In some cases, the lymph glands in the groin become enlarged and swollen. Up to one-third of males have very minor symptoms or none at all.

Most females with gonorrhea are asymptomatic. Those who do have symptoms often experience urinary pain, increased vaginal discharge, and severe menstrual cramps. Up to 40% of women with untreated gonorrhea develop PID. Women may also develop painful abscesses in the Bartholin's glands, a pair of glands located on either side of the opening of the vagina.

Gonorrhea can also infect the throat or rectum of people who engage in oral or anal sex. Gonorrhea symptoms in the throat may be a sore throat or pus on the tonsils, and those in the rectum may be pus or blood in the feces, or rectal pain and itching.

Diagnosis   Several tests—gram stain, detection of bacterial genes or DNA, or culture—may be performed; depending on the test, samples of urine or cervical, urethral, throat, or rectal fluids may be collected.

Treatment   A variety of new and relatively expensive antibiotics are usually effective in curing gonorrhea. Older, less expensive antibiotics such as penicillin and tetracycline are not currently recommended for treating gonor-

rhea because of widespread drug resistance. People with gonorrhea often also have chlamydia, so additional antibiotics are typically given to treat chlamydia. Follow-up tests are sometimes performed to make sure the infection has been eradicated.

Pelvic Inflammatory Disease

A major complication in 10–40% of women who have been infected with either gonorrhea or chlamydia and have not received adequate treatment is **pelvic inflammatory disease (PID)**. PID occurs when the initial infection with gonorrhea and/or chlamydia travels upward, often along with other bacteria, beyond the cervix into the uterus, oviducts, ovaries, and pelvic cavity. PID is often serious enough to require hospitalization and sometimes surgery. Even if the disease is treated successfully, about 25% of affected women will have long-term problems such as a continuing susceptibility to infection, ectopic pregnancy, infertility, and chronic pelvic pain.

PID is the leading cause of infertility in young women, often undetected until later, when the inability to become pregnant leads to further evaluation. Infertility occurs in 8% of women after one episode of PID, 20% after two episodes, and 40% after three episodes. The risk of ectopic pregnancy increases significantly in women who have had PID.

Young women under age 25 are much more likely to develop PID than older women. As with all STDs, the more sex partners a woman has had, the greater her risk of PID. Smokers have twice the risk of PID as nonsmokers. Using IUDs for contraception and vaginal douching also increase the risk of PID. In general, women should avoid douching because this practice may actually force bacteria up through the cervix and into the uterus and oviducts. Women who use oral contraceptives, barrier methods like condoms and diaphragms, and spermicides have a lower risk of PID.

Symptoms   Symptoms of PID vary greatly. Some women, especially those with PID from chlamydia, may be asymptomatic; others may feel very ill with abdominal pain, fever, chills, nausea, and vomiting. Early symptoms are essentially the same as those described earlier for chlamydia and gonorrhea. Symptoms often begin or worsen during or soon after a woman's menstrual period. Many women have abnormal vaginal bleeding—either bleeding between periods or heavy and painful menstrual bleeding.

Diagnosis   Diagnosis of PID is made on the basis of symptoms, physical examination, ultrasound, and laboratory tests. Laparoscopy may be used to confirm the diagnosis and obtain material for cultures. Cultures from the rectum or cervix may also be taken to help identify the specific organism. The symptoms of PID, ectopic pregnancy, and

TERMS   **gonococcal conjunctivitis**   An inflammation of the mucous membrane lining of the eyelids, caused by the gonococcus bacterium.

pelvic inflammatory disease (PID)   An infection that progresses from the vagina and cervix to the uterus, oviducts, and pelvic cavity.

genital warts   A sexually transmitted viral infection characterized by growths on the genitals; also called *genital HPV infection.*

human papillomavirus (HPV)   The pathogen that causes human warts, including genital warts.

appendicitis can be quite similar, so careful evaluation is required to make the correct diagnosis.

Treatment Starting treatment of PID as quickly as possible is important in order to minimize damage to the reproductive organs. Antibiotics are usually started immediately; in severe cases, the woman may be hospitalized and antibiotics given intravenously. It is especially important that an infected woman's partners be treated. As many as 60% of the male contacts of women with PID are infected but asymptomatic.

Genital Warts

Genital warts, also known as condyloma, are caused by infection with **human papillomavirus (HPV).** The CDC estimates that 24 million people in the United States have this persistent viral infection, and another 5.5 million people are infected each year. Condyloma is the most common STD for which diagnosis and treatment are sought in student health services (see the box "College Students and STDs," p. 508). The disease appears to be most prevalent in young people age 16–25.

HPV infection presents a challenge to the medical community because of its known relationship to cervical cancer. A precancerous condition known as cervical dysplasia often occurs among women with genital HPV infection (see Chapter 16). If untreated, women with this condition sometimes develop cervical cancer. Other factors that increase a woman's chance of getting cervical cancer include smoking, sexual activity at a young age, and multiple sex partners.

Human papillomaviruses cause many types of human warts. There are about 80 different strains of HPV, and different strains infect specific locations. More than 20 types are likely to cause genital infections, and five of these are often implicated in cervical cancer; other strains are linked to anal, penile, and other genital cancers.

Genital HPV infection is quite contagious. Condoms and other barrier methods can help prevent the transmission of HPV, but warts frequently occur in areas where condoms are not fully protective. These areas are the labia in women, the base of the penis and the scrotum in men, and around the anus in both men and women.

Controlling the current genital HPV epidemic is difficult for several reasons. First, many people who carry HPV have no visible warts or symptoms. And although people with visible genital warts may be more likely to transmit the disease, asymptomatic people can also infect others. Second, although current treatments can often (but not always) eliminate visible warts, HPV continues to infect healthy tissue nearby. So even after treatment, a person can still transmit HPV to someone else. Third, as mentioned above, condoms do not provide complete protection against the transmission of HPV.

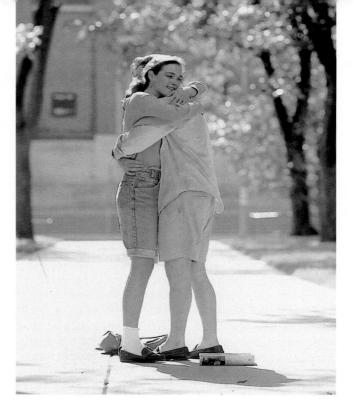

By taking a responsible attitude toward STDs, people show respect and concern for themselves and their partners. This couple's plans for the future could be seriously disrupted if one of them contracted an STD like gonorrhea or chlamydia. Either of these diseases, if untreated, could result in PID, the leading cause of infertility in young women.

Symptoms Genital warts can look like warts that are seen on other parts of the body. They are often dry, painless growths, rough in texture and gray or pink in color. They can be flat or raised, and they vary in size. Early on, genital warts look like small, barely noticeable bumps. Untreated warts can grow together to form a cauliflower-like mass. In males, they appear on the penis and often involve the urethra, appearing first at the opening and then spreading inside. The growths may cause irritation and bleeding, leading to painful urination and a urethral discharge. Warts may also appear around the anus or within the rectum.

In women, warts may appear on the labia, vulva, and may spread to the perineum, the area between the vagina and the rectum. They may also appear on the cervix. If warts occur only on the cervix, the woman will generally have no symptoms or awareness that she has HPV.

The incubation period is about 4–6 weeks from the time of contact, but it can be 6 months or longer before any symptoms are identified. People can be infected with the virus and be capable of transmitting it to their sex partners without having any symptoms at all. In addition, newborns can be infected during delivery.

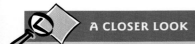

How many college students have STDs?

- By age 21, 25% of all people will have had an STD. More than half the people who contract STDs are under age 25.

- Among sexually active college students, 5–20% tests positive for chlamydia and nearly half are infected with HPV. Although incidence varies at different campuses, about 1 in 500 college students carries HIV.

Why do college students have high rates of STDs?

- Risky sexual behavior is common. One study of college students found that fewer than half used condoms consistently and one-third had had ten or more sex partners. Another study found that 19% of male students and 33% of female students had consented to sexual intercourse simply because they felt awkward refusing.

- College students underestimate their risk of STDs and HIV. Although students may have considerable knowledge about STDs, they often feel the risks do not apply to them—a dangerous assumption. One study of students with a history of STDs showed that more than half had unprotected sex while they were infected, and 25% of them continued to have sex without ever informing their partner(s).

What effect does alcohol or drug use have on my likelihood of getting an STD?

- Between one-third and one-half of college students report participating in sexual activity as a direct result of being intoxicated. All too often, sexual activity while intoxicated leads to unprotected intercourse.

- Students who binge drink are more likely to have multiple partners, use condoms inconsistently, and delay seeking treatment for STDs than students who drink little or no alcohol. Sexual assaults occur more frequently when either the perpetrator or the victim has been drinking.

What can students do to protect themselves against STDs?

- Limit the number of sex partners. Even people who are always in a monogamous relationship can end up with extensive potential exposure to STDs if, over the years, they have numerous relationships.

- Use condoms consistently, and don't assume it's safe to stop after you've been with a partner for several months. HIV infection, HPV infection, herpes, and chlamydia can be asymptomatic for months or years and can be transmitted at any time. If you haven't been using condoms with your current partner, start now.

- Think about how you use alcohol or other drugs. If alcohol or drug use is causing problems in your life, get help.

- Enjoy sexuality on your own terms. Don't let the expectations of friends and partners cause you to ignore your own feelings. Let your own wellness be your first priority. If you choose to be sexually active, learn about safer sex practices.

- Get to know your partner, and talk to him or her before becoming intimate. Be honest about yourself, and encourage your partner to do the same. Unfortunately, studies show that many people lie about their sexual past. So listen to your intuition, and practice safer sex no matter what.

Diagnosis   Genital warts are usually diagnosed based on the appearance of the lesions. Sometimes examination with a special magnifying instrument or biopsy is done to evaluate suspicious lesions. Frequently, HPV infection of the cervix is detected on routine Pap tests.

Treatment   Treatment focuses on individual lesions, but the currently available methods cannot ensure the eradication of HPV. Warts may be removed by cryosurgery (freezing), electrocautery (burning), or laser surgery. Direct applications of podophyllin or other cytotoxic acids may be used; newer treatments include injections of interferon or 5-FU (a chemotherapy agent). Two treatments may be applied by patients at home: imiquimod, an immune enhancer, and podofilox, a drug that destroys warts. The success rates of methods vary, and warts often recur despite initial improvement.

Recent research indicates that HPV infection often resolves on its own after a number of months, although this is unpredictable. Even after treatment and the disap-

pearance of visible warts, the individual may continue to carry HPV in healthy-looking tissue and can probably still infect others. Anyone who has ever had HPV should inform all partners. Condoms should be used, even though they do not provide total protection. Because of the relationship between HPV and cervical cancer, women who have had genital warts should have Pap tests at least every 12 months.

Genital Herpes

Genital herpes affects about 45 million people in the United States. Two types of herpes simplex viruses, HSV-1 and HSV-2, cause genital herpes and oral-labial herpes (cold sores). Genital herpes is usually caused by HSV-2, and oral-labial herpes is usually caused by HSV-1, although both virus types can cause either genital or oral-labial lesions. HSV can also cause rectal lesions, usually transmitted through anal sex. (Other types of herpesviruses cause different illnesses; see Chapter 17.)

people, especially women, have no symptoms.

- Pelvic inflammatory disease (PID), a complication of untreated gonorrhea or chlamydia, is an infection of the uterus and oviducts that may extend to the ovaries and pelvic cavity. It can lead to infertility, ectopic pregnancy, and chronic pelvic pain.
- Genital warts, caused by the human papillomavirus (HPV), are associated with cervical cancer. Treatment does not eradicate the virus, which can be passed on even by asymptomatic people.
- Genital herpes is a common incurable infection that can be fatal to newborns. After an initial infection, outbreaks may recur at any time. Most people acquire herpes from asymptomatic sex partners who are unaware that they are infected.
- Hepatitis B is a viral infection of the liver transmitted through sexual and nonsexual contact. Following an initial infection, most people recover; but some become chronic carriers of the virus who may develop serious, potentially fatal complications.
- Syphilis is a highly contagious bacterial infection that can be treated with antibiotics. If left untreated, it can lead to deterioration of the central nervous system and death.

Other STDs

- Less serious diseases that can be transmitted sexually or are linked to sexual activity include trichomoniasis, bacterial vaginosis, chancroid, pubic lice, and scabies. Any STD that causes sores or inflammation can increase risk for HIV transmission.

What You Can Do

- Education about STDs is critical to preventing their spread.
- Successful diagnosis and treatment of STDs involves being alert for symptoms, getting tested, informing partners, and following treatment instructions carefully.
- All STDs are preventable; the key is practicing responsible sexual behaviors. Those who are sexually active are safest with one mutually monogamous uninfected partner. Using a condom properly with every act of sexual intercourse helps protect against STDs.

TAKE ACTION

1. Go to a drugstore and examine the OTC contraceptives. Which ones provide protection against STDs? If you are sexually active, make sure you use the best protection available.

2. More and more communities have treatment and support programs for people with HIV infection. Look in the yellow pages or contact local health agencies to find out what services are available where you live. If any of

these agencies use volunteers, consider donating some of your time to help.

3. If you have ever engaged in unprotected sex or another behavior that puts you at risk for STDs, talk with your health care provider about being screened for common STDs. What tests are available and useful for your situation?

JOURNAL ENTRY

1. In your health journal, list the positive behaviors that help you avoid exposure to sexually transmitted diseases. Consider what additions you can make to this list or how you can strengthen your existing behaviors. Then list the behaviors that may block your positive behaviors or put you at risk of contracting an STD. Consider which ones you can change and how you can begin doing so.

2. In your health journal, write a brief script for four different ways you could bring up the subject of STDs and safer sex with a potential sex partner. Then write out a response you could use if a potential partner brought up the subject of safer sex.

3. *Critical Thinking* What responsibility do you think the federal government has for funding programs for the prevention and treatment of HIV infection? Do you think the government should pay for national prevention programs or increase financial aid to cities bearing the medical costs of caring for people with HIV? Or should these costs be borne by individuals, families, communities, or private insurance companies? Should the new, more effective (and expensive) drugs be available only to people who can afford them or who have private insurance? Write an essay describing what role, if any, you think the government should play; explain your reasoning.

Books

Bartlett, J. G., and A. K. Finkbeiner. 1998. *The Guide to Living with HIV Infection: Developed at the Johns Hopkins AIDS Clinic.* Baltimore, Md.: Johns Hopkins University Press. *Medical, scientific, social, and financial information about living with HIV/AIDS.*

Ebel, C. 1998. *Managing Herpes: How to Live and Love with a Chronic STD.* Durham, N.C.: American Social Health Association. *Helpful advice and support.*

Institute of Medicine. 1997. *The Hidden Epidemic: Confronting Sexually Transmitted Diseases.* Washington, D.C.: National Academy Press. *An examination of the scope of STDs in the United States and the nation's response to the epidemic.*

Marr, L. 1999. *Sexually Transmitted Disease: A Physician Tells You What You Need to Know.* Baltimore, Md.: Johns Hopkins University Press. *Provides practical information about protecting oneself against infection and obtaining appropriate medical care.*

Nevid, J. S. 1997. *Choices: Sex in the Age of STDs,* 2nd ed. New York: Allyn & Bacon. *Provides practical information about STDs and prevention.*

Schoub, B. D. 1999. *AIDS and HIV in Perspective: A Guide to Understanding the Virus and Its Consequences,* 2nd ed. New York: Cambridge University Press. *Provides information about the biology and treatment of HIV for the general reader.*

Organizations, Hotlines, and Web Sites

American College Health Association. Offers free brochures on STDs, alcohol use, acquaintance rape, and other college health issues.

> P.O. Box 28937
> Baltimore, MD 21240-8937
> 410-859-1500
> http://www.acha.org

American Social Health Association. Provides written information and referrals on STDs; sponsors support groups for people with herpes and HPV.

> P.O. Box 13827
> Research Triangle Park, NC 27709-3827
> 800-653-HEALTH; 800-230-6039
> http://www.ashastd.org

The Body/A Multimedia AIDS and HIV Information Resource. Provides basic information about HIV—prevention, testing, treatment—and links to related sites.

> http://www.thebody.com

CDC National HIV and AIDS Hotline. Provides confidential information and referrals for testing and treatment.

> 800-342-AIDS; 800-344-SIDA (Spanish);
> 800-243-7889 (TTY, deaf access)

CDC National Prevention Information Network. Provides extensive information and links on HIV/AIDS and other STDs.

> P.O. Box 6003
> Rockville, MD 20849
> 800-458-5231
> http://www.cdcnpin.org

CDC National STD Hotline. Provides confidential information and referrals.

> 800-227-8922

HIV InSite: Gateway to AIDS Knowledge. Provides information about prevention, education, treatment, statistics, clinical trials, and new developments.

> http://hivinsite.ucsf.edu

Joint United Nations Programme on HIV/AIDS (UNAIDS). Provides statistics and information on the international HIV/AIDS situation.

> http://www.unaids.org

Journal of the American Medical Association Information Centers. Provides daily news summaries, patient information, expert advice, and glossaries.

> http://www.ama-assn.org/special/hiv (HIV/AIDS Center)
> http://www.ama-assn.org/special/std (STDs Center)

Latex Love. Sponsored by the makers of Trojan condoms, this site includes directions for condom use and sample dialogues for overcoming excuses for not using condoms.

> http://www.loveandsex.com/sex/safer/latexlove

The NAMES Project Foundation AIDS Memorial Quilt. Includes the story behind the quilt, images of quilt panels, and information and links relating to HIV infection.

> http://www.aidsquilt.org

National Herpes Hotline. Provides counseling to people with herpes.

> 919-361-8488

National Institute of Allergies and Infectious Disease/STDs Information. Provides up-to-date fact sheets and brochures.

> http://www.niaid.nih.gov/publications/stds.htm

Safer Sex Page. Provides information on a variety of topics related to safer sex and STD prevention; includes audio of sample dialogues for talking about safer sex and condom use with partners. (Information is geared to people of all sexual orientations, and some is explicit.)

> http://www.safersex.org/safer.sex

See also the listings for Chapters 6 and 17.

SELECTED BIBLIOGRAPHY

Abdala, N., et al. 1999. Survival of HIV-1 in syringes. *Journal of Acquired Immune Deficiency Syndrome and Human Retrovirology* 20(1): 73–80.

Alexander, J. M., et al. 1999. Efficacy of treatment for syphilis in pregnancy. *Obstetrics and Gynecology* 93(1): 5–8.

Anderson, J. E., et al. 1999. Condom use and HIV risk behaviors among U.S. adults: Data from a national survey. *Family Planning Perspectives* 31(1): 24–28.

Borgatta, L., et al. 1998. A contemporary approach to curbing STDs. *Patient Care* 30(20): 30–42.

Bozzette, S. A., et al. 1998. The care of HIV-infected adults in the United States. *New England Journal of Medicine* 339(26): 1897–1904.

Branson, B. 1998. Home sample collection tests for HIV infection. *Journal of the American Medical Association* 280(19): 1699–1701.

Bucy, R. P., et al. 1999. *A New Steady State of HIV Infection After HAART. Abstract 157: Sixth Conference on Retroviruses and Opportunistic Infections* (retrieved February 10, 1999; http://www.retroconference.org/99/abstracts/157.htm).

Centers for Disease Control and Prevention. 1999. HIV testing—United States. *Morbidity and Mortality Weekly Report* 48(3): 52–55.

Centers for Disease Control and Prevention. 1999. Increases in unsafe sex and rectal gonorrhea among men who have sex with men. *Morbidity and Mortality Weekly Report* 48(3): 45–48.

Centers for Disease Control and Prevention. 1998. 1998 guidelines for treatment of sexually transmitted diseases. *MMWR Recommendations and Reports* 47(RR-1).

Centers for Disease Control and Prevention. 1998. *Draft Guidelines for National HIV Case Surveillance, Including Monitoring for HIV Infection and AIDS.* Atlanta, Ga.: Centers for Disease Control and Prevention.

Centers for Disease Control and Prevention. 1998. Management of possible sexual, injecting-drug-use, or other nonoccupational exposure to HIV, including considerations related to antiretroviral therapy. *MMWR Recommendations and Reports* 47(RR-17).

Centers for Disease Control and Prevention. 1998. *Rapid HIV Tests: Questions and Answers* (retrieved February 8, 1999; http://www.cdc.gov/nchstp/hiv_aids/pubs/rt/rapidqas.htm).

Cohen, O., and A. Fauci. 1998. The latest recommendations for antiretroviral therapy. *Patient Care* 32(130): 154–171.

Engel, J. P. 1998. Long-term suppression of genital herpes. *Journal of the American Medical Association* 280(10): 928–929.

Gao, F., et al. 1999. Origin of HIV-1 in the chimpanzee *Pan troglodytes troglodytes. Nature* 397: 436–441.

Gaydos, C. A., et al. 1998. *Chlamydia trachomatis* infections in female military recruits. *New England Journal of Medicine* 339(11): 739–744.

Goodnough, L. T., et al. 1999. Transfusion medicine: First of two parts—blood transfusion. *New England Journal of Medicine* 340(6): 438–447.

Haase, A., and T. Schacker. 1998. Potential for the transmission of HIV-1 despite highly active antiretroviral therapy. *New England Journal of Medicine* 339(25): 1846–1848.

Ho, G., et al. 1998. Natural history of cervicovaginal papillomavirus infection in young women. *New England Journal of Medicine* 338(7): 423–428.

International Perinatal HIV Group. 1999. The mode of delivery and the risk of vertical transmission of HIV-1: A meta-analysis of 15 prospective cohort studies. *New England Journal of Medicine—Early Release* (retrieved February 2, 1999; http://www.nejm.org/content/embargo/HIV.asp).

Joint United Nations Programme on HIV/AIDS (UNAIDS). 1999. *Early Data from Mother-to-Child HIV Transmission Study in Africa Finds Shortest Effective Regimen Ever* (retrieved February 6, 1999; http://www.unaids.org/highband/press/mtct99e.html).

Joint United Nations Programme on HIV/AIDS (UNAIDS). 1999. *Young People and HIV/AIDS: UNAIDS Briefing Paper.* Geneva: UNAIDS.

Kahn, O., and B. D. Walker. 1998. Acute HIV-1 infection. *New England Journal of Medicine* 339(1): 33–39.

Kaiser Family Foundation. 1998. *Sexually Transmitted Diseases in America: How Many Cases and at What Cost?* (retrieved December 16, 1998; http://www.kff.org/archive/repro/policy/std/std_rep.html).

Lot, F., et al. 1999. Probable transmission of HIV from an orthopedic surgeon to a patient in France. *Annals of Internal Medicine* 130: 1–6.

Martin, M. P., et al. 1998. Genetic acceleration of AIDS progression by a promoter variant of CCR5. *Science* 282(5395): 1907–1911.

Monk, B., et al. 1998. Advances in therapy for genital condyloma in women. *Patient Care* 32(17): 53–61.

Nakashima, A., et al. 1998. Effect of HIV reporting by name on use of HIV testing in publicly funded counseling and testing programs. *Journal of the American Medical Association* 280(16): 1421–1426.

National Institute of Allergy and Infectious Diseases. 1998. *Fact Sheet: Vaginitis Due to Vaginal Infections* (retrieved February 6, 1999; http://www.niaid.nih.gov/factsheets/stdvag.htm).

Paterson, D., et al. 1999. *How Much Adherence Is Enough? Abstract 92: Sixth Conference on Retroviruses and Opportunistic Infections* (retrieved February 10, 1999; http://www.retroconference.org/99/abstracts/92.htm).

Pomerantz, R. J., et al. 1999. *HIV-1 Reservoirs Exist in the Semen of Men Receiving HAART. Abstract 7: Sixth Conference on Retroviruses and Opportunistic Infections* (retrieved February 10, 1999; http://www.retroconference.org/99/abstracts/7.htm).

Rome, E. 1998. Pelvic inflammatory disease: The importance of aggressive treatment in adolescents. *Cleveland Clinic Journal of Medicine* 65(7): 369–376.

Rosen, A. D., and T. Rosen. 1999. Study of condom integrity after brief exposure to over-the-counter vaginal preparation. *Southern Medical Journal* 92: 305–307.

Rosenberg, P., et al. 1998. Trends in HIV incidence among young adults in the United States. *Journal of the American Medical Association* 279(23): 1894–1899.

Royce, R. A., et al. 1999. Bacterial vaginosis associated with HIV infection in pregnant women from North Carolina. *Journal of Acquired Immune Deficiency Syndrome and Human Retrovirology* 20(4): 382–386.

Sande, M. 1998. HIV and AIDS: 20 key questions for 1999. *Consultant* 38(11): 2599–2617.

Shain, R. N., et al. 1999. A randomized, controlled trial of a behavioral intervention to prevent sexually transmitted disease among minority women. *New England Journal of Medicine* 340(2): 93–100.

Siegal, H. A., et al. 1999. Under the influence: Risky sexual behavior and substance abuse among DUI offenders. *Sexually Transmitted Diseases* 26(2): 87–92.

Stein, M. D., et al. 1998. Sexual ethics: Disclosure of HIV-positive status to partners. *Archives of Internal Medicine* 158: 253–257.

U.S. Food and Drug Administration. 1999. *Approved Drugs for HIV/AIDS or AIDS-Related Conditions* (retrieved February 8, 1999; http://www.fda.gov/oashi/aids/stat_app.html).

Wegner, S., et al. 1999. *High Frequency of Antiretroviral Drug Resistance in HIV-1 from Recently Infected Therapy Naive Individuals. Abstract 9: Sixth Conference on Retroviruses and Opportunistic Infections* (retrieved February 10, 1999; http://www.retroconference.org/99/abstracts/lb9.htm).

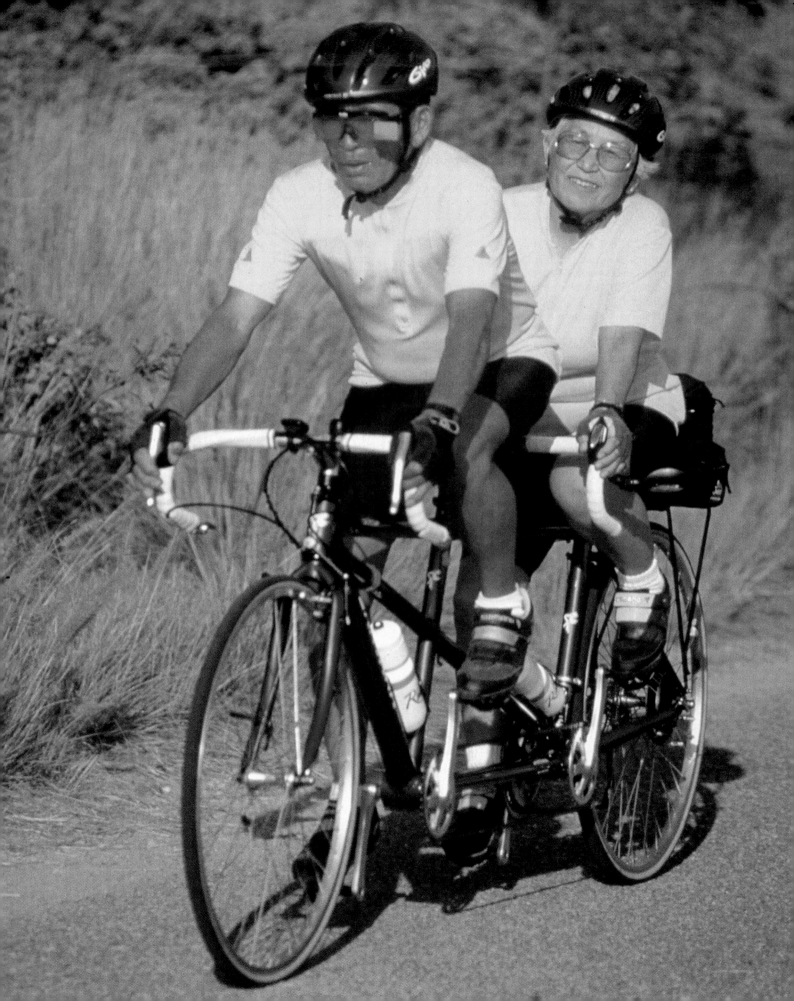

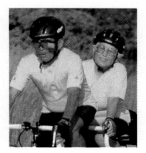

LEARNING OBJECTIVES

After reading this chapter, you should be able to:

- List strategies for healthful aging.

- Explain the physical, social, and mental changes that may accompany aging, and discuss how people can best confront these changes.

- Compare different theories on the causes of aging.

- Describe practical considerations of older adults, including housing, finances, health care, and transportation.

Aging: A Vital Process

19

TEST YOUR KNOWLEDGE

1. At any given time, about what percentage of older Americans live in nursing homes or other institutional settings?
    a. 5%
    b. 15%
    c. 30%

2. People over age 65 have the highest motor-vehicle-related death rate of any age group.
    True or false?

3. On average, a woman will spend more time caring for an aging relative than raising children.
    True or false?

4. Exercise is beneficial for older people because it
    a. protects against osteoporosis.
    b. maintains alertness and intelligence.
    c. prevents falls.

5. Alcohol abuse is rare among older adults.
    True or false?

Answers

1. a. Most older adults live in their own homes or with a family member.

2. False. Although the motor-vehicle-related death rate is high for older Americans, young adults age 16–24 have the highest rate. Older drivers are more likely to wear safety belts and less likely to drive while intoxicated than young drivers.

3. True. The average woman will spend 17 years raising kids and 18 years caring for an aging relative.

4. All three. Even for people over 80, exercise can improve physical functioning and balance and reduce falls and injuries.

5. False. Alcohol abuse affects about 10% of elderly people. It often goes undetected because its symptoms may mimic those of other conditions, such as Alzheimer's disease.

Many people would like to live for a long time and never grow old. When we see that old age has taken us in its grip, we're stunned. We regard old age as something foreign: Can I become a different person while I still remain myself? Yes. And no. Life is like a river. The flow is continuous, and you can never step in the same place twice.

Aging does not begin on the sixty-fifth birthday, and there is no precise age at which a person becomes "old." Rather, aging is a normal process of development that occurs over the entire lifetime. It happens to everyone, but at different rates for different people. Some people are "old" at 25, and others are still "young" at 75.

Although youth is not entirely a state of mind, your attitude toward life and your attention to your health significantly influence the satisfaction you will derive from life, especially when new physical, mental, and social challenges occur in later years. If you optimize wellness during young adulthood, you can exert great control over the physical and mental aspects of aging, and you can better handle your response to events that might be out of your control. With foresight and energy you can shape a creative, graceful, and even triumphant old age.

GENERATING VITALITY AS YOU AGE

As we age, we experience both gains and losses. Physical and mental changes occur gradually, over a lifetime. Biological aging includes all the normal, progressive, irreversible changes to one's body that begin at birth and continue until death. Psychological and social aging usually involve more abrupt changes in circumstance and emotion: relocating, changing homes, losing a spouse and friends, retiring, having a lower income, and changing roles and social status. These changes represent opportunities for growth throughout life.

Not all of them happen to everybody, and their timing varies, partly depending on how we have prepared for our later days. Some people never have to leave their homes and appear to be in good health until the day they die. Others have tremendous adjustments to make—to entirely new surroundings with fewer financial resources, to new acquaintances, to decreasing mobility, to the changing physical condition of their bodies and new health problems, and possibly to loneliness and loss of self-esteem.

Successful aging requires preparation. People need to establish good health habits in their teens and twenties. During their twenties and thirties, they usually develop important relationships and settle into a particular lifestyle. By their mid-forties, they generally know how much money they need to support the lifestyle they've chosen. At this point, they must assess their financial status and perhaps adjust their savings in order to continue enjoying that lifestyle after retirement. In their mid-fifties, they need to reevaluate their health insurance plans and

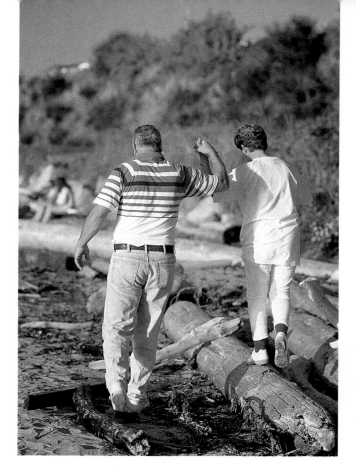

Middle age is a time of reassessment and readjustment in preparation for the second half of life. Many people in their forties and fifties who have cultivated healthy lifestyles will continue to lead vigorous lives well into old age.

may want to think about retirement housing. Throughout life, people should cultivate interests and hobbies they enjoy, both alone and with others, so they can continue to live an active and rewarding life in their later years.

PERSONAL INSIGHT   How do you envision your old age? How will it resemble the old age of older adults you know now, and how will it differ? What external events could affect your control of your lifestyle when you're older?

What Happens as You Age?

Many of the characteristics associated with aging are not due to aging at all. Rather, they are the result of neglect and abuse of our bodies and minds. These assaults lay the foundation for later psychological problems and chronic conditions like arthritis, heart disease, diabetes, hearing loss, and hypertension. We sacrifice our optimal health by smoking, having poor nutrition, overeating, abusing alcohol and drugs, bombarding our ears with excessive noise, and exposing our bodies to too much ultraviolet radiation

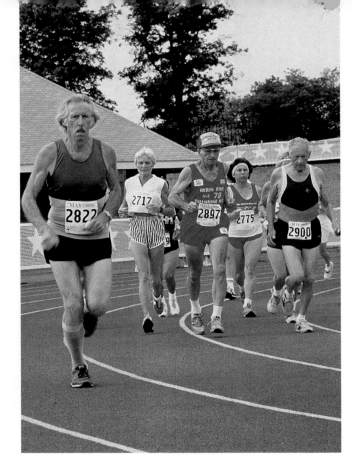

Regular exercise throughout life is an important key to successful aging. By keeping fit, these people have maintained a high level of physical functioning. Regular exercise also helps prevent depression, boredom, and losses in fluid intelligence typically associated with aging.

from the sun. We also jeopardize our bodies through inactivity, encouraging our muscles and even our bones to wither and deteriorate. And we endure abuse from the toxic chemicals in our environment.

But even with the healthiest behavior and environment, aging inevitably occurs. It results from biochemical processes we don't yet fully understand. The physiological changes in organ systems are caused by a combination of gradual aging and impairment from disease. Because of redundancy in most organ systems, the body's ability to function is not affected until damage is fairly extensive. Studies of healthy people indicate that functioning remains essentially constant until after age 70. See the box "Aging and Changing: Your Body Through Time" on pages 524 and 525 for a summary of the physical changes that accompany aging.

Life-Enhancing Measures: Age-Proofing

You can prevent, delay, lessen, or even reverse some of the changes associated with aging through good health habits. A few simple things you can do every day will make a vast difference to your appearance, level of energy,

and vitality—your overall wellness. The following suggestions have been mentioned throughout this text. But because they are profoundly related to health in later life, we highlight them here.

Challenge Your Mind   Creativity and intelligence remain stable in healthy individuals. Develop interests and hobbies you can enjoy throughout your life. Staying involved in learning as a lifelong process can help you remain alert and keep your mental abilities. Pablo Picasso, Margaret Mead, and Duke Ellington were productive well past their seventy-fifth birthdays.

Develop Physical Fitness   Exercise enhances both psychological and physical health. We cannot say enough about the positive effects of appropriate exercise throughout your life, particularly when weighed against the physical and mental deterioration of older people who have not kept their minds and bodies fit. The benefits of an active lifestyle include the following:

- Increased resiliency and suppleness of arteries.
- Lower blood pressure and healthier cholesterol levels.
- Better protection against heart attacks, and an increased chance of survival should one occur.
- Sustained capacity of the lungs and respiratory reserves.
- Weight control through less accumulation of fat.
- Maintenance of physical flexibility, balance, agility, and reaction time.
- Greatly preserved muscle strength.
- Protection against ligament injuries; dislocation strains in the knees, spine, and shoulders.
- Protection against osteoporosis and Type 2 diabetes.
- Increased effectiveness of the immune system.
- Maintenance of mental agility and flexibility, response time, memory, and hand-eye coordination.

The stimulus that exercise provides also seems to protect against the loss of **fluid intelligence,** the ability to find solutions when confronted with a new problem. Fluid intelligence depends on rapidity of responsiveness, memory, and alertness. Contrary to former notions that this capability necessarily declines with age, studies reveal that older people who are highly fit score better on tests of intelligence than their less fit counterparts. Many of the other functional losses associated with aging are also due to a lack of exercise.

Find a variety of activities that you enjoy and can do regularly. Accumulate at least 30 minutes of moderate-

fluid intelligence The ability to develop a solution when confronted with a new problem.	**TERMS**

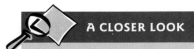

Skin

Skin becomes looser as you get older; it stretches more easily and is less resilient. Long-term exposure to UV radiation from the sun produces wrinkles and areas of spotty pigmentation ("age spots"). Hats, gloves, sunglasses, and sunscreen provide protection from the sun. Skin also becomes drier as you age, as sweat and oil glands gradually cease functioning. The overuse of soaps and antiperspirants can worsen dry skin.

Body Fat

You can expect an increase in body fat and reduction in body size from a decrease in muscle mass and body water content. However, changes in muscle tone and body composition (the ratio of fat to muscle) can be kept to a minimum through regular exercise. Deposits of fat in the waist are associated with a higher incidence of disease. Weight management is important throughout life.

Hearing

The ability to hear high-pitched and sibilant (hissing) consonant sounds such as *s, z, sh,* and *ch* declines for most people as they age, enough so that hearing loss is now the fourth most common chronic physical disability in the United States. Even by age 35, you may not hear as well as you did at 25. Most people don't notice the progressive muffling until their sixties, when they may begin to have difficulty comprehending speech. These losses may be due to abuse rather than to aging, however. Extremely loud noise, such as from stereo earphones or loud machines, may contribute to hearing loss. In certain developing societies, hearing is almost as keen in old age as it is in youth. A high-fat diet has been linked to clogging of the blood vessels that nourish the hearing organs.

Eyesight

Beginning in your forties, you will probably develop **presbyopia,** a gradual decline in the ability to focus on objects close to you. This occurs because the lens of the eye no longer expands and contracts as readily. You will need brighter lights for reading and close work. Slowed light-to-dark adaptation and distorted depth perception make night driving more difficult and require compensating driving techniques. **Cataracts,** a clouding of the lens caused by lifelong oxidation damage (a by-product of normal body chemistry), may dim vision by the sixties. Visual defects in older adults often go undetected. Annual eye exams can help prevent injury from falls and automobile crashes.

Taste and Smell

The senses of taste and smell diminish with age. About two-thirds of the taste buds in the mouth die by age 70, as do many of the sensory receptors in the nose. Some medications can further interfere with taste, and long-term exposure to smoke lessens the ability to smell.

Hair

As you age, cells at the base of hair follicles produce progressively less pigment and eventually die. By age 50, some 50% of Americans are partially gray, and hair loss in men becomes apparent. About 12% of men are balding by age 25; 65% by age 65. Thickest at age 20, individual hair shafts shrink after that; by age 70, your hair will probably be as fine as when you were a baby.

Bones, Muscles, and Teeth

Bones maintain themselves through a cyclic process called remodeling, in which old bone is absorbed and new bone develops. By the mid-thirties, more bone is being absorbed than developed. Loss of bone mass is generally not a problem for men because they have denser bones than women to begin with. For women, bone loss accelerates after menopause. One out of every four women over age 60 develops **osteoporosis,** a condition in which bones become weaker, more porous, and more prone to fractures. Adequate calcium in your diet and regular weight-bearing exercise will help build strong bones while you're young and slow the loss of bone as you age (see Chapter 12).

Muscles become weaker, too, although you can retard your loss of muscle strength and mass through regular physical work and play. As you age, more protein is being broken down and less is being synthesized, so muscle fibers atrophy and lose their ability to contract; some are lost; fat and collagen accumulate. Aging muscles are less flexible and more susceptible to strains, pulls, and cramps. After the mid-forties, strength usually declines: A man may lose 10–20% of his maximum strength by age 60, and a woman even more.

Height also decreases with age; about 1–4 inches are lost after young adulthood. Factors contributing to this decrease in height are a loss of bone mass, weakening back muscles, and deterioration of the discs between the bones in the spine (vertebrae).

Your teeth, with proper care, can last a lifetime. Not aging, but disuse, abuse, and chronic degenerative disease cause dental problems. Teeth and their support structures respond well to the stress and stimulation of chewing crunchy foods. **Periodontitis** is a common cause of tooth loss after age 35; it is caused by the buildup of plaque. You can prevent it with proper dental care, including brushing and flossing each day, as described in Chapter 21.

intensity physical activity every day, and begin a formal exercise program to develop cardiorespiratory endurance, muscular strength and endurance, and flexibility (see Chapter 13). Older individuals who have been sedentary should be encouraged to become more active. Studies have shown that it's never too late to start exercising. Even in people over 80, endurance and strength training can improve balance, flexibility, and physical functioning and reduce the potential for dangerous falls.

Eat Wisely   Good health at any age is enhanced by eating a varied diet, paying special attention to lower fat and calorie intake. A periodic dietary evaluation will keep your diet in line with your changing needs (see Chapter 12):

Heart

Your resting heart rate stays about the same throughout your life, but the heart pumps less blood with each beat as you get older. This effect is most pronounced during exercise because your pulse can no longer rise as high, nor return as rapidly to its resting rate, as it once did. The dramatic problems of the cardiovascular system associated with aging—heart attack and stroke—are usually caused by atherosclerosis and high blood pressure, which sometimes can be controlled with diet and exercise. People who have high blood cholesterol levels, who smoke, or who have diabetes or a family history of coronary heart disease may wish to discuss aspirin therapy with their physician.

Lungs

Your respiratory system resists change, and your respiratory tract actually grows stronger with age. After a lifetime of exposure to viruses, people build up immunity and catch fewer and less severe colds by middle age. Your vital capacity—the amount of air you can expel from your lungs—should not decline if you keep fit and don't smoke. Regular, vigorous exercise can increase vital capacity.

Digestive System and Kidneys

With age, your stomach will secrete less acid and smaller amounts of the enzymes that aid digestion. Digesting a meal takes longer and may be more difficult. The kidneys filter wastes more slowly, causing decreased drug clearance. Fewer calories are required to maintain body weight.

Immune System

With age, your immune system may become less efficient, but the decline varies greatly among people. Only the progressive atrophy of the thymus gland seems invariably linked to advancing age. The consequences of immune system decline are increased rates of cancer and autoimmune and infectious diseases but better tolerance of tissue and organ transplants. Good nutrition and exercise both benefit the immune system. People who are physically healthy recover from respiratory infections much faster than those who are not.

Brain and Nervous System

Only half as much blood travels to the brain of a 50-year-old as to that of a 10-year-old, with most of the reduction occurring before age 30. By age 85, the brain has lost 10–20% of its weight, mainly through nerve cell atrophy. These **neuron** losses are selective: Some sites show no loss, while in the **cerebral cortex**, the site of higher mental activities, loss is significant. Your mental ability will not necessarily decline with the loss of neurons, partly because the brain continues to extend new **dendrites**, communication lines to other neurons. They may be one way the brain compensates for neuron loss.

Sleep patterns change with age, although troubled sleep (insomnia or daytime drowsiness) may be a sign of an emotional or physical disorder rather than part of the aging process. The deepest stage of sleep decreases as you age, which may explain why older people are considered light sleepers. Reliance on sleeping medications should be avoided because they interfere with sleep patterns (see Chapter 2).

Sex Organs and Sexual Response

An active and satisfying sex life can continue as you age. Women do not ordinarily lose their capacity for orgasm nor men their capacity for erection and ejaculation. A slowing of response, especially in men, is considered a part of the normal aging process.

For women, menopause (cessation of menstruation) usually occurs around age 50. The common symptoms of menopause can be treated with hormone replacement therapy. Women may experience a drying and thinning of the vaginal walls due to lower levels of estrogen after menopause; the use of an estrogen cream and/or a water-soluble lubricant can usually solve the problem. A hysterectomy or mastectomy does not have to affect sexual activity. Monthly breast self-exams and mammograms are important.

As they age, men may take longer to attain an erection, and the erection may not be as firm or as large as when they were younger. The prostate gland may become enlarged after middle age, causing problems with urination. This condition can now usually be treated without affecting sexual response.

- Eat meals low in fat and high in complex carbohydrates. Concentrate on fresh fruits and vegetables, whole grains, and pasta.
- Eat fish and poultry (no skin) instead of eggs and fatty meats. Use nonfat or lowfat dairy products. Substitute olive oil for other oils and fats.
- If you frequently salt your food, reduce your intake.
- Maintain calcium and vitamin B-12 intake, with supplements if necessary (see Chapter 12).

Maintain a Healthy Weight   Weight management is especially difficult if you have been overweight most of your life. A sensible program of expending more calories through exercise, cutting calorie intake, or a combination of both will work for most people who want to lose weight, but

TERMS

presbyopia   The inability of the eyes to focus sharply on nearby objects, caused by a loss of elasticity of the lens that occurs with advancing age.

cataracts   Opacity of the lens of the eye that impairs vision and can cause blindness.

osteoporosis   The loss of bone density, causing bones to become weak, porous, and more prone to fractures.

periodontitis   A disease of the bone, tissue, and gum that support the teeth, caused by the accumulation of plaque.

neuron   A nerve cell.

cerebral cortex   The outer layer of the brain, which controls behavior and mental activity.

dendrite   An extension of a neuron that transmits nerve impulses toward the cell body.

there is no magic formula. Obesity is not physically healthy, and it leads to premature aging (see Chapter 14). Recommended calorie intake declines with age, to 1600 per day for women and 2050 for men over age 75. Protein, vitamin, and mineral requirements remain the same.

Control Drinking and Overdependence on Medications

Alcohol abuse ranks with depression as a common hidden mental health problem, affecting about 10% of older adults. (The ability to metabolize alcohol decreases with age.) The problem is often not identified because the effects of alcohol or drug dependence can mimic disease, such as Alzheimer's disease. Signs of potential alcohol or drug dependence include unexplained falls or frequent injuries, forgetfulness, depression, and malnutrition. Older people who retire or lose a spouse are especially at risk. Problems can be avoided by not using alcohol to relieve anxiety or emotional pain, and not taking medication when safer forms of treatment are available. Women taking hormone replacements should use alcohol cautiously because it appears to raise blood levels of estrogen to more than three times the intended dose.

Don't Smoke

The average pack-a-day smoker can expect to live about 12 years less than a nonsmoker. Furthermore, smokers suffer more illnesses that last longer, and they are subject to respiratory disabilities that limit their total vigor for many years before their death. Most older tobacco users started smoking between the ages of 15 and 25. Even young cigarette smokers suffer respiratory impairment, some within a year of starting to smoke. Premature balding, skin wrinkling, and osteoporosis have been linked to cigarette smoking. Smokers at age 50 often have wrinkles resembling those of a person of 60.

Schedule Physical Examinations to Detect Treatable Diseases

When detected early, many diseases, including hypertension, diabetes, and many types of cancer, can be successfully controlled by medication and lifestyle changes (see Chapter 21 for medical testing guidelines). Regular testing for **glaucoma** after age 40 can prevent blindness from this eye disease. Recommended immunizations including those for influenza and pneumococcus, can protect you from preventable infectious diseases (see Chapter 17).

Recognize and Reduce Stress

Stress-induced physiological changes increase wear and tear on your body. Cut down on the stresses in your life. Don't wear yourself out through lack of sleep, substance abuse or misuse, or over-work. Practice relaxation, using the techniques described in Chapter 2. If you contract a disease, consider it your body's attempt to interrupt your life pattern; reevaluate your lifestyle, and perhaps slow down.

The health behaviors you practice *now* are more influential in determining how long and how well you will live than your behaviors at a later age. Retiring from your life's occupation with a physically healthy body will allow far more options for enjoying yourself than will retiring with frail health or disabilities. Poor health that could have been prevented drains finances, emotions, and energy and contributes to poor psychological health. By enhancing your wellness today, you're buying some insurance for the future.

CONFRONTING THE CHANGES OF AGING

The changes that occur with aging have repercussions that must be grappled with and resolved. Just as you can act now to prevent or limit the physical changes of aging, you can also begin preparing yourself psychologically, socially, and financially for changes that may occur later in life. If you have aging parents, grandparents, and friends, the following information may give you insight into their lives and encourage you to begin cultivating appropriate and useful behaviors now.

Planning for Social Changes

Retirement marks a major change in the second half of life. As the longevity of Americans has increased, people spend a larger proportion of their lives in retirement: 17 years or more. This has implications for reestablishing important relationships, developing satisfying interests outside work, and saving for an adequate retirement income. People who have well-developed leisure pursuits adjust better to retirement than those with few interests outside of work.

Changing Roles and Relationships

Changes in social roles are a major feature of middle age. Children become young adults and leave home, putting an end to daily parenting. Parents experiencing this "empty nest syndrome" must adapt to changes in their customary responsibilities and personal identities. And while retirement may be a desirable milestone for most people, it may also be viewed as a threat to prestige, purpose, and self-respect—the loss of a valued or customary role—and will probably require a period of adjustment.

Retirement and the end of child rearing also bring about changes in the relationship between marriage partners. The amount of time a couple spend together will increase and activities will change. Couples may need a period of adjustment, in which they get to know each other as individuals again. Discussing what types of activ-

---

TERMS   **glaucoma**   A disease in which fluid inside the eye is under abnormally high pressure; can lead to blindness.

arthritis   Inflammation of a joint or joints, causing pain and swelling.

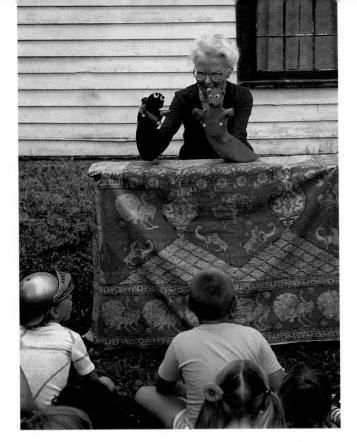

One of the challenges of aging is finding satisfying activities that provide meaningful connections with others. This retired woman helps out at an after school activity program by entertaining children.

ities each partner enjoys can help couples set up a mutually satisfying routine of shared and independent activities.

Increased Leisure Time Planning ahead for retirement is crucial. What kinds of things do you enjoy doing? How will you spend your days? Although retirement confers the advantages of leisure time and freedom from deadlines, competition, and stress, many people do not know how to enjoy their free time. If you have developed diverse interests, retirement can be a joyful and fulfilling period of your life. It can provide opportunities for expanding your horizons by giving you the chance to try new activities, take classes, and meet new people. Volunteering in your community can enhance self-esteem and allow you to be a contributing member of society (see the box "Help Yourself by Helping Others").

The Economics of Retirement Retirement is usually accompanied by a new economic situation. It may mean a severely restricted budget, or possibly even financial disaster if you don't take stock of your finances and plan ahead. Financial planning for retirement should begin early in life. People in their twenties and thirties should estimate how much money they need to support their standard of living, calculate their projected income, and

begin a savings program. The earlier such a program is begun, the more money they will have at retirement.

Financial planning for retirement is especially critical for women. American women are much less likely than men to be covered by pension plans, reflecting the fact that many women have lower-paying jobs or work part-time during their childbearing years. They tend to have less money vested in other types of retirement plans as well. Although the gap is narrowing, women currently outlive men by about 7 years, and they are more likely to develop chronic conditions that impair their daily activities later in life. The net result of these factors is that older women are almost twice as likely as older men to live in poverty. Women should investigate their retirement plans and take charge of their finances to be sure they will be provided for as they get older.

Adapting to Physical Changes

As described earlier in the chapter, there are many things a person can do to avoid or minimize the impact of the physical changes associated with aging. However, some changes in physical functioning are inevitable, and successful aging involves anticipating and accommodating these changes.

Decreased energy and changes in health mean that older people have to develop priorities for how to use their energy. Rather than curtailing activities to conserve energy, they need to learn how to generate energy. This usually involves saying "yes" to enjoyable activities and paying close attention to need for rest and sleep.

Adapting, rather than giving up, favorite activities may be the best strategy for dealing with physical limitations. For example, if **arthritis** interferes with piano playing, a person can continue to enjoy music by attending concerts or checking out music from the local library. Obtaining treatment for medical problems such as arthritis and glaucoma can also help limit the effects of aging on daily activities (see the box "Arthritis" for more information).

Hearing Loss The loss of hearing is a common physical disability that can have a particularly strong effect on the lives of older adults. Hearing loss affects a person's ability to interact with others and can lead to a sense of isolation and depression. If someone you know complains that words are difficult to understand, that another person's speech sounds slurred or mumbled, or that people are not speaking loudly enough, that person may have suffered some hearing loss. You may also notice that the person sets the volume of a radio or TV very high.

Hearing loss should be assessed and treated by a health care professional; in some cases, hearing can be completely restored by dealing with the underlying cause of hearing loss. In other cases, hearing aids may be prescribed. The following strategies can help improve communication with a hearing-impaired person:

Choosing to help others—whether as a volunteer for a community organization or through spontaneous acts of kindness—can enhance emotional, social, spiritual, and physical wellness. Surveys and studies indicate that the sense of purpose and service, and the feelings of generosity and kindness, that go with helping others may be as important a consideration for wellness as good nutrition and regular exercise. For example, in a study of nearly 3000 male residents of Michigan, those who volunteered for community organizations were two-and-a-half times less likely to die during the study than their nonhelping peers.

In a national survey of volunteers from all fields, helpers reported the following benefits:

- "Helper's high"—physical and emotional sensations such as sudden warmth, a surge of energy, and a feeling of euphoria that occur immediately after helping.

- Feelings of increased self-worth, calm, and relaxation.

- A perception of greater physical health.

- Fewer colds and headaches, improved eating and sleeping habits, and some relief from the pain of chronic diseases such as asthma and arthritis.

Just how might helping benefit the health of the helper? By helping others, we may relieve our own distress and guilt over their problems. We focus on things other than our own problems, and we get a special kind of attention from the people we help. Helping others can be effective at banishing a bad mood or a case of the blues. Helping may block physical pain because we can only pay attention to a limited number of things at a given time. Helping others can also expand our perspective and enhance our appreciation for our own lives. Helping may benefit physical health by providing a temporary boost to the immune system and by combating stress and hostile feelings linked to the development of chronic diseases.

Helping others doesn't require a huge time commitment or a change of career. To get the most out of helping, keep the following guidelines in mind:

- *Make contact.* Choose an activity that involves personal contact.

- *Help as often as possible.* If your schedule allows, volunteer at least once a week. However, as with many parts of a wellness lifestyle, any amount of time spent helping is better than none.

- *Make helping voluntary.* Voluntary helping has positive results, whereas obligatory helping situations can actually increase stress.

- *Volunteer with others.* Working with a group enables you to form bonds with other helpers who can support your interests and efforts. Studies have found that the health benefits of volunteering are strongest for people who otherwise have low levels of social interaction.

- *Focus on the process, not the outcome.* We can't always measure or know the results of our actions.

- *Practice random acts of kindness.* Smile, let people go ahead of you in line, pick up litter, and so on.

- *Adopt a pet.* Several studies suggest that pet owners enjoy better health, perhaps by feeling needed or by having a source of unconditional love and affection.

- *Avoid burnout.* Recognize your own limits, pace yourself, and try not to feel guilty or discouraged. Take pride in being a volunteer or caregiver, and give yourself frequent pats on the back.

You can experience the "helper's high" and the other personal rewards of volunteering as soon as you begin helping others. In addition to the benefits for you, volunteering has the added bonus of having a positive impact on the wellness of others. It fosters a sense of community and can provide some practical help for many of the problems facing our society today.

SOURCE: Adapted from Sobel, D. S., M.D., and R. Ornstein, Ph.D. 1996. *The Healthy Mind, Healthy Body Handbook* (Los Altos, Calif.: DRx) and *The Mind/Body Health Newsletter.* For further information about the book or newsletter subscriptions contact: Center for Health Sciences, P.O. Box 381069, Cambridge, MA 02238-1069 or call 1-800-222-4745.

- Speak at your normal rate; do not shout or over-articulate. This distorts speech sounds and makes visual cues more difficult to follow.

- Speak to the person at a distance of 3–6 feet. Stand near a good light so that your lip movements, facial expressions, and gestures may be seen more clearly.

- If the person does not understand you, rephrase your ideas. Use short, simple sentences.

- Don't leave hearing-impaired people out of conversations. Practice can improve their ability to communicate.

- Decrease the amount of extraneous noise in the environment.

Vision Changes   There are many strategies for dealing with the gradual decline in vision that occurs with aging. The first is to treat any underlying medical problems, such as cataracts or glaucoma. Older people may need about a 30% increase in light in order to work more effectively; increasing light sources and painting rooms in a lighter color can help. Improving the light in dark areas such as stairwells can reduce falls from the slower light-to-dark accommodation that occurs with age. Wearing a

Over half of all people age 65 and over have some form of arthritis. A chronic disease causing pain and the loss of movement in joints, its warning signs include the following:

- Swelling, pain, redness, warmth, or tenderness in one or more joints.

- Changes in joint mobility and early morning stiffness.

- Unexplained weight loss, fever, or weakness in combination with joint pain.

There are over 100 different types of arthritis; osteoarthritis (OA) is by far the most common. (Rheumatoid arthritis and lupus, both autoimmune disorders that affect joints, are described in Chapter 17.) OA is a degenerative joint disease most often affecting the hands and weight-bearing joints of the body—knees, ankles, and hips. OA affects an estimated 21 million Americans, 74% of whom are women. OA is second only to heart disease in disabling people so that they cannot work.

Strategies for reducing the risk of arthritis and, for those who already have OA, for managing it include the following:

- *Exercise* to lubricate joints and strengthen the muscles around them, protecting them from further damage.

- *Maintain an appropriate weight* to avoid placing excess stress on the hips, knees, and ankles.

- *Avoid joint injuries* from recreational or occupational activities that involve heavy or repetitive use of particular mus-

cles. "Tennis elbow" and "bus driver's shoulder" are examples of these types of injuries. Women are advised to wear comfortable, low-heeled shoes to avoid possible damage to knee joints from wearing high heels.

It's also important to visit a physician as soon as arthritis symptoms occur so appropriate treatment can begin—to reduce pain and swelling, keep joints moving safely, and prevent further joint damage. Many people with OA take nonsteroidal anti-inflammatory drugs (NSAIDs). NSAIDs block the action of the enzyme cyclooxygenase (COX), which is involved in the production of a family of hormones called prostaglandins. Traditional NSAIDs such as aspirin and ibuprofen block both COX-1 enzymes, which produce "good" prostaglandins that protect the lining of the stomach, and COX-2 enzymes, which make "bad" prostaglandins that cause pain and inflammation. For this reason, traditional NSAIDs can produce stomach irritation and even gastric ulcers and bleeding.

A major development in the treatment of arthritis occured in 1999, when a new type of NSAID became available. Known as COX-2 inhibitors, these new prescription NSAIDs block only the inflammatory COX-2 prostaglandins; COX-1 is unaffected, so the drugs shouldn't irritate the stomach. Another new type of drug designed to ease OA is a synthetic version of hyaluronic acid, a component of joint lubricating fluid. The synthetic hyaluronic acids are injected directly into affected joints. If joints become severely damaged and activity is limited, surgery to repair or replace joints may be considered.

---

hat and sunglasses outside helps reduce glare. If visual losses are more severe, large-print books, magnifying glasses, and a variety of electronic devices are available to help. Every state has an association for the blind or visually impaired.

Menopause A special concern for women is the changes accompanying menopause. During their forties or fifties, women's ovaries gradually stop functioning and menstruation ceases. About 85% of women experience symptoms related to menopause, such as hot flashes, vaginal dryness, and emotional changes (see Chapter 5).

One important decision women need to make after menopause is whether to start hormone replacement therapy (HRT). The advantages of HRT include significant protection against heart disease and osteoporosis and relief from many symptoms of menopause. However, for some women HRT increases the risk of breast cancer (Figure 19-1), and women should carefully review their personal risk factors with their physician before deciding whether to begin HRT. As described in earlier chapters, drugs called selective estrogen-receptor modulators (SERMs) mimic estrogen's effects on some body tissues while blocking its effects on others. Researchers hope to

develop SERMs that provide all estrogen's beneficial effects without the risks currently associated with HRT.

Handling Psychological and Mental Changes

Many people associate old age with forgetfulness, and slowly losing one's memory was once considered an inevitable part of growing old. However, we now know that most older adults in good health remain mentally alert and retain their full capacity to learn and remember new information. Slight confusion and occasional forgetfulness may indicate only a temporary information overload, or fatigue. Many people become smarter as they become older and more experienced.

Dementia Severe and significant brain deterioration in elderly individuals, termed **dementia,** affects about 7% of

dementia Deterioration of mental functioning (including memory, concentration, and judgment) resulting from a brain disorder; often accompanied by emotional disturbances and personality changes.

TERMS

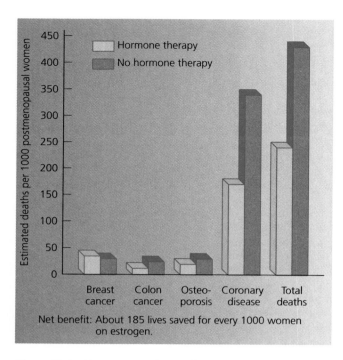

Figure 19-1 Hormones and mortality. Although hormone replacement therapy saves lives overall, women's individual risks vary greatly. SOURCE: Estrogen saves lives. 1998. *Consumer Reports on Health*, May. Copyright 1998 by Consumers Union of U.S., Inc., Yonkers, NY 10703-1057. Reprinted by permission from Consumer Reports on Health. No photocopying or reproduction permitted. To order a subscription, call 1-800-234-1645.

people under age 80 (the incidence rises sharply for people in their eighties and nineties). Early symptoms include slight disturbances in a person's ability to grasp the situation he or she is in. As dementia progresses, memory failure becomes apparent, and the person may forget conversations, the events of the day, or how to perform simple tasks. It is important to have any symptoms evaluated by a health care professional because some of the over 50 known causes of dementia are treatable (for example, depression, dehydration, vitamin B-12 deficiency, alcoholism, misuse of medications, and thyroid gland problems). The two most common forms of dementia among older people—**Alzheimer's disease** and multi-infarct dementia—are irreversible. Alzheimer's disease is characterized by changes in brain nerve cells. Multi-infarct dementia results from a series of small strokes or changes in the brain's blood supply that destroy brain tissue. Even for the incurable forms of dementia, however, appropriate treatment may greatly improve an affected person's qual-

ity of life (see the box "Alzheimer's Disease").

You can improve communication with a person suffering from dementia. Slow down and simplify what you are saying; dementia often means a person processes information more slowly. Avoid correcting mistakes in memory, and be patient with any repetition of ideas. Use structured approaches for routine tasks, such as laying out clothes in sequence to help with dressing. Listen to the meaning behind the communication, and be supportive.

Repeatedly telling stories about the past—something older people often do—doesn't necessarily indicate dementia. Reminiscence is a normal part of development and allows an older person to integrate life by making past events meaningful in the present. Reminiscing can be of great significance to members of the younger generations because it is a rich source of social, cultural, and family history.

Grief Another psychological and emotional challenge of aging is dealing with grief and mourning. Aging is associated with loss—the loss of friends, peers, physical appearance, possessions, and health. Grief is the process of getting through the pain of loss, and it can be one of the most lonely and intense times in a person's life. It can take a year or two or more to completely come to terms with the loss of a loved one. (See Chapter 20 for more information about responses to loss and how to support a grieving person.)

Unresolved grief can have serious physical and psychological or emotional health consequences and may require professional help. Signs of unresolved grief include hostility toward people connected with the death (physicians or nurses, for example), talking about the death as if it occurred yesterday, and unrealistic or harmful behavior (such as giving away all of one's own belongings). Many people become depressed after the loss of a loved one or when confronted with retirement or a chronic illness. But after a period of grieving, people are generally able to resume their lives.

Depression Unresolved grief can lead to depression, a common problem in older adults (see Chapter 3). If you notice the signs of depression in yourself or someone you know, consult a mental health professional. A marked loss of interest in usual pleasurable activities, decreased appetite, insomnia, fatigue, and feelings of worthlessness are signs of depression. Listen carefully when an older friend or relative complains about being depressed; it may be a request for help. Suicide rates are relatively high among the elderly, and depression should be taken seriously (see the box "Suicide Among Older Men").

It is a mistake to think that a depressed person will "snap out of it" or that people are too old to be helped. Both professional treatment and support groups can help people deal successfully with major life changes, such as retirement, moving, health problems, or loss of a spouse.

TERMS **Alzheimer's disease** A disease characterized by a progressive loss of mental functioning (dementia), caused by a degeneration of brain cells.

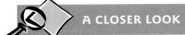

Alzheimer's disease (AD) is a fatal brain disorder that causes physical and chemical changes in the brain. As the brain's nerve cells are destroyed, the system that produces the neurotransmitter acetylcholine breaks down, and communication among parts of the brain deteriorates. Autopsies reveal that the diseased brain nerve cells are packed with shriveled filaments known as tangles, and the tips of their branches are mired in plaques, clusters of degenerating nerve fibers. More than 4 million Americans have Alzheimer's disease, and that number is expected to quadruple in the next 50 years, as more people live into their eighties and nineties. AD usually occurs in people over 60 but can occur in people as young as 40.

Symptoms

The first symptoms of AD are forgetfulness and inability to concentrate. A person may have difficulty performing familiar tasks at home and work and have problems with abstract thinking. As the disease progresses, people experience severe memory loss, especially for recent events. A person may vividly remember events from their childhood but be unable to remember the time of day or their location. Depression and anxiety are also common. In the later stages, people with AD are disoriented and may even hallucinate; some experience personality changes—becoming very aggressive or very docile. Eventually, they lose control of physical functioning and are completely dependent on caregivers. On average, a person will survive 8 years after the development of the first symptoms.

Causes

Scientists do not yet know what causes Alzheimer's disease. Age is the main risk factor, although about 10% of cases seem tied to inherited gene mutations. Inherited familial AD generally strikes people before age 65, while the more common late-onset AD occurs in people 65 and older. Other possible clues are provided by substances that appear to delay the onset or progression of the disease. People who regularly take nonsteroidal anti-inflammatory drugs (NSAIDS) like ibuprofen (often to control arthritis), women on HRT, and people who regularly consume fish rich in omega-3 fatty acids appear to have lower rates of AD, indicating a possible protective effect of substances that reduce inflammation. Some studies indicate that vitamin E and other antioxidants may reduce risk for AD or slow the progress of the disease, suggesting that oxidative stress caused by free radicals may play a role. (As described in Chapter 12, antioxidants block damage by free radicals.) Other possible risk factors include a high-fat diet, high blood levels of homocysteine, and brain damage from small strokes.

Diagnosis and Treatment

Currently, the only certain way to diagnose AD is to examine brain tissue during an autopsy. Physicians usually use a combination of physical, psychological, and neurological tests. New diagnostic techniques under study include specialized brain scans, blood tests for special types of proteins, and a 7-minute pencil-and-paper test that evaluates whether memory and related mental functions are appropriate for a person of a particular age. A behavior diary can also aid in diagnosis.

For people with mild to moderate AD, there are several drugs that provide modest improvements in memory. Tacrine and donepezil both work by inhibiting the breakdown of acetylcholine, thus raising levels of the neurotransmitter in the brain. People with AD may also be prescribed antidepressant or antianxiety medications. Many new treatments are under study, including selegiline, a drug used to treat Parkinson's disease; high doses of the antioxidant vitamin E; and the herbal compound *Ginkgo Biloba*, which may improve blood flow to the brain and act as an antioxidant. As scientists gain more insight into Alzheimer's disease, they hope to develop more effective treatments that will ease the burden of AD for both families and society.

One group of Americans is more than twice as likely to commit suicide than any other. From mass media accounts, you might imagine this group to be adolescents; however, suicide is much more common among the elderly—especially white males over the age of 65. Women and minorities of all ages have much lower rates of suicide than white men.

Why is this so? One explanation is that because white men generally have greater power and status in our society, aging and retirement represent a relatively greater loss for them. Women, more accustomed to "secondary" status, are not as threatened by the loss of economic and social power. Another theory is that white men tend to have weaker social ties than women or than men from other cultural groups, and as they retire, their increasing social isolation leads to depression and suicide. Indeed, depression is probably the single most significant factor associated with suicidal behavior in older adults.

Why are rates for other groups lower? In general, women are more likely than men to attempt suicide, but men are more likely to succeed, due in large part to their choice of more lethal methods. Some cultural groups, particularly Latinos and Native Americans, afford greater respect and status to older people, who are valued for their wisdom and experience. Cultural groups that emphasize family and social ties also seem to have lower rates of suicide.

The high rate of suicide among the elderly often fails to receive much attention. As a society, we are less disturbed about the deaths of older Americans from any cause than the deaths of younger people. What does it say about our society if, after a lifetime of contributions, an older person finds himself or herself in a position where suicide seems to be the best option?

TABLE 19-1	Life Expectancy		
Year		Men	Women
At birth:			
1900		46.3	48.3
1950		65.6	71.1
2000		73.0	79.7
2050 (projected)		79.7	84.3
At age 65:			
1900		11.5	12.2
1950		12.8	15.0
2000		15.9	19.5
2050 (projected)		20.3	22.4

SOURCE: U.S. Bureau of the Census (http://www.census.gov).

If someone refuses help, be reassuring and emphasize that treatment helps make people feel better; in some cases, a mental health professional can make a home visit.

One of the most important ways of dealing with the changes associated with aging is to adopt a flexible attitude toward whatever life brings you. Self-acceptance can help make the later years more meaningful and enjoyable. The right attitude can also help minimize the negative effects of some circumstances. Accepting limitations, having an optimistic outlook, and a sense of humor are tools that can help you cope with all of life's changes.

AGING AND LIFE EXPECTANCY

Life expectancy is the average length of time we can expect to live. It is calculated by averaging mortality statistics, the ages of death of a group of people over a certain period of time. A female born in the United States in 2000 has a longer life expectancy (79.7 years) than her male counterpart (73.0 years). Individuals who reach their sixty-fifth birthday can expect to live even longer—17 more years or longer—because they have already survived hazards to life in the younger years (Table 19-1).

Factors Influencing Life Expectancy

The reason for the gender gap in life expectancy is not known, but estrogen production and other factors during

TERMS **life expectancy** The average length of time a person is expected to live.

life span A theoretically projected length of life based on the maximum potential of the human body in the best environment.

a woman's fertile years appear to protect her from heart disease. Her risks increase after menopause. Increased male mortality can also be traced to smoking (lung cancer, heart and respiratory disease), more injuries, and more alcoholism. Where these factors are not operative, men live as long as women, as in the Amish, a religious sect with strict rules against smoking and drinking. Life expectancy also varies among ethnic groups; reasons for these differences include socioeconomic, genetic, and lifestyle factors.

Life expectancy in the United States has increased dramatically in this century, as described in Chapter 1. This does not mean that every American now lives longer than in 1900; rather, far fewer people die young now, because childhood and infectious diseases are better controlled and diet and sanitation are much improved. Only 30% of people born in 1900 would live to age 70; of those born in 2000, closer to 70% can expect to live that long.

How long can humans expect to live in the best of circumstances? It now seems possible that our maximum potential **life span** is 100–110 years. Failure to achieve that span in good health results to some degree from destructive environmental and behavioral factors—factors over which we can exert considerable control. Long life does not necessarily mean a longer period of disability, either. People often live longer because they have been well longer. A healthy, productive old age is very often an extension of a healthy, productive middle age. However, behavior changes cannot extend the maximum human life span, which seems to be built into our genes.

Theories on Aging

Throughout history, people have searched for and invented a great variety of "magic" preparations, devices, and practices for preserving youth. None has ever worked. More recently, science has entered the arena and directed research toward the aging process. Researchers would like to break through the riddles of hormones and the cell, to help enable people to live longer and maintain much of their youthful vigor.

What causes the eventual breakdown of the body? No existing theory on aging accommodates all the facts. Perhaps aging is caused by a variety of different processes and affected by a multitude of factors, both environmental and biological.

Biological theories can be divided into cellular and noncellular explanations for aging. Some aging processes may be built into individual cells; others seem to involve whole systems, such as the nervous system, the endocrine system, and the immune system. A cellular theory based on the genetic makeup of cells suggests that a cell contains "aging" genes that specify the exact number of times the cell can duplicate itself. The limiting number varies from species to species. This is why the maximum life span for fruit flies is about 100 days, for dogs 25–30 years, for humans about 110 years, and for giant tortoises about 180 years.

Another cellular theory is that the body generates free radicals, which undermine the integrity of cell membranes, damage DNA, and inactivate many enzymes and proteins required for normal cellular functioning. Environmental pollution also promotes free radical activity, but a diet rich in antioxidants can reduce it (see Chapter 12).

A theory of aging involving the immune system suggests that the body begins to make errors in protein synthesis, producing proteins that the immune system cannot recognize. The immune system then attacks them as it would any foreign substance, destroying cells and impairing body functions (see Chapter 17). Also, the immune system itself may weaken as we age, producing fewer antibodies to fight disease. Researchers are testing drugs that would reinforce faltering immune systems.

A theory of aging that focuses on metabolic function helps explain the immobility seen in old age. Connective tissue all over the body is given structural support by fibers of a class of proteins called collagen. Collagen becomes stiffer and chemically immobilized with age. This is because by-products of metabolism, called cross-links, form between parallel collagen fibers, making it impossible for the two fibers to slip past each other or stretch.

Some of the changes that accompany aging are due to declining levels of sex hormones. Hormone replacement therapy for women is now widely available to supply estrogen after menopause. A male hormone replacement therapy that raises levels of testosterone is currently being tested, but is not now generally available. There are concerns that supplementing testosterone in older men could increase the risk of heart disease, aggravate prostate problems, or promote tumor growth; however, for some men there are advantages to the therapy, including increased libido, muscle mass, and an overall sense of well-being.

Is aging associated with decline in all areas of functioning? Some social theorists maintain that while the biological processes tend to break down with aging, psychological and social development continues. In his theory of psychosocial development, Erik Erikson described the last phase of life as one in which people look back over their lives in an attempt to integrate and accept who they are and what they've accomplished. This review of life and integration of events can be a catalyst for personal growth. Despite possible physical limitations, many of your older friends and relatives may be role models for the successful personal integration of life's experiences and the ability to adapt to life's changes and challenges.

> **PERSONAL INSIGHT** Which theory of aging seems to describe the aging process of your grandparents, or other older people you know? What kind of social adjustments do you think your generation will face as you get older?

LIFE IN AN AGING AMERICA

As life expectancy increases, a larger proportion of the population will be in their later years. This change will necessitate new government policies and changes in our general attitudes toward older adults.

America's Aging Minority

People over 65 are a large minority in the American population—over 34 million people, about 13% of the total population in 2000 (Figure 19-2). As birth rates drop, the percentage increases dramatically. Many older people are happy, healthy, and self-sufficient. Changes that come with age, including negative ones, normally occur so gradually that most people adapt, some even gracefully.

Today the status of older adults is improving more than ever before. People now in their forties and fifties will probably benefit from new knowledge about the aging process. And the enormous increase in the over-55 population is markedly affecting our stereotypes of what it means to grow old. The misfortunes associated with aging—frailty, forgetfulness, poor health, isolation—occur in fewer people in their sixties and seventies and are shifting instead to burden the very old, those over 85.

The "younger" elderly who are in good physical and psychological health are gaining status in our society; politicians are listening to them, and advertisers have targeted them as a good market. In general, today's older adults are better off than they have ever been in the past. They have more money than they did 20 years ago. The poverty rate of the elderly has dropped from 28.5% to 10.8% since the 1960s, largely from the effects of Social Security payments and health care benefits from Medicare.

About 78% of older Americans own their homes. Their living expenses are lower after retirement because they no longer support children and have fewer work-related expenses; they consume and buy less food. They are more likely to continue practicing their expertise for years after retirement and to be paid in cash. Thousands of retired consultants, teachers, technicians, and craftspeople work until their middle and late seventies. They receive greater amounts of assistance, such as Medicare, pay proportionately lower taxes, and have greater net worth from lifetime savings.

As the aging population increases proportionately, however, the number of older people who are ill and dependent rises. Health care remains the largest expense for older adults. On average, they visit a physician 10–12 times a year and are hospitalized more frequently and require twice as many prescription drugs as the general population. Tens of thousands of older Americans live in poverty, particularly minorities and women living alone. These other elderly—poverty-stricken, isolated, lonely—are just as ignored as they ever were, and their numbers are increasing.

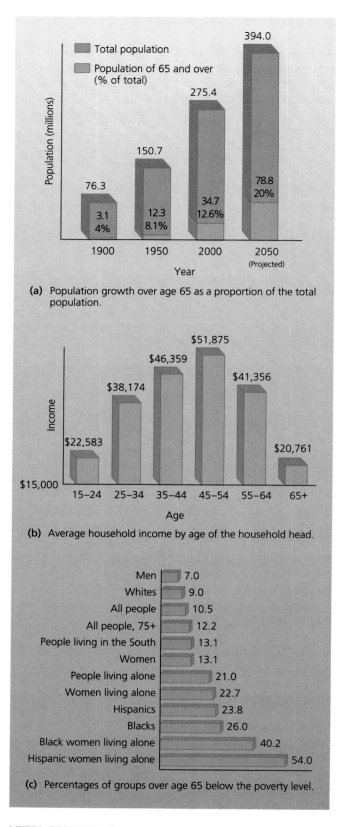

(a) Population growth over age 65 as a proportion of the total population.

(b) Average household income by age of the household head.

(c) Percentages of groups over age 65 below the poverty level.

Figure 19-2 A statistical look at older Americans. SOURCES: U.S. Bureau of the Census. U.S. Administration on Aging.

Retirement finds many older people with their incomes reduced to subsistence levels. This is especially true of the very old. The majority of older Americans live with fixed sources of income, such as pensions, that are eroded by inflation. Expenses tend to increase more rapidly, especially those due to circumstances over which people have little or no control, such as deteriorating health. Many Americans rely on **Social Security** payments as their only source of income; they are not covered by other types of retirement plans. Social Security was intended to serve as a supplement to personal savings and private pensions, not as a sole source of income. It is vital that people plan early for an adequate retirement income.

Family and Community Resources for Older Adults

With help from friends, family members, and community services, people in their later years can remain active and independent. About 66% of noninstitutionalized older Americans live with a spouse or other family member; the other 34% live alone or with a nonrelative. Only 4% live in nursing homes or other institutional settings at any point in time.

Family Involvement in Caregiving Most families do not abandon their aging relatives when they need help. Studies show that in about three out of four cases, a grown daughter or daughter-in-law assumes a caregiving role for elderly relatives. This may mean bringing them into the home, helping them remain in their own homes, or arranging for alternative housing. With more parents living into their eighties and with fewer children per family, many people, especially women, will face the choice of how to care for an aging relative. Recent surveys indicate that the average woman will spend about 17 years raising children and 18 years caring for an aging relative.

Caregiving can be rewarding, but it is also hard work. If the experience is stressful and long-term, family members may become emotionally exhausted. Caregivers should use available community services and consider their own needs for relaxation and relief from caregiving duties. Corporations are increasingly responsive to the needs of their employees who are family caregivers by providing such services as referrals, flexible schedules and leaves, and on-site adult care. Professional health care advice is another critical part of successful home care.

The best thing a family can do to prepare for the task of caring for aging parents is to talk frankly about the future. What does everyone expect will happen? What living and caring options are available, and which ones do family members prefer? What community resources are available? Planning ahead can reduce the stress on everyone involved and help ease difficult transitions (see the box "Caring for Older Adults").

Other Living and Care Options If aging parents and adult children living together is not possible, other living

At some point in their lives, many people will be called on to care for an older family member. There are advantages to caring for aging relatives in the home, including financial savings and family closeness. However, caregiving can be exhausting work. Primary caregivers must take time for themselves and their own needs to avoid burnout and feelings of hostility. Using all possible resources, becoming educated about the caregiving process, and involving the elder in decisions can relieve some of the stress of caregiving.

Mobilize Your Resources

- Enlist the help of other family members, neighbors, and friends.

- Look for an elder day-care program. These services, offered by many corporations and religious and community organizations, provide structured activities, meals, and medical services while primary caregivers are at work.

- Hire caregivers who can shop, cook, and help with personal care. Orient these people carefully in writing, and be sure they have all necessary information, including emergency phone numbers, medical needs, and dietary restrictions.

- Consider installing electronic communications equipment such as an automatic phone dialer or Medic Alert or intercom system.

Evaluate the Environment

- Check the home for possible safety concerns, such as slippery floors, throw rugs, and difficult stairs. Be sure the older person will be able to get around without being hurt.

- Add some functional aids, such as a grab bar, chair, and hand-held nozzle for the shower, a special elevated toilet seat, and stair railings.

Understand Medications

- Clarify with the physician or pharmacist the dose, timing, and possible side effects of all medications.

- Be alert for interactions between medications, including OTC drugs. Consider getting a consumer medication reference book; when in doubt, consult a pharmacist or physician.

- Get a medication organizer with compartments for each day or hour, or use an egg carton to keep drugs organized.

- Consult a physician about any changes in health or behavior; these may be due to medication side effects and not just disease or aging.

---

and care options are available. There are agencies that specialize in recruiting and matching like-minded individuals for shared living situations. Homesharing, as this is called, offers older adults who are in fairly good health the opportunity for new relationships, either with peers or with a younger family. Intergenerational homesharing may relieve elders of transportation problems and demanding physical tasks, which can be taken care of by younger household members. Conversely, elders in good health can help busy, working families with child care and household chores.

Retirement communities are an option for individuals in good health, with a good income, who want to maintain home ownership. These communities typically offer social and recreational activities and maintenance services to their residents. Other types of facilities are available for people who need more assistance with daily living (see the box "Choosing a Nursing Home").

Community Resources   Different kinds of community resources are available to help older adults remain active and in their own homes. The key to success is matching services with the needs of the individual person. Typical services include the following:

- *Senior citizens' centers or adult day-care centers,* which may provide meals, group social activities, and some health care services for those unable to be alone during the day.

- *Homemaker services,* which may include light housekeeping, cooking, running errands, doing shopping, and providing escort service.

- *Visiting nurses,* who provide some basic health care services.

- *Household services,* which may include basic household repairs and seasonal work.

- *Friendly visitor or daily telephone reassurance services,* which provide daily contacts for older people who live alone and may feel isolated.

- *Home food delivery services,* which provide daily meals to homebound people.

- *Adult day hospital care,* which provides day care plus physical therapy and treatment for chronic illnesses.

- *Low-cost legal aid,* which can help in managing finances and health care.

Sometimes elderly people refuse services. They may worry about the cost, be confused about what the service

Social Security   A government program that provides financial assistance to people who are unemployed, disabled, or retired (and over a certain age); financed through taxes on business and workers.   TERMS

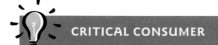
The decision to place a loved one in a nursing home is often a difficult one. Families may worry about whether or not the elder will get quality care, and how they will afford the cost of nursing home care. Indeed, the cost, $3500–$5500 per month, is as much as, or more than, many people's entire household income. Because long-term care is covered only briefly by Medicare and often not at all by private insurance, the cost is often borne by families.

There are several options available in nursing home care. Residential care facilities provide room and board, and some offer social and recreational programs. Continuing care communities include room and board plus personal and health care, and social activities. Assisted living facilities include retirement homes and board and care homes. Services range widely from place to place, but they usually include meals and help with personal care. Skilled nursing facilities provide 24-hour nursing care and supervision, with emphasis on improving or maintaining personal care skills.

Finding a good nursing home takes some investigation. Because the best homes often have a waiting list, plan ahead, and don't wait until your family member is too sick to function. A good starting place is the ombudsperson service in your state, which at no cost helps families find the right nursing home. Once you have an initial list of facilities in your area, start visiting the homes, keeping the following evaluation points in mind:

- Read the state inspection reports and state survey on each facility. These reports detail violations of laws regarding health, safety, and quality of life on unannounced inspec-

tions conducted every 12–15 months. By law, nursing homes must make their latest reports available and accessible to the public; be suspicious if the report is unavailable, hidden, or out-of-date. Contact your state ombudsperson for copies of the reports, or visit the Nursing Home Compare page of the Medicare Web site (http://www.medicare.gov).

- Tour the facility unannounced. Check to see that the residents are clean and well groomed. Get a feel for the way residents spend their time and are treated.

- Ask about bedsore, infection, and incontinence rates. Do you see signs of untreated bedsores? What percentage of residents are restrained?

- Ask about staff turnover. Many nursing homes are chronically understaffed, with turnover rates as high as 100%.

- Watch residents involved in activities. Is an effort made to engage all the residents? Do they seem passive or active? Do residents talk with each other?

- Watch how nurses interact with the residents. Do they call residents by name, and speak to them with warmth and caring? Is there a lot of yelling or scolding going on? Do residents in distress receive prompt attention?

Once you have placed a family member in a nursing home, visit often, and notice the quality of care. Say something nice when care is good, and speak up when care is poor. If you have trouble resolving a complaint, your local ombudsperson or citizen advocacy groups may be able to help.

---

offers, be unwilling to accept "charity," or want to avoid feeling dependent on others. You can help an older friend or relative accept needed services by providing accurate information about the services, explaining that they are designed to help the person remain independent. It may help to have an older friend of your relative suggest the service. When cost is a problem, some people offer to make arrangements for payment or to pay part or all of the cost of the service as a gift. Services can usually be located by looking in the phone book under local government agencies or in the yellow pages under Senior Citizens' Services.

Transportation   Older drivers usually have safe driving records compared with young adults because they tend to be more cautious; however, crashes in the older age group are more likely to be fatal. Many states require special driver's testing for people over age 70 and may restrict some drivers as to the time, area, and distances they may drive. Because of changes in vision or other health problems, some older drivers may be required to give up their license before they feel ready. Elderly people report that the loss of a driver's license and the loss of independence that it brings is one of the most severe hardships they face.

Older people who no longer have a driver's license must investigate and use other forms of transportation. These include buses, some of which are specially designed for people with disabilities; friends and family members with cars; taxis; dial-a-ride services; and volunteer drivers for seniors. Community agencies can also help.

Whatever their circumstances, older adults have the same needs as people at any other stage of life, including the need to feel that their lives have meaning. Becoming dependent on others for daily care and transportation is difficult for many people to accept. Most caregivers are motivated by love and responsibility and want to do the best they can for their aging friend or relative. However, some situations can lead to abuse, physical or economic (see the box "Elder Abuse"). Assistance is available, including respite care for caregivers and legal and protective services for abused elders.

PERSONAL INSIGHT   How do you think you would react if you had to care for an elderly parent or grandparent? Could you be patient, or would you lose your temper frequently? What experiences make you answer the way you do?

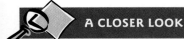

Abuse of the elderly is a serious problem in the United States. Each year, at least 500,000 older persons are abused, and for every reported incident, five go unreported. Most victims are 75 or older, and most abusers are family members who are serving as caregivers.

Elder abuse can take different forms:

- *Physical abuse:* The use of physical force that may result in bodily injury, physical pain, or impairment.

- *Sexual abuse:* Nonconsensual sexual contact of any kind.

- *Emotional abuse:* Inflicting anguish, pain, or distress through verbal or nonverbal acts.

- *Financial exploitation:* The illegal or improper use of an elder's funds, property, or assets.

- *Neglect:* The refusal or failure to fulfill any part of one's obligations or duties toward an older person.

- *Abandonment:* The desertion of an elderly person by an individual who has responsibility for providing care.

- *Self-neglect:* Behaviors of an elder that threaten that person's health or safety.

Neglect by caregivers is the most common form of elder abuse, accounting for about 55% of reported cases (excluding self-neglect). Elders who have lost some mental or physical functions and must rely on others for care are most at risk for neglect. The victim may suffer malnutrition, dehydration, mismanaged medication, or infection due to poor hygiene. Physical abuse accounts for about 15% of reported cases, and financial exploitation accounts for about 13%. Elder abuse is associated with an increased risk of death.

Why does abuse occur? Caring for a dependent adult can be stressful, especially if the elder is incontinent, has suffered mental deterioration, or is violent. Abuse may become an outlet for frustration. Risk factors for abuse include caregiver stress, severe impairment in the dependent elder, a history of violence or physical abuse in the family, and substance abuse or mental illness in the caregiver.

Depending on the laws of a particular state, elder abuse may or may not be a crime; most physical, sexual, and financial abuses are considered crimes. In most states, Adult Protective Services (APS) is the public agency responsible for investigating elder abuse. Many states have a toll-free number for reporting cases of abuse.

Many authorities believe that the solution to elder abuse is support in the form of greater social and financial assistance. Adult day-care centers, for example, provide needed relief for caregivers. Financial help can enable caregivers to earn a living while simultaneously providing round-the-clock care. Education and public care programs are necessary steps for preventing abuse.

SOURCE: U.S. Administration on Aging. 1998. *The National Elder Abuse Incidence Study: Final Report* (retrieved February 13, 1999; http://www.aoa.gov/abuse/report); National Center on Elder Abuse (http://www.gwjapan.com/NCEA).

Government Aid and Policies

The federal government helps older Americans through several programs, such as food stamps, housing subsidies, Social Security, Medicare, and Medicaid. Social Security, the life insurance and old-age pension plan, has saved many from destitution, although it is intended not as a sole source of income but as a supplement to other income. Social Security funds have been used to cover other government financial deficits, so the future solvency of the program is uncertain.

Medicare is a major health insurance program for the elderly and the disabled. It has two parts: Part A is financed by part of the payroll (FICA) tax that also pays for Social Security; Part B is financed by monthly premiums paid by people who choose to enroll. Part A helps pay for inpatient hospital care, some inpatient care in a skilled nursing facility, and some types of home and hospice care. Medicare Part B helps pay for physicians' services and other medical supplies and services not covered by Part A.

Medicare pays about 30% of the medical costs of older Americans. It provides basic health care coverage for acute episodes of illness that require skilled professional care; it does not pay for custodial or preventive care, including most expenses for routine checkups, dental care and dentures, immunizations, and prescription drugs. Over 1 million older people currently live in nursing homes, but Medicare pays less than 2% of nursing home costs, and private insurers pay less than 1%, creating a tremendous financial burden for nursing home residents and their families. Because of these gaps in coverage, many older people are joining managed health care plans to get more care for their money.

When their financial resources are exhausted, they may apply for Medicaid. A 1965 amendment to the Social Security Act, Medicaid provides medical insurance to low-income people of any age. Funded by state and federal contributions, the services vary from state to state but typically include hospital, nursing home and home health care, physician services, and some medical supplies and services. The portion of federal Medicaid spending attributed to the elderly has declined since 1980 from about 37% to about 30%.

A crucial question regarding aid for the elderly is: Who will pay for it? The government picks up much of the health care expenses, primarily through Medicare and Medicaid. Total health care expenditures are about 13.5%

The following is excerpted from an article written by Dr. Robert Coles, a professor of psychiatry and medical humanities at Harvard Medical School.

Why are so many Americans afraid of growing old? This question occurred to me often during the three years my wife and I lived in New Mexico and Arizona. Not a day went by when we weren't reminded of how much Native American and Hispanic families value old age. These are cultures that grant dignity and authority to their elders.

One young Hispanic woman described to us her relationship with her parents, both in their seventies, in this way: "When I am wondering what to do about a problem, I turn to my mother or my father. Even if they are not here, I still turn to them. I picture them in my mind and I hear them saying words that make good sense." One day, this woman's father made a show of his humorous and practical good sense before his young grandson. "You know what my son said to me that night when he was going to bed?" the woman asked. "He told me he wished he could be old like his grandpapa!"

To be old is to "last" oneself—to go through ups and downs, to survive bad luck and avoid all sorts of hazards. To be old is to

be blessed by fate, by chance and circumstance. Pueblo Indians know that. One Hopi child drew me a picture of an old woman shaking hands with the moon. Then she explained, "When you're old, you're a full moon; you make the night a little less dark." For Hopi children, an older person is a source of encouragement, instruction, inspiration, a part of nature's awesome presence.

For many young people living in other parts of America, old age is regarded not as a major achievement but rather as a last, sad, brief way station. One boy in Boston commented, "It's no fun to be old; it's the worst thing in the world, except to die." To many of us, old age means abandonment, rejection, loneliness, a loss of respect from others, and subsequently a loss of self-respect. This is not the case, though, in Hispanic and Native American cultures. The elders we met in New Mexico and Arizona showed a great deal of self-confidence, and in general they seemed contented with their lives. In their contentment and harmony with nature lies a lesson for all of us.

SOURCE: Adapted from Coles, R. 1989. Full-moon wisdom. *New Choices for the Best Years,* September. Reprinted with permission of Robert Coles, James Agee Professor of Social Ethics, Harvard University.

---

of the U.S. gross national product; about one-third of these expenditures go to care for older Americans.

Many health care policy planners believe that instead of adding temporary measures to Medicare and Medicaid, the government should address the issue of health insurance for the elderly in the context of an overall national health care policy. Many difficult and complex issues need attention, including the lack of health insurance for more than 43 million Americans and the rising costs of nursing home care and prescription drugs. Because resources are ultimately limited, difficult decisions have to be made and priorities have to be established.

In the meantime, health care policy planners hope that rising medical costs for older adults will dwindle dramatically through education and prevention. Health care professionals, including **gerontologists** and **geriatricians,** are beginning to practice preventive medicine, just as pediatricians do. They advise older people about how to avoid and, if necessary, how to manage disabilities. They try to instill an ethic of physical and psychological maintenance that will prevent chronic disease and enable older people to live long, healthy, vigorous lives.

TERMS **gerontologist** One who studies the biological, psychological, and social phenomena associated with aging and old age.

geriatrician A physician specializing in the diseases, disabilities, and care of older adults.

Changing the Public's Idea of Aging

Aging people may be one of our least used and least appreciated resources. (For another view, see the box "Multicultural Wisdom About Aging.") How can we use the knowledge and productivity of our growing numbers of older citizens, particularly those now leaving the workforce through mandatory early retirement?

First, we must change our thinking about what aging means. We must learn to judge productivity rather than age. Capacity to function should replace age as a criterion for usefulness. Instead of singling out 65 as a magic number, we could consider ages 50–75 as the third quarter of life. Changes occur around 50 that signal a new era: Children are usually grown and gone; a person has often achieved a level in career, earnings, and accomplishments that is satisfactory in terms of his or her ambitions. The upper end of the quarter is determined by the fact that most people today are vigorous, in good health, mentally alert, and capable of making a productive contribution until they are at least 75 years old. That age estimate may be a bit high for some, but not for most. About 21% of the population—57 million people—falls within the third quarter. But 25 years from now, about 93 million will be in their third quarter.

Other formulas have been suggested for drawing the boundary line between middle and old age. Rather than counting from birth, we could count back a fixed number of years from the expected age at death. Using a current life table, we could calculate the age at which the average

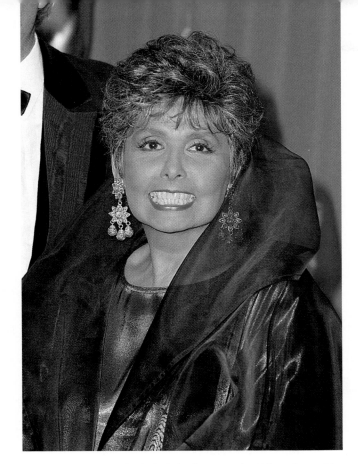

Some extraordinary individuals defy all preconceived ideas about old age. Singer and actress Lena Horne, now in her eighties, continues to live an intensely vigorous and creative life.

number of remaining years of life is 15. That would place old age around 67 today and 72 in the year 2030. Another way to decide who is old would be to limit the group to the most elderly 10% of the population, which would fix the age at 75 in 2030.

Whatever way we define old age, the costs of losing what these people can contribute to our national productivity and quality of life are too high. Through their early retirement we forfeit substantial income tax and Social Security tax revenues on their earnings. Those who retire at 62 start using their Social Security benefits earlier than otherwise.

A far better arrangement would be to make available full-time and part-time volunteer and paid employment. We would benefit by providing retraining programs for both occupational and leisure time activities. We need more community-sponsored classes in remunerative activities such as real estate selling and management, horticulture, and library work, and in recreational and self-improvement activities such as music, writing, and health maintenance. Volunteer opportunities, such as preparing recordings for the blind, helping with activities for the disabled, and performing necessary tasks in hospitals, could be expanded. At the same time, we could possibly change both public and private pension programs to make partial retirement possible. In such cases we could allow people to borrow against their Social Security benefits to finance retraining or enrollment in new educational programs.

There can be benefits to aging, but they don't come automatically. They require planning and wise choices earlier in life. One octogenarian, Russell Lee, founder of a medical clinic in California, perceived the advantages of aging as growth: "The limitations imposed by time are compensated by the improved taste, sharper discretion, sounder mental and esthetic judgment, increased sensitivity and compassion, clearer focus—which all contribute to a more certain direction in living. . . . The later years can be the best of life for which the earlier ones were preparation."

SUMMARY

- People who take charge of their health during their youth have greater control over the physical and mental aspects of aging.

Generating Vitality as You Age

- Biological aging takes place over a lifetime, but some of the other changes associated with aging are more abrupt. The more people prepare for aging, the more likely they are to be satisfied with their middle and old age.
- Many characteristics traditionally considered to be consequences of aging are due rather to neglect and abuse of body and mind.
- A lifetime of interests and hobbies helps maintain creativity and intelligence.
- Exercise throughout life enhances physical and psychological health; it may prevent deterioration of fluid intelligence with age.
- A lowfat, high-carbohydrate diet that includes a variety of foods promotes health at every age. Obesity leads to premature aging.
- Alcohol abuse is a common but often hidden problem, as is overdependence on medications. Tobacco use not only shortens life but also may cause severe health impairment for many years.
- Regular physical examinations help detect conditions that can shorten life and make old age less healthy. Immunizations protect against preventable infectious diseases.
- Stress increases wear and tear on the body; getting enough sleep, avoiding drugs, and practicing relaxation help reduce stress.

Confronting the Changes of Aging

- Retirement can be a fulfilling and enjoyable time of life for those who adjust to their new roles, enjoy participating in a variety of activities, and have planned ahead for financial stability.

- Successful aging involves anticipating and accommodating physical limitations.
- Slight confusion and forgetfulness are not signs of a serious illness; severe symptoms may indicate Alzheimer's disease or another form of dementia.
- Resolving grief and mourning and dealing with depression are important tasks for older adults; adopting a flexible attitude can help.

Aging and Life Expectancy

- Life expectancy, which has risen dramatically since the 1900s, is generally longer for women.
- Theories on aging examine the influences of cellular changes, free radicals, inappropriate immune responses, and changes in metabolism.
- Older adults can be role models for the successful integration of life's experiences and the ability to adapt to challenges.

Life in an Aging America

- People over 65 form a large minority in the United States, and their status is improving.
- Those who are ill and dependent—often those who were already poor—experience major social and economic problems.
- About 66% of all noninstitutionalized older people are cared for by their spouse or by family members, usually daughters and daughters-in-law.
- Community resources can help older adults stay active and independent.
- Government aid to the elderly includes food stamps, housing subsidies, Social Security, Medicare, and Medicaid.
- Older people represent an underused resource; society should consider productivity and the capacity to function, rather than age.

TAKE ACTION

1. Interview your parents or grandparents to find out how they want to spend their later years. Do they want to live at home, in a retirement community, with a relative? Do they plan to live on a pension, retirement account, Social Security? Have they made any concrete plans, or have they not yet confronted those decisions?

2. Investigate and, if possible, visit the different facilities in your community for the elderly—nursing homes, hospitals, senior citizen centers, recreational programs. What do you like about them, and what do you dislike? Do you have suggestions for improvement?

3. Interview several people from different cultural backgrounds about their attitudes toward aging and older people. How do they view the aging process? How are elderly people treated or viewed in their culture? Do you notice any significant differences between their attitudes and yours?

JOURNAL ENTRY

1. Imagine that you are very old and are looking back on your life. What will have given you satisfaction—a successful career, parenthood, happiness, travel, self-knowledge? Make a list in your health journal of your life goals and priorities. What actions can you take now to work toward your goals? Choose one goal, and take an action this week that moves you toward it.

2. *Critical Thinking* Assuming that government funding for medical care is limited, should more money be allocated for children's services or for medical care for older adults? Write a brief essay making a case for each side of the debate. Provide evidence to support each position.

FOR MORE INFORMATION

Books

Cassel, C. K., and G. A. Vallasi, eds. 1999. *The Practical Guide to Aging.* New York: New York University Press. *A practical guide to medical, financial, and legal aging issues.*

Kausler, D. H., and B. C. Kausler. 1996. *The Graying of America: An Encyclopedia of Aging, Health, Mind and Behavior.* Urbana-Champaign, Ill.: University of Illinois Press. *Contains a variety of information about the mental, physical, behavioral, and social aspects of aging.*

Rowe, J. W., and R. L. Kahan. 1998. *Successful Aging.* New York: Pantheon Books. *Provides practical advice for maintaining physical and mental health throughout life; based on the MacArthur Foundation Study of Aging in America.*

Wilkinson, J. A. 1999. *A Family Caregiver's Guide: Planning and Decision Making for the Elderly.* Minneapolis, Minn.: Fairview Press. *Provides information and advice for people caring for an aging family member.*

Organizations and Web Sites

Access America for Seniors. A gateway to government resources on the Internet for older Americans.
http://www.seniors.gov

Aging Well. A practical resource for seniors that includes information on diet, exercise, safety, and medical care.

    http://agingwell.state.ny.us

Alzheimer's Association. Offers tips for caregivers and patients, as well as information on research into the causes and treatment of Alzheimer's disease.

    800-272-3900

    http://www.alz.org

American Association of Homes and Services for the Aging (AAHSA). Provides information about living and care arrangements available for older adults.

    202-783-2242

    http://www.aahsa.org

American Association of Retired Persons (AARP). Provides information on all aspects of aging, including health promotion, health care, and retirement planning.

    601 E St., N.W.

    Washington, DC 20049

    800-424-2277

    http://www.aarp.org

Arthritis Foundation. Provides information about arthritis, including free brochures, referrals to local services, and research updates.

    800-283-7800

    http://www.arthritis.org

ElderWeb. A gateway to aging resources on the Internet, with information about health, housing, and financial issues.

    http://www.elderweb.com

Exercise: A Guide from the National Institute on Aging and the National Aeronautics and Space Administration. Provides practical advice on fitness for seniors; includes animated instructions for specific exercises.

    http://weboflife.arc.nasa.gov/exerciseandaging

The Interactive Aging Network/Senior Resources. Provides practical information and resources for seniors, including career development, discussion groups, financial planning, health promotion, and volunteering opportunities.

    http://www.ianet.org/resource

National Center on Elder Abuse Develops and disseminates information and statistics relating to elder abuse.

    http://www.gwjapan.com/NCEA

National Council on Aging. Promotes the well-being of older persons through research and advocacy; Web site provides helpful information on retirement planning, health promotion, and lifelong learning.

    http://www.ncoa.org

National Institute on Aging. Provides fact sheets and brochures on aging-related topics.

    http://www.nih.gov/nia

U.S. Administration on Aging. Provides fact sheets, statistical information, and Internet links to other resources on aging.

    330 Independence Ave., S.W.

    Washington, DC 20201

    202-619-0556

    http://www.aoa.gov

SELECTED BIBLIOGRAPHY

Agüero-Torres, H., et al. 1998. Dementia is the major cause of functional dependence in the elderly. *American Journal of Public Health* 88: 1452–1456.

Arthritis. 1999. *Mayo Clinic Health Letter: Special Supplement,* February.

Arthritis Foundation. 1998. The new drugs: The latest information. *Arthritis Today,* November/December.

Burkhardt, J. E., et al. 1998. *Mobility and Independence: Changes and Challenges for Older Drivers* (retrieved December 16, 1998; http://www.aoa.dhhs.gov/research/drivers.html).

Centers for Disease Control and Prevention. 1996. Suicide among older persons—United States, 1980–1992. *Morbidity and Mortality Weekly Report* 45(1): 3–6.

Evans, W. J. 1999. Exercise training guidelines for the elderly. *Medicine and Science in Sports and Exercise* 31(1): 12–17.

Ewbank, D.C. 1999. Deaths attributable to Alzheimer's disease in the United States. *American Journal of Public Health* 89(1): 90–92.

Giacobini, E. 1998. Aging, Alzheimer's disease, and estrogen therapy. *Experimental Gerontology* 33(7–8): 865–869.

Hingley, A. T., 1998. Alzheimer's: Few clues on the mysteries of memory. *FDA Consumer,* May/June.

Kerrigan, D. C., M. K. Todd, and P. O. Riley. 1998. Knee osteoarthritis and high-heeled shoes. *Lancet* 351(9113): 1399–1401.

Leventhal, K. 1999. Aging and medications. An overview. *ASHA* 41(1): 34–38.

Menopause: A guide to smart choices. 1999. *Consumer Reports,* January.

National Highway Traffic Safety Administration. 1998. *Traffic Safety Facts*. Washington, D.C.: U.S. Department of Transportation.

Pardes. H., et al. 1999. Effects of medical research on health care and economy. *Science* 283(5398): 36–37.

Reed, D. M., et al. 1998. Predictors of healthy aging in men with high life expectancies. *American Journal of Public Health* 88: 1463–1468.

Shadlen, M. F., and E. B. Larson. 1999. What's new in Alzheimer's disease treatment? Reasons for optimism about future pharmacologic options. *Postgraduate Medicine* 105(1): 109–118.

Singh, M. A. 1998. Combined exercise and dietary intervention to optimize body composition in aging. *Annals of the New York Academy of Science* 854: 378–393.

U.S. Administration on Aging. 1998. *Profile of Older Americans: 1998* (retrieved December 16, 1998; http://www.aoa.dhhs.gov/aoa/stats/profile).

U.S. Food and Drug Administration. 1999. *Consumer Drug Information: Celebrex* (retrieved February 13, 1999; http://www.fda.gov/cder/consumerinfo).

Vita, A. J., et al. 1998. Aging, health risks, and cumulative disability. *New England Journal of Medicine* 338(15) 1035–1041.

Wannamethe, S. G., A. G. Shaper, and M. Walker. 1998. Changes in physical activity, mortality, and incidence of CHD in older men. *Lancet* 351(9116): 1603–1608.

Whooley, M. A., and W. S. Browner. 1998. Association between depressive symptoms and mortality in older women. *Archives of Internal Medicine* 158: 2129–2135.

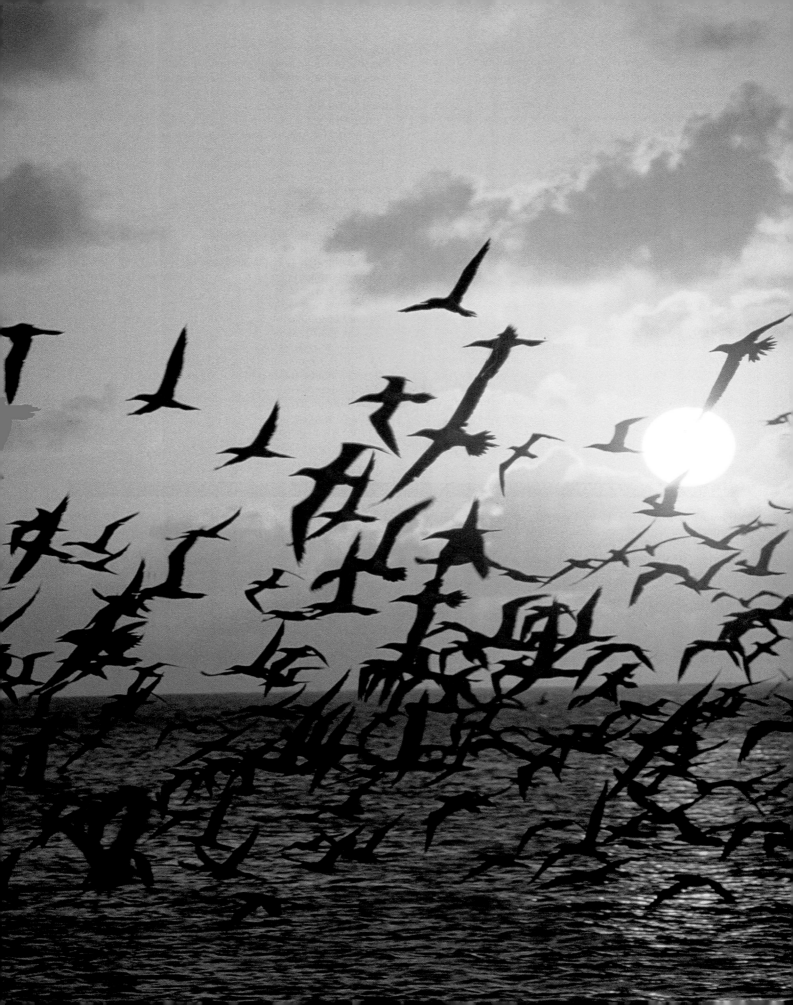

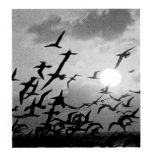

LEARNING OBJECTIVES

After reading this chapter, you should be able to:

- Explain the physical, emotional, social, and spiritual dimensions of death.

- Discuss legal considerations in planning for death, including wills, advance directives, and organ donation.

- Understand personal considerations in preparing for death, such as deciding where to die, deciding whether to prolong life, and making funeral arrangements.

- Describe the stages or process that a dying person may go through, and list ways you can support a person who is dying.

- Explain the grieving process and ways you can support a person who has suffered a loss.

Dying and Death

20

TEST YOUR KNOWLEDGE

1. If you die in a car crash, your organs will automatically be donated to people waiting for transplants.
    True or false?

2. How many Americans die without leaving a will?
    a. 1 in 10
    b. 4 in 10
    c. 7 in 10

3. The majority of Americans are in favor of legalizing physician-assisted suicide.
    True or false?

4. The average cost of a traditional funeral, not including cemetery costs, is about
    a. $1500
    b. $2500
    c. $5500

5. The best way to help a friend who is grieving is to distract her or him from the loss by talking about sports, gossip, or other light-hearted topics.
    True or false?

Answers

1. *False.* For your organs to be donated, you must have authorized it prior to your death (such as by completing an organ donor card), or the donation must be authorized by relatives at the time of your death.

2. *c.* In such cases, the estate is distributed according to state law, which may not reflect what the individual would have wanted.

3. *True.* In recent surveys, about 70% of Americans are in favor of a law that would allow a physician to prescribe a lethal dose of drugs to a terminally ill patient who requests it.

4. *c.* Depending on the type of casket and burial chosen, the full costs of a funeral and burial can range from about $600 to $20,000 or more.

5. *False.* Most people who are grieving need to talk about their loss, and a friend who will let them talk freely is very valuable. The best strategy is simply to be a good listener.

A man hiking a high mountain trail suddenly lost his footing and found himself hurtling toward certain death. As he plummeted past a small bush growing out of the sheer rock wall, he caught a berry in his hand and ate it. It was the most delicious berry he had ever eaten. Each of us is that man, hurtling toward certain death. How we deal with our mortality has a lot to do with how we live our lives.

If you suddenly discovered you had a terminal illness, how would you spend your last year or months? What kind of final ceremony would your family have? How would you wish to dispose of your possessions? Have you ever discussed these things with your family?

WHAT IS DEATH?

Death, like life, is change. When the body is no longer able to resist unhealthy changes in itself or is mechanically broken beyond repair, it ceases to function and dies.

Defining Death

Traditionally, death has been defined in clinical terms as occurring when the heart stops beating and breathing ceases. Defining death in this way—as cessation of the flow of vital body fluids—is adequate for determining death in most cases. However, the use of respirators and other **life-support systems** in modern medicine allows some body functions to be artificially sustained. Determining death in such cases requires investigating the presence or absence of a physical response other than the heartbeat or breathing.

Medical scientists now agree that the brain is the physical locus for determining whether a person is alive or dead. Thus, when a body is being kept alive on a respirator, for example, death is determined by measuring brain wave activity. According to the standards published in 1968 by a Harvard Medical School committee, four characteristics describe **brain death:** (1) lack of receptivity and response to external stimuli, (2) absence of sponta-

neous muscular movement and spontaneous breathing, (3) absence of observable reflexes, and (4) absence of brain activity, signified by a flat **electroencephalogram (EEG).** The Harvard criteria call for a second set of tests to be performed after 24 hours have elapsed. They also exclude cases of hypothermia (body temperature below 90°F), as well as situations involving the presence of central nervous system depressants, such as barbiturates. Most states have adopted legislation that redefines death according to these criteria when conventional methods of determining death prove inconclusive.

In contrast to **clinical death,** which is determined according to the criteria just discussed, **cellular death** refers to a gradual process that takes place when heartbeat, respiration, and brain activity have stopped. It encompasses the breakdown of metabolic processes in the cells, resulting in the complete cessation of function at the cellular level. Death can be defined biologically as the cessation of life resulting from irreversible changes in cell metabolism.

The definition of death can have legal and social consequences in areas such as criminal prosecution, inheritance, taxation, treatment of the corpse, even mourning. It also directly affects the practice of organ transplantation. Some organs—hearts, most obviously—must be taken from a human being whose heart is undamaged but who is legally determined to be dead. Critical timing is needed to remove a heart from someone who has been declared dead and to transplant it into a person whose life can thereby be saved. The definitions of death currently in use provide strict safeguards to ensure that the determination of death takes place without regard to any subsequent transplantation of the deceased's organs.

Why Is There Death?

Ultimately, no answer to the question of why death exists can be completely satisfying. Although we acknowledge that every living thing eventually dies, that recognition is of little comfort. Nor are we comforted by being told that matter and energy are never destroyed but simply changed. Most of us want our conscious self to continue. The notion of being reborn, with another consciousness, is not especially attractive.

Looking at the big picture, we can see that death promotes variety by permitting the renewal and evolution of species. The average human life span is long enough to allow us to reproduce ourselves and to ensure that the lineage of our species continues. Yet it is brief enough to allow for new genetic combinations. As a species, this mechanism provides a means of adaptation to changing conditions in the environment. Thus, looked at from the perspective of species survival and evolution, the cycle of life and death makes sense. From a personal point of view, however, death challenges our sense of emotional and intellectual security—especially when it involves seem-

TERMS **life-support systems**   Medical technologies, such as the artificial respirator, used to keep alive patients who would otherwise die.

brain death   A medical definition of death that indicates final cessation of activity in the central nervous system as determined by the use of various diagnostic criteria, particularly a flat EEG reading.

electroencephalogram (EEG)   A record of the electrical activity of the brain (brain waves).

clinical death   A determination of death made according to accepted medical criteria.

cellular death   The total breakdown of metabolic processes at the level of the cell.

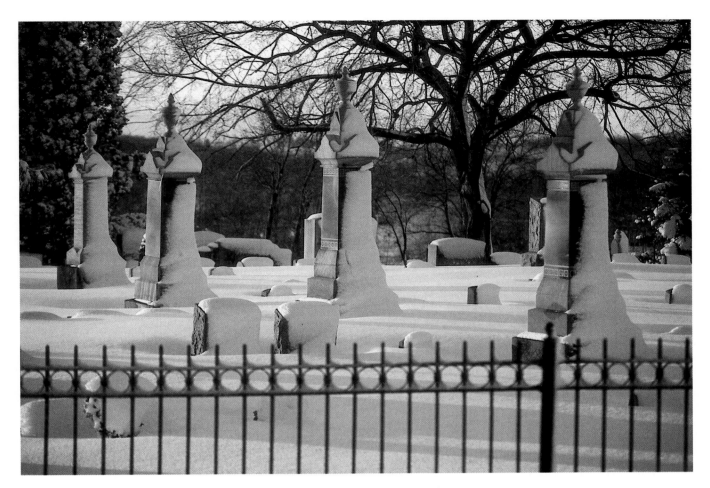

Death awaits all of us at the end of our lives, and accepting and dealing with death are difficult but important tasks. Some people have found that facing the prospect of death makes them more aware of the preciousness of life.

ingly needless, accidental, or sudden death of children or adults in the prime of life.

Consequently, theories abound concerning what happens when we die. Most religions are founded on the issue of death and what, if anything, follows. Some promise a better life after death if adherents accept the beliefs and behave according to the rules of the group and its god(s). Other religions or philosophies teach that everyone is evolving toward divinity and is reborn over and over again until they eventually reach perfection. Other views suggest that we cannot know what happens after death, and that any judgment about whether life is worth living must be made on the basis of rewards we find or create for ourselves in this life.

Attitudes Toward Death

Death is absolute loss. The death of a best friend, parent, mate, or child typically evokes feelings of confusion and pain. The prospect of our own death can be emotionally

devastating. We prefer not to think about it—not so much because we don't know what will happen after death, but because death is the letting go of everything and everyone dear to us. Death forces us to puzzle out an understanding of its meaning in our lives. We may choose not to ponder some issues, such as the possibility of an afterlife, but we cannot refrain from facing the reality of death itself. Regardless of our explanations and efforts to minimize its effect, death is painful—both to the person who is dying and to those left behind.

Our attitudes toward death change as we grow and mature, as does our understanding of it. Very young children recognize death as an interruption and an absence, but their lack of a mature time perspective means they don't understand that death is final. This view of death evolves considerably from about age 5 to 9. Children come to understand that death is final, although initially this recognition applies only to others, not to themselves. They think they will somehow escape the universality of death (an illusion that even adults sometimes display by their risk-taking activities). By age 10 or so, most children do recognize that death is universal, inescapable, and irreversible. The conscious recognition of these facts is said to reflect a mature understanding of death. During the years of adolescence and young adulthood, the mature understanding of death is further refined by contemplating the impact of death on close relationships and the value of religious or philosophical answers to the enigma of death.

Based on work done by Mark Speece and Sandor Brent, a formal statement of the empirical, or observable, facts about death includes four components:

1. *Universality.* All living things eventually die. Death is all-inclusive, inevitable (unavoidable), and unpredictable with respect to its exact timing.

2. *Irreversibility.* Organisms that die cannot be made alive again.

3. *Nonfunctionality.* Death involves the cessation of all physiological functioning, or signs of life.

4. *Causality.* There are biological reasons for the occurrence of death.

It is important to add, however, that nonempirical ideas about death—that is, ideas that are not subject to scientific proof—are also held by people who possess a mature understanding of the observable facts. Such nonempirical ideas deal mainly with the notion that human beings survive in some form beyond the death of the physical body. Questions and concerns about the possibility of an "afterlife" are important for adults as well as children. What happens to an individual's "personality" after he or she dies? Does the self or soul continue to exist in some form after the death of the physical body? Finding personally satisfying answers to such questions, which involve what Speece and Brent term **noncorporeal continuity**, is also part of the process of acquiring a mature understanding of death.

Having an understanding of death does not mean that one never experiences anxiety about the deaths of loved ones or the prospect of one's own death. Between couples who have shared nearly a lifetime together, thoughts of death may elicit fears about being left alone. The news of a friend's or loved one's terminal illness can shock us into an encounter with mortality, creating the need to cope not just with the painful reality of our friend's or loved one's illness, but also with the prospect of our own death. In these and many other situations, our ability to find meaning and comfort depends not only on our understanding the facts of death, but also on our attitude toward it.

Denying Death Over the past several generations, Americans have generally engaged in denial about death. We know that death is an unavoidable reality, yet we try fervently to avoid any thought or mention of it. Rather than speak the words "die" or "dead," we describe the deceased with euphemisms like "passed away" or "gone to glory." As if acknowledging the fact of death might prove to be traumatic for us, the sick and old are isolated in hospitals or nursing homes. Few Americans have been present at the death of a loved one. Death is rarely a home event. Usually, we don't want to be told the details, or we are happy to allow the details to be tastefully edited. Such practices foster the notion that death happens to others—but not to you or me.

The reality of death—its finality and its aftermath of grief—is largely a taboo subject in our culture. Instead of facing it directly, we amuse ourselves with unrealistic portrayals. When death is faked on television and movie screens, it is often presented as reversible. The fictitious deaths of characters we barely know do not force us to confront the reality of death as it is experienced in real life. Our children watch a daily fare of superhuman heroes and robots, invincible to bullets and other weapons, as well as characters traveling through time to thwart inevitable death. In their games, children reenact these ideas of death—falling down "dead" and jumping up again. Video games, like cartoons, present death in a two-dimensional world where one can "die" and then be "reborn" to play another day. (For another perspective on death, see the box "*Día de los Muertos:* The Day of the Dead.")

Welcoming Death Although a denial of death constitutes the predominant attitude in American society, death is sometimes welcomed as a relief or release from insufferable pain. This attitude toward death is associated with people who suffer mental and emotional anguish related to depression or physical pain caused by terminal illness. The physical debility and social isolation that may accompany old age can also give rise to a welcoming attitude toward death. It is important to recognize that individuals may hold conflicting or ambivalent attitudes toward death—denying its reality while simultaneously seeking the release or relief it seems to offer.

This ambivalence toward death is seen most clearly in cases of suicide, the intentional taking of one's own life. The motive for suicide commonly involves despair over one's life situation coupled with a sense of hopelessness about the future. Often, the specific motives that lead to a person's decision to end his or her life are not altogether clear, and a **psychological autopsy** is needed to uncover them. Initiated by a coroner or medical examiner when the circumstances surrounding a death are unclear, the psychological autopsy provides a method for determining the thoughts, feelings, and actions of the victim prior to his or her death. Information is gathered by interviewing the deceased's friends and relatives, with particular atten-

TERMS   **noncorporeal continuity**   The notion that humans survive in some form after the death of the physical body.

psychological autopsy   An investigation to determine the thoughts, feelings, and actions of a suicide victim prior to his or her death.

In contrast to the solemn attitude toward death so prevalent in the United States, a familiar and even ironic attitude is more common among Mexicans and Mexican Americans. In the Mexican worldview, death is another phase of life, and those who have passed into it remain accessible. Ancestors are not forever lost, nor is the past dead. This sense of continuity has its roots in the culture of the Aztecs, for whom regeneration was a central theme. When the Spanish came to Mexico in the sixteenth century, their beliefs about death, along with such symbols as skulls and skeletons, were absorbed into the native culture.

Today, symbols of death are visible everywhere in Mexico and in the Mexican American communities of the United States. Mexican artists and writers confront death with humor and even sarcasm, depicting it as the inevitable fate that all—even the wealthiest—must face. At no time is this attitude toward death livelier than at the beginning of each November on the holiday known as *Día de los Muertos*, "the Day of the Dead." This holiday coincides with All Soul's Day, the Catholic commemoration of the dead, and represents a unique blending of indigenous ritual and religious dogma.

Festive and gay, the celebration in honor of the dead typically spans two days—one day devoted to dead children, one to adults. It reflects the belief that the dead return to Earth in spirit once a year to rejoin their families and partake of holiday foods prepared especially for them. The fiesta usually begins at midday on October 31, with flowers and food—candies, cookies, honey, milk—set out on altars in each house for the family's dead children. The next day, family groups stream to the graveyards, where they have cleaned and decorated the graves of their loved ones, to celebrate and commune with the dead. They bring games, music, and special food—chicken with *mole* sauce, enchiladas, tamales, and *pan de muertos*, the "bread of the dead," sweet rolls in the shape of bones. People sit on the graves, eat, sing, and talk with the departed ones. Tears may be shed as the dead are remembered, but mourning is tempered by the festive mood of the occasion.

Perhaps the greatest contrast between the solemn North American attitude toward death and the livelier Mexican way is found in the colors associated with death. In Mexico it is yellow, not black, that colors the rituals of death. During the season of the dead, graveyards and family altars are decorated with yellow candles and yellow marigolds—the "flower of death." In some Mexican villages, yellow flower petals are strewn along the ground, connecting the graveyard with all the houses visited by death during the year.

As families cherish memories of their loved ones on this holiday, the larger society satirizes death itself—and political and public figures. The impulse to laugh at death finds expression in what are called *calaveras,* a word meaning "skeletons" or "skulls" but also referring to humorous newsletters that appear during this season. The *calaveras* contain biting, often bawdy, verses caricaturing well-known public figures, often with particular reference to their deaths. Comic skeletal figures march or dance across these pages, portraying the wealthy and influential as they will eventually become.

Wherever Mexican Americans have settled in the United States, *Día de los Muertos* celebrations keep the traditions alive, and the cultural practices associated with the Day of the Dead have found their way into the nation's culture. Books and museum exhibitions have brought to the public the "art of the dead," with its striking blend of skeletons and flowers, bones and candles. Even the schools in some areas celebrate the holiday. Students create paintings and sculptures depicting skeletons and skulls with the help of local artists.

Does this more familiar attitude toward death help people accept death and come to terms with it? Keeping death in the forefront of consciousness may provide solace to the living, reminding them of their loved ones and assuring them that they themselves will not be forgotten when they die. Yearly celebrations and remembrances may help people keep in touch with their past, their ancestry, and their roots. The festive atmosphere may help dispel the fear of death, allowing people to look at it more directly. Although it is possible to deny the reality of death even when surrounded by images of it, such natural practices as *Día de los Muertos* may help people face death with more equanimity.

SOURCES: Adapted from Puente, T. 1991. Día de los Muertos. *Hispanic*, October. Milne, J. 1965. *Fiesta Time in Latin America.* Los Angeles: Ward Ritche Press. Despelder, L., and A. Strickland. 1999. *The Last Dance*, 5th ed. Mountain View, Calif.: Mayfield.

tion to the role of stressful circumstances, psychological and medical histories, and lifestyle. Both social context and individual factors are examined. The goal of such an investigation is to provide a picture of a person's state of mind prior to committing suicide.

Analysis of suicidal behavior often reveals the presence of conflicting forces that compete for the greater share of the person's mental energies. Given this ambivalence, one way to help people who are experiencing a suicidal crisis is to help them discover something about themselves that matters, however small or insignificant it may seem. Suicidal thoughts and behaviors indicate a critical loss of a person's belief in himself or herself. Nevertheless, the desire to help a suicidal person should be tempered by the recognition that the sustaining motive to survive cannot come from outside; it must be generated from within the potentially suicidal person. For a discussion of assistance and treatment for suicidal people, see Chapter 3.

Suicide reminds us of the awesome fact that each of us has the power to choose whether we continue to live. It forces us to contemplate our own mortality and to assess our attitudes toward death. Few people wholly avoid death or wholly seek death. The fear of death and the wish to deny its reality usually coexist more or less peace-

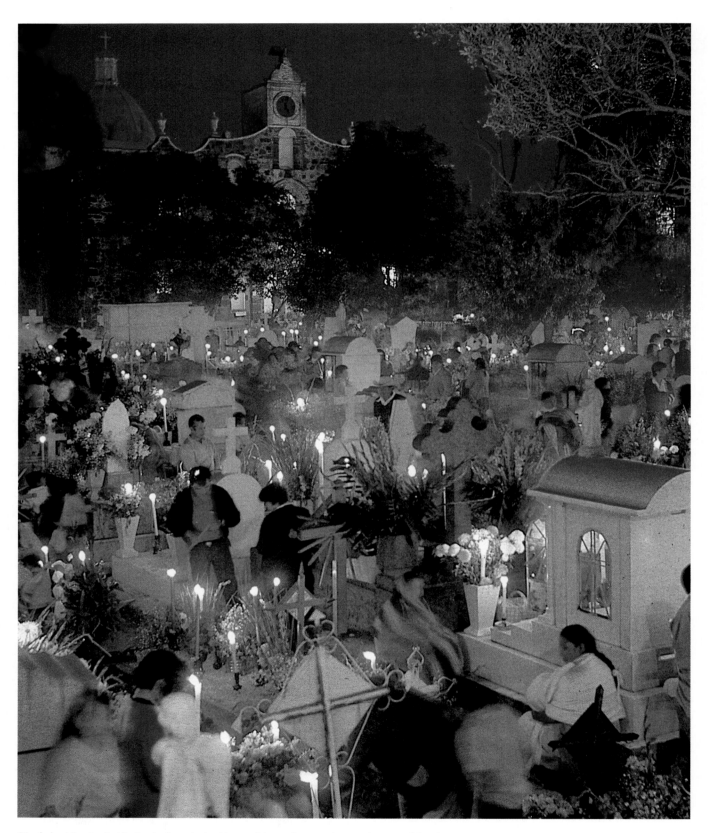

Día de los Muertos in Mexico is characterized by a mixture of reverent remembrance of the departed, festivity to make them happy upon their return, and irony and mockery to defy the fear of death itself. After cleaning the graves and decorating them with candles and flowers, these families will spend the night in the graveyard—eating, singing, praying, and talking with the departed.

ably with a sense of resignation, even acceptance. While perhaps consciously wishing to postpone the inevitable, our behavior—especially in the context of taking risks—reveals that we actually hold a considerable range of attitudes toward death.

Religious Beliefs About Death

Even in modern secular societies, religion plays a major role in shaping our attitudes and behaviors toward death. Religion may provide solace to the extent that it suggests some meaning in dying. Mourning rituals associated with religious practice ease the pangs of grief for many bereaved people. A young Filipino American man whose father died, for example, talked about the comfort he felt in connection with a funeral mass held in the church where his family worshiped. Commenting on the use of Latin during the service, he said, "You know, I've never known exactly what those prayers are all about, but the soothing rhythms of the chants and the pungent smell of the incense made me feel that my dad is taken care of, that he's really OK."

Dying and death are more than biological events; they have social and spiritual dimensions. Our religious beliefs can be a key to how we relate to the prospect of our own death, as well as the deaths of others.

PLANNING FOR DEATH

Once we acknowledge the inevitability of death, we can plan for it and thereby ease what otherwise could be difficult decisions for both our survivors and ourselves. Preparing for death requires completing unfinished business, dealing with medical care needs, allocating our time and other resources, and helping our survivors plan tasks that will be carried out after we die. People who unexpectedly find themselves in the midst of a painful and debilitating terminal illness may be so drained physically and emotionally that they are unable to make prudent decisions that could have easily been made before the onset of crisis.

Indeed, some decisions can be made while you are young. Decisions about a will, for example, can and should be made as early as the college years. Adequate planning can help ensure that a sudden, unexpected death is not made even more difficult for survivors.

Although some decisions cannot be made until one is actually in a particular situation, other decisions can be anticipated and discussed with close relatives and friends.

Making a Will

It is estimated that 7 out of 10 Americans die without leaving a will. Perhaps the failure to make a will is attributable to the discomfort we feel about death. Whatever the reason, dying without a will creates added hardships for survivors, even when an estate is quite modest. If the estate is substantial, the complications can be formidable.

A **will** is a legal document expressing a person's intentions and wishes for the disposition of his or her property after death. It is a declaration of how a person's estate—everything he or she owns—will be distributed upon that person's death. During the life of the **testator** (the person making the will), a will can be changed, replaced, or revoked. Upon the testator's death, it becomes a legal instrument governing the distribution of the testator's estate.

When a person dies **intestate**, without having left a valid will, his or her property is distributed according to rules set up by the state. The failure to provide a will may cause the welfare of one's spouse and children to be considered separately, resulting in a distribution of property that may not be compatible with one's own wishes or best suited to the interests and needs of heirs.

Choosing Where to Die

Would you prefer to spend your last days at home, tended by relatives and friends? Or would you rather have access to the sophisticated medical techniques available in a hospital setting? Would hospice care, with its emphasis on family involvement and alleviating pain, be your choice for care at the end of life? Although the place where we die is not always something we can choose, we can and should consider the alternatives.

Home   Until well into the early decades of this century, virtually everyone died at home. Now, however, most deaths occur in an institutional setting, usually a hospital or nursing home. Advocates of home care believe that a person's home is the preferred setting for terminal care at the end stage of an illness. Compared to institutional settings such as hospitals and nursing homes, home care makes it easier to sustain relationships with loved ones and to exercise self-determination about the details of care.

will   A legal document expressing a person's intentions and wishes for the disposition of his or her property after death.

testator   A person who dies with a will in force.

intestate   Referring to the situation in which a person dies having made no legal will.

TERMS

The advantages of home care come at a price, however. Support must be available not only from the patient's family and friends, but also from skilled, professional caregivers who both supervise the care at home and provide relief when necessary. If a patient requires sophisticated medical procedures, cannot afford the professional staff needed to make home care work, or intends to donate organs, hospital care may be more appropriate. Similarly, unless family members or friends can dedicate themselves to the necessary continuity of care, other alternatives should be considered. Still, for those who wish to provide home care to a loved one, resources are available for educating oneself about every facet of tending a dying patient. When appropriate, home care is probably the most satisfying option for caring for a loved one as his or her life comes to a close.

Hospital   Hospitals are organized to provide short-term intensive treatment for acute injury and illness. Highly specialized care is provided to patients who usually stay in the hospital only briefly before returning to normal life. Because of this emphasis on acute care, hospitals are generally not well suited to meet the needs of patients expected to die from terminal disease. In addition, a highly trained staff and expensive medical technologies make the cost of hospital care high.

Nevertheless, some medical institutions have instituted **palliative care** programs to care for patients who are not expected to recover. Palliative care focuses on providing relief from pain while acknowledging that further treatment would be futile. A comprehensive program of hospital-based palliative care offers counseling support to dying patients and their families, as well as care by specially trained staff.

Hospice   The concept of **hospice** care grew out of the perception that care of the dying within conventional hospital settings was inadequate. An alternative to both home care—especially when families need relief—and hospital care, the hospice philosophy of care has met with rapid and widespread acceptance (see the box "Hospice: Comfort and Care for the Dying").

Most hospice organizations provide support services—including nursing care, social services, pain medication, counseling, and volunteer caregivers—to patients who are either at home or in an institutional care setting. The most recent survey of hospices carried out by the National Center for Health Statistics revealed that the vast majority of hospice users have terminal cancer and are cared for in their homes; other common diagnoses for hospice patients are congestive heart failure, emphysema, stroke, Alzheimer's disease, and HIV infection. In addition, some hospice programs have been developed specifically to provide care for terminally ill children. In a relatively brief time, the hospice philosophy of care, with an emphasis on alleviation of pain and acceptance of death, has made important contributions to the care of dying patients and their families.

Asking for Help: Granting Power of Attorney

Just as making a will is a responsible way to plan for the eventuality of one's own death, a person may delegate authority over certain matters to a trusted friend or relative who can thereby act on his or her behalf. This trusted person, or agent, is granted **power of attorney,** the legal authority to act in another person's name. Depending on the authority being delegated, it may be important to acquaint one's agent with any survivor benefits that are expected (such as Social Security, pensions, and life insurance), as well as with important documents such as a will, birth and marriage certificates, insurance policies, bank account records and other financial documents, and deeds. You can complete a durable power of attorney for health care, designating someone who will make health care decisions for you if you are unable to act on your own behalf. (See the section on advance directives below.)

Deciding Whether to Prolong Life

If you were diagnosed with a terminal illness, would you want to be kept alive on life-support systems? Many people are alive today because of advanced medical technology, such as the heart pacemaker and the kidney dialysis machine. In spite of successes, however, modern medical innovations do not always clearly confer benefits. Should a patient without any hope of recovery be kept alive by means of artificial life support? What if the patient has fallen into a **persistent vegetative state,** a state of profound unconsciousness, lacking any sign of normal reflexes and unresponsive to external stimuli, with no reasonable hope of improvement?

Ethical questions about the "right to die" have become widespread in American society since the landmark case of Karen Ann Quinlan in 1975. At age 22, she was admitted in a comatose state to an intensive care unit where her breathing was soon being sustained by a respirator. When she remained unresponsive in a persistent vegetative

---

TERMS   **palliative care**   Measures taken to reduce the intensity of a disease, especially those involving control of pain and other symptoms.

hospice   A facility or program designed to provide care and support for terminally ill patients.

power of attorney   A legal instrument allowing one person to act as the agent of another person.

persistent vegetative state   A condition of profound unconsciousness caused by disease or injury in which a person lacks normal reflexes and is unresponsive to external stimuli, lasting for an extended period with no reasonable hope of improvement.

Hospice is a special kind of care for people in the final phase of a terminal illness. Instead of being in a hospital, where the emphasis is on curing disease, most hospice patients stay in their home or another homelike setting surrounded by family and friends. The goals of hospice care include the following:

- To make every terminally ill patient as pain-free as possible.

- To support the patient and family as a unit.

- To respect the feelings and beliefs about death held by patients and their families.

- To involve patients in decision making regarding their care.

- To help patients and family members deal with feelings of loneliness and fears of abandonment.

- To counsel family members after a patient's death.

Although institutions dedicated to the care of the dying have existed throughout history, the modern hospice movement began in 1967, when Dr. Cicely Saunders founded St. Christopher's Hospice near London. The first hospice program in the United States began in 1974. Today there are over 3000 such programs, serving an estimated 450,000 terminally ill patients and their families each year. Once a patient can no longer benefit from medical treatment based on curing disease, the primary physician may refer the patient to hospice. Referrals can also be made by family members, friends, clergy, or health professionals.

Most patients receive care at home, with the primary caregiver often a partner or family member. Providing medical care and other types of support to the patient, family, and caregivers is a team of trained professionals—physicians, nurses, counselors, therapists, social workers, home health aides, and volunteers. The emphasis of care is on enhancing the quality of life rather than extending its length. Most hospice patients have a life expectancy of 6 months or less at the time they enter hospice, and about two-thirds of them are over 65 years old.

Hospice care is often less expensive than conventional care—high-cost technology is much less likely to be used, and family, friends, and volunteers provide much of the day-to-day patient care at home. Because a principle of hospice is to offer services based on need rather than the ability to pay, many hospices rely on grants, donations, and a large volunteer staff. In the 1970s, hospice care relied heavily on professional and lay volunteers, and today over 70,000 volunteers serve in hospice programs. At the same time, hospice has grown into a more formal, regulated industry. Hospice care is a covered benefit under most private insurance plans, Medicare, and, in many states, Medicaid. Medicare-certified hospice programs meet quality standards set by the federal government, including 24-hour access to professional care.

Some experts believe hospice could serve over twice as many patients as it currently does. There are several stumbling blocks to an increase in usage, however. Physicians may be reluctant to stop treatment and tell patients and their families that there's no hope. Patients and family members may also have trouble conceding that death is on its way. And under Medicare rules, a physician must certify that the patient has only 6 months or less to live. This requirement makes it hard for any patients to be eligible other than those having late-stage cancer. Many experts call for an expansion of hospice programs and the development of new ways of using the hospice approach in conventional settings.

SOURCES: National Hospice Organization. 1998. *The Basics of Hospice* (retrieved January 11, 1999; http://www.nho.org/basics.htm). Hospice care. 1997. *Mayo Clinic Health Letter*, July.

state, her parents requested that the respirator be disconnected, but this request was denied by the medical staff responsible for Karen's care. Eventually, the request reached the New Jersey Supreme Court, which ruled that artificial respiration could be discontinued.

More recently, courts in various parts of the country have ruled on requests to remove other forms of life support, including artificial feeding mechanisms that provide nutrition and hydration to comatose patients who are able to breathe on their own. The case of Nancy Beth Cruzan was heard before the U.S. Supreme Court in 1990. As a result of injuries she received in 1983, Cruzan was in a persistent vegetative state. Physicians had implanted a feeding tube to provide nourishment, the only form of life support she was receiving. As in the case of Karen Quinlan, when Nancy Cruzan's parents requested that artificial life support be withdrawn, hospital staff members refused, arguing that the state had an inherent interest in preserving life.

The Supreme Court ruled that states are justified in making a requirement that only the patient can decide to withdraw treatment. Since Nancy apparently had not provided a clear expression of her wishes on the matter before her injury, the state was not bound to honor the wishes of her parents. However, a few months later, in light of new testimony from several of Nancy's friends that she had expressed her wishes "not to live like a vegetable," a state court ruled that the "clear and convincing" evidence standard now had been met, and permission was granted for removal of the feeding tube. This case highlights the value of expressing one's wishes regarding life-sustaining measures, preferably in writing, before the need for such a statement arises.

Allowing Someone to Die When suffering outweighs the benefits of continued existence, many people argue that individuals have a "right to die," whether or not they choose to exercise that right. Withdrawing or not initiating treatments that could potentially sustain life is sometimes termed **passive euthanasia,** although many medical practitioners and ethicists reject this term because it tends to confuse the generally unacceptable and unlawful practice of actively causing death with the fairly well-established practice of withholding or withdrawing useless treatments. It is increasingly considered good medical practice not to artificially prolong the life and suffering of a person whose condition is inevitably fatal. Courts also seem to be coming to a consensus that mentally competent, informed patients have the right to refuse medical treatment, including life support provided by mechanical or artificial means.

Assisted Suicide and Active Euthanasia In contrast to withdrawing or withholding treatment, assisted suicide and active euthanasia refer to practices that intentionally hasten the death of a terminally ill patient. Assisted suicide refers to the act of providing someone with the means to commit suicide. In **physician-assisted suicide (PAS),** a physician provides medications to a patient knowing that the patient plans to use them to end her or his life. In **voluntary active euthanasia,** someone else administers the fatal treatment; "voluntary" indicates the fact that the act is performed at the request of the patient. In most cases, a physician is involved, and death is brought about by **lethal injection.** The distinction between passive euthanasia and assisted suicide or voluntary active euthanasia is sometimes characterized as the difference between "letting die" and "killing" (although

advocates of PAS and voluntary active euthanasia prefer the phrase "helping to die").

In the United States, taking active steps to end someone's life is a crime, even if the motive is to alleviate suffering. No U.S. laws currently authorize voluntary active euthanasia, and, as of 1998, Oregon was the only state that allowed PAS (see the box "Helping Terminally Ill Patients Die: Is It Legal? Is it Ethical?"). Because of the legal status of assisted suicide and active euthanasia, family members and physicians are unlikely to report their involvement, and there are no good statistics on the number of cases that occur each year. Also, because dying patients are often heavily dosed with drugs that have potentially lethal side effects, the immediate cause of death may not be certain.

The greatest acceptance of PAS and active euthanasia is currently found in the Netherlands. Decisions made during the 1970s and 1980s by Dutch courts and upheld by the Dutch parliament in 1993 formed a consensus that assisted suicide and active euthanasia would not be prosecuted as long as certain conditions were met. As a result, physicians are permitted to take active steps to end the lives of patients who request a "dignified death." The criteria established by Dutch courts and affirmed by the parliament include the presence of a confirmed terminal diagnosis; the patient's unwavering desire, confirmed in writing, of his or her wish to die; the presence of unbearable and incurable physical suffering; and a second medical opinion. It is estimated that about 3% of the approximately 130,000 deaths that occur annually in the Netherlands involve PAS or related practices.

Many people who endorse the philosophy of hospice and palliative care argue that adequate treatment for pain and depression usually eliminates the need to consider active measures to end a patient's life. According to this view, the distinction between allowing to die and helping to die ought to be maintained. If we wish to avoid the burden on ourselves and on medical practitioners of actively hastening patients' deaths, we must actively seek better ways of lifting the burden of suffering experienced by the dying.

Advance Directives

Living wills, natural death directives, and durable powers of attorney for health care—known collectively as **advance directives**—are increasingly important in medical decision making. Advance directives express the desire that medical heroics be avoided when death is imminent, that life-sustaining devices and extraordinary medical procedures not be used when there is no chance of recovery. Advance directives also protect physicians and hospitals from malpractice accusations and from civil liability or criminal prosecution when following a patient's directive to forgo medical heroics.

TERMS

passive euthanasia The practice of withholding (not initiating) or withdrawing (removing) life-prolonging but ultimately futile treatment, thereby allowing a terminally ill person to die naturally.

physician-assisted suicide The practice of a physician providing the means for a patient to commit suicide knowing that the patient intends to use it to end her or his life.

voluntary active euthanasia The practice of administering —at the request of a patient—medication or another intervention that causes death.

lethal injection The injection of a drug intended to result in death.

advance directive A document, such as a living will or durable power of attorney for health care, that is typically used to express a person's desire that life-sustaining devices or other medical heroics not be used when there is no chance of recovery and death is imminent.

living will A type of advance directive that enables individuals to provide instructions about the kind of medical care they wish to receive if they become incapacitated or otherwise unable to participate in treatment decisions at the end of life.

durable power of attorney for health care A legal instrument allowing one person to act as the agent of another person in making health care decisions regarding the withholding or withdrawal of life-sustaining treatment.

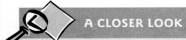 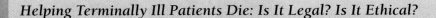

In September 1998, Michigan physician Dr. Jack Kevorkian used a lethal injection of drugs to end the life of Thomas Youk, a 52-year-old man with amyotrophic lateral sclerosis (Lou Gehrig's disease) who had requested Kevorkian's help in dying. A videotape of Youk's death was later shown on the television program *60 Minutes*. Although Kevorkian has admitted to participating in over 130 cases of physician-assisted suicide (PAS), the Youk case was the first instance where he administered the lethal drugs himself. For this case of voluntary active euthanasia, Kevorkian was convicted of second-degree murder. Kevorkian's participation in Youk's death and in earlier cases of PAS has been hotly debated in the medical and legal communities, fueling the arguments for and against legalized euthanasia.

Many patients facing a terminal illness may wish to end their pain and suffering by refusing medical treatment that prolongs life. As of 1990, this choice is sanctioned by law. In the case of *Cruzan v. Missouri*, the Supreme Court decided that a person has the right to refuse life-sustaining medical treatment. Subsequently, Congress passed the Patient Self-Determination Act (PSDA), which requires that all government-funded health care providers inform patients of their right to refuse medical treatment. Hospitals and physicians, then, are permitted to withhold or withdraw treatment when a patient is in a persistent vegetative state, with no chance of recovery, and when there is evidence that the person wants no life-prolonging treatment—for example, if the person communicated these wishes through an advance directive. Perhaps as a result of the *Cruzan v. Missouri* case, advance directives have become more popular.

Although the 1990 Supreme Court ruling permits withdrawal or noninitiation of treament, it does not allow people to assist actively in a patient's choice to die. In 1997, the U.S. Supreme Court upheld bans on PAS in New York and Washington, finding that terminally ill people do not have a broad constitutional right to a physician's help in dying. However, their decision left the door open for actions by states and for future lawsuits by terminally ill people. The only state that currently allows PAS is Oregon. First passed in 1994 but not implemented until 1997, the Oregon Death with Dignity Act allows a physician to prescribe life-ending drugs for a terminally ill patient. The law requires that the patient be a "capable" adult resident of Oregon who has less than 6 months to live and who voluntarily requests a prescription for lethal drugs. In the year after the law went into effect, 23 patients received prescriptions for lethal drugs under the Act.

The issue of suicide, whether assisted or not, is a complex one. On the whole, Americans value quality of life, humane treatment for pain and suffering, and the right of free choice for individuals. At the same time, society places a high value on the very nature of life, and Americans tend to fear the consequences of condoning suicide. To many people, it simply seems unethical to accept death as a solution, because it devalues human life. Attitudes toward suicide are also shaped by religion. Christian doctrine holds that humans have no inherent right to control their own death. So suicide, whether assisted or not, runs contrary to most religious belief in America.

Attitudes are also shaped by our views toward physicians and the health care system in America. Some people fear that if assisted suicide or active euthanasia becomes legal, health care workers may abuse patients' trust or that errors in judgment will result in unnecessary deaths. Many people believe that sanctioning assisted suicide will negate the advances in medical science that offer hope to terminally ill patients. Cures may arrive before a patient dies, or advances in pain management may sufficiently relieve a patient's discomfort and enhance his or her quality of life. Finally, there is concern that the growing "right to die" movement may be a response to rising health care costs: Patients may look to death as a solution only because the expense of medical treatment may be burdensome.

In spite of these attitudes, many Americans seem to believe that people have the right to terminate their lives and to seek help in doing so. A 1998 poll found that nearly 70% of Americans approved of the Oregon law and wanted a similar law in their own state. In view of the strong feelings on both sides of this issue, assisted suicide and active euthanasia are likely to remain the subject of heated debate in the years ahead.

Originally, **living wills** had no force in law. They were merely an expression of a person's wishes. During the late 1970s, however, state legislatures began to consider laws that would require physicians to honor patients' desires at the end of life. Most states now have some type of legislation regarding advance directives, although laws vary from state to state. Whether the wishes expressed by a patient are followed may depend on the policies of a given health care institution and standard practices within a community or state jurisdiction. Uncertainty about the projected course of an illness or a disease may cause physicians to be wary of declaring that a patient is terminal.

Completing a **durable power of attorney for health care** provides an additional safeguard that an individual's preferences about life-sustaining treatment will be followed (Figure 20-1). This document allows a person to designate an agent who is empowered to make health care decisions with respect to the withholding or withdrawal of life-sustaining treatment. The designated person might be a spouse, adult offspring, or friend with whom one has discussed treatment preferences. An agent must act in accordance with a patient's wishes as specifically stated in the document or as otherwise made known.

Although advance directives can safeguard a patient's autonomy and minimize conflict in a critical care situation, these directives are useless if physicians and hospital staff members do not know of their existence. Some advocates suggest that hospitals have a policy to routinely ask patients whether they have completed an advance

FLORIDA LIVING WILL

Declaration made this _____ day of _____, 19___.

I, _____, willfully and voluntarily make known my desire that my dying not be artificially prolonged under the circumstances set forth below, and I do hereby declare:

If at any time I have a terminal condition and if my attending or treating physician and another consulting physician have determined that there is no medical probability of my recovery from such condition, I direct that life-prolonging procedures be withheld or withdrawn when the application of such procedures would serve only to prolong artificially the process of dying, and that I be permitted to die naturally with only the administration of medication or the performance of any medical procedure deemed necessary to provide me with comfort care or to alleviate pain.

It is my intention that this declaration be honored by my family and physician as the final expression of my legal right to refuse medical or surgical treatment and to accept the consequences for such refusal.
In the event that I have been determined to be unable to provide express and informed consent regarding the withholding, withdrawal, or continuation of life-prolonging procedures, I wish to designate, as my surrogate to carry out the provisions of this declaration:

Name: _____
Address: _____
_____ Zip Code: _____
Phone: _____

I wish to designate the following person as my alternate surrogate, to carry out the provisions of this declaration should my surrogate be unwilling or unable to act on my behalf:

Name: _____
Address: _____
_____ Zip Code: _____
Phone: _____

Additional instructions (optional):

I understand the full import of this declaration, and I am emotionally and mentally competent to make this declaration.

Signed: _____

Witness 1:
    Signed: _____
    Address: _____
Witness 2:
    Signed: _____
    Address: _____

Figure 20-1   Sample advance directives. The document on the left is a living will; the document on the right is a durable power of attorney for health care. Because of differences in state law, each state has its own format for advance directives; the samples shown here are for Florida.   SOURCE: Reprinted by permission of Choice in Dying, 200 Varick St., New York, NY 10014 (212-366-5540). © 1996 Choice in Dying, Inc.

directive. Not only would such a policy bring existing documents to light, it would also give the patient an opportunity to revise those portions of the directives that no longer accurately express his or her treatment preferences. Another suggestion is the use of wallet cards and bracelets (similar to those used for Medic Alert) to signify that an individual has completed an advance directive. This could be especially worthwhile in situations when life-sustaining treatment is routinely initiated (as by paramedics at a car crash scene) or when a person is unable to express his or her wishes about the desirability of such treatment.

The Patient Self-Determination Act (PSDA) of 1990 requires that health care providers who receive federal Medicare funds—including hospitals, skilled nursing facilities, home health agencies, hospice programs, and health maintenance organizations (HMOs)—take specific actions relative to advance directives. These actions in-clude informing patients in writing of their rights regarding advance directives and treatment decisions, and documenting the existence of an advance directive in a patient's medical record. The PSDA has been described as a "medical Miranda warning" (referring to the requirement that police officers advise arrested suspects of their rights) because of its insistence that patients be advised of their rights regarding advance directives and life-sustaining treatment.

PERSONAL INSIGHT   How do you think you'd feel if someone you loved were terminally ill and in pain and asked to be allowed to die? What would you do? How do you think you'd feel if a friend told you he or she wanted to die because of depression and an inability to cope with life's problems? What would you do?

FLORIDA DESIGNATION OF HEALTH CARE SURROGATE

Name: _____
      (Last)   _(First)_   _(Middle Initial)_

In the event that I have been determined to be incapacitated to provide informed consent for medical treatment and surgical and diagnostic procedures, I wish to designate as my surrogate for health care decisions:

Name: _____
Address: _____
_____ Zip Code: _____
Phone: _____

If my surrogate is unwilling or unable to perform his duties, I wish to designate as my alternate surrogate:

Name: _____
Address: _____
_____ Zip Code: _____
Phone: _____

I fully understand that this designation will permit my designee to make health care decisions and to provide, withhold, or withdraw consent on my behalf; to apply for public benefits to defray the cost of health care; and to authorize my admission to or transfer from a health care facility.

Additional instructions (optional):

I further affirm that this designation is not being made as a condition of treatment or admission to a health care facility. I will notify and send a copy of this document to the following persons other than my surrogate, so they may know who my surrogate is:

Name: _____
Address: _____

Name: _____
Address: _____

Signed: _____
Date: _____

Witness 1:
Signed: _____
Address: _____

Witness 2:
Signed: _____
Address: _____

Figure 20-1 Sample advance directives (continued).

Donating Organs

A human body is a valuable resource. Of all the recent advances in medical techniques for helping patients who were formerly considered beyond recovery, probably the best known and most widely accepted is the transplantation of human organs. Eye corneas can be transplanted to give sight to persons who are blind. Donated kidneys can give years of vigorous life to people whose own have stopped working. Human skin is the best dressing for burn wounds. Perhaps the most dramatic organ transplants are those involving the heart. The increasing success of transplants has made them a feasible option for more patients, and more people are on waiting lists for organs than ever before (Figure 20-2, p. 557). Although some people may find the thought of donating organs unsettling, the procedures are not very different from those used in routine autopsies and normal preparation for burial.

A widely used method for donating body parts is through the **Uniform Donor Card,** which is available from the National Kidney Foundation (Figure 20-3, p. 557). In some states, the desire to donate organs can be communicated by use of a card attached to a person's driver's license. Besides specifying how one's body may be used after death, the donor may also specify the final disposition of his or her remains once the donation has been completed. Many donations are authorized by relatives at the time of a loved one's death. Plans for organ or body donation should be discussed with members of your family so that they are aware of your wishes and can help see that they are fulfilled.

Uniform Donor Card A consent form authorizing the use of the signer's body parts for transplantation or medical research upon his or her death. **TERMS**

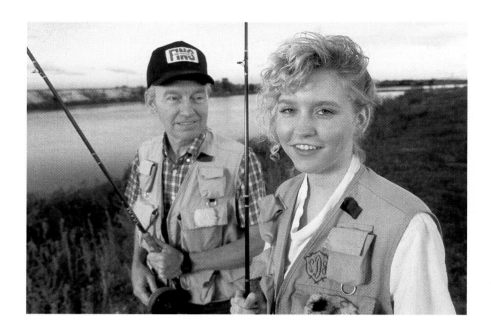

Organ transplants give hope to those who would otherwise have died. After recovering from a heart-lung transplant, this young woman is on a camping trip with her father.

Certification of Death

Following death, the deceased's family must obtain copies of the death certificate signed by a physician, medical examiner, or **coroner.** Required by all legal jurisdictions in the United States, the death certificate constitutes legal proof of death and affects the disposition of property rights, life insurance benefits, pension payments, and so on. The typical death certificate now in use includes four different *modes* of death: accident, suicide, homicide, and natural. The *cause* of death is not necessarily the same as the mode of death. For example, if a death is caused by asphyxiation due to drowning, it can be classified as an accident, a suicide, or a homicide. Any of these modes might apply.

If a person dies unexpectedly (even of natural causes), or from a rare or highly researched disease, the medical staff may request an **autopsy,** which involves surgically opening the body, examining the organs of interest, and perhaps removing certain body parts for further study. If the cause of death occurred under questionable or suspicious circumstances, the coroner will require an autopsy.

Otherwise, permission from the next of kin must be obtained before an autopsy can be performed.

Deciding What to Do with the Body

Most people have a preference about how their body will be disposed of when they die. For Americans, this decision usually involves either burial or cremation. *Burial* can be in a single grave dug into the soil or entombment in a multitiered mausoleum. *Cremation* involves burning a body to its bones by intense heat. Cremated remains can be buried, entombed, kept by the family, or scattered at sea or on land, in accordance with state and local laws. If a body or organ donation has been made, burial or cremation will take place once the donation procedures have been completed. Depending on the type of funeral ceremony desired, a body destined for burial or cremation may or may not be embalmed.

Decisions about how one's body will be disposed of after death are best considered early in life while a person is healthy and able to gather the necessary information about available choices. If no such plans are made, decisions must be made by family or friends (see the box "Tasks for Survivors" on page 558).

Thought should also be given to how funeral and body disposition costs will be paid. Depending on the options selected, the cost of a funeral ranges upward from about $600. The least expensive choices involve direct cremation or immediate burial, with no viewing of the body and no funeral ceremony. The average cost of a traditional funeral, not including cemetery costs, is about $5500. Cemetery plots have a wide range of prices, from less than $100 to more than $5000. The cost of entombment in a mausoleum or outdoor crypt averages about $2000. Vet-

TERMS **coroner** A public official who investigates the causes of deaths and helps police with crimes involving death.

autopsy Dissection and examination of a dead body to determine cause of death or to investigate the extent and nature of changes caused by disease; also performed in connection with medical research and training.

memorial society A nonprofit membership group that provides no-frills, economical burial or cremation.

embalming Removing blood and other fluids from a body and replacing them with chemicals to disinfect and temporarily retard deterioration of the corpse.

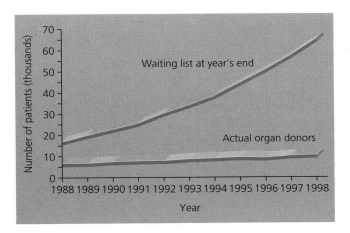

Figure 20-2 The need for organ donors. As organ transplants have become an option for more and more patients, the number of people waiting for transplants has increased. The number of actual donations has not grown nearly so significantly. SOURCE: United Network for Organ Sharing (http://www.unos.org).

UNIFORM DONOR CARD

of_____
(print or type name of donor)

In the hope that I may help others, I hereby make this anatomical gift, if medically acceptable, to take effect upon my death. The words and marks below indicate my wishes.

I give: ☐ _____ any needed organs or parts
☐ _____ only the following organs or parts

_____
(specify the organ(s), tissue(s) or part(s))

for the purposes of transplantation, therapy, medical research or education;

☐ _____ my body for anatomical study if needed

Limitations or special wishes, if any: _____

Signed by the donor and the following two witnesses in the presence of each other:

_____   _____
Signature of Donor   Date of Birth of Donor

_____   _____
Date Signed   City and State

_____   _____
Witness   Witness

This is a legal document under the Anatomical Gift Act or similar laws.
☐ Yes, I have discussed my wishes with my family.
For further information consult your physician or

NKF **National Kidney Foundation**
30 East 33rd Street, New York, NY 10016

Figure 20-3 A sample organ donor card. SOURCE: Uniform Donor Card. Copyright © 1996 the National Kidney Foundation, Inc. Reprinted with permission.

erans may be eligible for burial in a national cemetery, an option that can reduce costs.

Of all funeral costs, people usually feel the most important is that of the casket because of its symbolic and emotional value in honoring the deceased. The choices range from inexpensive cardboard containers to solid mahogany, copper, or bronze caskets costing $10,000 or more. Caskets made of plywood and covered with cloth typically cost about $300–$1000. Gasketed steel caskets, the most popular option with Americans, are available at prices ranging from $1000 to $8000.

In the United States, most people choose some form of traditional funeral service followed by burial. However, concerns about the cost of this traditional approach to body disposal have created an interest in alternatives. One response has been the rise of **memorial societies,** nonprofit groups that help members prearrange simple, economical burial or cremation. Those who choose this plan often prefer a no-frills funeral service or perhaps only a simple memorial service. Conventional funeral establishments have also responded to the widespread desire for a less costly alternative to the traditional funeral by offering burial and cremation plans similar to those available through memorial societies. The result is a wide range of choices to meet the diverse needs and wishes of consumers.

Planning a Funeral or Memorial Service

Survivors generally benefit from participating in a ceremony to mark the death of a loved one. The choice of funeral rites may involve a traditional funeral ceremony or a simple memorial service. Although some people prefer no service, bereaved friends and relatives usually want

an opportunity to mark their grief through ritual and ceremony. Ideally, last rites and body disposition will be planned in agreement with the wishes and needs of the survivors.

A typical American Christian funeral ceremony involves **embalming** the corpse, viewing the body in the funeral home before the funeral service, a religious ceremony with the body present, and a processional to the graveside where a brief final ceremony is held. Other religious traditions follow different practices, as do other ethnic groups. There are many ways of constructing a meaningful funeral or memorial service.

Funeral practices in Hawaii are a good example of cultural diversity. Historically, each of the ethnic groups in Hawaii added its own distinctive customs to a unique cultural mix. For example, the native Hawaiian tradition of feasting at important ceremonial events is widespread among Hawaii's residents. Mourners often gather after the funeral ceremony to share food and conversation. Similarly, most funeral announcements in Hawaii include the notice "Aloha attire requested," and mourners respond by wearing colorful clothing, as well as fragrant and beautiful flower leis. In traditional Hawaiian culture, such leis carry symbolic meanings. The *hala* lei is associated with

Some of the following tasks must be attended to soon after a death occurs; others take weeks or months to complete. Many of these tasks, especially those that need to be dealt with in the first hours and days following the death, can be taken care of by friends and relatives of the immediate survivors.

- Prepare a list of relatives, close friends, and business colleagues, and arrange to telephone them about the death as soon as possible. Friends can help with the notification process.

- Find out whether the deceased left instructions or made plans for disposition of the body or for a funeral or memorial service.

- If no prior plan exists, contact a mortuary or memorial society for help in making arrangements. Clergy, friends, and other family members can be asked to help decide what is most appropriate.

- If flowers are to be omitted from the funeral or memorial service, choose an appropriate charity or other memorial to which gifts can be made.

- Write the obituary. Include the deceased's age, place of birth, cause of death, occupation, academic degrees, memberships, military service record, accomplishments, names and relationships of nearest survivors, and an announcement of the time and place of the funeral or memorial service.

- Arrange for family members or close friends to take turns welcoming those who come to express their condolences

in person and responding to those who telephone their condolences.

- Ask friends to help coordinate the supplying of meals for the first few days following the death, as well as the management of other household tasks and child care, if necessary.

- Arrange hospitality for relatives and friends who are visiting from out of town.

- If a funeral ceremony is planned, choose the individuals who are to be pallbearers, and notify them that you would like their participation.

- Notify the lawyer, accountant, and other personal representatives who will be helping to settle the deceased's estate.

- Send handwritten or printed notes of acknowledgment to the people who have provided assistance or who have sent flowers, contributions, or their condolences.

- With the help of a lawyer or an accountant, review all insurance policies as well as other sources of potential death benefits, such as Social Security, military service, fraternal organizations, and unions.

- Review all debts, mortgages, and installment payments. Some may carry clauses that cancel debt in the event of death. If payments must be delayed, contact creditors to arrange for a grace period.

---

the breath (*ha*) and connotes passing away or dying; the ginger or *'awapuhi* lei symbolizes things that pass too soon. By merging funeral customs with their own distinctive cultural traditions, Hawaii's residents create a unique expression of local identity and community feeling.

THE EXPERIENCE OF LIFE-THREATENING ILLNESS

People with life-threatening illnesses face costly medical care coupled with their own loss of income, repeated and often lengthy hospitalization, and the emotional havoc that accompanies the news of a potentially terminal condition. The emotional response to life-threatening illness can include anguish, a sense of hopelessness, depression, and feelings of isolation and loneliness. Gathering information about the disease and its treatment, sharing one's experience in settings where mutual support can be provided, and finding ways of communicating more clearly with caregivers as well as with family and friends—these are all examples of positive approaches to dealing with life-threatening illnesses.

Coping with Dying

How do people come to terms with the prospect of dying? When death confronts us squarely, even if we have come to some degree of acceptance, we may yet hope for a last-minute reprieve. The way each of us copes with dying will likely resemble the ways we have coped with living and with other losses in our lives.

Kübler-Ross's Stage Theory   After talking with hundreds of dying people, Dr. Elisabeth Kübler-Ross identified several common, although not inevitable, psychological stages that people experience while coping with the prospect of imminent death. She described this coping process in her landmark 1968 book, *On Death and Dying*. In an idealized model, an early period of shock, disbelief, and denial eventually gives way to some degree of acceptance. It should be emphasized that not everyone experiences each of the psychological stages, or states, listed below, nor are they necessarily experienced in the same order or for the same duration. Indeed, some reactions may be experienced simultaneously, and there is a cycling between the various states during different phases of the

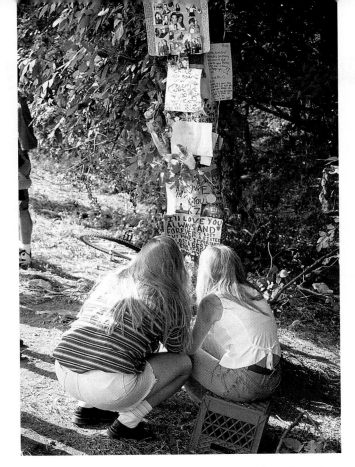

Death can challenge our sense of emotional and intellectual security, particularly the sudden death of a young person. This roadside marker was placed in memory of people killed in an automobile crash at this site.

illness. Dealing with these intense emotions can enable the dying person eventually to arrive at a personal sense of acceptance with respect to his or her impending death.

• *Denial and isolation.* The initial stage of coping with terminal illness is characterized as a temporary state of shock in which people deny the fact of death and isolate themselves from further confrontation with it. They say "Not me" and insist "It can't be." Denial is a useful coping mechanism because it acts as a buffer against shock and allows time for the mobilization of other defenses.

• *Anger.* When the truth can no longer be denied, anger often follows. People ask "Why me?" and may lash out at family members, their physicians, and the hospital staff—blaming them for the situation. Anger is a normal response to disability and the loss of control over one's life and situation.

• *Bargaining.* As a means of marshaling what hope remains, people often try to find a way out. A common scenario involves making promises to God in exchange for a prolonged life. The intense desire to find an "out" can also cause people to become vulnerable to medical quackery.

• *Depression.* When people begin to accept their fate and face the reality of their impending death, they may become depressed about things that will be left unfinished in their lives and all they are leaving behind. Depression is a natural part of grief as a person strives to prepare for separation from this world.

• *Acceptance.* People facing their own death may eventually come to some resolution about their situation. It often seems that they are able to suspend judgment or expectations about the future and simply appreciate the present. Acknowledging that they are ultimately not in control of their future, they seem content to make the best of what comes their way. At the end, when death is near, they may choose not to talk much with visitors, even family members and close friends. This, too, is part of letting go.

A Task-Based Approach The stage-based model of coping with dying devised by Kübler-Ross has been an important stimulus to increasing our understanding of dying and death. It has directed caregivers and lay people alike to a thoughtful consideration of issues related to dying. We should be aware, however, that a person's way of coping with dying will differ according to his or her individual traits and particular situation. It can be useful to examine the perspective offered by a task-based approach. As described by theorist Charles Corr, this approach distinguishes four primary tasks in coping with dying:

1. *Physical:* Satisfying bodily needs and minimizing physical distress.
2. *Psychological:* Maximizing a sense of security, autonomy, and richness in living.
3. *Social:* Sustaining significant relationships and addressing the social implications of dying.
4. *Spiritual:* Identifying, developing, or reaffirming sources of meaning and, in so doing, fostering hope.

There is no single "right" way to cope with dying. But better or worse models, from the standpoint of those involved, may exist. Any model is a general description of the coping process, not a schedule to be strictly followed or imposed on a particular situation. In actuality, the way a person will live his or her final weeks and days cannot be predicted. Changing circumstances may make it seem as if the dying person is tossed from one emotion to another and then back again. The point to remember is that a dying person will not and should not behave in some prescribed fashion; rather, each person's patterns of coping should be respected.

Supporting a Dying Person

Most people feel somewhat uncomfortable in the presence of a person who has been diagnosed with a terminal illness. What can we say? How should we act? It may

These suggestions can help you provide effective support for someone facing a life-threatening illness:

- Be honest about your own thoughts, concerns, and feelings.

- When in doubt, ask questions: "How is that for you?" "Can you tell me more about that?" "Am I intruding?"

- When you are responding to a person facing a crisis situation, be sure to use statements such as "I feel . . ." "I believe . . ." or "I would want . . ." rather than "You should . . ." "That's wrong" or "Everything will be OK." Give the person the opportunity to express her or his own unique needs and feelings.

- Stay in the present as much as possible. Ask, "How do you feel right now?" or "What do you need right now?"

- Listening is profoundly healing. You don't have to make it better. You don't have to have the answers. You don't have to take away the pain.

- People in crisis need to know they have decision-making power. It may be appropriate to point out alternatives.

- Offer any practical assistance you feel comfortable providing. If appropriate, refer the individual to a counselor or agency for more help.

SOURCE: Adapted from the Centre for Living with Dying (554 Mansion Park Dr., Santa Clara, CA 95050; 408-980-9801).

seem that any attempt to provide comfort results in words that are little more than stale platitudes. Nevertheless, we want to express our concern and make meaningful contact. Perhaps the most important gift we can bring to the person who is confronting his or her own death is the gift of listening. Giving the person an opportunity to speak honestly and openly about his or her experience is crucial, even though talking about death may be painful at first (see the box "Your Caring Presence").

Although we sometimes tend to place dying people in a special category, the reality is that their needs are not fundamentally different from anyone else's, although their situation is perhaps more urgent. As is true of anyone, dying people want to know that they are valued, that they are not alone, that they are not being unfairly judged, and that those close to them are also trying to come to terms with a difficult situation. As with any relationship, there are opportunities for growth on both sides.

Besides friends and family, the dying person may want access to other supportive resources. These might include the family physician, counselors, and clergy. Many hospitals, hospices, and other health care organizations sponsor group programs for dying patients. These groups are usually chaired by a professional counselor and are designed to help patients express their concerns in a supportive atmosphere. You can make contact with groups of this kind by inquiring among hospital staff members or other health care workers. In addition, local chapters of support groups affiliated with organizations such as the American Cancer Society and Make Today Count can be found in many cities.

COPING WITH LOSS

Even if we have not experienced the death of someone close, all of us are survivors of the various losses that have occurred in our lives. Death is not the only kind of loss that calls upon our resources for coping; everyone experiences the losses that accompany changes and endings. The loss of a job, the ending of a relationship, transitions from one neighborhood or school to another—all these are examples of the kinds of losses that fill our lives. Some people call these losses "little deaths," and our response to them, although less painful perhaps, includes many of the mental and emotional reactions that occur in connection with the death of loved ones.

Experiencing Grief

Grief encompasses a person's response to the event of loss; it includes emotions, mental perceptions, and physical reactions. Among the emotions that may be part of a survivor's grief are not only sorrow and sadness, but also relief, anger, disgust, and self-pity. Limiting our definition of grief reduces the chances of accepting all of the responses that may be present. When we recognize that many kinds of feelings occur in grief—not just feelings of sadness—then we are likely to be better able to accept our grief and move toward its resolution. Grieving is the means to healing.

The type of death—whether natural, accidental, homicide, or suicide—influences experience of grief, as does the survivor's previous experience with that type of death. Consider the ways in which people die: the aged grandmother, dying quietly in her sleep; the young child pronounced DOA after a bicycle crash; the innocent bystander caught in the crossfire of violence; the chronically ill person who dies a "lingering death"; the despon-

TERMS   **grief** The emotions, mental perceptions, and physical reactions a person experiences in response to a loss.

dent executive who commits suicide. The mode and circumstances of a death influence a survivor's manner of dealing with the loss. Sudden deaths that occur in the context of specific kinds of events—war, for example—result in a particular set of circumstances that affects how survivors deal with the loss.

Some people believe that, when death is anticipated, as in the case of chronic illness, it is easier to cope with than when death occurs without warning. But this is not always true. When a person dies after a long period of illness, survivors often experience both relief that the ordeal is over and anguish because a beloved relationship has come to an end. Thus, having foreknowledge that a death is likely to occur does not necessarily mean that grief will be diminished when the loss becomes real.

Talking and crying, even yelling in rage, are ways of resolving the intense feelings of grief. Don't try to hold back feelings or be "strong" and "brave." Those who offer such advice do not understand the dynamics of grief, nor the necessity for grief to be expressed as a way of healing. On the other hand, you needn't pretend to grieve or exaggerate your emotions if the strong feelings that often accompany grief simply aren't present in your particular experience.

Although various models have been proposed to summarize the processes associated with grief, each person's actual experience is highly individual. We can use such models as an aid to understanding grief, but it is important that we do not try to superimpose a rigid structure on our own or another's experience.

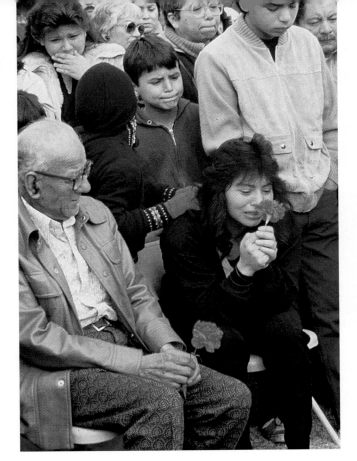

Funeral or memorial services give friends and relatives of the deceased the opportunity to mark their grief through ritual and ceremony.

Phases of Grief   In the aftermath of a death, the early period of grief is characterized by shock and numbness, often with strong feelings of disbelief and denial. The sense of disorganization that pervades our mental and emotional life during this period is challenged by the need to attend to the various actions and decisions surrounding the disposition of the deceased's body. Being forced to engage in such activities is therapeutic; it helps us accept the reality of the death, thereby taking us beyond the initial period of shock and into the intense adjustment that is at the heart of coping with loss.

The middle phase of grief is a period of deeply experiencing the pain of separation. The bustle of activities that takes place immediately after a death begins to lessen, and friends are usually not as accessible as they had been during the initial crisis. This is often a time of intense yearning for the lost loved one, an intense reexamination of the whole relationship as the bonds of attachment are slowly relinquished. Survivors experience fantasies of somehow "undoing" the loss, making everything as it was before. This phase of grief generally lasts from several weeks to several months. It is during this period that many physiological symptoms associated with intense grief are experienced: lethargy, restlessness, disturbed sleep, lack of appetite, and weight loss.

As survivors and as caring helpers, we need to keep in mind that social support is every bit as critical during this phase of grief as during the early days following the loss. To go through the psychological process of mourning, the bereaved person needs to express his or her feelings. As the reality of the loss is absorbed, the predominant feeling will likely be sadness. By gradually undoing the bonds of the lost relationship through intense grieving, emotions are slowly freed for reinvestment in life (see the box "Coping with Grief" on page 562).

The last phase of "active" grief is characterized as a period of resolution, a time of reestablishing our physical and emotional balance, of reintegration. The acute feelings and emotional turmoil of grief are no longer experienced constantly. Our sadness doesn't go away completely, but it recedes into the background. Reminders will stimulate the pain of loss from time to time, but we begin to move ahead with life and focus more on present concerns, not past memories. This newfound sense of freedom can be difficult to admit at first; it may feel like a betrayal of the deceased loved one. In fact, it indicates a healthy willingness to engage once again in the outside world. Coming to terms with grief does not mean forgetting the loved one or denying the significance of the lost relationship. At var-

- Realize and recognize the loss.
- Take time for nature's slow, sure process of healing.
- Give yourself massive doses of restful relaxation and routine busy-ness.
- Know that powerful, overwhelming feelings will change with time.
- Be vulnerable, share your pain, and be humble enough to accept support.
- Surround yourself with life: plants, animals, and friends.
- Use mementos to help your mourning, not to live in the past.
- Avoid rebound relationships, big decisions, and substances that could cause dependence.

- Keep a diary, and record your successes, memories, and struggles.
- Prepare for change, new interests, new friends, solitude, creativity, and growth.
- Recognize that forgiveness (of ourselves and others) is a vital part of the healing process.
- Know that holidays and anniversaries can bring up the painful feelings you thought you had successfully worked through.
- Realize that any new death-related crisis will bring up feelings about past losses.

SOURCE: The Centre for Living with Dying (554 Mansion Park Dr., Santa Clara, CA 95050; 408-980-9801).

ious times throughout our lives, reminders of the loss can stimulate a recurrence of grief; as time passes, however, this happens with diminishing frequency and intensity.

The Tasks of Grief A model devised by psychologist William Worden provides a summary overview of the process of coping with loss. This model encompasses four tasks:

1. *Accepting the reality* of the loss, and making the transition from present to past tense.

2. *Working through the pain* of grief, without "deadening" the pain through the abuse of alcohol or drugs.

3. *Adjusting to a changed environment* in which the deceased is missing, a task that may take considerable time, especially when a relationship was of long duration and exceptional closeness.

4. *Emotionally relocating the deceased and moving on with life.*

The fourth task can seem problematic, because it seems to involve a dishonoring of the deceased's memory or because of anxiety about investing emotional energy into another relationship that could also end in loss. Working through this task involves the recognition that, although one does not love the deceased person any less, there are also other people to be loved. Thus, grief is a process by which the bereaved incorporates a loss into his or her ongoing life. In some cultural settings, this occurs in the context of rituals that locate the deceased in the realm of beloved ancestors. In others, it means keeping a special place for the deceased in one's heart and mind. In this sense, keeping a continuing bond with the deceased is not viewed as an aberration in grieving that needs to be rectified; rather, it is testimony to the enduring strength of love.

Supporting a Grieving Person

A variety of activities, rituals, and social institutions can help survivors cope with loss. Social support provided by relatives and friends can be a major source of strength for the bereaved. The simple gift of listening can be extremely helpful, because talking about a loss is an important way that survivors cope with their changed reality. The key to being a good listener is to refrain from making judgments about whether the feelings expressed by the survivor are "right" or "wrong," "good" or "bad." The feelings generated by a loss are not necessarily the ones we might expect, but they are valid in terms of a particular survivor's total response to loss.

Funerals and similar leave-taking rituals can provide a sense of closure on the deceased person's life and can help survivors integrate the loss into their ongoing lives. In some societies, funerals provide an opportunity for the bereaved not only to express their sadness at losing a loved one, but also to vent their anger at the deceased's abandonment of them: "Why did you leave me? I need you!" This practice of scolding the corpse stands in contrast to the Western cultural notion that one should not speak ill of the dead. In modern American society, there are different styles of mourning behavior among different regional or ethnic groups. For one group, funerals are occasions of weeping and wailing; for another, stoic expressions and subdued emotions are the rule.

Although family and friends may be very supportive during the initial period following a death, the extended need for support that continues throughout the first year or two of mourning may not be met by relying solely on those traditional sources of support. Organized support groups offer a helpful way for bereaved people to share their concerns and empathy with one another as they come to terms with loss. Perhaps the best known of the organized support groups are those that focus on the concerns of widows and widowers. Other support groups provide support for particular types of loss. The Compassionate Friends organization, for example, serves parents who have experienced a child's death. Hospital or hospice social workers and community service organizations can provide referrals to appropriate support groups.

Helping Children Cope with Loss

How can we offer help to a bereaved child? Adults are sometimes uncomfortable about exposing children to painful or disturbing news, but a child's natural curiosity usually eliminates the option of withholding information. Children tend to cope more easily with death when they are allowed to be part of their family's experience of grief and mourning. Sharing the reality of what is happening teaches a child to begin to understand and cope with the experience.

In responding to a child's questions about death, one should not overwhelm the child with excessive detail, nor talk down to the child as if he or she were incapable of comprehending at all. Responses should be framed in a way that addresses the child's concerns within the context of his or her own ability to understand. Keep the explanation simple, stick to basics, and always verify what the child has understood.

Children generalize from known concepts to make new experiences fit. This may result in a very literal-minded interpretation of new information, especially among young children. Avoid metaphorical explanations that might lead to confusion in the child's mind. When religious beliefs are important to parents' understanding of death, they will naturally want to share these beliefs with their children. Although children may be comforted by such notions, they need to be told that these are *beliefs*. An adult's concept of an afterlife, for example, may be quite different from what a child is able to understand from a metaphorical explanation.

When children are asked about their experiences of crises involving death, many say that the most difficult times occurred when they did not know what was happening. Sudden changes in family communication patterns can alarm a child and heighten anxiety. The best gauge of a child's readiness to be informed about a potentially painful situation is the child's own interest, usually expressed through questions. Above all, children in crisis situations need to be reassured that they are loved.

COMING TO TERMS WITH DEATH

For many of us, death has been kept out of view, a fearful possibility that we avoid at all costs. With the death of a friend or a relative, or perhaps with the news of a major disaster, we are forced to confront our emotions, our rela-

tionship with the experience that awaits all of us at the end of life. Encountering death can help make us more aware of the preciousness of life. Survivors of the Nazi death camps during World War II have repeatedly expressed this theme in their writings. Many had been condemned to death and were awaiting execution. Yet they found that the confrontation with death liberated them from petty personal concerns that had once seemed overwhelming. People who have come near death as a result of serious illness or injury or other catastrophes report a similar awakening to what is ultimately valuable in life.

In facing death, we find that relationships are more important than things; priorities are reordered, as we cope with the painful reality of loss. Realizing that life offers no guarantees, we find ourselves able to overcome our own anxieties and petty concerns, as well as the social structures that stop us from living more fully.

Examining our assumptions about death leads us to a discovery of its meaning in our own lives. Denying death eventually results in denying life. This denial is inherent in our news reports, where only the deaths of the famous or violent deaths get attention, and then only for a moment. In societies where each individual is considered important and irreplaceable, death is not ignored but is marked by community-wide grief for a genuine social loss. When we stop avoiding death, we find that it is an event whose significance touches not only the individual and his or her immediate family and friends, but also the wider community of which we are all part.

> **PERSONAL INSIGHT** If you were told you had a short time to live, what would you do—withdraw, try to tie up loose ends, try to satisfy unfulfilled desires or have new experiences, try to take care of others, make no changes? Why do you think you would react this way?

SUMMARY

What Is Death?

- The traditional criteria for defining death focus on vital signs such as breathing and heartbeat.

- Brain death is characterized by a lack of receptivity and response to external stimuli; the absence of spontaneous muscular movement and spontaneous breathing; the absence of observable reflexes; and the absence of brain activity, signified by a flat EEG.

- Clinical death refers to a determination of death made according to either the traditional signs of death or the criteria used in defining brain death. Cellular death refers to the breakdown of metabolic processes in the cells when heartbeat, respiration, and brain activity cease.

- Although death makes logical sense in terms of species survival and evolution, to many people, no answer to the question of why death exists can ever be completely satisfying.
- From about age 10, most children understand that death is universal, inescapable, and irreversible.
- Ambivalence toward death is a common component of suicide. A psychological autopsy is used to uncover the factors that led to a particular suicide.
- Religion plays a major role in shaping people's attitudes and behaviors toward death.

Planning for Death

- Some decisions about death can and should be made while one is young.
- A will is a legal instrument governing the distribution of a person's property after his or her death.
- Dying at home requires considerable time and energy from relatives or friends who must also learn the techniques of home care.
- Palliative care devoted to making dying patients comfortable and pain-free is available in many hospitals.
- The hospice philosophy of care stresses a team approach in providing palliative care to dying patients and relies to a large extent on volunteer help.
- A terminal patient can grant power of attorney to a trusted friend or relative to handle matters affecting the patient if he or she becomes incapacitated or otherwise unable to attend to legal matters.
- Passive euthanasia refers to the practice of withdrawing or withholding life-sustaining treatment.
- Assisted suicide involves providing a patient with the means of taking her or his own life; in active voluntary euthanasia, someone other than the patient administers the fatal treatment (at the patient's request).
- Advance directives are vehicles for expressing one's wishes about the use of life-sustaining measures.

- People can donate their bodies or individual organs for use after death.
- For Americans, the decision about what to do with the body after death usually involves either burial or cremation.
- It is generally agreed that bereaved people benefit from participating in a funeral ceremony or memorial service to commemorate a loved one's death.

The Experience of Life-Threatening Illness

- Facing death is a difficult and painful experience. Although the dying must find their own way of adapting to the changes they face, they can benefit from the help of others.
- Responses to one's own imminent death vary greatly, although periods of denial and isolation, anger, bargaining, depression, and acceptance are commonly experienced.
- Those who wish to offer support to a dying person should consider that person's unique needs. Giving the dying person opportunities to speak openly is crucial.

Coping with Loss

- Grief encompasses a person's response to the event of loss, and it can include a variety of feelings.
- Social support provided by relatives and friends is a major source of strength for the bereaved.
- Children tend to cope with death more easily when they are allowed to be part of their family's experience of grief and mourning.

Coming to Terms with Death

- Encountering death can help make a person more aware of the preciousness and precariousness of life.
- Death touches not only the individual and his or her family and friends, but also the wider community.

TAKE ACTION

1. In some states, the Department of Motor Vehicles provides organ donor forms. If your state doesn't provide them, you can request a donor card from the National Kidney Foundation (800-622-9010; http://www.kidney.org), the Coalition on Donation (800-355-7427), or the Department of Health and Human Services (http://www.organdonor.gov). When you receive the donor form, consider the advantages and disadvantages of being a donor. If you decide to be a donor, fill out the card, and keep it with your driver's license.

2. Obtain sample copies of advance directives that are appropriate for the state you live in. Check with your local hospital or health services organization for these forms, or request them from Choice in Dying (800-989-WILL; http://www.choices.org). Review the forms, and consider the advantages and disadvantages of using them. If you decide to execute a living will or durable power of attorney for health care, discuss your decision with members of your family to make them aware of your wishes.

3. Talk with your spouse, parents, grandparents, or other family members about their wishes for how they would want things to be at the end of their lives. Ask if they have made out wills or advance directives. If they do not wish to discuss these matters, let them know that you are open to such a discussion in the future.

4. Investigate the services available in your community to care for the dying, including hospitals, hospices, and counseling resources. Visit one or more of them, and evaluate their services.

1. What do you believe happens after death—heaven or hell, eternal sleep, nothingness, return to life in another form, union with a higher consciousness, something mysterious and unknowable? Write a brief essay explaining your concept or belief. Where did it come from? Is it what you wish would happen after death?

2. *Critical Thinking* Research the issue of physician-assisted suicide. Write a brief essay that presents the main arguments on both sides of the issue, and conclude with a statement of your own opinion. Be sure to explain your reasoning. What are the most important factors in your decision? Why do you think you have the opinion you do?

FOR MORE INFORMATION

Books

Anderson, P. 1998. *All of Us: Americans Talk About the Meaning of Death*. New York: Dell. *A compilation of interviews about dying conducted with a wide cross section of Americans.*

Byock, I. 1998. *Dying Well: Peace and Possibilities at the End of Life*. New York: Riverhead. *An eminent hospice physician provides a blueprint for making the end of life as precious and meaningful as the beginning.*

DeSpelder, L. A., and A. L. Strickland. 1999. *The Last Dance: Encountering Death and Dying*, 5th ed. Mountain View, Calif.: Mayfield. *A comprehensive text covering legal, medical, and emotional aspects of death.*

Doka, K. J. 1998. *Living with Life-Threatening Illness: A Guide for Patients, Their Families, and Caregivers*. San Francisco: Jossey-Bass. *Provides a practical, comprehensive view of life-threatening illness from the crisis of diagnosis through various treatment options to eventual recovery or impending death.*

Emanuel, L. L. 1998. *Regulating How We Die: The Ethical, Medical, and Legal Issues Surrounding Physician-Assisted Suicide*. Cambridge, Mass.: Harvard University Press. *Provides a historical and legal perspective on both sides of the issue of physician-assisted suicide.*

Filene, P. G. 1998. *In the Arms of Others: A Cultural History of the Right-to-Die In America*. Chicago: Ivan Dee. *A survey of how American attitudes about end-of-life issues have changed over the past 30 years.*

Mitford, J. 1998. *The American Way of Death Revisited*. New York: Knopf. *An update of a landmark exposé of the funeral industry.*

Webb, M. 1999. *The Good Death: The New American Search to Reshape the End of Life*. New York: Bantam. *An examination of how Americans think about and confront death.*

Organizations, Hotlines, and Web Sites

Association for Death Education and Counseling. Provides resources for education, counseling, and caregiving related to dying, death, grief, and loss.

342 N. Main St.
West Hartford, CT 06117
860-586-7503
http://www.adec.org

Bereavement and Hospice Support Netline. Supplies a national directory of bereavement support groups, listed by state and type of bereavement.

http://www.ubalt.edu/www/bereavement

Choice in Dying. Provides information about right-to-die issues and supplies advance directives that meet specific state requirements.

1035 30th St., NW
Washington, DC 20007
800-989-WILL
http://www.choices.org

DeathNet. Provides information about right-to-die issues.

http://www.islandnet.com/deathnet

The End of Life: Exploring Death in America. Information and links relating to end-of-life issues; based on a National Public Radio series.

http://www.npr.org/programs/death

Growth House. A gateway to Internet resources on life-threatening illness and end-of-life issues.

http://www.growthhouse.org

Hospice Foundation of America. Provides information about hospice care and selecting a local hospice.

2001 S St., N.W., Suite 300
Washington, DC 20009
202-638-5419
http://www.hospicefoundation.org

Kearl's Guide to Sociological Thanatology. Provides resources related to sociocultural aspects of death.

http://www.trinity.edu/~mkearl/death.html

Longwood College Library Physician-Assisted Suicide Page. Information about physician-assisted suicide and links to related sites.

http://web.lwc.edu/administrative/library/suic.htm

National Funeral Directors Association. Provides consumer resources related to funeral costs, arranging funerals and memorial services, and bereavement support.

> 13625 Bishops Dr.
> Brookfield, WI 53005
> 414-789-1880; 800-228-6332
> http://www.nfda.org

National Hospice Organization. Provides information about hospice care and supplies a national directory of hospices listed by state and city.

> 1901 N. Moore St., Suite 901
> Arlington, VA 22209
> 703-243-5900
> http://www.nho.org

Oregon Health Division. Provides information about Oregon's Death with Dignity Act, which allows physician-assisted suicide in certain cases.

> http://www.ohd.hr.state.or.us

Project on Death in America. Promotes an understanding of issues related to the culture and experience of dying.

> http://www.soros.org/death.html

The following organizations provide information about organ donation and blank organ donor cards:

Coalition on Donation
> 800-355-7427

National Kidney Foundation
> 800-622-9010
> http://www.kidney.org

United Network for Organ Sharing
> 888-894-6361
> http://www.unos.org

U.S. Department of Health and Human Services
> http://www.organdonor.gov

SELECTED BIBLIOGRAPHY

Alexander. G. C., and A. R. Sehgal. 1998. Barriers to cadaveric renal transplantation amoung blacks, women, and the poor. *Journal of the American Medical Association* 280: 1148–1152.

Ariès, P. 1985. *Images of Man and Death.* Cambridge, Mass.: Harvard University Press.

Arras, J. D., and B. Steinbock. 1999. *Ethical Issues in Modern Medicine,* 5th ed. Mountain View, Calif.: Mayfield.

Bai, M. 1998. Death wish. *Newsweek,* 7 December.

Bower, J. E., et al. 1998. Cognitive processing, discovery of meaning, CD4 decline, and AIDS-related mortality among bereaved HIV-seropositive men. *Journal of Consulting and Clinical Psychology* 66(6): 979–986.

Bowker, J. 1991. *The Meanings of Death.* New York: Cambridge University Press.

Carney, M. T., and R. S. Morrison. 1997. Advance directives: When, why, and how to start talking. *Geriatrics* 52: 65–66, 69–74.

Chin, A. E., et al. 1999. Legalized physician-asissted suicide in Oregon—The first year's experience. *New England Journal of Medicine* 340(7): 577–583.

Choice in Dying. 1999. *Issues: Background on the Right to Die* (retrieved January 11, 1999; http://www.choices.org/issues. htm).

Choice in Dying. 1998. *Physician-Assisted Suicide:* Vacco v. Quill, Washington v. Glucksberg (retrieved January 11, 1999; http://www.choices.org/sctdec.htm).

Clark, D., ed. 1993. *The Sociology of Death: Theory, Culture, Practice.* Cambridge, Mass.: Blackwell.

Corr, C. A. 1995. "A Task-Based Approach to Coping with Dying." In *The Path Ahead: Readings in Death and Dying,* ed. L. A. DeSpelder and A. L. Strickland. Mountain View, Calif.: Mayfield.

Counts, D. R., and D. A. Counts, eds. 1991. *Coping with the Final Tragedy: Cultural Variation in Dying and Grieving.* Amityville, N.Y.: Baywood.

DeSpelder, L. A., and A. L. Strickland. 1999. *The Last Dance: Encountering Death and Dying,* 5th ed. Mountain View, Calif.: Mayfield.

Fischer, G. S., et al. 1997. Can goals of care be used to predict intervention preferences in an advance directive? *Archives of Internal Medicine* 157: 801–807.

Fried, T. R., et al. 1999. Who dies at home? Determinants of site of death for community-based long-term care patients. *Journal of the American Geriatrics Society* 47: 25–29.

Fulton, R., and R. Bendiksen, eds. 1994. *Death and Identity,* 3rd ed. Philadelphia: The Charles Press.

Ganzini, L., et. al. 1999. Attitudes of patients with amyotrophic lateral sclerosis and their caregivers toward assisted suicide. *New England Journal of Medicine* 339(14): 967–973.

Haupt, B. J. 1998. *Characteristics of Hospice Care Users: Data from the 1996 National Home and Hospice Care Survey. Advance Data from Vital and Health Statistics.* No. 299. Hyattsville, Md.: National Center for Health Statistics.

Iserson, K. V. 1994. *Death to Dust: What Happens to Dead Bodies?* Tucson: Galen Press.

Kastenbaum, R., and B. Kastenbaum, eds. 1989. *Encyclopedia of Death.* Phoenix: Oryx Press.

Klass, D., P. R. Silverman, and S. Nickman, eds. 1996. *Continuing Bonds: New Understandings of Grief.* Washington, D.C.: Taylor and Francis.

Kübler-Ross, E. 1968. *On Death and Dying.* New York: Macmillan.

National Funeral Directors Association. 1999. *Funeral Price Information* (retrieved January 11, 1999; http://www.nfda. org/resources/funeralprice.html).

Oregon Health Division. 1998. *Death with Dignity Preliminary Summary Issued* (retrieved January 11, 1999; http://www. ohd.hr.state.or.us/news/0818pas.htm).

Osterweis, M., F. Solomon, and M. Green, eds. 1984. *Bereavement: Reactions, Consequences, and Care.* Washington, D.C.: National Academy Press.

Poll shows strong support for assisted suicide. 1998. *Washington Post,* 30 July.

Singer, P. A., D. K. Martin, and M. Kelner. 1999. Quality end-of-life care. Patients' perspectives. *Journal of the American Medical Association* 281: 163–168.

Speece, M. W., and S. B. Brent. 1996. "The Development of Children's Understanding of Death." In *Helping Children Cope with Death and Bereavement,* ed. C. A. Corr and D. M. Corr. New York: Springer.

Stroebe, M. S., W. Stroebe, and R. O. Hansson, eds. 1993. *Handbook of Bereavement: Theory, Research, and Intervention.* New York: Cambridge University Press.

United Network for Organ Sharing. 1999. *U.S. Facts About Transplantation* (retrieved February 13, 1999; http://www.unos.org/Newsroom/critdata_main.htm).

U.S. Department of Health and Human Services. 1999. *Report Shows Significant Waiting Time Disparities for Organ Transplant Recipients* (retrieved January 22, 1999; http://www.hhs.gov/news/press/1999pres/990122a.html).

van der Maas, P. J., et al. 1996. Euthanasia, physician-assisted suicide, and other medical practices involving the end of life in the Netherlands, 1990–1995. *New England Journal of Medicine* 335: 1699–1705.

Volkan, V. D., and E. Zintl. 1994. *Life After Loss: The Lessons of Grief.* New York: Collier.

Walter, T. 1994. *The Revival of Death.* London: Routledge.

Williamson, J. B., and E. S. Shneidman. 1995. *Death: Current Perspectives,* 4th ed. Mountain View, Calif.: Mayfield.

Worden, J. W. 1991. *Grief Counseling and Grief Therapy: A Handbook for the Mental Health Practitioner,* 2nd ed. New York: Springer.

Worsnop, R. L. 1992. Assisted suicide. *CQ Researcher,* 21 February.

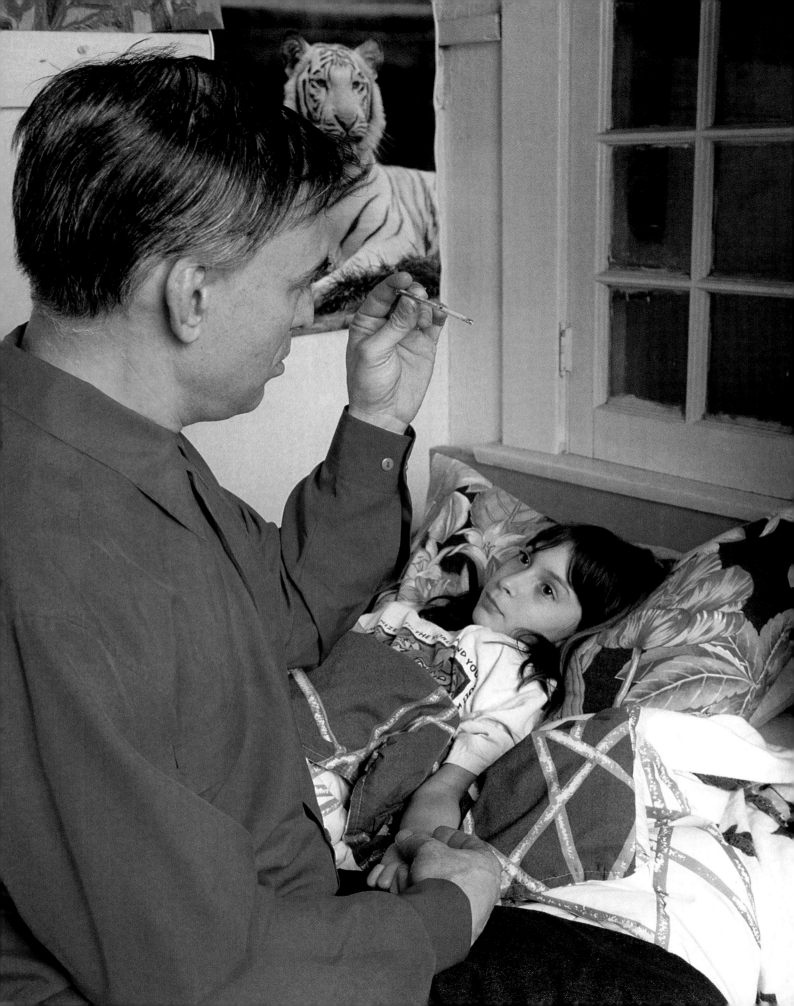

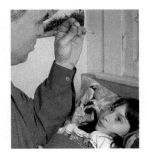

LEARNING OBJECTIVES

After reading this chapter, you should be able to:

- Describe your role as your own primary health care provider.

- Explain the self-care decision-making process, including how to decide whether to see a physician.

- Discuss options for self-treatment.

- Explain the physician-patient partnership, including how to communicate effectively with a health care professional.

- Describe how medical problems are diagnosed, tested, and treated, and list ways that patients can participate fully in each step.

Medical Self-Care: Skills for the Health Care Consumer

21

TEST YOUR KNOWLEDGE

1. About what percentage of medical symptoms are self-diagnosed and self-treated?
   - a. 40%
   - b. 60%
   - c. 80%

2. Generic drugs are generally less effective than brand-name drugs. True or false?

3. Which pain reliever is best for menstrual cramps, toothaches, and rheumatoid arthritis?
   - a. aspirin
   - b. ibuprofen
   - c. acetaminophen (Tylenol)

4. You can buy a nonprescription test for HIV at your local drugstore. True or false?

5. How long can medications be expected to be potent?
   - a. for 1 year from when they're opened, if stored properly
   - b. for 5 years from when they're opened, if stored properly
   - c. until their expiration date

Answers

1. c. The health care system would be overwhelmed if people started visiting their physicians for even a small proportion of the symptoms they now treat themselves.

2. False. Price is often the only difference. The generic version of a drug has the same active ingredient as the brand-name drug, but it may have different inactive ingredients.

3. b. Ibuprofen interferes with the body's production of prostaglandins, hormone-like substances that promote inflammation and are involved in certain types of pain.

4. True. Since 1996, consumers have been able to test themselves at home and receive the results anonymously over the phone.

5. a. The expiration date is the manufacturer's estimate of how long the *unopened* medication is likely to be potent.

When you think of the health care system, do you envision physicians, nurses, clinics, hospitals, and medical laboratories? This is an accurate picture as far as it goes, but don't forget your own role in the health care system—as a self-care provider. Even with today's dazzling medical technology, highly effective medications, and wide variety of skilled practitioners, the individual plays a crucial role in the health care system. In fact, the professional medical care system depends on the functioning of nonprofessional care. If people were to stop practicing self-care and seek professional care for even a small percentage of the complaints they usually manage themselves—colds, backaches, stomach aches, headaches, fatigue, and so on—the professional health care system would be overwhelmed. The average person has about four new medical symptoms each *month,* yet consults a physician only four times a *year.* At least 80% of medical symptoms are self-diagnosed and self-treated.

Until recently, this critical role of people as the *primary* providers of health care for themselves and their families went largely unnoticed. With attention focused on the "delivery" of professional services, many people remained unaware of how important a part they played in their own health care. Today, people are becoming more confident of their own ability to solve personal health problems. With increased knowledge of when and how to self-treat and when to seek professional care, they can become even more competent in self-care.

Even a small increase in appropriate self-care could result in billions of health care dollars saved. For example, in one study, simply providing people with a book of information about self-care and when to contact a health care professional reduced overall visits to physicians by 17% and visits for minor illnesses by 35%. When people are provided with clear, simple information, they can prevent and treat most common health problems in their own homes—earlier, more cheaply, and often better than health care professionals.

The key element in this transition is the recognition that people can *manage* their own health care. Managers don't do everything themselves; they use others—consultants, advisers, experts—to help them get the job done. Once they have all the information they need, they make decisions and take responsibility for follow-through. People who manage their own health care gather information and learn skills from physicians, friends, classes, books, magazines, or self-help groups; solicit opinions and advice; make decisions; and take action. They recognize that everyday choices about diet, exercise, and other habits are critical determinants of health. They participate in every phase of their health care and accept personal responsibility for it. They realize that the choices are theirs.

Health promotion and a healthy lifestyle include being an informed partner in medical care and practicing safe, effective self-care. How can you develop this self-care attitude and take a more active role in your health care? The first step is to learn the skills you need to identify and manage medical problems. The second step is to learn how to make the health care system work effectively for you. This chapter provides information that will help you become competent in both these areas.

MANAGING MEDICAL PROBLEMS

Effectively managing medical problems involves developing several skills. First, you need to learn how to be a good observer of your own body and assess your symptoms. You also must be able to decide when to seek professional advice and when you can safely deal with the problem on your own. You need to know how to safely and effectively self-treat common medical problems. Finally, you need to know how to develop a partnership with physicians and other care providers, and how to carry out treatment plans.

Self-Assessment

Self-care begins with careful observation of your own body. We are constantly observing our bodies, scanning for unusual sensations, aches, or pains. Symptoms are signals from our bodies. They alert us that something may be wrong.

Observing Symptoms   Symptoms are often an expression of the body's attempt to heal itself. For example, the pain and swelling that occur after an ankle injury immobilize the injured joint to allow healing to take place. A fever may be an attempt to make the body less hospitable to infectious agents. A cough can help clear the airways and protect the lungs. Understanding what a symptom means and what is going on in your body helps reduce anxiety about symptoms and enables you to practice safe self-care that supports your body's own healing mechanisms.

Carefully observing symptoms also lets you identify those signals that suggest you need professional assistance to help your body heal. You should begin by noting when the symptom began, how often and when it occurs, what makes it worse, what makes it better, and if you have any associated symptoms. You can also monitor your body's vital signs, such as temperature and heart rate. These signs may give important clues to how your body is managing an illness.

Medical Self-Tests   Not too long ago, the thermometer was the only tool available for evaluating medical problems at home. Now a new generation of medical self-tests are available: home blood pressure machines, home blood sugar tests for diabetics, pregnancy tests, self-tests for urinary tract infections, and over a dozen other do-it-yourself kits and devices. All these tools are designed to help you make a more informed decision about when to

Before the mid-1970s, a woman who thought she was pregnant had to see her physician, provide a urine sample, and wait several days before she would know whether or not "the rabbit died." These days, most women who suspect they may be pregnant buy a home pregnancy test at the drugstore or grocery store and have a highly accurate answer in minutes. Home testing kits are also available to predict ovulation; monitor blood pressure, cholesterol, and blood sugar levels; and detect the presence of blood in the urine. It is even possible to test for HIV infection and hepatitis C at home. Americans now spend about $1 billion per year on medical self-tests.

There are many benefits to the consumer of self-test kits. They are usually accurate—about as accurate as professional ones (as required by the FDA). And many of the home tests are less expensive than similar tests done by a lab. A home pregnancy test is available for less than $15, while a lab test usually costs $35–$45. There is a public health benefit as well: Self-test kits may be used by people who might not get tested otherwise. For example, a recent government survey found that only 20% of people at high risk for HIV infection planned to be tested for the disease in the next year, but 42% said they would be likely to use a self-test kit. Self-tests also give individuals a greater sense of control over their health.

However, there are some drawbacks to using home tests. Like all tests, they can give occasional inaccurate results. **False positive** results—in which the test indicates that a person has a disease or condition when he or she really doesn't—can be caused by a variety of unrelated conditions. **False negatives**—in which tests fail to accurately detect a disease or condition—could lead people to think they don't need to see a physician. Home tests are subject to user error; most are fairly simple to use, but be sure to follow the directions carefully.

Results of a home self-test won't answer all your questions. If the result is positive, you'll probably need to visit a physician. Manufacturers of home HIV tests have addressed the need for counseling by having people phone in for test results; callers whose result is positive or inconclusive are routed to a trained HIV counselor.

If you are shopping for a home self-test kit, follow these suggestions for the most accurate result:

- Compare brands before you buy. Some are very simple to use, others are more complex. Some include only one test per package, others have several. Price can vary considerably, and a higher price doesn't necessarily mean a more accurate test.
- Check the expiration date and storage information on the package.
- Read the instructions carefully before you begin, and follow them exactly.
- Be sure to time the test carefully with a watch or clock with a second hand. Don't delay reading the result; it can become inaccurate in as little as 10–20 extra minutes.
- If you will be using a test frequently, like a blood sugar meter or blood pressure monitor, see if you can try several before you buy one. Your physician or health clinic may have several models you can try.
- Remember that false negative and false positive results are possible. If you get a negative result from a home test but symptoms persist, see your physician.
- Follow up a positive result with a visit to a physician when appropriate. If you are pregnant or have a medical condition, you'll need to find out the next steps as soon as possible.

seek medical help and when to self-treat (see the box "Choosing and Using Medical Self-Tests").

Careful self-observation and the selective use of self-tests may help provide you with the type of information you need to make informed self-care decisions and participate more actively in your care.

PERSONAL INSIGHT How do you feel about taking responsibility for your health care? Do you feel confident about self-care? Are there ways you can increase your confidence?

Decision Making: Knowing When to See a Physician

To self-treat or not self-treat? That is the question. When confronted with a symptom, a person must ask a series of questions: "What's going on in my body?" "Is this dangerous?" "Have I or anyone else I know had something like this before?" Some of the answers you give to these questions are conscious and rational; others are more unconscious, emotional responses.

Evaluating Symptoms People often make two kinds of mistakes in deciding what to do when faced with symptoms. They may rush to their physician too often or too quickly for minor complaints they could easily and effectively manage on their own. Or they may ignore symptoms and self-treat when they should be seeking professional help.

Your decision to seek professional assistance for a symptom is generally guided by your history of medical problems and the nature of the symptom you are experiencing. In general, you should check with a physician for symptoms that are described as follows:

false positive A test result that incorrectly detects a disease or condition in a healthy person. TERMS

false negative A test result that fails to correctly detect a disease or condition.

1. *Severe.* If the symptom is very severe or intense, medical assistance is advised. Examples include severe pains, major injuries, and other emergencies.

2. *Unusual.* If the symptom is peculiar and unfamiliar, it is wise to check it out with your physician. Examples include unexplained lumps, changes in a mole, problems with vision, difficulty swallowing, numbness, weakness, unexplained weight loss, and blood in sputum, urine, or stool.

3. *Persistent.* If the symptom lasts longer than expected, seek medical advice. Examples in adults include fever for more than 5 days, a cough lasting longer than 2 weeks, a sore that doesn't heal within a month, and hoarseness lasting longer than 3 weeks.

4. *Recurrent.* If a symptom tends to return again and again, medical evaluation is advised. Examples include recurrent headaches, stomach pains, and backache.

Sometimes a single symptom is not a cause for concern, but when the symptom is accompanied by other symptoms, the combination suggests a more serious problem. For example, a fever with a stiff neck suggests meningitis. A cough with green sputum and a high fever might mean pneumonia.

Getting Professional Assistance   If you evaluate your symptoms and think that you need professional help, you must decide how urgent the problem is. If it is a true emergency, then you should go (or be taken) to the nearest emergency room (ER). Emergencies would include:

- Major trauma or injury, such as head injury, suspected broken bone, deep wound, severe burn, eye injury, or animal bite.
- Uncontrollable bleeding or internal bleeding, as indicated by blood in the sputum, vomit, or stool.
- Intolerable and uncontrollable pain or severe chest pain.
- Severe shortness of breath.
- Persistent abdominal pain, especially if associated with nausea and vomiting.
- Poisoning or drug overdose.
- Loss of consciousness or seizure.
- Stupor, drowsiness, or disorientation that cannot be explained.
- Severe or worsening reaction to an insect bite or sting, or to a medication, especially if breathing is difficult.

TERMS   **over-the-counter (OTC) medication**   A medication or product that can be purchased by the consumer without a prescription.

Unfortunately, many visits to the ER are not true emergencies. And there are many reasons not to go there if it is not a true emergency. You may have to wait hours while more critically ill patients are seen before you. Your medical records are usually not available at an ER, and it is harder to get appropriate follow-up care. Also, many insurance policies do not cover nonemergency visits to emergency rooms, so if you go to an ER with a mild symptom, you could end up paying the bill. And ER medical bills are much higher than office or urgent care center visits.

If your problem is not an emergency but still requires medical attention, consider a call to your physician's office. Often you can be given medical advice over the phone without the inconvenience of a visit. If you do require a visit, it can often be arranged at the most convenient and appropriate time and place. Nearly 16% of all outpatient medical advice and 30% of pediatric advice is now dispensed by telephone.

To help you make wise medical decisions, a Self-Care Guide for Common Medical Problems is provided in Appendix B. This guide includes some specific suggestions on when to call a physician for certain medical problems and on when and how to self-treat. Of course, you should also see a health care professional for help with preventive care, including lifestyle counseling, immunizations, and screening tests.

Self-Treatment: Many Options

When confronted with a new symptom, many people try to find some pill or potion that will relieve or cure it. However, other self-treatment options are available.

Watchful Waiting   In most cases, your body can itself relieve your symptoms and heal the disorder. The prescriptions filled by your body's internal pharmacy are frequently the safest and most effective treatment. So patience and careful self-observation are often the best choices in self-treatment.

Nondrug Options   Nondrug options are often easy, inexpensive, safe, and highly effective. For example, massage, ice packs, and neck exercises may be at times more helpful than drugs in relieving headaches and other pains. Adequate rest, increasing exercise, drinking more water, eating more or less of certain foods, using humidifiers, changes in ergonomics when working at desks, and so on are just some of the hundreds of nondrug options for preventing or relieving many common health problems. For a variety of disorders either caused or aggravated by stress, relaxation, visualization, humor, assertive communication, changing negative thoughts, and other stress-management strategies may be the treatment of choice (see Chapter 2). Before reaching for medications, consider all your self-treatment options.

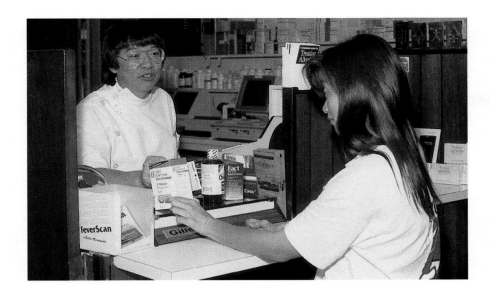

Home pregnancy test kits are just one type of self-test that can be obtained without a prescription in a pharmacy or even your supermarket. Using one of these kits, a woman can determine whether she is pregnant within a week of having missed her period.

Self-Medication   Self-treatment with nonprescription medications is an important part of our health care system. Nonprescription or **over-the-counter (OTC) medications** are medicines that the Food and Drug Administration (FDA) has determined are safe for use without a physician's prescription. There are about 100,000 OTC drugs on the market; about 60% of all medications are sold over the counter. Within every 2-week period, nearly 70% of Americans use one or more OTC drug.

Many OTC drugs are highly effective in relieving symptoms and sometimes in curing illnesses. In fact, many OTC drugs were formerly prescription drugs: More than 600 products sold over the counter today use ingredients or dosage strengths available only by prescription 20 years ago. With this increased consumer choice, however, comes increased consumer responsibility (see the box "What's Your Medicine Cabinet IQ?" on page 574).

Consumers also need to be aware of the barrage of OTC drug advertising aimed at them. The implication of such advertising is that every symptom can and should be relieved by a drug. Although many OTC products are effective, others are unnecessary or divert attention from better ways of coping. Many ingredients in OTC drugs— perhaps 70%—have not been proven to be effective, a fact the FDA does not dispute.

In addition to OTC drug advertising, consumers are now the target of multibillion-dollar "direct-to-consumer" (DTC) advertising campaigns for *prescription* drugs. Proponents of DTC advertising claim that it enhances public health by providing educational information to consumers (about such underdiagnosed conditions as diabetes, high cholesterol, and depression) and motivating them to seek medical care. Opponents claim the DTC advertising is more promotional than educational; that it is misleading and omits important precautions; that it is designed to create consumer demand; and that it causes

patients to pressure physicians to prescribe particular drugs. In general, physicians' attitudes toward DTC advertising are negative, whereas consumers' attitudes are positive.

When you see a DTC ad for a prescription drug, remember to use your critical thinking skills. Look for common advertising strategies such as overpromising results; omitting or hiding important information, especially negative information like side effects; failing to mention other possible treatments, especially nondrug treatments like lifestyle and behavioral changes; and creating problems and needs you didn't know you had.

Remember too that any drug, whether OTC or prescription, can have side effects. Follow these simple guidelines to self-medicate safely:

1. Always read labels, and follow directions carefully. By 2001, the information on most OTC drug labels will appear in a standard format developed by the FDA (Figure 21-1, p. 575); ingredients, directions for safe use, and warnings will be clearly indicated. If you have any questions, ask a pharmacist or physician before using a product.

2. Do not exceed the recommended dosage or length of treatment unless you discuss this change with your physician.

3. Use caution if you are taking other medications, because OTC and prescription drugs can interact. If you have questions about drug interactions, ask your physician or pharmacist *before* you mix medicines.

4. Try to select medications with one active ingredient rather than combination ("all-in-one") products. A product with multiple ingredients is likely to include drugs for symptoms you don't even have, so why risk the side effects of medications

True False

_____ _____ 1. Acetaminophen (Tylenol) is safer for children than aspirin.

_____ _____ 2. It's a good idea to keep some prescription antibiotics on hand in case you start to come down with a cold.

_____ _____ 3. Hydrogen peroxide is a safe, effective antiseptic for cleaning cuts and scrapes.

_____ _____ 4. Vitamin pills containing iron can be very toxic to children.

_____ _____ 5. Taking vitamin C can help prevent you from catching a cold.

_____ _____ 6. It's OK to share prescription medications with other people you know with the same physical complaints.

_____ _____ 7. Calamine lotion is a good product for relieving minor itching.

_____ _____ 8. Everyone should take vitamin supplements to boost his or her health.

Answers

1. True. Aspirin can cause a dangerous condition known as Reye's syndrome in children.

2. False. It is very dangerous to keep old antibiotics on hand. If you get a prescription for antibiotics, you should finish taking them even if you start to feel better.

3. True. Hydrogen peroxide is just as effective and less expensive than many other OTC antiseptics.

4. True. Consuming iron-containing vitamins is the leading cause of poisoning in children under age 6. Be sure they are stored where children can't get them.

5. False. But some studies indicate that taking vitamin C may slightly diminish the severity of symptoms once a cold develops.

6. False. Taking someone else's prescription medicine can be very dangerous.

7. True. Calamine lotion can relieve itching from poison ivy or oak, insect bites, sunburn, and minor forms of dermatitis (skin irritations).

8. False. Most people who eat a healthy diet don't need vitamin supplements. There are some exceptions; ask your physician.

Scoring Add the number of questions you answered correctly.

7–8 Congratulations! You are very knowledgeable about self-care. Continue to educate yourself about home health issues.

4–6 You have some knowledge about self-care issues, but you need to be careful to read and follow all medication instructions.

0–3 Your lack of knowledge about self-care could put your health at risk. Read this chapter carefully, and look for other ways to educate yourself about home health care issues.

---

you don't need? Using single-ingredient products also allows you to adjust the dosage of each medication separately for optimal symptom relief with minimal side effects.

5. When choosing medications, try to buy **generic drugs**, which contain the same active ingredient as the brand-name product but generally at a much lower cost. (Brand-name and generic drugs are discussed in more detail later in the chapter.)

6. Never take or give a drug from an unlabeled container or in the dark when you can't read what the label says.

7. If you are pregnant, nursing, or have a chronic condition such as kidney disease, consult your physician before self-medicating.

8. The expiration date marked on many medications is an estimate of how long the *unopened* medication is likely to be potent. Once the package is opened, the medication will probably be potent for about a

year if stored properly. Mark the date on the package when you open it, and dispose of it safely after a year by taking it to a pharmacy or hospital.

9. Store your medications in a cool, dry place that is out of the reach of children. Poisoning with medications is a common and preventable problem. The bathroom medicine chest is usually not a secure or dry place to store medications. Consider a lockable tool chest or fishing box that can be stored out of the reach of children, preferably not in a bathroom or other location where dampness or heat might ruin medications.

10. Use special caution with aspirin. Because of an association with a rare but serious problem known as Reye's syndrome, aspirin should not be used by children or adolescents who may have the flu, chicken pox, or any other viral illness.

The Home Pharmacy If you were to survey home medicine cabinets, what would you find? On average, there would be 22 medications, including 17 OTC products. You would probably find an oversupply of expired medications and leftover prescription drugs. At the same time, certain essential medications and equipment would

TERMS **generic drug** A drug that is not registered or protected by a trademark; a drug that does not have a brand name.

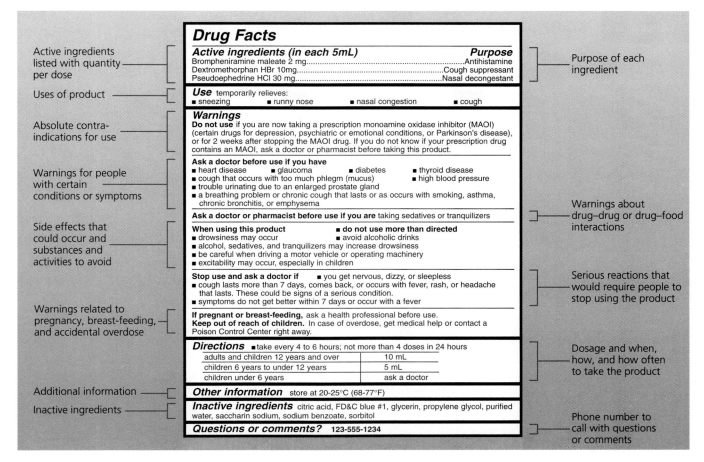

Active ingredients listed with quantity per dose

Uses of product

Absolute contra-indications for use

Warnings for people with certain conditions or symptoms

Side effects that could occur and substances and activities to avoid

Warnings related to pregnancy, breast-feeding, and accidental overdose

Additional information

Inactive ingredients

Purpose of each ingredient

Warnings about drug–drug or drug–food interactions

Serious reactions that would require people to stop using the product

Dosage and when, how, and how often to take the product

Phone number to call with questions or comments

Drug Facts

Active ingredients (in each 5mL) | **Purpose**
Brompheniramine maleate 2 mg...Antihistamine
Dextromethorphan HBr 10mg...Cough suppressant
Pseudoephedrine HCl 30 mg..Nasal decongestant

Use temporarily relieves:
■ sneezing   ■ runny nose   ■ nasal congestion   ■ cough

Warnings
Do not use if you are now taking a prescription monoamine oxidase inhibitor (MAOI) (certain drugs for depression, psychiatric or emotional conditions, or Parkinson's disease), or for 2 weeks after stopping the MAOI drug. If you do not know if your prescription drug contains an MAOI, ask a doctor or pharmacist before taking this product.

Ask a doctor before use if you have
■ heart disease   ■ glaucoma   ■ diabetes   ■ thyroid disease
■ cough that occurs with too much phlegm (mucus)   ■ high blood pressure
■ trouble urinating due to an enlarged prostate gland
■ a breathing problem or chronic cough that lasts or as occurs with smoking, asthma, chronic bronchitis, or emphysema

Ask a doctor or pharmacist before use if you are taking sedatives or tranquilizers

When using this product   ■ **do not use more than directed**
■ drowsiness may occur   ■ avoid alcoholic drinks
■ alcohol, sedatives, and tranquilizers may increase drowsiness
■ be careful when driving a motor vehicle or operating machinery
■ excitability may occur, especially in children

Stop use and ask a doctor if   ■ you get nervous, dizzy, or sleepless
■ cough lasts more than 7 days, comes back, or occurs with fever, rash, or headache that lasts. These could be signs of a serious condition.
■ symptoms do not get better within 7 days or occur with a fever

If pregnant or breast-feeding, ask a health professional before use.
Keep out of reach of children. In case of overdose, get medical help or contact a Poison Control Center right away.

Directions ■take every 4 to 6 hours; not more than 4 doses in 24 hours

adults and children 12 years and over	10 mL
children 6 years to under 12 years	5 mL
children under 6 years	ask a doctor

Other information store at 20-25°C (68-77°F)

Inactive ingredients citric acid, FD&C blue #1, glycerin, propylene glycol, purified water, saccharin sodium, sodium benzoate, sorbitol

Questions or comments? 123-555-1234

Figure 21-1   Reading and understanding OTC drug labels. By 2001, most OTC drug labels will present information in the format shown here. SOURCE: Food and Drug Administration. 1999. Over-the-counter human drugs; labeling requirements; final rule. *Federal Register* 64, no. 51 (17 March): 13254–13303.

be absent. Most people wait until a crisis arises. They then search frantically through a poorly stocked medicine cabinet and often have to make an inconvenient midnight dash to a pharmacy, if they can find one open.

Only a few supplies are essential; additional items depend upon the particular health problems you or your family are likely to have (Table 21-1). Because many medications deteriorate, buy small quantities of infrequently used medications, and replace them about every 3 years.

PERSONAL INSIGHT   How were you cared for when you were sick or injured as a child? Would you care for family members and friends in the same way or differently?

GETTING THE MOST OUT OF YOUR MEDICAL CARE

Self-care involves more than self-diagnosis and self-treatment. It includes knowing when to seek professional care and how to get the most out of your medical care. The key

to making the health care system work for you lies in good communication with your physician and other members of the health care team. Studies show that patients who are more active in interacting with physicians, who ask more questions, enjoy better health outcomes.

Unfortunately, many people are intimidated by their physicians and afraid to communicate freely. Medical jargon can be very confusing. One survey revealed that 20–30% of college-educated people had significant misunderstandings about the meaning of such common medical terms as *hypertension, virus, herpes, tumor, Pap test, strep throat,* and *uterus.* Yet some patients tend not to ask their physicians what such medical jargon means, because they fear appearing stupid. Others are afraid to ask why a test or treatment is needed for fear of appearing to challenge the authority of the physician. Patients often conceal personal concerns about sexuality, drug abuse, emotional problems, and cancer. All these fears and others block open communication with the physician.

Physicians share the responsibility for poor communication. They may feel they are too busy or too important to take time to talk with patients. They may ignore questions, use incomprehensible medical jargon, and respond

TABLE 21-1	*Your Home Self-Care Kit*
Symptom or Problem	**Medication or Supplies**
Allergies or hay fever	Antihistamine
Coughs	Expectorant or cough suppressant (dextromethorphan)
Constipation	Milk of magnesia; bulk laxative (psyllium seed)
Diarrhea	Kaolin/pectate; loperamide HCl (Imodium A-D)
Eye irritations	Eyedrops and artificial tears; eyecup
Fever	Thermometer; acetaminophen; aspirin (adults only); ibuprofen; naproxen sodium
Fungal infections of skin (athlete's foot, ringworm)	Antifungal preparations
Heartburn and indigestion	Antacids (nonabsorbable, such as magnesium hydroxide or aluminum hydroxide); acid reducer (Tagamet, Pepcid, Zantac)
Hemorrhoids	Hemorrhoid preparations
Nasal congestion	Decongestant tablets, nose sprays, or drops
Pain (minor)	Aspirin, acetaminophen, ibuprofen, or naproxen sodium
Poisoning (to induce vomiting if necessary)	Syrup of ipecac
Skin rashes and irritations	Hydrocortisone cream; sodium bicarbonate (baking soda); Burrow's solution
Sore throat	Anesthetic lozenges, gargle, or spray
Splinters	Needle-nosed tweezers
Sprains and strains	Elastic bandages; ice pack; heating pad or hot water bottle
Sunburn (preventive)	Sunscreen (15+ SPF)
Wounds (minor)	Povidone iodine (Betadine); antibacterial creams/ointments; adhesive bandages; gauze; cotton balls; adhesive tape

in an unsupportive way to patients' attempts to assert themselves.

The Physician-Patient Partnership

The physician-patient relationship is undergoing an important transformation. The image of the all-knowing physician and the passive patient is slowly fading. What is emerging is more of a physician-patient *partnership,* in which the physician acts more like a consultant and the patient participates more actively. The necessary ingredients in a successful physician-patient partnership are a sympathetic, caring physician and a prepared, assertive patient. As one observer commented, "It is not enough for the doctor to stop playing God. You've got to get off your knees."

You should try to remember that physicians are human: They have off days, and they make mistakes just as everyone else does. You don't have to "love" your physician as a best friend, but you should expect someone who is attentive, caring, able to listen, and able to clearly explain things to you. You also have to do your part. You need to be assertive in a firm but not aggressive manner. You need to express your feelings and concerns, ask questions, and, if necessary, be persistent. If your physician is unable to communicate clearly with you in spite of your best efforts, then you probably need to change physicians. Remember, the best medical care requires a healthy partnership (see the box "Patient Rights and Responsibilities").

Of course, not everyone can be an active partner all of the time. Depending on the situation, you may wish to shift more of the responsibility for decision making onto your physician, entrusting yourself to her or his judgment and skills. It is important to find a comfortable, flexible way of interacting with your physician—one that suits both your personal preferences and your medical and psychological condition.

Patient Rights

- You have the right to considerate and respectful care.

- You have the right to have access to treatment or accommodations that are available and medically indicated without consideration as to race, color, creed, national origin, disability, or the nature of the source of payment for your care.

- You have the right to privacy concerning your medical care. You have the right to expect that all communications and records pertaining to your care will be treated as confidential, except when restricted by law.

- You have the right to communicate with the physician(s) and other members of the health care team responsible for your medical care.

- You have the right to receive information concerning the diagnosis, nature, and extent of your medical problem. In addition, you have the right to be informed about the nature and purpose of any procedure (test or treatment) that is to be performed, by whom it is to be performed, the risks associated with such procedure(s), the reasonable alternatives, and their accompanying risks and benefits.

- You have the right to make decisions about your plan of care prior to and during the course of testing and/or treatment, and to refuse a recommended treatment or plan of care to the extent permitted by law and clinic or hospital policy, and to be informed of the medical consequences of this action.

- You have the right to have your personal values and beliefs respected and to exercise your cultural and spiritual beliefs in a manner that does not interfere with the care and treatment of you or other patients.

- You have the right to designate another individual to make medical decisions for you if you are unable to do so through an advance directive (see Chapter 20).

- You have the right to review the records pertaining to your medical care and to have the information explained or interpreted as necessary, except when restricted by law.

- You have the right to decide whether to participate in research projects after receiving a full explanation.

- You have the right to request and receive a complete, itemized bill for services rendered.

- You have the right to be informed of the clinic's or hospital's rules and regulations.

Patient Responsibilities

- You have the responsibility to monitor your health on an ongoing basis, identify symptoms, and know when it is appropriate to seek professional care and when and how to safely self-manage medical conditions.

- You have the responsibility to become informed about how to maintain your health and how to manage medical conditions by seeking appropriate information from books, online services, other patients, care providers, and other sources.

- You have the responsibility to provide, to the best of your knowledge, accurate, concise, and complete information about present complaints, past illnesses, hospitalizations, medications, and other health matters and to report unexpected changes in your condition to your care providers.

- You have the responsibility for asking questions if you do not understand tests, treatments, or actions, or do not understand what is expected of you.

- You have the responsibility for following an agreed-upon treatment plan negotiated with your physician or other care providers, or communicating to your care providers any problems you have in following a treatment plan.

- You have the responsibility to call the health care professional to cancel an appointment or treatment as a courtesy to allow other patients to be seen in your absence.

- You have the responsibility to follow the rules and regulations of the clinic or hospital.

- You have the responsibility to be considerate of the rights and needs of other patients and clinic, office, or hospital personnel; to assist in the control of noise and number of visitors; and to respect the property of other people and of the facility where you are receiving care.

- You have the responsibility to pay your portion of any reasonable bills associated with the care received and to provide required information for insurance claims.

SOURCE: Patient rights © 1992 American Hospital Association. Reprinted with permission.

How to Communicate with Your Physician

One of the realities of medical care today is that physicians are often pressed for time. We all wish they had more time to discuss things, explain things, and explore options. The constraints of time make it even more essential that you prepare for your visit to the physician and use your time to maximum advantage. Although the advice that follows is written to support communication with your physician, it applies to your interactions with nurses, pharmacists, dentists, physical therapists, psychotherapists, or any member of your health care team.

Before Your Visit

- *Prepare a list of concerns, questions, and observations.* Have you ever thought to yourself after you walked out

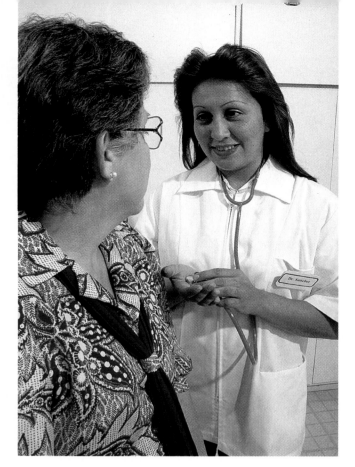

Good communication is a crucial factor in a satisfactory physician-patient partnership.

of the office, "Why didn't I ask about . . . ?" Preparing a list of your observations, concerns, and questions *ahead of time* helps ensure that they get addressed. Here are some things to do:

Decide what you want to get out of this visit to the physician.

Before a visit, make a written list of your most important questions or concerns. Be realistic. If you have a dozen problems and questions, the physician probably can't adequately deal with them all in one visit. So prioritize them.

Prepare notes about your symptoms: when they started, how long they last, exactly where they are located, what makes them worse and what makes them better, what treatments you have already tried, and what you think might be causing the problem.

If you have questions that you are uneasy about, practice discussing them ahead of time, or even write them down and hand the paper to your physician.

Bring a list of all the medications (both prescription and nonprescription) you are taking, or bring all the containers and show them to your physician.

If you have previous medical records or test results

that might be relevant to your condition, bring them along, or arrange to have them sent.

During the Visit

• *Present your concerns at the beginning.* The first few moments of the visit are the most important. A study of medical visits found that physicians allowed patients to talk an average of only 23 *seconds* before interrupting them with questions. Take the initiative, and use this time to briefly list your concerns. They will then form the agenda for the visit. For example, you might say, "I have several things that I'd like to discuss with you today if there is time. The things that most concern me are my shoulder pain, my dizziness, and the possible side effects from my allergy medication." Be direct and honest. If you are concerned about a sexually transmitted disease, for example, don't disguise your concern or wait until the end of the visit to bring it up.

• *Be specific and concise.* Studies show that in over 70% of cases, patients' descriptions of their symptoms lead to a correct diagnosis. You are the expert about how you feel and how you experience symptoms. By telling your own story, you can share your expertise with the physician and help increase the chances of a speedy and accurate diagnosis.

When the physician asks a question, try to answer it as concisely and specifically as you can. If asked when the symptom started, saying "a while ago" is not very helpful. Was it a few minutes ago, or hours, days, years, or decades? If you've been having numbness in your right thumb and index finger, say that, rather than "My hands are numb." The more specific you can be (without overdoing it with irrelevant details), the clearer a picture the physician will have of your problem and the less time you will waste for both of you.

• *Be open and honest.* Try to be as open as you can in sharing your thoughts, feelings, and fears. Remember, your physician is not a mind reader. If you are worried, try to explain why. For example, "I'm worried that what I have is contagious." Also share your hunches about what might be causing your symptoms: "I think I picked up my illness on a recent camping trip." Your guesses can often provide vital clues; even if they aren't correct, they will give your physician the opportunity to reassure you or address your hidden concerns.

If, for some reason, you don't think you can (or will) follow the physician's advice, say so. For example, "I don't think I will take the aspirin because it badly upsets my stomach," or "I don't think I can afford that medication; it isn't covered by my insurance." If your physician knows why you are unlikely to follow advice, he or she may be able to suggest alternatives to help you overcome the barriers.

• *Ask questions.* Your most powerful tool in the physician-patient partnership is the question. You can

Dental diseases can be prevented through proper self-care and regular visits to the dentist. For healthy teeth and gums, follow these guidelines.

Brushing

Brushing the outer, inner, and biting surfaces of your teeth removes food particles and plaque (a thin sticky film of bacteria that grows on teeth and produces an acid that causes tooth decay). Brush twice a day using a soft brush that is sized and shaped to allow you to reach every tooth. The following is one of several effective brushing methods for removing plaque.

1. Place the head of your toothbrush beside your teeth, with the bristle tips at a 45-degree angle against the gumline.

2. Move the brush back and forth in short (half-tooth-width) strokes several times, using a gentle "scrubbing" motion.

3. Brush the outer surfaces of each tooth, upper and lower, keeping the bristles angled against the gumline.

4. Use the same method on the inside surfaces of all teeth, still using short back-and-forth strokes.

5. Scrub the chewing surfaces of the teeth.

6. To clean the inside surfaces of the front teeth, tilt the brush vertically and make several gentle up-and-down strokes with the "toe" (the front part) of the brush.

7. Brushing your tongue will help freshen your breath and clean your mouth by removing bacteria.

Flossing

Flossing removes plaque and food particles from between the teeth and under the gumline, areas where your toothbrush can't reach. It is essential for preventing gum disease. When flossing, follow the instructions given to you by your dentist or dental hygienist. Here are some suggestions:

1. Break off about 18 inches of floss, and wind most of it around one of your middle fingers. Wind the remaining floss around the same finger of the opposite hand. This finger will "take up" the floss as you use it.

2. Hold the floss tightly between your thumbs and forefingers, with about an inch of floss between them. There should be no slack. Using a gentle sawing motion, guide the floss between your teeth. Never "snap" the floss into the gums.

3. When the floss reaches the gumline, curve it into a C-shape against one tooth. Gently slide it into the space between the gum and the tooth until you feel resistance.

4. Hold the floss tightly against the tooth. Gently scrape the side of the tooth, moving the floss away from the gum.

5. Repeat this method on the rest of your teeth. Don't forget the back side of your last tooth.

SOURCE: Adapted from the American Dental Association.

---

fill in vital missing pieces of information, and close gaps in communication, with *your* questions. And asking questions reflects your engagement and active participation in the process of care—two critical ingredients to restoring your health. Don't be afraid to ask what you may consider a "stupid" question. It may indicate an important concern or misunderstanding. Later in this chapter you'll find suggestions for questions to ask whenever medical tests are ordered, medications are prescribed, or surgery is recommended.

• *Alert your physician.* Let your physician know if you are taking any medications (prescription, OTC, or street drugs), have a history of allergic or unusual reactions to any medications, are breastfeeding, or might be pregnant.

• *Share in medical decisions.* Many decisions in medical care are not clear-cut, and often there is more than one option. Except in the case of a life-threatening emergency, the best decisions depend on your values and preferences and should not be left solely to your physician. For example, if you mention that you are having trouble sleeping and your physician offers to prescribe sleeping pills, you might say, "I'm conservative about taking medicines. I'd like to try avoiding caffeine first."

• *Clarify instructions.* When appropriate, ask your physician to write down instructions. Or ask how to get more information on a particular subject. If you tend to have trouble remembering instructions, take notes during the visit or bring someone else along to act as a second listener. Another set of eyes and ears can help you remember the details, and you can discuss them together when you leave the office.

At the End of the Visit

• *Repeat key points.* Briefly repeat five key points to your physician at the end of your visit:

The diagnosis (the nature and cause of your symptoms or what might be causing your symptoms).

The prognosis (the expected duration, course, and outcome of the condition).

The physician's treatment recommendations and instructions.

The follow-up plan.

What you are going to do.

This repetition confirms that you clearly understand the most important information and gives the physician a

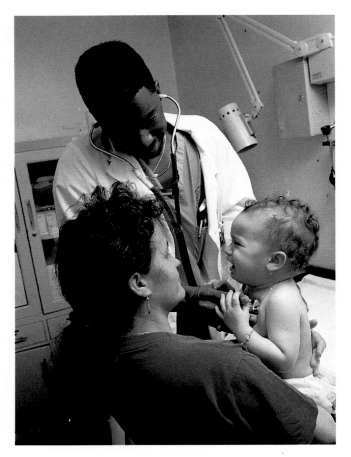

Physical examinations are particularly important for infants and are scheduled at regular intervals during the first few years of life. In addition to vaccinating the child against many diseases, the physician has the opportunity to spot any problems that may be developing, and the parents have the chance to discuss their concerns.

chance to correct any misunderstanding. If you don't understand or remember something the physician said, admit that you need to go over it again. You might say, for example, "I'm pretty sure you told me this before, but I'm not clear about it."

• *Know the follow-up plan.* Before you leave the office, make sure you understand the next steps:

Should you return for a visit?

If so, when and why?

Should you phone for test results?

Are there any signs or symptoms you should watch for and report back to your physician?

• *Give feedback to your physician.* Your physician needs to know how satisfied you are with your care. If you don't like the way you have been treated by your physician or someone else on the team, let him or her know. If you have been unable to follow the physician's

advice or had problems with a treatment, give him or her feedback.

Also let your physician know if you are very pleased. You might say, "I really appreciate your taking the time to explain that so clearly to me," or drop a note to express your thanks. Most physicians very much appreciate compliments and positive feedback.

The Diagnostic Process

Solving a medical problem is sometimes like solving a mystery. The problem is presented, clues are discovered, evidence is sought, possibilities are tracked down, and finally (we hope) a correct diagnosis is made.

There are three main sources of clues and information on which to base a diagnosis: the medical history, the physical exam, and test results. All this information is evaluated to reach a diagnosis that names and explains the problem and guides treatment.

The Medical History   The most important part of medical diagnosis is usually the medical history. This is the description that you give the physician of your problem, concerns, and background. Depending on the nature of the problem, you may be asked about the following: your primary reason for visiting the physician, your present symptoms, your past medical history, and your social history (job, living conditions, family life, major stressors, and health habits).

Your ability to describe your illness clearly, concisely, and accurately is an essential first step in the diagnostic process. Refer to the guidelines in the last section for communicating effectively with your physician.

The Physical Examination   The next step in the diagnostic process is the physical examination. Often, a physical exam begins with a review of vital signs: your heart rate (pulse), breathing rate, temperature, and blood pressure. Depending on your primary complaint, the examination may be a complete head-to-toe exam or may be directed to certain areas. If you have a sore throat and earache, for example, the physician may look into your throat and ear canals, listen with a stethoscope while you breathe, and feel your neck for swollen lymph nodes.

If you notice any pain or unusual sensations during the examination, say so. Your response may provide important information. Also, if you are curious about what is being done during the exam or why, ask your physician (but not while the stethoscope is in his or her ears!).

Medical Testing   In addition to the medical history and physical examination, diagnostic testing now provides a wealth of new information to help solve medical problems. High-tech and high-cost medical testing now accounts for nearly one-third of our national health bill.

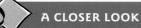

Preventive Medicine for Healthy Adults

While many people associate medical care solely with an illness or injury, preventive medicine can help healthy people stay healthy. Good preventive care includes:

1. Counseling and support to develop healthy habits and reduce health risks.

2. Selective screening tests based on your age, gender, and medical or family history (see the chart below).

3. Appropriate immunizations (see Chapter 17) and use of medications to prevent disease.

The prevention recommendations below are based on scientific research. They apply to generally healthy adults. If you have ongoing health problems, if certain diseases run in your family, or if you have other special health needs or risks, your prevention plan may be somewhat different. Your health care providers can help you design a personalized plan for staying healthy based on your individual needs. And remember, don't rely just on medical exams, tests, and treatments to protect your health. Developing and maintaining a wellness lifestyle is the cornerstone of disease prevention and health promotion.

SOURCES: U.S. Preventive Services Task Force. 1996. *Guide to Clinical Preventive Services: Report of the U.S. Preventive Services Task Force,* 2nd ed. Baltimore: Williams & Wilkins.

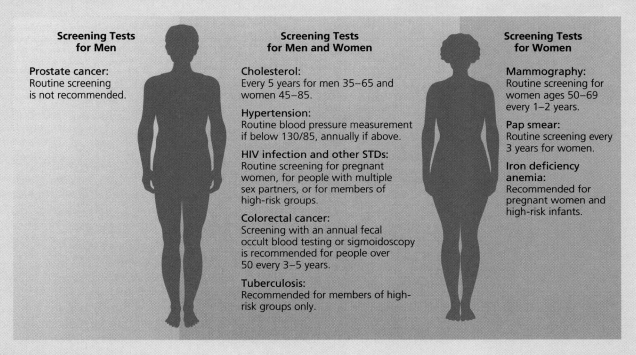

Screening Tests for Men

Prostate cancer: Routine screening is not recommended.

Screening Tests for Men and Women

Cholesterol: Every 5 years for men 35–65 and women 45–85.

Hypertension: Routine blood pressure measurement if below 130/85, annually if above.

HIV infection and other STDs: Routine screening for pregnant women, for people with multiple sex partners, or for members of high-risk groups.

Colorectal cancer: Screening with an annual fecal occult blood testing or sigmoidoscopy is recommended for people over 50 every 3–5 years.

Tuberculosis: Recommended for members of high-risk groups only.

Screening Tests for Women

Mammography: Routine screening for women ages 50–69 every 1–2 years.

Pap smear: Routine screening every 3 years for women.

Iron deficiency anemia: Recommended for pregnant women and high-risk infants.

The recommendations of the U.S. Preventive Services Task Force differ from those of the American Heart Association, American Cancer Society, and other organizations. See Chapters 15–17 for other sets of testing guidelines, and check with your physician about which tests are best for you.

No body fluid, orifice, or cavity is beyond the reach of a medical probe: blood and urine tests, X rays, biopsies, taps, scans, electronic monitors, and a wide array of **endoscopies** (bronchoscopy, arthroscopy, sigmoidoscopy, and so on), the procedures that can view nearly every part of the body.

More than 10 billion medical tests are performed in the United States each year—over 40 tests per person—at a staggering cost of $140 billion, or $600 for each of us. There are many good reasons for medical tests: to help your physician diagnose symptoms accurately, monitor the progress of a known disease, or screen for a hidden one (see the box "Preventive Medicine for Healthy Adults"). Unfortunately, numerous tests are performed for other reasons. Physicians may order tests to protect themselves from malpractice or because patients ask for particular tests. Careful scientific studies reveal that at least 25% of all medical tests are unnecessary. Tests provide patients with a measure of reassurance, but more tests

endoscopy   A medical procedure in which a viewing instrument is inserted into a body cavity or opening. Specific procedures are named for the area viewed: inside joints (arthroscopy), inside airways (bronchoscopy), inside the abdominal cavity (laparoscopy), and inside the lower portion of the large intestine, or sigmoid colon (sigmoidoscopy).

TERMS

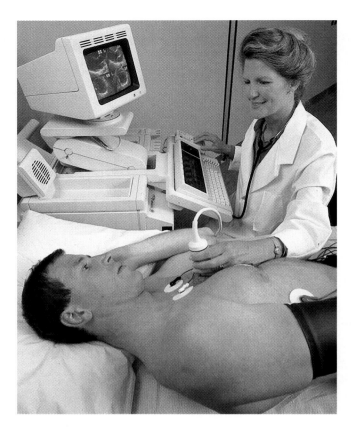

Physicians get information they need from medical tests, but patients have the right to know what the test is for, why they need it, what it will involve, and what the results will indicate. This man is undergoing an echocardiogram to assess the condition of his heart and arteries.

don't necessarily mean better care. A diagnosis can be made 80–90% of the time from a thorough history and physical examination.

When you visit a physician, you can help assure that you get the medical tests you need by asking some of the questions below. While it is not realistic to ask all these questions for every minor blood or urine test, you should consider such questions whenever an expensive, uncomfortable, or potentially risky test is recommended.

• *Why do I need the test?* Is the test necessary to diagnose your problem or determine your treatment? If not, you probably don't need the test. "Because you need it" or "because we usually do it" are not satisfactory answers. Here's an example of a better explanation: "I'm recommending this test because you have persistent stomach pain and indigestion. Your symptoms may be due to lifestyle factors, but they could also indicate a treatable bacterial infection. This test will help diagnose your condition and determine the appropriate treatment."

Ask about alternatives. For example, if you have already had the proposed test, can those earlier results be used? To this end, it is wise to keep a record of all your medical tests—when and where they were done, and the results. Also, ask your physician about the risk of waiting and not testing. Monitoring the symptoms under a physician's supervision for a specific period of time may provide the necessary diagnostic clue, or the symptoms may simply resolve on their own.

• *What are the risks?* No test is completely risk-free. Begin by weighing the potential benefits against the risks. Physical risks vary, depending on the nature of the test, your age, past medical history, general state of health and your ability to cooperate, and the skill and experience of your physician.

• *How do I prepare for the test?* For some tests, preparation is very important. Be sure to remind your physician about any allergies, especially to medications, anesthetics, or X ray contrast materials (substances introduced into the body to make structures visible in an X ray). Mention medications you may be taking, bleeding problems, or whether you might be pregnant. Ask whether you should do anything special before the test, such as fasting or discontinuing medications.

• *What will the test be like?* Knowing how the test is done and how it will feel can decrease your anxiety and discomfort. During and after the procedure, let the physician or technician know what you are feeling. If you're uncomfortable, something can usually be done.

• *What do the results mean?* No test is 100% accurate. False positives and false negatives do occur.

Medical tests often give the impression of objectivity and precision. Yet some tests, such as X rays, electrocardiograms, and scoping procedures, require subjective interpretation. Therefore, getting an experienced second opinion on diagnosis may be important. Above all, remember that medical tests are only part of the diagnostic puzzle. Such clues must always be considered in the context of other information about you: medical history, family, age, habits, medications, symptoms, and physical examination. Good physicians treat patients—not test results.

Medical and Surgical Treatments

Once a diagnosis is made, the treatment options can be considered. The treatments offered for diseases should reflect the wide variety of physical, chemical, and psychosocial factors that cause or aggravate the disease condition. Although some diseases can be cured or ameliorated by medical or surgical treatment, other diseases require no treatment at all or may be aggravated by attempts at therapy. Ask the following questions to help ensure that you are getting the best possible care:

• *What are my treatment options?* Many conditions can be treated in a variety of ways, and your physician should be able to explain the alternative choices to you. In some cases, lifestyle changes, including exercise, diet, and stress management, should be considered alongside medication or surgery before making a choice. When any treatment is recommended, also ask what the consequences are likely to be if you postpone treatment.

• *What are the risks, costs, and expected benefits of each treatment option?* To make an informed choice, you need to know about possible risks and side effects, as well as the likelihood that the proposed treatment will relieve your condition. You need to know how much your health insurance will pay. No one can tell you which choice is right for you, and informed *choice,* not merely informed *consent,* is an essential ingredient in quality medical care.

Prescription Medications Thousands of lives are saved each year by **antibiotics,** heart medications, insulin, and scores of other drugs. But we pay a price for having such powerful tools. Of all admissions to hospitals, nearly 10% are due primarily to drug reactions, and 20% of these patients are likely to have a second drug reaction during their hospital stay. In fact, a 1998 study found that over 100,000 hospital patients died from toxic reactions to properly administered prescription drugs, ranking adverse drug reactions somewhere between the fourth and sixth leading cause of death in the United States. Another 2 million patients suffered serious side effects.

Responsibility for adverse drug reactions is shared by pharmaceutical companies, physicians, pharmacists, and patients. Although pharmaceutical companies carry out extensive trials on new drugs, even the most extensive studies involve just a few thousand people. A large natural experiment begins when the drug is approved and physicians start prescribing it to people in the general population. Side effects that did not show up in premarket studies often become apparent when more people begin taking a drug. For this reason, be especially alert when taking drugs that are new to the market because physicians have less experience with them.

Physicians may overprescribe drugs, sometimes in response to pressure by patients, or they may misprescribe drugs or combinations of drugs. At the pharmacy, patients may receive the wrong drug because of a physician's poor handwriting, misinterpretation of an abbreviated drug name, an incorrect data entry into the computer, or similarities between the names and packaging of different drugs. One in four prescribing errors by pharmacists is thought to be caused by similar drug names, such as Prozac (an antidepressant) and Prilosec (an ulcer drug) and Accupril (for high blood pressure) and Accutane (for severe acne). Pharmacists may also neglect to warn patients of drug interactions.

Medication mishaps may also occur when patients do not receive adequate information about medications. Good communication between patients and their physicians and pharmacists is essential, but written informa-

tion about drugs can provide an important backup to personal advice. The FDA requires written patient information in the form of package inserts for some drugs, and manufacturers voluntarily provide it for others. A 1997 FDA survey found that 67% of consumers were getting some written information with their prescription drugs. A goal of *Healthy People 2010* is that useful prescription drug information, including directions for taking the drug correctly and possible side effects, reach at least 95% of patients by the year 2006. Physicians or pharmacists can add information about "off-label" use based on an individual patient's needs. (Off-label use occurs when a physician prescribes a drug for a use other than the one for which it was approved by the FDA. For example, minoxidil was approved to treat high blood pressure, but once its hair-growing properties were discovered, physicians started prescribing it to treat male pattern baldness. Other examples include the use of antihistamines as sleep aids and the use of retin-A, developed to treat acne, for wrinkles.)

Finally, patients themselves also share responsibility for adverse drug reactions and medication errors. Many people don't take their medications properly, skipping doses, taking incorrect doses, stopping too soon, or not taking the medication at all. An estimated 30–50% of the 2 billion medications prescribed annually in the United States are not taken correctly and thus do not produce the desired results. Consumers can increase their chances of avoiding adverse drug reactions and medication errors by asking the following questions:

• *Do I really need this prescription?* Sometimes physicians prescribe drugs because they think patients want or expect them. Ask about the risks and benefits of the drug and if there are any nondrug alternatives.

• *What is the name of the medication, and what is it supposed to do?* Find out why the medication is being prescribed, how it is expected to help you, and how soon you can expect results.

• *How and when do I take the medication, how much, and for how long? What should I do if I miss a dose?* Be sure your physician provides specific directions on how to take the medication (the label may simply state, "Take as directed"). Also be sure your physician is aware of any chronic conditions you have that may affect dosage. For example, liver and kidney disease may slow metabolism, increasing the toxic effects of some drugs.

• *What other medications, foods, drinks, or activities should I avoid?* Tell your physician or pharmacist about any other drugs you're taking and if you are pregnant or breastfeeding. Other drugs, including alcohol and OTC drugs, can interact with medications, diminishing or increasing their effect (Figure 21-2). For example, certain antibiotics, including ampicillin and tetracycline, may prevent oral contraceptives from working. The presence or absence of food in the stomach can also

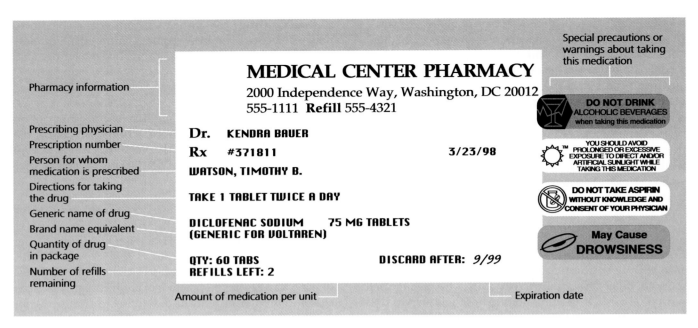

Pharmacy information

Prescribing physician

Prescription number

Person for whom
medication is prescribed

Directions for taking
the drug

Generic name of drug

Brand name equivalent

Quantity of drug
in package

Number of refills
remaining

Special precautions or
warnings about taking
this medication

MEDICAL CENTER PHARMACY

2000 Independence Way, Washington, DC 20012
555-1111 **Refill** 555-4321

Dr. KENDRA BAUER

Rx #371811   3/23/98

WATSON, TIMOTHY B.

TAKE 1 TABLET TWICE A DAY

DICLOFENAC SODIUM   75 MG TABLETS
(GENERIC FOR VOLTAREN)

QTY: 60 TABS   DISCARD AFTER: 9/99
REFILLS LEFT: 2

DO NOT DRINK
ALCOHOLIC BEVERAGES
when taking this medication

YOU SHOULD AVOID
PROLONGED OR EXCESSIVE
EXPOSURE TO DIRECT AND/OR
ARTIFICIAL SUNLIGHT WHILE
TAKING THIS MEDICATION

DO NOT TAKE ASPIRIN
WITHOUT KNOWLEDGE AND
CONSENT OF YOUR PHYSICIAN

May Cause
DROWSINESS

Amount of medication per unit

Expiration date

Figure 21-2   Reading and understanding prescription medication labels.

affect the action of some drugs. Ask whether there are any special precautions to observe while taking the drug, such as staying out of the sun.

• *What are the side effects, and what do I do if they occur?* All medications have side effects, ranging from minor annoyances to life-threatening allergic reactions. Find out what to watch for and what action to take if they occur. If you have a drug allergy or other medical condition (such as epilepsy or diabetes) that may require special attention in case of an emergency, wear a medical ID necklace or bracelet or carry a medical ID card. For comprehensive emergency medical service, consider joining Medic Alert. Call 1-800-ID-ALERT for more information.

• *Can I take a generic drug rather than a brand-name drug?* When a drug is first developed, it's given a patent and a generic name. The patent gives an exclusive right for the pharmaceutical company that developed the drug to sell it, usually under a brand name. When the patent expires (usually in about 17 years), the drug becomes public property, and other companies can make and sell the drug under its generic name or their own brand name.

Generic drugs contain the exact same FDA-approved ingredients as the original brand-name drug, but may contain different inactive ingredients. Generic drugs usually cost less than their brand-name counterparts, and they can often be substituted at a substantial savings to the patient. In certain cases, your physician may have a special reason for preferring a particular brand.

• *Is there any written information about the medication?* Even if your physician takes the time to carefully answer all your questions, you will probably find it difficult to remember all the information. Fortunately, there are now many sources of information, from FDA-approved package inserts to pamphlets and books, where you can read more about the medications you are taking (see Appendix C, Resources for Self-Care).

Remember, never share your prescription medication with anyone else, and never take someone else's. Store your drugs in a cool, dry place, out of direct light, and never use an old prescription for a new ailment.

Surgery   Surgical procedures are performed more often in the United States than anywhere else in the world. Each year, over 70 million operations and related procedures are performed. About 20% of these are in response to an emergency such as a severe injury, while 80% are **elective surgeries,** meaning the patient can generally choose when and where to have the operation, if at all.

Worldwide, the number of operations performed varies widely from country to country, city to city, and even surgeon to surgeon. The most important factor predicting the rates of surgery in a given community is the number of surgeons, not the amount of disease: The more

TERMS   **elective surgery**   A nonemergency operation that the patient can choose to schedule.

mortality rate   The number of deaths occurring in a population of a given size in a given time period.

morbidity rate   The number of illnesses or injuries occurring in a population of a given size in a given time period.

outpatient   A person receiving medical attention without being admitted to the hospital.

surgeons, the more surgery. All this suggests that you would do well to ask some questions when surgery is recommended for you or a family member, to help ensure that the operation is really necessary:

• *Why do I need surgery at this time?* Your physician should be able to explain to you the reason for the surgery, alternatives to surgery, and what is likely to happen if you don't have the operation. You should also be sure you understand how the surgery is likely to benefit you.

With most surgery, getting a *second opinion* is advised, and many health insurance plans now require a second opinion before all or certain elective operations. Consulting a nonsurgeon may also be helpful in exploring alternatives to surgery.

• *What are the risks and complications of the surgery?* All surgical procedures carry some risk. The overall risk varies, depending on the type of operation performed, the surgeon, and your general state of health. You should ask about the **mortality rate** (risk of death) and **morbidity rate** (risk of nonlethal complications). Also ask how often the surgeon has performed the operation because surgical teams with more experience tend to have lower rates of complications. Some state governments and consumer organizations publish "report cards" on individual physicians or hospitals that show comparative complication rates for various surgical procedures.

• *Can the operation be performed on an outpatient basis?* More than 40% of all procedures are now performed on an **outpatient** (ambulatory) basis without requiring an overnight stay in the hospital. Outpatient surgery has many advantages, including lower costs and less family disruption and psychological trauma. In addition, it decreases the opportunities for the patient to develop a hospital-acquired medical complication such as an infection.

• *What can I expect before, during, and after surgery?* Knowing what to expect can help you prepare psychologically and physically for the operation. Preparation also appears to decrease postoperative discomfort and the need for pain medications, and to shorten postoperative hospital stays. Also ask about the length of the recovery period, and what you can do to accelerate it. You should also be informed about what symptoms to expect after surgery, and which ones might signal a complication and should be reported.

You are an important part of the health care system—not only as a *consumer* of medical care but also as a primary health care *provider*. Managing common medical problems; knowing when and how to self-treat and when to seek professional care; communicating clearly and concisely with your physician; asking questions about medical tests, medications, and surgery; and knowing how to get more information on health topics—these are some of the essential skills of an informed consumer of the health care system. Developing these skills will not only result in

better health care but will also help you develop a real sense of competence and confidence about managing your health.

PERSONAL INSIGHT   People often feel overawed or intimidated by their physicians. Do you tend to accept everything your physician says? Do you assume he or she is always right? Do you feel comfortable saying that you would like to seek a second opinion? If not, what can you do to increase your feelings of partnership with your physician?

SUMMARY

Managing Medical Problems

• Self-care involves assessing the body for significant symptoms, which may indicate the need for professional assistance.

• Home medical tests allow cost savings, convenience, privacy, an increased sense of control, and sometimes more comprehensive information.

• Informed self-care requires knowing how to evaluate symptoms so that you don't go to a physician too soon or too late. It's necessary to see a physician if symptoms are severe, unusual, persistent, or recurrent.

• Conditions that require emergency room treatment include major trauma or injury, such as broken bones or burns; uncontrollable or internal bleeding; intolerable or uncontrollable pain; severe chest pain; severe shortness of breath; and loss of consciousness.

• Self-treatment doesn't necessarily require medication. The body can heal itself; massage, ice or heat, exercises, and relaxation techniques can help.

• OTC drugs are a necessary and helpful part of self-care but should not be substituted for nondrug coping techniques. Strategies for effective use include reading drug labels carefully and following the directions.

• A home medicine cabinet should contain small quantities of the medicines needed for an individual family as well as essential supplies.

Getting the Most Out of Your Medical Care

• Good communication with the physician and other members of the health care team is essential. The ideal relationship should be more like a partnership, in which the physician acts like a consultant and the patient actively participates.

• Preparation for a visit to a physician should include making a written list of questions or concerns and bringing a list of all medications. During the visit, it's

Even though we sometimes have to entrust ourselves to the care of medical professionals, that doesn't mean we give up responsibility for our own behavior. Following medical instructions and advice often requires the same kind of behavioral self-management that's involved in quitting smoking, losing weight, or changing eating patterns. For example, if you have an illness or injury, you may be told to take medication at certain times of the day, do special exercises or movements, or change your diet.

The medical profession recognizes the importance of patient adherence, or compliance, and encourages different strategies to support it, such as the following:

1. Use reminders placed at home, in the car, at work, or elsewhere that improve follow-through in taking medication and keeping scheduled appointments. To help you remember to take medications:

   - Link taking the medication with some well-established routine, like brushing your teeth or at mealtimes.

   - Use a medication calendar, and check off each pill.

   - Use a medication organizer or pill dispenser.

   - Plan ahead; don't wait until the last pill to get a prescription refilled.

2. Use a journal and other forms of self-monitoring to keep a detailed account of health-related behaviors, such as pill taking, diet, exercise, and so on.

3. Use self-reward systems so that desired behavior changes are encouraged, with a focus on short-term rewards.

Successful medical care involves more than following physicians' orders; it also has to accommodate the individual's habits and preferences. The next time you have to follow a treatment plan for an illness or injury, use the suggestions given here and in Chapter 1 to help you comply.

---

important to be open, to ask questions, and request clarification.

- The diagnostic process involves a medical history, a physical exam, and medical tests.

- The patient should ask questions about the need for the medical test, the risks, preparation, what the test will be like, and what the results mean.

- Patients should understand the reasons for treatments, options, risks, and expected benefits.

- Safe use of prescription drugs requires knowledge of what the medication is supposed to do, how and when to take it, and what the side effects are.

- All surgical procedures carry risk; patients should ask about alternatives and get a second opinion. Some operations can be performed on an outpatient basis.

TAKE ACTION

1. Examine all the medications in your medicine cabinet. Discard any that have expired or are unlabeled. Ask your physician or pharmacist whether you should keep any medications you are uncertain about. Compare the contents of your medicine cabinet with the list of medications in Table 21-1, and expand your supplies if you need to.

2. Before your next visit to your physician, prepare a written list of your concerns. Be prepared to ask questions. After the visit, review how it went. Were your concerns satisfactorily addressed? Were you able to communicate your needs? Did you feel involved and in con-

trol? What aspects would you like to handle better the next time?

3. Review the box "Preventive Medicine for Healthy Adults" (p. 581). Are there any tests you need to have done? If so, make an appointment at your clinic or medical office, and have the test.

4. Ask your physician whether you have any medical condition that may require special attention in an emergency. If you do, complete a medical ID card for your wallet, or obtain a medical ID bracelet or necklace. More complete emergency service can be obtained by joining Medic Alert (call 1-800-ID-ALERT for information).

JOURNAL ENTRY

1. **Critical Thinking**   Studies have shown that people often ignore the warnings and instructions on labels for OTC drugs; for example, they drive after taking an antihistamine that causes drowsiness or take more than the recommended dosage of a cold remedy or a stimulant. Do people have a responsibility to use medications as directed, or do they have the right to choose any course of action affecting their

own bodies or health, even if their choices have potential negative consequences for others, such as an automobile crash? In your health journal, write a brief essay outlining your opinion about individual responsibility for the correct use of medications. Explain your reasoning.

2. Write a self-care profile in your health journal. Include your age, weight, and height, any conditions or diseases you have and any treatments or medications you take, any conditions or diseases that run in your family or are common in your ethnic group, any surgery you have had and the date, diseases against which you have been immunized and dates of your last booster shots, and any drug or food allergies you have. Include names and telephone numbers of your health care practitioners and pharmacy; information about prescriptions you take (including prescription number, number of refills remaining, and phone number of the pharmacy that filled each one); and information about your health insurance (including policy number and telephone number for someone who can answer questions about it). Keep your self-care profile current, and use it for reference.

FOR MORE INFORMATION

See Appendix C for self-care resources.

SELECTED BIBLIOGRAPHY

Farley, D. 1998. Label literacy for OTC drugs. *FDA Consumer,* September.

Ferguson, T. 1993. Working with your doctor. In *Mind/Body Medicine,* ed. D. Goleman and J. Gurin. Yonkers, N.Y.: Consumers Union.

Graves, E. J., and M. F. Owings. 1998. 1996 Summary: National hospital discharge survey. *Advance Data from Vital and Health Statistics.* No. 301. Hyattsville, Md.: National Center for Health Statistics.

Hafen, B. Q., K. J. Karren, K. J. Frandsen, and N. L. Smith. 1996. *Mind/Body Health: The Health Effects of Attitudes, Emotions, and Relationships.* Boston: Allyn & Bacon.

Hall, M. J., and L. Lawrence. 1998. Ambulatory surgery in the United States, 1996. *Advance Data from Vital and Health Statistics.* No. 300. Hyattsville, Md.: National Center for Health Statistics.

Hollon, M. F. 1999. Direct-to-consumer marketing of prescription drugs: Creating consumer demand. *Journal of the American Medical Association* 281: 382–384.

Holmes, A. F. 1999. Direct-to-consumer prescription drug advertising builds bridges between patients and physicians. *Journal of the American Medical Association* 281: 380–382.

How drug savvy are you? 1999. *Consumer Reports on Health.* January.

Kalb, C. 1998. When drugs do harm. *Newsweek,* 27 April.

Kasper, J. F., A. G. Mulley, and J. E. Wennberg. 1992. Developing shared decision-making programs to improve the quality of health care. *Quality Review Bulletin* (June): 183–190.

Kemper, D. W., K. Lorig, and M. Mettler. 1993. The effectiveness of medical self-care interventions: A focus on self-initiated responses to symptoms. *Patient Education and Counseling* 21: 29–39.

Lazarou, J., B. H. Pomeranz, and P. N. Corey. 1998. Incidence of adverse drug reaction in hospitalized patients: A meta-analysis of prospective studies. *Journal of the American Medical Association* 279: 1200–1205.

Making sense of prescription-drug ads. 1997. *Consumer Reports on Health,* May.

Makoul, G., P. Arntson, and T. Schofield. 1995. Health promotion in primary care: Physician-patient communication and decision making about prescription medications. *Social Science and Medicine* 41(9): 1241–1254.

Marvel, M. K., et al. 1999. Soliciting the patient's agenda: Have we improved? *Journal of the American Medical Association* 281: 283–287.

Nonprescription Drug Manufacturers Association. 1996. *Nonprescription Medicines: What's Right for You?* Washington, D.C.: Nonprescription Drug Manufacturers Association.

Off-label drug use. 1997. *Harvard Women's Health Watch,* October.

Prescription drugs: Playing it safe. 1998. *HealthNews,* July.

Riessman, F., and D. Carroll, 1995. *Redefining Self-Help.* San Francisco: Jossey-Bass.

Steiner, J. F., and A. V. Prochazka. 1997. The assessment of refill compliance using pharmacy records. *Journal of Clinical Epidemiology* 50: 105–116.

Thom, D. H., and B. Campbell. 1997. Patient-physician trust: An exploratory study. *Journal of Family Practice* 44: 169–176.

U.S. Preventive Services Task Force. 1996. *Guide to Clinical Preventive Services: Report of the U.S. Preventive Services Task Force,* 2nd ed. Baltimore: Williams & Wilkins.

Woodward, C. A., et al. 1996. Do female primary care physicians practise preventive care differently from their male colleagues? *Canadian Family Physician* 42: 2370–2379.

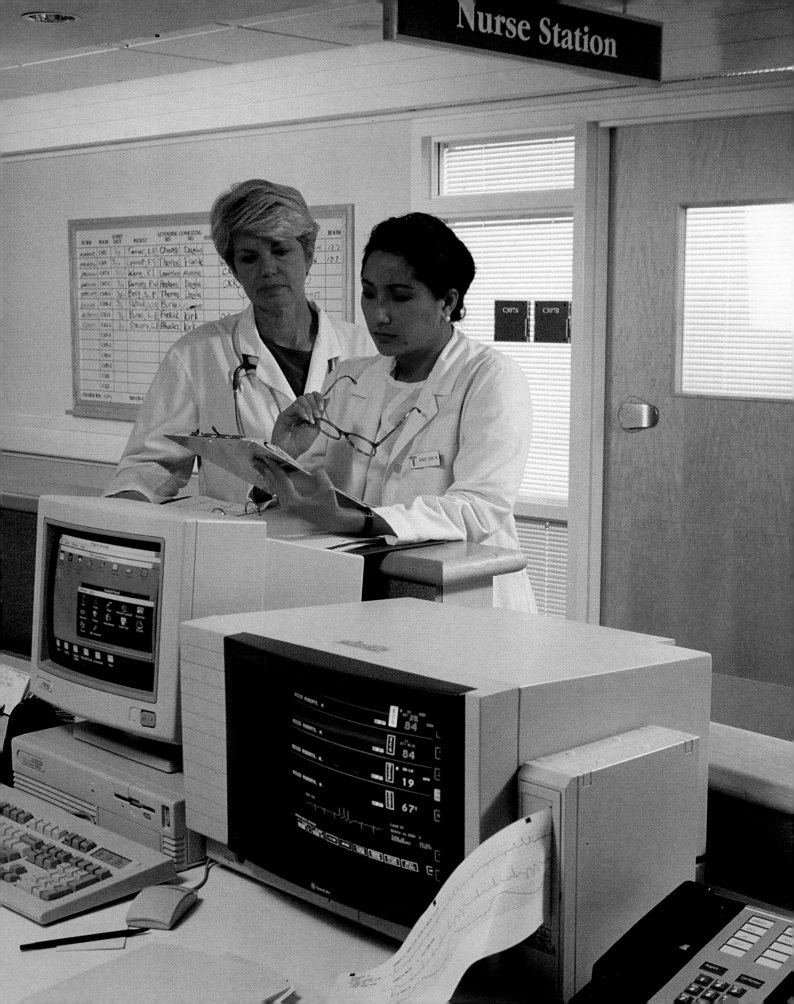

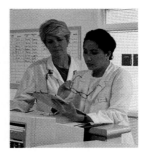

LEARNING OBJECTIVES

After reading this chapter, you should be able to:

- List different types of health care providers, and discuss strategies for choosing a primary care physician.

- Describe unconventional treatment methods, and know how to avoid quackery.

- Explain the current system of health care payments in the United States.

- Describe different types of health insurance plans, and list questions to ask when evaluating different plans.

The Health Care System 22

TEST YOUR KNOWLEDGE

1. On average, how many times do Americans contact their physicians each year, either on the phone or in person?
   - a. 3
   - b. 6
   - c. 12

2. What proportion of Americans do not have health insurance?
   - a. 1 in 6
   - b. 1 in 10
   - c. 1 in 20

3. Including payments made by individuals, insurance companies, and the government, about how much is spent on health care for each American?
   - a. $500 per year
   - b. $2000 per year
   - c. $4000 per year

4. About two-thirds of users of alternative therapies discuss their use of these therapies with their physicians.
   True or false?

Answers

1. **b.** People over age 65 have the most physician contacts, 10–12 per year.

2. **a.** More than 43 million Americans have no health insurance. People age 18–24, minorities, and those with low incomes and less than a high school education are much more likely than other Americans to be uninsured.

3. **c.** Costs are expected to increase to $7,100 by 2007.

4. **False.** Less than 40% disclose their use of alternative therapies. As many as 15 million American adults are at risk for potentially adverse interactions involving prescription drugs and herbs or high-dose vitamin supplements.

The health care system in the United States consists of a network of individuals and organizations involved in providing health services. The participants include independent practitioners, allied health care providers, hospitals, outpatient clinics, nursing homes, voluntary agencies, and public and private insurance programs.

The United States is said to be undergoing a "health care crisis" as a result of skyrocketing costs and inequalities in the distribution of services. More than 40 million Americans have no health insurance coverage, and millions more are underinsured. Part of the high cost of health care is due to the cost of new technology. But critics of the health care system believe that high costs are also due to waste, inefficiency, and fraud. Corrective legislation has been stymied by both the complexity of the problems and the competing demands of special-interest groups.

This chapter provides information on the health care system, as well as guidelines for choosing health care providers and paying for your health care.

HEALTH CARE PROVIDERS

When you seek medical care, how should you go about it? Should you go to a general practitioner? A specialist? A hospital emergency room? An urgent care center? Whom should you see—a physician, a nurse, a therapist? And what about the chiropractors and acupuncturists listed in the phone book? The process of finding appropriate treatment can seem overwhelming, until you understand some basics about health care providers.

Conventional Practitioners

The term *conventional health care* as used in this book refers to the prevention, diagnosis, and treatment of disease based on currently accepted scientific information.

TERMS

medical doctor   An independent practitioner who holds a doctor of medicine degree from an accredited medical school.

independent practitioner   A physician or other health professional who is legally permitted to provide health care services without direction from another health professional.

osteopathic physician   A medical practitioner who has graduated from an osteopathic medical school. Osteopathy incorporates the theories and practices of scientific medicine but focuses on musculoskeletal problems.

podiatrist   A nonmedical practitioner whose practice is limited to the feet and legs.

optometrist   A nonmedical practitioner who primarily examines the eyes and prescribes corrective lenses.

dentist   A nonmedical practitioner specializing in the prevention and treatment of diseases and injuries of the teeth, mouth, and jaws.

allied health care provider   A health care professional who typically provides services under the supervision and/or control of independent practitioners.

This information is based on research and observations gathered by practitioners and researchers throughout the world.

Health professionals who provide conventional health care are regulated by state licensing laws. To become licensed, they must graduate from an accredited professional school, have additional clinical experience, and pass a licensing examination given by a state or national board. Competent professionals continue their education throughout their careers by attending seminars, talking with colleagues, reading journals, and other activities.

Independent Practitioners   This section looks at five types of health professionals who are permitted by law to practice independently in the United States: medical doctors, osteopaths, podiatrists, optometrists, and dentists.

• **Medical doctors** are **independent practitioners** who hold an M.D. (doctor of medicine) degree from an accredited medical school. Once licensed, they are legally authorized to administer any type of medical or surgical treatment. What they actually do depends on their training, their inclinations, and the available facilities. Because the scope of medicine is so vast, most physicians take additional full-time training after graduation. (A partial list appears in the box "Selected Medical Specialties.") Those choosing to become specialists take 3 or more years of hospital-based specialty training, after which they can become "board-certified" by taking a rigorous examination. Most specialty boards require periodic recertification to ensure current skills and knowledge. Some specialists require a referral by a primary care physician, while others will see patients without a referral. To work in a hospital, physicians must apply for staff privileges, which are based on training and experience and are reviewed annually.

• **Osteopathic physicians** are independent practitioners who have received a D.O. (doctor of osteopathy) degree. Osteopathic practice is virtually identical to medical practice except that osteopaths tend to have greater interest in musculoskeletal problems and manipulative therapy.

• **Podiatrists** are independent practitioners whose care is limited to problems of the feet and legs. They hold a D.P.M. (doctor of podiatric medicine) degree. The length of their training is similar to that of physicians. Podiatrists can prescribe drugs and do minor surgery in their offices. Those who wish to perform major surgery must secure hospital privileges.

• **Optometrists** are independent practitioners who are trained to examine the eyes and related structures to detect vision problems, eye diseases, and related disorders. They hold an O.D. (doctor of optometry) degree. All states allow them to use drugs for diagnostic purposes, and nearly all states permit them to use drugs to treat minor ailments.

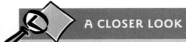
Allergy and immunology   The management of asthmatic, allergic, immunological, and related disorders.

Anesthesiology   The administration of drugs to prevent pain or to induce unconsciousness during surgical operations or diagnostic procedures.

Cardiology   A subspecialty of internal medicine that deals with the heart and blood vessels.

Cardiovascular surgery   The surgical treatment of diseases of the heart and blood vessels.

Dermatology   The diagnosis and treatment of skin diseases.

Emergency medicine   The diagnosis and treatment of emergencies.

Endocrinology   A subspecialty of internal medicine that deals with glandular and metabolic disorders.

Family practice   General medical services for patients and their families.

Gastroenterology   A subspecialty of internal medicine that deals with disorders of the digestive tract (esophagus, stomach, and intestines).

General surgery   Surgery for parts of the body that are not in the domain of specific surgical specialties (there are some overlapping areas).

Geriatrics   A subspecialty of family practice and internal medicine that deals with the medical problems of older adults.

Hematology/oncology   A subspecialty of internal medicine concerned with blood disorders and cancers.

Internal medicine   The diagnosis and nonsurgical treatment of internal organs of the body of adults.

Nephrology   The diagnosis and treatment of kidney diseases.

Neurology   The diagnosis and nonsurgical treatment of diseases of the brain, spinal cord, and nerves.

Neurosurgery   The diagnosis and surgical treatment of diseases of the brain, spinal cord, and nerves.

Nuclear medicine   The use of radioactive substances for diagnosis and treatment.

Obstetrics and gynecology   The care of pregnant women and disorders of the female reproductive system.

Ophthalmology   Medical and surgical care of the eye, including the prescribing of corrective lenses.

Orthopedics   The care of diseases of the muscles, and diseases, fractures, and deformities of the bones and joints.

Otolaryngology   The care of diseases of the head and neck, except for those of the eyes or brain.

Pathology   The examination and diagnosis of organs, tissues, body fluids, and excrement.

Pediatrics   The care of children from birth through adolescence. Subspecialties include allergy, cardiology, hematology/oncology, nephrology, and surgery.

Physiatry   The treatment of convalescent and physically handicapped patients.

Plastic surgery   Surgery to correct or repair deformed or mutilated parts of the body, or to improve facial or body features.

Proctology   Medical and surgical treatment of disorders of the intestines and rectum.

Psychiatry   The treatment of psychological and emotional problems.

Pulmonary disease   A subspecialty of internal medicine that deals with diseases of the lungs.

Radiology   The use of radiation for the diagnosis and treatment of disease.

Rheumatology   A subspecialty of internal medicine that deals with arthritis and related disorders.

Urology   The treatment of the male sex organs, and the male and female urinary tracts.

SOURCE: © 1996 Stephen Barrett, M.D.

• **Dentists** form another group of practitioners who can practice without medical supervision. They hold either a D.D.S. (doctor of dental surgery) or D.M.D. (doctor of medical dentistry) degree. Those who wish to become specialists complete 2 or more years of specialty training after graduation from dental school. Dentists are permitted to perform certain types of surgery and to prescribe a limited number of drugs within the scope of their training.

Allied Health Care Providers   In addition to these independent practitioners, millions of other trained practitioners, known as **allied health care providers,** deliver health care in the United States. These practitioners include registered nurses (R.N.), licensed vocational nurses (L.V.N.), registered dietitians (R.D.), psychologists, social workers, physician assistants (P.A.), physical therapists, and occupational therapists. Licensing laws, which vary from state to state, permit many of these practitioners to work independently. Others must be medically supervised or must have a medical referral in order to treat patients. The health care team also includes many types of technicians who work in hospitals and physicians' offices.

Choosing a Primary Care Physician   Most experts believe it is best to have a primary care physician, one who gets to know you and can treat you or coordinate referrals to specialists. Physicians who are board-certified in family practice (for adults and children), internal medicine (for adults only), or pediatrics (for children only) are good

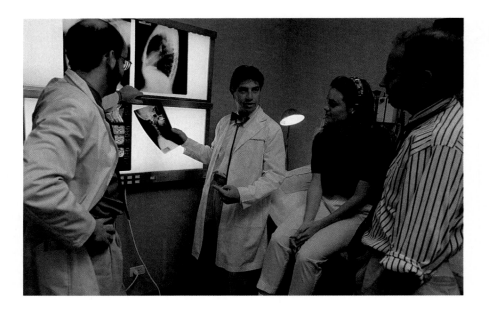

The health care system in the United States includes many different kinds of physicians and other health care workers. A physician can become a board-certified specialist in a particular field, such as orthopedics or radiology, by taking 3 or more years of special training and passing a rigorous examination.

choices; some women prefer to have an obstetrician-gynecologist as their primary care physician.

Staff affiliation with a hospital connected with a medical school or a program that trains residents indicates that a physician is apt to have current skills and information. Less favorable is affiliation with only privately owned hospitals, especially small ones, unless they are the only ones in the area. The absence of any hospital affiliation may be a sign of substandard care. Information on a physician's credentials can be obtained from her or his office, the local medical society, a local hospital, a directory at a medical or public library, or the World Wide Web (see For More Information at the end of the chapter).

The best time to look for a physician is before you are ill. Start by considering whether you would prefer your primary care physician to be an individual or a group, whether age or gender matters, and whether you have a complicated health problem for which a specialist would be an appropriate choice. Next, ask for recommendations from friends and acquaintances, other health care professionals, the local medical society, and hospital referral services. If you join a managed-care plan, the plan will issue a list of available physicians. Some health care providers and managed-care systems have their own Web sites, where you can get information about services, review physicians' credentials, and find answers to frequently asked questions.

After selecting a few prospects, telephone the physician's office to inquire about availability, fees, insurance participation, emergency and off-hours coverage, and any special concerns that you have. If your health problems are complicated, it may be useful to schedule a brief "get-acquainted visit" before making a final decision. After the first visit, consider whether: (1) the office appears to be run efficiently, (2) you were given adequate time to describe your problem, (3) the physician seemed thor-

ough, (4) the physician seemed receptive to your concerns, (5) your questions were answered, and (6) you received sufficient explanation of your problem and any recommended treatment.

Choosing a Medical Facility   If you become ill, the best choice of facility depends on the type and urgency of the problem, as well as your health insurance coverage and other financial considerations. For college students, the most practical choice will be the student health service. People with a primary care physician can telephone that practitioner's office. Ambulatory care centers provide an alternative for people who do not have a regular physician, who wish to be seen for an acute problem outside their regular physician's working hours, or who are traveling away from home. For chronic conditions, or for conditions where familiarity with the patient is important for making a diagnosis or for designing a treatment plan, a primary care physician is a better choice.

Table 22-1 summarizes the advantages and disadvantages of various sources of medical care.

> **PERSONAL INSIGHT**   In general, how do you feel about conventional medical practices—confident, reverent, resigned, skeptical, suspicious, apprehensive? How about unconventional practices? Why do you think you feel the way you do?

Unconventional Practitioners

The term *unconventional practitioners* refers to individuals whose philosophy and methods either clash with accepted knowledge about health and disease or are both unproven

TABLE 22-1	*Outpatient Health Care Facilities*	
Facility	**Advantages**	**Disadvantages**
Private medical office	Maximum personal attention; relatively low cost per visit	Limited hours
Multispecialty group	Relatively low cost per visit; consultations may be more readily available	Same physician may not always be seen (varies with setup of group)
Student health service	Convenient location; minimal cost	Hours and scope of practice may be limited
Ambulatory care center	Cost similar to medical office; much less than hospital emergency department; open long hours; no appointment needed	When care is episodic, physician does not get to know the patient as an individual; extra tests may be ordered because records are unavailable or physician does not know patient well
Hospital emergency department	Open 24 hours a day; can handle serious emergencies; sophisticated equipment available	Highest cost; nonemergency cases may not receive much attention; follow-up care may be minimal; care is episodic and less personal
Hospital outpatient clinic	Fees may be reduced for individuals who cannot afford private care	Patients may have to wait a long time to be seen; tend to have high staff turnover so different physicians may be seen
Ambulatory surgery center	Surgery costs less than it would in a hospital	Unsuitable for major surgery

SOURCE: © 1996 Stephen Barrett, M.D.

and unlikely. Reliance on unscientific practitioners may delay effective care and can involve financial exploitation. Except for chiropractic and acupuncture, most unconventional practices are not covered by health insurance.

Common Unconventional Practices   The approaches to health care discussed in this section are based on theories that are unproven or rejected by the scientific community. But the fact that an approach is unconventional does not mean its practitioners never help people or that everything they do should be considered quackery. Many people whose symptoms are bodily responses to tension (such as fatigue or headaches) may feel better following attention by anyone they believe in. Moreover, many of the practitioners described here might persuade patients to develop healthier living habits. Some also recommend appropriate medical care for patients who need it.

Many of the practitioners described in this section refer to themselves as "holistic," meaning that they treat the whole patient, giving attention to emotions and lifestyle in addition to physical problems. Good medical doctors have always practiced in this manner.

Unconventional methods are sometimes called "alternative" approaches to health care. This term can be misleading because it implies that the methods are *equivalent* or equally logical choices, which they are not. "Alternative" approaches have become newsworthy since the National Institutes of Health established the Office of Alternative Medicine (now the National Center for Complementary and Alternative Medicine) to stimulate research into unconventional treatment methods (see the

box "Complementary and Alternative Medicine," p. 594). This has been taken by some to indicate that "alternative" methods are becoming more acceptable in the scientific community. However, it is difficult to see how the underlying principles of many of these approaches could be reconciled with scientific thinking.

- **Chiropractic** is based on the late nineteenth-century teachings of Daniel David Palmer, who concluded that the main cause of disease is misplaced spinal bones. He believed that the body would be able to heal itself if vertebrae were restored to their proper places through spinal manipulation. There is no scientific evidence to justify this belief. Today, some chiropractors closely follow Palmer's ideas, while others acknowledge that germs, hormones, and other factors also play a role in disease. Some completely reject Palmer's theories and limit their practice to musculoskeletal disorders; chiropractors in this group are likely to work in tandem with medical doctors.

Chiropractors today are licensed in all 50 states. Their schools are accredited, and they hold a doctor of chiropractic degree (D.C.). Chiropractors are not licensed to prescribe drugs or perform surgery. Chiropractic manipulation for musculoskeletal problems is covered by many insurance plans.

chiropractic   A system of health care based on the premise that misalignments of the vertebrae contribute to most diseases and ailments.   TERMS

If you have ever gone to a chiropractor for back pain, taken herbal medicine for a cold, or had acupuncture for hay fever, you are among the estimated 4 in 10 Americans who have used at least one alternative therapy. According to a 1998 national survey, Americans made 629 million visits to herbalists, massage therapists, energy healers, and other alternative medicine practitioners in 1997, an increase of nearly 50% from 1991. Visits to such practitioners cost Americans $21.2 billion in 1997, at least $12.2 billion of it paid out of pocket; the number of such visits now exceeds the number of visits to primary care physicians. One reason offered for this trend is patients' disillusionment with the often hurried and impersonal care given by conventional physicians.

In recognition of the interest in alternative medicine, Congress funds the National Center for Complementary and Alternative Medicine (formerly the Office of Alternative Medicine) at the National Institutes of Health to evaluate alternative health practices. (The use of the word *complementary* suggests that alternative treatments may complement, rather than replace, conventional medicine.) The center facilitates and conducts basic and applied research and disseminates information on complementary and alternative medicine to practitioners and the public. Among the treatments being investigated are massage therapy for postsurgical recovery, hypnosis for chronic low-back pain, guided imagery for asthma, acupuncture for

depression, biofeedback and relaxation for diabetes, and Ayurvedic medicine for Parkinson's disease.

Despite the funding of the center, alternative medicine continues to be controversial. In 1998, the prestigious *Journal of the American Medical Association* devoted an issue to alternative treatments, but the equally prestigious *New England Journal of Medicine* launched a stinging attack on alternative medicine, denouncing it as unproven, unregulated, and sometimes dangerous. The potential for harm is borne out by the finding that less than 40% of the people who use alternative treatments tell their physicians that they are doing so, even when they are taking both prescription drugs and herbal remedies or high-dose vitamin supplements. In light of such findings and the rapidly growing use of alternative medicine, many researchers are urging the federal government and academic institutions to take a more proactive stance toward clinical research into alternative treatments, as well as toward quality control, credentialing, and surveillance in relation to alternative medicine.

SOURCES: Eisenberg, D. M., et al. 1998. Trends in alternative medicine use in the United States, 1990–1997. *Journal of the American Medical Association* 280: 1569–1575. Angell, M., and J. P. Kassirer. 1998. Alternative medicine: The risks of untested and unregulated remedies. *New England Journal of Medicine* 339(12): 839–841. Rising use of alternative medicine. 1999. *Healthline*, February.

Most people who consult chiropractors suffer from backaches or other musculoskeletal disorders. Although one recent study found no difference in back pain between subjects who received chiropractic treatment and subjects who read an educational booklet on back pain, numerous other studies have suggested that chiropractic manipulation can help some people with lower back pain, especially pain caused by a lack of mobility of bony segments of the spine. However, seeing a chiropractor regularly for "preventive maintenance" of the spine is a practice with no medical justification.

• **Acupuncture,** a technique dating from ancient China, involves the insertion of needles into the skin at one or more "acupuncture points." These points, said to represent various internal organs, are generally located along "meridians" on the surface of the body. Proponents claim that good health is produced by a harmonious mixture of yin and yang (thought of as "energy modes"), and that the stimulation of acupuncture points can balance them so that internal organs can return to normal functioning. Similar concepts underlie **acupressure (shiatsu),** but no needles are used.

Although there is no evidence that acupuncture can affect the course of any physical illness, a panel of independent experts convened by the NIH in 1997 concluded that it is an effective treatment for nausea caused by chemotherapy, anesthesia, or pregnancy and for some

postoperative and other kinds of pain. Scientists speculate that the effects may be due to the secretion of hormones or neurotransmitters or to changes in blood flow.

• **Homeopathy** is based on the theories of Samuel Hahnemann, a nineteenth-century German physician who theorized that the symptoms of disease can be cured by substances that produce similar symptoms in healthy people. The word *homeopathy* is derived from the Greek words *homeo,* meaning similar, and *pathos,* meaning suffering or disease.

Hahnemann believed that diseases represent a disturbance in the body's ability to heal itself, and that only a small stimulus is needed to trigger the healing process. After experimenting on himself and others, he concluded that the smaller the dose, the more powerful the effect—just the opposite of what pharmacologists have demonstrated in dose-response studies.

Homeopathic remedies are plant products, minerals, or other substances diluted to an extreme degree. Homeopathic remedies were recognized as drugs by the 1938 amendment to the federal Food, Drug, and Cosmetic Act. Unlike many other drugs, homeopathic remedies have been allowed to remain on the market without proof of their effectiveness being presented to the FDA.

• **Naturopathy** is based on the idea that disease is caused by a violation of nature's laws. Naturopaths believe that diseases are the body's effort to purify itself

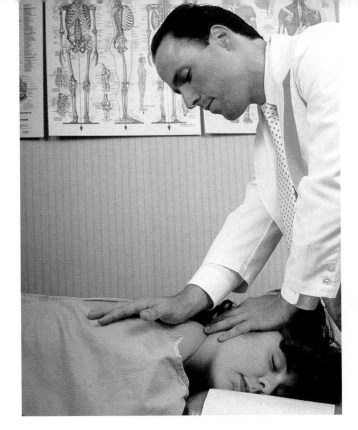

The primary treatment used by chiropractors is spinal manipulation. Properly applied, manipulation can benefit people with some types of musculoskeletal disorders.

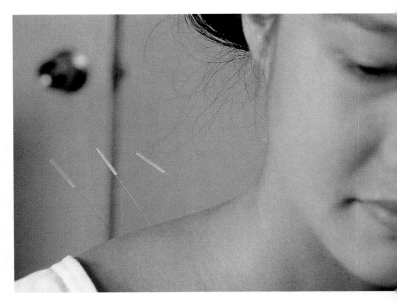

Acupuncture is based on the notion that illness results from an imbalance of vital energy flowing through the body along 14 meridians, each of which corresponds to a vital organ. The acupuncturist inserts needles at certain points and rotates them.

and that cures result from increasing the patient's "vital force" by ridding the body of toxins. Naturopathic treatments can include natural food diets, vitamins, herbs, manipulation, and massage. Naturopaths hold a doctor of naturopathy (N.D.) degree. They are licensed in 11 states, and one of their three schools is accredited.

• **Ayurvedic medicine** is based on a traditional Indian approach that includes meditation, "purification procedures," "rejuvenation therapies," herbal and mineral preparations, exercises, and dietary advice, all related to "Ayurvedic body type." The approach asserts that disease is caused by underlying "imbalances" in the principles that regulate body functions. Proponents claim that Ayurvedic medicine corrects such imbalances.

• **Clinical ecology** is practiced by a few hundred medical and osteopathic physicians. It is not a recognized specialty but is based on the notion that hypersensitivity to common foods and chemicals can cause depression, difficulty in thinking, headaches, muscle and joint pains, and many other common symptoms. Clinical ecologists speculate that the immune system can become "overloaded," producing what they call environmental illness. Many clinical ecologists claim their patients are suffering from hypersensitivity to the common yeast *Candida albicans*. The American Academy of Allergy and Immunology, the nation's largest professional organization of allergists, regards the concepts of environmental illness and yeast hypersensitivity as "speculative and unproven."

Other unconventional practices include iridology, applied kinesiology, reflexology, and faith healing.

Evaluating Unconventional Practices Given the relatively advanced state of medical science and the fairly high level of consumer awareness among Americans, why do unconventional practices persist—and even thrive? Proponents of unconventional practices—and especially promoters of quackery—appeal to people in many ways. They often offer hope to people who feel desperate, including people with incurable diseases. Some exploit

TERMS

acupuncture A technique based on the theoretical healing power of inserting needles into points on the skin.

acupressure (shiatsu) A technique based on the theory that pressing on various body parts can promote healing.

homeopathy A treatment method based on the theory that tiny doses of certain substances can exert powerful healing effects within the body.

naturopathy A treatment approach based on the belief that the basic cause of disease is a violation of nature's laws.

Ayurvedic medicine An adaptation of a traditional Indian approach based on "Ayurvedic body types" and on correcting imbalances in the principles that supposedly regulate body functions.

clinical ecology A treatment approach based on the concept that symptoms can be triggered by hypersensitivity to common foods and chemicals when the immune system becomes "overloaded."

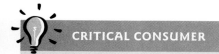

1. *Remember that quackery seldom looks outlandish.* Its promoters often use scientific terms and quote (or misquote) from scientific references. Some actually have reputable scientific training but have diverged from it.

2. *Ignore any practitioner who says that most diseases are caused by faulty nutrition or can be remedied by taking supplements.* Although some diseases are related to diet, most are not. Moreover, in most cases where diet actually is a factor in a person's health problem, the solution is not to take vitamins but to alter the diet.

3. *Be wary of anecdotes and testimonials.* If someone claims to have been helped by an unorthodox remedy, ask yourself and possibly your physician whether there might be another explanation. Most single episodes of disease recede with the passage of time, most chronic ailments have symptom-free periods, and many people giving testimonials have undergone conventional as well as unconventional therapies.

4. *Be wary of pseudomedical jargon.* Instead of offering to treat your disease, some quacks will promise to "detoxify" your body, "balance" its chemistry, release its "nerve energy," "bring it into harmony with nature," or correct supposed "weaknesses" of various organs. The use of concepts that are impossible to measure permits a claim of success, even though nothing has actually been accomplished.

5. *Don't fall for paranoid accusations.* Unorthodox practitioners often claim that the medical profession, drug companies, and the government are conspiring to suppress whatever method they espouse. It defies logic to believe that large numbers of people would oppose the development of treatment methods that might someday help themselves or their loved ones.

6. *Forget about "secret cures."* No one who actually discovered a cure would have reason to keep it secret. If a method works—especially for a serious disease—the discoverer would gain enormous fame, fortune, and personal satisfaction by sharing the discovery with others.

7. *Be wary of herbal remedies.* Many herbs contain hundreds or even thousands of chemicals that have not been completely cataloged. While some may turn out to be useful, others could well prove toxic. With safe and effective treatment available, treatment with herbs rarely makes sense.

8. *Be skeptical of any product claimed to be effective against a wide range of unrelated diseases, particularly diseases that are serious.* There is no such thing as a panacea or "cure-all."

9. *Ignore appeals to your vanity.* One of quackery's most powerful appeals is the suggestion to "think for yourself" instead of following the collective wisdom of the scientific community. A similar appeal is that although a remedy has not been proven to work for others, it still might work for you.

10. *Don't let desperation cloud your judgment.* If you feel that your physician isn't doing enough to help you, or if you have been told that your condition is incurable and don't wish to accept this fate without a struggle, don't stray from scientific health care in a desperate attempt to find a solution. Instead, discuss your feelings with your physician, and consider a consultation with a recognized expert.

SOURCE: © 1996 Stephen Barrett, M.D.

---

strains in the relationship between patient and physician, promising to cure those who are dissatisfied with the course of their treatment.

Some take advantage of current health threats, such as cancer and AIDS. Some attack the medical establishment, suggesting it is trying to suppress effective treatments. Some foster anxiety by suggesting that many people have problems that are actually uncommon, such as vitamin deficiencies and low blood sugar. And many promise new, quick, or easy ways to stay slim, strong, and young.

How can you protect yourself against quackery? Most important is maintaining an appropriate level of suspicion. For example, don't assume that health claims made in advertisements on the Internet or on radio or television talk shows must be true or would not have been allowed—that is not necessarily the case. Be especially wary of "cyberdocs" offering free medical consultation on the Internet.

To take advantage of the best that medical science can offer and to avoid being led astray, you must make reasoned, informed decisions about what to believe. Many resources exist to help people assess the claims made for a product or treatment. You can consult a physician, registered dietitian, or other reputable professional; do some reading at a public library (preferably with some professional guidance); get information from a reputable Internet source, such as an academic medical center or government agency; contact a consumer group or local health organization; or ask your insurance company whether they will pay for the treatment. The specific strategies listed in the box "Ten Ways to Avoid Being Quacked" will help you know what to do the next time you encounter a treatment that seems too good to be true. Several books listed at the end of this chapter provide more comprehensive advice.

In addition, Table 22-2 lists places where you can obtain information or express any concerns you may have about questionable health matters. Remember that people who make responsible complaints not only may help themselves, but also may help protect others.

TABLE 22-2	*Where to Complain or Seek Help*

Problem	Agencies to Contact*
False advertising	FTC Bureau of Consumer Protection Regional FTC office National Advertising Division, Council of Better Business Bureaus Editor or station manager of media outlet where ad appeared
Product marketed with false or misleading claims	Regional FDA office State attorney general State health department Local Better Business Bureau Congressional representatives
Bogus mail-order promotion	Chief Postal Inspector, U.S. Postal Service State attorney general
Improper treatment by licensed practitioner	Local or state professional society (if practitioner is a member) Local hospital (if practitioner is a staff member) State professional licensing board National Council Against Health Fraud Task Force on Victim Redress
Improper treatment by unlicensed individual	Local district attorney State attorney general National Council Against Health Fraud Task Force on Victim Redress
Advice needed about questionable product or service	National Council Against Health Fraud Local, state, or national professional or voluntary health groups

*Addresses:
FTC Bureau of Consumer Protection, Washington, DC 20580. 202-326-2222 (http://www.ftc.gov).
National Advertising Division, Council of Better Business Bureaus, 845 Third Ave., New York, NY 10022. 212-754-1320.
FDA, 5600 Fishers Lane, Rockville, MD 20857. 301-443-1240 or 800-532-4440 (http://www.fda.gov/medwatch).
Chief Postal Inspector, U.S. Postal Service, 475 L'Enfant Plaza, S.W., Washington, DC 20260. 202-268-4267.
Consumer Health Information Resource Institute, 300 E. Pink Hill Rd., Independence, MO 64057. 816-228-4595.
National Council Against Health Fraud, P.O. Box 1276, Loma Linda, CA 92354. 909-824-4690 (http://www.ncahf.org).
NCAHF Task Force on Victim Redress, P.O. Box 1747, Allentown, PA 18105. 610-437-1795.
For regional offices of federal agencies, consult the telephone directory under U.S. Government. When more than one agency might be appropriate, contact all of them.

SOURCE: © 1996 Stephen Barrett, M.D.

PAYING FOR HEALTH CARE

The American health care system is one of the most advanced and comprehensive in the world, but it is also the most expensive. In 1997, the nation spent more than $1 trillion on health care, or $4000 per person. Health care costs are expected to nearly double in the first decade of the twenty-first century, reaching $2.1 trillion, or about $7100 per person, by 2007. Numerous factors contribute to the high cost of health care in the United States, including the cost of advanced equipment and new technology; expensive treatments for some illnesses and conditions, such as cancer, heart disease, HIV infection, injuries, and low birth weight in infants; the aging of the population; and high earnings by some people in the health care industry and, in some cases, the demand for profits by investors.

The Current System

Health care is currently financed by a combination of private and public insurance plans, patient out-of-pocket payments, and government assistance (Figure 22-1). In 1997, private insurance and individual patients paid about 55% of the total; the government paid the remaining 45%, mainly through Medicare and Medicaid (discussed below). Most nonelderly Americans receive their health insurance through their employers.

Despite high spending, not everyone is included in this financing system. More than 43 million people (16% of the population), the vast majority of them employed, have no health care insurance at all. Many more are underinsured and thus either pay for medical services out of pocket or forgo medical care altogether. The uninsured include 10.6 million children—15% of all American

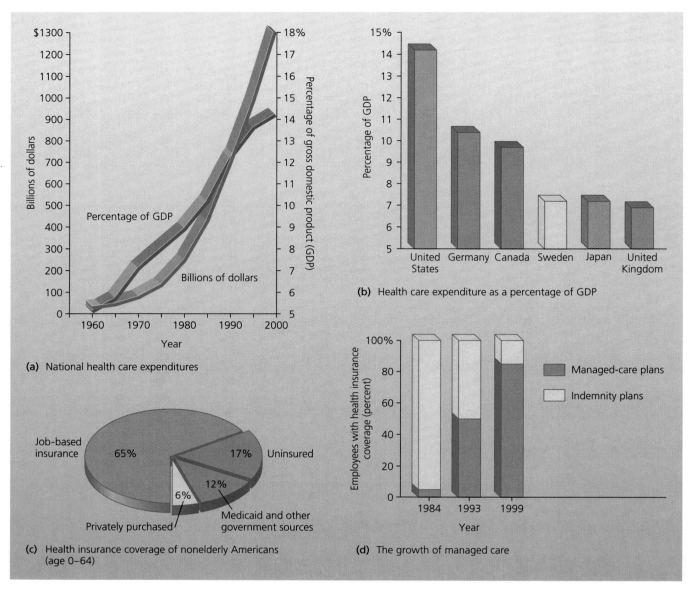

VITAL STATISTICS

Figure 22-1   A statistical look at health care expenditures and health insurance.

SOURCES: Kuttner, R. 1999. The American health care system: Employer-sponsored health coverage. *New England Journal of Medicine* 340(3): 248–252. U.S. National Center for Health Statistics. 1998. *Health, United States, 1998.* Hyattsville, Md.: U.S. Public Health Service. Health Care Financing Administration (http://www.hcfa.gov).

children—most in working, low-income families. In a trend contrary to the *Healthy People* goal of health insurance coverage for all Americans, the number of uninsured Americans has risen since 1990, largely because of a deterioration in employer-provided coverage.

Lack of insurance affects both access to care and quality of care. People without insurance use health services less often and receive poorer care when they do use the services. Children without insurance are less likely to have screening tests and immunizations. They have fewer checkups, are less likely to be treated for injuries and for

chronic conditions such as asthma, and are more likely to go without eyeglasses and prescribed drugs.

Another problem is that national health spending is growing faster than the rest of the economy, consuming an ever-increasing share of the U.S. gross domestic product (GDP). Health care spending represented 13.5% of the GDP in 1997 and is projected to reach 16.6% by 2007. Health care costs soared in the 1980s and then were contained to some extent in the 1990s by a large-scale switch from private insurance to managed care (discussed below), which is designed to achieve cost economies. But the savings from this switch were likely a one-time phenomenon, since 85% of working Americans are now covered by managed-care plans. Experts predict that health costs will double in the next 10 years; due to restrictions on government spending, much of the increase will be borne by private insurers and individuals.

Over the past several years, dozens of health care reform plans have been presented to Congress in attempts to solve the problems of cost and unequal access to services. To date no single plan has received widespread endorsement from politicians, the health care industry, and consumers. What does the future hold? Experts see countertrends emerging in reaction to the cost cutting of the 1990s, including a renewed focus on quality of care, more interest in consumer choice, and greater demands for physician autonomy—as well as higher health care costs for individual Americans.

Health Insurance

Health insurance enables people to receive health care they might not otherwise be able to afford. Hospital care costs hundreds of dollars a day, and surgical fees can cost thousands. Health insurance is important for everyone, especially as health care costs continue to rise.

Health insurance plans are either indemnity (or fee-for-service) or managed care. With both types the individual or the employer pays a basic premium, usually on a monthly basis; there are often other payments as well. Insurance policies are sold to both groups and individuals; group plans tend to cover more services and cost less. Group coverage is often available through employers to workers and their families. People who are self-employed or whose employers don't offer group policies may need to buy individual plans. Americans who are 65 or older, have disabilities, or have a low income may receive health insurance through government programs.

Indemnity Plans In an indemnity or fee-for-service plan, you can use any medical provider (such as a physician or a hospital) you choose. You or the provider sends the bill to your insurance company, which pays part of it. Usually you have to pay a "deductible" amount each year, ranging from $100 up to several hundred dollars, before the insurer starts covering your expenses. Once you meet the deductible, most plans pay a percentage—often 80%—of what they consider the "usual and customary" charge for covered services. You pay the remaining 20%, which is known as coinsurance. Most indemnity plans cover hospital, surgical, and many medical services, but coverage varies widely from one plan to another, so it is important to read your policy carefully.

Managed-Care Plans Managed-care plans have agreements with certain physicians, hospitals, and health care providers to give a range of services to plan members at reduced cost. In general, you have lower out-of-pocket costs and less paperwork with a managed-care plan than with an indemnity plan, but you also have less freedom in choosing health care providers. There are three types of managed-care plans: HMOs, PPOs, and POS plans.

• **Health maintenance organizations (HMOs)** offer members a range of health benefits for a set monthly fee. When you use the service, you pay either nothing or a small copayment of $5 or $10. If you go outside the HMO, you have to pay for the service yourself. The HMO provides you with a list of physicians from which you choose your primary care physician, usually a family physician, internist, obstetrician-gynecologist, or pediatrician. Your primary care physician manages your care and refers you to specialists if you need them. Physicians in the HMO agree to accept a monthly per patient fee, or **capitation,** or to charge according to a lower-than-standard fee schedule. This arrangement encourages physicians to avoid unnecessary services. Physicians may be located in a central office or clinic and be salaried employees, or they may have private offices and be under contract to the HMO.

• **Preferred provider organizations (PPOs)** are plans that have arrangements with physicians, hospitals, and other care providers who have agreed to accept lower fees for their services. If you go to a provider within the PPO network, you pay a copayment that is lower for members of the plan. If you go outside the network, you have to meet the deductible and pay coinsurance based on higher charges. You may also have to pay the difference between what the provider charges and what the plan will pay.

• **Point-of-service (POS) plans** are options offered by many HMOs, in which you can see a physician outside the plan and still be partially covered. If your primary care physician refers you to a specialist outside

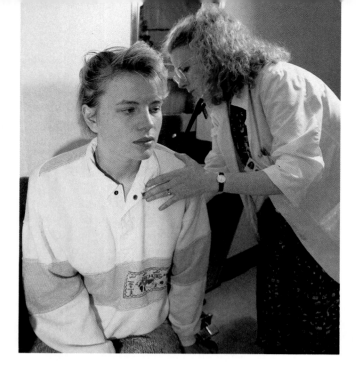

Physicians who work for a health maintenance organization usually receive a salary or monthly payment rather than fees from patients. The advantage of HMOs for patients is that their medical care is pre-paid; the disadvantage is that the choice of physicians is narrowed.

the network, the plan pays all or most of the bill. If you refer yourself to a provider outside the network for a covered service, you have to pay coinsurance.

Government Programs   Americans who are 65 or older and younger people with certain disabilities can be covered by **Medicare,** a federal health insurance program with two parts. Part A provides hospital insurance and is financed by mandatory contributions by all working Americans. Part B helps pay for physician and other medical services and is financed through general tax revenues and monthly premiums paid by those who wish to subscribe. Private insurance companies also sell "medigap" policies to supplement Medicare coverage. Under Medicare, physicians who "accept assignment" are paid directly by the government and may not bill the patient for the difference between their usual fee and the amount the government pays (except for amounts that involve deductibles and coinsurance). As a result of limits placed on Medicare payments, some physicians have stopped accepting patients with this type of insurance coverage.

Medicaid is a joint federal-state health insurance program run by the states. It covers some low-income people, especially children and pregnant women, and people with certain disabilities. The Balanced Budget Act of 1997 established the Children's Health Insurance Program (CHIP), designed to protect children from loss of Medicaid coverage as a result of welfare reform laws. CHIP provides the states with billions of dollars for health care services for children; in the first year of its implementation, nearly a million children were enrolled in CHIP.

Indemnity Plans Versus Managed-Care Plans   Different types of plans have advantages and disadvantages for consumers. Indemnity plans collect a premium from you or your employer up front. Then, as you use medical services, you pay a set deductible and a percentage of the expenses thereafter. You can see any physician you choose, including specialists. Your physician is paid based on the service he or she provides. Critics point to the fee-for-service payment system as a contributing factor in the rapid growth of health care costs in the United States because physicians have a financial incentive to order more tests and treatments for their patients.

In a managed-care plan, you or your employer pay the premium plus, in many cases, a small per-visit fee. When services are used, the fixed fees remain the same, regardless of the amount or level of services provided. Many plans try to reduce costs over the long term by paying for routine preventive care, such as regular checkups, routine screening tests, and prenatal care; they may also encourage prevention by offering health education and lifestyle modification programs for members. (Many indemnity plans also stress preventive care.)

Other cost-cutting measures are less consumer-oriented. Patients' choices are limited: They have to choose health care providers from the plan list or network, and they may have to wait longer for appointments and travel farther to get to participating clinics or offices. Due to consumer demand for more flexibility, many HMO plans now include a point-of-service option.

Managed-care plans also try to control costs by discouraging overtreatment through the use of "gatekeepers." Once a patient has chosen a primary care physician, he or she must get this physician's preapproval for diagnostic tests and referrals to specialists; in some plans, physicians themselves must receive approval from a plan representative prior to treating or referring a patient. Patients may also be required to get a plan representative's preapproval for any hospital treatment not involving an emergency. If a patient violates the rules for obtaining services, the plan typically will not cover the cost of the services in question. Plans based on a capitation system give physicians a financial incentive to limit the number of tests and treatments they offer patients, the reverse of the financial incentive in indemnity plans. Critics claim that physicians in managed-care plans deny patients needed services in their efforts to keep costs down. Recently there has been a broad shift of patients from traditional HMOs to PPOs and POS plans. For strategies on getting the most from a managed-care plan, see the box "Managing with Managed Care."

PERSONAL INSIGHT   Do you believe that physicians and hospitals have a responsibility to treat and care for patients who can't pay? Do you think medical care is a right or a privilege? What is the basis for your beliefs and opinions?

Managed-care plans can save insurers and patients money, but they can also be costly for those who don't follow the plan's rules. The key to getting the most from managed care is knowing how your plan works. The following guidelines can help you work successfully within a managed-care plan.

- *Consider your options.* If you have the option of choosing among several managed-care plans, read through the materials for each. Look especially at the cost of the plan and the types of services covered. What is the copayment for physician visits? How much do prescriptions cost? If you go to an emergency room for something that turns out to be a nonemergency, what is the plan's policy for covering the cost? For plans with a point-of-service option, find out what percentage of the cost is covered when you visit a physician outside the plan. If services you think you'll need are not covered (for example, physical therapy or psychotherapy), it may be worthwhile to choose a plan with a higher premium that offers more comprehensive coverage.

- *Investigate.* Talk with a physician who works with each of the plans you're considering. Ask the physician how happy he or she is with the plan. Are there bureaucratic hassles or delays? Find out how approval for treatments and specialist referrals are handled. Does the individual physician make the determination, or must the decision go before a plan representative or utilization committee? How does the plan pay its physicians? Are there financial incentives for restricting care?

- *Know how each plan will affect your current health care situation.* Is your current physician a participant? Will the plan approve the continuation of any current treatments you are receiving, such as a drug regimen for allergies or asthma? Find out exactly how each plan will affect the type and level of care you receive.

- *Learn the rules of the plan you choose.* Know what payments are required and what the process is for making an

appointment or obtaining a referral. Find out what facilities in your area are covered by your plan and what restrictions apply. Know how to obtain care when you're away from home, including when you are out of the country.

- *Choose a physician carefully.* If you will be choosing a new physician when you join a plan, follow the strategies on pp. 591–592. The health plan's office can provide you with information about participating physicians; in addition, ask your friends, family, and colleagues for recommendations. If you are going to shop around and change physicians within a plan, do it soon and not too often; continuity is an important part of good health care. However, there is no need to settle on a physician with whom you don't feel comfortable. Schedule an initial examination; don't wait until you're ill to see your physician for the first time.

- *Take advantage of wellness programs.* Find out what types of lifestyle management and wellness programs your managed-care plan offers. In addition to programs for losing weight, quitting smoking, and reducing stress, your plan may offer discounts on health club memberships, eyeglass frames, and other such items. Take full advantage of opportunities to make positive changes in your lifestyle.

- *Speak up if you're not happy.* If you're not satisfied with the care you receive, or if you don't get an appointment or a referral when you think you need one, complain to the plan's administrative office. Don't let the inconvenience of the complaint process dissuade you. Also, discuss your problem with your company's benefits manager. Unless your employer hears about problems with a particular plan, the health insurance options you are offered won't change.

SOURCES: In search of quality health care. 1998. *Consumer Reports,* October. How good is your health plan? 1996. *Consumer Reports,* August. Managing your care. 1994. *Harvard Women's Health Watch,* September.

Choosing a Policy

Choosing health insurance can be a complicated process. There are many types of plans, and contracts can vary greatly from company to company, and even within the same company. It's important to evaluate the coverage provided by different plans and choose the one that's best for you. (The box "A Glossary of Health Insurance Terms" can help you understand different policies.)

Colleges typically provide outpatient services through a student health center. Some also require students to purchase additional insurance to cover hospitalization or other outside services. Students covered under their family's policy may not be required to purchase additional insurance. It is usually most economical to remain covered under a family policy for as long as possible, rather than obtain a separate policy.

After college, it is usually best to see whether group coverage is available through work or membership in an organization. If you work for a large company, several plans may be available. If no group coverage is available, contact Blue Cross/Blue Shield and agents for several other insurance companies, including some that provide managed-care plans.

Managed-care plans tend to have lower premiums and result in fewer out-of-pocket costs, particularly for young adults and families with young children. Traditional indemnity policies tend to cost more and involve more

Medicare A federal health insurance program for people 65 **TERMS** or older and for younger people with certain disabilities.

Medicaid A federally subsidized state-run plan of health care for people of low income.

Because health insurance policies are legal contracts, they use precise legal language. Some of these terms appear in all policies, while others appear just in some. Understanding them will help you figure out how a policy works and what it actually covers. Below are terms not defined elsewhere in this chapter.

assignment of benefits   By signing a form (usually the insurance claim form), you authorize the insurance company to pay the physician directly. Otherwise, payment must be made directly to you. Most physicians will ask you to sign the form if you don't want to pay your bill before the insurance company pays its share.

coinsurance   An arrangement whereby you and the insurance company share costs. Typically, the insurer pays 75–85% of covered costs and you pay the rest. Some policies set an upper limit to coinsurance expense, after which the company pays all additional charges.

conversion privilege   A provision that enables those insured by group contracts to obtain an individual policy under various circumstances, such as leaving the job that provided the group coverage.

coordination of benefits   A provision that prohibits you from collecting identical benefits from two or more policies, thereby profiting when you are ill. After the primary company pays, other companies will calculate their coverage of the remainder. All group policies contain a coordination clause, but some individual policies do not.

copayment   A fixed dollar amount paid whenever an insured person receives specified health care services.

deductible   The amount you must pay before the insurance company starts paying.

endorsement or rider   An attachment to the basic insurance policy that changes its coverage.

exclusion   A specified condition or circumstance for which the policy does not provide benefits.

gatekeeper   A health care provider, usually a primary care physician, who supervises all aspects of a patient's care and must authorize care (except in emergencies) from other providers before the plan will pay for it.

grace period   The number of days that you may delay payment of your premium without losing your insurance.

guaranteed renewability   A provision whereby the company agrees to continue insuring you up to a certain age (or for life), as long as you pay the premium. Under this provision, the premium structure cannot be raised unless it is raised for all members of a group or class of insured, such as all people living in your state with the same kind of policy.

indemnity insurance   A policy that provides benefits specified within a framework of fee schedules, exclusions, and limitations.

inpatient services   Services received while hospitalized.

notice of claim   Written notice the company must receive when a claim exists. Typically, it must be received within 20 days or as soon thereafter as reasonably possible.

outpatient services   Services obtained at a hospital by people who are not confined to the hospital.

participating physician   A physician who agrees to abide by the rules of a plan in return for direct payment by the insurance company. The agreement includes acceptance of a fixed fee schedule, a monthly fee per eligible patient, or other fee limitation.

portability   The right, after employment terminates, to transfer from a group insurance plan to another group or individual plan.

preexisting condition   A health problem the policyholder had before becoming insured. Some policies exclude these conditions, while others do not.

provider   Any source of health care services, such as a hospital, physician, pharmacist, or laboratory.

reasonable charge   The amount a company will pay for a given service based on what most providers charge for it.

subscriber   An individual who contracts for health insurance coverage.

utilization review   Case review to determine whether the care rendered was necessary and appropriate.

waiting period   A specified time between issuance of a policy and coverage of certain conditions. Typically, there are waiting periods for preexisting conditions and maternity benefits.

---

paperwork (in filing claims) but provide a greater choice of providers, which may be important for people who are chronically or seriously ill. People inclined toward managed care should investigate whether a suitable primary physician is available to them in any plan they consider. Some HMOs provide data on subscriber satisfaction with their primary care physicians.

The following questions are designed to help you choose the most appropriate insurance for you:

- What services are covered? Different policies may

cover any of the following: physicians' office visits, X ray examinations, outpatient diagnostic tests, medications, inpatient medical and hospital costs, surgical costs, physical therapy, maternity fees, vision care, emergency room care, mental health services, skilled nursing home care, and alcohol and drug dependency treatment.

- Which of these services am I most likely to need?
- Are there exclusions for any preexisting conditions or chronic problems?

- What preventive health services are covered?
- How do the various policies compare in cost?
- Are the deductible and copayments (coinsurance provisions) suitable?
- Are the maximum limits high enough?
- Will I be able to see the physicians I prefer?
- Does my present physician participate?

Most of the time, you can take care of yourself without personally consulting an expert. You can learn to manage stress, eat sensibly, get adequate exercise, minimize contact with contagious disease, and so on. When you do need professional care (Chapter 21 provides guidelines to help you identify those situations), you can continue to take responsibility for yourself by making reasoned decisions about the care and health insurance you obtain.

Because so many people are involved in the health care field and because human knowledge has its limits, you are bound to have a frustrating or unpleasant experience now and then, as can happen in any area of your life. Take setbacks in stride and be persistent about getting good care.

SUMMARY

- The U.S. health care system is a network of individuals and organizations that provide health services. The system is in crisis today because of high costs and unequal distribution of services.

Health Care Providers

- Conventional health care is the prevention, diagnosis, and treatment of disease based on currently accepted scientific information. Conventional practitioners are regulated by state licensing laws; many are permitted to practice independently.

- Medical doctors have degrees from accredited medical schools and are licensed to administer medical and surgical treatment; specialists have additional training and can become board-certified.

- Osteopathic practice incorporates all the theories and practices of medicine but focuses on musculoskeletal problems.

- Podiatrists specialize in the care of feet and legs. Optometrists examine the eyes to detect vision problems and eye diseases.

- Dentists are permitted to perform certain types of surgery on the mouth and prescribe certain drugs.

- Allied health care providers include registered nurses, licensed vocational nurses, registered dietitians, psychologists, physical therapists, occupational therapists, and many other kinds of trained practitioners.

- When seeking medical care, people should usually find a primary physician, who can refer them to specialists when necessary.

- Choice of a facility for health care depends on the type and urgency of the problem and on health insurance coverage and other financial considerations.

- Unconventional practitioners are individuals whose philosophy and methods are not based on scientifically accepted knowledge.

- Chiropractic is based on the idea that the main cause of disease is misplaced spinal bones.

- Acupuncture involves the insertion of needles into the skin at various points said to represent internal organs. Acupressure is a similar technique that doesn't use needles.

- Homeopathy is based on the belief that the symptoms of disease can be cured by substances that produce similar symptoms in healthy people, and that the smaller the dose, the more powerful the effect.

- Other unconventional practices include naturopathy, Ayurvedic medicine, and clinical ecology.

- Proponents of certain unconventional methods, especially quackery, offer hope to the desperate and exploit people's needs, anxieties, and desperation. The best protection against quackery is a skeptical mind.

Paying for Health Care

- Health care is financed through a combination of public and private sources. Health care reforms have been proposed because health care costs are increasing rapidly and a large number of Americans do not have health insurance.

- Health insurance plans are usually described as either indemnity (or fee-for-service) or managed-care plans. The three types of managed-care plans are HMOs, PPOs, and POS plans. Indemnity plans allow consumers more choice in medical providers, but managed-care plans are less expensive.

- Government programs include Medicaid, for the poor, and Medicare, for those who are 65 and over or chronically disabled.

- Group insurance usually offers the best coverage. The choice of a policy should depend on services covered, services needed, exclusions for preexisting conditions or chronic problems, deductibles, maximum limits, and choice of physicians.

1. Visit the student health center on your campus or another health care facility. Evaluate the quality and kinds of services available. Consider such things as hours, waiting time, health literature available, the scope of services, the availability of specialists, and so on. Do you think there is room for improvement? What recommendations would you make?

2. Talk to a practitioner of one or more of the unconventional practices described in this chapter. Ask what training they have, what conditions they treat most often, how they make diagnoses, what treatments they give, and whether they have any pamphlets you can read. What questions do you have about these practices? Where would you go to find the answers?

1. Using the insurance guidelines in the chapter, evaluate your current coverage. In your health journal, make a list of the services it covers and does not cover; put a check mark next to the services you are most likely to need. Examine the cost of the policy, including the deductibles and copayments and the maximum limits on coverage. Also look at the rules governing your choice of physicians. Does your current plan meet your needs? Does it lack any services that are important for you or cover any unnecessary ones?

2. *Critical Thinking* Examine and evaluate a TV or printed advertisement for a health-related product or service. What methods are used in the ad to make the product or service appeal to consumers? Does it contain any hidden messages? Are there any aspects of the ad you feel are misleading? Write a short essay describing your findings.

Books, Newsletters, and Articles

Alternative Medicine Alert: A Clinician's Guide to Alternative Therapies (American Health Consultants: 800-688-2421; http://www.ahcpub.com). *Costly but useful, this newsletter presents scientific information and opinion on alternative medicine.*

The American Health Care System Revisited. 1999. *New England Journal of Medicine.* January 7–February 25. *An eight-part series of articles that reviewed the current state of the U.S. health care system; issues covered include expenditures, insurance coverage, Medicare, and quality of care.*

Barrett, S., and W. T. Jarvis, eds. 1993. *The Health Robbers.* Amherst, N.Y.: Prometheus. *A comprehensive look at quackery in America.*

Callahan, D. 1999. *False Hopes: Why America's Quest for Perfect Health Is a Recipe for Disaster.* New York: Simon & Schuster. *A critical review of the values and goals of modern medicine by a medical ethicist.*

Cassileth, B. R. 1998. *The Alternative Medicine Handbook: The Complete Reference Guide to Alternative and Complementary Therapies.* New York: Norton. *A reference summarizing each approach and analyzing research-based evidence of efficacy.*

Consumer Reports magazine frequently publishes articles that help consumers make informed decisions about health care, including the following: Alternative medicine: The facts (January 1994); Homeopathy (March 1994); Chiropractors (June 1994); Can HMOs help solve the health-care crisis? (October 1996); Acupuncture (September 1998); In search of quality health care (October 1998).

Humber, J. M., and R. F. Almeder, eds. 1998. *Alternative Medicine and Ethics.* Totowa, N.J. Humana Press. *Six essays on issues facing policymakers relating to alternative medicine.*

Korczyk, S. M., and H. A. Witte. 1998. *The Complete Idiot's Guide to Managed Health Care.* New York: Macmillan. *Provides consumer-oriented information about how to understand options and get the best care possible.*

Organizations, Hotlines, and Web Sites

Agency for Health Care Policy and Research. Provides practical, science-based information to health care providers and consumers.

    800-358-9295

    http://www.ahcpr.gov

Alternative Health News Online. Provides a selection of Web pages on complementary and alternative health.

    http://www.altmedicine.com

American Council on Science and Health. Provides consumer education materials relating to food, chemicals, lifestyle, environment, and health.

    212-362-7044

    http://www.acsh.org

American Medical Association (AMA). Provides information about physicians, including their training, licensure, and board certification; the Web site provides recent medical news, AMA policy statements, and links to related sites.

    515 N. State St.

    Chicago, IL 60610

    312-464-5000

    http://www.ama-assn.org

Electronic Policy Network Idea Central/Health Policy Page. A "virtual" magazine with articles on managed care, the uninsured, the future of Medicare, and other issues.

    http://www.epn.org/idea/health.html

Health Care Financing Administration. Provides information, statistics, and other material on Medicare, Medicaid, and the Children's Health Insurance Program.

800-638-6833; 877-KIDSNOW

http://www.hcfa.gov

National Center for Complementary and Alternative Medicine (NCCAM)/National Institutes of Health. Provides general information packets, answers to frequently asked questions about alternative therapies, research abstracts, and bibliographies.

P.O. Box 8218

Silver Spring, MD 20907

888-644-6226

http://nccam.nih.gov

National Consumers League. Represents consumers on a variety of issues, including health care and food and drug safety; provides a variety of brochures on health-related topics.

1701 K Street, N.W., Suite 1201

Washington DC 20006

202-835-3323

http://www.nclnet.org

National Council for Reliable Health Information. Provides news and information about health fraud and quackery and links to related Web sites.

300 E. Pink Hill Rd.

Independence, MO 64057

816-228-4595

http://www.ncahf.org

Physician Credentials. To check the credentials of a medical doctor or osteopathic physician who advertises as a "specialist," call the appropriate board:

American Board of Medical Specialties

800-776-2378

http://www.certifieddoctor.org

American Osteopathic Association

800-621-1773

Quackwatch. Provides information on health fraud, quackery, and health decision making.

http://www.quackwatch.com

U.S. Food and Drug Administration. Provides information on FDA activities and publishes *FDA Consumer* magazine, which frequently includes helpful strategies for evaluating health products and services.

5600 Fishers Lane

Rockville, MD 20857

888-INFOFDA

http://www.fda.gov

See also the listings in Chapter 1 and Appendix C; resources relating to dietary supplements are provided in Chapter 12.

SELECTED BIBLIOGRAPHY

Acupuncture: What the experts think now. 1998. *Consumer Reports,* September.

Acupuncture: NIH Consensus Development Panel on Acupuncture. 1998. *Journal of the American Medical Association* 280: 1518–1524.

Agency for Health Care and Policy Research. 1997. *Choosing and Using a Health Plan* (retrieved February 25, 1999; http://www.ahcpr.gov/consumer/hlthpln1.htm).

Barrett, S., et al. 1997. *Consumer Health: A Guide to Intelligent Decisions,* 6th ed. Madison, Wis.: Brown and Benchmark.

Bodenheimer, T. 1999. The American health care system: Physicians and the changing medical marketplace. *New England Journal of Medicine* 340(7): 584–588.

Chen, J., et al. 1999. Do "America's Best Hospitals" perform better for acute myocardial infarction? *New England Journal of Medicine* 340(4): 286–292.

Cherkin, D. C., et al. 1998. A comparison of physical therapy, chiropractic manipulation, and provision of an educational booklet for the treatment of patients with low-back pain. *New England Journal of Medicine* 339(15): 1021–1029.

Dold, C. 1998. Needles and nerves. *Discover,* September.

Eisenberg, D. M., et al. 1998. Trends in alternative medicine use in the United States, 1990–1997. *Journal of the American Medical Association* 280: 1569–1575.

Fact and fiction about chiropractic. 1999. *Harvard Health Letter,* January.

Ferguson, T. 1998. Digital doctoring—Opportunities and challenges in electronic patient-physician communication. *Journal of the American Medical Association* 280: 1361–1362.

Health Care Financing Administration. 1998. *Highlights of the National Health Expenditure Projections,* 1997–2007 (retrieved September 15, 1998; http://www.hcfa.gov/stats.nhe-proj/hilites.htm).

If it ducks like a quack . . . 1999. *U.C. Berkeley Wellness Letter,* February.

Iglehart, J. K. 1999. The American health care system: Expenditures. *New England Journal of Medicine* 340(1): 70–76.

Kuttner, R. 1999. The American health care system: Health insurance coverage. *New England Journal of Medicine* 340(2): 163–168.

Lewis, C. 1998. Sizing up surgery. *FDA Consumer,* November/December.

National Center for Complementary and Alternative Medicine. 1998. *Considering Alternative Therapies?* (retrieved March 1, 1999; http://altmed.od.nih.gov/nccam/what-is-cam/consider.shtml).

National Center for Health Statistics. 1998. *Health, United States, 1998.* Hyattsville, Md.: U.S. Public Health Service.

National Council Against Health Fraud. 1995. *Position Paper on Over-the-Counter Herbal Remedies.* Loma Linda, Calif.: National Council Against Health Fraud.

Public Citizen Health Research Group. 1998. The pitfalls of untested "alternative medicine" remedies. *Health Letter,* November.

Raso, J. 1996. *Dictionary of Metaphysical Healthcare: Alternative Medicine, Paranormal Healing, and Related Methods.* Loma Linda, Calif.: National Council Against Health Fraud.

U.S. Preventive Services Task Force. 1996. *Guide to Clinical Preventive Services,* 2nd ed. Baltimore, Md.: Williams & Wilkins.

Yaeger, S. 1998. A consumer's guide to alternative medicine. *Prevention,* February.

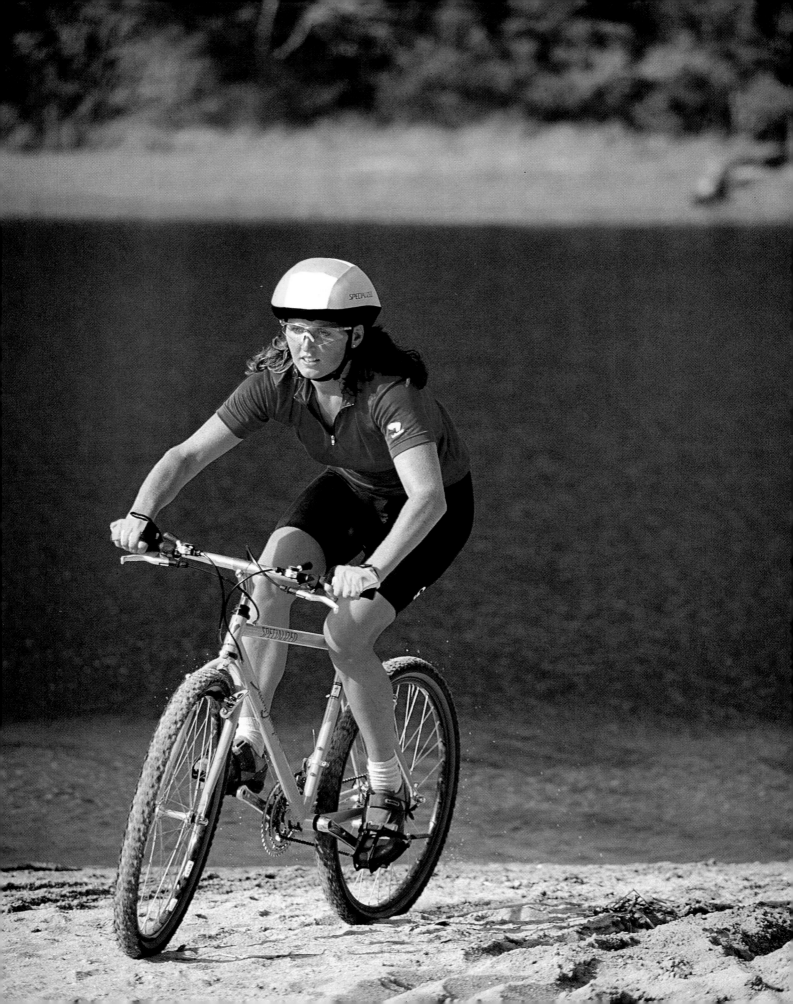

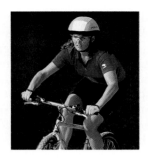

LEARNING OBJECTIVES

After reading this chapter, you should be able to:

- Discuss factors that contribute to unintentional injuries.

- List the most common types of unintentional injuries and strategies for preventing them.

- Describe factors that contribute to violence and intentional injuries.

- Discuss different forms of violence and how to protect yourself from intentional injuries.

- List strategies for helping others in an emergency situation.

Personal Safety: Protecting Yourself from Unintentional Injuries and Violence 23

TEST YOUR KNOWLEDGE

1. More people are injured each year through intentional acts of violence than through unintentional injuries (accidents).
   True or false?

2. A person who wears a safety belt is three to four times more likely to survive an automobile crash than someone who does not.
   True or false?

3. The recent introduction of higher speed limits on highways and freeways has not affected motor vehicle death rates.
   True or false?

4. What proportion of injured in-line skaters are not wearing appropriate safety gear when they crash?
   a. 25%
   b. 45%
   c. 65%

5. What percentage of sexual assaults against women are committed by strangers?
   a. 20%
   b. 40%
   c. 80%

Answers

1. *False.* Far more people are injured and killed each year through unintentional injuries than through violence; unintentional injuries are the leading cause of death for people between the ages of 15 and 24.

2. *True.* It is estimated that 60–70% of unbelted drivers killed in crashes would have survived if they had buckled up.

3. *False.* In states that have increased speed limits since 1995, motor vehicle death rates have increased 15%; in states without increases, rates have remained constant.

4. *c.* There are about 100,000 emergency room visits per year because of in-line skating injuries; most injuries would be prevented if skaters wore safety gear.

5. *a.* The vast majority of sexual assaults against women are committed by friends, acquaintances, or intimate partners.

E ach year, more than 140,000 Americans die from injuries, and many more are temporarily or permanently disabled. Injuries can be intentional or unintentional. An **intentional injury** is one that is purposely inflicted, by either oneself or another person; examples are homicide, suicide, and assault. If an injury occurs when no harm is intended, it is considered an **unintentional injury**. Motor vehicle crashes, falls, and fires often result in unintentional injuries. (The word *accidents* was formerly used to describe unintentional injuries, but it is now considered inaccurate because it suggests events beyond human control. *Injuries* are predictable outcomes of factors that can be controlled or prevented.) Although Americans tend to express more concern about intentional injuries, unintentional injuries are actually more common (see the box "Violence and the News Media: Perception Versus Reality"). The following occur on an average day in the United States:

- 50 homicides
- 80 suicides
- 250 deaths from unintentional injuries
- 3000 suicide attempts
- 18,000 interpersonal assaults
- 100,000 unintentional injury–related emergency room visits

Unintentional injuries are the fifth leading cause of death among all Americans and the leading cause of death and disability among children and young adults. Heart disease, cancer, and stroke are responsible for more deaths each year than injuries, but because unintentional injuries are so common among people, they account for more **years of potential life lost** than any other cause of death. Suicide and homicide rank eighth and thirteenth respectively on the list of leading causes of death among Americans; because they often affect young people, they also account for many years of potential life lost. Injuries affect all segments of the population, but they are particularly common among men, minorities, and people with low incomes, primarily due to social, environmental, and economic factors. Although rates of both unintentional and intentional injuries have fallen in recent years, they remain a major area of concern.

The economic cost of injuries is high, with more than $500 billion spent each year for medical care and rehabil-itation of injured people. But injuries also cause emotional suffering for injured people and their families, friends, and colleagues. Luckily, there are many steps that can be taken to reduce the risk of injuries. Engineering strategies such as safety belts can help lower injury rates, as can the passage and enforcement of safety-related laws, such as those requiring tamper-proof containers for OTC medications. Public education campaigns about risky behaviors such as driving under the influence of alcohol or smoking in bed can also help prevent injuries.

Ultimately, though, it is up to each individual to take responsibility for his or her actions and make wise choices about safety behaviors. Many of the same sensible attitudes, responsible behaviors, and informed decisions that optimize your wellness can improve your chances of avoiding injuries. This chapter explains how you can protect yourself and those around you from becoming the victims of unintentional and intentional injuries.

UNINTENTIONAL INJURIES

Unintentional injuries are the leading cause of death in the United States for people under age 45. Injury situations are generally categorized into four general classes, based on where they occur: motor vehicle injuries, home injuries, leisure injuries, and work injuries. The greatest number of deaths occur in motor vehicle crashes, but the greatest number of disabling injuries occur in the home (Table 23-1). In all of these arenas, the action you take can mean the difference between injury or death and no injury at all.

What Causes an Injury?

Most injuries are caused by a combination of human and environmental factors. Human factors are inner conditions or attitudes that lead to an unsafe state, whether physical, emotional, or psychological. Environmental factors are external conditions and circumstances, such as poor road conditions, a slippery surface, or the undertow of the ocean at the beach.

A common human factor that leads to injuries is risk-taking behavior. People vary in the amount of risk they tend to take in life; young men are especially prone to taking risks. Some people take risks to win the admiration of their peers; other people simply overestimate their physical abilities. Using alcohol or drugs is another common risk factor that leads to many injuries and deaths.

Psychological and emotional factors can also play a role in injuries. People sometimes act on the basis of inadequate or inaccurate beliefs about what is safe or unsafe. For example, a person who believes that safety belts trap people in cars when a crash occurs and who therefore decides not to wear a safety belt is acting on an inaccurate belief. Young people often have unsafe attitudes, such as

TERMS **intentional injury** An injury that is purposely inflicted, by either oneself or another person.

unintentional injury An injury that occurs without harm being intended.

years of potential life lost The difference between an individual's life expectancy and his or her age at death.

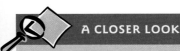 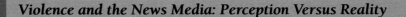 *Violence and the News Media: Perception Versus Reality*

When Americans are asked to name the most important problems facing the United States today, most mention violent crime. In the polls, the majority of Americans say they feel more threatened today by crime than they did 5 years ago and feel that violent crime is increasing at the national level. How do these beliefs stack up against actual statistics? In reality, the overall rate of violent crime in the United States is at its lowest level since 1973; the murder rate, although high in comparison to other developed nations, hit a 30-year low in 1998.

What explains the difference between the perception and the reality of rates of violence in the United States? One possible explanation is mass media reporting. Crime stories account for about 10–20% of all newspaper and television news stories, and the number of crime stories has increased dramatically since 1990, even as U.S. rates of violence and crime have fallen.

Politicians also frequently focus on violent crime. Heightening the public's fears about an issue and then offering simple solutions is a common political strategy for getting sound bites on the evening news and for getting votes. To capture the attention of the public, reporters and politicians are likely to focus on unusual and particularly violent or sensational crimes. Criminologist Ray Surette likens this to learning geology from a volcanic eruption—the information does not reflect the daily reality. For example, a study comparing news coverage of homicides in Los Angeles with actual homicide statistics found that the crimes received more coverage if they were statistically unusual—if the suspect was a stranger to the victim; if the victim was a female, a child, or an elderly person; or if the crime occurred in a wealthy neighborhood. Other homicides—those in which the victim knew the suspect; the victim was black or Latino or had less than

a high school education; or a weapon other than a firearm was used—were underrepresented in news coverage.

Disproportionate coverage of violence by the media may help explain why Americans tend to overestimate their risk of being a victim of many types of violence, including being shot or seriously injured by a stranger. Such overestimation is productive when it motivates people to make safer lifestyle choices and to be better prepared for emergency situations. It is counterproductive when it triggers anxiety and causes the public to demand expensive but unnecessary policies on crime. (The only type of violence for which Americans do not overestimate their risk is intimate violence—being assaulted by a spouse or partner.)

As with other areas of wellness, critical thinking is essential. Get the facts about violence and its risk factors so you can make informed personal lifestyle choices and promote effective community and national strategies for combating violence. The For More Information section at the end of the chapter lists sources of statistics for all types of injuries and violence.

SOURCES: Harris Poll. 1999. *Perceptions of Risk* (retrieved February 22, 1999; http://www.louisharris.com/poll/1999pols/Jan2799.html). Gallup Poll. 1998. *Crime Issues* (retrieved February 22, 1999; http://www.gallup.com/congressandpub/issues/crime.htm). Sorenson, S. G., J. G. Manz, and R. A. Berk. 1998. News media coverage and the epidemiology of homicide. *American Journal of Public Health* 88(1): 1510–1514. Surette, R. 1998. *Media, Crime, and Criminal Justice: Images and Realities,* 2nd ed. Belmont, Calif.: Wadsworth. Morris, N. 1997. Crime, the media, and our public discourse. In *Perspective on Crime and Justice: 1996–1997 Lecture Series.* Washington, D.C.: U.S. Department of Justice.

VITAL STATISTICS

TABLE 23-1	*Fatal and Disabling Injuries in the United States*	
	Deaths	**Disabling Injuries**
Motor vehicle	43,200	2,300,000
Home	28,400	6,800,000
Leisure	19,400	6,500,000
Work	5,100	3,800,000
All classes*	93,800	19,300,000

*Deaths and injuries for the four separate classes total more than the "All classes" figures because of rounding and because some deaths and injuries are included in more than one class.

SOURCE: National Safety Council. 1998. *Accident Facts.* Chicago: National Safety Council.

"I won't get hurt." Attitudes like this can lead to risk taking and ultimately to injuries.

Environmental factors leading to injury may be natural (weather conditions), social (a drunk driver), work-

related (defective equipment), or home-related (faulty wiring). Making the environment safer is an important aspect of safety. Laws are often passed to try to make our environment safer, such as speed limits on roads and highways and workplace safety requirements.

When unsafe human states and unsafe environmental factors interact, an injury is often the result. A good example might be an inexperienced person borrowing a rifle to go hunting with his friends on a cold, rainy afternoon. The group drinks alcohol because they mistakenly believe it will keep them warmer. It is not difficult to imagine how the interaction of these human and environmental factors could lead to an injury. Again, it is important to realize that injuries do not "just happen." With hindsight, we can almost always pinpoint the internal and external factors that combined to cause an injury situation.

PERSONAL INSIGHT Think back to the last time you were injured. What would you say caused the injury? Do you have a tendency to blame other people or environmental factors for things that happen to you?

To find out if you are an aggressive driver, check any of the following statements that are true for you:

____ I consistently exceed the speed limit; I'm often unaware of both my speed and the speed limit.

____ I frequently follow closely behind the car in front of me.

____ If I feel the car in front of me is going too slowly, I tailgate.

____ I change lanes frequently to pass people.

____ I seldom use my turn signal when changing lanes or turning.

____ I often run red lights or roll through stop signs.

____ I react to what I feel as another driver's mistake by cursing, shouting, or making rude gestures; by blocking a car from passing or changing lanes; by using high beams; or by braking suddenly in front of a tailgater.

____ My personality changes and I become more competitive when I get behind the wheel.

____ I often get angry or impatient with other drivers and with pedestrians.

____ I would consider pulling over for a personal encounter with a bad driver.

Each of these statements is characteristic of aggressive drivers; the more items you checked, the greater your road rage. If you checked even one statement, consider taking some of the following steps to reduce your hostility behind the wheel:

- Allow enough time for your trip to reach your destination without speeding.

- Avoid driving during periods of heavy traffic.

- Don't drive when you are angry, tired, or intoxicated.

- Imagine that the other drivers are all people that you know and like. Be courteous and forgiving.

- Listen to soothing music or a book on tape, or practice a relaxation technique such as deep breathing (see Chapter 2).

- Take a course in anger management.

Even if you are successful at controlling your own aggressive driving impulses, you may still encounter an aggressive driver on the road. The AAA Foundation for Traffic Safety recommends the following strategies to avoid being a victim of an aggressive driver:

- Avoid behaviors that may enrage an aggressive driver; these include cutting cars off when merging, driving slowly in the left lane, tailgating, and making rude gestures.

- If you make a mistake while driving, apologize. In surveys, the most popular and widely understood gestures for apologies include raising or waving a hand and touching or knocking the head with the palm of your hand (to indicate "What was I thinking?").

- Refuse to join in a fight. Avoid eye contact with an angry driver, and put distance between your car and his or her vehicle. If you think another driver is following you or trying to start a fight, call the police on a cellular phone or drive to a public place.

SOURCES: AAA Foundation for Traffic Safety. 1997. *Road Rage: How to Avoid Aggressive Driving.* Washington, D.C.: AAA Foundation for Traffic Safety. Citizens Against Speeding and Aggressive Driving (http://www.aggressivedriving.org).

Motor Vehicle Injuries

Motor vehicle crashes are the leading cause of death for Americans between the ages of 1 and 25. **Motor vehicle injuries** also result in the majority of cases of paralysis due to spinal injuries, and they are the leading cause of severe brain injury in the United States.

Factors Contributing to Motor Vehicle Injuries   The common causes of motor vehicle injuries are bad driving, the failure to use safety belts, driving while under the influence of alcohol and drugs, and dangerous environmental conditions.

DRIVING HABITS   Nearly two-thirds of all motor vehicle crashes are caused by bad driving, especially speeding. As speed increases, momentum and the force of impact increase, and the time allowed for the driver to react (reaction time) decreases. Speed limits are posted to

establish the safest *maximum* speed limit for a given area under *ideal* conditions; if visibility is limited or the road is wet, the safe maximum speed may be considerably lower.

Speeding is also a hallmark of aggressive drivers—those who operate a motor vehicle in an unsafe and hostile manner without regard for others. Aggressive driving, also known as "road rage," has increased more than 50% since 1990, and one in four U.S. drivers admits to driving aggressively at least some of the time. Other characteristics of aggressive driving include frequent, erratic, and abrupt lane changes, tailgating, running red lights or stop signs, passing on the shoulder, and blocking other cars trying to change lanes or pass. Aggressive drivers increase the risk of crashes for themselves and others; injuries may also occur if aggressive drivers stop their vehicles and confront each other following an incident on the road. For more on aggressive driving, take the quiz and review the strategies in the box "Are You an Aggressive Driver?"

Inattentiveness and a failure to yield or observe posted

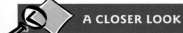
Myth If I wore a safety belt, I might get trapped in my car if it caught on fire or were submerged in water.

Fact Only 0.5–1% of motor vehicle crashes involve fire or submersion. If that does happen, safety belts will help prevent you from being knocked unconscious, so you'll have a better chance of escaping from your car.

Myth I would be better off if I were thrown clear of the car in a crash.

Fact The chances of being killed are 25 times *greater* if you're thrown out of the vehicle. Hitting a tree or the pavement can cause severe injuries, which won't occur if you stay buckled inside the car. Also, people who are thrown out of their cars are sometimes crushed or hit by their own vehicles or those of others.

Myth I can brace myself in a crash, so I don't need to bother with a safety belt.

Fact The force of an impact at just 10 mph can be equivalent to catching a 200-pound bag of cement thrown from a 10-foot ladder. At 35 mph, the force of impact is even more brutal. There's no way your arms and legs can brace against that kind of force—even if you could react in time.

Myth A safety belt couldn't possibly hold me in place during a sudden stop or collision. When I yank it by hand, it doesn't work.

Fact Most safety belts are designed to lock automatically when the car stops suddenly or changes direction quickly. Belts normally expand and contract to allow freedom of movement.

Myth I'm not going far or driving fast, so I don't need to wear a safety belt.

Fact It's smart to wear a safety belt no matter where you're going because 75% of all crashes occur within 25 miles of home. Most deaths and injuries (80%) occur in automobiles traveling less than 40 mph. People have been killed in crashes at speeds of less than 12 mph.

Myth Pregnant women are not supposed to wear safety belts.

Fact According to the American Medical Association, both a pregnant woman and her unborn child are much safer with belts than without, provided the lap belt is worn as low as possible on the pelvic area.

Myth I am a good driver, so I'll never be in a crash. I don't need to wear a safety belt.

Fact Safety belts are the most effective defense against a drunken driver. No matter how well you drive, you can't control what other drivers are going to do.

SOURCE: *Buckle Up,* a publication of Traffic Safety Now, Inc., Detroit, MI.

---

warnings are other common causes of motor vehicle crashes. Anything that distracts a driver—sleepiness, bad mood, children or pets in the car—can increase the risk of a motor vehicle injury. One study found that use of a cellular phone while driving *quadruples* the risk of having a collision. When driving tasks are complex, such as at intersections, inattention is especially dangerous.

> **PERSONAL INSIGHT** Some otherwise mild-mannered people become hostile and aggressive behind the wheel of a car. Does this ever happen to you? If so, what do you think accounts for it?

SAFETY BELTS AND AIR BAGS   A second factor contributing to injury and death in motor vehicle crashes is the decision not to wear a safety belt (see the box "Myths About Safety Belts"). A person who doesn't wear a safety belt is twice as likely to be injured in a crash as a person who does wear one. If you wear a combination lap and shoulder belt, your chances of surviving a crash are three to four times better than those of a person who doesn't wear one. Of drivers not wearing a safety belt who have been killed in automobile crashes, an estimated 60–70% would have survived had they been wearing one.

Safety belts not only prevent you from being thrown from the car at the time of the crash but also provide protection from the "second collision." If a car is traveling at 65 mph and hits another vehicle, the car stops first; then the occupants stop because they are traveling at the same speed. The second collision occurs when the occupants of the car hit something inside the car, such as the steering column, dashboard, or windshield. The safety belt stops the second collision from occurring and spreads the stopping force of the collision over the body.

Since 1998, all new cars have been equipped with dual air bags—one for the driver and one for the front passenger. Although air bags provide supplementary protection in the event of a collision, most are useful only in head-on collisions (Figure 23-1). They also deflate immediately after inflating and therefore do not provide protection in collisions involving multiple impacts.

Air bags deploy forcefully and can injure a child or short adult who is improperly restrained or sitting too close to the dashboard. To ensure that air bags work safely, always follow these basic guidelines: place infants

motor vehicle injuries Unintentional injuries and deaths involving motor vehicles in motion, both on and off the highway or street; incidents causing motor vehicle injuries include collisions between vehicles and collisions with objects or pedestrians.   **TERMS**

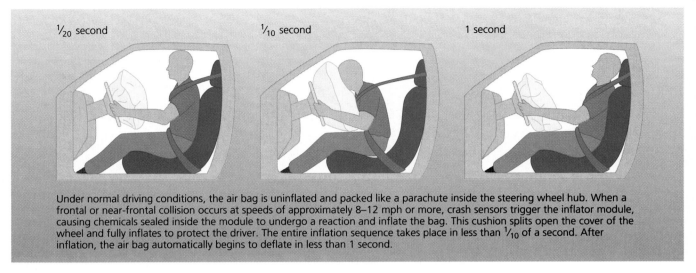

| $\frac{1}{20}$ second | $\frac{1}{10}$ second | 1 second |

Under normal driving conditions, the air bag is uninflated and packed like a parachute inside the steering wheel hub. When a frontal or near-frontal collision occurs at speeds of approximately 8–12 mph or more, crash sensors trigger the inflator module, causing chemicals sealed inside the module to undergo a reaction and inflate the bag. This cushion splits open the cover of the wheel and fully inflates to protect the driver. The entire inflation sequence takes place in less than $\frac{1}{10}$ of a second. After inflation, the air bag automatically begins to deflate in less than 1 second.

Figure 23-1   How an air bag works.   SOURCE: *Consumer Information.* 1989. U.S. Department of Transportation, National Highway Traffic Safety Administration.

in rear-facing infant seats in the back seat; transport children age 12 and under in the back seat; always use safety belts or appropriate safety seats; and keep 10 inches between the air bag cover and the breastbone of the driver or passenger. If necessary, adjust the steering wheel or use seat cushions to ensure that an inflating air bag will hit a person in the chest and not in the face.

In the rare event that a person cannot comply with these guidelines, permission to install an on-off switch that temporarily disables the air bag can be applied for from the National Highway Traffic Safety Administration (NHTSA). Air bags currently prevent far more injuries than they cause and are expected to save at least 3200 lives each year once they are installed in all vehicles. The NHSTA has proposed that by 2002, all new cars can be equipped with advanced air bags that include such risk-reduction technologies as sensors to detect and respond to crash severity, seat position, passenger size, and whether a passenger is wearing a safety belt.

ALCOHOL AND OTHER DRUGS   Alcohol is involved in about half of all fatal crashes. Alcohol-impaired driving, defined by blood alcohol concentration (BAC), is illegal in all states. The legal BAC limit varies by state from 0.08% to 0.10%, but people are impaired at much lower BACs. Because alcohol affects reason and judgment as well as the ability to make fast, accurate, and coordinated movements, a person who has been drinking will be less likely to recognize that he or she is impaired. All psychoactive drugs have the potential to impair driving ability. (For a full discussion of the effects of alcohol and other drugs on users, refer to Chapters 9 and 10.)

Preventing Motor Vehicle Injuries   About 75% of all motor vehicle collisions occur within 25 miles of home

and at speeds lower than 40 mph. Strategies for preventing motor vehicle injuries include the following:

- Obey the speed limit. If you have to speed to get there on time, you're not allowing enough time. Try leaving 10–15 minutes earlier.

- Always wear a safety belt. Fasten the lap belt, even if the vehicle has automatic shoulder belts. Strap infants and toddlers into government-approved car seats in the back seat of the vehicle.

- Never drive under the influence of alcohol or other drugs. Never ride with a driver who has been drinking or using drugs.

- Keep your car in good working order. Regularly inspect the tires, oil and fluid levels, windshield wipers, spare tire, and so on.

- Always allow enough following distance. Use the "3-second rule": When the vehicle ahead passes a reference point, count out 3 seconds. If you pass the reference point before you finish counting, drop back and allow more following distance.

- Always increase your following distance and slow down if weather or road conditions are poor.

- Choose interstate highways rather than rural roads. Highways are much safer because of better visibility, wider lanes, fewer surprises, and other factors.

- Always signal when turning or changing lanes.

- Stop completely at stop signs. Follow all traffic laws.

- Take special care at intersections. Always look left, right, and then left again. Make sure you have plenty of time to complete your maneuver in the intersection.

- Don't pass on two-lane roads unless you're in a designated passing area and have a clear view ahead.

Motorcycles and Mopeds   About one out of every ten traffic fatalities among people age 15–34 involves someone riding a motorcycle. Injuries from motorcycle collisions are generally more severe than those involving automobiles because motorcycles provide little, if any, protection. Because head injuries are the major cause of death, the use of a helmet is critical for rider safety. Learning the skills to operate the motorcycle safely is another key injury-prevention strategy; operator error is a factor in 75% of fatal crashes involving motorcycles.

Moped riders face additional challenges. Mopeds usually have a maximum speed of 30–35 mph and have less power for maneuverability, especially in an emergency. Moped riders should use caution and take the time to develop the skills needed to handle the vehicle in traffic.

Additional strategies for preventing motorcycle and moped injuries include the following:

- Maximize your visibility by wearing light-colored clothing, driving with your headlights on, and correctly positioning yourself in traffic.

- Develop the necessary skills. Lack of skill, especially when evasive action is needed to avoid a collision, is a major factor in motorcycle and moped injuries. Skidding from improper braking is the most common cause of loss of control.

- Wear a helmet. Helmets should be marked with the symbol DOT, certifying that they conform to federal safety standards established by the Department of Transportation.

- Protect your eyes with goggles, a face shield, or a windshield.

- Drive defensively, and never assume that you've been seen by other drivers.

Bicycles   Injuries to bicyclists and pedestrians are considered motor-vehicle-related because they are usually caused by motor vehicles. Bicycle injuries result primarily from riders not knowing or understanding the rules of the road, failing to follow traffic laws, and not having sufficient skill or experience to handle traffic conditions. Bicycles are considered vehicles; bicycle riders must obey all traffic laws that apply to automobile drivers, including stopping at traffic lights and stop signs.

Head injuries are involved in about two-thirds of bicycle-related deaths, yet studies indicate that less than 50% of cyclists wear helmets (see the box "Bicycle Helmets," p. 614). Safe cycling strategies include the following:

- Wear safety equipment, including a helmet, eye protection, gloves, and proper footwear. Secure the bottom of your pant legs with clips, and secure your shoelaces so they don't get tangled in the chain.

- Maximize your visibility by wearing light-colored, reflective clothing. Equip your bike with reflectors, and use lights, especially at night or when riding in

wooded or other dark areas.

- Ride with the flow of traffic, not against it, and follow all traffic laws. Use bike paths when they are available.

- Ride defensively; never assume that drivers have seen you. Be especially careful when turning or crossing at corners and intersections. Watch for cars turning right.

- Stop at all traffic lights and stop signs. Know and use hand signals.

- Continue pedaling at all times when moving (no coasting) to help keep the bike stable and to maintain your balance.

- Properly maintain the working condition of your bike.

Pedestrians   Pedestrians are no match for the speed, size, and weight of motor vehicles. About one in eight motor vehicle deaths involves pedestrians, and more than 80,000 pedestrians are injured each year. The highest rates of death and injury occur among the very young and the elderly. Most injuries occur in urban settings, primarily after dark, and between intersections, where people may walk or dart into traffic. Alcohol intoxication plays a significant role in up to half of all adult pedestrian fatalities.

The following strategies can help prevent injuries when you're walking or jogging:

- Walk or jog in daylight.

- Maximize your visibility by wearing light-colored, reflective clothing.

- Face traffic when walking or jogging along a road, and follow traffic laws.

- Avoid busy roads or roads with poor visibility.

- Cross only at marked crosswalks and intersections.

- Don't listen to a radio or tape on headphones while walking.

- Don't hitchhike; it places you in a potentially dangerous situation.

Home Injuries

A person's place of residence, whether it be a house, an apartment, a trailer, or a dormitory, is considered home. People spend a great deal of time at home and feel that they are safe and secure there. However, home can be a dangerous place. The most common fatal **home injuries** are falls, fires, poisoning, suffocation, and unintentional firearm injuries.

home injuries   Unintentional injuries and deaths that occur in the home and on home premises to occupants, guests, domestic servants, and trespassers; falls, burns, poisonings, suffocations, unintentional shootings, drownings, and electrical shocks are examples.   **TERMS**

Every year, nearly 50,000 bicyclists suffer serious head injuries, and 60% of cyclists killed in crashes die as a result of head injuries. The brain is extremely sensitive to any impact, even bicycling at a very low speed. On a concrete surface, a fall from a distance of less than 1 foot can cause a concussion. A helmet can reduce your risk of head injury by about 80% if you are involved in a collision or fall. In addition to preventing injuries, helmets provide other advantages:

- *Visibility.* You are easier to see with a white or yellow helmet on, especially at dusk, in rain or fog, or after dark. Putting reflective trim tape on the helmet makes you even more visible.

- *Climate protection.* A helmet will help keep your head dry in the rain or snow; if you do have to cycle in bad weather, it will be more enjoyable.

- *Emergency data.* Put your name, address, and phone number, and the name and number of an emergency contact, on a piece of tape inside the brim of your helmet. If you have a medical emergency condition, include that information as well. Also, tape change inside for an emergency phone call.

Helmets are designed to cushion a blow to your head and must pass special safety tests to be certified. A good helmet will have a hard outer shell to spread the force of a blow over a larger area and to shield against any sharp objects. A helmet should also have a crushable liner (usually polystyrene foam) to absorb the shock of a collision and a strong strap and buckle to keep the helmet securely on your head (see the figure).

Every good bicycle shop carries a supply of helmets for adults and children. Ask someone who works at the shop to help you select a helmet that's right for you. Since 1999, all bike

helmets sold in the United States have met federal safety standards established by the U.S. Consumer Product Safety Commission. These standards ensure that helmets adequately protect the head and that chin straps are strong enough to prevent the helmet from coming off during a fall or crash.

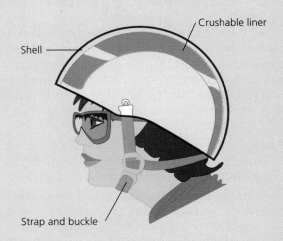

SOURCES: U.S. Consumer Product Safety Commission (CPSC). 1998. *CPSC Issues New Safety Standards for Bike Helmets* (retrieved April 13, 1998; http://www.cpsc.gov/gophroot/pre%5Frel/pre%5Frel/98%5Fpre/98062.txt). Thompson, D. C., R. P. Rivera, and R. S. Thompson. 1996. Effectiveness of bicycle safety helmets in preventing head injuries: A case-controlled study. *Journal of the American Medical Association* 276(24): 1968–1973. Art and text from *Get Into the Helmet Habit,* copyright © 1986 Outdoor Empire Publishing, Inc. Used with permission.

Falls About 85% of fatal falls involve people age 45 and over, but falls are the fifth leading cause of unintentional death for all people under 25. Most falls occur as a result of common activities in the home, with nearly two-thirds of deaths occurring from falls at floor level (tripping, slipping, and so on) rather than from a height. Alcohol is a contributing factor in many falls. Strategies for preventing falls include the following:

- Place skidproof backing on rugs and carpets.
- Install handrails and nonslip applications in the shower and bathtub.
- Keep floors clear of objects or conditions that could cause slipping or tripping, such as heavy wax coating, electrical cords, and toys.
- Put a light switch by the door of every room so no one has to walk across a room to turn on a light. Use night lights in bedrooms, halls, and bathrooms.
- Outside the house, clear dangerous surfaces created by ice, snow, fallen leaves, or rough ground.
- Install handrails on stairs. Keep stairs well lit and clear of objects.

- When climbing a ladder, use both hands. Never stand higher than the third step from the top. When using a stepladder, make sure the spreader brace is in the locked position. With straight ladders, set the base out 1 foot for every 4 feet of height.

- Don't use chairs to reach things; they are meant to be sat on, not stood on.

- If there are small children in the home, place gates at the top and bottom of stairs. Never leave a baby unattended on a bed or table. Install window guards to prevent children from falling out of windows.

Fires Each year in the United States, approximately 80% of fire deaths and 65% of fire injuries occur in the home; a death caused by a residential fire occurs every 2 hours. The ignition of furniture, combustible liquid or gas, and bedding accounts for 60% of home fires. Most fires begin in the kitchen, living room, or bedroom. Careless smoking accounts for about 25% of fire deaths, followed by arson (20%) and problems with heating equipment (16%). Strategies for preventing fires include the following:

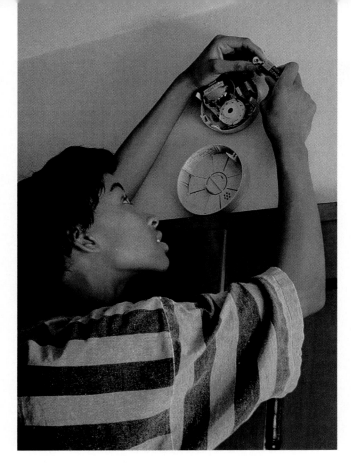

The risk of dying in a fire is reduced by half if you use a smoke detector. Install detectors on every floor, check them monthly, and replace the batteries at least once a year.

- Dispose of all cigarettes in ashtrays. Never smoke in bed.
- Do not overload electrical outlets. Do not place extension cords under rugs or where people walk. Replace worn or frayed extension cords.
- Place a wire screen in front of fireplaces and wood stoves. Remove ashes carefully and store them in airtight metal containers, not paper bags.
- Properly maintain electrical appliances, kerosene heaters, and furnaces, and clean flues and chimneys annually.
- Keep portable heaters at least 3 feet away from curtains, bedding, towels, or anything that might catch fire. Never leave heaters on when you're out of the room or sleeping.

It's important to be adequately prepared to handle fire-related situations. Plan at least two escape routes out of each room, and designate a location outside the home as a meeting place. For practice, stage a home fire drill; do it at night, since that's when most deadly fires occur.

Install smoke detectors on every level of your home. Your risk of dying in a fire is almost twice as high if you do not use them. Clean the detectors and check the batteries once a month, and replace the batteries at least once a year. (More than 90% of U.S. homes have at least one smoke alarm, but about half are no longer functioning a year after installation.) Be sure that all residents are familiar with the sound of the smoke detector's alarm; when it goes off, take it seriously.

If a fire does occur, following these strategies can help prevent injuries:

- Get out as quickly as possible, and go to the designated meeting place. Don't stop for a keepsake or a pet. Never hide in a closet or under a bed. Once outside, count heads to see if everyone is out. If you think someone is still inside the burning building, tell the firefighters. Never go back inside a burning building.
- If you're trapped in a room, feel the door. If it is hot, or if smoke is coming in through the cracks, don't open it; use the alternative escape route. If you can't get out of a room, go to the window and shout or wave for help.
- Smoke inhalation is the largest cause of death and injury in fires. To avoid inhaling smoke, crawl along the floor away from the heat and smoke. Cover your mouth and nose, ideally with a wet cloth, and take short, shallow breaths.
- If your clothes catch fire, don't run. Drop to the ground, cover your face, and roll back and forth to smother the flames. Remember: stop-drop-roll.

Although house fires cause the most deaths, hot water causes the most nonfatal burns. Young children are particularly at risk. Place barriers around stoves and radiators, and keep young children out of the kitchen where they might be burned by spills. Put pans on rear burners, and turn pot handles toward the back of the stove. Keep hot foods away from the edge of counters and tables, and don't put them on a tablecloth that a small child can pull. Set your water heater no higher than 120°F. Always test the contents of a baby bottle; when bottles are heated in microwave ovens, the liquid can become scalding before the outside of the bottle gets very hot.

Poisoning More than 1 million poisonings occur every year in the United States. The home is the site of about 80% of deaths by poisonous solids and liquids and over 60% of those from poisonous gases and vapors. A majority of cases involve children under age 5, although rates have increased recently among people age 15–44.

Poisons come in many forms, some of which are not typically considered poisons. For example, medications are safe when used as prescribed, but overdosing and incorrectly combining medications with another substance may result in poisoning. Other poisonous substances in the home include cleaning agents, petroleum-based products, insecticides and herbicides, cosmetics, nail polish and remover, and many houseplants.

Be Prepared

Take a moment now to look up the phone number of the nearest Poison Control Center; place it in a convenient location. Poison Control Centers are staffed by certified poison information specialists. They provide confidential, free, 24-hour emergency service. Don't hesitate to call for any possible poisoning.

Should a poisoning occur, the most important item you can have in your home is syrup of ipecac, a nonprescription plant extract that causes vomiting. While it can minimize the effects of certain poisons or actually save a life, it is dangerous for some types of poisonings. *Use syrup of ipecac only on the advice of the Poison Control Center or your physician.*

Emergency First Aid for Poisonings

If you are faced with a case of poisoning, your immediate response is critical.

1. Remove the poison from contact with eyes, skin, or mouth, or remove the victim from contact with poisonous fumes or gases.

2. Do not follow emergency instructions on labels. Some may be out of date and carry incorrect treatment information.

3. Call the Poison Control Center immediately for instructions. Depending on the circumstances, you may be asked the following:

   - The name of the substance and its ingredients (you may need to bring the container to the phone).

   - The amount of substance involved.

   - When exposure occurred and how long it lasted.

   - Whether any symptoms are present.

   - Characteristics of the person exposed, including name, age, weight, and general health history; you should mention any episodes of allergy, seizure, asthma, diabetes, or other chronic or recurring conditions.

   - Information about yourself, including name, relationship to the victim, and the phone number from which you are calling.

4. If you are instructed to go to an emergency room, take the poisonous substance or container with you.

5. Administer syrup of ipecac to induce vomiting—*but only if advised by the Poison Control Center or your physician.*

Guidelines for Specific Types of Poisonings

- *Swallowed poisons:* If the person is awake and able to swallow, give water only; then call the Poison Control Center or your physician for advice.

- *Poisons on the skin:* Remove any affected clothing. Flood affected parts of the skin with warm water, wash with soap and water, and rinse. Then call for advice.

- *Poisons in the eye:* For children, flood the eye with lukewarm water poured from a pitcher held 3–4 inches above the eye for 15 minutes; alternatively, irrigate the eye under a faucet. For adults, get in the shower and flood the eye with a gentle stream of lukewarm water for 15 minutes. Then call for advice.

- *Inhaled poisons:* Immediately carry or drag the person to fresh air and, if necessary, give mouth-to-mouth resuscitation. If the victim is not breathing easily, call 9-1-1 for help. Ventilate the area. Then call for advice.

SOURCE: Adapted from Alsop, J., and C. Niezabitowska. 1995. *The U.C. Davis Poison Center Answer Book* (http://www.ucdmc.ucdavis.edu/health/index.html). © 1995 UCDMC Regional Poison Control Center. Used with permission.

The most common type of poisoning by gases is carbon monoxide poisoning. Carbon monoxide gas is emitted by motor vehicle exhaust and some types of heating equipment. The effects of exposure to this colorless, odorless gas include headache, blurred vision, and shortness of breath, followed by dizziness, vomiting, and unconsciousness. Carbon monoxide detectors similar to smoke detectors are available for home use; they should be used according to the manufacturer's instructions.

Strategies for preventing poisonings in the home include the following:

- Store all medications out of reach of children. Use medicines only as directed on the label or by a physician.

- Use cleaners, pesticides, and other dangerous substances only in areas with proper ventilation. Store them out of the reach of children.

- Never operate a vehicle in an enclosed space. Have your furnace inspected yearly, and use caution with any substance that produces potentially toxic fumes, such as kerosene. If appropriate, install carbon monoxide detectors.

- Keep poisonous plants out of reach of young children. These include azalea, oleander, rhododendron, wild mushrooms, daffodil and hyacinth bulbs, mistletoe berries, apple seeds, morning glory seeds, wisteria seeds, and the leaves and stems of potato, rhubarb, and tomato plants.

If a poisoning does occur, it's important that you act quickly (see the box "What to Do in Case of Poisoning").

Suffocation and Choking Suffocation accounts for nearly 4000 deaths annually in the United States. Young children account for nearly half of these deaths. Children can suffocate if they put small items in their mouths, get tangled in their crib bedding, or get trapped in airtight appliances like old refrigerators. Keep small objects out of reach of children under age 3, and don't give them raw carrots, hot dogs, popcorn, or hard candy. Examine toys carefully for small parts that could come loose; don't give plastic bags or balloons to small children.

Adults can also become choking victims, especially if they fail to chew food properly, eat hurriedly, or try to talk and eat at the same time. Many choking victims can be saved with the **Heimlich maneuver** (Figure 23-2, p. 618). Until 1986, the American Red Cross recommended blows to the upper back for choking, but since then it has adopted the Heimlich maneuver (which it also calls "abdominal thrusts") as the easiest and safest thing to do when an adult is choking. Back blows administered in conjunction with abdominal thrusts are an acceptable procedure for dislodging an object from the throat of an infant.

Firearms Firearms pose a significant threat, especially to people age 15–24. People who use firearms should remember the following:

- Never point a loaded gun at something you do not intend to shoot.
- Store unloaded firearms under lock and key, in a place separate from the ammunition.
- Always inspect firearms carefully before handling.
- Behave in the safe and responsible manner advocated in firearms safety courses.

Proper storage is critical. Do not assume that young children cannot fire a gun: About 25% of 3–4-year-olds and 70% of 5–6-year-olds have enough finger strength to pull a trigger. Every year, about 120 Americans are unintentionally shot to death by children under 6.

Probably the best advice for anyone who picks up a gun is to assume it is loaded. Too many deaths and injuries occur when someone unintentionally shoots a friend while under the impression that the gun he or she is handling is not loaded. In addition, if you plan to handle a gun, you should avoid the use of alcohol and drugs, which may affect your judgment and coordination. (Firearms and intentional injuries are discussed later in the chapter.)

Leisure Injuries

Leisure activities encompass a large part of our free time, so it is not surprising that **leisure injuries** are a significant health-related problem in the United States. Leisure injuries have been identified in the areas of boating, playground activities, all-terrain vehicles, in-line skating, and sports.

Drowning and Boating Injuries Over 4000 drownings occur annually in the United States. Males drown at a rate two to four times that of females; children under age 5 and people between ages 15 and 24 have the highest drowning rates. Although most drownings are reported in lakes, ponds, rivers, and oceans, more than half the drownings of young children take place in residential pools. Among adolescents and adults, alcohol plays a significant role in many drownings.

Over 800 recreational boating fatalities and nearly 4000 injuries are reported each year. Most injuries occur when a boat strikes another object, such as another boat, but most deaths occur when people fall overboard and drown. Alcohol use is a major contributing factor in boating injuries.

Strategies for preventing drowning and boating injuries include the following:

- Develop adequate swimming skill, and make sure children learn to swim.
- Make sure residential pools are fenced and that children are never allowed to swim without supervision.
- Don't swim alone or in unsupervised places.
- Use caution when swimming in unfamiliar surroundings or for an unusual length of time. Avoid being chilled by water colder than 70°F.
- Don't swim or boat under the influence of alcohol or other drugs. To prevent choking, don't chew gum or eat while in the water.
- Check the depth of water before diving.
- When on a boat, use a **personal flotation device** (life jacket). The U.S. Coast Guard recommends six different types, each keyed to particular water conditions.

Playground Injuries More than 600,000 injuries occur on American playgrounds each year. Most are not severe and do not require medical attention; deaths are usually the result of head injuries. Most injuries occur on swings, monkey bars or climbers, or slides, usually as a result of falling or striking a piece of equipment. Equipment design, installation, and condition can also influence injuries on the playground, as can the surface beneath the equipment. The misuse of equipment is a common cause of injuries.

TERMS

Heimlich maneuver A maneuver developed by Henry J. Heimlich, M.D., to help force an obstruction from the airway.

leisure injuries Unintentional injuries and deaths that occur in public places or places used in a public way, not involving motor vehicles; includes most sports and recreation deaths and injuries; falls, drownings, burns, and heat and cold stress are examples.

personal flotation device (PFD) A device designed to save a person from drowning by buoying up the body while in the water; also called a *life jacket*.

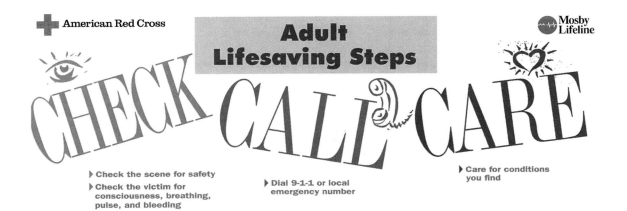

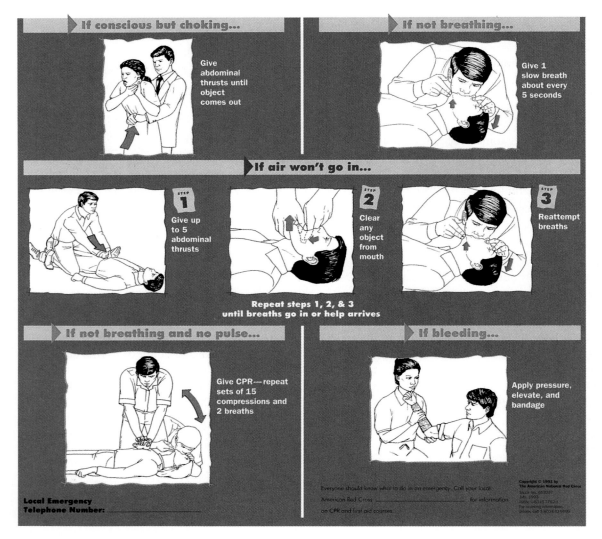

Figure 23-2   Rescue breathing, first aid for choking, and ways to control bleeding; procedures recommended by the American Red Cross.   SOURCE: Courtesy of the American Red Cross. All rights reserved in all countries.

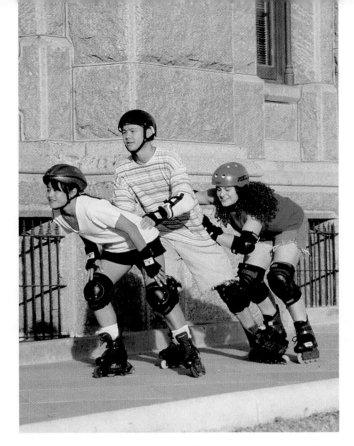

Leisure activities injure more than 6 million people each year, including 200,000 in-line skaters. The use of proper safety equipment—helmet, wrist guards, and elbow and knee pads—is critical for injury prevention.

All-Terrain Vehicle Injuries Most injuries involving **all-terrain vehicles (ATVs)** occur during recreational use; males under the age of 16 are those most often injured. Most of the injuries associated with ATVs are to the head; about 70% of the deaths are the result of head injuries. As in the case of motorcycles, a lack of experience, the use of alcohol, and a failure to use safety equipment like helmets are common contributors to ATV injuries. Other factors include excessive speed, stunt riding, and carrying passengers when inappropriate and unsafe to do so.

In-Line Skating Injuries In-line skating, or rollerblading, has become a very popular recreational activity for people of all ages. More than 22 million Americans use in-line skates, and nearly 100,000 are injured badly enough each year to wind up in an emergency room. Injuries to the wrist and head are most common; many occur because users do not wear appropriate safety gear. Researchers estimate that more than one-third of all serious injuries could be prevented if all skaters wore helmets and wrist and elbow protection.

To reduce your risk of being injured while rollerblading, wear a helmet, elbow and knee pads, wrist guards, a long-sleeved shirt, and long pants. Alcohol use appears to be a significant factor in in-line skating injuries that occur on college campuses. Because in-line skating involves skill, judgment, and coordination, it makes sense not to mix skating and drinking.

Sports Injuries Sports also contribute to leisure injuries, especially since more people are participating in community, recreational, and intramural activities to improve their health and physical fitness. The following can help you prevent injuries when you participate in sports:

- Develop the skills required for the activity. Recognize and guard against the hazards associated with it.
- Warm up before you exercise, and cool down afterward.
- Make sure facilities are safe.
- Follow the rules, and practice good sportsmanship.
- Use proper safety equipment, including, where appropriate, helmets; eye protection; knee, elbow, and wrist pads; and correct footwear.
- When it is excessively hot and humid, drink plenty of fluids, rest frequently in the shade, and slow down or stop if you feel uncomfortable. Danger signals of heat stress include excessive perspiration, dizziness, headache, muscle cramps, nausea, weakness, rapid pulse, and disorientation.

For more on exercise safety, refer to Chapter 13.

Work Injuries

Since 1912, when industrial records were first kept in the United States, the work site has become a much safer place, as evidenced by a reduction in the unintentional death rate of nearly 76%. That figure becomes even more impressive when one realizes that the size of the labor force has more than doubled and production has increased more than tenfold. One very significant factor to account for such a marked decline in **work injuries** has been the Occupational Safety and Health Act of 1970. As a result of that act, the Occupational Safety and Health Administration (OSHA) was created within the U.S. Department of Labor to ensure a safer and healthier environment for workers. The employer has a legal obligation to inform employees of safety standards, but the employee has a responsibility to read safety materials, comply with safety standards, wear or use protective equipment, and report hazardous conditions.

all-terrain vehicle (ATV) A small open vehicle designed for recreational use on rugged terrain; usually seats one person.   **TERMS**

work injuries Unintentional injuries and deaths that arise out of and in the course of gainful work, such as falls, electrical shocks, exposure to radiation and toxic chemicals, burns, cuts, back sprains, and loss of fingers or other body parts in machines.

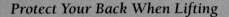
Almost everyone has to lift a heavy object at one time or another. Doing it the right way can protect your back from serious injury. Follow these simple guidelines:

- Know your own strength, and don't try to lift beyond it. Get help if necessary.

- Avoid bending at the waist. Try to remain in an upright, but not stiffly straight, position. If you need to lower yourself to grasp the object, crouch down. Bending at the knees and hips rather than at the waist is the key to safe lifting.

- Get a firm footing, with feet about shoulder-width apart. Get a firm grip on the object with the palms of your hands. If the object or your hands are slippery, wipe them off.

- Lift gradually, keeping your arms straight. Avoid quick, jerky motions, which put a strain on your muscles. Lift by standing up or by pushing up with your leg muscles.

- Don't twist. Twisting is a common and dangerous cause of injury when you're moving something. If you have to turn with the object, change the position of your feet.

- Keep the object close to your body. Your ability to lift safely will be greatly increased.

- Put the object down gently, reversing the rules for lifting.

- Plan ahead. Make sure doors are open and your pathway is clear before you pick up the object.

Back injuries are among the most common, painful, and long-lasting of all the injuries you can sustain. If you hurt your back when you're young, you may have a "bad back" your whole life. It pays to take precautions to make sure your back will be strong when you need it to be.

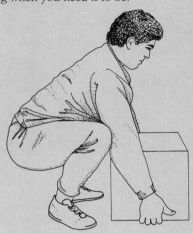

Today, every state has a worker's compensation law. Provisions vary from state to state, but assistance is typically available for medical and hospital services, rehabilitation, and income compensation. The definition of a work-related disability has also been extended beyond physical injury and illness to include stress-related disorders. To be eligible for benefits, a worker must notify his or her employer and provide documentation as evidence for the illness or injury.

The highest risk of injury or illness occurs among laborers. Although laborers make up less than half of the workforce, they account for more than 75% of all work-related injuries and illnesses. Such jobs usually involve extensive manual labor and lifting, neither of which is addressed in OSHA safety standards. Consequently, back problems are the most frequently cited injury and account for over 20% of work injuries. (For guidelines on safe lifting techniques, see the box "Protect Your Back When Lifting.") Skin disorders account for nearly 40% of

reported occupational illnesses; the introduction of more hazardous chemicals and other substances at the work site means that these disorders are of increasing concern. Most fatal occupational injuries involve crushing injuries, severe lacerations, burns, and electrocutions.

Other new workplace problems are related to musculoskeletal injuries and disorders, particularly **repetitive-strain injuries (RSIs)**. RSIs are caused by repeated strain on a particular part of the body. Twisting, vibrations, awkward postures, and other stressors may contribute to RSIs. **Carpal tunnel syndrome** is one type of RSI that has increased in recent years due to increased use of computers, both at work and in the home. This condition is characterized by pain and swelling in the tendons of the wrists and sometimes numbness and weakness. Computer users can protect themselves from carpal tunnel syndrome and other problems by maintaining good posture, positioning the computer screen at eye level, positioning the keyboard so that hands and wrists are straight, using a chair that provides support for the back, and placing the feet flat on the floor or on a footrest. Periodic breaks are also recommended to lessen the cumulative effects of stress. In response to growing concerns about RSIs and related problems, OSHA is developing workplace ergonomics standards. (OSHA defines ergonomics as the science of fitting the job to the worker.)

Whatever the working conditions, employees should make a conscious effort to avoid hazardous situations.

TERMS   **repetitive-strain injury (RSI)**   A musculoskeletal injury or disorder caused by repeated strain to the hand, arm, wrist, or other part of the body; also called cumulative trauma disorder (CTD).

carpal tunnel syndrome   Compression of the median nerve in the wrist, often caused by repetitive use of the hands, such as in computer use; characterized by numbness, tingling, and pain in the hands and fingers; can cause nerve damage.

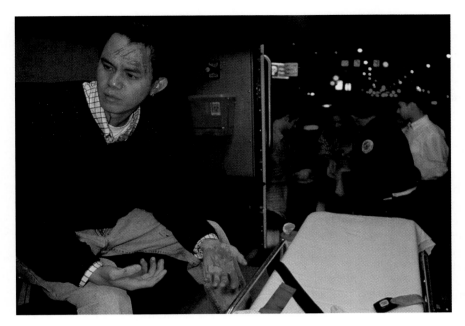

For every violent death that occurs in the United States, there are at least 100 nonfatal injuries caused by violence. The victims of most types of violence are statistically likely to be young (under 25 years), poor, in a minority, urban, and—except for rape and domestic violence—male.

VIOLENCE AND INTENTIONAL INJURIES

Violence—the use of physical force with the intent to inflict harm, injury, or death upon oneself or another—is a major public health concern in the United States. More than 2 million Americans are victims of violent injury each year; about three violent crimes occur every minute. Examples of types of violence are assault, homicide, sexual assault, domestic violence, suicide, and child abuse.

It is difficult to determine the overall level of violence in our society because the major sources of data, which are police reports and victim surveys, are often at odds. In general, the overall violent crime rate increased between the 1950s and 1970s and then leveled off until the mid-1980s, when it again began to rise. Since 1993, however, the rate of violent crime has declined by over 20%; the homicide rate in 1998 was at its lowest level in three decades. Possible factors cited for this decline include the aging of the population, reduced unemployment, the decline of the crack cocaine trade, law enforcement strategies to get guns off the street, violence prevention programs for youth, and longer prison sentences. In comparison to other industrialized countries, U.S. rates of violence are abnormally high in only two areas—homicide and firearm-related deaths. The U.S. homicide death rate is four to ten times that of similar countries, and the firearm death rate in the United States exceeds that of other developed countries eightfold.

Factors Contributing to Violence

Everyone gets angry sometimes, but few people translate their angry and aggressive impulses into action. Most intentional injuries and deaths are associated with an argument or the committing of another crime. However, there are a great many forms of violence, and no single factor can explain all of them.

Social Factors Rates of violence are not the same throughout society; they vary by geographic region, neighborhood, socioeconomic level, and many other factors. In the United States, violence is highest in the West, followed by the South, and among those who are disadvantaged in some way. Neighborhoods that are disadvantaged in status, power, and economic resources are typically the ones with the most violence. Rates of violence are highest among young people and minorities, groups that have relatively little power. People under age 25 account for nearly half the arrests for violent crimes in the United States and about 40% of the arrests for homicide.

People who feel a part of society (have strong family and social ties), who are economically integrated (have a reasonable chance at getting a decent job), and who grow up in areas where there is a feeling of community (good schools, parks, and neighborhoods) are significantly less likely to engage in violence. American society, where more than one-third of all children live in poverty and where the gap between rich and poor keeps growing, should be expected to breed violence. Many criminologists feel we have a growing underclass of people who cannot expect to have even the worst permanent jobs. That absence of hopes and dreams, when combined with family devastation and poverty, certainly contributes to violent behavior.

The mass media play a major role in exposing audiences of all ages to violence as an acceptable and effective means of solving problems. Children may view as many as 10,000 violent acts on television and in movies each year. The consequences of violence, on both perpetrator and victim, are shown much less frequently. People may model their behavior on the acts of family members and peers, as well as on what the mass media portray.

Studies have shown that the environment on college campuses can contribute to violence. The nature of college campuses—transitory communities rather than permanent places where people work and live together over the long term—means that there is less incentive for people to cooperate and coexist amicably. Some campus groups even promote the ideas of bigotry and bias toward others, particularly toward individuals about whom they know little or with whom they have had little contact. Ignorance and insensitivity to differences can be precursors to acts of violence. College students must become more familiar with concepts like inclusion, tolerance, and diversity if the problem is to be addressed.

Gender In most cases, violence is committed by men. (Figure 23-3). Males are more than nine times more likely than females to commit murder. Some researchers have suggested that the male hormone testosterone is in some way linked to aggressive behavior. Others point to prevailing cultural attitudes about male roles (men as dominant and controlling) as an explanation for the high rate of violence among men. However, these theories do not explain just why it is that violent men are more likely to live in the West, belong to minorities, be poor, and be young.

Women do commit acts of violence, including a small but substantial proportion of murders of spouses. This fact has been used to argue that women have the same capacity to commit violence as men, but most researchers feel that there are substantial differences. Men often kill their wives as the culmination of years of violence or after stalking them; they may kill the entire family and themselves at the same time. Women virtually never kill in these circumstances; rather, they kill their husbands after repeated victimization or while being beaten.

Interpersonal Factors Although most people fear attack from strangers, the majority of victims are acquainted with their attacker (see Figure 23-3). Approximately 60% of murders of women and 80% of sexual assaults are committed by someone the woman knows. In many cases, the people we need to fear the most live in our own household. Crime victims and violent criminals tend to share many characteristics—that is, they are likely to be young, male, in a minority, and poor.

Alcohol and Other Drugs Substance abuse and dependence are consistently associated with interpersonal violence and suicide. Intoxication affects judgment and may increase aggression in some people, causing a small argument to escalate into a serious physical confrontation. On college campuses, alcohol is involved in about 95% of all violent crimes.

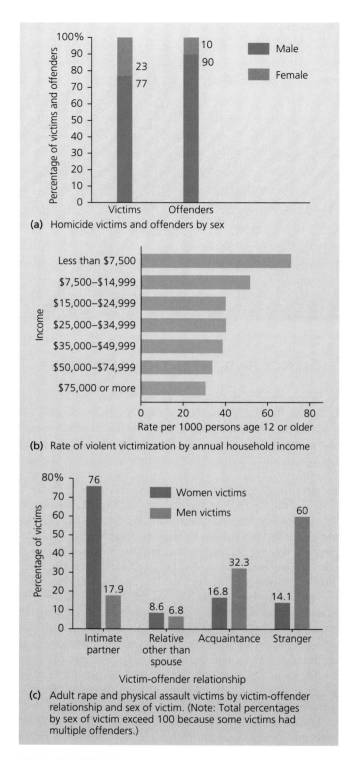

(a) Homicide victims and offenders by sex

(b) Rate of violent victimization by annual household income

(c) Adult rape and physical assault victims by victim-offender relationship and sex of victim. (Note: Total percentages by sex of victim exceed 100 because some victims had multiple offenders.)

VITAL STATISTICS

Figure 23-3 Facts about violence in the United States.
SOURCES: Bureau of Justice Statistics. 1998. *National Crime Victimization Survey: Criminal Victimization 1997.* Washington, D.C.: U.S. Department of Justice. Tjaden, P., and N. Thoennes. 1998. *Prevalence, Incidence, and Consequences of Violence Against Women.* Washington, D.C.: U.S. Department of Justice. Federal Bureau of Investigation. 1998. *Crime in the United States. Uniform Crime Reports, 1997.* Washington, D.C.: U.S. Department of Justice.

Firearms Many criminologists feel that the high rate of homicide in the United States is directly related to the fact that we are the only industrialized country in which handguns are widespread and easily available. Simply put, most victims of assaults with other weapons don't die, but the death rate from assault by handgun is extremely high. The possession of a handgun can change a suicide attempt to a completed suicide and a violent assault to a murder. Every hour, guns are used to kill four people in the United States.

Over 100,000 deaths and injuries occur in the United States each year as a result of the use of firearms. Firearms are used in more than two-thirds of homicides, and studies reveal a strong correlation between the incidence of gun ownership and homicide rates for a given area of the country. Over half of all suicides involve a firearm, and people living in households in which guns are kept have a risk of suicide that is five times greater than that of people living in households without guns. Men between the ages of 15 and 34 have the highest risk of death from homicide and suicide when guns are the weapon used.

Research indicates that of all firearms, handguns are the murder weapon of choice, used in about 80% of homicides involving firearms. People at particularly high risk of being murdered by handguns are teenagers and young adults. The following sequence of events often leads to gun murder: Someone obtains a firearm, two or more people come within reach of that firearm, a dispute escalates into an attack, the firearm is fired, and an injury occurs, resulting in death.

> **PERSONAL INSIGHT**   Have you ever witnessed or been involved in a violent incident? What events led up to the violence? What contributing factors do you think were most important?

Assault

Assault is the use of physical force by a person or persons to inflict injury or death on another; homicide, aggravated assault, and robbery are examples of assault. Research indicates that the victims of assaultive injuries and their perpetrators tend to resemble one another in terms of ethnicity, educational background, psychological profile, and reliance on weapons. In many cases, the victim actually magnifies the confrontation through the use of a weapon. Rates of injury from violent and abusive behavior are highest for males, African Americans, people age 16–19, people who have been never married or are separated or divorced, people of low income, and residents of inner cities.

Homicide

Homicide is the thirteenth leading cause of death in the United States. Men, teenagers, young adults, and members of minority groups, particularly African Americans and Latinos, are most likely to be murder victims.

Although homicide rates for African Americans have declined dramatically in the last 25 years, no other cause of death so greatly differentiates African Americans from other Americans: Among black males, the rate of death from homicide is about six times higher than the rate for the U.S. population as a whole. Poverty and unemployment have been identified as key factors in homicide, and this may account for the high rates of homicide among blacks and other minority groups.

Most homicides are committed with a firearm, occur during an argument, and occur among people who know one another. Intrafamilial homicide, where the perpetrator and victim are related, accounts for about one out of every eight homicides. About 40% of family homicides are committed by spouses, usually following a history of physical and emotional abuse directed at the woman. Wives are more likely to be murdered than husbands, and when a wife kills her husband, it is usually in self-defense.

Gang-Related Violence

Violence results from more than just individual acts, as evidenced by the number of injuries and deaths resulting from gang activities. Gangs are most frequently associated with large cities, but gang activity also extends to the suburbs and even to rural areas. It is estimated that more than 800,000 Americans belong to gangs; the average age for joining a gang is 14. Most gangs control a particular territory and will oppose other gangs, as well as police and community efforts to eliminate them. Gangs may be involved in illegal drug trade, extortion, and "protection" schemes. Gang members are more likely than non-gang members to possess weapons, and violence may result from conflicts over territory or illegal activities.

Gangs are more common in areas that are poor and suffer from high unemployment, population density, and crime. In these areas, an individual may feel that his or her chance of legitimate success in life is out of reach and know that involvement in the drug market makes some gang members rich. Often, gangs also serve as a mechanism for companionship, self-esteem, support, and security; indeed, in some areas, gang membership may be viewed as the only possible means of survival.

To prevent gang violence, individuals, communities, and lawmakers must work together to address factors linked to gang membership and activities. A successful program for combating gangs in Los Angeles includes mediators to help handle disputes or negotiate truces between gangs, job skill development for ex-gang members, and programs for at-risk youths that incorporate tutoring, counseling, and recreational activities. The program helps create an anti-gang community infrastructure by promoting neighborhood watch groups, community-based anti-gang activities, and economic development.

Hate Crimes

When bias against another person's race or ethnicity, national origin, religion, sexual orientation, or disability motivates a criminal act, then the offense is classified as a hate crime. Hate crimes may be committed against people or property; those against people may include intimidation, assault, and even rape or murder. Crimes against property most frequently involve graffiti, the desecration of churches or synagogues, cross burnings, and other acts of vandalism or property damage.

About 10,000 hate crimes are reported every year; many more go unreported, so the actual total is much higher. Crimes against people make up about 70% of all incidents; intimidation and assault are the most common offenses. Racial or ethnic bias was cited as the motivating bias in 59% of the hate crimes reported in 1997; religion was cited in 17% of the cases, sexual orientation in 14%, national origin in 10%, and disability in less than 1%.

Hate crimes may be extremely brutal acts perpetrated at random on total strangers by multiple offenders. Suspects are frequently not identified, but research indicates that a substantial number of hate crimes are committed by males under age 20. Hate crimes are frequently, but not always, associated with fringe groups that have extremist ideologies, such as the Ku Klux Klan and neo-Nazi groups. In 1999, the Southern Poverty Law Center counted more than 500 hate groups and group chapters active in the United States; the rapid growth of hate sites on the Internet is another area of concern.

A variety of factors lead to the prejudice and intolerance that is a major force behind hate crimes. A social context of unemployment and hard economic times, an influx of immigrants, and the growth of visible minority rights movements have been associated with the recent increases in hate crimes in the United States. To combat hate crimes, individuals and communities must foster tolerance, understanding, and an appreciation of differences among people.

School Violence

A recent series of high-profile school shootings brought national attention to the problem of school violence. According to the National School Safety Center, more than 250 school-associated violent deaths of students, faculty, and administrators have occurred since 1992. A majority of these deaths occurred in urban areas and involved use of a firearm; as with other types of violence, both victims and offenders were predominantly young men. Homicide and suicide are the most serious and least

common types of violence in schools; an estimated 400,000 less serious incidents of violence and crime occur each year, including theft, vandalism, and fights not involving weapons.

How risky is the school environment for students? Research indicates that children are actually much safer at school than away from it. Less than 1% of all homicides among youths age 5–19 occur at school, and 90% of schools report no incidents of serious violence. Children and adolescents are far more likely to be killed by an adult in their own home or away from school than they are to die as a result of school-associated violence. According to the CDC, the overall number of violent incidents has decreased steadily since 1992; however, the number of multiple victim events may have increased. Recent school shootings received so much attention in part because they were unusual—they took place in predominantly white suburban or rural schools and involved multiple victims.

Although schools are basically safe places overall, there are steps that can be taken to identify at-risk youths and improve safety for all students. Characteristics associated with youths who have caused school-associated violent deaths include a history of uncontrollable angry outbursts, violent and abusive language and behavior, isolation from peers, depression and irritability, access to and preoccupation with weapons, and lack of support and supervision from adults. Recommendations for reducing school violence include offering classroom training in anger management and improved self-control, providing mental health and social services for students in need, developing after school programs that help students build self-esteem and make friends, and keeping guns out of the hands of children and out of schools.

Workplace Violence

Each year U.S. workers experience an average of 1.5 million minor assaults, 400,000 serious assaults, 85,000 robberies, 50,000 sexual assaults, and 1000 homicides. In about 60% of cases, workplace violence is committed by strangers; acquaintances account for nearly 40% of cases, and intimates for 1%. Police and corrections officers have the most dangerous jobs, followed by taxi drivers, security guards, bartenders, mental health professionals, and workers at gas stations and convenience and liquor stores. Middle school teachers are nearly three times more likely than high school teachers and twenty times more likely than college or university teachers to experience workplace violence.

Most of the perpetrators of workplace violence are white males over 21 years of age. Firearms are used in more than 80% of workplace homicides, and the majority of these homicides occur during the commission of a robbery or other crime. General crime prevention strategies, including controls on firearms, may help reduce the rate of workplace-violence injuries and deaths.

There are no sure ways to tell whether someone will become abusive or violent toward an intimate partner, but there are warning signs that you can look for. If you are concerned that a man you are involved with has the potential for violence, observe his behavior, and ask yourself these questions:

- What is this person's attitude toward women? How does he treat his mother and his sister? How does he work with female students, female colleagues, or a female boss? How does he treat your women friends?

- What is his attitude toward your autonomy? Does he respect the work you do and the way you do it? Or does he put it down, or tell you how to do it better, or encourage you to give it up? Does he tell you he'll take care of you?

- How self-centered is he? Does he want to spend leisure time on your interests or his? Does he listen to you? Does he remember what you say?

- Is he possessive or jealous? Does he want to spend every minute with you? Does he cross-examine you about things you do when you're not with him?

- What happens when things don't go the way he wants them to? Does he blow up? Does he always have to get his way?

- Is he moody, mocking, critical, or bossy? Do you feel as if you're "walking on eggshells" when you're with him?

- Do you feel you have to avoid arguing with him?

- Does he drink too much or use drugs?

- Does he refuse to use condoms or take other precautions for safer sex?

Listen to your own uneasiness, and stay away from any man who disrespects women, who wants or needs you intensely and exclusively, and who has a knack for getting his own way almost all the time.

If you are in a serious relationship with a controlling person, you may already have experienced abuse. Consider the questions on the following list:

- Does your partner constantly criticize you, blame you for things that are not your fault, or verbally degrade you?

- Does he humiliate you in front of others?

- Is he suspicious or jealous? Does he accuse you of being unfaithful or monitor your mail or phone calls?

- Does he "track" all your time? Does he discourage you from seeing friends and family?

- Does he prevent you from getting or keeping a job or attending school? Does he control your shared resources or restrict your access to money?

- Has he ever pushed, slapped, hit, kicked, bitten, or restrained you? Thrown an object at you? Used a weapon on you?

- Has he ever destroyed or damaged your personal property or sentimental items?

- Has he ever forced you to have sex or to do something sexually you didn't want to do?

- Does he anger easily when drinking or taking drugs?

- Has he ever threatened to harm you or your children, friends, pets, or property?

- Has he ever threatened to blackmail you if you leave?

If you answered yes to one or more of these questions, you may be experiencing domestic abuse. If you believe you or your children are in imminent danger, look in your local telephone directory for a women's shelter, or call 9-1-1. If you want information, referrals to a program in your area, or assistance, contact one of the organizations listed in For More Information at the end of the chapter.

SOURCES: Family Violence Prevention Fund. 1996. *Take Action Against Domestic Violence.* San Francisco, Calif.: Family Violence Prevention Fund. How to tell if you're in an abusive situation. 1994. *San Francisco Chronicle,* 24 June. Jones, A. 1994. *Next Time She'll Be Dead.* Boston: Beacon Press.

Family and Intimate Violence

Violence in families challenges some of our most basic assumptions about the family. Family violence generally refers to any rough and illegitimate use of physical force, aggression, or verbal abuse by one family member toward another. Such abuse may be physical and/or psychological in nature. Each year, an estimated 5–7 million women and children are abused in the United States.

Battering Studies reveal that 95% of domestic violence victims are women; 20–35% of women who visit medical emergency rooms are there for injuries related to ongoing abuse. Violence against wives/intimate partners, or battering, occurs at every level of society but is more common at lower socioeconomic levels. It occurs more frequently in relationships with a high degree of conflict—an apparent inability to resolve arguments through negotiation and compromise. Nearly 25% of women report having been physically assaulted or raped by an intimate partner.

At the root of much of this abusive behavior is the need to control another person: Abusive partners are controlling partners. They not only want to have power over another person, they believe they are entitled to it, no matter what the cost to the other person. Abuse includes behavior that physically harms, arouses fear, prevents a person from doing what she wants, or compels her to behave in ways she does not freely choose. Controlling

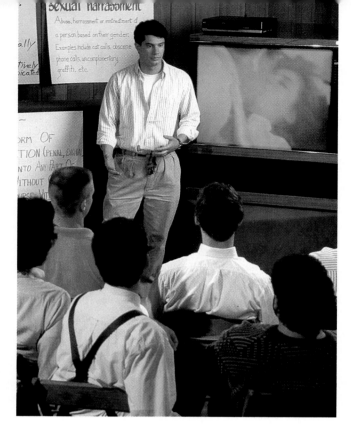

Date rape and sexual harassment are important issues for college students. The goals of this college workshop are to raise men's awareness of the double standard about appropriate sexual behavior for men and women and to examine the differences in how men and women may perceive each other's comments and actions.

people use a variety of psychological, emotional, and physical tactics to keep their partners bound to them, including the following:

- Using criticism, moodiness, anger, or threats.
- Being overprotective and "caring."
- Ignoring the other person's needs and opinions.
- Making all the decisions and controlling the money.
- Limiting contact with other people.
- Using physical or sexual intimidation or violence.

Early in a relationship, a person's tendency to be controlling may not be obvious. If you are a woman concerned about whether a man you are dating has the potential to be abusive, review the guidelines in the box "Recognizing the Potential for Abusiveness in a Partner" on p. 625.

In abusive relationships, the man usually has a history of violent behavior, traditional beliefs about gender roles, and problems with alcohol abuse. He has low self-esteem and seeks to raise it by dominating and imposing his will on another person. Research has revealed a three-phase cycle of battering, consisting of a period of increasing tension, a violent explosion and loss of control, and a period of contriteness, in which the man begs forgiveness and promises it will never happen again. The batterer is drawn back to this cycle over and over again, but he never succeeds in changing his feelings about himself.

Battered women often stay in violent relationships for years. They may be economically dependent on their husbands, believe their children need a father, or have low self-esteem themselves. They may love or pity their husbands, or they may believe they'll eventually be able to stop the violence. They usually leave the relationship only when they become determined that the violence must end. Battered women's shelters offer physical protection, counseling, support, and other types of assistance.

Many battering husbands are arrested, prosecuted, and imprisoned. Treatment programs for men are helpful in some cases, but not all. Programs focus on stress management, communication and conflict resolution skills, behavior change, and individual and group therapy. A crucial factor in changing men's violent behavior seems to be their partner's adamant insistence that the abuse stop.

Battering is closely associated with stalking, characterized by harassing behaviors such as following or spying on a person and making verbal, written, or implied threats. In the United States, it is estimated that 1 million women and 400,000 men are stalked each year; about 87% of stalkers are men. About half of female victims are stalked by current or former intimate partners; of these, 80% had been physically or sexually assaulted by that partner during the relationship. A stalker's goal may be to control or scare the victim or to keep her or him in a relationship. Most stalking episodes last a year or less, but victims may experience social and psychological effects long after the stalking ends

Violence Against Children Violence is also directed against children. At least 1 million American children are physically abused by their parents every year. Parental violence is one of the five leading causes of death for children age 1–18. Parents who abuse children tend to have low self-esteem, to believe in physical punishment, to have a poor marital relationship, and to have been abused themselves (although many people who were abused as children do not grow up to abuse their own children). Poverty, unemployment, and social isolation are characteristics of families in which children are abused. Single parents, both men and women, are at especially high risk for abusing their children. Very often one child, whom the parents consider different in some way, is singled out for violent treatment.

When government agencies intervene in child-abuse situations, their goals are to protect the victims and to assist and strengthen the families. The most successful programs are those that emphasize education and early intervention, such as home visits to high-risk first-time mothers. Educational efforts focus on stress management, money management, job-finding skills, and information about child behavior and development. Parents may also receive counseling and be referred to substance-abuse treatment programs. Support groups like Parents Anonymous are effective for parents committed to changing their behavior.

Sexual Violence

The use of force and coercion in sexual relationships is one of the most serious problems in human interactions. The most extreme manifestation of sexual coercion—forcing a person to submit to another's sexual desires—is rape, but sexual coercion occurs in many more subtle forms, including sexual harassment.

Sexual Assault: Rape

Sexual coercion that relies on the threat and use of physical force or takes advantage of circumstances that render a person incapable of giving consent (such as when drunk) constitutes **sexual assault** or **rape.** When the victim is younger than the legally defined "age of consent," the act constitutes **statutory rape,** whether or not coercion is involved. Coerced sexual activity in which the victim knows or is dating the rapist is often referred to as **date rape** (or acquaintance rape).

Any woman—or man—can be a rape victim. It is conservatively estimated that at least 3.5 million females are raped annually in the United States. Some men are raped by other men, perhaps 10,000 annually—and not all of these rapes are committed in prison.

WHO COMMITS RAPE? Men who commit rape may be any age and come from any socioeconomic group. Some rapists are exploiters in the sense that they rape on the spur of the moment and mainly want immediate gratification. Some attempt to compensate for feelings of sexual inadequacy and an inability to obtain satisfaction otherwise. Others are more hostile and sadistic and are primarily interested not in sex but in hurting and humiliating a particular woman or women in general.

Most women are in much less danger of being raped by a stranger than of being sexually assaulted by a man they know or date. Surveys suggest that as many as 25% of women have had experiences in which the men they were dating persisted in trying to force sex despite pleading, crying, screaming, or resisting. Research also shows that of every 6–15 women, one has been raped by a man she knew or was dating.

Most cases of date rape are never reported to the police, partly because of the subtlety of the crime. Usually no weapons are involved, and direct verbal threats may not have been made. Rather than being terrorized, the victim usually is attracted to the man at first. Victims of date rape tend to shoulder much of the responsibility for the incident, questioning their own judgment and behavior rather than blaming the aggressor.

Sometimes husbands rape their wives. Strong evidence suggests that 15% of American women who have ever married have been raped by their husbands or ex-husbands; as many as 60% of battered women may have been raped by their husbands. A charge of mate rape can now be taken to court in nearly all states.

FACTORS CONTRIBUTING TO DATE RAPE One factor in date rape appears to be the double standard about appropriate sexual behavior for men and women. Although the general status of women in society has improved, it is still a commonly held cultural belief that nice women don't say yes to sex (even when they want to) and that real men don't take no for an answer.

There are also widespread differences between men and women in how they perceive romantic encounters and signals. In one study, researchers found that men tend to interpret women's actions on dates, such as smiling or talking in a low voice, as indicating an interest in having sex, while the women interpreted the same actions as just being "friendly." Men's thinking about forceful sex also tends to be unclear. One psychologist reports that men find "forcing a woman to have sex against her will" more acceptable than "raping a woman," even though the former description is the definition of rape.

Aside from the double standard and unclear perceptions and thinking about sex, men who rape their dates tend to have certain attributes, including hostility toward women, a belief that dominance alone is a valid motive for sex, and an acceptance of sexual violence. They may feel that force is justified in certain circumstances, such as if they are sexually involved with a woman and she refuses to "go all the way," if the woman is known to have slept with other men, or if the woman shows up at a party where people are drinking and taking drugs. The man often primes himself to force himself sexually on his date by drinking, which lowers his ordinary social inhibitions. Many college men who have committed date rape tried to seduce their dates by plying them with alcohol first.

Recently, there has been an increase in the reported use of Rohypnol pills and other "date-rape drugs." Rohypnol is a tasteless tranquilizer 10–20 times more powerful than Valium that some rapists have used on victims, causing them to pass out and have little memory of what happens next. In 1996, President Clinton signed a bill outlawing Rohypnol and adding 20 years to the prison sentence of any rapist who uses a narcotic to incapacitate his victim. Supporters of the new law likened dropping a pill in a victim's drink to putting a knife to her throat. (The makers of

TERMS

sexual assault or **rape** The use of force to have sex with someone against that person's will.

statutory rape Sexual interaction with someone under the legal age of consent.

date rape Sexual assault by someone the victim knows or is dating; also called *acquaintance rape.*

Guidelines for Women

- Believe in your right to control what you do. Set limits, and communicate these limits clearly, firmly, and early. Say "no" when you mean "no."

- Be assertive with someone who is sexually pressuring you. Men often interpret passivity as permission.

- If you are unsure of a new acquaintance, go on a group date or double date. If possible, provide your own transportation.

- Remember that some men assume sexy dress and a flirtatious manner mean a desire for sex.

- Remember that alcohol and drugs interfere with clear communication about sex.

- Use the statement that has proven most effective in stopping date rape: "This is rape, and I'm calling the police."

Guidelines for Men

- Be aware of social pressure. It's OK not to "score."

- Understand that "no" means "no." Don't continue making advances when your date resists or tells you she wants to stop. Remember that she has the right to refuse sex.

- Don't assume sexy dress and a flirtatious manner are invitations to sex, that previous permission for sex applies to the current situation, or that your date's relationships with other men constitute sexual permission for you.

- Remember that alcohol and drugs interfere with clear communication about sex.

Rohypnol are modifying the pills so they will be a more noticeable color and will dissolve more slowly, thereby reducing the likelihood that Rohypnol can be used as a date-rape drug.)

Date rape is largely a result of sexual socialization in which the man develops an exaggerated sexual impulse and puts a premium on sexual conquests. Sex and violence are linked in our society, and coercion is accepted by some adolescents as an appropriate form of sexual expression. Both males and females can take actions that will reduce the incidence of acquaintance rape; see the box "Preventing Date Rape" for specific suggestions.

DEALING WITH A SEXUAL ASSAULT   Experts disagree about whether a woman who is faced with a rapist should fight back or give in quietly to avoid being injured or gain time in the hope of escaping. Some rapists say that if a woman had screamed or resisted loudly, they would have run; others report they would have injured or killed her. (If a rapist is carrying a weapon, most experts advise against fighting unless absolutely necessary.) A woman who is raped by a stranger is more likely to be physically injured than a woman raped by someone she knows. Each situation is unique, and a woman should respond in whatever way she thinks best. If a woman chooses not to resist, it does not mean that she has not been raped.

If you are threatened by a rapist and decide to fight back, here is what Women Organized Against Rape (WOAR) recommends:

- Trust your gut feeling. If you feel you are in danger, don't hesitate to run and scream. It is better to feel foolish than to be raped.

- Yell—and keep yelling. It will clear your head and start your adrenaline going; it may scare your at-

tacker and also bring help. Don't forget that a rapist is also afraid of pain and afraid of getting caught.

- If an attacker grabs you from behind, use your elbows for striking the neck, his sides, or his stomach.

- Try kicking. Your legs are the strongest part of your body, and your kick is longer than his reach. Kick with your rear foot and with the toe of your shoe. Aim low to avoid losing your balance.

- His most vulnerable spot is his knee; it's low, difficult to protect, and easily knocked out of place. Don't try to kick a rapist in the crotch; he has been protecting this area all his life, and will have better protective reflexes there than at his knees.

- Once you start fighting, keep it up. Your objective is to get away as soon as you can.

- Remember that ordinary rules of behavior don't apply. It's OK to vomit, act "crazy," or claim to have a sexually transmitted disease.

If you are raped, tell what happened to the first friendly person you meet. Call the police, tell them you were raped, and give your location. Try to remember as many facts as you can about your attacker; write down a description as soon as possible. Don't wash or change your clothes, or you may destroy important evidence. The police will take you to a hospital for a complete exam; show the physician any injuries. Tell the police simply, but exactly, what happened. Be honest, and stick to your story.

If you decide that you don't want to report the rape to the police, be sure to see a physician as soon as possible. You need to be checked for pregnancy and STDs.

THE EFFECTS OF RAPE   Rape victims suffer both physical and psychological injury. For most, physical wounds are

---

not severe and heal within a few weeks. Psychological pain may endure and be substantial. Even the most physically and mentally strong are likely to experience shock, anxiety, depression, shame, and a host of psychosomatic symptoms after being victimized. These psychological reactions following rape are called rape trauma syndrome, which is characterized by fear, nightmares, fatigue, crying spells, and digestive upset. (Rape trauma syndrome is a form of post-traumatic stress disorder; see Chapter 3.) Self-blame is very likely; society has contributed to this tendency by perpetuating the myths that women can actually defend themselves and that no one can be raped if she doesn't want to be. Fortunately, these false beliefs are dissolving in the face of evidence to the contrary.

Many organizations offer counseling and support to rape victims. Look in the telephone directory under Rape or Rape Crisis Center for a hotline number to call. Your campus may have counseling services or a support group.

Child Sexual Abuse

Child sexual abuse is a sexual act imposed on a minor. Adults and older adolescents are able to coerce children into sexual activity because of their authority and power over them. Threats, force, or the promise of friendship or material rewards may be used to manipulate a child. Sexual contacts are typically brief and consist of genital manipulation; genital intercourse is much less common.

Sexual abusers are usually male, heterosexual, and known to the victim. The abuser may be a relative, a friend, a neighbor, or another trusted adult acquaintance. Child abusers are often pedophiles, people who are sexually attracted to children. With other adults, they may have poor interpersonal and sexual relationships and feel socially inadequate and inferior.

One highly traumatic form of sexual abuse is **incest**, sexual activity between people too closely related to legally marry. The most common forms of incest are father-daughter (which includes stepfather-stepdaughter) abuse, brother-sister abuse (usually an adolescent boy abusing a preadolescent girl), and uncle-niece abuse; mother-son sexual activity is rare. Adults who commit incest may be pedophiles, but very often they are simply sexual opportunists or people with poor impulse control and emotional problems.

Most sexually abused children are between ages 8 and 12 when the abuse first occurs. More girls are sexually abused than boys. The degree of trauma for the child can be very serious, but it varies with the types of encounters, their frequency, the child's age and relationship to the abuser, and the parents' response. Father-daughter abuse may be the most traumatic form, in part because it is a violation of the basic parent-child relationship and because the abuse tends to be more frequent.

Sexual abuse is often unreported. Surveys suggest that as many as 27% of women and 16% of men were sexually abused as children. An estimated 150,000–200,000 new cases of child sexual abuse occur each year. It can leave lasting scars, and adults who were abused as children are more likely to suffer from low self-esteem, depression, anxiety, eating disorders, self-destructive tendencies, sexual problems, and difficulties in intimate relationships.

If you were a victim of sexual abuse as a child and feel it may be interfering with your functioning today, you may want to address the problem. A variety of approaches may help, such as joining a support group of people who have had similar experiences, confiding in a partner or friend, or seeking professional help. Some people have experienced tremendous relief by confronting the person who abused them years earlier, but the possible consequences of this course of action have to be carefully considered, preferably with the help of a professional.

Sexual Harassment

Unwelcome sexual advances, requests for sexual favors, and other verbal, visual, or physical conduct of a sexual nature constitute **sexual harassment** if such conduct explicitly or implicitly does any of the following:

- Affects academic or employment decisions or evaluations
- Interferes with an individual's academic or work performance
- Creates an intimidating, hostile, or offensive academic, work, or student living environment

Extreme cases of sexual harassment occur when a manager, professor, or other person in authority uses his or her ability to control or influence jobs or grades to coerce people into having sex or to punish them if they refuse. A hostile environment can be created by such conduct as sexual gestures, displaying of sexually suggestive objects or pictures, derogatory comments and jokes, sexual remarks about clothing or appearance, obscene letters, and unnecessary touching or pinching. Sexual harassment can occur between people of the same or opposite sex. Although forbidden by law, many cases of sexual harassment go unreported. In a survey of 17,000 federal employees, 42% of women and 15% of men reported having been sexually harassed.

If you have been the victim of sexual harassment, you can take action to stop it. Be assertive with anyone who uses language or actions you find inappropriate. If possible, confront your harasser in writing, over the telephone,

incest Sexual activity between close relatives, such as siblings or parents and their children. **TERMS**

sexual harassment Unwelcome sexual advances, requests for sexual favors, and other conduct of a sexual nature that affects academic or employment decisions or evaluations; interferes with an individual's academic or work performance; or creates an intimidating, hostile, or offensive academic, work, or student living environment.

At Home

- Secure your home with good lighting and effective locks, preferably deadbolts.

- Make sure that all doors and windows are securely locked. Always lock windows and doors, including sliding glass doors, whenever you go out.

- Get a dog, or post "Beware of Dog" signs.

- Don't hide keys in obvious places. Don't give anyone the chance to duplicate your keys; for example, don't give your entire set of keys to a parking attendant, only the car key.

- Install a peephole in your front door. Don't open your door to people you don't know.

- If you or a family member owns a weapon, store it securely. Guns and ammunition should be stored separately.

- If you are a woman living alone, use your initials rather than your full name in the phone directory. Don't use an answering-machine greeting that implies that you live alone or are not home.

- Teach everyone in the household how to obtain emergency assistance.

- Know your neighbors. Work out a system for alerting each other in case of an emergency.

- Establish a neighborhood watch program.

On the Street

- Avoid walking alone, especially at night. Stay where people can see and hear you.

- Dress sensibly, in clothing that allows you freedom of movement.

- Walk purposefully. Act alert and confident. Walk on the outside of the sidewalk, facing traffic.

- Know where you are going. Appearing to be lost increases your vulnerability.

- Don't hitchhike.

- Carry valuables in a fanny pack, pants pocket, or shoulder bag strapped diagonally across the chest. Conceal small purses inside a tote or shopping bag. Keep at least one hand free.

- Always have your keys ready as you approach your vehicle or home.

- Carry enough change so that you can make a telephone call or take public transportation. Carry a whistle to blow if you are attacked or harassed.

- If possible, allow at least two arm lengths between yourself and a stranger. Be aware of suspicious behavior.

- If you feel threatened, run and/or yell. Go into a store or knock on the door of a home. If someone grabs you, yell "Help!" or "Fire!"

In Your Car

- Keep your car in good working condition, carry emergency supplies, and keep the gas tank at least half full.

- When driving, keep doors locked and windows rolled up at least three-quarters of the way.

- Park your car in well-lighted areas or parking garages, preferably those with an attendant or security guard.

- Lock your car when you leave it, and check the interior before opening the door when you return.

- Don't pick up strangers. Don't stop for vehicles in distress; drive on and call for help.

- Notice the location of emergency call boxes along highways and in public facilities. If you travel alone frequently, consider using a cellular phone.

- If your car breaks down, raise the hood, and tie a white cloth to the antenna or door handle. Wait in the car, with the doors locked and windows rolled up. If someone approaches to offer help, open a window only a crack and ask the person to call the police or a towing service.

- If you are involved in a minor automobile crash and you think you have been bumped intentionally, do not leave your car. Motion to the other driver to follow you to the nearest police station. If confronted by a person with a weapon, give up your car.

- Don't get into disputes or arguments with drivers of other vehicles.

On Public Transportation

- While waiting, stand in a populated, well-lighted area.

- Sit near the driver or conductor in a single seat or an outside seat.

- If traveling to an unfamiliar location, call the transit agency for the correct route and time. Make sure that the bus, subway, or train is bound for your destination before you board it.

- If you flag down a taxi, make sure it is from a legitimate service. When you reach your destination, ask the driver to wait until you are safely inside the building.

On Campus

- Ensure that door and window locks are secure and that halls and stairwells have adequate lighting.

- Don't give dorm or residence keys to anybody.

- Don't leave your door unlocked or allow strangers into your room.

- Avoid solitary late-night trips to the library or laundry room. Take advantage of on-campus escort services.

- Don't jog or exercise outside alone at night. Don't take shortcuts across campus that are unfamiliar or seem unsafe.

- If security guards patrol the campus, know the areas they cover, and stay where they can see or hear you.

SOURCES: Fike, R. 1994. *Staying Alive! Your Crime Prevention Guide.* Washington, D.C.: Acropolis Books. Dimona, L., and C. Herndon, eds. 1994. *The 1995 Information Please® Women's Sourcebook.* Boston: Houghton Mifflin. Out of harm's way. 1994. *Harvard Women's Health Watch*, April. Reducing your risk of becoming a carjacking victim. 1993. *Healthline*, August.

or in person, informing him or her that the situation is unacceptable to you and you want the harassment to stop. Be clear: "Do not *ever* make sexual remarks to me" is an unequivocal statement. If assertive communication doesn't work, assemble a file or log documenting the harassment, noting the details of each incident and information about any witnesses who may be able to support your claims. You may discover others who have been harassed by the same person, which will strengthen your case. Then file a grievance with the harasser's supervisor or employer, such as someone in the dean's office if you are a student or someone in the human resources office if you are an employee.

If your attempts to deal with the harassment internally are not successful, you can file an official complaint with your city or state Human Rights Commission or Fair Employment Practices Agency, or with the federal Equal Employment Opportunity Commission. You may also wish to pursue legal action under the Civil Rights Act or under local laws prohibiting employment discrimination. Very often, the threat of a lawsuit or other legal action is enough to stop the harasser.

What You Can Do About Violence

It is obvious that violence in our society is not disappearing and that it is a serious threat to our collective health and well-being. This is especially true on college campuses, which in a sense are communities in themselves but which sometimes lack the authority or guidance to tackle the issue of violence directly. Although government and law enforcement agencies are working to address the problem of violence, individuals must take on a greater responsibility to bring about change. New programs are being developed at the grass-roots level to deal with problems of violence directly. Schools are now providing training for conflict resolution and are educating people about the diverse nature of our society, thereby encouraging tolerance and understanding.

Looking at the problem of violence from a public health perspective points to the importance of the social environment. As with any public health problem, one potential approach is to identify and target high-risk groups for intervention. Violence prevention programs currently focus on conflict resolution training and the development of social skills. These measures have proven effective, but for behavior change to be lasting, the focus of such programs must expand beyond individual intervention to include social and environmental factors.

Reducing gun-related injuries may require changes in the availability, possession, and lethality of the 12 million firearms sold in the United States each year. As part of the Brady gun control law, computerized instant background checks are preformed for most gun sales to prevent purchases by convicted felons, people with a history of mental instability, and certain other groups. In some states,

waiting periods are required in addition to the background checks. Some groups advocate a complete and universal federal ban on the sale of all handguns.

Safety experts also advocate the adoption of consumer safety standards for guns, including features such as childproofing, personalization (to prevent unauthorized use), and indicators to show if a gun is loaded. Education about proper storage is also important: Surveys indicate that more than 40% of homes with children contain guns; in about 23% of gun-owning households, the weapon is stored loaded, and in 28%, the gun is kept hidden but not locked. To be effective, any approach to firearm injury prevention must have the support of law enforcement and the community as a whole.

Change will take time, but it must start somewhere. There are many steps you can take to prevent harm or injury to yourself and to others from violence (see the box "Protecting Yourself Against Violence").

PROVIDING EMERGENCY CARE

By following the safety guidelines described in this chapter and being aware of the potential risks associated with different activities, you can avoid many injuries on the road, at home, at work, and in public places. However, some injuries will inevitably occur. Therefore, it is also important to prepare for situations when you may need to provide emergency care for yourself or others. If you are prepared to help, you can improve someone else's chances of surviving or of avoiding permanent disability.

A course in **first aid** can help you respond appropriately when someone is injured. One important benefit of first aid training is that you learn what *not* to do in certain situations. For example, a person with a suspected neck or back injury should not be moved unless other life-threatening conditions exist. A knowledgeable person can assess emergency situations accurately before acting. An emergency first aid guide is provided inside the back cover of this book.

Emergency rescue techniques can save the lives of people who are choking, who have stopped breathing, or whose hearts have stopped beating. As described earlier, the Heimlich maneuver is used when a victim is choking. Pulmonary resuscitation (also known as rescue breathing, artificial respiration, or mouth-to-mouth resuscitation) is used when a person is not breathing (see Figure 23-2). **Cardiopulmonary resuscitation (CPR)** is used when a

first aid Emergency care given to an ill or injured person until medical care can be obtained. **TERMS**

cardiopulmonary resuscitation (CPR) An emergency first aid procedure that combines artificial respiration and artificial circulation; used in first aid emergencies where breathing and blood circulation have stopped.

pulse cannot be found. Training is required before a person can perform CPR. Courses are offered by the American Red Cross and the American Heart Association. A new feature of some of these courses is training in the use of automatic external defibrillators (AEDs), which monitor the heart's rhythm and, if appropriate, deliver an electrical shock to restart the heart. Because of the importance of early use of defibrillators in saving heart attack victims, these devices are being installed in public places, including casinos, airports, and certain office buildings.

As a person providing assistance to someone, you are the first link in the **emergency medical services (EMS) system.** Your responsibility may be to render first aid as needed, provide emotional support for the victim, or just call for help. Here are some tips:

- Remain calm, and act sensibly. The basic pattern for providing emergency care is check-call-care.
- *Check the situation:* Make sure the scene is safe for both you and the injured person. Don't put yourself in danger; if you get hurt too, you will be of little help to the injured person.
- *Check the victim:* Conduct a quick head-to-toe examination. Assess the victim's signs and symptoms, such as level of responsiveness, pulse, and breathing rate. Look for bleeding and any indications of broken bones or paralysis.
- *Call for help:* Call 9-1-1 or a local emergency number. Identify yourself and give as much information as you can about the condition of the victim and what happened.
- *Care for the victim:* If the situation requires immediate action (no pulse, shock, etc.), provide first aid if you are trained to do so (see Figure 23-2).

Like other kinds of behavior, avoiding and preventing injuries and acting safely involve choices you make every day. If you perceive something to be a serious personal threat, you tend to take action to protect yourself. Ultimately, your goal is healthy, safe behavior. You can motivate yourself to act in the safest way possible by increasing your knowledge and level of awareness, by examining your attitudes to see if they're realistic, by knowing your capacities and limitations, by adjusting your responses when environmental hazards exist, and, in general, by taking responsibility for your actions. You can't eliminate all risks and dangers from your life—no one can do that—but you can improve your chances of avoiding injuries and living to a healthy, ripe old age.

PERSONAL INSIGHT　How do you feel about being trained to handle emergency situations by taking courses in CPR or first aid? Does it make you feel more confident and in control to know you could help? Or does it feel like a possibly frightening responsibility? What is the basis for your feelings?

SUMMARY

Unintentional Injuries

- Injuries are caused by a dynamic interaction of human and environmental factors. Risk-taking behavior is associated with a high rate of injury.
- Key factors in motor vehicle injuries include bad driving (especially speeding), a failure to wear safety belts, and alcohol and drug intoxication.
- Motorcycle and moped injuries can be prevented by developing appropriate skills, driving defensively, and wearing proper safety equipment, especially a helmet.
- Bicyclists can increase safety by following all traffic laws, increasing visibility, using bicycle paths, and wearing helmets.
- Poor decision making, lack of visibility, and alcohol or drug intoxication contribute to pedestrian injuries and deaths.
- Most fall-related injuries are a result of falls at floor level, but stairs, chairs, and ladders are also involved in a significant number of falls.
- Careless smoking and problems with heating equipment are common causes of home fires. Being prepared for fire emergencies means planning escape routes and installing smoke detectors.
- The home can contain many poisonous substances, including medications, cleaning agents, plants, and fumes from cars and appliances.
- Performing the Heimlich maneuver can prevent someone from dying from choking.
- The proper storage and handling of firearms can help prevent injuries; assume that a gun is loaded.
- Alcohol use is a major factor in drownings and boating injuries among adults. Proper supervision of children and the use of personal flotation devices can help prevent drownings.
- Many injuries during leisure activities and sports result from the misuse of equipment, lack of experience, and a failure to wear proper safety equipment.
- Most work-related injuries involve extensive manual labor when lifting. Back problems are most common; newer problems include repetitive-strain injuries.

Why do you get injured? What human and environmental factors contribute to injuries? Identifying those factors is one step toward making your lifestyle safer. Changing unsafe behaviors *before* they lead to injuries is an even better way of improving your chances.

For the next 7–10 days, keep track of any mishaps you are involved in or injuries you receive, recording them on a daily behavior record like the one shown in Chapter 1. Count each time you cut, burn, or injure yourself, fall down, run into someone, or have any other potentially injury-causing mishap, no matter how trivial. Also record any risk-taking behaviors, such as failing to wear your safety belt or bicycle helmet, drinking and driving, exceeding the speed limit, putting off home or bicycle repairs, and so on. For each entry (injury or incidence of unsafe behavior), record the date, time, what you were doing, who else was there and how you were influenced by him or her, what your motivations were, and what you were thinking and feeling at the time.

At the end of the monitoring period, examine your data. For each incident, determine both the human factors and the environmental factors that contributed to the injury or unsafe behavior. Were you tired? Distracted? Did you not realize this situation was dangerous? Did you take a chance? Did you think this incident couldn't happen to you? Was visibility poor? Were you using defective equipment? Then consider each contributing factor carefully, determining why it existed and how it could

have been avoided or changed. Finally, consider what preventive actions you could take to avoid such incidents or change your behaviors in the future.

As an example, let's say that you usually don't use a safety belt when you run local errands in your car, and that several factors contribute to this behavior: You don't really think you could be involved in a crash so close to home, you only go on short trips, you just never think to use it, and so on. One of the contributing factors to your unsafe behavior is inadequate knowledge. You can change this factor by obtaining accurate information about auto crashes (and their usual proximity to a victim's home) from this chapter and from library research. Just acquiring information about auto crashes and safety belt use may lead you to examine your beliefs and attitudes about safety belts and motivate you to change your behavior.

Once you're committed, you can use behavior change techniques described in Chapter 1, such as completing a contract, asking family and friends for support, and so on, to build a new habit. Put a note or picture reminding you to buckle up in your car where you can see it clearly. Recruit a friend to run errands with you and to remind you about using your safety belt. Once your habit is established, you may influence other people—especially people who ride in your car—to use safety belts all the time. By changing this behavior, you have reduced the chances that you or your passengers will suffer a serious injury or even die in a vehicle crash.

Violence and Intentional Injuries

- Factors contributing to violence include poverty, the absence of strong social ties, the influence of the mass media, cultural attitudes about gender roles, problems in interpersonal relationships, abuse of alcohol and other drugs, and the widespread availability of firearms.

- Assault is the use of physical force to inflict injury or death. Most homicides are committed with a firearm and occur during an argument between people who know each other.

- Other types of violence include gang-related violence, hate crimes, school violence, and workplace violence.

- Wife battering and child abuse occur at every socioeconomic level. The core issue is the abuser's need to control other people. Stalking is closely associated with battering.

- Most rape victims are women, and most know their attackers. Factors in date rape include different standards of appropriate sexual behavior for men and women and different perceptions of signals and

actions. Rape victims suffer both physical and psychological pain.

- Child sexual abuse often results in serious trauma for the victim; usually the abuser is a relative, friend, or other trusted adult acquaintance.

- Sexual harassment is unwelcome sexual advances or other conduct of a sexual nature that affects academic or employment performance or evaluations or that creates an intimidating, hostile, or offensive academic, work, or student living environment.

- Strategies for reducing violence include conflict resolution training, social skills development, and education programs that foster tolerance and understanding among diverse groups.

Providing Emergency Care

- By taking first aid courses, people can learn how to help others who are injured.

- Steps in giving emergency care include making sure the scene is safe for you and the injured person, conducting a quick examination of the victim, calling for help, and providing emergency first aid.

1. Contact your local fire department, and obtain a checklist for fire safety procedures. What would you do if a fire started in your home? What types of evacuation procedures would be necessary? Do a practice fire drill at home to see what problems might arise in a real emergency.

2. Look up the nearest Poison Control Center in your telephone book, and post the number near your telephone. Contact the center, and ask them to send you information on poisonings. Read it carefully so you know what to do in case of poisoning.

3. Contact the American Red Cross or American Heart Association in your area, and ask about first aid and CPR classes. These courses are usually given frequently and at a variety of times and locations. They can be invaluable in saving lives. Consider taking one or both of the courses.

4. Find out what resources are available on your campus or in your community for victims of rape, hate crimes, or other types of violence. Does your campus sponsor any violence prevention programs or activities? If so, consider participating in one.

JOURNAL ENTRY

1. In your health journal, list the positive behaviors that help you avoid injuries and keep yourself safe. What can you do to reinforce and support these behaviors? Then list the behaviors that keep you from following safety guidelines or that put you at risk of being injured. How can you change one or more of them?

2. *Critical Thinking*   Federal, state, and local governments have passed many regulations and laws to enforce a certain level of safety among citizens, such as laws regulating safety belts, helmets, and firearms. Some people believe that government should not be involved in issues of individual safety and injury prevention; others feel the government has a right to demand certain behaviors for the public good. How do you feel about this issue? Write a brief essay outlining your opinion; be sure to explain your reasoning.

FOR MORE INFORMATION

Books

Bever, D. L. 1996. *Safety: A Personal Focus,* 4th ed. St. Louis, Mo.: Mosby, Year Book. *An overview of injury prevention, including automobile, fire, and recreational safety.*

Hafen, B. Q., K, J. Karren, and K. J. Frandsen. 1999. *First Aid for Colleges and Universities.* 7th ed. Needham Heights, Mass.: Allyn & Bacon. *Provides basic information about first aid.*

Harteau, J., and H. Keegel. 1998. *A Woman's Guide to Personal Safety.* Minneapolis, Minn.: Fairview Press. *A guide to safety in the car and at work, school, and home.*

Henderson, H. 1999. *Domestic Violence Sourcebook.* Detroit, Mich.: Omnigraphics. *Provides information about domestic physical, emotional, and sexual abuse, with resources for help.*

Parrot, A. 1999. *Coping with Date Rape and Acquaintance Rape.* Rev. ed. New York: Rosen Group. *Information about date rape, geared toward young adults.*

Organizations, Hotlines, and Web Sites

American Automobile Association Foundation for Traffic Safety. Provides consumer information about all aspects of traffic safety; Web site has online quizzes and extensive links.
   1440 New York Ave., N.W., Suite 201
   Washington, DC 20005
   800-305-SAFE
   http://www.aaafts.org

American Bar Association: Domestic Violence. Provides information on statistics, research, and laws relating to domestic violence.
   http://www.abanet.org/domviol/home.html

National Center for Injury Prevention and Control. Provides consumer-oriented information about preventing unintentional injuries and violence.
   4770 Buford Highway N.E.
   Atlanta, GA 30341-3724
   770-488-1506
   http://www.cdc.gov/ncipc

National Highway Traffic Safety Administration. Supplies materials about reducing deaths, injuries, and economic losses from motor vehicle crashes.
   400 Seventh St., S.W.
   Washington, DC 20590
   800-424-9393
   http://www.nhtsa.dot.gov

National Safety Council. Provides information and statistics about preventing unintentional injuries.
   1121 Spring Lake Dr.
   Itasca, IL 60143
   630-285-1121
   http://www.nsc.org

National Center for Victims of Crime. An advocacy group for crime victims; provides statistics, news, safety strategies, tips on finding local assistance, and links to related sites.

800-FYI-CALL
http://www.nvc.org

National Violence Hotlines. Provide information, referral services, and crisis intervention.

800-799-SAFE (domestic violence); 800-422-4453 (child abuse); 800-656-HOPE (sexual assault)

Outdoor Empire Publishing, Inc. Publishers of bicycle safety materials for K–3, middle school, and teen/adult; coloring/activity books, student manuals, and bicyclist's guides and brochures.

800-645-5489

Prevent Child Abuse America. Provides statistics, information, and publications relating to child abuse, including parenting tips.

312-663-3520
http://www.childabuse.org

Sexual Assault Information Page. Provides information on a wide variety of topics relating to sexual violence.

http://www.cs.utk.edu/~bartley/saInfoPage.html

The following sites provide statistics and background information on violence and crime in the United States:

Bureau of Justice Statistics
http://www.ojp.usdoj.gov/bjs

Federal Bureau of Investigation
http://www.fbi.gov

Justice Information Center
http://www.ncjrs.org

SELECTED BIBLIOGRAPHY

Bureau of Alcohol, Tobacco, and Firearms. 1998. *Brady Handgun Violence Prevention Act: Questions and Answers* (retrieved February 6, 1999; http://www.atf.treas.gov/core/firearms/information/brady/q_abrady.htm).

Bureau of Justice Statistics. 1998. *National Crime Victimization Survey: Criminal Victimization 1997.* Washington, D.C.: U.S. Department of Justice.

Centers for Disease Control and Prevention. 1999. *Facts About Violence Among Youth and Violence in Schools* (retrieved April 28, 1999; http://www.cdc.gov/od/oc/media/pressrel/r990421.htm).

Centers for Disease Control and Prevention. 1999. National Child Passenger Safety Week. *Morbidity and Mortality Weekly Report* 48(4): 83–84.

Centers for Disease Control and Prevention. 1998. International comparative analysis of injury mortality. *Advance Data* No. 303.

Centers for Disease Control and Prevention. 1998. Deaths resulting from residential fires and prevalence of smoke alarms—United States, 1991–1995. *Morbidity and Mortality Weekly Report* 47(38): 803–807.

Center to Prevent Handgun Violence. 1998. *Parents, Kids, and Guns: A Nationwide Survey* (retrieved February 28, 1999; http://www.handguncontrol.org/press/oct31-98c.htm).

Cole, T. B. 1999. Ebbing epidemic: Youth homicide rate at a 14-year low. *Journal of the American Medical Association* 281: 25–26.

Federal Bureau of Investigation. 1998. *Crime in the United States. Uniform Crime Reports, 1997.* Washington, D.C.: U.S. Department of Justice.

Krug, E. G., K. E. Powell, and L. L. Dahlberg. 1998. Firearm-related deaths in the United States and 35 other high- and upper-middle-income countries. *International Journal of Epidemiology* 27(2): 214–221.

Moore, J. P., and C. P. Terrett. 1998. *Office of Juvenile Justice and Delinquency Prevention: Highlights of the 1996 Youth Gang Survey* (retrieved February 28, 1999; http://www.ncjrs.org/txtfiles/fs-9886txt).

National Center for Education Statistics. 1998. *Indicators of School Crime and Safety, 1998.* Washington, D.C.: National Center for Education Statistics Pub. NCES 98-251.

National Highway Traffic Safety Administration. 1999. *Strategies for Aggressive Driver Enforcement.* Washington, D.C.: U.S. Department of Transportation.

National Highway Traffic Safety Administration. 1998. *Notice of Proposed Rulemaking: Occupant Crash Protection* (retrieved February 22, 1999; http://www.nhtsa.dot.gov/airbag/proposed/advbag.html).

National School Safety Center. 1999. *Report on School Associated Violent Deaths* (retrieved April 28, 1999; http://nssc1.org/savd/savd.pdf).

Occupational Safety and Health Administration. 1999. *Background on the Working Draft of OSHA's Proposed Ergonomics Program Standard* (retrieved February 22, 1999; http://www.osha-slc.gov/SLTC/ergonomics/backgroundinfo.html).

Seldes, R. M., et al. 1999. Predictors of injury among adult recreational in-line skaters. A multi-city study. *American Journal of Public Health* 89: 238–241.

Southern Poverty Law Center. 1999. *The Year in Hate: Hate Group Count Tops 500, Internet Sites Soar* (retrieved February 24, 1999: http://www.splcenter.org/intelligenceproject/ip-4i1.html).

Strasburger, V. C., and E. Donnerstein. 1999. Children, adolescents, and the media: Issues and solutions. *Pediatrics* 103(1): 129–139.

Teran-Santos, J., et al. 1999. The association between sleep apnea and the risk of traffic accidents. *New England Journal of Medicine* 340(11): 847–856.

Tjaden, P., and N. Thoennes. 1998. P*revalence, Incidence, and Consequences of Violence Against Women.* Washington, D.C.: U.S. Department of Justice.

U.S. Consumer Product Safety Commission. 1999. *Childproofing Your Home: 12 Safety Devices to Protect Your Children* (retrieved February 24, 1999; http://www.cpsc.gov/cpscpub/pubs/grand/12steps/12steps.html).

U.S. Department of Justice. 1999. *1999 National Crime Victims' Rights Weeks Resource Guide: Homicide* (retrieved February 25, 1999; http://www.ojp.usdoj.gov/ovc/ncvrw/1999/homic.htm).

U.S. Equal Employment Opportunity Commision. 1998. *Facts About Sexual Harassment* (retrieved September 29, 1998; http://www.eeoc.gov/facts/fs-sex.html).

Warchol, G. 1998. Workplace violence. 1992–1996. *Bureau of Justice Statistics Special Report.* Washington D.C.: U.S. Department of Justice.

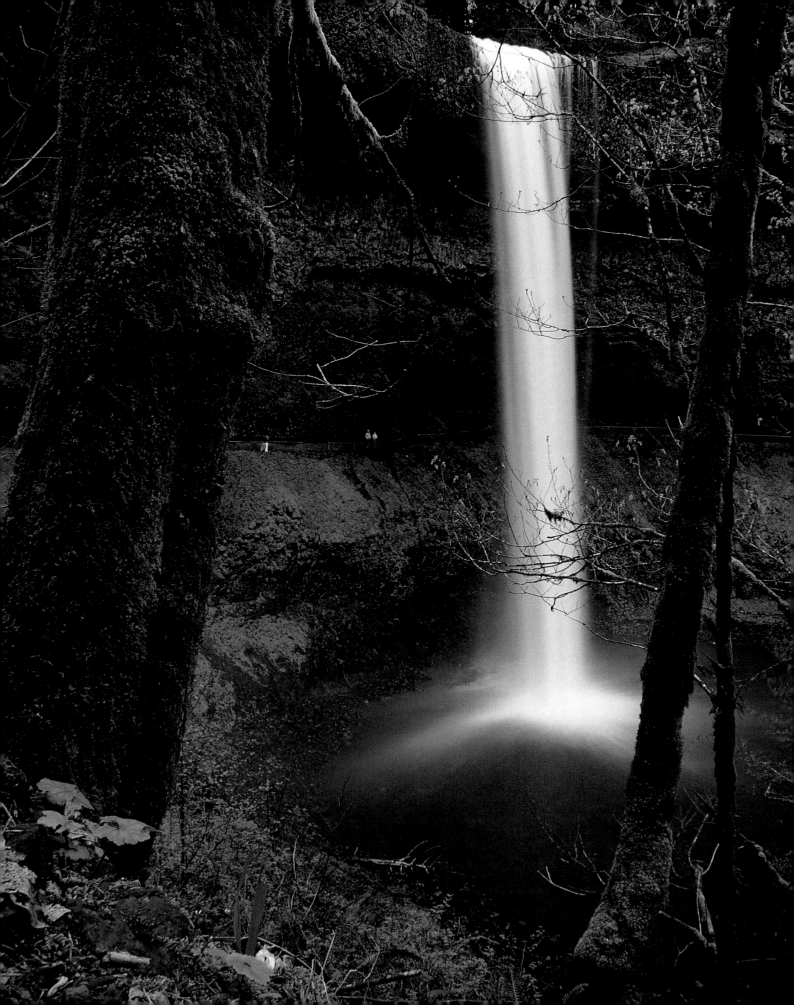

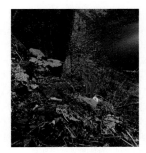

LEARNING OBJECTIVES

After reading this chapter, you should be able to:

- Describe the methods used to deal with the classic environmental concerns of clean water and waste disposal.

- Discuss the effects of rapid increases in human population, and list factors that may limit or slow world population growth.

- Describe the short- and long-term effects of air, chemical, and noise pollution and exposure to radiation.

- Outline strategies that individuals, communities, and nations can take to preserve and restore the environment.

Environmental Health

24

TEST YOUR KNOWLEDGE

1. The world's population, currently at about 6 billion, is increasing by about _____ people every minute?
    a. 50
    b. 100
    c. 150

2. One serving of which of the following requires the most water to produce?
    a. apple
    b. wheat bread
    c. chicken
    d. steak

3. Which of the following statements about sport utility vehicles is true?
    a. They currently account for about half of all new vehicles sold.
    b. They get relatively poor gas mileage.
    c. They currently have weaker pollution standards than regular cars and so pollute more.

4. Most oil pollution comes from large spills that occur when tankers run aground or ships clean out their holds at sea.
    True or false?

5. Most of the energy used by a standard incandescent light bulb is converted into light.
    True or false?

Answers

1. c. Although birth rates are declining, the world's population is expected to nearly double by 2200.

2. d. It takes about 15 gallons of water to produce an apple or a slice of bread, 400 to produce a serving of chicken, and 2600 to produce a steak.

3. All three. Sport utility vehicles use more nonrenewable fuels and release more pollutants than more energy-efficient vehicles.

4. False. More than twice as much oil pollution comes from individual cars and boats. More than 200 million gallons of oil are dumped each year by people changing their own auto engine oil. Put discarded oil in a sturdy container and take it to a service station for disposal.

5. False. About 90% of the energy used by a standard bulb is wasted because it is given off as heat, not light. If each American replaced one incandescent bulb with a compact fluorescent, the yearly energy savings would equal the total production of four nuclear power plants.

We are constantly reminded of our intimate relationship with all that surrounds us—our environment. Although the planet supplies us with food, water, air, and everything else that sustains life, it also presents us with natural occurrences—earthquakes, hurricanes, drought, climate changes—that destroy life and disrupt society. In the past, humans have frequently had to struggle against the environment to survive. Today, in addition to dealing with natural disasters, we also have to find ways to protect the environment from the by-products of our way of life.

Environmental health has historically focused on preventing infectious diseases spread by water, waste, food, rodents, and insects. Although these problems still exist, the focus of environmental health has expanded and become more complex, for several reasons. First, we now recognize that environmental pollutants contribute not only to infectious diseases but to many chronic diseases as well. In addition, technological advances have increased our ability to affect and damage the environment. And finally, rapid population growth, which has resulted partly from past environmental improvements, means that far more people are consuming and competing for resources than ever before, magnifying the effect of humans on the environment (see the box "Environmental Index").

Environmental health is therefore seen as encompassing all the interactions of humans with their environment and the health consequences of these interactions. Fundamental to this definition is a recognition that we hold the world in trust for future generations and for other forms of life. Our responsibility is to pass on to the next generation an environment no worse, and preferably better, than the one we enjoy today (see the box "Nature and the Human Spirit"). Although many environmental problems are complex and seem beyond the control of the individual, there are ways that people can make a difference in the future of the planet.

CLASSIC ENVIRONMENTAL HEALTH CONCERNS

The field of environmental health originally grew out of efforts to control communicable diseases. When certain insects and rodents were found to carry microorganisms that cause disease in humans, campaigns were undertaken to eradicate or control these animal vectors. It was also recognized that pathogens could live and be transmitted in sewage, drinking water, and food. These discoveries led to the development of such practices as systematic garbage collection, sewage treatment, filtration and chlorination of drinking water, food inspection, and the establishment of public health enforcement agencies.

These successful efforts to control and prevent communicable diseases changed the health profile of the developed world (see Chapter 1). Americans now only rarely contract **cholera,** typhoid fever, plague, diphtheria, or other diseases that once killed entire populations. But that doesn't mean these diseases have been eradicated worldwide or that no efforts are required to keep them under control in the United States. Recently there have been more than 2 million cases of cholera in South and Central America, spread by contaminated seafood and poor sewage disposal.

In the United States, a huge, complex health system is constantly at work behind the scenes attending to the details of these concerns. Every time this system is disrupted, danger recurs. Every time a flood, a hurricane, an earthquake, a tornado, or some other natural disaster damages a community, these areas again become of prime importance. And every time we venture beyond the boundaries of our everyday world, whether traveling to a less developed country or camping in a wilderness area, we are reminded of the importance of these basics: clean water, sanitary waste disposal, safe food, and insect and rodent control.

Clean Water

Few parts of the world have adequate quantities of safe, clean drinking water, and yet few things are as important to human health.

Water Contamination and Treatment   Many cities rely at least in part on wells that tap local groundwater, but often it is necessary to find lakes and rivers to supplement wells. Because such surface water is more likely to be contaminated with both organic matter and pathogenic microorganisms, it is purified in water-treatment plants before being piped into the community. At treatment facilities, the water is subjected to various physical and chemical processes, including screening, filtration, and disinfection (often with chlorine), before it is introduced into the water supply system. **Fluoridation,** a water-treatment process that reduces tooth decay by 20–40%, is common in many communities.

In most areas of the United States, water systems have adequate, dependable supplies, are able to control water-borne disease, and provide water without unacceptable color, odor, or taste. However, problems do occur. In 1993, 400,000 people became ill and 100 died when Milwaukee's drinking water was contaminated with the bacterium *Cryptosporidium.* The Centers for Disease Control

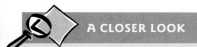

Environmental Index

Some of the Bad News

- The 15 warmest years since global records of air temperature were first kept in the 1800s have all occurred since 1979; 1998 was the hottest year to date. Antarctica is warmer now than at any time in the past 4000 years.

- The atmospheric concentration of carbon dioxide, one of the gases that contributes to global warming, is higher than it has been in at least 160,000 years. Per-capita U.S. carbon dioxide emissions are five times the global average.

- Some 73% of American commuters drive alone to work; 13% carpool, 5% take public transportation, and 4% walk. U.S. energy consumption has more than doubled since 1960.

- Between 50 and 100 species become extinct every day.

- One-third of Americans live in areas where the air exceeds pollution standards.

- The world is losing about 50 million acres of rainforest each year. At current rates, all the remaining rainforest will be destroyed in 50 years; in some countries, it will be gone within a decade.

- The number of autos is growing three times faster than the rate of population growth.

- World population continues to skyrocket, increasing by about 9000 people every hour. It is expected to grow by more than a billion people between 2000 and 2013.

Some of the Good News

- Levels of air pollution in the United States have decreased by nearly 30% over the past 25 years, despite an almost doubling of the economy. Lead levels are down 78%.

- The proportion of garbage that is recycled more than doubled between 1985 and 2000. About half of all Americans are served by curbside recycling programs.

- Energy use from renewable sources such as solar, wind, and hydroelectric is at an all-time high. Wind energy is the fastest growing energy source.

- Sales of energy efficient compact fluorescent lights soared from 80 million units in 1990 to 350 million in 1997.

- Since the Montreal Protocol of 1987, the worldwide release of ozone-damaging CFCs has fallen by 88%.

- The number of nuclear warheads worldwide is down more than 40% from its 1986 peak.

- Birth rates are dropping worldwide, from an average of 3.7 children per woman in 1980 to 3.2 in 1990 and 2.7 in 2000.

SOURCES: International Association for Energy-Efficient Lighting. NASA Goddard Institute for Space Studies. National Resources Defense Council. U.S. Department of Health and Human Services. U.S. Environmental Protection Agency. United Nations Environmental Programme. United Nations Population Division. Worldwatch Institute.

SOUND MIND, SOUND BODY *Nature and the Human Spirit*

In this excerpt from her book *The Sense of Wonder,* noted scientist and author Rachel Carson affirms the nurturing power of the natural world and urges us to appreciate the deep relationship between nature and the human spirit.

> What is the value of preserving and strengthening this sense of awe and wonder, this recognition of something beyond the boundaries of human existence? Is the exploration of the natural world just a pleasant way to pass the golden hours of childhood or is there something deeper?
>
> I am sure there is something much deeper, something lasting and significant. Those who dwell, as scientists or laymen, among the beauties and mysteries of the earth are never alone or weary of life. Whatever the vexations or concerns of their personal lives, their thoughts can find paths that lead to inner contentment and to renewed excitement in living. Those who contemplate the beauty of the earth find reserves of strength that will endure as long as life lasts. There is symbolic as well as actual beauty in the migration of the birds, the ebb and flow of the tides, the folded bud ready for spring. There is something infinitely healing in the repeated refrains of nature—the assurance that dawn comes after night, and spring after the winter.

SOURCE: Carson, R. 1956. *The Sense of Wonder.* New York: Harper & Row. Copyright © 1956 by Rachel Carson. Copyright © renewed 1984 by Roger Christie.

and Prevention (CDC) estimates that 1 million Americans become ill and 900–1000 die each year from microbial illnesses from drinking water. Pollution by hazardous chemicals from manufacturing, agriculture, and household wastes is another concern. (Chemical pollution is discussed later in the chapter.)

The *Healthy People 2010* report sets the goal of increasing from 80% to 95% the proportion of Americans with drinking water that meets standards set by the U.S. Environmental Protection Agency (EPA). More stringent testing and treatment of water is one strategy for meeting this objective. Another is to change our water distribution sys-

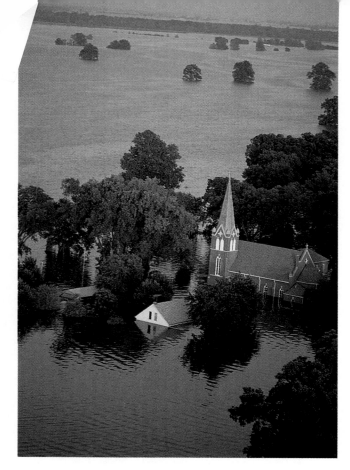

We often take for granted the well-organized system responsible for environmental health in our society, but natural disasters remind us of its fragility. In addition to forcing people from their homes, flooding can cause widespread disruption in essential services such as the delivery of electricity, gas, and clean drinking water.

tem. Most cities have one water-treatment system that supplies water to homes, industry, and agriculture alike. However, much of that water does not have to be made as pure and safe as drinking water. For example, the water you use to wash your car does not need to meet the same standards as the water you drink. As treatment becomes more difficult and expensive, a multilevel distribution system based on intended use may help to save money and improve drinking water supplies.

Water Shortages   Water shortages are also a growing concern. Some parts of the United States are experiencing rapid population growth that outstrips the ability of local systems to provide adequate water to all. Many proposals are being discussed to relieve these shortages, including long-distance transfers, conservation, and the recycling of some water, such as the water in office-building air conditioning towers.

According to the World Health Organization (WHO), only about 35% of the world's people have an adequate water supply. Groundwater pumping and the diversion of water from lakes and rivers for irrigation are further reducing the amount of water available to local communities. In some areas, groundwater is being removed at twice the rate it is replaced. The Aral Sea, located in Kazakhstan and Uzbekistan, was once one of the world's largest inland seas. Since the 1960s, it has lost two-thirds of its volume to irrigation. People living in the area have experienced severe water shortages and increased rates of respiratory disease and throat cancer linked to dust storms from the dry seabed. Due to agricultural diversions, the Yellow River ran dry for the first time in China's 3000-year history in 1972, failing to reach the sea for 15 days that year; by 1998, this period had grown to 226 days. In the United States, the Colorado River is now diverted to the extent that it no longer flows into the ocean.

What You Can Do to Protect the Water Supply

- Take showers, not baths, to minimize your water consumption. Don't let water run when you're not actively using it while brushing your teeth, shaving, or hand-washing clothes. Don't run a dishwasher or washing machine until you have a full load.

- Install sink faucet aerators and water-efficient shower heads, which use two to five times less water with no noticeable decrease in performance.

- Purchase a water-saver toilet, or put a displacement device in your toilet tank to reduce the amount of water used with each flush.

- Fix any leaky faucets in your house. Leaks can waste thousands of gallons of water per year.

- Don't overfertilize your lawn or garden; the extra could end up in the groundwater.

- Don't pour toxic materials such as cleaning solvents, bleach, or motor oil down the drain. Store them until you can take them to a hazardous waste collection center.

PERSONAL INSIGHT   Are you ever tempted to throw toxic substances down the drain or in the trash? If so, what do or can you tell yourself in order to resist?

Waste Disposal

Humans generate large amounts of waste, which must be handled in an appropriate manner if the environment is to be safe and sanitary. Some of this waste is sewage composed of human excrement, some is garbage from food materials, and some is solid waste, a by-product of our "throw-away" society. This last category, consisting of packaging, newspapers, "junk mail," insulated fast-food wrappers, aluminum cans, and other trash, accounts for an ever-growing proportion of solid waste generated in the United States.

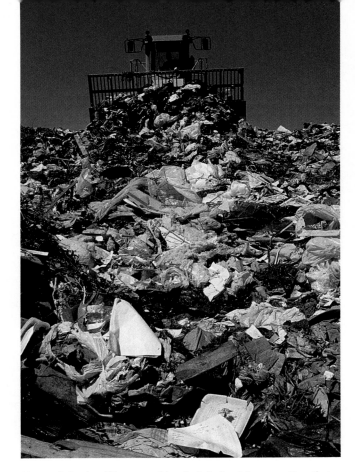

Many existing landfills are reaching their limits at the same time that people are becoming more resistant to the opening of new ones in their communities. The solution to the waste problem lies in less consumption of disposable items and more recycling.

Sewage Prior to the mid-nineteenth century, many people contracted diseases such as typhoid, cholera, and hepatitis A by direct contact with human feces, which were simply disposed of at random. Once the links between sewage and disease were discovered, practices began to change. People learned how to build sanitary outhouses and how to locate them so they would not contaminate water sources. As plumbing moved indoors, sewage disposal became more complicated. In rural areas, the **septic system**, a self-contained sewage disposal system, worked quite well; today, many rural homes still rely on septic systems.

Different approaches became necessary as urban areas developed. Most cities have sewage-treatment systems that separate fecal matter from water in huge tanks and ponds and stabilize it so that it cannot transmit infectious diseases. Once treated and biologically safe, the water is released back into the environment. The sludge that remains behind may be spread on fields as fertilizer if it is free from **heavy metal** contamination, or it may be burned or buried. If incorporated into the food chain, heavy metals, such as lead, cadmium, copper, and tin, can

cause illness or death; therefore, these chemicals must be prevented from being released into the environment when sludge is burned or buried.

In addition to regulating industrial discharge, many cities have now begun expanded sewage-treatment measures to remove heavy metals and other hazardous chemicals. This action has resulted from many studies linking exposure to such chemicals as mercury, lead, and **polychlorinated biphenyls (PCBs)** with long-term health consequences, including cancer and damage to the central nervous system. The technology to effectively remove heavy metals and chemicals from sewage is still developing, and the costs involved are immense.

Solid Waste The bulk of the organic food garbage produced in American kitchens is now dumped in the sewage system by way of the mechanical garbage disposal. The garbage that remains is not very hazardous from the standpoint of infectious disease because there is very little food waste in it, but it does represent an enormous disposal and contamination problem.

WHAT'S IN OUR GARBAGE? The biggest single component of household trash (38.9% by weight) is paper products, including junk mail, glossy mail-order catalogs, and computer printouts. Yard waste is the next biggest source by weight (14.6% before recycling). Plastics make up 9.5% of all trash by weight but take up about 18% of landfill space. Most of this plastic waste is in the form of packaging, which accounts for about one-third of the 6 million tons of plastics produced each year in the United States. Other significant sources of trash include metals (7.6% by weight), wood (7.0%), food (6.7%), and glass (6.3%). About 1% of the solid waste is toxic. Burning, as opposed to burial, reduces the bulk of solid waste, but it may release hazardous material into the air.

Solid waste is not limited to household products. Manufacturing, mining, and other industries all produce large amounts of potentially dangerous materials that cannot simply be dumped. The experiences of communities like Love Canal near Buffalo, New York, and Times Beach, Missouri, clearly demonstrated the dangers of the careless disposal of toxic wastes. At Love Canal, toxic industrial wastes had been dumped into a waterway for years until, in the 1970s, nearby residents began to suffer from associated birth defects and cancers. Human health was

septic system A self-contained sewage disposal system, often used in rural areas, in which waste material is decomposed by bacteria.

heavy metal A metal with a high specific gravity, such as lead, copper, or tin.

polychlorinated biphenyl (PCB) An industrial chemical used as an insulator in electrical transformers and linked to certain human cancers.

TERMS

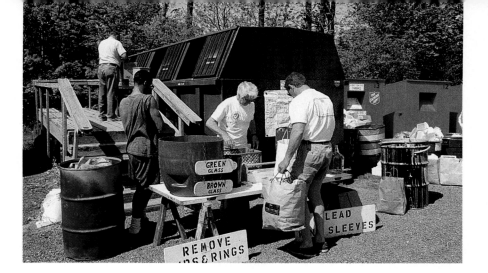

Recycling paper, cans, bottles, and plastics conserves resources, saves energy, and keeps large amounts of solid wastes out of landfills. Some communities have curbside pickup recycling, while others have drop-off sites.

affected, the government had to step in, people had to move from homes, and huge costs were incurred.

DISPOSING OF SOLID WASTE   Since the 1960s, much solid waste has been buried in **sanitary landfill** disposal sites. Careful site selection and daily management are an essential part of this approach to disposal. First, the site is thoroughly studied to ensure that it is not near groundwater, streams, or any other source of water that could be contaminated by leakage from the landfill. Soil composition under and around the site is studied to make sure that materials cannot leach, or seep, from the area. Sometimes protective liners are used around the site, and nearby monitoring wells are now required in most states. Layers of solid waste are regularly covered with thin layers of dirt until the site is filled. Some communities then plant grass and trees and convert the site into a park. Landfill is relatively stable; almost no decomposition occurs in the solidly packed waste.

Burying solid waste in sanitary landfills has several disadvantages. Much of this waste contains chemicals, ranging from leftover pesticides to nail polish remover to paints and oils, which should not be released indiscriminately into the environment. Despite precautions, buried contaminants do leak into the surrounding soil and groundwater. Burial is also expensive and requires huge amounts of space.

Industrial toxic waste poses an even greater disposal problem. In 1980, Congress enacted the Superfund program to clean up inactive hazardous waste sites that are a threat to human health and the environment. Because many such sites are in areas with high population density, 60 million Americans live within 4 miles of a priority Superfund site. By 1998, clean-up was complete at 35% of priority sites, but further action was still needed at 900 priority sites and nearly 10,000 other sites.

Because of the expense and potential chemical hazards of any form of solid waste disposal, many communities today encourage individuals and businesses to recycle their trash. Some cities offer curbside pickup of recyclables; others have recycling centers to which people can bring their waste. These materials are not limited to paper, glass, and cans but also include such things as discarded tires and used oils. Recycling programs have been successful in reducing the proportion of solid waste sent to landfills: in 1980, 81% went to landfills; in 1998, 63%. However, the total amount of garbage Americans generate will probably continue to rise as the population increases, and researchers estimate that 80% of the nation's landfills will be closed within 20 years.

What You Can Do to Reduce Garbage

- Buy products with the least amount of packaging you can, or buy products in bulk (see the box "How to Be a Green Consumer"). For example, buy large jars of juice, not individually packaged juice drinks. Buy products packaged in glass, paper, or metal containers; avoid plastic and aluminum (unless it's recycled). Reuse glass containers to store products bought in bulk or other household items.

- Buy recycled or recyclable products. Avoid disposables; instead, use long-lasting or reusable products such as refillable pens and rechargeable batteries.

- When shopping, take along your own bag. Reuse paper and plastic bags.

- Avoid using foam or paper cups and plastic stirrers by bringing your own china coffee mug and metal spoon to work or wherever you drink coffee or tea.

- To store food, use glass jars and reusable plastic containers rather than foil and plastic wrap.

- Recycle your newspapers, glass, cans, paper, and other recyclables. If your sanitation department doesn't pick up recyclables, take them to a local recycling center. If you receive something packaged with foam pellets, take them to a commercial mailing center that accepts them for recycling.

- Start a compost pile for your organic garbage (nonanimal food and yard waste) if you have a yard.

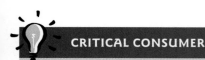
If you live in an apartment, you can create a small composting system using earthworms, or take your organic wastes to a community composting center.

- Stop junk mail. To cancel your junk mail, write a request to: Mail Preference Service, Direct Marketing Association, P.O. Box 9008, Farmingdale, NY 11735.

Food Inspection

Diseases and death associated with foodborne illnesses and toxic food additives have decreased substantially ever since the passage of the Pure Food and Drug Act of 1906. Many agencies inspect food at various points in production. On the federal level, the U.S. Department of Agriculture (USDA) inspects grains and meats, and the U.S. Food and Drug Administration (FDA) is responsible for ensuring the wholesomeness of foods and regulating the chemicals that can be used in foods, drugs, and cosmetics. On the state level, public health departments inspect dairy herds, milking barns, storage tanks, tankers that transport milk, and processing plants. Local health departments inspect and license restaurants.

Overall, the food distribution system in the United States is safe and efficient, but cases of foodborne illness do occur. It is estimated that every American suffers an average of two or three episodes of foodborne illness every year. Recent outbreaks of serious illness have been traced to contaminated and undercooked fast-food hamburgers, unpasteurized juice, and imported berries. In response to these and other outbreaks, new federal rules passed in 1996 require meat and poultry processing plants to begin using microbiological testing in addition to visual inspections to check for the presence of pathogens. Many cases of foodborne illness can be prevented through the proper storage and preparation of food. (For guidelines on avoiding foodborne illness, see Chapter 12.)

Insect and Rodent Control

A great number of illnesses can be transmitted to humans by animal and insect vectors. In recent years, we have seen outbreaks of **encephalitis** transmitted by mosquitoes, **Lyme disease** from ticks in the Northeast, Midwest,

sanitary landfill　A disposal site where solid wastes are buried.　**TERMS**

encephalitis　An inflammation of the brain sometimes caused by insect-borne diseases.

Lyme disease　A disease spread by a deer tick that can lead to fever and arthritis-like conditions if untreated.

VITAL STATISTICS

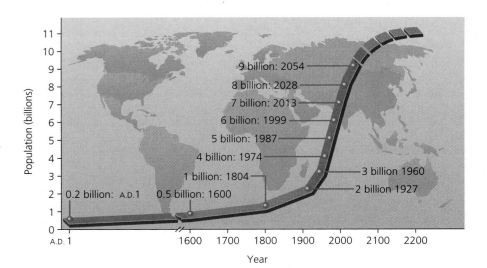

Figure 24-1 World population growth.
The United Nations estimates that the world's population will continue to increase dramatically until it stabilizes at about 11 billion people in 2200.   SOURCE: United Nations Population Division. 1998. *Revision of the World Population Estimates and Projections* (retrieved March 2, 1999; http://www.popin.org/pop1998).

and West, **Rocky Mountain spotted fever** from another type of tick in the Southeast, and **bubonic plague** from fleas on wild mammals in the West. Rodents carry forms of hantavirus, tapeworms, and *Salmonella*.

Disability and death from these diseases can be prevented by spraying insecticides when necessary, wearing protective clothing, and exercising reasonable caution in infested areas. Individuals should be concerned about possible exposure to rodent-borne illnesses if they see rodents or rodent droppings in the home. In public facilities, such sightings should be reported to the local or state health department. Children should be warned to never play with sick animals. Travelers should be careful about mosquito bites, especially in developing countries and where disease warnings have been posted. For tips on avoiding tickborne illnesses, see the discussion of Lyme disease in Chapter 17.

POPULATION GROWTH

Throughout most of history, humans have been a minor pressure on the planet. About 200 million people were alive in the year A.D. 1; by the time Europeans were set-

tling in the United States 1600 years later, the world population had increased gradually to 500 million. But then it began rising exponentially—zooming to 1 billion by about 1830, more than doubling by 1950, then doubling again in just 40 years (Figure 24-1).

The world's population, currently about 6 billion, is increasing at a rate of about 78 million per year—150 people every minute. The United Nations projects that world population will reach nearly 9 billion by 2050 and will continue to increase until it levels off at about 11 billion in 2200. About 97% of this increase takes place in less developed regions; each year, the population of Asia increases by 50 million, that of Africa by 17 million, and that of Latin America by nearly 8 million. In 1950, Europe and North America accounted for 28.5% of the world's population; their share dropped to 17.5% in 2000 and is expected to further decline to 11.5% in 2050. Changes are also projected for the world's age distribution: The proportion of people age 60 and over will increase from 10% in 2000 to about 22% in 2050, and by 2050, there will be more older persons than children.

This rapid expansion of population, particularly in the last 50 years, is generally believed to be responsible for most of the stress humans put on the environment. A large and rapidly growing population makes it more difficult to provide the basic components of environmental health discussed earlier, including clean and disease-free food and water. It is also a driving force behind many of the newer environmental health concerns, including chemical pollution, global warming, and the thinning of the atmosphere's ozone layer.

How Many People Can the World Hold?

No one knows how many people the world can support, but most scientists agree that there is a limit. The primary factors that may eventually put a cap on human population are the following:

TERMS   **Rocky Mountain spotted fever**   A tickborne disease causing high fever; occurs primarily in the southeastern U.S.

bubonic plague   A virulent infectious disease carried by fleas on wild mammals, marked by characteristic discolored swellings; one of the great plagues of the European Middle Ages.

ecosystem   The community of organisms (plants and animals) in an area, and the nonliving physical factors with which they interact.

food chain   The transfers of food energy and other substances in which one type of organism consumes another.

biodiversity   The variety of living things on the earth, including all the different species of flora and fauna and the genetic diversity among individuals of the same species.

Our world supports an abundant variety of life. Scientists have identified some 1.75 million species, but they suspect that there are probably 10–80 million more. Different environments generate diverse life strategies, so that each **ecosystem**—from desert to tropical rainforest—contains a unique, close-knit community of organisms, linked together in a **food chain** or web. Plants use sunlight and soil for their needs. In turn, they sustain herbivores (plant eaters), which may themselves succumb to predators. When predators and surviving herbivores die, they become food for scavengers, then insect larvae, and finally bacteria, which break them down into organic substances. These, drawn from the soil by plants, help maintain the cycle. A similar system, based on plankton, exists in the oceans. Disruption at any point in this intricate, balanced cycle can alter or destroy an entire ecosystem.

Natural ecosystems provide humans with a wide variety of essential services. They maintain the climate and the composition of the atmosphere, cycle water and nutrients, produce food, dispose of organic wastes, generate and maintain soils, control pests, and pollinate crops; in addition, ecosystems support biological diversity, or **biodiversity,** represented by both the millions of different species on the earth and the genetic diversity within these species. (A 1997 study estimated the value of these essential services at $16–54 trillion per year.)

Biodiversity is critical, as the basis for the future evolution of new species and as a genetic bank from which humans can draw useful genetic material and compounds. Although thus far we have examined few of these resources, the ones we have used provide many benefits, including medicines and pest and disease resistance for crops. For example, many children with leukemia can now be saved by drugs developed from the rosy periwinkle plant, and species of wild rice in India and wild tomato in Peru have provided domestic species with the disease resistance they need to be productive.

Human activity—driven by poverty and population growth in the developing world and excessive consumerism in the industrial nations—threatens biodiversity. Some species and populations are being lost through direct action, such as the overharvesting of whales, elephants, and certain fish. But the major danger comes indirectly, from habitat destruction: We are paving over, chopping down, digging up, draining, and poisoning many areas. The destruction of tropical rainforests, which are disappearing at the rate of an acre every second, is of particular concern. Rainforests cover only about 7% of the planet but are thought to harbor more than half the world's species. Extinction is irreversible, and species are disappearing far faster (50–100 a day) than they can be identified and assessed for useful properties.

Some scientists fear that humans are precipitating a wave of mass extinction so great that the diminished stock of species will not be an adequate base on which natural selection can work to rebuild biodiversity. Even if adequate, it could take several million years for biodiversity to "bounce back." And because of the many ties between organisms and the physical environment, mass extinction could also threaten the functioning of the entire biological world.

What can be done to maintain biodiversity? The United States has laws that protect specific endangered species, which by indirectly preserving natural communities help maintain biodiversity. International laws and conventions also protect certain rare species, although enforcement continues to be a problem. The Convention on Biological Diversity, signed by more than 170 countries (but *not* the United States) since the 1992 Earth Summit in Rio de Janeiro, deals specifically with the issue of biodiversity. It commits countries to preserving and managing biological resources and to integrating plant and animal preservation into economic planning. It also allows countries that are rich in species but poor in cash to share in the profits from the sale of medicines or other products derived from their biological resources. Although much still needs to be done to protect the biodiversity of our world, these actions are a step in the right direction.

• *Food.* Enough food is currently produced to feed the world's entire population, but economic and sociopolitical factors have led to food shortages and famine. Food production can be expanded in the future, but better distribution of food will be needed to prevent even more widespread famine, as the world's population continues to grow. For all people to receive adequate nutrition, the makeup of the world's diet may also need to change. Because animal products require more resources to produce, the world could support nearly twice as many vegetarians as people eating a typical American diet, which is based heavily on animal products.

• *Available land and water.* Rural populations rely on trees, soil, and water for their direct sustenance, and a growing population puts a strain on these resources—forests are cut for wood, soil is depleted, and water is withdrawn at ever-rising rates. These trends contribute to local hardships and to many global environmental problems, including habitat destruction and species extinction (see the box "Natural Ecosystems and Biodiversity").

• *Energy.* Currently, most of the world's energy comes from nonrenewable sources: oil, coal, natural gas, and nuclear power. As nonrenewable sources are depleted, the world will have to shift to renewable energy sources, such as hydropower, solar, geothermal, wind, biomass, and ocean power. Supporting a growing population, maintaining economic productivity, and preventing further environmental degradation will require greater energy efficiency and an increased use of renewable energy sources.

• *Minimum acceptable standard of living.* The mass media have exposed the entire world to the American lifestyle and raised people's expectations of living at a comparable level. But such a lifestyle is supported by

.vels of energy consumption that the earth cannot support worldwide. The United States has 5% of the world's population but uses 25% of the world's energy. By contrast, India has 16% of the population but uses only 3% of the energy. An average American consumes 280 times the amount of energy that the average Ethiopian does. If *all* people are to enjoy a minimally acceptable standard of living, the population must be limited to a number that the available resources can support.

Factors That Contribute to Population Growth

Although it is apparent that population growth must be controlled, population trends are difficult to influence and manage. A variety of interconnecting factors fuel the current population explosion:

- *High fertility rates.* The combination of poverty, very high child mortality rates, and a lack of social provisions of every type is associated with high fertility rates in the developing world. Perhaps families have to have more children to ensure that enough survive childhood to work for the household and to care for parents in old age.
- *Lack of family planning resources.* Half the world's couples don't use any form of family planning, and 300 million couples worldwide say they want family planning services but cannot get them.
- *Lower death rates.* Although death rates remain relatively high in the developing world, they have decreased in recent years because of public health measures and improved medical care.

Changes in any of these factors can affect population growth, but the issues are complex. Increasing death rates through disease, famine, or war might slow population growth, but few people would argue in favor of these as methods of population control. Although the increased availability of family planning services is a crucial part of population management, cultural, political, and religious factors also need to be considered. (For more information on contraceptive use around the world, see the box in Chapter 6.)

To be successful, population management must change the condition of people's lives to remove the pressures for having large families, especially poverty. Research indicates that the combination of improved health, better education, and increased literacy and em-

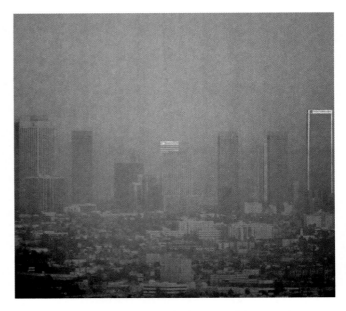

Smog tends to form over Los Angeles because of the natural geographical features of the area and because of the tremendous amount of motor vehicle exhaust in the air. The health effects of smog are most noticeable in people who already have some respiratory impairment.

ployment opportunities for women works together with family planning to decrease fertility rates. Unfortunately, in the fastest-growing countries, the needs of a rapidly increasing population use up financial resources that might otherwise be used to improve lives and ultimately slow population growth.

POLLUTION

As mentioned earlier, the classic environmental health concerns are not just historical. They still have the potential to cause serious problems today under certain circumstances, and they take on added significance as our population grows. At the same time, new problems are arising, and some long-standing problems are gaining increased public attention. Many of these modern problems are problems of pollution. The term *pollution* refers to any unwanted contaminant in the environment that may pose a health risk. When we are talking about health risks, the level of concentration of a particular pollutant is very important. In typical concentrations, many environmental pollutants do not seem to harm our general health in the short term. The long-term effects are harder to evaluate.

Air Pollution

Air pollution is not a human invention or even a new problem. The air is "polluted" naturally with every forest fire, pollen bloom, and dust storm, as well as with count-

---

TERMS **fossil fuels** Buried deposits of decayed animals and plants that are converted into carbon-rich fuels by exposure to heat and pressure over millions of years; oil, coal, and natural gas are fossil fuels.

temperature inversion A weather condition in which a cold layer of air is trapped by a warm layer so that pollutants cannot be dispersed.

London-type smog A form of smog caused by coal burning.

TABLE 24-1

TABLE 24-1 *Sources and Effects of Common Air Pollutants*

Pollutant	Sources	Effects
Sulfur dioxide (SO_2)	Burning of coal and fossil fuels	Irritates the respiratory tract; aggravates the symptoms of heart and lung diseases; damages plants; produces acid precipitation.
Carbon monoxide (CO)	Combustion, especially fossil fuel combustion by motor vehicles	Deprives body of oxygen, causing headaches, fatigue, and impaired judgment; aggravates heart and vascular diseases.
Nitrogen dioxide (NO_2)	Motor vehicles, power stations, industrial boilers, manufacture of fertilizers and other chemicals	Irritates the respiratory tract; causes bronchitis, pneumonia, and lowered resistance to respiratory infections; produces acid precipitation.
Particulates	Fossil fuel combustion	Carry heavy metals and carcinogens into the lungs; corrode metal; lessen visibility.
Hydrocarbons (volatile organic compounds)	Incomplete fossil fuel combustion, evaporation of solvents and oil, natural sources	React with sunlight and other pollutants to form respiratory irritants and potential carcinogens.
Ozone	Photochemical reactions (interaction of nitrogen oxides and hydrocarbons in the presence of sunlight)	Irritates mucous membranes; inflames eyes and respiratory tract; aggravates heart and lung diseases; damages plants and slows their growth.

less other natural pollutants. To these natural sources, humans have always contributed the by-products of their activities. During the Industrial Revolution, English cities had far more daily air pollution than we can observe or even imagine today. However, we now live long enough to experience both the short-term and the long-term consequences of air pollution. Also, increased population growth, combined with more industrialization using old technologies, concentrates the problems and makes them more visible to the public—and possibly more dangerous.

Temperature Inversions and Smog   Air pollution can cause illness and death if pollutants become concentrated for a period of several days or weeks. Increased amounts of carbon monoxide and airborne acids and decreased amounts of oxygen all put excess strain on people suffering from asthma, congestive heart failure, and chronic obstructive pulmonary diseases, such as chronic bronchitis and emphysema. Air pollution especially affects very young children and older adults.

For an air pollution emergency to occur, three conditions must be present. First, there must be a source of pollution. Today, this is most frequently the burning of **fossil fuels,** such as coal in industry or gasoline in cars (Table 24-1). Second, there must be a topographical feature, such as a mountain range or a valley, that prevents the prevailing winds from pushing stagnant air out of the region. Third, there must be a weather event called a temperature inversion.

A **temperature inversion** occurs when there is little or no wind and a layer of warm air traps a layer of cold air next to the ground. Normally, the sun heats the earth, making the air closest to the ground warmer than that just above it. Warm air rises and is replaced by cooler air, which in turn is warmed and rises, thereby producing a natural circulation. This circulation, combined with horizontal wind circulation, prevents pollutants from reaching dangerous levels of concentration.

When there is a temperature inversion, this replacement and cleansing action cannot occur. The effect is like covering an area with a dome that traps all the pollutants and prevents vertical dispersion. If this condition persists for several days, the buildup of pollutants may reach dangerous levels and threaten people's health. Many cities have plans for shutting down certain industries and even curtailing transportation if unsafe levels are approached. State and federal governments have "clean air" legislation that has helped improve U.S. air quality in the past 20 years. However, it is estimated that 100 million people in North America and Europe are still exposed to unsafe air.

The buildup of pollutants that occurs during a temperature inversion may be visible as smog. There are two types of smog: London-type smog and Los Angeles-type smog, distinguished primarily by the source of the pollution. **London-type smog** results from the burning of fossil fuels such as coal. At one time, coal was the major source of heat for homes as well as the major energy source for factories. Now that many homes and factories se oil, steam, gas, and electricity, this source of pollution has been minimized in developed countries. However, coal burning is increasing in developing countries.

Los Angeles-type smog, also known as photochemical smog, is a more complex phenomenon. Here the source of pollution is primarily motor vehicle exhaust that contains oxides of nitrogen and hydrocarbons. When sunlight acts on these products (a photochemical reaction), the result is a characteristic brown smog. Large cities with a high ratio of cars to people and with poorly developed public transportation are more likely to experience Los Angeles-type smog. The health effects are very similar to those resulting from London-type smog: eye irritation, impairment of respiratory and cardiovascular functioning in vulnerable individuals, and possibly cancers.

The Greenhouse Effect and Global Warming The temperature of the earth's atmosphere depends on the balance between the amount of energy the planet absorbs from the sun (mainly as high-energy ultraviolet radiation) and the amount of energy radiated back into space as lower-energy infrared radiation. Key components of temperature regulation are carbon dioxide, water vapor, methane, and other "greenhouse gases"—so named because, like a pane of glass in a greenhouse, they let through visible light from the sun but trap some of the resulting infrared radiation and reradiate it back to the earth's surface. This reradiation causes a buildup of heat that raises the temperature of the lower atmosphere, a natural process known as the **greenhouse effect.** Without it, the atmosphere would be far cooler and much more hostile to life.

Human activity may be tipping this balance toward **global warming** (Figure 24-2). The concentration of greenhouse gases is increasing because of human activity, especially the combustion of fossil fuels. Carbon dioxide levels in the atmosphere have increased rapidly since the onset of the Industrial Revolution, and current levels are higher than at any time in the past 160,000 years. Deforestation, often by burning, also sends carbon dioxide into the atmosphere and reduces the number of trees available to convert carbon dioxide into oxygen. But energy use in

TABLE 24-2	*Sources of Greenhouse Gases*
Greenhouse gas	**Sources**
Carbon dioxide	Fossil fuel and wood burning, factory emissions, car exhaust, deforestation
Chlorofluorocarbons (CFCs)	Refrigeration and air conditioning, aerosols, foam products, solvents
Methane	Cattle, wetlands, rice paddies, landfills, gas leaks, coal and gas industries
Nitrous oxide	Fertilizers, soil cultivation, deforestation, animal feedlots and wastes
Ozone and other trace gases	Photochemical reactions, car exhaust, power plant emissions, solvents

the developed world is the primary cause of increases in the concentrations of greenhouse gases (Table 24-2). The United States alone is responsible for over 20% of the world's total emission of greenhouse gases.

Experts predict that the increase in greenhouse gases will cause global temperatures to rise by about 1.8–6.3°F (1.0–3.5°C) by 2100, with a corresponding rise in sea level of 6 to 37 inches (15 to 95 cm). Although the full implications of climate change are unknown, possible consequences include the following:

- Increased rainfall and flooding in some regions, increased drought in others. Coastal zones, where half the world's people live, would be severely affected.

- Increased mortality from heat stress, urban air pollution, and tropical diseases (due to the spread of disease-carrying organisms like mosquitoes).

- A poleward shift of about 50–350 miles (150–550 km) in the location of vegetation zones, affecting crop yields, irrigation demands, and forest productivity.

Since record-keeping began in the mid-1800s, 15 of the hottest years have occurred since 1979; 1998 was the hottest year to date. Data from tree rings and other sources suggest that recent temperatures are the warmest in 1000 years. What can be done? The Kyoto Protocol to the UN Convention on Climate Change calls for industrialized countries to cut greenhouse gas emissions to about 5.2% below 1990 levels by 2008–2012; U.S. emissions, however, have actually increased by 10% since 1990.

Thinning of the Ozone Layer A second air pollution problem is the thinning of the **ozone layer** of the atmosphere, a fragile, invisible layer about 10–30 miles above

TERMS

Los Angeles-type smog A characteristic brown smog caused by sunlight reacting with chemicals produced by the burning of transportation fuels; also called *photochemical smog.*

greenhouse effect A warming of the earth due to a buildup of carbon dioxide and certain other gases.

global warming An increase in the earth's atmospheric temperature when averaged across seasons and geographical regions.

ozone layer A layer of ozone molecules (O_3) in the upper atmosphere that screens out UV rays from the sun.

chlorofluorocarbons (CFCs) Chemicals used as spray-can propellants, refrigerants, and industrial solvents, implicated in the destruction of the ozone layer.

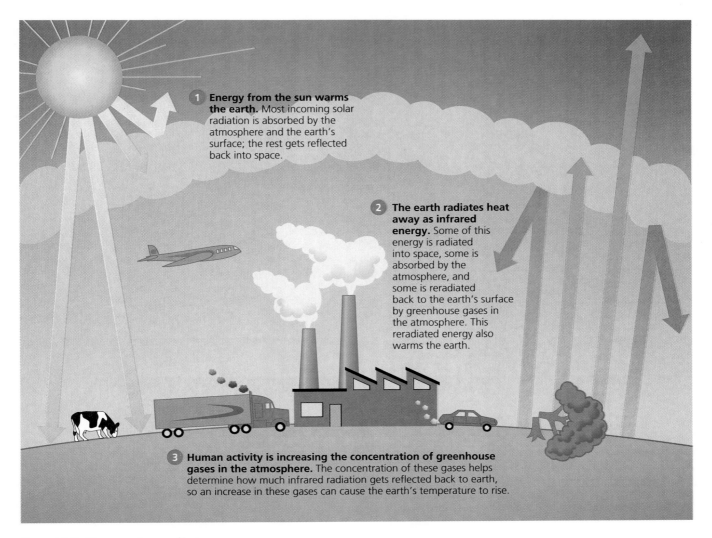

Figure 24-2   The greenhouse effect.

Inside the figure:

1 Energy from the sun warms the earth. Most incoming solar radiation is absorbed by the atmosphere and the earth's surface; the rest gets reflected back into space.

2 The earth radiates heat away as infrared energy. Some of this energy is radiated into space, some is absorbed by the atmosphere, and some is reradiated back to the earth's surface by greenhouse gases in the atmosphere. This reradiated energy also warms the earth.

3 Human activity is increasing the concentration of greenhouse gases in the atmosphere. The concentration of these gases helps determine how much infrared radiation gets reflected back to earth, so an increase in these gases can cause the earth's temperature to rise.

the earth's surface, shielding the planet from the sun's hazardous ultraviolet (UV) rays. Since the mid-1980s, scientists have observed the seasonal appearance and growth of a "hole" in the ozone layer over Antarctica. More recently, thinning over other areas—including Canada, Scandinavia, the northern United States, Russia, Australia, and New Zealand—has been noted.

The ozone layer is being destroyed primarily by **chlorofluorocarbons (CFCs),** industrial chemicals used as coolants in refrigerators and in home and automobile air conditioners; as foaming agents in some rigid foam products, including insulation; as propellants in some kinds of aerosol sprays (most such sprays were banned in 1978); and as solvents. When CFCs rise into the atmosphere, winds carry them toward the polar regions. During winter, circular winds form a vortex that keeps the air over Antarctica from mixing with air from elsewhere. Ice crystals form in the Antarctic clouds during the cold, sunless months; chemical reactions taking place on these crystals, which wouldn't take place in air, free chlorine atoms from

CFCs. When stimulated by the reappearance of the sun, the chlorine atoms begin destroying ozone (Figure 24-3). When the polar vortex weakens in the summer, winds richer in ozone from the north replenish the lost Antarctic ozone, but the ozone hole's growth each year may be contributing to the general thinning of the global ozone layer.

Since 1979, about 15% of Antarctic ozone has been destroyed, although locally and seasonally up to 95% of the ozone disappears (forming the "hole"). The hole above Antarctica in late 1998 was larger and persisted longer than any previous ozone hole. In the Northern Hemisphere, ozone levels have declined about 10% since 1980, and certain areas may be temporarily depleted in late winter and early spring by as much as 40%.

The loss of ozone is of concern because without the ozone layer to absorb the sun's UV radiation, life on earth would be impossible. The potential effects of increased long-term exposure to UV light for humans include skin cancer, wrinkling and aging of the skin, cataracts and blindness, and reduced immune response. The United

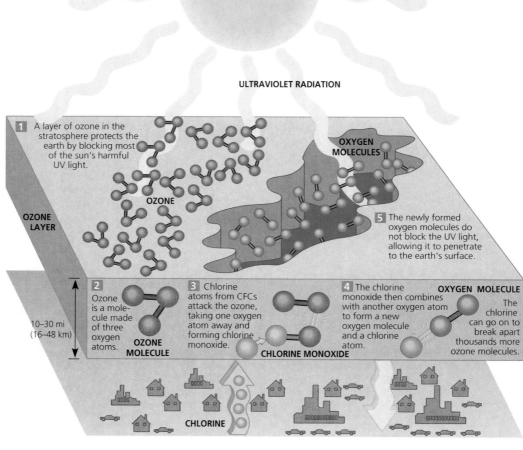

ULTRAVIOLET RADIATION

1 A layer of ozone in the stratosphere protects the earth by blocking most of the sun's harmful UV light.

OZONE LAYER

OZONE

OXYGEN MOLECULES

5 The newly formed oxygen molecules do not block the UV light, allowing it to penetrate to the earth's surface.

10–30 mi (16–48 km)

2 Ozone is a molecule made of three oxygen atoms.

OZONE MOLECULE

3 Chlorine atoms from CFCs attack the ozone, taking one oxygen atom away and forming chlorine monoxide.

CHLORINE MONOXIDE

4 The chlorine monoxide then combines with another oxygen atom to form a new oxygen molecule and a chlorine atom.

OXYGEN MOLECULE

The chlorine can go on to break apart thousands more ozone molecules.

CHLORINE

Figure 24-3   Destruction of the ozone layer of the atmosphere.   SOURCE: *Time,* 17 February 1992, p. 63. Copyright © 1992 Time, Inc. Reprinted by permission.

Nations Environmental Program predicts that a drop of 10% in overall ozone levels would cause a 26% rise in the incidence of nonmelanoma skin cancer. Some scientists blame ozone loss over Australia for a recent rise in melanoma cases there.

UV light may interfere with photosynthesis and cause lower crop yields; it may also kill phytoplankton and krill, the basis of the ocean food chain. And because heat generated by the absorption of UV rays in the ozone layer helps create stratospheric winds, the driving force behind weather patterns, a drop in the concentration of ozone could potentially alter the earth's climate systems.

Worldwide production and use of CFCs has declined rapidly since the danger to the ozone layer was recognized. Industrialized nations agreed to eliminate CFC production and use by 2000, and limits have also been placed on other agents that destroy ozone. By the late

1990s, metered-dose inhalers for conditions like asthma were the only significant commercial product to contain CFCs; and CFC-free inhalers are already available for some medications. In addition, use of some ozone depleting agents, including halon-1211, is still increasing. Future ozone losses are inevitable, however, because CFCs persist in the atmosphere for 50–150 years.

Acid Precipitation   A by-product of many industrial processes, **acid precipitation** occurs when atmospheric pollutants combine with moisture in the air and fall to earth as highly acidic rain, snow, sleet, or hail. It occurs especially when coal containing large amounts of sulfur is burned and sulfur dioxide, sulfur trioxide, nitrogen dioxide, nitric acid, and other chemicals are released into the atmosphere. These concentrations can be carried great distances by the prevailing winds and form a highly acidic mixture containing sulfuric acid and nitric acid. Most of the pollutants in acid precipitation are produced by coal-burning electric power plants. Other sources are motor vehicles and certain industrial activities, such as smelting.

Acidification of lakes and streams due to acid precipitation has completely eradicated fish and other aquatic species in some areas. Trees are also affected because acid precipitation damages leaves, strips the soil of key nutrients, and releases toxic substances such as heavy metals from the soil; in some areas of central Europe, entire forests are dying. The air pollutants that cause acid precipitation reduce visibility and cause respiratory problems in some people. Acid precipitation also corrodes metals and damages stone and paint on buildings, monuments, and cars; repairs can cost billions of dollars. Acid precipitation appears to be causing the most damage in Canada, the northeastern United States, Scandinavia, and parts of central Europe. In the United States, the areas most affected are the Adirondacks, the mid-Appalachian highlands, the upper Midwest, and high elevations in the West.

Energy Use and Air Pollution

Americans are the biggest energy consumers in the world. We use energy to create electricity, transport us, power our industries, and run our homes. About 75% of the energy we use comes from fossil fuels—oil, coal, and natural gas; the remainder comes from nuclear power and renewable energy sources (such as hydroelectric, wind, and solar power).

Energy consumption is at the root of many environmental problems, especially those relating to air pollution. Automobile exhaust and the burning of oil and coal by industry and by electricity-generating plants are primary causes of smog, acid precipitation, and the greenhouse effect. The mining of coal and the extraction and transportation of oil cause pollution on land and in the water; coal miners often suffer from serious health problems related to their jobs. Nuclear power generation creates hazardous wastes and carries the risk of dangerous releases of radiation.

Two key strategies for controlling energy use are conservation and the development of nonpolluting, renewable sources of energy. Although the use of renewable energy sources has increased in recent years, renewables still supply only a small proportion of our energy, in part because of their cost. Some countries have chosen to promote energy efficiency by removing subsidies or adding taxes on the use of fossil fuels. This strategy is reflected in the varying prices drivers pay for gasoline. According to a 1999 report from the U.S. Energy Information Agency, the average per gallon price of premium gas is about $1.10 in the United States, $1.90 in Canada, $2.50 in Taiwan, and $3.50 in France and Britain. It is not surprising that per-capita energy use in the United States is twice that of many European countries. The International Center for Technology Assessment estimates that the actual price of gasoline—including tax breaks, government subsidies, and environmental, health, and social costs of gas usage—is as high as $15.14 per gallon.

Actions that individuals can take to promote energy efficiency and cut their use of energy are listed in the section "What You Can Do to Prevent Air Pollution."

Indoor Air Pollution

Although most people associate air pollution with the outdoors, your home may also harbor potentially dangerous pollutants. Some of these compounds trigger allergic responses, and others have been linked to cancer. Common indoor pollutants include the following:

- *Environmental tobacco smoke (ETS),* a human carcinogen that also increases the risk for asthma, bronchitis, and cardiovascular disease (see Chapter 11).

- *Carbon monoxide and other combustion by-products,* which can cause chronic bronchitis, headaches, dizziness, nausea, fatigue, and even death. Common sources in the home are wood stoves, fireplaces, kerosene heaters and lamps, and gas ranges.

- *Formaldehyde gas,* which can cause eye, nose, and throat irritation; shortness of breath; headaches; nausea; lethargy; and, over the long term, cancer. This gas can seep from resins used in particle board, plywood paneling, and some carpeting and upholstery; it is also emitted by certain paints and floor finishes, permanent press clothing, and nail polish.

- *Biological pollutants,* including bacteria, dust mites, mold, and animal dander, which can cause allergic reactions and other health problems. These allergens need nutrients and moisture to survive and are typically found in bathrooms, damp or flooded basements, humidifiers, air conditioners, and even some carpets and furniture.

Asbestos and radon, two other dangerous indoor pollutants, are discussed later in the chapter.

What You Can Do to Prevent Air Pollution

- Cut back on driving. Ride your bike, walk, use public transportation, or carpool in a fuel-efficient vehicle.

- Keep your car tuned up and well-maintained. Use only unleaded gas, and keep your tires inflated at recommended pressures. To save energy when driving, avoid quick starts, stay within the speed limit, don't use air conditioning when opening a

---

acid precipitation   Rain, snow, sleet, or hail with a low pH (acid), caused by atmospheric moisture combining with products of industrial combustion to form acids such as sulfur dioxide; harmful to forests and lakes, which cannot tolerate changes in acidity/alkalinity.   **TERMS**

dow would suffice, and don't let your car idle unless absolutely necessary. Have your car's air conditioner checked and serviced by a station that recycles CFCs; consider having your car's air conditioner retrofitted with a safer refrigerant.

- Buy energy-efficient appliances, and use them only when necessary. Run the washing machine, dryer, and dishwasher only when you have full loads, and do laundry in warm or cold water instead of hot; don't overdry your clothes. Clean refrigerator coils and clothes dryer lint screens frequently. Towel or air-dry your hair rather than using an electric dryer.

- Replace incandescent bulbs with compact fluorescent bulbs (not fluorescent tubes). Although they cost more initially, they'll save you money over the life of the bulb. They produce a comparable light, last longer, and use only 25–35% of the energy of a regular bulb, thereby lowering carbon dioxide emissions from electric power plants.

- Make sure your home is well-insulated with ozone-safe agents; use insulating shades and curtains to keep heat in during winter and out during summer. Seal any openings that produce drafts. In cold weather, put on a sweater and turn down the thermostat. In hot weather, wear lightweight clothing and, whenever possible, use a fan instead of an air conditioner to cool yourself.

- Plant and care for trees in your own yard and neighborhood. Because they recycle carbon dioxide, trees work against global warming. They also provide shade and cool the air, so less air conditioning is needed.

- Before discarding a refrigerator, air conditioner, or humidifier, check with the waste hauler or your local government to ensure that ozone-depleting refrigerants will be removed prior to disposal. If you use a metered-dose inhaler, ask your physician if an ozone-safe inhaler is available for your medication.

- To prevent indoor air pollution, keep your house adequately ventilated, and buy some houseplants; they have a natural ability to rid the air of harmful pollutants.

- Keep paints, cleaning agents, and other chemical products in their original, tightly sealed containers.

- Don't smoke, and don't allow others to smoke in your room, apartment, or home. If these rules are too strict for your situation, limit smoking to a single, well-ventilated room.

- Clean and inspect chimneys, furnaces, and other appliances regularly. Install carbon monoxide detectors.

PERSONAL INSIGHT If you found out you could get a smog certificate without having to get your car fixed, what would you do? Would the convenience be worth the pollution?

Chemical Pollution

Chemical pollution is by no means a new problem. The ancient Romans were plagued by lead poisoning, which damages the central nervous system, in part because they stored sugar solutions in lead containers. Over 200 years ago in Europe, the phrase "mad as a hatter" came from the hatters' practice of preparing felt hats with mercury, which also destroyed the central nervous system.

The difference today is that new chemical substances are constantly being created and introduced into the environment—as pesticides, herbicides, solvents, cleaning fluids, flame retardants, and hundreds of other products. We have many more chemicals, in more concentrated forms and in wider use, and larger numbers of people are exposed and potentially exposed to them than ever before.

Chemical pollutants have been responsible for several environmental disasters. The Hudson River in New York and the Housatonic River in Massachusetts have both been contaminated with PCBs, carcinogenic compounds used in the manufacture of electrical appliances. In 1984, thousands of people in Bhopal, India, were killed or injured when a powerful chemical used in manufacturing the insecticide Sevin was released from a plant. Catastrophes illustrate the short-term potential for disaster, but the long-term health consequences may be just as deadly. The following are brief descriptions of just a few current problems.

Asbestos A mineral-based compound, asbestos was widely used for fire protection and insulation in buildings until the late 1960s. When first introduced, asbestos was hailed as a great advance in fire safety. As long as it stayed where it was applied and its protective coating was not disturbed, there was no problem. However, microscopic asbestos fibers can be released into the air when this material is applied or when it later deteriorates or is damaged. These fibers can lodge in the lungs, causing **asbestosis,** lung cancer, and other serious lung diseases. Similar conditions are risks in the coal mining industry, from exposure to coal dust (black lung disease), and in

TERMS **asbestosis** A lung condition caused by inhalation of microscopic asbestos fibers, which inflame the lung and can lead to lung cancer.

pesticides Chemicals used to prevent the spread of diseases transmitted by insects and to maximize food production by killing insects that eat crops.

Residents of poor and minority communities are often exposed to more environmental toxins than residents of wealthier communities, and they are more likely to suffer from health problems caused or aggravated by pollutants. Poor neighborhoods are often located near highways and industrial areas that have high levels of air pollution; they are also common sites for hazardous waste production and disposal. Residents of substandard housing are more likely to come into contact with lead, asbestos, carbon monoxide, and other hazardous pollutants associated with peeling paint, old plumbing, and poorly maintained insulation and heating equipment. And poor people are more likely to have jobs that expose them to asbestos, silica dust, and pesticides.

The most thoroughly researched and documented link among poverty, the environment, and health is lead poisoning in children. Many studies have shown that children of low-income black families are much more likely to have elevated levels of lead in their blood than white children. One survey found that two-thirds of urban African American children from families earning less than $6000 a year had elevated lead levels.

The CDC and the American Academy of Pediatrics recommend annual testing of blood lead levels for all children under age 6, with more frequent testing for children at special risk.

Asthma is another health threat that appears to be linked with both environmental and socioeconomic factors. The number of Americans with asthma grew by more than 6 million between 1985 and 1995, an increase of nearly 75%. Most of the increase occurred in children, with African Americans and the poor hardest hit. Researchers are not sure what accounts for this increase, but suspects include household pollutants, pesticides, air pollution, cigarette smoke, and allergens like cockroaches. These risk factors are likely to cluster in poor urban areas where inadequate health care may worsen asthma's effects.

A new push for research on the health effects of exposure to toxins on low-income communities is being called for by the environmental justice movement. New studies are investigating the links between environmental factors and respiratory problems, skin diseases, and cancer. While health researchers seek to quantify the health impacts, neighborhood activists continue to fight against the "dumping" of pollution in poor communities.

---

the textile industry, from exposure to cotton fibers (brown lung disease).

Asbestos can pose a danger in homes and apartment buildings, about 25% of which are thought to contain some asbestos. Areas where it is most likely to be found are insulation around water and steam pipes, ducts, and furnaces; boiler wraps; vinyl flooring; floor, wall, and ceiling insulation; roofing and siding; and fireproof board. An experienced contractor can pinpoint asbestos-containing materials in a home, which can then be analyzed by a laboratory. If any of these materials begin to release asbestos fibers, the asbestos must be sealed off, encapsulated, or removed by a professional.

Lead Lead poisoning continues to be a serious problem, particularly among children living in older buildings and adults who are exposed to lead in the workplace. When lead is ingested or inhaled, it can damage the central nervous system, cause mental impairment, hinder oxygen transport in the blood, and create digestive problems. Severe lead poisoning may cause coma or even death. Some symptoms of lead poisoning, including anemia, headaches, and abdominal pain, may cease if exposure stops, but neurological damage can be permanent. Lead damage to the brain can start even before birth if a pregnant woman has elevated levels of lead in her body.

The CDC estimates that 890,000 children under age 6 may have unsafe lead levels in their blood. Many of these children live in poor, inner-city areas (see the box "Poverty and Environmental Health"). Long-term expo-

sure to low levels of lead may cause kidney disease; it can also cause lead to build up in bones, where it may be released into the bloodstream during pregnancy or when bone mass is lost from osteoporosis. Little is known about the effect of lead stored in or freed from bone.

Young children can easily ingest lead from their environment by picking up dust and dirt on their hands and then putting their fingers in their mouth. Lead-based paints are believed to be the chief culprit in lead poisoning of children. They were banned from residential use in 1978, but as many as 57 million American homes still contain lead paint. The use of lead in plumbing is now also banned, but some old pipes and faucets contain lead that can leach into drinking water. Recently it was discovered that some imported window blinds have high lead levels.

Lead gets into the air from industrial and vehicle emissions, from tobacco smoke and paint dust, and from the burning of solid wastes that contain lead. Levels of lead in the air have dropped sharply as leaded gas use has declined, but many vehicles still use leaded fuel. Lead occurs naturally in soil, which also collects lead from the air and other sources. Other sources of lead are foods stored or served in lead-glazed pottery or lead crystal and processed foods sold in lead-soldered cans.

Pesticides Pesticides are used primarily for two purposes: to prevent the spread of insect-borne diseases and to maximize food production by killing insects that eat crops. Both uses have risks as well as benefits. Take, for example, the pesticide DDT. Recognized as a powerful

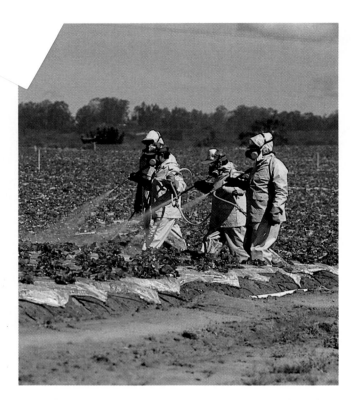

Although some pesticide residues may remain in or on produce when it reaches the consumer, the most serious health effects of pesticides are seen in agricultural workers. Special clothing and equipment help protect these workers from toxic chemicals as they spray strawberries.

pesticide in 1939, DDT was extremely important in efforts to control widespread insect-borne diseases in tropical countries and increase crop yields throughout the world. But in 1962, biologist Rachel Carson questioned the safety of DDT in her book *Silent Spring,* pointing out that the pesticide disrupts the life cycles of birds, fish, and reptiles. DDT also builds up in the food chain, increasing in concentration as larger animals eat smaller ones, a process known as **biomagnification.** Despite its effectiveness as a pesticide, DDT was banned in the United States in 1972 because the costs associated with its use—to wildlife and potentially to humans—were too high. Most pesticide hazards to date have been a result of overuse, but there are concerns about the health effects of long-term exposure to small amounts of pesticide residues in foods, especially for children.

The list of real and potential chemical pollution problems may well be as long as the list of known chemicals. To the preceding list we can add recent concern about mercury in fish, formaldehyde in synthetic building materials, and other by-products of our industrial age. As mentioned earlier, hazardous wastes are also found in the home and should be handled and disposed of properly. They include automotive supplies (motor oil, antifreeze,

transmission fluid), paint supplies (turpentine, paint thinner, mineral spirits), art and hobby supplies (oil-based paint, solvents, acids and alkalis, aerosol sprays), insecticides, batteries, and household cleaners containing sodium hydroxide (lye) or ammonia. These chemicals are dangerous when inhaled or ingested, when they contact the skin or the eyes, or when they are burned or dumped. Many cities provide guidelines about approved disposal methods and have hazardous waste collection days. Look in the government pages of your phone book under Environmental Health or Hazardous Waste.

What You Can Do to Prevent Chemical Pollution

- When buying products, read the labels, and try to buy the least toxic ones available. Choose nontoxic nonpetrochemical cleansers, disinfectants, polishes, and other personal and household products.

- Dispose of your household hazardous wastes properly. If you are not sure whether something is hazardous or don't know how to dispose of it, contact your local environmental health office or health department. Don't burn trash.

- Buy organic produce or produce that has been grown locally. Wash, scrub, and, if appropriate, peel fruits and vegetables. Consider eating less meat; animal products require more pesticides, fertilizer, water, and energy to produce.

- If you must use pesticides or toxic household products, store them in a locked place where children and pets can't get to them. Don't measure chemicals with food-preparation utensils, and wear gloves whenever handling them.

- If you have your house fumigated for pest control, be sure to hire a licensed exterminator. Keep everyone, including pets, out of the house while they work, and if possible for a few days after.

Radiation

Many people are afraid of **radiation,** in part because they don't understand what it is. Basically, radiation is energy. It can come in different forms, such as ultraviolet rays, microwaves, or X rays, and from different sources, such as the sun, uranium, and nuclear weapons. Although radiation cannot be seen, heard, smelled, tasted, or felt, its health effects at high doses can include **radiation sickness** and death and at lower doses, chromosome damage, sterility, tissue damage, cataracts, and cancer. Current health concerns about radiation focus on nuclear weapons and nuclear energy, the medical uses of radiation, and the sources of radiation in the home and workplace.

Nuclear Weapons and Nuclear Energy   Nuclear weapons pose a health risk of the most serious kind to all species. Public health associations have stated that in the event of an intentional or accidental discharge of these weapons, the casualties would run into the hundreds of thousands or millions. Reducing these stockpiles is a challenge and a goal for the twenty-first century.

Power-generating plants that use nuclear fuel also pose health problems. When **nuclear power** was first developed as an alternative to oil and coal, it was promoted as clean, efficient, inexpensive, and safe. In general, this has proven to be the case. Power systems in several parts of the world rely on nuclear-generating plants. However, despite all the built-in safeguards and regulating agencies, accidents in nuclear power plants do happen, and the consequences of such accidents are far more serious than similar accidents in other types of power-generating plants. The 1986 fire and explosion at the Chernobyl Nuclear Power Station in Ukraine caused hundreds of deaths and increased rates of genetic mutation and cancer; the long-term effects are not yet clear. The zone around Chernobyl has been sealed off to human habitation and could be unsafe for the next 24,000 years.

An additional, enormous problem is disposing of the radioactive wastes these plants generate. They cannot be dumped in a sanitary landfill because the amount and type of soil used to cap a sanitary landfill is not sufficient to prevent radiation exposure. Deposit sites have to be developed that will be secure not just for a few years but for tens of thousands of years—longer than the total recorded history of human beings on this planet. To date, no storage method has been devised that can provide infallible, infinitely durable shielding for nuclear waste.

Medical Uses of Radiation Another area of concern is the use of radiation in medicine, primarily the X ray. The development of machines that could produce images of internal bone structures was a major advance in medicine, and applications abounded. Chest X rays were routinely given to screen for tuberculosis, and children's feet were even X rayed in shoe stores to make sure their new shoes fit properly. But, as is often the case, this new technology had disadvantages. As time passed, studies revealed that X ray exposure is cumulative and that no exposure is absolutely safe.

Early X ray machines are no longer used because of the high amounts of radiation they give off. Each "generation" of X ray machines has used less radiation more effectively. From a personal health point of view, individuals should never have a "routine" X ray examination; each one should have a definite purpose, and its benefits and risks should be carefully weighed.

Radiation in the Home and Workplace Recently, there has been concern about electromagnetic radiation associated with such common modern devices as microwave ovens, computer monitors, microwave telephones, and even high-voltage power lines. These forms of radiation do have effects on health, but research results are inconclusive.

Another recent area of concern is **radon**, a naturally occurring radioactive gas found in certain soils, rocks, and building materials. When the breakdown products of radon are inhaled, they cling to lungs and bombard sensitive tissue with radioactivity. Among miners, exposure to high levels of radon has been shown to cause lung cancer. Radon can enter a home by rising though the soil into the basement through dirt floors, cracks, and other openings. Research into whether exposure to low levels of radon significantly increases the risk of lung cancer has yielded mixed results. However, the EPA recommends that people test their homes for radon and take appropriate actions—sealing cracks in basement walls and installing ventilation systems—to bring elevated levels down.

What You Can Do to Avoid Radiation

- If your physician orders an X ray, ask why it is necessary. Only get X rays that you really need, and keep a record of the date and location of every X ray exam.
- Check with your local or state health department to find out if there are radon problems in your area. If there are, consider buying a home radon testing kit.
- Find out if there are radioactive sites in your area. If you live or work near such a site, form or join a community action group to get the site cleaned up.

Noise Pollution

We are increasingly aware of the health effects of loud or persistent noise in the environment. Concerns focus on two areas: hearing loss and stress. Prolonged exposure to sounds above 80–85 **phons** (a measure of the volume of sound) can cause permanent hearing loss (Figure 24-4). The scream of an infant, the noise in a machine shop, and freeway traffic sounds can all exceed the safe range. Two common potential sources of excessive noise are (1) the workplace and (2) large gatherings of people at sporting events and rock concerts. The Occupational Safety and Health Administration (OSHA) sets legal standards for noise in the workplace, but no laws exist regulating noise

---

biomagnification The accumulation of a substance in a food chain. **TERMS**

radiation Energy transmitted in the form of rays, waves, or particles.

radiation sickness An illness caused by excess radiation exposure, marked by low white blood cell counts and nausea; possibly fatal.

nuclear power The use of controlled nuclear reactions to produce steam, which in turn drives turbines to produce electricity.

radon A naturally occurring radioactive gas emitted from rocks and natural building materials that can become concentrated in insulated homes, causing lung cancer.

phon A unit for expressing the relative intensity of sounds; 0 is least perceptible, and 120 is the average pain threshold.

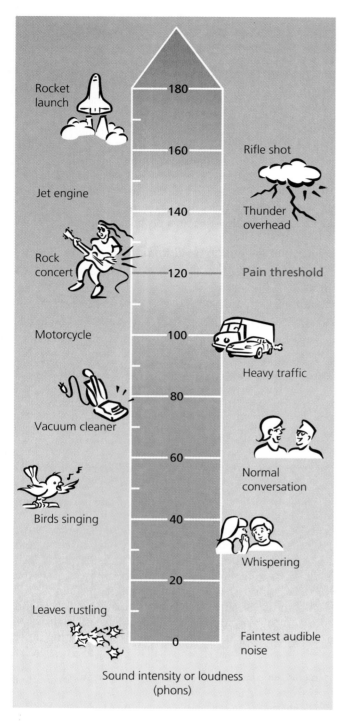

Figure 24-4 **The intensity of selected sounds.** Hearing damage can occur after 8 hours of exposure to sounds louder than 80 phons; regular exposure to more than 100 phons for longer than 1 minute can cause permanent hearing loss.

Sound intensity or loudness (phons)

Rocket launch — 180
Rifle shot — 160
Jet engine
Thunder overhead — 140
Rock concert
Pain threshold — 120
Motorcycle — 100
Heavy traffic
— 80
Vacuum cleaner
— 60
Normal conversation
Birds singing — 40
Whispering
— 20
Leaves rustling
Faintest audible noise — 0

levels at rock concerts, which often exceed OSHA standards for the workplace.

Most hearing loss occurs in the first 2 hours of exposure, and hearing usually recovers within 2 hours after the noise stops. But if exposure continues or is repeated frequently, hearing loss may be permanent. The employees of a club where rock music is played loudly are at much greater risk than the patrons of the club, who might be exposed for only 2 hours at a time. Another possible effect of exposure to excessive noise is **tinnitus**, a condition of more or less continuous ringing or buzzing in the ears.

Excessive noise is also an environmental stressor, producing the typical stress response described in Chapter 2: faster heart rate, increased respiration, higher blood pressure, and so on. A chronic and prolonged stress response can have serious effects on health.

What You Can Do to Avoid Noise Pollution

- Wear ear protectors when working around noisy machinery.

- When listening to music on a headset with a volume range of 1–10, keep the volume no louder than 4; your headset is too loud if you are unable to hear people around you speaking in a normal tone of voice.

- Avoid loud music. Don't sit or stand near speakers or amplifiers at a rock concert, and don't play a car radio or stereo so high that you can't hear the traffic.

- Avoid any exposure to painfully loud sounds, and avoid repeated exposure to any sounds above 80 phons.

HEALING THE ENVIRONMENT

Faced with a vast array of confusing and complex environmental issues, you may feel overwhelmed and conclude that there isn't anything you can do about global problems. But this is not true. If everyone made individual changes in his or her life, the impact would be tremendous. (To assess your current lifestyle, refer to the box "Environmental Health Checklist.")

At the same time, it is important to recognize that large corporations and manufacturers are the ones primarily responsible for environmental degradation. Many of them have jumped on the "environmental bandwagon" with public relations and advertising campaigns designed to make them look good, but they haven't changed their practices nearly enough to make a difference. To influence them, people have to become educated, demand changes in production methods, and elect people to office who consider environmental concerns along with sound business incentives.

Large-scale changes and individual actions complement each other. What you do every day *does* count. Following the suggestions in the What You Can Do sections throughout this chapter will help you make a difference

The following list of statements relates to your impact on the environment. Put a check mark next to the statements that are true for you.

———— I ride my bike, walk, carpool, or use public transportation whenever possible.

———— I keep my car tuned up and well maintained.

———— My residence is well insulated.

———— Where possible, I use compact fluorescent bulbs instead of incandescent bulbs.

———— I turn off lights and appliances when they are not in use.

———— I avoid turning on heat or air conditioning whenever possible.

———— I run the washing machine, dryer, and dishwasher only when they have full loads.

———— I run the clothes dryer only as long as it takes my clothes to dry.

———— I dry my hair with a towel rather than a hair dryer.

———— I keep my car's air conditioner in good working order and have it serviced by a service station that recycles CFCs.

———— When shopping, I choose products with the least amount of packaging.

———— I choose recycled and recyclable products.

———— I avoid products packaged in plastic and unrecycled aluminum.

———— I store food in glass jars and waxed paper rather than plastic wrap.

———— I take my own bag along when I go shopping.

———— I recycle newspapers, glass, cans, and other recyclables.

———— When shopping, I read labels and try to buy the least toxic products available.

———— I dispose of household hazardous wastes properly.

———— I take showers instead of baths.

———— I take short showers and switch off the water when I'm not actively using it.

———— I do not run the water while brushing my teeth, shaving, or hand-washing clothes.

———— My sinks have aerators installed in them.

———— My shower has a low-flow showerhead.

———— I have a water-saver toilet or a water displacement device in my toilet.

———— I snip or rip plastic six-pack rings before I throw them out.

———— When hiking or camping, I never leave anything behind.

Statements you have not checked can help you identify behaviors you can change to improve environmental health.

---

in the environment. In addition, you can become a part of larger community actions to work for a healthier world:

- Share what you learn about environmental issues with your friends and family.

- Join, support, or volunteer your time to organizations working on environmental causes that are important to you.

- Contact your elected representatives and communicate your concerns. For guidelines on how to be heard, see the box "Making Your Letters Count."

PERSONAL INSIGHT   Do you recycle? If you do not, why don't you? How convenient would it have to be to get you to recycle?

SUMMARY

Classic Environmental Health Concerns

- Water used in municipal systems must be purified because it's likely to be contaminated with organic matter and pathogenic microorganisms.

- Concerns with water quality focus on hazardous chemicals from industry and households, as well as on water shortages.

- Sewage treatment prevents pathogens from contaminating drinking water; it must also often deal with heavy metals and hazardous chemicals.

- The amount of garbage is growing all the time; paper is the biggest component. Recycling can help solid waste disposal problems.

- Illness and death associated with foodborne disease have decreased substantially because of food inspection standards.

Population Growth

- The world's population is increasing rapidly, especially in the developing world.

- Factors that may eventually limit human population are food, availability of land and water, energy, and minimum acceptable standard of living.

- Many factors influence population growth, including high fertility rates, lack of family planning resources, and decreasing death rates.

It takes only a few minutes to write to an elected official, but it can make a difference on an environmental issue you care about. When elected officials receive enough letters on an issue, it does influence their vote—they want to be reelected, and your vote counts! To give your letter the greatest possible impact, use these guidelines:

- Use your own words and your own stationery.

- Be clear and concise. Keep your letter to one or two paragraphs, never more than one page.

- Focus on only one subject in each letter, and identify it clearly. Refer to legislation by its name or number.

- Request a specific action—vote a particular way on a piece of legislation, request hearings, cosponsor a bill—and state your reasons for your position.

- If you live or work in the legislator's district, say so.

- Courteous letters work best. Don't be insulting or unnecessarily critical.

Your phone book has addresses of all state and local representatives. You can write to the president or vice president at the White House:

President (Vice President) _____
White House
Washington, D.C. 20500
president@whitehouse.gov
vice.president@whitehouse.gov

United States senators and representatives can be reached at the following addresses:

The Honorable _____   The Honorable _____
U.S. Senate   U.S. House of Representatives
Washington, D.C. 20510   Washington, D.C. 20515

Members of Congress also have e-mail addresses and many have Web sites; you can find a directory of this information at: http://lcweb.loc.gov/global/legislative/email.html.

Pollution

- In terms of health risks, the level of concentration of a particular pollutant is very important. Long-term effects of pollutants are difficult to evaluate.

- Increased amounts of air pollutants are especially stressful to those with heart and lung problems. Air pollution emergencies occur when (1) fossil fuels are burned, (2) a topographic feature prevents prevailing winds from pushing stagnant air away, and (3) a temperature inversion exists.

- Smog is human-made air pollution caused by the burning of fossil fuels (London-type) or by motor vehicle exhausts containing oxides of nitrogen (Los Angeles-type).

- Carbon dioxide and other natural gases act as a "greenhouse" around the earth, increasing the temperature of the atmosphere. Levels of these gases are rising through human activity; as a result, the world's climate could change.

- The ozone layer that shields the earth's surface from the sun's UV rays has thinned and developed holes in certain regions. One cause is the release of CFCs, which break down into chlorine in the atmosphere.

- Acid precipitation occurs when certain atmospheric pollutants combine with moisture in the air.

- Environmental damage from energy use can be limited through energy conservation and the development of nonpolluting, renewable sources of energy.

- Indoor pollutants can trigger allergies and illness in the short term and cancer in the long term.

- Potentially hazardous chemical pollutants include asbestos, lead, pesticides, and many household products. Proper handling and disposal is critical.

- Radiation can cause radiation sickness, chromosome damage, and cancer, among other health risks. Sources of radiation include nuclear power, nuclear weapons, medical X rays, and radon gas.

- Loud or persistent noise can lead to hearing loss and/or stress; two common sources of excessive noise are the workplace and rock concerts.

Healing the Environment

- Most health advances today must come from lifestyle changes and improvements in the global environment. The impact of personal changes made by every concerned individual could be tremendous.

TAKE ACTION

1.   Prepare an inventory to find out what hazardous chemicals you have in your household. Read the labels for disposal instructions. If there aren't any instructions, call your local health department and ask how to dispose of specific chemicals. Also ask if there are hazardous waste disposal sites in your community or special pickup days. If possible, get rid of some or all of the hazardous wastes in your home.

2. Junk mail is an environmental hazard coming and going; millions of trees are cut down to produce the paper it's printed on, and millions of pieces of junk mail clog the nation's landfills. Keep your name from being sold to any more mailing list companies by writing to Mail Preference Service, Direct Marketing Association, P.O. Box 9008, Farmingdale, NY 11735. Recycle the junk mail you still get.

3. Investigate the recycling facilities in your community. Find out how materials are recycled and what they are used for in their recycled state. If recycling isn't available in your community, contact your local city hall to find out how a recycling program can be started.

4. Keep track of exactly how many bags (or gallons) of trash your household produces per week. Is it more or less than the national weekly average of 6.73 bags (87.5 gallons) per three-person household? In either case, try to reduce it by recycling, composting, and buying and using fewer disposable products.

JOURNAL ENTRY

1. In your health journal, list the positive behaviors that help you protect the environment. What can you do to reinforce and support these behaviors? Then list the behaviors that may harm the environment. How can you change one or more of them?

2. *Critical Thinking* Some developing nations want to "catch up" with the West in terms of economic development and standard of living by using the same kinds of industrial practices that developed nations have used to get where they are. They are cutting down forests to raise cattle for beef, using pesticides that have been banned in the developed nations on export crops, and polluting their water and air with industrial and agricultural wastes. Do you think it's fair to expect them to be environmentally conscious when the developed nations were not? Do they have a right to the same standard of living that Americans have, no matter what the environmental costs? Write a short essay that makes a case for or against their continuing use of these practices.

FOR MORE INFORMATION

Books

Athanasiou. 1998. *Divided Planet: The Ecology of Rich and Poor.* Athens: Univerity of Georgia Press. *Discusses environmental issues in the context of the economic inequality between developed and developing nations.*

Cunningham, W. P., and B. W. Saigo. 1999. *Environmental Science: A Global Concern,* 5th ed. New York: McGraw-Hill. *A basic text in environmental science for the nonscientist.*

Getis, J. 1999. *You Can Make a Difference: Be Environmentally Responsible,* 2nd ed. New York: McGraw-Hill. *Describes environmental problems and suggestions for individual action.*

Goudie, A. 1998. *The Earth Transformed.* Malden, Mass.: Blackwell. *An introduction to the ways humans affect the environment.*

Houghton, J. T. 1997. *Global Warming: The Complete Briefing.* New York: Cambridge University Press. *An introduction to the science and politics of global warming.*

Useful annual or biennial publications include the following:

Brown, L., et al. 1999. *State of the World 1999.* New York: Norton.

National Wildlife Federation. 1999. *1999 Conservation Directory.* Washington, D.C.: National Wildlife Federation.

World Resources Institute. 1998. *World Resources 1998–1999: A Guide to the Global Environment.* New York: Oxford University Press.

Organizations, Hotlines, and Web Sites

The Earth Times. An international online newspaper devoted to global environmental issues.
http://www.earthtimes.org

Energy Efficiency and Renewable Energy Network (EREN). U.S. Department of Energy. Provides information about alternative fuels and tips for saving energy at home and in your car.
http://www.eren.doe.gov

Environmental Health Clearinghouse (EHC). An information clearinghouse that provides fact sheets and answers to frequently asked questions on many environmental problems.
http://infoventures.com/e-hlth

Environmental News Network. Provides daily environmental news and special reports in print, audio, and video.
http://www.enn.com

Garbage. Provides information and links about ways to reduce solid and hazardous waste.
http://www.learner.org/exhibits/garbage

Indoor Air Quality Information Hotline. Answers questions, provides publications, and makes referrals.
800-438-4318

National Lead Information Center. Provides information packets and specialist advice.
800-LEAD-FYI

National Safety Council Environmental Health Center. Provides information on lead, radon, indoor air quality, hazardous chemicals, and other environmental issues.
1025 Connecticut Ave., Suite 1200
Washington, DC 20036
800-55-RADON (Radon Hotline)
http://www.nsc.org/ehc.htm

Ozone Hole Tour. An illustrated look at the science behind the Antarctic ozone hole.

http://www.atm.ch.cam.ac.uk/tour

Student Environmental Action Coalition (SEAC). A coalition of student and youth environmental groups; Web site has contact information for local groups.

P.O. Box 31909
Philadelphia, PA 19104
215-222-4711
http://www.seac.org

United Nations. Several UN programs are devoted to environmental problems on a global scale; the Web sites provide information on current and projected trends and on international treaties developed to deal with environmental issues.

http://www.undp.org/popin (Population Division)
http://www.unep.org (Environment Programme)

U.S. Environmental Protection Agency (EPA). Provides information about EPA activities and many consumer-oriented materials. The Web site includes special sites devoted to global warming, ozone loss, pesticides, and other areas of concern.

401 M St., S.W.
Washington, DC 20460
202-260-2090
http://www.epa.gov

The following are a few of the specific EPA Web sites:

http://www.epa.gov/ozone
http://www.epa.gov/globalwarming
http://www.epa.gov/acidrain
http://www.epa.gov/pesticides

Worldwatch Institute. A public policy research organization focusing on emerging global environmental problems and the links between the world economy and the environment.

http://www.worldwatch.org

There are many national and international organizations working on environmental health problems. A few of the largest and best known are listed below:

Greenpeace
202-462-1177; http://www.greenpeace.org
National Audubon Society
212-979-3000; http://www.audubon.org
National Wildlife Federation
202-797-6800; http://www.nwf.org
Nature Conservancy
703-841-5300; http://www.tnc.org
Sierra Club
415-977-5500; http://www.sierraclub.org

SELECTED BIBLIOGRAPHY

Alward, R. D., J. K. Detling, and D. G. Milchunas. 1999. Grassland vegetation changes and nocturnal global warming. *Science* 283: 229–231.

Brown, L. R., et al. 1999. *State of the World 1999.* New York: Norton.

Environmental myths. 1999. *Discover,* March.

Eulitz, D., et al. 1998. Mobile phones modulate response patterns of human brain activity. *Neuroreport* 9(14): 3229–3232.

Intergovernmental Panel on Climate Change. 1998. *The Regional Impacts of Climate Change: An Assessment of Vulnerability. Summary for Policymakers.* New York: Cambridge University Press.

International Center for Technology Assessment. 1998. *The Real Price of Gas* (retrieved March 3, 1999; http://www.icta.org/projects/trans/rlprexsm.htm).

Lin, J. L., H. H. Ho, and C. C. Yu. 1999. Chelation therapy for patients with elevated body lead burden and progressive renal insufficiency. A randomized, controlled trial. *Annals of Internal Medicine* 130(1): 7–13.

Mann, M. E., R. S. Bradley, and M. K. Hughes. 1999. Northern hemisphere temperatures during the past millennium: Inferences, uncertainties, and limitations. *Geophysical Research Letters* 26(6): 759.

Miller, R. C., et al. 1999. The oncogenic transforming potential of the passage of single α particles through mammalian cell nuclei. *Proceedings of the National Academy of Sciences* 96: 19–22.

NASA Goddard Institute for Space Studies. 1999. *Global Temperature Trends: 1998 Global Surface Temperature Smashes Record* (retrieved March 3, 1999; http://www.giss.nasa.gov/research/observe/surftemp).

National Oceanic and Atmospheric Administration Climate Prediction Center. 1999. *Stratosphere: Southern Hemisphere Winter Summary—1998* (retrieved March 3, 1999; http://nic.fb4.noaa.gov/products/stratosphere/winter_bulletins/sh_98).

National Oceanic and Atmospheric Administration Climate Prediction Center. 1998. *Northern Hemisphere Winter Summary 1997–1998* (retrieved March 3, 1999; http://nic.fb4.noaa.gov/products/stratosphere/winter_bulletins/nh_97-98/index.html)

Pacini, F., et al. 1998. Prevalence of thyroid autoantibodies in children and adolescents from Belarus exposed to the Chernobyl radioactive fallout. *Lancet* 352(9130): 763–766.

Pimental, D., et al. 1998. Ecology of increasing disease. *Bioscience* 48(10): 817.

Tong, S., et al. 1998. Declining blood lead levels and changes in cognitive function during childhood. *Journal of the American Medical Association* 280: 1915–1919.

United National Population Division. 1998. *World Population Prospects: The 1998 Revision* (retrieved March 2, 1999; http://www.popin.org/pop1998).

U.S. Energy Information Agency. 1999. *Weekly Retail Premium Gasoline Prices* (retrieved March 3, 1999; http://www.eia.doe.gov/emeu/international/gas1.html).

U.S. Environmental Protection Agency. 1999. *Global Warming Slides: Potential Climate Change Impacts* (retrieved March 3, 1999; http://www.epa.gov/globalwarming/reports/slides/cc&ri/f-impct.html).

U.S. Environmental Protection Agency. 1999. *Characterization of Municipal Solid Waste Management: 1996 Update.* Washington, D.C.: U.S. Environmental Protection Agency.

U.S. Environmental Protection Agency. 1998. *Superfund Cleanup Figures* (retrieved March 2, 1999; http://www.epa.gov/superfund/whatissf/mgmtrpt.htm).

World Resources Institute, et al. 1998. *World Resources 1998–99: A Guide to the Global Environment.* New York: Oxford University Press.

Nutritional Content of Popular Items from Fast-Food Restaurants

Arby's

	Serving size	Calories	Protein	Total fat	Saturated fat	Total carbohydrate	Sugars	Fiber	Cholesterol	Sodium	Vitamin A	Vitamin C	Calcium	Iron	% calories from fat
	g		g	g	g	g	g	g	mg	mg	% Daily Value				
Regular roast beef	154	388	23	19	7	33	N/A	3	43	1009	N/A	N/A	N/A	N/A	44
Super roast beef	247	523	25	27	9	50	N/A	5	43	1189	N/A	N/A	N/A	N/A	46
Light roast beef deluxe	182	296	18	10	3	33	N/A	6	42	826	N/A	N/A	N/A	N/A	30
Roast chicken deluxe	216	433	24	22	5	36	N/A	2	34	763	N/A	N/A	N/A	N/A	46
French dip	195	475	30	22	8	40	N/A	3	55	1411	N/A	N/A	N/A	N/A	41
Turkey sub	277	550	31	27	7	47	N/A	2	65	2084	N/A	N/A	N/A	N/A	44
Light roast turkey deluxe	195	260	20	7	2	33	N/A	4	33	1262	N/A	N/A	N/A	N/A	21
Grilled chicken BBQ	201	388	23	13	3	47	N/A	2	43	1002	N/A	N/A	N/A	N/A	30
Cheddar curly fries	120	333	5	18	4	40	N/A	0	3	1016	N/A	N/A	N/A	N/A	49
Potato cakes	85	204	2	12	2	20	N/A	0	0	397	N/A	N/A	N/A	N/A	53
Red ranch dressing	14	75	0	6	1	5	N/A	0	0	115	N/A	N/A	N/A	N/A	72
French-toastix	124	430	10	21	5	52	N/A	3	0	550	N/A	N/A	N/A	N/A	44
Jamocha shake	340	384	15	10	3	62	N/A	0	36	262	N/A	N/A	N/A	N/A	23

N/A: not available.

SOURCE: Arby's, http://www.arbysrestaurant.com.

Burger King

	Serving size	Calories	Protein	Total fat	Saturated fat	Total carbohydrate	Sugars	Fiber	Cholesterol	Sodium	Vitamin A	Vitamin C	Calcium	Iron	% calories from fat
	g		g	g	g	g	g	g	mg	mg	% Daily Value				
Whopper®	270	640	27	39	11	45	8	3	90	870	N/A	N/A	N/A	N/A	55
Whopper Jr.®	164	420	21	24	8	29	5	2	60	530	N/A	N/A	N/A	N/A	51
Double Whopper® with cheese	375	960	52	63	24	46	8	3	195	1420	N/A	N/A	N/A	N/A	59
BK Big Fish™ sandwich	252	720	23	43	9	59	4	3	80	1180	N/A	N/A	N/A	N/A	54
BK Broiler® chicken sandwich	247	530	29	26	5	5	4	2	105	1060	N/A	N/A	N/A	N/A	44
Chicken Tenders® (8 piece)	123	350	22	22	7	17	0	1	65	940	N/A	N/A	N/A	N/A	57
Ranch dipping sauce	28	170	0	17	3	2	1	0	0	200	N/A	N/A	N/A	N/A	90
Barbecue dipping sauce	28	35	0	0	0	9	7	0	0	400	N/A	N/A	N/A	N/A	0
Broiled chicken salad (no dressing)	302	190	20	8	4	9	5	3	75	500	N/A	N/A	N/A	N/A	38
Garden salad (no dressing)	215	100	6	5	3	8	4	4	15	115	N/A	N/A	N/A	N/A	45
Bleu cheese salad dressing	30	160	2	16	4	1	0	<1	30	260	N/A	N/A	N/A	N/A	90
French fries (medium, salted)	116	400	3	21	8	50	0	4	0	820	N/A	N/A	N/A	N/A	47
Onion rings	124	310	4	14	2	41	6	6	0	810	N/A	N/A	N/A	N/A	41
Chocolate shake (medium)	284	320	9	7	4	54	48	3	20	230	N/A	N/A	N/A	N/A	20
Croissan'wich® w/sausage, egg, and cheese	176	600	22	46	16	25	3	1	260	1140	N/A	N/A	N/A	N/A	69
French toast sticks	141	500	4	27	7	60	11	1	0	490	N/A	N/A	N/A	N/A	49
Dutch apple pie	113	300	3	15	3	39	22	2	0	230	N/A	N/A	N/A	N/A	45

N/A: not available.

SOURCE: Burger King, http://www.burgerking.com.

Domino's Pizza

(1 serving = 2 of 12 slices or 1/6 of 14-inch pizza; 2 of 8 slices or 1/4 of 12-inch pizza; 1 6-inch pizza)

	Serving size (g)	Calories	Protein (g)	Total fat (g)	Saturated fat (g)	Total carbohydrate (g)	Sugars (g)	Fiber (g)	Cholesterol (mg)	Sodium (mg)	Vitamin A	Vitamin C	Calcium	Iron	% calories from fat
											% Daily Value				
14-inch lg. hand-tossed cheese	137	317	13	10	5	45	3	3	14	669	10	9	17	18	28
14-inch lg. thin crust cheese	99	253	11	11	5	29	2	2	14	757	9	4	20	5	39
14-inch lg. deep dish cheese	173	455	18	20	8	54	5	3	18	1029	11	5	22	21	39
12-inch med. hand-tossed cheese	149	347	14	11	5	50	3	3	15	723	11	8	18	20	29
12-inch med. thin crust cheese	106	271	12	12	5	31	3	2	15	509	10	4	22	5	40
12-inch med. deep dish cheese	180	477	18	22	8	55	5	3	19	1085	12	5	23	21	42
6-inch deep dish cheese	215	595	23	27	11	68	6	4	24	1300	13	5	28	26	41
Toppings: pepperoni	*	66	3	6	2	<1	<1	<1	14	212	†	†	†	†	82
ham	*	17	2	1	<1	<1	<1	0	7	156	†	†	†	†	53
Italian sausage	*	44	2	3	1	1	<1	<1	9	137	†	†	†	†	61
bacon	*	75	4	6	2	<1	<1	0	11	207	†	7	†	†	72
beef	*	44	2	4	2	<1	<1	<1	8	123	†	†	†	†	82
anchovies	*	23	3	1	<1	0	0	0	9	395	†	†	3	3	39
extra cheese	*	45	3	4	2	<1	<1	<1	7	140	3	†	12	†	80
cheddar cheese	*	48	3	4	2	<1	<1	0	12	73	3	†	9	†	75
Barbeque wings	25	50	6	2	1	2	1	<1	26	175	†	†	†	†	38
Hot wings	25	45	6	2	1	<1	<1	<1	26	354	3	†	†	†	40
Breadsticks (1 piece)	22	78	2	3	1	11	<1	<1	0	158	†	†	†	3	35
Cheesy bread (1 piece)	28	103	3	5	2	11	<1	<1	6	187	†	26	†	4	44

* Topping information is based on minimal portioning requirements for one serving of a 14-inch large pizza; add the values for toppings to the values for a cheese pizza. The following toppings supply fewer than 15 calories per serving: green and yellow peppers, onion, olives, mushrooms, pineapple.

† Contains less than 2% of the Daily Value of these nutrients.

SOURCE: Domino's Pizza, http://www.dominos.com.

Jack in the Box

	Serving size (g)	Calories	Protein (g)	Total fat (g)	Saturated fat (g)	Total carbohydrate (g)	Sugars (g)	Fiber (g)	Cholesterol (mg)	Sodium (mg)	Vitamin A	Vitamin C	Calcium	Iron	% calories from fat
											% Daily Value				
Breakfast Jack®	126	280	17	12	5	30	3	1	195	920	8	4	15	20	39
Supreme croissant	163	520	21	32	13	39	6	2	245	1240	15	20	10	20	57
Hamburger	97	280	13	11	4	31	5	1	45	560	2	2	10	20	39
Jumbo Jack®	263	590	25	36	11	42	6	4	80	720	8	20	15	35	55
Sourdough Jack	229	690	31	46	15	38	3	3	110	1180	10	15	30	20	60
Chicken fajita pita	187	280	24	9	4	25	5	3	75	840	25	0	15	15	29
Grilled chicken fillet	231	520	27	26	6	42	9	4	140	1240	8	15	20	25	45
Chicken supreme	235	680	23	45	11	46	8	4	85	1500	10	15	20	15	60
Chicken Caesar sandwich	232	490	24	26	6	41	6	3	55	1050	15	15	20	20	48
Garden chicken salad	253	200	23	9	4	8	4	3	65	420	70	20	20	4	41
Blue cheese dressing	57	210	1	15	2.5	11	4	0	25	750	0	0	2	0	64
Chicken teriyaki bowl	502	670	26	4	1	128	27	3	15	1730	130	40	10	10	5
Monster taco	125	270	12	17	6	19	2	4	30	678	8	2	20	10	57
Egg rolls (3 pieces)	170	440	15	24	6	40	5	4	35	1020	15	20	8	15	49
Chicken breast pieces (5)	150	360	27	17	3	24	0	1	80	970	4	2	2	6	39
Stuffed jalapeños (10 pieces)	240	750	20	44	17	65	7	5	80	2470	30	50	45	4	53
Barbeque dipping sauce	28	45	1	0	0	11	7	0	0	310	0	0	0	0	0
Seasoned curly fries	125	410	6	23	5	45	0	4	0	1010	6	0	4	8	50
Onion rings	120	460	7	25	5	50	3	3	0	780	4	30	4	10	49
Cappuccino ice cream shake	16*	630	11	29	17	80	58	0	90	320	15	0	35	0	41

*Fluid ounces

SOURCE: Jack in the Box, 1998, *Jack's Nutrition Facts,* http://www.jackinthebox.com.

KFC

	Serving size	Calories	Protein	Total fat	Saturated fat	Total carbohydrate	Sugars	Fiber	Cholesterol	Sodium	Vitamin A	Vitamin C	Calcium	Iron	% calories from fat
	g		g	g	g	g	g	g	mg	mg	% Daily Value				
Original Recipe®: breast	153	400	29	24	6	16	0	1	135	1116	*	*	4	6	54
thigh	91	250	16	18	4.5	6	0	1	95	747	*	*	2	4	65
Extra Tasty Crispy™: breast	168	470	31	28	7	25	0	1	80	930	*	*	4	6	54
thigh	118	370	19	25	6	18	0	2	70	540	*		2	4	61
Hot & Spicy: breast	180	530	32	35	8	23	0	2	110	1110	*	*	4	6	59
thigh	107	370	18	27	7	13	0	1	90	570	*	*	*	4	66
Tender Roast™: breast (as served)	139	251	37	11	3	1	<1	0	151	830	*	*	*	*	39
breast (skin removed)	118	169	31	4	1	1	0	0	112	797	*	*	*	*	21
thigh (as served)	90	207	18	12	4	<2	<1	0	120	504	*	*	*	*	52
thigh (skin removed)	59	106	13	6	2	<1	<1	0	84	312	*	*	*	*	51
Hot Wings™ Pieces	135	471	27	33	8	18	0	2	150	1230	*	*	4	8	63
Colonel's Crispy Strips™ (3)	92	261	20	16	4	10	0	3	40	658	*	*	*	3	55
Chunky chicken pot pie	368	770	29	42	13	69	8	5	70	2160	80	2	10	10	49
Corn on the cob	162	150	5	2	0	35	8	2	0	20	2	6	*	*	12
Mashed potatoes w/gravy	136	120	1	6	1	17	0	2	<1	440	*	*	*	2	45
Mean Greens™	152	70	4	3	1	11	1	5	10	650	60	10	20	10	39
BBQ baked beans	156	190	6	3	1	33	13	6	5	760	8	*	8	10	14
Potato salad	160	230	4	14	2	23	9	23	15	540	10	*	2	15	55
Cole slaw	142	180	2	9	1.5	21	20	3	5	280	*	60	4	4	45
Biscuit (1)	56	180	4	10	2.5	20	2	<1	0	560	*	*	2	6	50

*Contains less than 2% of the Daily Value of these nutrients.

SOURCE: KFC, http://www.kfc.com.

McDonald's

	Serving size	Calories	Protein	Total fat	Saturated fat	Total carbohydrate	Sugars	Fiber	Cholesterol	Sodium	Vitamin A	Vitamin C	Calcium	Iron	% calories from fat
	g		g	g	g	g	g	g	mg	mg	% Daily Value				
Hamburger	107	260	13	9	3.5	34	7	2	30	580	*	4	15	15	31
Cheeseburger	121	320	15	13	6	35	7	2	40	820	6	4	20	15	37
Quarter-Pounder®	172	420	23	21	8	37	8	2	70	820	2	4	30	25	45
Quarter-Pounder® w/cheese	200	530	28	30	13	38	9	2	95	1290	10	4	15	25	51
Big Mac®	216	560	26	31	10	45	8	3	85	1070	6	4	25	25	50
Arch Deluxe™	239	550	29	31	11	39	8	4	90	1010	10	10	15	25	51
Fish Filet Deluxe™	228	560	23	28	6	54	5	4	60	1060	6	4	8	15	45
Grilled Chicken Deluxe™	223	440	27	20	3	38	8	4	60	1040	4	8	6	15	41
French fries (large)	147	450	6	22	4	57	0	5	0	290	*	30	2	6	44
Chicken McNuggets® (6 pieces)	106	290	18	17	3.5	15	0	0	60	510	*	*	2	6	53
Barbeque sauce	28	45	0	0	0	10	10	0	0	250	*	6	*	*	0
Garden salad (no dressing)	177	35	2	0	0	7	3	3	0	20	120	40	4	6	0
Grilled chicken salad (no dressing)	257	120	21	1.5	0	7	3	3	45	240	120	25	4	8	1
Ranch dressing (1 pkg.)	N/A	230	1	21	3	10	6	0	20	550	*	2	4	*	82
Fat-free herb vinaigrette (1 pkg.)	N/A	50	0	0	0	11	9	0	0	330	*	2	*	2	0
Egg McMuffin®	136	290	17	12	4.5	27	3	1	235	790	10	2	20	15	37
Hash browns	53	130	1	8	1.5	14	0	1	0	330	*	4	*	2	55
Hotcakes w/margarine & syrup	222	570	9	16	3	100	42	2	15	750	8	*	10	15	25
Chocolate shake, small	N/A	360	11	9	6	60	54	1	40	250	6	2	35	4	23
Baked apple pie	77	260	3	13	3.5	34	13	<1	0	200	*	40	2	6	45

*Contains less than 2% of the Daily Value of these nutrients.

SOURCE: McDonald's, March, 1998, *Nutrition Facts*, http://www.mcdonalds.com.

Taco Bell

	Serving size (g)	Calories	Protein (g)	Total fat (g)	Saturated fat (g)	Total carbohydrate (g)	Sugars (g)	Fiber (g)	Cholesterol (mg)	Sodium (mg)	Vitamin A	Vitamin C	Calcium	Iron	% calories from fat
											\% Daily Value				
Taco	2.75	180	9	10	4	12	1	3	25	330	10	0	8	6	50
Taco Supreme®	4	220	10	14	6	14	2	3	35	350	15	6	10	6	57
Double Decker Taco Supreme®	7	390	15	19	8	40	3	9	35	760	15	6	15	10	44
BLT soft taco	4.5	340	11	23	8	22	3	2	40	610	4	6	10	4	61
Burrito Supreme®	9	440	17	19	8	51	4	10	35	1230	50	8	15	15	39
Big Beef Burrito Supreme®	10.5	520	17	23	10	54	4	11	55	1520	60	8	15	15	40
Chili cheese burrito	5	330	10	13	6	37	2	5	35	870	60	0	20	8	35
Beef Gorditas Supreme®	5	300	21	13	6	31	3	3	35	390	10	4	8	15	39
Chicken Gorditas Supreme®	5	290	14	12	5	30	4	2	55	420	10	4	8	10	37
Big Beef MexiMelt®	4.75	290	21	15	7	23	0	4	45	850	25	6	20	6	47
Taco salad	19	850	9	52	15	65	1	16	60	1780	160	40	30	35	55
Taco salad w/o shell	16.5	420	5	21	11	32	1	15	60	1520	160	35	25	25	47
Chicken Fajita Wrap™	8	470	9	21	6	51		4	60	1290	35	6	15	8	42
Veggie Fajita Wrap™	8	420		19	5	53		3	20	980	35	6	15	8	41
Steak Fajita Wrap™ Supreme	9	510		25	8	52		3	50	1200	30	10	15	10	44
Big Beef Nachos Supreme	7	450		24	8	45		9	30	810	10	6	15	15	48
Nachos BellGrande®	11	720		39	11	84		17	35	1310	15	6	20	20	46
Pintos 'n cheese	4.5	190		9	4	18		10	15	650	50	0	15	10	43
Mexican rice	4.75	190		9	3.5	23	1		15	760	100	2	15	8	43
Fiesta breakfast burrito	3.5	280		16	6	25		2	25	580	15	0	8	4	51

SOURCE: Taco Bell, 1997, *Nutritional Guide,* http://www.tacobell.com.

Wendy's

	Serving size (g)	Calories	Protein (g)	Total fat (g)	Saturated fat (g)	Total carbohydrate (g)	Sugars (g)	Fiber (g)	Cholesterol (mg)	Sodium (mg)	Vitamin A	Vitamin C	Calcium	Iron	% calories from fat
											\% Daily Value				
Single w/everything	219	420	25	20	7	37	9	3	70	920	6	10	13	26	43
Big Bacon Classic	282	580	34	30	12	46	11	3	100	1460	15	25	25	30	47
Jr. hamburger	118	270	15	10	3.5	34	7	2	30	610	2	2	11	17	33
Jr. bacon cheeseburger	166	380	20	19	7	34	7	2	60	850	8	10	17	19	45
Grilled chicken sandwich	189	310	27	8	1.5	35	8	2	65	790	4	10	10	15	23
Caesar side salad (no dressing)	92	110	10	5	2.5	7	1	1	15	650	35	25	15	6	41
Grilled chicken salad (no dressing)	338	200	25	8	1.5	9	6	3	50	720	120	60	19	11	36
Taco salad (no dressing)	468	380	26	19	10	28	9	7	65	1040	45	45	37	23	45
Blue cheese dressing (2T)	28	180	1	19	3	0	0	0	15	180	2	0	2	0	95
Ranch dressing, reduced fat (2T)	28	60	1	5	1	2	1	0	10	240	0	0	1	0	75
Soft breadstick	44	130	4	3	0.5	23	N/A	1	5	250	0	0	4	9	21
French fries, medium	130	390	5	19	3	50	0	5	0	120	0	10	2	6	44
Baked potato w/broccoli & cheese	411	470	9	14	2.5	80	6	9	5	470	35	120	21	25	27
Baked potato w/chili & cheese	439	630	20	24	9	83	7	9	40	770	20	60	35	28	34
Chili, small, plain	227	210	15	7	2.5	21	5	5	30	800	8	6	8	16	30
Chili, large w/cheese & crackers	363	405	28	16.5	7	37	8	7	60	1380	14	10	25	26	37
Chicken nuggets (5)	75	230	11	16	3	11	0	0	30	470	0	2	2	2	63
Barbeque sauce	28	45	1	0	0	10	7	0	0	160	0	0	1	3	0
Frosty dairy dessert, medium	298	440	11	11	7	73	56	0	50	260	20	0	41	8	23
Chicken club sandwich	216	470	31	20	4	44	6	2	70	970	4	10	11	17	38

N/A: not available.

SOURCE: Wendy's, 1998, *Nutrition/Ingredient Guide,* http://www.wendys.com.

A Self-Care Guide for Common Medical Problems

This self-care guide will help you manage some of the most common symptoms and medical problems:

- Fever
- Sore throat
- Cough
- Nasal congestion
- Ear problems
- Nausea, vomiting, or diarrhea

- Heartburn and indigestion
- Headache
- Low-back pain
- Strains and sprains
- Cuts and scrapes

Each symptom is described here in terms of what is going on in your body. Most symptoms are part of the body's natural healing response and reflect your body's wisdom in attempting to correct disease. Self-care advice is also given, along with some guidelines about when to seek professional advice. In most cases, the symptoms are self-limiting; that is, they will resolve on their own with time and simple self-care strategies.

No medical advice is perfect. You will always have to make the decision about whether to self-treat or get professional help. This guide is intended to provide you with more information so you can make better, more informed decisions. If the advice here differs from that of your physician, discuss the differences with him or her. In most cases, your physician will be able to customize the advice to your individual medical situation.

The guidelines given here apply to *generally healthy adults*. If you are pregnant or nursing, or if you have a chronic disease, particularly one that requires medication, check with your physician for appropriate self-care advice. Additionally, if you have an allergy or suspected allergy to any recommended medication, check with your physician before using it.

If you have several symptoms, read about your primary symptom first, and then proceed to secondary symptoms. Use your common sense when determining self-care. If you are particularly concerned about a symptom or confused about how to manage it, call your physician to get more information.

FEVER

A fever is an abnormally high body temperature, usually over 100°F (37.7°C). It is most commonly a sign that your body is fighting an infection. Fever may also be due to an inflammation, an injury, or a drug reaction. Chemicals released into your bloodstream during an infection reset the thermostat in the hypothalamus of your brain. The message goes out to your body to turn up the heat. The blood vessels in your skin constrict, and you curl up and throw on extra blankets to reduce heat loss. Meanwhile, your muscles begin to shiver to generate additional body heat. The resulting rise in body temperature is

a fever. Later, when your brain senses that the temperature is too high, the signal goes out to increase sweating. As the sweat evaporates, it carries heat away from the body surface.

A fever may not be all bad; it may even help you fight infections by making the body less hospitable to bacteria and viruses. A high body temperature appears to bolster the immune system and may inhibit the growth of infectious microorganisms.

Most generally healthy people can tolerate a fever as high as 103–104°F (39.5–40°C) without problems. Therefore, if you are essentially healthy, there is little need to reduce a fever unless you are very uncomfortable. Older adults and those with chronic health problems such as heart disease may not tolerate the increased metabolic demand of a high fever, and fever reduction may be advised.

Most problems with fevers are due to the excessive loss of fluids from evaporation and sweating, which may cause dehydration.

Self-Assessment

1. If you are sick, take your temperature several times throughout the day. Oral temperatures should not be measured for at least 10 minutes after smoking, eating, or drinking a hot or cold liquid. When using an oral glass thermometer, first clean it with rubbing alcohol or cool soapy water (hot water may break it). Then shake it down until it reads 95°F or lower. Place the thermometer under your tongue, and leave it in place for a *full 3 minutes*. (If you leave it in for only 2 minutes, the temperature reading will be off by at least half a degree.) To read the thermometer, notice where the silver or red column ends, and compare it with the degrees marked in lines on the thermometer. If you are using an electronic digital thermometer, follow the directions that came with it.

   "Normal" temperature varies from person to person, so it is important to know what is normal for you. Your normal temperature will also vary throughout the day, being lowest in the early evening. If you exercise or if it is a hot day, your temperature may normally rise. Women's body temperature typically varies by a degree or more through the menstrual cycle, peaking around the time of ovulation. Rectal temperatures normally run about 0.5–1.0°F higher than oral temperatures. If your recorded temperature is more than 1.0–1.5°F above your normal baseline temperature, you have a fever.

2. Watch for signs of dehydration: excessive thirst; very dry mouth; infrequent urination with dark, concentrated urine; and light-headedness.

Self-Care

1. Drink plenty of fluids to prevent dehydration—at least 8 ounces of water, juice, or broth every 2 hours.

2. Take a sponge bath using lukewarm water; this will increase evaporation and help reduce body temperature naturally.

3. Don't bundle up. This decreases the body's ability to lose excess heat.

4. Take aspirin or aspirin substitute (acetaminophen, ibuprofen, or naproxen sodium). For adults, two standard-size tablets every 4–6 hours can be used to reduce the fever and the associated headache and achiness. Do not use aspirin if you have a history of allergy to aspirin, ulcers, or bleeding problems. In addition, pediatricians warn that aspirin should usually not be used for fever in children and adolescents because some children with chicken pox, influenza, or other viral infections have developed a life-threatening complication, Reye's syndrome, after taking aspirin.

When to Call the Physician

1. Fever over 103°F (39.5°C), or 102°F (38.8°C) if over 60 years old.

2. Fever lasting more than 5 days.

3. Recurrent unexplained fevers.

4. Fever accompanied by a rash, stiff neck, severe headache, cough with brown or green sputum, severe pain in the side or abdomen, painful urination, convulsions, or mental confusion.

5. Fever with signs of dehydration.

6. Fever after starting a new medication.

SORE THROAT

A sore throat is caused by inflammation of the throat lining resulting from an infection, allergy, or irritation (especially from cigarette smoke). If you have an infection, you may also notice some hoarseness from swelling of the vocal cords and "swollen glands," which are enlarged lymph nodes that produce white blood cells to help fight the infection. The lymph nodes, part of your body's defense system, may remain swollen for weeks after the infection subsides.

   Most throat infections are caused by viruses, so antibiotics are not effective against them. However, about 20–30% of throat infections are due to streptococcal bacteria. This type of microbe can cause complications such as rheumatic fever and rheumatic heart disease and therefore should be diagnosed by a physician and treated with antibiotics. Strep throat is usually characterized by very sore throat, high fever, swollen lymph nodes, a whitish discharge at the back of the throat, and the absence of other cold symptoms such as a cough and runny nose (which suggest a viral infection). Allergy-related sore throats are usually accompanied by running nose and watery, itchy eyes.

Self-Assessment

1. Take your temperature.

2. Look at the back of your throat in a mirror. Is there a whitish, puslike discharge on the tonsils or in the back of the throat?

3. Feel the front and back of your neck. Do you feel enlarged, tender lymph nodes?

Self-Care

1. If you smoke, stop smoking to avoid further irritation of your throat.

2. Drink plenty of liquids to soothe your inflamed throat.

3. Gargle warm salt water ($1/4$ tsp salt in 4 oz water) every 1–2 hours to help reduce swelling and discomfort.

4. Suck on throat lozenges, cough drops, or hard candies to keep your throat moist.

5. Use throat lozenges, sprays, or gargles that contain an anesthetic to temporarily numb your throat and make swallowing less painful.

6. Try aspirin or aspirin substitute to ease throat pain.

7. For an allergy-related sore throat, try an antihistamine such as chlorpheniramine.

When to Call the Physician

1. Great difficulty swallowing saliva or breathing.

2. Sore throat with fever over 101°F (38.3°C), especially if you do not have other cold symptoms such as nasal congestion or a cough.

3. Sore throat with a skin rash.

4. Sore throat with whitish pus on the tonsils.

5. Sore throat and recent contact with a person who has had a positive throat culture for strep.

6. Enlarged lymph nodes lasting longer than 3 weeks.

7. Hoarseness lasting longer than 3 weeks.

COUGH

A cough is a protective mechanism of the body to help keep the airways clear. There are two types of cough: a dry cough (without mucus) and a productive cough (with mucus). Common causes of cough include infection (viral or bacterial), allergies, and irritation from smoking and pollutants. If you have a cold, the cough may be the last symptom to improve, because the airways may remain irritated for several weeks after the infection has resolved.

   Your airways are lined with hairlike projections called cilia, which move back and forth to help clear the airways of mucus, germs, and dust. Infections and cigarette smoking paralyze and damage this vital defensive mechanism.

Self-Assessment

1. Take your temperature.

2. Observe your mucus. Thick green, brown, or bloody mucus suggests a bacterial infection.

Self-Care

1. If you are a smoker, stop smoking. Smoking irritates the airways and undermines your body's immune defenses, leading to more serious infections and longer-lasting

symptoms. Most people do not feel like smoking when they have a cold with a cough. If you want to quit, a cold may provide an excellent opportunity to do so.

2. Drink plenty of liquids (at least six 8-ounce glasses a day) to help thin mucus and loosen chest congestion.

3. Use moist heat from a hot shower or vaporizer to help loosen chest congestion.

4. Suck on cough drops, throat lozenges, or hard candy to keep your throat moist and help relieve a dry, tickling cough.

5. If you have a dry, nonproductive cough or the cough keeps you from sleeping, you can use a cough syrup or lozenge that contains the nonprescription cough suppressant dextromethorphan. Because a cough that produces mucus is protective, it is generally not advisable to suppress a productive cough.

When to Call the Physician

1. Cough with thick green, brown, or bloody sputum.

2. Cough with high fever—above 102°F (38.8°C)—and shaking chills.

3. Severe chest pains, wheezing, or shortness of breath.

4. Cough that lasts longer than 2 weeks.

NASAL CONGESTION

Nasal congestion is most commonly caused by infection or allergies. With infection, the nasal passages become congested because of increased blood flow and mucus production. This congestion is actually part of the body's defense to fight infection. The increased blood flow raises the temperature of the nasal passages, making them less hospitable to germs. The nasal secretions are rich in white blood cells and antibodies to help fight and neutralize the invading organisms and flush them away. Nasal congestion associated with sore throat, cough, and fever usually indicates a viral infection.

Nasal congestion caused by allergies is often accompanied by a thin, watery discharge, sneezing, and itchy eyes; it is sometimes associated with a seasonal pattern. In an allergic reaction, the offending allergen (such as pollen, dust, mold, or dander) triggers the release of histamine and other chemicals from the cells lining the nose, throat, and eyes. These chemicals cause swelling, discharge, and itching. Antihistamine drugs block the release of these irritating chemicals.

Self-Assessment

1. Take your temperature.

2. Observe the color and consistency of your nasal secretions. A thick green, brown, or bloody discharge suggests a bacterial sinus infection.

3. Tap with your fingers over the sinus cavities above and below the eyes. If the tapping causes increased pain, you may have a bacterial sinus infection.

Self-Care

1. If you smoke, stop smoking to prevent continuing irritation of the nasal passages.

2. Use moist heat from a hot shower or vaporizer to help liquefy congested mucus.

3. Use a decongestant nasal spray or drops to temporarily relieve congestion. However, if these decongestants are used for more than 3 days, they can cause "rebound congestion" that actually creates more nasal congestion. As an alternative, use saltwater nose drops (¼ tsp salt in ½ cup of boiled water, cooled before using).

4. Try an oral decongestant such as pseudoephedrine (60 mg every 6 hours) to help shrink swollen mucous membranes and open nasal passages. In some people, these medications can cause nervousness, sleeplessness, or heart palpitations. If you have uncontrolled high blood pressure, heart disease, or diabetes, check with your physician before using decongestants.

When to Call the Physician

1. Nasal congestion with severe pain and tenderness in the forehead, cheeks, or upper teeth and a high fever (above 102°F or 38.8°C).

2. Thick green, brown, or bloody nasal discharge.

3. Nasal congestion and discharge unresponsive to self-care treatment and lasting longer than 3 weeks.

EAR PROBLEMS

Ear symptoms include earache, discharge, itching, stuffiness, and hearing loss. They may be caused by problems in the external ear canal, eardrum, middle ear, or eustachian tube (the passageway that connects the middle ear space to the back of the throat). The ear canal can be become blocked by excess wax, producing hearing loss and a sense that the ear is plugged. An infection of the external ear canal due to excessive moisture and trauma is often referred to as "swimmer's ear." It can cause pain, a sense of fullness, discharge, and itching. Congestion and blockage of the eustachian tube by a cold or allergy can result in pain, a sense of fullness, and hearing loss. A middle ear infection often produces severe pain, hearing loss, and fever.

Self-Assessment

1. Take your temperature. A fever may be a sign of infection.

2. Have someone look into the ear canal with a flashlight or otoscope. Look for wax blockage or a red, swollen canal indicating an external ear infection.

3. Wiggle the outer part of the ear. If this increases the pain, an infection or inflammation of the external canal is the likely cause.

Self-Care

1. If blockage of the ear canal with wax is the problem, first try a hot shower to liquefy the wax, and use a wash cloth to wipe out the ear canal. You can also use a few drops of an over-the-counter wax softener and then flush the canal gently with warm water in a bulb syringe. Do not use sharp objects or cotton swabs; they can scratch the canal or push the wax in deeper.

2. To treat mild infections of the external ear canal, you must thoroughly dry the ear canal. A few drops of a drying agent (Burrow's solution) on a piece of cotton gently inserted into the canal can act as a wick to dry the canal.

3. To relieve congestion and blockage of the eustachian tube, try a decongestant like pseudoephedrine, a nasal spray (but for no longer than 3 days), or an antihistamine. Hot showers or a vaporizer may help loosen secretions, and yawning or swallowing may help open the eustachian tube. For a mild plugging sensation without fever or pain, pinch your nostrils and blow gently to force air up the eustachian tube and "pop" your ears.

When to Call the Physician

1. Severe earache with fever.
2. Puslike or bloody discharge from the ear.
3. Sudden hearing loss, especially if accompanied by ear pain or recent trauma to the ear.
4. Ringing in the ears or dizziness.
5. Any ear symptom lasting longer than 2 weeks.

NAUSEA, VOMITING, OR DIARRHEA

Nausea, vomiting, and diarrhea usually are defensive reactions of your body to rapidly clear your digestive tract of irritants. These symptoms are most commonly caused by the "stomach flu," a viral infection, but they may also be caused by foodborne illness, medications, or other types of infection. Vomiting dramatically ejects irritants from your stomach, and nausea discourages eating to allow the stomach to rest. In diarrhea, overstimulated intestines flush out the offending irritants.

The major complications of vomiting and diarrhea are dehydration from fluid losses and decreased fluid intake, as well as a risk of bleeding from irritation of the digestive tract.

Self-Assessment

1. Take your temperature. A fever is often a clue that an infection is causing the symptoms.
2. Note the color and frequency of vomiting and diarrhea. This will help you estimate the severity of fluid losses and check for bleeding (red, black, or "coffee grounds" material in the stool or vomit; iron tablets and Pepto-Bismol can also cause black stools).
3. Watch for signs of dehydration: very dry mouth; excessive thirst; infrequent urination with dark, concentrated urine; and light-headedness.
4. Look for signs of hepatitis, an infection of the liver: a yellow color in the skin and the white parts of the eyes.

Self-Care

1. To replace fluids, take frequent, small sips of clear liquids such as water, noncitrus juice, broths, flat ginger ale, or ice chips.
2. When the vomiting and diarrhea have subsided, try nonirritating, constipating foods like the BRAT diet:

bananas, rice, applesauce, and toast.

3. For several days, avoid alcohol, milk products, fatty foods, aspirin, and other medications that might irritate the stomach. Do not stop taking regularly prescribed medications without discussing this change with your physician.

4. Medications are not usually advised for vomiting. For diarrhea, over-the-counter medications containing kaolin, pectin, or attapulgite may help thicken the stool. Loperamide, now available without a prescription, can be used to ease diarrhea. Medications containing paregoric may help decrease painful intestinal spasms.

When to Call the Physician

1. Inability to retain any fluids for 12 hours or signs of dehydration.
2. Severe abdominal pains not relieved by the vomiting or diarrhea.
3. Blood in the vomit (red or "coffee grounds" material) or in the stool (red or black tarlike material).
4. Vomiting or diarrhea with a high fever (above 102°F or 38.8°C).
5. Yellow color in skin or white parts of the eyes.
6. Vomiting with severe headache and a history of a recent head injury.
7. Vomiting or diarrhea that lasts 3 days without improvement.
8. If you are pregnant or have diabetes.
9. Recurrent vomiting and/or diarrhea.

Recurrent diarrhea, constipation, or alternating bouts of both may indicate irritable bowel syndrome (IBS), also known as irritable or spastic colon. This condition, which affects three times as many women as men, is characterized by a disruption of the normal pattern of muscular contractions that move waste through the intestines. Other symptoms include abdominal pain or swelling, feelings of excessive fullness, gas, and painful bowel movements. Since these symptoms can occur with other disorders, diagnosis by a physician is important. The causes of IBS are still under investigation; treatments include stress management, antispasmodic medications, antidepressants, and changes in diet to eliminate foods that provoke symptoms.

HEARTBURN AND INDIGESTION

Indigestion and heartburn are usually a result of irritation of the stomach or the esophagus, the tube that connects the mouth to the stomach. The stomach lining is usually protected from stomach acids, but the esophagus is not. Therefore, if stomach acids "reflux" or back up into the esophagus, the result is usually a burning discomfort beneath the breastbone. The esophagus is normally protected by a muscular valve that allows food to enter the stomach but prevents stomach contents from flowing upward into the esophagus. Certain foods (such as chocolate), medications, and smoking can loosen and open this protective sphincter valve. Overeating, lying down, or bending over can also cause the stomach acids to gain access to the sensitive lining of the esophagus.

Self-Assessment

1. Look for a pattern in the symptoms. Do they occur after eating certain foods, taking certain medications, or when you bend over or lie down? Do certain foods or an antacid relieve the symptoms?

2. Observe your bowel movements. Black tarlike stools may indicate bleeding in the stomach (iron tablets and Pepto-Bismol can also cause black stools).

Self-Care

1. Avoid irritants such as smoking, aspirin, ibuprofen, naproxen sodium, alcohol, caffeine (coffee, tea, cola), chocolate, onions, carbonated beverages, spicy or fatty foods, acidic foods (vinegar, citrus fruits, tomatoes), or any other foods that seem to make your symptoms worse.

2. Take nonabsorbable antacids such as Maalox, Mylanta, or Gelusil every 1–2 hours and especially before bedtime, or try an acid reducer, now available without a prescription (Pepcid, Tagamet, or Zantac).

3. Avoid tight clothing.

4. Avoid overeating; eat smaller, more frequent meals.

5. Don't lie down for 1–2 hours after a meal. Elevate the head of your bed with 4- to 6-inch blocks of wood or bricks. Adding extra pillows usually makes things worse by creating a posture that increases pressure on the stomach. Using a waterbed also usually makes reflux worse.

6. If you are overweight in the abdominal area, weight loss may help. Abdominal obesity can increase pressure on the stomach when lying down.

When to Call the Physician

1. Stools that are black and tarlike or vomit that is bloody or contains material that looks like coffee grounds.

2. Severe abdominal or chest pain.

3. Pain that goes through to the back.

4. No relief from antacids.

5. Symptoms lasting longer than 3 days.

Recurrent or persistent abdominal pain may be a symptom of an ulcer, a raw area in the lining of the stomach or duodenum (the first part of the small intestine). About 1 in 5 men and 1 in 10 women develop an ulcer at some time in their lives. Most ulcers are linked to infection with the bacterium *Helicobacter pylori*; people who regularly take nonsteroidal anti-inflammatory drugs like aspirin or ibuprofen are also at risk for ulcers because these drugs irritate the lining of the stomach. *H. pylori* infection is relatively easy to diagnose and treat, and other medications are available to treat ulcers linked to other causes. Many of the self-care measures described above are also frequently recommended for people with ulcers.

HEADACHE

Headache is one of the most common symptoms. There are three major types of headache: muscle tension (the most common type), vascular (related to the blood vessels), and sinus (involving blocked sinus cavities). Muscle tension headaches are often due to emotional stress or physical stress, such as poor posture. The muscles in the neck, scalp, and jaws tighten, producing a dull, aching sensation or band of tension around the head. Vascular headaches, which include the common migraine, are thought to be due to a constriction and then dilation of blood vessels in the head; they are more common in women than in men. Vascular headaches are usually severe, one-sided, throbbing headaches often associated with nausea, vomiting, and visual disturbances (flashing lights or stars). Sinus headaches are caused by blockage of the sinus cavities with resulting pressure and pain in the cheeks, forehead, and upper teeth. These headaches are often associated with nasal congestion. Sometimes a combination of these types of headaches will occur. Headache caused by elevated blood pressure is very uncommon and occurs only with very high pressures.

Self-Assessment

1. Take your temperature. The presence of fever may indicate a sinus infection. Fever, severe headache, and a very stiff neck suggest meningitis, a rare but serious infection around the brain and spinal cord.

2. Tap with your fingers over the sinus cavities in your cheeks and forehead. If this causes increased pain, it may indicate a sinus infection.

3. For recurrent headaches, keep a headache journal. Record how often and when your headaches occur, associated symptoms, activities that precede the headache, and your food and beverage intake. Look for patterns that may provide clues to the cause(s) of your headaches.

Self-Care

1. Try applying ice packs or heat on your neck and head.

2. Gently massage the muscles of your neck and scalp.

3. Try deep relaxation or breathing exercises.

4. Take aspirin or aspirin substitute for pain relief. Recently, over-the-counter products containing a combination of aspirin, acetaminophen, and caffeine were approved by the FDA for treating migraines.

5. If pain is associated with nasal congestion, try a decongestant medication like pseudoephedrine.

6. Try to avoid emotional and physical stressors (like poor posture and eyestrain).

7. Try avoiding foods that may trigger headaches, such as aged cheeses, chocolate, nuts, red wine, alcohol, avocados, figs, raisins, and any fermented or pickled foods.

When to Call the Physician

1. Unusually severe headache.

2. Headache accompanied by fever and a very stiff neck.

3. Headache with sinus pain, tenderness, and fever.

4. Severe headache following a recent head injury.

5. Headache associated with slurred speech, visual disturbance, or numbness or weakness in the face, arms, or legs.

6. Headache persisting longer than 3 days.

7. Recurrent unexplained headaches.

8. Increasing severity or frequency of headaches.

9. Severe migraine headaches. In recent years, many new prescription medications have been approved for the prevention and treatment of migraines.

LOW-BACK PAIN

Pain in the lower back is a very common condition; it is most often due to a strain of the muscles and ligaments along the spine, often triggered by bending, lifting, or other activity. Low-back pain can also result from bone growths (spurs) irritating the nerves along the spine or pressure from ruptured or protruding discs, the "shock absorbers" between the vertebrae. Sometimes back pain is caused by an infection or stone in the kidney. Fortunately, however, simple muscular strain is the most common cause of low-back pain and can usually be effectively self-treated.

Self-Assessment

1. Take your temperature. Back pain with high fever may indicate a kidney or other infection.

2. Check for blood in your urine or frequent, painful urination, which may also indicate a kidney problem.

3. Observe for tingling or pain traveling down one or both legs below the knee with bending, coughing, or sneezing. These symptoms suggest a disc problem.

Self-Care

1. Lie on your back or in any comfortable position on the floor or a firm mattress, with knees slightly bent and supported by a pillow. Rest for 24 hours or longer if the pain persists.

2. Use ice packs on the painful area for the first 24 hours, and then continue with cold or change to heat, whichever gives more relief.

3. Take aspirin or aspirin substitute for pain relief as needed.

4. After the acute pain has subsided, begin gentle back and stomach exercises. Practice good posture and lifting techniques to protect your back. Try to resume gentle, everyday activities like walking as soon as possible. Bed rest beyond 24–48 hours is no longer advised. To learn more about proper back exercises and use of your back, consult a physical therapist or your physician.

When to Call the Physician

1. Back pain following a severe injury such as a car crash or fall.

2. Back pain radiating down the leg below the knee on one or both sides.

3. Persistent numbness, tingling, or weakness in the legs or feet.

4. Loss of bladder or bowel control.

5. Back pain associated with high fever (above 101°F or 38.3°C), frequent or painful urination, blood in the urine, or severe abdominal pain.

6. Back pain that does not improve after 1 week of self-care.

STRAINS AND SPRAINS

Missteps, slips, falls, and athletic misadventures can result in a variety of strains, sprains, and fractures. A strain occurs when you overstretch a muscle or tendon (the connective tissue that attaches muscle to bone). Sprains are caused by overstretching or tearing ligaments (the tough fibrous bands that connect bone to bone). Depending on the severity and location, a sprain may actually be more serious than a fracture, because bones generally heal very strongly while ligaments may remain stretched and lax after healing. After a sprain, it may take 6 weeks for the ligament to heal.

After most injuries, you can expect pain and swelling. This is the body's way of immobilizing and protecting the injured part so that healing can take place. The goal of self-assessment is to determine whether you have a minor injury that you can safely self-treat or a more serious injury to an artery, nerve, or bone that should be treated by your physician.

Self-Assessment

1. Watch for coldness, blue color, or numbness in the limb beyond the injury. These may be signs of damage to an artery or a nerve.

2. Look for signs of a possible fracture, which would include a misshapen limb, reduced length of the limb on the injured side compared to the uninjured side, an inability to move or bear weight, a grating sound with movement of the injured area, extreme tenderness at one point along the injured bone as you press with your fingers, or a sensation of snapping at the time of the injury.

3. Gently move the injured area through its full range of motion. Immobility or instability suggests a more serious injury.

Self-Care

1. Immediately immobilize, protect, and rest the injured area until you can bear weight on it or move it without pain. Remember: If it hurts, don't do it.

2. To decrease pain and swelling, immediately apply ice (a cold pack or ice wrapped in a cloth) for 15 minutes every hour for the first 24–48 hours. Then apply ice or heat as needed for comfort.

3. Immediately elevate the injured limb above the level of your heart for the first 24 hours to decrease swelling.

4. Immobilize and support the injured area with an elastic wrap or splint. Be careful not to wrap so tightly as to cause blueness, coldness, or numbness.

5. Take aspirin or aspirin substitute for pain as needed.

When to Call the Physician

1. An injury that occurred with great force such as a high fall or motor vehicle crash.

2. Hearing or feeling a snap at the time of the injury.

3. A limb that is blue, cold, or numb.

4. A limb that is bent, twisted, or crooked.

5. Tenderness at specific points along a bone.

6. Inability to move the injured area.

7. A wobbly, unstable joint.

8. Marked swelling of the injured area.

9. Inability to bear weight after 24 hours.

10. Pain that increases or lasts longer than 4 days.

CUTS AND SCRAPES

Cuts and scrapes are common disruptions of the body's skin. Fortunately, the vast majority of these wounds are minor and don't require stitches, antibiotics, or a physician's care. An abrasion involves a scraping away of the superficial layers of skin. Abrasions, though less serious, are often more painful than cuts because they disrupt more skin nerves. There are two types of cuts: lacerations (narrow slices of the skin) and puncture wounds (stabs into deeper tissues).

Normal healing of a cut or abrasion is a remarkable process. After the bleeding stops, small amounts of serum, a clear yellowish fluid, may leak from the wound. This fluid is rich in antibodies to help prevent an infection. Redness and swelling may normally occur as more blood is shunted to the area, bringing white blood cells and nutrients to speed healing. There may also be some swelling of nearby lymph nodes, which are another part of your body's defense against infection. Finally, a scab forms. This is "nature's bandage," which protects the area while it heals.

The main concerns about cuts are the possibilities of damage to deeper tissues and the risk of infection. Damage to underlying blood vessels may lead to severe bleeding as well as blueness and coldness in areas beyond the wound. Injured nerves may produce numbness and a loss of the ability to move parts of the body beyond the injured area. Damaged muscles, tendons, and ligaments can also result in inability to move areas beyond the cut.

Wound infection usually does not take place until 24–48 hours after an injury. Signs of infection include increasing redness, swelling, pain, pus, and fever. One of the most serious, though fortunately uncommon, complications of puncture wounds is tetanus ("lockjaw"). This bacterial infection thrives in areas not exposed to oxygen, so it is more likely to develop in deep puncture wounds or dirty wounds. Tetanus is not likely to develop in minor cuts or wounds caused by clean objects like knives. You need a tetanus immunization shot following a cut under the following conditions:

- If you have never had the basic series of three tetanus immunization injections.

- If you have a dirty or contaminated wound and it has been longer than 5 years since your last injection.

- If you have a clean, minor wound and it has been longer than 10 years since your last injection.

Self-Assessment

1. Look for warning signs of complications: persistent bleeding, numbness, an inability to move the injured area, or the later development of pus, increasing redness, and fever.

2. Measure the size of the cut. If your cut is shallow, less than an inch long, not in a high-stress area (such as a joint, which bends), and you can easily hold the edges of the wound closed, it probably won't need stitches.

Self-Care

1. Apply direct pressure over the wound until the bleeding stops. The only exception is puncture wounds, which should be encouraged to bleed freely (unless spurting a large amount of blood) for a few minutes to flush out bacteria and debris.

2. Try to remove any dirt, gravel, glass, or foreign material from the wound with tweezers or by gentle scrubbing.

3. Wash the wound vigorously with soap and water, followed by an application of hydrogen peroxide solution as an antiseptic.

4. If it is an abrasion, cover the area with a sterile adhesive bandage until a scab forms. For minor lacerations, close the cut with a butterfly bandage or a sterile adhesive tape, drawing the edges close together but not overlapping. If there is an extra flap of clean skin, leave it in place for extra protection. Do not attempt to close a puncture wound. Instead, soak the wound in warm water for 15 minutes several times a day for several days. Soaking helps keep the wound open and thus prevents infection.

When to Call the Physician

1. Bleeding that can't be controlled with direct pressure.

2. Numbness, weakness, or an inability to move the injured area.

3. Any large, deep wound.

4. A cut in an area that bends and with edges that cannot easily be held together.

5. Cuts on the hands or face unless clean and shallow.

6. A contaminated wound in which you cannot remove the foreign material.

7. Any human or animal bite.

8. If you need a tetanus immunization (see indications noted earlier).

9. Development of increasing redness, swelling, pain, pus, or fever 24 hours or more after the injury.

10. If the wound is not healing well after 3 weeks.

Resources for Self-Care

BOOKS AND AUDIOTAPES

Clarke, P., and S. H. Evans. 1998. *Surviving Modern Medicine: How to Get the Best from Doctors, Family, and Friends.* Piscataway, N.J.: Rutgers University Press. *Provides practical consumer advice for navigating the health care system.*

The Diagram Group. 1999. *Woman's Body: An Owner's Manual.* Chicago: Contemporary Books. *Provides the latest scientific information on many aspects of women's health.*

Griffith, H. W. 1998. *Complete Guide to Prescription and Nonprescription Drugs, 1999 Edition.* New York: Perigee. *A comprehensive guide to side effects, warnings, and precautions for the safe use of over 4000 brand-name and generic drugs.*

Huddleston, P., and C. Northrup. 1998. *Prepare for Surgery, Heal Faster: A Guide to Mind-Body Techniques.* Cambridge, Mass.: Angel River Press. *Presents mind-body techniques to help patients better prepare for surgery; audiotape also available.*

Inlander, C. B. 1997. *The Savvy Medical Consumer.* Rev. ed. Allentown, Pa.: People's Medical Society. *Provides information about getting the most out of medical care; topics range from physician visits to managed care.*

Inlander, C. B., K. Morales, and the People's Medical Society. 1999. *Family Health for Dummies.* Foster City, Calif.: IDG. *Addresses a wide range of health topics.*

Inlander, C., and the People's Medical Society. 1999. *Men's Health for Dummies.* Foster City, Calif.: IDG. *An easy-to-understand reference on a variety of health topics.*

Isler, C. 1997. *The Patient's Guide to Medical Terminology.* Los Angeles: Health Information Press. *A layperson's guide to over 1500 medical terms and abbreviations.*

Kemper, D. W. 1997. *Healthwise Handbook: A Self-Care Manual for You.* Boise, Id.: Healthwise. *Practical guidelines for home care of common medical problems in adults and children.*

Patient Comfort, Inc. 141618 Tyler Foote Rd., Nevada City, CA 95959 (800-213-3223; http://www.patientcomfort.com). *Provides a selection of audiotapes for surgical preparation.*

The PDR Family Guide Encyclopedia of Medical Care. 1999. New York: Ballantine. *A home guide to hundreds of medical problems.*

Rybacki, J. J., and J. W. Long. 1999. *The Essential Guide to Prescription Drugs.* New York: HarperCollins. *A comprehensive drug reference that includes descriptions of how each drug works, possible side effects, and other precautions.*

Shapiro, M. B. 1998. *What You Need to Know About Surgery.* Freedom, Calif.: Crossing Press. *Describes tests, anesthesia and other medications, and what to expect while in the hospital; also includes a medical dictionary.*

Sullivan, D. 1998. *The American Pharmaceutical Association's Guide to Prescription Drugs.* New York: Signet. *A reference covering the most commonly prescribed drugs.*

U.S. Pharmacopeia. 1998. *Consumer Reports Complete Drug Reference.* Yonkers, N.Y.: Consumers Union. *A comprehensive reference book on medications available in the United States.*

Vickery, D. M., and J. F. Fries. 1996. *Take Care of Yourself: The Consumer's Guide to Medical Care,* 6th ed. Reading, Mass.: Addison-Wesley. *An excellent self-care guide that includes easy-to-follow decision charts outlining when to see a physician and how to apply safe and effective home treatment.*

White, B., and E. Madara, eds. 1998. *The Self-Help Sourcebook: Your Guide to Community and Online Support Groups,* 5th ed. Denville, N.J.: Northwest Covenant Medical Center. *Includes listings for groups in many different categories and advice on how to develop your own group.*

See Chapter 1 for a list of general health-related newsletters and magazines.

HEALTH INFORMATION CENTERS

Consumer Information Center (P.O. Box 100, Pueblo, CO 81002, 888-8PUEBLO; http://www.pueblo.gsa.gov).

National Health Information Center (P.O. Box 1133, Washington, DC 20013, 800-336-4797; http://nhic-nt.health.org or http://www.healthfinder.gov).

Office of Minority Health Resource Center (P.O. Box 37337, Washington, DC 20013, 800-444-6472; http://www.omhrc.gov).

SELF-HELP AND MUTUAL AID GROUPS

Self-help groups provide information and peer support for nearly every conceivable medical condition or problem. Look in the telephone book for a local chapter, or contact one of the following self-help clearinghouses for the names of self-help groups in your community.

American Self-Help Clearinghouse (St. Clare's Hospital, 25 Pocono Road, Denville, NJ 07834, 973-625-3037; http://www.cmhc.com/selfhelp).

National Self-Help Clearinghouse (25 West 43rd Street, Room 620, New York, NY 10036, 212-354-8525; http://www.selfhelpweb.org).

TELEPHONE HOTLINES

For hotlines relating to the main topics of this text, see the For More Information sections at the end of each chapter. Additional hotlines are listed below. Extensive lists of health-related hotlines and clearinghouses are available from the National Health Information Center (800-336-4797; http://nhic-nt.health.org or http://www.healthfinder.gov), the American Self-Help Clearinghouse (973-625-3037; http://www.cmhc.com/selfhelp/fonenums/helpline.htm), and Johns Hopkins Info-Net (http://infonet.welch.jhu.edu/advocacy.html).

Blindness: American Foundation for the Blind, 800-232-5463; National Library Service for the Blind and Physically Handicapped, 800-424-8567; Recording for the Blind and Dyslexic, 800-221-4792.

Chronic fatigue syndrome: CFIDS Association, 800-442-3437.

Consumer products: U.S. Consumer Product Safety Commission, 800-638-2772; FDA National Hotline, 888-463-6332.

Deafness/hearing problems: American Speech Language and Hearing Association, 800-638-8255; Dial-a-Hearing Screening Test, 800-222-EARS; National Institute on Deafness and Other Communication Disorders, 800-241-1044, 800-241-1055 (TTY).

Down syndrome: National Down Syndrome Society, 800-221-4602.

Endometriosis: Endometriosis Association, 800-992-3636.

Epilepsy: Epilepsy Foundation of America, 800-EFA-1000; Epilepsy Information Service, 800-642-0500.

Gambling: National Council on Compulsive Gambling, 800-522-4700.

Headache: National Headache Foundation, 800-843-2256.

Immunization: National Immunizations Information Hotline, 800-232-2522, 800-232-0233 (Spanish).

Incontinence: Incontinence Information Center, 800-543-9632.

Irritable bowel syndrome: International Foundation for Functional Gastrointestinal Disorders, 888-964-2001.

Kidney disease: American Kidney Fund, 800-638-8299; National Kidney Foundation, 800-622-9010.

Lung disease/respiratory disorders: Lung Line, sponsored by the National Jewish Medical and Research Center, 800-222-LUNG, 800-552-LUNG (recorded information, 24 hours); American Lung Association, 800-LUNG-USA.

Lupus: Lupus Foundation of America, 800-558-0121.

Lyme disease: Lyme Disease Foundation, 800-886-LYME.

Multiple sclerosis: Multiple Sclerosis Foundation, 800-441-7055.

Rare disorders: National Organization for Rare Disorders, 800-999-6673.

Self-abuse and self-mutilation: SAFE (Self-Abuse Finally Ends), 800-DONT-CUT.

Sickle cell disease: Sickle Cell Disease Association of America, 800-421-8453.

Spinal cord injury: National Spinal Cord Injury Hotline, 800-526-3456.

Sports and sports injuries: Women's Sports Foundation, 800-227-3988.

Sudden infant death: American SIDS Institute, 800-232-SIDS; National SIDS Resource Center, 703-821-8955.

ELECTRONIC RESOURCES

A wide variety of electronic resources is available on health-related topics, including research aids, self-care guides, and support networks.

OPACs (Online Public Access Catalogs)

OPACs are library catalogs displayed on a computer terminal; their use can increase the speed and scope of research into a particular topic. Many libraries also include periodical indexes, full-text encyclopedias, and other databases and documents on their OPACs. Ask the reference librarian what services are available at your college or community library.

CD-ROM (Compact Disc–Read Only Memory)

CD-ROMs can hold large amounts of information, including text, sound, and video. Databases containing bibliographic references and abstracts or the complete text of journal and newspaper articles are often available in libraries on CD-ROM. Health-related databases include MEDLINE, Consumer Health and Nutrition Index, Health Reference Center, and Health Source. For a fee, document delivery services can provide you with copies of articles or periodicals not available at your local library.

Reference books such as the *Mayo Clinic Family Health Book* and the *Physician's Desk Reference* are also available on CD-ROM, as are multimedia self-care guides such as *Family Doctor* (Creative Multimedia), *Family Medical Guide* (DK Multimedia), *Vital Signs: The Good Health Resource* (Texas Caviar), *Home Medical Advisor Pro* (Pixel Perfect), and *Medical Housecall* (Applied Medical Infomatics). For more on CD-ROMs, consult the annual directory *CD-ROMs in Print* (Gale Research).

The Internet

The Internet is a global network of computers that links together commercial online communication services, such as America Online and CompuServe, with tens of thousands of university, government, and corporate networks. The Internet is composed of many parts, including World Wide Web documents, e-mail, newsgroups, mailing lists, and chat rooms. With access to the Internet, you can obtain in-depth information about hundreds of wellness topics and keep up with the latest research; you can also connect with people worldwide who share a medical problem or another challenge to wellness.

To reach the Internet, you need a computer, a modem, access to the network through a provider, and browser software, which allows you to navigate. Internet access is often available to students at little or no cost through college computer centers. If you have to obtain access through a commercial Internet service provider, choose one that suits your needs and your budget. Bare-bones access is available at low cost, but you may need to obtain additional software, including a browser such as Netscape Navigator. Online services such as America Online, CompuServe, and Microsoft Network are often more expensive, but they provide all the necessary software and offer many features, including e-mail, newsgroups, and Web browsers.

The World Wide Web The World Wide Web is made up of computer files called Web pages or Web sites that have been created by individuals, companies, and organizations. The Web is considered a user-friendly part of the Internet because it offers easy access and navigation and has media capabilities, such as audio, video, and animation.

Each Web site is identified by an address or uniform resource locator (URL), such as http://www.healthfinder.gov. To access a site, you can type the URL into the appropriate screen of your browser or you can click on a *hyperlink,* a shortcut to another Web page or to a different part of the current page. When you view a Web page, hyperlinks may appear as images or as text that is a different color and/or is underlined. By clicking on links, you can jump quickly from one Web site to related sites, even if they are located on the other side of the world.

To search out information on a particular topic, you need to use a search engine, such as one of the following:

AltaVista	http://www.altavista.com
Excite	http://www.excite.com
Hotbot	http://www.hotbot.com
Infoseek	http://infoseek.go.com
Lycos	http://www.lycos.com
Magellan	http://magellan.excite.com
Northern Light	http://www.northernlight.com
WebCrawler	http://webcrawler.com
Yahoo!	http://www.yahoo.com

These search engines search a unique database of Web pages, so you will obtain different results from different search engines. A meta-search engine like one of the following simultaneously submits your search to multiple search engines:

Dogpile	http://www.dogpile.com
Inference Find	http://www.infind.com
MetaCrawler	http://www.go2net.com/search.html

To use a search engine, you may need to enter key words or navigate through a series of increasingly more specific directories; some search engines offer both key word and directory searches. Within seconds, the search engine will generate a list of sites (with hyperlinks) that match your search parameters, often with a brief description of each site.

When you are searching, it's best to make your searches as specific as possible. Searching for key words such as "AIDS" or "cancer" will yield thousands or even millions of matches. Use more specific phrases, such as "HIV vaccine" or "cervical cancer treatment." If the search engine has a help section, take a look at it. Different engines have different rules for how best to enter key words. For example, you may need to enclose phrases in quotation marks or put plus or minus signs between words to obtain an appropriate result. If you don't find the information you are looking for using one search engine, try another. In addition, there are search engines and directories that specialize in health and medicine:

Achoo	http://www.achoo.com
Health A to Z	http://www.healthatoz.com
Health on the Net	http://www.hon.ch
Karolinska Institutet	http://micf.mic.ki.se/Diseases
Medical Matrix	http://www.medmatrix.org
MedWeb	http://www.medweb.emory.edu
MedWorld: Medbot	http://www-med.stanford.edu/medworld/medbot
NLM Medline Plus	http://www.nlm.nih.gov/medlineplus

Listed below is a sampling of Web sites that contain information on a variety of wellness topics and/or links to many other appropriate sites. For Web sites dealing with a specific health topic, refer to the For More Information section in the appropriate chapter. Hyperlinks to all the sites in this text can be accessed from the *Core Concepts* Web page (http://www.mayfieldpub.com/insel).

American Academy of Family Physicians
http://www.aafp.org

American Medical Association Health Insight
http://www.ama-assn.org/consumer.htm

CDC Health Information A to Z
http://www.cdc.gov/health/diseases.htm

Clinical Tool's Health-Center.Com
http://www.health-center.com

Dr. Koop's Community
http://www.drkoop.com

Duke University Healthy Devil On-Line
http://gilligan.mc.duke.edu/h-devil

Go Ask Alice
http://www.goaskalice.columbia.edu

Healthfinder
http://www.healthfinder.gov

HealthTouch Online
http://www.healthtouch.com

HealthWorld Online
http://www.healthworld.com

InteliHealth: Johns Hopkins Health Information
http://www.intelihealth.com

iVillage Better Health
http://www.betterhealth.com

Mayo Health Oasis
http://www.mayohealth.org

MedicineNet
http://www.medicinenet.com

National Center for Health Statistics
http://www.cdc.gov/nchswww

National Women's Health Resource Center
http://www.healthywomen.org

NetWellness
http://www.netwellness.org

New York Online Access to Health
http://www.noah.cuny.edu

NIH Health Information Index
http://www.nih.gov/health

Thrive Online
http://www.thriveonline.com

U.S. Consumer Gateway: Health
http://www.consumer.gov/health.htm

WellnessWeb
http://wellweb.com

Newsgroups Newsgroups consist of archived messages, articles, and postings about a particular topic; they are similar to bulletin boards. Commercial online services maintain members-only newsgroups, but many more are available on the Internet. To locate a newsgroup on a particular topic, use a search engine or visit one of several Web sites devoted to newsgroups:

Deja.com	http://www.deja.com
Reference.COM	http://www.reference.com

You are free to browse any newsgroup's articles. Postings on related topics are often grouped together in a "thread," consisting of an original message that began a discussion and all the replies to that message. A busy newsgroup can receive thousands of postings a day, and older articles are deleted to make room for new ones. If you find an article of interest, print it or save it to your computer—it may be deleted from the newsgroup by your next visit.

In addition to browsing, reading, and saving newsgroup postings, you can also be an active participant. You can reply to a message, either to the person who posted it or to the entire newsgroup, or you can post a new message that starts a new thread of discussion. To ensure that your postings are appropriate, it's often a good idea to observe a newsgroup for a while or look at its "frequently asked questions" page prior to becoming an active member.

Listserv Mailing Lists

Listservs are similar to newsgroups, except that messages are delivered by e-mail to all subscribers to the mailing list rather than posted at a public site. Once you subscribe to a mailing list, you receive messages posted by other subscribers and you can post your own messages. As with newsgroups, it's a good idea to read messages for a while before joining the discussion. You can stop subscribing to a mailing list at any time.

To locate listservs for a particular topic, do a key-word search using a search engine by entering the topic and the word *listserv*. There are also several search engines and Web sites that deal specifically with mailing lists, including the following:

Liszt	http://www.liszt.com
InterLinks	http://alabanza.com/kabacoff/Inter-Links
Reference.COM	http://www.reference.com

Real-Time Communication: Chat Rooms

With access to the Internet, you may also have the opportunity to participate in real-time communication with people from around the world. You can sign on to a particular chat group and communicate with others who are signed on to the same group at that time. You can have a "public" conversation, in which everyone in the chat room is included, or a "private" conversation between you and one other person. Many chat groups have a moderator who can kick people off and/or refuse them further access if they don't behave appropriately. For reasons of privacy and security, many people suggest that chat room participants avoid divulging too much personal information.

Evaluating Information from the Internet

Anyone can post information and advice on the Internet—true or false, good or bad. When evaluating information from the Internet, ask the following questions:

- *What is the source of the information? Who is the author or sponsor of the Web page?* Web sites maintained by government agencies, professional associations, or established academic or medical institutions are likely to present trustworthy information. Many other groups and individuals post accurate information, but it is important to watch your sources carefully. Many sites will describe their sponsor on the home page; alternatively, they may have an "about us" or "who we are" link that provides this information. Take a look at the backgrounds, qualifications, and credentials of the people who are behind the information at the site. Beware of sites that don't indicate

the sources of the information they post; if you don't know where it comes from, you can't assess its validity.

As you click on links and move from page to page, also pay attention to where you are. Even if you start out at a trustworthy site, the click of a button can catapult you into a completely different site. Learn how to read your current Web address so that you know when you've left one site and entered another. Look at the abbreviation in the server name in the URL, which will change according to the sponsor's purpose—for example, "org" for organizational, "gov" for governmental, "edu" for educational, and "com" for commercial.

- *How often is the site updated?* Most Web pages will indicate the date of their most recent modifications. Major organizations may update their Web sites on a daily or weekly basis. Look for sites that are updated frequently.

- *What is the purpose of the page? Does the site promote particular products or procedures? Are there obvious reasons for bias?* The same common sense you'd use to evaluate any factual claim applies to the Internet. Be wary of sites that sell specific products, use testimonials as evidence, appear to have a social or political agenda, or ask for money. Many sites sponsored by commercial companies and lay organizations do provide sound, useful information; however, it's a good idea to consider possible sources of bias in the information they present.

- *What do other sources say about a topic?* To get a broad perspective on a piece of information, check out other online sources or ask a professional. You are more likely to obtain and recognize quality information if you use several different sources. Be wary of claims that appear at only one site.

- *Does the site conform to any set of guidelines or criteria for quality and accuracy?* A number of organizations, including the American Medical Association and the Health on the Net Foundation, have developed codes of conduct for health-related sites; these codes include criteria such as use of information from respected sources and disclosure of the site's sponsors. Look for sites that identify themselves as conforming to some code or set of principles. (A recent article in the *British Medical Journal* reviewed many of these sets of criteria: Kim, P., et al. 1999. Published criteria for evaluating health-related Web sites: Review. *British Medical Journal* 318: 647–649; http://www.bmj.com/cgi/content/full/318/7184/647.)

- *Is the site easy to use? Does it have links to other sites?* In addition to strong content, good Web pages should be easy to use, be clearly organized, and have a good search capability.

For more on finding and evaluating online wellness-related information, check out the following Web sites:

California Medical Association (select Health Care Links)
  http://www.cmanet.org
Oncolink Source Reliability Information
  http://www.oncolink.upenn.edu/resources/reliability
Science Panel on Interactive Communication and Health
  http://www.scipich.org
Search Engine Watch
  http://www.searchenginewatch.com
UC Berkeley Library Internet Tutorial
  http://www.lib.berkeley.edu/TeachingLib/Guides/Internet/FindInfo.html

Index

Boldface numbers indicate pages on which glossary definitions appear.

"*t*" indicates that the information is in a table.

AA (Alcoholics Anonymous), 19, 236–237, 261–262
abortifacient, **138**
abortion, 162–181, **164**
   complications of, 175–177
   current trends, 170–172
   deaths, risk of, 132*t*, 176*t*
   decision making and, 177–178
   history in the U.S., 164
   legal status, 164–165
   methods of, 172, 174–175
   moral considerations, 165–166, 167
   personal considerations, 169–170, 177
   public opinion about, 166, 168–169
   rates, 171, 173
   worldwide daily occurrence, 132*t*
absorption of alcohol, 248–249
abstinence from sex, 123, **146–148**, 149*t*
abuse
   abusive partners, recognizing potential for, 625
   of children, 626–627, 629
   domestic violence, 625–626
   elder abuse, 537
academic stressors, 36
accidents. *See* unintentional injuries
Accutane, birth defects and, 202, 203*t*
acetaldehyde, 250
acetaminophen, 253, 482
acid precipitation, 650–**651**
acquaintance rape. *See* date rape
acquired immunity, **470**, 471
acquired immunodeficiency syndrome. *See* AIDS
ACTH (adrenocorticotropic hormone), **27**
active immunity, 473
acupressure (shiatsu), 594, **595**
acupuncture, 594, **595**
acyclovir, 483, 509
addiction/dependency, **217**, 221
   alcohol, **257–258**, 259–264
   behavior change strategy for, 242
   characteristics of people with, 217–218
   codependency and, 236, 238
   development of, 217
   drugs, 219–227, 234–240
   families and, 234–235
   gambling, 218
   Internet, 219
   nicotine, 274–275
   physical, **221**
   prevention of, 237–239
   sex and love, 218–219
   spending or shopping, 219
   symptoms of, 216–217, 220–221, 239
   treatment of, 236–237
   See also alcoholism; psychoactive drugs; *specific drug names*
additives and preservatives in foods, 333–334, 452–453
Adequate Intake (AI), 314
adoption, 171
adrenal glands, **27**, **107**
adrenocorticotropic hormone (ACTH), **27**
advance directives, **552–555**
advertising
   alcohol, 266

nonprescription medication, 573
   prescription drugs, 573
   tobacco, 276–277, 288
   See also media
AEDs (automatic external defibrillators), 632
aerobic exercise. *See* cardiorespiratory endurance
AFP (alpha-fetoprotein) screening, **199**
African Americans
   alcohol abuse, 263
   assault rates, 623
   asthma and, 475
   cardiovascular disease among, 414
   death, leading causes of, 9
   diabetes and, 187
   fetal alcohol syndrome (FAS) rates, 200
   health issues for, 9
   heart disease death rate, 415
   HIV infection, 496
   homicide rates, 623
   lactose intolerance, 187
   life expectancy, 5
   lupus and women, 484
   obesity prevalence among women, 375*t*
   prostate cancer rate, 439
   regular physical activity, 343*t*
   sickle-cell disease, 186
   single-parent families, 96
   skin cancer rate, 443
   smokers, percentage of, 278*t*
   thalassemia, 187
African sleeping sickness, **484**
aging, 520–541
   body changes through time, 524–525
   cardiovascular disease and, 410
   dietary challenges for older adults, 326
   driving and, 536
   life-enhancing measures, 523–526
   life expectancy, **532–533**
   ovarian cancer and, 442
   physical changes, 527–529
   prostate cancer and, 439
   psychological and mental changes, 529–532
   sexuality and, 111–112
   social changes, 526–527
AI (Adequate Intake), 314
AIDS, **492-504**
   deaths, 132*t*, 429, 475*t*
   diagnosing, 498
   injecting drug use and, 225, 496, 497, 504
   prevention, 502–504
   reporting of cases, 498
   virus illustrated, 479
   worldwide distribution of, 494
   See also HIV infection
AIDS dementia, 499*t*
air pollution, 453, 646–652
Al-Anon, 262
Alaska Natives. *See* Native Americans
alcohol, 246–271, **249**
   absorption of, 248–249
   abstinence rate, 236
   assessing use of, 12
   behavioral effects, 251*t*
   cancer risk and, 255, 434*t*, 450
   cardiovascular disease risk and, 422
   chemistry of, 248
   chronic use, 254–255
   college student drinking, 217*t*, 259
   colon and rectal cancer, 437
   deaths per year, 274*t*
   diet and, 322
   drunk driving, 253–254, 255, 612
   estrogen levels increased by, 438
   fetal alcohol syndrome (FAS), **200**, **255–256**
   fetus or infant problems, 203*t*

health effects, 251–257
   metabolism of, **249**, 250
   myths about, 250
   nutritional value of, 300
   oral cancer and, 445
   osteoporosis and, 312
   pregnancy and, 185, 200, **255–257**
   responsible use of, 264–267
   triglyceride levels and, 410
alcohol abuse, **257–258**
   aging and, 526
   ethnicity and, 263–264
   gender and, 263
   violence and, 622
   warning signs of, 258
   See also alcoholism; binge drinking
Alcoholics Anonymous, 19, 236–237, 261–262
alcoholism, **257**, 259–263
   causes of, 261
   patterns of, 259
   treatment for, 261–263
   See also alcohol abuse
alcohol poisoning, 252
alendronate, 312
allergen, **474**
allergies, **474**
   indoor air pollution, 651
   stress and, 34
   symptoms of, 483
allied health care providers, **590**, 591
allostatic load, 32
all-terrain vehicle (ATV), **619**
allyl sulfides, potential anticancer effects of, 452*t*
alpha-fetoprotein (AFP) screening, **199**
altered states of consciousness, **233**
alternative medical care, 592–596
Alzheimer's disease, **530**, 531
amenorrhea, **376**, 396
American Cancer Society early detection tests, 456*t*
American Indians. *See* Native Americans
American Public Health Association, 155–156
amino acids, 300, **301**
amnesia (anterograde), date rape drugs, 227
amniocentesis, 198–**199**
amniotic sac, 174, **175**, 196, **197**, 198
amoebic dysentery, **484**
amphetamines, 217*t*, 222, 229–230
anabolic steroids, **357**
anal intercourse, 123–124
anaphylactic shock, 474
androgens, **107**
androgyny, **117**
anemia, 135, 185, **310**, 591
anesthetics, 228, **229**
aneurysm, 420, **421**
angel dust. *See* PCP
anger
   cardiovascular disease and, 410
   and intimate relationships, 87–88
   managing, 411
   and psychological health, 63–64
angina pectoris, 280, **281**, **417**
angiogenesis, 439
angiograms, 418, **419**
angioplasty, 418–419
anorexia nervosa, **395–396**
Antabuse, 250, 262
anti-angiogenesis drugs, 456
antibiotics, 477–478, **582**, 583
   colds and, 482
   fetal or infant problems and, 203*t*
   resistant bacteria, 478, 481
   yeast infections and, 484
antibodies, **468**, 469
   binding with antigen, 470

Braxton Hicks contractions, 194, **195**
BRCA1 and BRCA2 gene, 449, 450
breast cancer, 438–439, 440
    alcohol and, 256
    clinical exam, 456t
    Depo-Provera injections and, 138
    ethnicity and, 9
    genes, 449, 450
    genetic testing for, 450
    hormone therapy and death rates, 530
    incidence and deaths, 435
    oral contraceptives and, 135
    self-exam, 440, 456t
breastfeeding, 209–210
bronchiole, smoker and nonsmoker compared, 283
bronchitis. *See* chronic bronchitis
bubonic plague, **644**
bulbourethral glands, 106–107
bulimia nervosa, **395**, 396
buprenorphine, 236
burial of body, 556–557
burnout, **37**
BV (bacterial vaginosis), 114, **510**, 511

CA 125 tumor marker test, 442
caffeine
    as CNS stimulant, 230–231
    dependence ranking, 222
    eliminating for stress management, 40
    osteoporosis and, 312
    pregnancy and, 185, 202
    sources of, 40, 231t
    strategy for eliminating, 242
calcitonin, 312
calcium
    cardiovascular disease risk reduction, 423
    DRIs for, 316t, 317t
    facts about, 311t
    osteoporosis and, 310, 312
    women and, 324
calendar method, 148
calories
    activities and calorie cost, 360t–361t
    burned by various activities, 387t
    how many are needed, 385
    sources of, 300
    weight management and, 384
Campylobacter jejuni, 332
cancer, 432–463, **435**
    alcohol and, 255, 434t, 450
    benign versus malignant tumors, 434, **435**
    causes of, 434t, 446–454
    common cancers, 436–446
    curing and smoking of foods and, 322–323
    deaths from, 3, 7t, 415, 435, 530
    Depo-Provera injections and, 138
    detecting, 454–455, 456t
    diagnosing, 455
    dietary factors, 304–305, 306, 307, 313, 321,
        322–323, 437, 438, 439, 449–452, 453, 458,
        460, 461
    early detection tests, 456t
    ethnicity and, 9
    exercise and, 346
    incidence of, 436
    living with, 457, 458
    malignant versus benign tumors, 434, **435**
    metastasis, 434–**435**
    microbes that cause, 442
    obesity and, 375
    oral contraceptives and, 135
    preventing, 457–459
    quackery, avoiding, 457
    screening test recommendations, 456, 456t, 459
    smoking and, 281

stress and, 34
support groups, 457, 459
treatments, 455–456
types of, 435–436
visiting a cancer patient, 458
warning signs of, 455
See also specific types of cancer
Candida albicans (yeast infection), 114, 483–484,
    595
cannabis. *See* marijuana and cannabis products
capillaries, **405**
capitation, **599**
capsaicin, potential anticancer effects of, 452t
carbohydrates, 305, 306–**307**, 385
carbon dioxide, 648t
carbon monoxide
    as air pollutant, 647t
    in cigarette smoke, 278–279
    indoor air pollution by, 651
    poisoning from gas, 616
carcinogens, **279**, **436**
    anticarcinogens, **451**
    avoiding, 459
    in cigarette smoke, 278, 279t, 436–437
    DNA mutations and, 449
    environmental tobacco smoke, 285, 437
    ingested chemicals, 452–453
    pollution, 453
    in sidestream smoke, 285
    in the workplace, 454t
    See also cancer
carcinomas, **436**, 444
cardiac myopathy, alcohol and, **255**
cardiology, 591
cardiopulmonary resuscitation (CPR), **417**, 618,
    631–632
cardiorespiratory endurance, **342–343**
    exercise, **351**, 352t, 353–354
    physical activity pyramid, 350
cardiovascular disease, **344**, **405**
    assess your risk for, 427
    dietary factors, 303–304, 306, 307, 313, 321,
        408, 422–423
    exercise and physical activity, 345–346
    reducing your risk, 422–426
    risk factors for, 406–414
    smoking and, 280–281, 406
    statistical overview of, 415
    stress and, 34
    types of, 414–422
    weight cycling and death from, 381
    See also heart disease
cardiovascular health, 402–431
cardiovascular surgery, 591
cardiovascular system, 404–405
    alcohol and, 255, 256
    anorexia nervosa and, 396
carotenoids, **451**, 452t
carotid endarterectomy, 420
carpal tunnel syndrome, **620**
cars. *See* motor vehicles
cataracts, 283, 524, 525
Caucasians
    cystic fibrosis, 186–187
    heart disease death rate, 415
    life expectancy, 5
    regular physical activity, 343t
    smokers, percentage of, 278t
    testicular cancer risk, 446
CAUTION warning signs of cancer, 455
CCR-5 gene and HIV, 499–501
CD4 T cell, **492**
celibacy, **123**
cell-mediated immune response, 470
cellular death, **544**

central nervous system, **227**
central nervous system depressants, 227–228
central nervous system stimulants, 228–231
cerebral cortex, **279**, **525**
cerebral embolism, **419**
cerebral hemorrhage, **419–420**
cerebral thrombosis, **419**
certification of death, 556
cervical cancer, 441, 442
    condoms for protection, 140
    diaphragms with spermicide for protection, 144
    HIV/AIDS and, 499t
    human papillomavirus (HPV), 441, 442, 507
cervical caps, **145**, 157
    costs of, 157t
    death risk from, 137t
    failure rate, 150
    STD protection, 149t
cervical dysplasia, 441
cervix, **104**, 105, 198
    dilation during labor, 206–207
    pregnancy symptoms and, 191, 193
cesarean section, 208, **209**
CFCs (chlorofluorocarbons), **648**, 648t, 649, 650
chancre, **510**
chancroid, **510**, 511
CHD. *See* coronary heart disease (CHD)
chemical pollution, 652–654
chemotherapy, **436**, 437, 439, 442–443, 446, 455
chest breathing, 44
chewing tobacco. *See* spit tobacco
chicken pox, 473t, 479
childbirth, 206–208
    death risk from, 137t, 176t
    deaths, worldwide daily occurrence, 132t
children
    aspirin and Reye's syndrome, 482
    cost of raising a child, 184
    death and loss, coping with, 563
    death, attitudes toward, 545–546
    dietary challenges for, 325–326
    DRIs for, 316t–317t
    and environmental tobacco smoke (ETS), 286
    gender roles, 116
    heart disease in, 421–422
    incest, **629**
    of mothers who smoked, 286–287
    obesity prevalence, 375t
    playground injuries, 617
    RDAs for, 315t
    sexual abuse of, 629
    sexual behavior, 118
    suffocation and choking, 616–617
    violence against, 626–627
children of alcoholics, 260
chiropractic, **593**
chlamydia, **476**, 477, **504–505**
    diaphragms with spermicide for protection, 144
    fetal or infant problems and, 203t
    oral contraceptives, 136
    PID and, 114
Chlamydia pneumoniae and cardiovascular disease,
    412
chloral hydrate, 227
chlorofluorocarbons (CFCs), **648**, 648t, 649, 650
choking, 616–617, 618
cholera, 481, **638**
cholesterol, **303**
    blood cholesterol recommendations, 407, 409t
    cardiovascular disease and, 407–408, 422
    diet and, 303–304, 321–322, 422–423
    exercise and, 346
    managing levels of, 425–426
    obesity and, 375
    screening tests for, 425, 581

cholesterol (continued)
  smoking and, 281, 406
  See also high-density lipoprotein (HDL); low-
      density lipoprotein (LDL)
choline, 317t
chorionic villus sampling (CVS), **199**
chromosomes, **107**, **447**
chronic bronchitis, smoking and, **282**
chronic disease, 3, 5, 34, 119
  See also specific diseases
chronic fatigue syndrome, 483
chronic obstructive lung disease (COLD)
  deaths from, 7t, 415
  smoking and, 281–282
cigarettes. *See* smoking
cigars, 284–285
  carcinogenic particles in smoke, 286
  oral cancer and, 445–446
  See also smoking
cilia, **468**
circumcision, 106, **107**, 116–117
cirrhosis of the liver, 7t, 9, 254, **255**
climate and the greenhouse effect, 648, 649
clinical death, **544**
clinical ecology, **595**
clitoris, **104**, 105
clonazepam, 227
cloning, 192, **193**
Clostridium botulinum, 332
"clot-busting" drugs, 417
CMV. *See Cytomegalovirus* (CMV)
CNS depressants, 227–228
CNS stimulants, 228–231
coarctation of the aorta, 421
cocaine, 228–229
  alcohol and, 253
  college student use of, 217t
  dependence ranking, 222
  fetal or infant problems and, 203t
cocarcinogen, 278, **279**
coccidioidomycosis, 484
codeine, alcohol and, 252
codependency, **236**, 238
coffee, 231t
  See also caffeine
cognitive distortion, **60**, 61
cognitive techniques, 42–43
cohabitation, **90**, 92
coitus, 124
Coke Enders, 19
COLD. *See* chronic obstructive lung disease
colds, 34, 479, 482, 483
cold sores. *See* herpes simplex
college stressors, 36
college students
  alcohol use by, 217t, 259
  binge drinking, 258t
  dietary challenges for, 326
  dietary strategies for, 327
  drug use among, 217t
  STDs and, 508
colon, 301
colon and rectal cancer, 437–438
  dietary fat intake and, 304–305
  exams for, 456t
  exercise and, 346
  hormone therapy and death rates, 530
  incidence and deaths by gender, 435
  screening tests for, 581
colonoscopy, 456t
colorectal cancer. *See* colon and rectal cancer
colostrum, 194, **195**, 209
communication
  contraception discussions, 155
  effective communication tips, 88

family success and, 97
gender and, 87
intimate relationships and, 62–63, 86–89
nonverbal communication, 86–87
with physician, 577–580
sexuality and responsible behavior, 125, 126
for stress management, 39
compulsions, **64**, 65
compulsive addictive behaviors, 218–219
compulsive overeating. *See* binge-eating disorder
computed tomography (CT), 420, **421**, **455**
conception, **187**–189
condoms, 140–143
  for anal intercourse, 123
  costs of, 157t
  death risk from, 137t
  female condoms, 142–143, 157
  genital wart transmission and, 507
  HIV transmission and, 503
  male condoms, **140**–142
  STD protection, 149t
  talking about with your partner, 516
  worldwide use of, 151
congenital heart disease, **421**
congenital malformation, **200**
congestive heart failure, **421**
constipation, insoluble fiber in diet and, 307
consumer guidelines
  agencies to contact for complaints, 597
  birth plans, 208
  condom purchase and use, 142
  contraceptives, 136
  dietary supplement labels, 331
  drug treatment programs, 238
  environmentally friendly product selection, 643
  exercise footwear, 362–363
  fat substitutes, 386
  food labels, 329
  health information evaluation, 14
  health news evaluation, 424
  mental health professionals, choosing, 75
  nursing homes, choosing, 536
  quackery, avoiding, 596
  self-test kits, 517
  smoking cessation, 293
  spermicide purchase and use, 142
  sugar substitutes, 386
  weight-loss programs (commercial), 391
contagious disease, **478**
contaminated food. *See* foodborne illness
contaminated needles, 225, 496, 497, 504
continuation rate, contraceptives, 134, **135**
contraception 130–161
  abstinence, **146**–148
  education for teenagers, 156
  fertility awareness method (FAM), 148
  issues in, 154–156
  myths about, 133
  new methods, 152–154
  principles of, 133–134
  responsible sexual behavior and, 125
  reversible contraceptives, 134–149
  sterilization, **149**–152
contraceptive immunization, 153–154
contraceptives, 132, **133**
  cervical cap, **145**
  choosing a method, 156–158
  continuation rate, 134, **135**
  costs of various methods, 157t
  death risk by method type, 137t
  Depo-Provera injections, 137–138
  diaphragms, **143**–145
  effectiveness of, 133–134
  emergency contraception, 138
  failure rates, 133–134, **135**, 150

female condoms, 142–143
intrauterine devices (IUDs), **138**–139
male condoms, 140–142
Norplant implants, 136–137
oral contraceptives, 134–136, **135**
spermicides, vaginal, 145–146
sponge, **152**, 153, 157
STD protection, 149t
worldwide use of various methods, 151
contract, for behavior change, 16, 17, 369
contractions, 194, 195, **206**
Copper T-380A IUD, 139, 157t
coronary arteries, **405**, 406
coronary bypass surgery, **419**
coronary heart disease (CHD)
  exercise and, 346
  obesity and, 375
  plaque buildup and, 416
  smoking and, 280–**281**
  steroids and, 357
  See also heart disease
coronary occlusion, 416, **417**
coronary thrombosis, 416, **417**
coroner, **556**
corpus luteum, **109**
corpus spongiosum, 106
corticosteroids, 486
cortisol, **27**, 32, 34
Cowper's glands, 106–107
COX-1 and COX-2, 529
CPR, **417**, 618, **631**–632
crabs (pubic lice), **512**
crack, 217t, 222, 228–229
crank, 222, 229–230
"crash diet" caution, 384
C-reactive protein and CVD risk, 412–413
cremation, 556
Creutzfeldt-Jakob disease (CJD), 480
Crixivan (indinavir), 483
cross-training, **366**
cruciferous vegetables, **313**, 319, 452t, 453
cryptosporidiosis, 499t
Cryptosporidium, 481, 638
crystal meth (methamphetamine), 222
CT (computed tomography), 420, **421**, **455**
culture
  abortion and, 173
  alcohol use patterns and, 262
  attitudes toward aging and, 531, 538
  attitudes toward death, 547, 557–558
  body image and, 394
  contraceptive use and, 151
  courtship and, 118
  drug abuse treatment and, 237
  gender roles and, 116–117, 118
  intercultural relationships, 91
  role in health, 8
  stress and, 31
  See also ethnicity
cunnilingus, **123**
CVD. *See* cardiovascular disease
CVS (chorionic villus sampling), **199**
cystic fibrosis, 8, 186–187
cytokines, **456**, **470**, 472
Cytomegalovirus (CMV), 203t, 412, 479, 499t

Daily Values, **317**
Dalkon Shield, 139
D & E (dilation and evacuation), 174, **175**
DASH (diet), 423
date rape, **627**–628
date-rape drugs, **217**t, 227, 228, 627–628
Day of the Dead, 547–548
DDT, 653–654
death rates. *See* mortality rates

deaths
  abortion, 176*t*
  cancer, 434*t*, 435
  cardiovascular disease, 404, 415, 421, 422
  causes of, 3, 4, 7*t*, 9, 274*t*, 415
  drowning, 617
  drug abuse, 235
  falls, 614
  firearms, 623
  foodborne illness in U.S., 330
  hepatitis B and C, 481
  infectious diseases, worldwide, 475*t*
  injuries, 609*t*
  sexual behavior, 132*t*, 274*t*
  See also dying and death; infant mortality; mortality rates
decision making
  about abortion, 177–178
  abstinence from sex, 147
  sexual, 119, 121
  and unintended pregnancy, 177–178
deep breathing technique, 44, 45
deep muscle relaxation, 43
deer tick (*Ixodes*), 476, 477
DEET, 445, 477
defense mechanisms, 60, 62*t*
defibrillators, 632
delirium tremens (DTs), 260, **261**
dementia, 499*t*, **529**–530
demoralization, 59–60, 66
dendrite, **525**
denigration, 62*t*
dental diseases, 283, 396, 412, 524, 579
  See also oral cancer
dentists (D.D.S. or D.M.D.), **590**, 591
deoxyribonucleic acid. *See* DNA
dependence. *See* addiction/dependency
depersonalization, 223, **230**, 231
Depo-Provera injections, 137–138, 157*t*
depressants, **227**
depression, **66**–68
  aging and, 526, 530, 532
  alcoholism and, 261
  cardiovascular disease and, 410
  eating disorders and, 396
  exercise and, 347
  genes and, 70
  obesity and, 376
  osteoporosis and, 312
  postpartum depression, **210**
  self-test for, 67
  stress and, 34
  treatments for, 68
  See also anti-depressant drugs; suicide
DES daughters, 186, 189, 443
DES sons, 189, 443, 446
Dexedrine, 229
diabetes, 377
  cardiovascular disease and, 409
  deaths from, 7*t*, 415
  diet and nutrition for, 326
  erectile dysfunction and, 115
  ethnicity and, 9
  exercise and, 346
  fetal or infant problems and, 203*t*
  genes and, 187
  obesity and, 375
  pregnancy and, 185, 199, 377
  prevention, 377
  smoking and, 283
  stress and, 34
  treatment for, 377
  types of, 377
  warning signs of, 377
  weight distribution and, 376

Dia de los Muertos, 547–548
diaphragms, **143**–145, 157
  costs of, 157*t*
  death risk from, 137*t*
  failure rate, 150
  STD protection, 149*t*
diastole, **405**
diet
  aging and, 524–525
  assess your diet, 324–325
  breast cancer and, 438
  cancer prevention and, 458
  cancer risk and, 434*t*, 449–452
  cardiovascular disease risk reduction, 422–423
  changing your diet, 336
  for college students, 327
  colon and rectal cancer, 437
  diabetes prevention, 377
  exercise and, 363–364
  food group serving suggestions, 317–320
  Food Guide Pyramid, **313**–314
  pancreatic cancer and, 446
  phytochemicals, 452*t*
  prostate cancer and, 439
  reducing saturated fat in diet, 428–429
  vegetarian, 323
  weight management and, 384–385
  See also nutrition
Dietary Approaches to Stop Hypertension (DASH), 423
Dietary fiber, **307**
  breast cancer and, 438
  cancer risk and, 450–451
  colon and rectal cancer, 437
  increasing for CVD risk reduction, 422
Dietary Guidelines for Americans, 314, **315**, 320–323
Dietary Reference Intakes (DRIs), **313**
dietary supplements, 314–317, 327–331
  anabolic steroids, **357**
  FDA and, 330
  iron supplement caution, 413
  reading the labels, 331
  for vitamins and minerals, 314–317
  for weight loss, 390
diethylstilbestrol. *See* DES daughters; DES sons
dieting
  books about, 389–390
  as cause of weight problems, 381–382
  "crash diet" caution, 384
  high-protein diet caution, 389–390
  rates of, 393
  "yo-yo dieting," 381
  See also eating disorders
diet pills and aids, 390–391
digestion, 300, **301**
digestive system, 254, 256, 301, 525
digital rectal exam, 456*t*
dilation and evacuation (D & E), 174, **175**
diphtheria vaccine, 473*t*
disabilities
  exercise and, 348
  sexuality and, 119
disease prevention, 13, 345–346
displacement, 62*t*
distress, **32**
disulfiram, 250, 262
diversity. *See* culture; ethnicity; gender; socioeconomic status
diverticulitis, **307**
divorce, 94–95, 96
DMT, 232, 233
DNA, **447**, 448–449
domestic violence, 625–626
donepezil, 531

dose-response function, 224, **225**, 253
douche, **145**, 506
Down syndrome, 185, 198–199
drinking water contamination, 481, 638–640
DRIs. *See* Dietary Reference Intakes (DRIs)
driving. *See* motor vehicles
drug abuse
  addictive behavior, 216–219, **217**
  changing your habits, 242
  dependence rankings for various drugs, 222
  economic cost of, 234
  Native Americans and treatment programs, 237
  preventing, 237, 239
  problem assessment, 224
  society and families, impact on, 234–235
  tactics and tips for dealing with, 239
  treatment for dependence, 236–237, 238
  See also addiction/dependency; psychoactive drugs
drugs and medications, 583–584
  abortion, drugs to induce, 175
  adverse reactions to, 583
  alcohol abuse, 250, 262–263
  Alzheimer's disease, 531
  aspirin for CVD, 413, 426
  caffeine in, 231*t*
  cancer, new and experimental drugs, 456
  erectile dysfunction, 115
  fetus or infant problems with, 203*t*
  generic drugs, 584
  HIV infection, 498–502
  home self-care kit contents, 576*t*
  labels on prescription drugs, 584
  nicotine withdrawal, 293
  obesity and weight loss, 391–392
  off-label use, 584
  osteoarthritis, 529
  osteoporosis, 312
  overprescribing of, 583
  over-the-counter (OTC) medication, **572**–575
  pregnancy and, 185, 200, 202
  sexual dysfunction and, 114
  tips for taking, 583–584
  viral illnesses, 483
  weight loss, 390–391
  See also antibiotics; anti-depressant drugs; chemotherapy; psychoactive drugs; *specific drug names*
drug substitution programs, 236
drug testing in the workplace, 235–236
drunk driving, 253–254, 255, 612
DTs (delirium tremens), 260, **261**
dual disorders, **223**, 261
dying and death, 542–567
  attitudes toward death, 545–549
  body disposition, 556–558
  certification of death, 556
  death defined, 544
  Kübler-Ross on, 558–559
  life-threatening illness, 558–560
  loss, coping with, 560–563
  planning for death, 549–558
  "right to die," 550–552, 553
  supporting a dying person, 559–560
  survivors, tasks for, 558
  where to die, 549–550
  See also deaths
dysentery, amoebic, **484**
dysmenorrhea, 109–110

EAR (Estimated Average Requirement), 314
ears and noise pollution, 655–656
  See also hearing loss
eating disorders, **393**–397
  anorexia nervosa, **395**–396

eating disorders (*continued*)
  binge-eating disorder, **395**, 396–397
  bulimia nervosa, **395**, 396
  factors in developing, 395
  stress and, 34
  treating, 397
eating habits, 383, 384–385
ebola hemorrhagic fever, 480
EBV. *See* Epstein-Barr virus
ECG (electrocardiogram), **351**, **418**, **419**
eclampsia, **205**
E. coli, 332, 334, 478, 480, 481
ecosystems, **644**, 645
ECT (electroconvulsive therapy), 68
ectopic pregnancy, 204, **205**
  chlamydia and, 504
  condoms for protection, 140
  oral contraceptives and, 135
  PID and, 506
  smoking and, 286
EEG (electroencephalogram), **544**
Effexor, 70
EFM (electronic fetal monitoring), 208, **209**
eggs, 319, 321*t*
ejaculation, 113, 114, **140**
  condoms and, 140
  nocturnal emissions, **119**
  problems with, 115
ejaculatory duct, 106
EKG (electrocardiogram), **351**, **418**, **419**
elder abuse, 537
electrical impedance analysis, 379
electrocardiogram (ECG or EKG), **351**, **418**, **419**
electroconvulsive therapy (ECT), 68
electroencephalogram (EEG), **544**
electronic fetal monitoring (EFM), 208, **209**
ELISA test, 498, **499**
embalming, **556**, 557
embolic stroke, 419
embolus, **419**
embryo, 107–108, **195**
emergency care. *See* first aid
emergency contraception, 138
emergency medical services (EMS) system, **632**
emergency medicine, 591
emotional wellness, 2
  assessment of, 12–13
  exercise and, 346–348
  stress and, 29–31
  See also psychological health
emphysema, smoking and, **281–282**
EMS system, **632**
encephalitis, **643**
endemic, **481**
endocrine glands, **107**
endocrine system, **27–28**, 34, 396
endocrinology, 591
endometrial cancer. *See* uterine or endometrial
  cancer
endometriosis, 114, 189
endometrium, 108, 109, 188, **189**, **441**
endorphins, **27**, **346**, 347
endoscopy, **581**
environmental changes, infectious disease and, 481
environmental contaminants, 332–333
environmental health, 636–660, **638**
  assess your impact on the environment, 657
  clean water, 638–640
  facts about our environment, 639
  food inspection, 643
  healing the environment, 656–657
  insect and rodent control, 643–644
  pollution, 646–656
  population growth, 644–646
  and poverty, 653

waste disposal, 640–643
  writing to elected officials, 658
environmental stressors, 37–38
environmental tobacco smoke (ETS), **285–286**
  avoiding, 287
  cardiovascular disease and, 286, 406
  deaths per year, 274*t*
  indoor air pollution, 651
  See also smoking
enzyme, **468**
ephedrine, 230
epidemic, **481**
epididymis, 106
epididymitis, **504**
epilepsy, pregnancy and, 185
epinephrine, **27**, 34
episiotomy, 208, **209**
epithelial layer, **436**
Epstein-Barr virus, 442, **478**, 479–480
erectile dysfunction, **115**, 282, **441**
erogenous zone, **112**
erotic fantasy, **123**
Escherichia coli, 332, 334, 478, 480, 481
esophagus, 301
essential fat, **374**
essential nutrients, 300, **301**
Estimated Average Requirement (EAR), 314
estradiol, 108–109
estrogen, **107**
  autoimmune diseases and, 484
  breast cancer and, 438
  as a cancer promoter, 449
  cardiovascular disease and, 413
  menopause and, 111
  puberty and, 108
  uterine cancer and, 441
  See also hormone replacement therapy (HRT)
ethchlorvynol, 227
ethnicity
  aging, attitudes about, 538
  alcohol abuse, 263–264
  alcohol metabolism, 250
  alcohol use and, 262
  asthma and, 475
  attracting a partner compared, 118
  body image and, 394
  cardiovascular disease and, 410–411, 415
  circumcision and, 107, 116–117
  death, attitudes toward, 547–548
  eating disorder rates, 395
  funeral practices, 557–558
  genetic diseases and, 186–187
  health issues and, 8–9
  intercultural friendships and relationships, 91
  lupus and, 484
  regular physical activity, 343*t*
  smokers and, 9, 278*t*
  stress and, 31, 37
ethyl alcohol, 248
ETS. *See* environmental tobacco smoke (ETS)
euphoria, **227**
eustress, **32**
euthanasia, 552, 553
exercise, 340–371
  activities and calorie cost, 360*t*–361*t*
  assessment of, 12, 365
  benefits of, 344–348
  cancer prevention and, 458
  cardiorespiratory endurance, **351**, 353–354
  cardiovascular disease and, 408–409, 423
  cool down, 354
  diabetes prevention, 377
  diet and, 363–364
  disabled people and, 348
  duration of, 352

equipment selection, 362–363
  facilities for, 362–363
  flexibility, 357, 358–359
  footwear for, 362–363
  frequency of, 351–352
  injury prevention and management, 364–366,
    A-10–A-11
  intensity of, 352
  managing your program, 364–367
  medical clearance before beginning, 351
  muscular strength and endurance, 354–357
  osteoporosis and, 312
  personal program plan, 368–369
  physical activity pyramid, 350
  pregnant women, 202, 203–204
  principles of training, 351–352
  programs for fitness, 349–353
  recommendations, 352*t*
  for stress management, 39–40
  triglyceride levels and, 409
  warm up, 353–354
  water and, 364
  weight management and, 385–387
  See also physical activity
exposure, **71**
eyesight, 524, 528–529
  See also cataracts

failure rate, contraceptives, 133–134, **135**, 150
fallopian tubes, 105, 153, 188, **189**
false negative, **571**
false positive, **571**
FAM. *See* fertility awareness method (FAM)
family health tree, create your own, 190
family life, 95–97
  assess family strengths, 98
  violence in families, 625–627
FAS (fetal alcohol syndrome), **200**, **255–256**
fast-food restaurants, eating in, 327, A-1–A-4
fat calories, 384–385
fat cell theory, weight gain and, 381
fats, 301–306
  cancer risk and, 450
  decreasing for CVD risk reduction, 422
  Food Pyramid, 319–320, 321*t*
  intake goals for, 305
  reducing in your diet, 321–322
  substitutes for, 386
  See also blood fat levels; body fat
fat-soluble vitamins, 308, 309*t*
fears, phobias about, 64–65
fellatio, **123**
female circumcision, 116–117
female condoms. *See* condoms
female sex organs, 104–105
fertility, **135**, 187–191, 282
fertility awareness method (FAM), 148, **149**
  death risk from, 137*t*
  failure rate, 150
  STD protection, 149*t*
  worldwide use of, 151
fertility drugs, and intrauterine insemination, 192
fertilization, **187–189**
fertilized egg, 188, **189**
fetal alcohol syndrome (FAS), **200**, **255–256**
fetus, 185, 198
  1st trimester development, 195–197
  2nd trimester development, 197–198
  3rd trimester development, 198
  3rd trimester illustration, 194
  chronology of development, 196
  diagnosing abnormalities, 198–199
  environmental hazards and, 200
  lightening process, 194, **195**
  See also pregnancy

fiber. *See* dietary fiber
fibrinogen levels, 413
fight-or-flight reaction, 28, **29**
firearms
    deaths per year, 274*t*
    injury prevention, 617
    violence and, 623
fire(s), 614–615
first aid, **631–632**
    bleeding control, 618
    for choking, 618
    (CPR), **417**, 618, **631–632**
    Heimlich maneuver, **617**
    for poisonings, 616
fish oils. *See* omega-3 fatty acids
fitness assessment of, 12, 364, 365
Flagyl, 511
flashbacks, **233**
flavonoids, potential anticancer effects of, 452*t*
flesh-eating bacteria, 476, 480
flexibility, **342**, 343–344
    exercise program, 357, 358–359
    exercise recommendations, 352*t*
    physical activity pyramid, 350
fluid intelligence, **523**
fluid retention, toxemia, **205**
flukes, 484, 485
flunitrazepam. *See* Rohypnol
fluoridation, **638**
fluoride, 311*t*, 312, 316*t*, 317*t*
flushing syndrome, alcohol metabolism and, 250
folate, 309*t*, 317*t*
folic acid, 200, 314–315, 423
follicle, 188, **189**
follicle-stimulating hormone (FSH), 108, 109
foodborne illness, 330, 332, 485, 486, 643
    See also E. coli
food chain, **644**, 645
Food Guide Pyramid, **313–314**
    average American diet compared to, 321*t*
    food group serving suggestions, 318–320
food labels, reading, 326–327, 329
foods and food groups
    additives in foods, 333–334
    certified organic, 332–**333**
    daily requirements for pregnant women, 201*t*
    genetically altered foods, 334
    irradiation of food, 334
    safe food handling, 332, 333
    serving sizes for, 319
    vegetarian diets, 323
    See also diet; Food Guide Pyramid
footwear for exercise, 362–363
foreplay, **123**
foreskin. *See* prepuce
formaldehyde gas, 651
fossil fuels, **646**, 647
fraternal twins, **189**
free radicals, **313**, **451**
friendships, 83, 84, 91
fruit group, 319, 321*t*, 451
FSH (follicle-stimulating hormone), 108, 109
funerals, 556–558
fungus, **483–484**

gallbladder, 301
gallbladder disease, 9, 375, 381
gambling, as addictive behavior, 218
gamete intrafallopian transfer (GIFT), 192, **193**
gamma globulin, **474**
gamma hydroxy butyrate (GHB), 227
gang-related violence, 623–624
garbage management, 641–643
GAS (general adaptation syndrome), 32
gastric resection, 392

gastroenterology, 591
gastroplasty, 392
gay relationships. *See* homosexual relationships
gender
    alcohol abuse and, 263
    bipolar disorder, incidence of, 68
    body image and, 394
    cancer incidence and deaths by site and, 435
    communication differences, 87
    contraception and gender differences, 155–156
    and depression, 68–69
    health issues and, 8
    heart attack incidence, 415
    heart disease death rates, 415
    HIV infection, 497
    illicit drug use and, 222
    media and, 118
    medical research and, 412
    motivations for engaging in sex, 120
    muscle size and strength differences, 356–357
    stress and, 31
    violence and, 622
    See also men; women
gender identity, 116, **117**
gender role, 31, **82**, 116–**117**
general adaptation syndrome (GAS), **32**
general anesthetic, 174, **175**
general surgery, 591
generic drugs, 584
genes and heredity, **189**, **447**
    Alzheimer's disease and, 531
    breast cancer and, 438, 449, 450
    cancer risks and heredity, 434*t*, 449
    cardiovascular disease and, 410
    CCR-5 gene and HIV, 499–501
    DNA mutations and cancer, 448–449
    egg and sperm and, 188
    obesity and, 380–381
    oncogenes, 448, **449**
    prostate cancer and, 439
    schizophrenia and depression, 70
    sexual orientation and, 112
    suppressor genes, 448, **449**
    Syndrome X, 413–414
genetically altered foods, 334
genetic diseases
    amniocentesis for diagnosis, 198–**199**
    ethnicity and, 8, 186–187
    family health tree, create your own, 190
genital herpes, **508–509**
    diaphragms with spermicide and, 144
    HSV-2 and, 508, 509
    pregnancy and, 202
    stress and, 34
genital self-exams, 447, 514
genital warts, 507–508
    See also human papillomavirus (HPV)
geriatrician, **538**
German measles. *See* rubella
germ cells, **104**
gerontologists, **538**
gestational diabetes, 185, 199, 377
giardiasis, 485
GIFT (gamete intrafallopian transfer), 192, **193**
gingivitis, cardiovascular disease and, 412
Ginkgo biloba, Alzheimer's disease and, 531
glans, 104, 105, **107**
glass (methamphetamine), 222, 229–230
glaucoma, 9, **526**
global warming, **648**, 649
glucose, 306, **307**
glycogen, 306, **307**
gonads, **104**
gonococcal conjunctivitis, **506**
gonorrhea, **504**, 505–506

anal intercourse and, 123–124
diaphragms with spermicide for protection, 144
fetal or infant problems and, 203*t*
oral contraceptives and, 136
PID and, 114, 505
pregnancy and, 202
"good" cholesterol. *See* high-density lipoprotein
gram-negative bacteria, 476
gram-positive bacteria, 476
grass. *See* marijuana and cannabis products
greenhouse effect, **648**, 649
grief, 530, 560–563
gum disease, cardiovascular disease and, 412
guns. *See* firearms

HAART and HIV treatment, 499, 502
Haemophilus ducreyi, 511
hair, 524. *See also* baldness
hair dyes, workplace carcinogen, 454*t*
hallucinations, 69, 73, **259**, 260, **261**
hallucinogens, 232–**233**
hantavirus, 480, 481, 644
hashish. *See* marijuana and cannabis products
hate crimes, 624
hatha yoga, 44–45
HCG (human chorionic gonadotropin), 109, **191**
HCV (hepatitis C virus). *See* hepatitis C
HDL. *See* high-density lipoprotein
headaches, 34, A-9–A-10
head injuries, helmets and, 613, 614
health care system, 588–605
    agencies to contact for complaints, 597
    expenditures and health insurance, 598
    paying for health care, 597–603
    providers, types of, 590–597
    See also medical care
health insurance, 599–603
    choosing a policy, 601–603
    coverage of nonelderly Americans, 598
    Medicaid, 537–538, 600, **601**
    Medicare, 537–538, 600, **601**
    uninsured Americans, 597–598
    See also managed care
health journal, sample entries, 15
health maintenance organizations (HMOs), **599**
    See also managed care
Healthy People 2010
    antibiotic prescriptions, reducing, 482
    on binge drinking, 258
    calcium intake for women, 324
    cesarean deliveries, 208
    drinking water standards, 639
    goals of, 5–6
    health insurance coverage goals, 598
    high blood pressure management, 425
    obesity prevalence goals, 375*t*
    Pap testing, 441
    physical activity, 342
    pregnant women and smoking, 287
    prescription drug information for patients, 583
    selected objectives of, 7*t*
hearing loss, 288, 544, 527–528, 655–656
heart, 404–405, 406, 421, 525
heart attacks
    helping a victim of, 417, 418
    high blood pressure and, 407
    incidence by gender, 415
    oral contraceptives and, 134, 135
    reducing cholesterol levels, 407
    smoking and, 280, 281
    symptoms of, 418
    types of, 416–417
heart disease, 416–421
    cardiorespiratory endurance, 343
    in children, 421–422

heart disease (continued)
  deaths from, 3, 6, 7t, 415
  detecting, 417–418
  dietary fat intake and, 303–304, 422, 428–429
  environmental tobacco smoke (ETS), 286
  erectile dysfunction and, 115
  ethnicity and, 9, 415
  exercise and, 345–346
  hormone therapy and, 413, 530
  personality and risk for, 30
  treating, 418–419
  See also cardiovascular disease; coronary heart disease
heart rate, target, 353, 354
heavy metal, 641
Hegar's sign, 193
height-weight charts, 378
Heimlich maneuver, 617
Helicobacter pylori, 412, 442
helper T cells, 468, 469, 470
hematology/oncology, 591
hemochromatosis (iron overload), 187
hemophilia, 496, 497
hemorrhagic stroke, 419–420
hemorrhoids, insoluble fiber in diet and, 307
hepatitis, 509
hepatitis A (HAV), 473t, 480–481
hepatitis B (HBV), 480–481, 509–510
  ethnicity and, 9
  liver cancer, 442
  pregnancy and, 185
  vaccine, 473t
hepatitis C (HCV), 480–482
HER2 protein, 439
Herceptin, 439
heredity. See genes and heredity
heroin, 217t, 227, 236, 253
herpes simplex
  herpesviruses and, 479
  HSV-1, 508–509
  HSV-2, 508–509
  pregnancy and, 202, 203t, 509
  See also genital herpes
herpesvirus, 478, 479–480, 483, 508–509
heterocyclics, 70
heterosexuality, 92, 93, 121
high, marijuana and, 226, 227
high blood pressure (hypertension), 407, 414–416
  cardiovascular disease and, 406–407, 424
  classification of blood pressure readings, 416t
  diet and nutrition for, 326, 423
  Dietary Approaches to Stop Hypertension, 423
  exercise and, 346
  obesity and, 375
  oral contraceptives and, 135
  pregnancy and, 185
  screening tests for, 581
  stress and, 34
  toxemia, 205
  walking to reduce, 39
  weight distribution and, 376
high-density lipoprotein, 304, 305, 346, 407
  cardiovascular disease and, 407–408
  estrogen and, 413
  guidelines for, 409t
  managing levels of, 425
  smoking and, 406
high-protein diet caution, 389–390
H. influenzae type b (Hib) vaccine, 473t
histamine, 468, 469, 474
histoplasmosis, 484
HIV antibody test, 498, 499
HIV infection, 492–504
  anal intercourse and, 123–124
  condoms, 140, 143, 149t, 503, 505, 516

contraceptives and, 149t
cost of treatment, 502
diagnosing, 498
ethnicity and, 9, 496–497
fetal or infant problems and, 203t
gender and, 496–497, 501–502
immune system and, 472
injecting drug use and, 225, 496, 497, 504
opportunistic infections, 499t, 501
pregnancy and, 186, 202, 501–502
prevention, 149t, 502–504
prostitutes and, 125
reporting of cases, 498
screening tests for, 581
self-test kits for, 571
sexual activities, risk ratings, 503
sexual orientation and, 121
stress and, 34
symptoms, 497–498
testing for, 498, 500, 571
transmitting, 495–496
treatment, 483, 498–502
worldwide daily occurrence, 132t
worldwide distribution of, 494
See also AIDS
HIV-positive, 498, 499
HIV RNA assay test, 498, 499
HMOs (health maintenance organizations), 599
  See also managed care
Hodgkin's disease, 442, 446
  See also lymphomas
"holiday heart" syndrome, 255
home injuries, 609t, 613–617
homeopathy, 594, 595
homeostasis, 28–29
home pregnancy test kits, 191, 571
home self-test kits, 191, 570–571
homicide, 9, 623
  See also violence
homocysteine levels, 411–412
homophobia, 121
homosexuality, 92, 93, 121
homosexual relationships, 92, 121
  HIV transmission, 496, 497
hookworms, 475t, 484, 485
hormone replacement therapy (HRT), 529
  breast cancer and, 438
  cardiovascular disease and, 413
  colon and rectal cancer, 437
  death rates and, 530
  fibrinogen levels, 413
  osteoporosis and, 312
  See also estrogen
hormones, 27
  reproductive cycle and, 107–112
  sex hormones, 104, 107
  stress and, 33, 34
hospice, 550, 551
host, 466
HPV. See human papillomavirus (HPV)
H. pylori. See Helicobacter pylori
HRT. See hormone replacement therapy (HRT)
HSV-1. See herpes simplex
HSV-2. See genital herpes
HTLV-1 virus, 482–483
human chorionic gonadotropin (HCG), 109, 191
Human Genome Project, 447
human immunodeficiency virus. See HIV infection
human papillomavirus (HPV)
  cervical cancer and, 441, 442, 507
  genital warts and, 506, 507
hydrocarbons, 647t
hydrogenation, 302–303
hydrostatic weighing, percent body fat and, 379
hymen, 104

hypertension. See high blood pressure
hypothalamus, 27, 107
hysterectomy, 137t, 152

ibuprofen, 252–253, 437, 482
  See also NSAIDs
ice (methamphetamine), 222, 229–230
ICSI (intracytoplasmic sperm injection), 192
identical twins, 189
identity crisis, 58
IDU. See injecting drug use
immune system, 468–472
  aging and, 525
  allergies and, 474
  exercise and, 348
  immune response, 469–470, 471
  obesity and, 375
  steroids and, 357
  stress and, 32–33, 34, 485
  supporting your immune system, 486–487
immunity and infection, 464–489
  autoimmune diseases, 485–486
  bacteria, 475–478
  emerging infectious diseases, 480–481
  fungi, protozoa, and parasitic worms, 483–485
  immunity, 470
  infection, 466
  pathogens and disease, 474–486
  top infectious diseases, worldwide, 475t
  viruses, 478–483
immunization, 472–474
  contraceptive, 153–154
  schedule for, 473t
impotence. See erectile dysfunction
incest, 629
income level
  environmental health and poverty, 653
  infectious diseases and poverty, 481
  obesity and, 382
  and regular physical activity, 343t
  See also socioeconomic status
incontinence, 441
incubation, 470, 471
independent practitioner, 590–591
Indians, American. See Native Americans
indinavir. See Crixivan
indoor air pollution, 651
induction chemotherapy, 455
infant mortality
  coping with loss, 205–206
  ethnicity and, 9
  socioeconomic status and, 8
  U.S. rate of, 205
infants
  Apgar score for, 206, 207
  chlamydia and, 504–505
  congenital syphilis, 511
  DRIs for, 316t–317t
  and environmental tobacco smoke (ETS), 286
  genital herpes infection, 509
  gonococcal conjunctivitis, 506
  low birth weight (LBW), 205
  newborns, vitamin K for, 316
  RDAs for, 315t
  sudden infant death syndrome (SIDS), 205
  thrush, 484
  See also birth defects
infatuation, 84, 85
infection, 466–467
  See also immunity and infection
infectious disease. See immunity and infection
inferior vena cava, 405, 406
infertility, 189
  causes of, 189
  condoms for protection from, 140

Quaalude, 222, 227
quackery, 457, 596
quitting smoking, 289, 290–292, 293

rabies vaccine, 473t
race. *See* ethnicity
radiation, 654–655
  as carcinogen, 453–454
  fetal or infant problems and, 203t
  workplace carcinogens, 454t
  See also ultraviolet radiation
radiation sickness, 654, **655**
radiation therapy, 455–456
radiology, 591
radionuclide imaging, 418, **419**
radon gas, 453–454, **655**
raloxifene, 312, 439
range of motion, and flexibility, 343–344
rape, **627–629**
Rational Recovery, 262
RDAs. *See* Recommended Dietary Allowances
Reality (female condom), 142, 143
recessive genes, 186
Recommended Dietary Allowances (RDAs), **313**, 314, 315t
rectal cancer. *See* colon and rectal cancer
rectum, 105, 106, 301, 456t
recycling to reduce garbage, 642–643
refined carbohydrates, 385
refractory period, 114
regional anesthetic, 174, **175**
reinforcement, **71**
relationships, intimate. *See* intimate relationships
relaxation response, **43**
relaxation techniques, 43–46
religion
  and death, 545, 549
  spiritual wellness and, 59
  wellness and, 426
  See also spiritual wellness
REM and non-REM sleep, 40–41
remission, **436**, 437
repetitive-strain injury (RSI), **620**
repression, 60, 62t
reproductive system, 104–107, 256, 282–283
reproductive technology, and infertility, 192
resistance exercise, **354**
respiratory damage, smoking and, 281–282
respiratory infections, and ETS, 286
response, **71**
re-stenosis, treatment for, 418–419
resting metabolic rate (RMR), **381**
resveratrol, potential anticancer effects of, 452t
retarded ejaculation, **115**
retirement, planning for, 526–527
reverse transcriptase inhibitors, 498, **499**, 501
  See also AZT
Reye's syndrome, 482
rheumatic fever, 421–422
rheumatic heart disease, 421–422
rheumatoid arthritis, women and, 484
Rh incompatibilities, 200
rhinovirus, 479. *See also* colds
riboflavin, 309t, 316t
rice, 317–318, 321t
R-I-C-E principle for sports injury, 365
rickettsia, **476**, 477
Rift Valley Fever, 481
"right to die," 550–552, 553
ringing in the ears, tinnitus, **656**
ringworm, fungal infection, 483, 484
Ritalin, 230
RMR (resting metabolic rate), **381**
road rage, aggressive driving, 610–611
Rocky Mountain spotted fever, **644**

rickettsias and, **476**, 477
rodent control, 643–644
Rohypnol, 227–228, 627–628
rollerblading injuries, 619
"roofies." *See* Rohypnol
rooming-in, mother and infant, 208, **209**
rotavirus vaccine, 473t
roundworms, deaths per year, worldwide, 475t
RSI (repetitive-strain injury), **620**
RU-486. *See* mifepristone
rubella (German measles)
  deaths per year, worldwide, 475t
  fetal or infant problems and, 203t
  pregnancy and, 185, 200, 202
  vaccine for, 473t

SADD (Students Against Drunk Driving), 266–267
safe food handling, 332, 333
safer sex, 125, 502–503, 505, 516
safety, assessment of, 13
  See also unintentional injuries; violence
safety belts, 610, 611
saline instillation, 174–175
Salmonella bacteria, 332, 644
salt, 322, 423
  See also sodium
salt-cured foods, 322–323
sanitary landfill, 642, **643**
sarcoma, **436**
saturated fat, 302, **303**, 321, 428–429
scabies, **512**
schizophrenia, 69, 70, 261
schools, violence in, 624
scleroderma, women and, 484
screening tests
  for adults, 581
  for cancer, 456, 456t, 459
scrotum, **104**, 105–106, 152
scurvy, **308**
Seconal, 227
secondary reinforcers, nicotine addiction, **276**
secondhand smoke. *See* environmental tobacco smoke
sedation, **227**
sedative-hypnotic, **227**
selective estrogen receptor modulators, 312, 439, 529
selective serotonin reuptake inhibitors (SSRIs), 70, 110
  See also anti-depressant drugs
selenium, 311t, 315t
self-actualization, 54–56, **55**
self-care skills, 568–587, A-5–A-11
  assess your knowledge of medications, 574
  dental self-care, 579
  home self-care kit contents, 576t
  self-assessment, 570–571
  treatment options, 572–575
  when to see a physician, 571–572
  See also medical care
self-esteem, **55**
  achieving, 58–60
  challenges to, 59–60
  intimate relationships and, 82–83
  obesity and, 376
  weight problems and, 388
self-help groups, 236–237
  See also support groups
self-medication, 573–575
self-talk, 42, 60, 61, 65, 388
self-test kits, 191, 570–571
semen, 106, 114, **115**
seminal vesicle, 106
semivegetarian, **323**
separation and divorce, 94–95

septic system, **641**
SERMs. *See* selective estrogen receptor modulators
seroconversion, 500, **501**
sewage issues, 641
sex chromosomes, 108, **109**
sex education for teenagers, 146
sex hormones, **104**, 107
sex toys, and atypical sexual behavior, 124
sexual anatomy, 104–107
sexual assault, **627–629**
sexual attitude assessment, 120
sexual behavior, 116–126
  addiction to sex, 218–219
  atypical types, 124
  commercial sex, 124–125
  date rape and, 627–628
  deaths resulting from, 132t, 274t
  development of, 116–121
  HIV and various sexual activities, 503
  problematic types, 124
  responsible behavior, 125–126
  sexual orientation, 121–123
  varieties of, 123–124
sexual coercion, **124**
sexual contact, HIV transmission, 495–496
sexual dysfunctions, 114–116, **115**
sexual functioning, 112–116
  aging and, 524
  alcohol and, 251, 256
  dysfunctions, 114–116
  response cycle, 112–114
sexual harassment, **629**, 630
sexual intercourse, **124**, 496, 497
sexuality, **104**, 111–112, 118
sexually transmitted diseases (STDs), **133**, 490–519, **492**
  assess your attitudes and behaviors, 513
  cervical cancer and, 441, 442
  chlamydia, 504–505
  circumcision and, 107
  college students and, 508
  contraceptive methods and, 132, 149t, 515
  diagnosis and treatment, 513–514
  fetus or infant problems, 203t, 496, 504–505, 509, 510
  genital herpes, 508–509
  genital self-exam, 514
  genital warts, 507–508
  gonorrhea, 505–506
  hepatitis B, 509–510
  HIV/AIDS, 492–504
  pelvic inflammatory disease (PID), 114, 506–507
  pregnancy and, 186, 202, 496, 501–502, 509, 510
  prevention, 502–503, 514–515
  safer sex practices and, 125, 502–503, 505
  screening tests for, 500, 581
  syphilis, 510–511
  talking with your partner about, 516
  treatment tips, 511
  worldwide daily occurrence, 132t
sexual maturation, 108–111
sexual orientation, 92, **93**, 121–123
sexual relationships, 83–85, 154–155
sexual response cycle, 112–114
sexual violence, 627–631
shiatsu (acupressure), 594, **595**
shingles, herpesviruses and, 479
shoes for exercise, 362–363
shopping, compulsive, 219
shyness, 64, 65, 69–72
sibutramine, 391
sickle-cell disease, 8, 9, 186
sidestream smoke, **285**